Operative Brachial Plexus Surgery

Alexander Y. Shin • Nicholas Pulos
Editors

Operative Brachial Plexus Surgery

Clinical Evaluation and Management Strategies

Springer

Editors
Alexander Y. Shin
Department of Orthopedic Surgery
Mayo Clinic
Rochester, MN
USA

Nicholas Pulos
Department of Orthopedic Surgery
Mayo Clinic
Rochester, MN
USA

ISBN 978-3-030-69516-3 ISBN 978-3-030-69517-0 (eBook)
https://doi.org/10.1007/978-3-030-69517-0

This Springer imprint is published by the registered company Springer Nature Switzerland AG
The registered company address is: Gewerbestrasse 11, 6330 Cham, Switzerland

Foreword

Injuries to the brachial plexus are the worst of all peripheral nerve lesions because of the frequency of associated injury to the spinal cord and the common complication of severe pain. Two distinguished clinical scientists from the Mayo Clinic, Alexander Shin and Nicholas Pulos, have brought together outstanding workers in the field to create this important book *Operative Brachial Plexus Surgery*. Whilst there are powerful contributions from the Mayo team, the thoughts, wisdom and experience are international. It is an honour to be invited to write this foreword.

The book opens with impressive chapters that set a high standard for what follows. "Anatomy", described from a surgical perspective, emphasises variation. "Mechanism of Injury" reminds us of the "skip" or double-level (or even multiple-level) lesion. A wide range of iatropathic injuries, occurring or inflicted during treatment, are considered. The "Biology of Nerve Injury" chapter challenges our current concepts. There are thorough chapters on epidemiology and on associated concomitant injuries. All these inform, all enlighten.

The next part of four chapters is a bridge between fundamental aspects and their application to treatment. These chapters are wide in scope and they provide clear conclusions and advice. "Evaluation" draws together diagnosis by clinical, electrophysiological and imaging examination. "Determinants of Treatment" sets out indications and contraindications to operation. "Priorities of Treatment and Rationale" gives a balanced and reflective appreciation of the principles guiding treatment planning.

"Treatment Options" is a monumental piece. In it, nerve grafting and transfer are rightly considered as complementary methods. There is, throughout the whole chapter, a welcome emphasis on elbow extension. Free functioning muscle transfer is discussed by experts. The essential role of musculotendinous transfer and arthrodesis is thoroughly considered. "Surgical Approaches" provides a clear and comprehensive guide to operative exposure.

The application of these options and possibilities is set out in "Management of Specific Injury Patterns", considering first the partial upper lesions, then the total and the C8-T1 lesions. The last two of these take us inexorably to the seemingly insoluble problem of the restoration of hand function, which is analysed in two extensive chapters, "Restoration of Hand Function in Pan Plexus Injuries" and "Sensory Reinnervation in Pan Plexus Injuries". Both of these contain much good matter.

The essential, central challenge of rehabilitation is reviewed in the last three chapters: "Management of Neuropathic Pain"; "The Role of Amputation and Prosthetic Fitting"; "The Role of Therapy". These are well set out, informative, and provide a great deal of guidance and advice, which is clearly derived from a considerable and wide experience.

Alas, so often initial high hopes must be tempered by further experience. The inability to understand the lesion was a major obstacle to repair efforts in the 1950s. George Bonney introduced and proved the concept of pre- and post-ganglionic injury, defined the natural history, and developed methods of diagnosis. His demonstration, with Roger Gilliatt (1958), of persisting conduction in preganglionic lesion led to so much subsequent work, and it seemed to open the path to effective repair. From 1962, 41 repairs were performed at St Mary's Hospital. Results were so bad that these operations were abandoned! They restarted in 1975, inspired by the example of Algimantas Narakas, who contributed so much to the field of with brachial plexus injuries.

Rehabilitation of patients after these often-catastrophic injuries requires an accurate diagnosis, and so prognosis, followed by urgent intervention to improve that prognosis. For many, pain will obtrude throughout the process. This book will guide aspirants and will inform those already established in this arduous field of work.

London, United Kingdom Rolfe Birch

Foreword

Brachial plexus injury in the newborn is an extremely complex condition. It is difficult to assess the extent of the injury, to predict the potential for recovery, to know which methods of treatment will predictably improve outcomes over the natural history, and to determine when to intervene. The neurological and biological effects on a growing musculoskeletal system make this injury in children even more burdensome.

Reports in the literature are most often not "pure" in that the outcomes are the result of interventions at multiple levels and with multiple techniques. Teasing out the details of when to do what for a condition that you cannot easily image, in an infant that cannot cooperate, and in which results require long-term follow-up, has been the challenge.

The pediatric part of *Operative Brachial Plexus Surgery* is a masterful compilation of what has been learned, presented in a cohesive and understandable manner by experts in this field. It is not simply a rehash of what has been published before.

The chapter "Historical Perspectives" details the early attempts to treat birth-related brachial plexus injuries. These occurred often in women with "rickety" pelves, a common condition in places where there was little sunlight and inadequate vitamin D in the diet. Public health measures to supplement milk with vitamin D and provide it to school children played a major role in eliminating this risk factor. Today's risk factor and public health challenge is obesity.

The chapter on the biology of brachial plexus injuries in children brings us to a new level of understanding of the differences between the adult and infant. What we had thought were contractures due to mechanical forces are now being explained at a molecular level. Prevention of some of the secondary changes to the growing limb is a goal that may someday be realized.

Details of the surgical care of each level of nerve injury are presented clearly and strategies are thoughtfully presented. The international perspective on the management of the child greatly enhances this section. Late complications and procedures to rebalance the shoulder are also outlined.

Although this is a textbook on the surgical management of these devastating injuries, we must always remind ourselves that these have occurred in "children," and not just "cases." Surgeons are part of the team that must address the psychosocial components of the child who is growing into maturity with a limb difference. Deformity, physical impairment, bullying, and altered lifetime expectations are often more important to our patients than the sometimes meager results we attain from our surgery. We, as surgeons, are privileged to be able to offer this comprehensive care.

Dallas, TX, USA Marybeth Ezaki

Preface

The field of peripheral nerve surgery and brachial plexus has grown so large in the past two decades that relegating it to a single chapter in a larger textbook of hand, microvascular, plastics, or neurosurgery is no longer adequate. While daunting to compile a definitive surgical reference for those managing brachial plexus injuries, our mentors fomented in us a passion of education and learning which inspired the creation of this textbook. To this end, experts in the disciplines of orthopedic surgery, plastic surgery, and neurosurgery from over 40 different institutions across 16 countries were invited to share their knowledge of brachial plexus.

As a first edition, we were free of the biases associated with prior editions but risked the incorporation of our own biases. We were delighted and amazed by the broad latitude the contributors took with their topic and how their approach balanced any potential bias. The result is a textbook of chapters written in the voice of authors who are true experts in not only in brachial plexus surgery, but leaders in the fields of biology of nerve injuries, neurodiagnostic testing, radiographic imaging, therapy, nerve transfers, and free functioning muscles.

We recognize the sacrifice and accomplishments of the pioneers of brachial plexus surgery, who mentored and taught our mentors. It is upon the shoulders of these giants and the cumulative knowledge they advanced that we humbly introduce the first edition of *Operative Brachial Plexus Surgery.*

Rochester, MN, USA

Alexander Y. Shin
Nicholas Pulos

Acknowledgments

A special thanks to Allen T. Bishop, MD, and Robert J. Spinner, MD, our partners of the Mayo Clinic Brachial Plexus Team – who continue to inspire and awe us with their incredible skill and knowledge.

AYS & NP

To my wife, Patti, and my children who sacrificed their time and needs to allow me to become the surgeon I am today.

AYS

To my children, who are too young to know how much they inspire me. And to my Bridge, for supporting me beyond what I could have ever fairly asked.

NP

Contents

Contributors

Abdullah Alawadhi Department of Orthopedic Surgery, Ogori Daiichi General Hospital, Yamaguchi City, Yamaguchi Prefecture, Japan

Abdullah Albazzaz Department of Orthopedic Surgery, Ogori Daiichi General Hospital, Yamaguchi City, Yamaguchi Prefecture, Japan

Leonardo Lopez Almejo Brachial Plexus International School, Barcelona, Spain

Department of Brachial Plexus and Microsurgery, Universidad Autonoma de Coahuila, Hospital Universitario, Torreon, Coahuila, Mexico

Navapong Anantavorasakul Upper Extremity and Reconstructive Microsurgery Unit, Institute of Orthopaedics, Lerdsin Hospital, Bangkok, Thailand

Anthony J. Archual Indiana University, Indianapolis, IN, USA

Jörg Bahm Section for Plexus Surgery, Clinic for Plastic, Hand and Burn Surgery, RWTH University Hospital Aachen, Aachen, Germany

Andrea S. Bauer Department of Orthopaedic Surgery, Boston Children's Hospital, Boston, MA, USA

Zoubir Belkheyar Clinique du Mont Louis, Paris, France

Keith A. Bengtson Physical Medicine and Rehabilitation, Mayo Clinic, Rochester, MN, USA

John C. Benson Department of Radiology, Division of Neuroradiology, Mayo Clinic, Rochester, MN, USA

Jayme Augusto Bertelli Center of Biological and Health Sciences, Department of Neurosurgery, University of the South of Santa Catarina (Unisul), Tubarão, SC, Brazil

Department of Orthopedic Surgery, Governador Celso Ramos Hospital, Florianópolis, SC, Brazil

Anil Ghanshyam Bhatia The International School of Brachial Plexus Surgery, Pune, Maharashtra, India

Brachial Plexus International School, Barcelona, Spain

Department of Brachial Plexus Surgery, Deenanath Mangeshkar Hospital, Pune, Maharashtra, India

Allen T. Bishop Department of Orthopedic Surgery, Mayo Clinic, Rochester, MN, USA

José L. Borrero University of Central Florida, College of Medicine, Orlando, FL, USA

Arnold Palmer Hospital for Children, Orlando Health, Orlando, FL, USA

Juan Manuel Breyer Orthopedic Surgery – Hand Surgery Unit, Hospital del Trabajador, Santiago, RM, Chile

Orthopedic Surgery – Hand Surgery Unit, Clinica Alemana de Santiago, Santiago, RM, Chile

Adeline Cambon-Binder Sorbonne University, Orthopaedic and Traumatology Surgery Department, Saint-Antoine Hospital, Paris, France

Rafael Reynoso Campo Brachial Plexus International School, Barcelona, Spain

Department of Plastic Surgery and Microsurgery, Hospital General de México, Ciudad de México, Mexico

Joaquin Casañas Department of Traumaunit, Brachial Plexus and Peripheral Nerve, Hospital Teknon, Barcelona, Spain

Rowan M. Chandler Section of Plastic Surgery, Department of Surgery, Winnipeg, MB, Canada

Peter Chang Department of Orthopedic Surgery, Washington University School of Medicine, St. Louis, MO, USA

David Chwei-Chin Chuang, MD Department of Plastic Surgery, Chang Gung Memorial Hospital, Taipei-Linkou, Taiwan

Tod A. Clark Plastic Surgery, University of Manitoba, Department of Orthopedic Surgery, Winnipeg, MB, Canada

Howard M. Clarke Department of Plastic and Reconstructive Surgery, Hospital for Sick Children, Toronto, ON, Canada

Department of Surgery, University of Toronto, Toronto, ON, Canada

Roger Cornwall Orthopaedic Surgery and Developmental Biology, Cincinnati Children's Hospital Medical Center, Cincinnati, OH, USA

Jorge Francisco Clifton Correa Brachial Plexus International School, Barcelona, Spain

Department of Hand, Micro and Nerve Surgery, Universidad Autonoma De Guadalajara, Universidad Autonoma de Coahuila Sede Torreon, Real San Jose: UAG, Guadalajara Jalisco, Hospital Universitario Dr. Joaquin Del Valle Sanchez, Torreon Coahuila, Zapopan, Jalisco, Mexico

The International School of Brachial Plexus Surgery, Guadalajara, Mexico

Robla Costales Department of Neurosurgery. Hospital HM Regla /HM San Francisco, León, Spain

Brian A. Crum Mayo Clinic, Rochester, MN, USA

Charles A. Daly Department of Orthopaedic Surgery, Emory University, Atlanta, GA, USA

Agnes Z. Dardas Department of Orthopaedic Surgery, University of Pennsylvania, Philadelphia, PA, USA

Jana Dengler Division of Plastic and Reconstructive Surgery, Sunnybrook Health Sciences Centre, University of Toronto, Toronto, ON, Canada

Felix E. Diehn Department of Radiology, Division of Neuroradiology, Mayo Clinic, Rochester, MN, USA

Kazuteru Doi Department of Orthopedic Surgery, Ogori Daiichi General Hospital, Yamaguchi City, Yamaguchi Prefecture, Japan

Lauren Dutton Naval Hospital Jacksonville, Jacksonville, FL, USA

Christopher J. Dy Department of Orthopedic Surgery, Washington University School of Medicine, St. Louis, MO, USA

Laurence J. Eckel Department of Radiology, Division of Neuroradiology, Mayo Clinic, Rochester, MN, USA

Tarek Abdalla El-Gammal Hand and Reconstructive Microsurgery Unit, Assiut University Hospitals and School of Medicine, Assiut, Egypt

Brachial Plexus International School, Barcelona, Spain

Department of Brachial Plexus and Microsurgery, Assiut University Hospitals, Assiut, Egypt

Bassem T. Elhassan Shoulder Fellowship at MGH, Boston, MA, USA

Brittany N. Garcia University of Utah, Department of Orthopaedic Surgery, Salt Lake City, UT, USA

Idris S. Gharbaoui Texas Orthopedic Hospital, Houston, TX, USA

Jennifer L. Giuffre Plastic Surgery, University of Manitoba, Section of Plastic Surgery, Department of Surgery, Winnipeg, MB, Canada

Julie B. Guerin Department of Radiology, Division of Neuroradiology, Mayo Clinic, Rochester, MN, USA

Yasunori Hattori Department of Orthopedic Surgery, Ogori Daiichi General Hospital, Yamaguchi City, Yamaguchi Prefecture, Japan

Kota Hayashi Department of Orthopedic Surgery, Ogori Daiichi General Hospital, Yamaguchi City, Yamaguchi Prefecture, Japan

Tim Hems Scottish National Brachial Plexus Injury Service, Queen Elizabeth University Hospital and Royal Hospital for Children, Glasgow, UK

Jonathan E. Isaacs Division of Hand Surgery, Department of Orthopedic Surgery, Virginia Commonwealth University Health System, Richmond, VA, USA

Michelle A. James Department of Orthopedic Surgery, Shriners Hospital for Children—Northern California, University of California, Davis, Sacramento, CA, USA

Kimberly Jensen Physical Medicine & Rehabilitation, Mayo Clinic, Rochester, MN, USA

Stephanie Kannas Physical Medicine & Rehabilitation, Mayo Clinic, Rochester, MN, USA

Dong Kun Kim Department of Radiology, Division of Neuroradiology, Mayo Clinic, Rochester, MN, USA

Piyabuth Kittithamvongs Upper Extremity and Reconstructive Microsurgery Unit, Institute of Orthopaedics, Lerdsin Hospital, Bangkok, Thailand

Pelagia Kouloumberis Plastic & Orthopedic Surgery, Peripheral Nerve/ Brachial Plexus Clinic, Mayo Clinic College of Medicine, Mayo Clinic Arizona, Phoenix, AZ, USA

Scott H. Kozin Shriners Hospitals for Children, Philadelphia, PA, USA

Sarah M. Lamont Division of Hand Surgery, Department of Orthopedic Surgery, Virginia Commonwealth University Health System, Richmond, VA, USA

Alejandro Muset Lara Brachial Plexus and Birth Palsy Surgery, Muset Institute and Brachial Plexus International School, Barcelona, Spain

Somsak Leechavengvongs Upper Extremity and Reconstructive Microsurgery Unit, Institute of Orthopaedics, Lerdsin Hospital, Bangkok, Thailand

Feng Li The Department of Hand Surgery, Beijing Jishuitan Hospital, Beijing, China

Peng-cheng Li The Department of Hand Surgery, Beijing Jishuitan Hospital, Beijing, China

Wen-jun Li The Department of Hand Surgery, Beijing Jishuitan Hospital, Beijing, China

Manuel Llusá Hospital Vall d'Hebron, Brachial Plexus and Peripheral Nerve, Barcelona, Spain

Johnny Chuieng-Yi Lu, MD, MSCI Department of Plastic Surgery, Chang Gung Memorial Hospital, Taipei-Linkou, Taiwan

Andrés A. Maldonado Peripheral Nerve and Brachial Plexus Unit, Department of Plastic Surgery, University Hospital Getafe, Madrid, Spain

Department of Plastic, Hand and Reconstructive Surgery, BG Unfallklinik Frankfurt, Frankfurt, Germany

Kanchai Malungpaishrope Upper Extremity and Reconstructive Microsurgery Unit, Institute of Orthopaedics, Lerdsin Hospital, Bangkok, Thailand

M. Claire Manske Department of Orthopedic Surgery, Shriners Hospital for Children—Northern California, University of California, Davis, Sacramento, CA, USA

Amy M. Moore Department of Plastic and Reconstructive Surgery, The Ohio State University Wexner Medical Center, Columbus, OH, USA

Ana Moratona Muset Institute, Barcelona, Spain

Marie Morris Department of Orthopaedic Surgery, Washington University School of Medicine, Saint Louis, MO, USA

M. Rosa Morro Department of Human Anatomy and Embriology, Faculty of Medicine, University of Barcelona, Barcelona, Spain

Nikhil K. Murthy Department of Neurological Surgery, Northwestern Memorial Hospital, Chicago, IL, USA

Andrew Nelson Prosthetics and Orthotics, Limb Lab, Rochester, MN, USA

Shelley S. Noland Plastic & Orthopedic Surgery, Peripheral Nerve/Brachial Plexus Clinic, Mayo Clinic College of Medicine, Mayo Clinic Arizona, Phoenix, AZ, USA

Christophe Oberlin Clinique du Mont Louis, Paris, France

Andrew L. O'Brien Department of Plastic and Reconstructive Surgery, The Ohio State University Wexner Medical Center, Columbus, OH, USA

Christine Oh Department of Orthopedic Surgery, Mayo Clinic, Rochester, MN, USA

Daniel Oliveras Muset Institute, Barcelona, Spain

Neehar Patel Bombay Hospital Institute of Medical Sciences, New Marine Lines, Mumbai, Maharashtra, India

Alfonso Perez Orthopedic Surgery – Hand Surgery Unit, Hospital del Trabajador, Santiago, RM, Chile

Orthopedic Surgery – Hand Surgery Unit, Clinica Las Condes, Santiago, RM, Chile

Willem Pondaag Department of Neurosurgery, Leiden University Medical Center, Leiden, The Netherlands

Louis H. Poppler Private Practice, Boise, ID, USA

Ross C. Puffer Mayo Clinic, Department of Neurologic Surgery, Rochester, MN, USA

Nicholas Pulos Department of Orthopedic Surgery, Mayo Clinic, Rochester, MN, USA

Detchporn Putthiwara Upper Extremity and Reconstructive Microsurgery Unit, Institute of Orthopaedics, Lerdsin Hospital, Bangkok, Thailand

Sotetsu Sakamoto Department of Orthopedic Surgery, Ogori Daiichi General Hospital, Yamaguchi City, Yamaguchi Prefecture, Japan

Brandon Sampson Prosthetics and Orthotics, Limb Lab, Rochester, MN, USA

Apurva S. Shah Division of Orthopaedic Surgery, Children's Hospital of Philadelphia, Philadelphia, PA, USA

Yun-Dong Shen Department of Hand Surgery, Huashan Hospital, Shanghai Medical College, Fudan University, Shanghai, China

Alexander Y. Shin Department of Orthopedic Surgery, Mayo Clinic, Rochester, MN, USA

V. Michelle Silvera Department of Radiology, Division of Neuroradiology, Mayo Clinic, Rochester, MN, USA

Brandon Smith University of Michigan, Ann Arbor, MI, USA

M. Socolovsky Peripheral Nerve & Brachial Plexus Surgery Program, Department of Neurosurgery, University of Buenos Aires School of Medicine, Buenos Aires, Argentina

Francisco Soldado Pediatric Hand Surgery and Microsurgery Unit, Barcelona University Children's Hospital HM Nens, HM Hospitales, Barcelona, Spain

Pediatric Hand Surgery and Microsurgery Unit, Vall d'Hebron Barcelona Hospital Campus, Barcelona, Spain

Robert J. Spinner Mayo Clinic, Department of Neurologic Surgery, Rochester, MN, USA

Jeff Strommen Abbott Northwester Hospital, Allina Health, Minneapolis, MN, USA

Chris Stutz Department of Orthopedics, Pediatric Orthopedic, Hand, and Microvascular Surgery, Texas Scottish Rite Hospital for Children, UT Southwestern School of Medicine, Dallas, TX, USA

Martijn R. Tannemaat Department of Neurology and Clinical Neurophysiology, LUMC, Leiden, The Netherlands

Chairoj Uerpairojkit Upper Extremity and Reconstructive Microsurgery Unit, Institute of Orthopaedics, Lerdsin Hospital, Bangkok, Thailand

Pamela Vergara Orthopedic Surgery – Hand Surgery Unit, Hospital del Trabajador, Santiago, RM, Chile

Orthopedic Surgery – Hand Surgery Unit, Clinica Las Condes, Santiago, RM, Chile

Eric Richard Wagner Department of Orthopaedic Surgery, Emory University, Atlanta, GA, USA

Lindley Wall Department of Orthopaedic Surgery, Washington University School of Medicine, Saint Louis, MO, USA

Angela A. Wang University of Utah, Department of Orthopaedic Surgery, Salt Lake City, UT, USA

Shu-feng Wang The Department of Hand Surgery, Beijing Jishuitan Hospital, Beijing, China

Ayobami Ward University of Michigan, Ann Arbor, MI, USA

Peter M. Waters Department of Orthopaedic Surgery, Boston Children's Hospital, Boston, MA, USA

Kitty Wu Department of Plastic and Reconstructive Surgery, Western University, London, ON, Canada

Wen-Dong Xu Department of Hand Surgery, Huashan Hospital, Shanghai Medical College, Fudan University, Shanghai, China

Yun-hao Xue The Department of Hand Surgery, Beijing Jishuitan Hospital, Beijing, China

Lynda Yang University of Michigan, Ann Arbor, MI, USA

Pablo Zancolli Fundacion Favaloro, Buenos Aires, Argentina

Dan A. Zlotolow Shriners Hospitals for Children, Philadelphia, PA, USA

Adult Brachial Plexus Injuries: A Historical Perspective

1

Johnny Chuieng-Yi Lu
and David Chwei-Chin Chuang

The history of brachial plexus injury (BPI) reconstruction has evolved over the nineteenth and twentieth centuries and has had a dramatic change in attitude from pessimism to optimism in the twenty-first century. This change started from recognizing brachial plexus as the source of palsy in the upper limb (such as infraclavicular BPI after reduction of shoulder dislocation, birth brachial plexus palsy due to improper neonatal delivery, and adult BPI due to traction injury) to significantly improve the surgical outcomes through advances in diagnosis and microsurgical nerve repair techniques. We divide the evolution to different "Periods" to detail the changes.

History Background

"Period of Recognizing" Brachial Plexus Injury: Before 1900

Galen (A.D.130–200), a Roman scholar, described nerve transection could result in motor and sensory lesions in the literature [1, 2]. During the next two millennia, brachial plexus was viewed only as a part of the peripheral nervous system. Smellie (1764) [3] described partial brachial plexus palsy in a newborn. Flaubert (1827) [4] and Duplay and Reclus (1895) [5] attributed neurovascular damages to sudden onset of traction with great force, such as axillary artery and the adjacent nerve tearing. Delbert (1910) [6] documented infraclavicular BPI associated with shoulder subluxation and noted favorable return of function even when no exploration or nerve surgery was performed. The mainstay of the nineteenth century recognized upper limb paralysis is an injury to the brachial plexus, and it is not the previously believed multiple isolated lesions of the terminal branches. Duchenne (1872) [7] described four children with upper brachial plexus lesion caused by forceful delivery of the shoulder and coined the term obstetric brachial plexus palsy (OBPP). Erb (1876) [8] recognized adult palsies of the shoulder and elbow injuries involving the C5 and C6 spinal nerves, with the same characteristics described by Duchenne. Thus, the term Erb-Duchenne palsy implies upper plexus palsy. Klumpke (1885) [9], a female medical intern, attributed palsies of the hand and forearm with associated Horner's sign to injuries to the C8 and T1 roots. The term Klumpke palsy is now synonymous with lower plexus palsy. Neurologists Duval and Guillain [10] (1898) further calculated the angle of spinal root emergence and demonstrated how forceful sudden stretch on the shoulder results in tearing of the upper roots. During this period, surgical treatment for nerve injuries was still in an exploratory and experimental state. Although Laugier (1864) [11]

J. C.-Y. Lu · D. C.-C. Chuang (✉)
Department of Plastic Surgery, Chang Gung Memorial Hospital, Taipei-Linkou, Taiwan

A. Y. Shin, N. Pulos (eds.), *Operative Brachial Plexus Surgery*,
https://doi.org/10.1007/978-3-030-69517-0_1

described successful nerve repair using suture technique, and shortly thereafter Phillipeaux and Vulpian (1870) [12], as well as Albert (1885) [13] experimented with nerve grafts in peripheral nerve gaps, none were used for brachial plexus injury.

"Period of Pessimism" for Clinical Brachial Plexus Injury Repair: Before Microscope Assistance (1964)

Unsatisfactory results for brachial plexus surgery in the early twentieth century brought forth pessimism. William Thorborne (1900) [14], a British surgeon, published the results of surgically repairing a brachial plexus lesion in a 16-year-old girl with flail arm. He was able to identify the level of injury distal to the suprascapular nerve, which was different from root avulsions, and he excised the neuroma while reportedly "secondarily suturing the two stumps directly without tension." At 4 years after surgery, the girl demonstrated good elbow and wrist flexion, but no shoulder or hand functions. This was considered the first documented attempt of surgically repairing a brachial plexus injury. Attention then shifted to repair in birth-related brachial plexus injuries. Kennedy (1903) [15] attempted surgical repair in C5 and C6 roots with birth-related injuries, while Taylor (1920) [16] expanded surgery from the pediatric population to the adults. In addition to excising the neuroma and attempting to suture the defect directly, the concept of shoulder immobilization was introduced to relieve tension on the sutured nerves. Unfortunately, documentation of the outcomes is absent and would most likely have been unfavorable. As seen in Sever's series (1925) [17] of 1100 obstetric patients, the author concluded no distinguishable benefits from surgery compared to nonoperative management. The common pessimism shared among surgeons was the realization that surgical exploration did not elucidate the true extent of the nerve injury. Most surgeons during this period preferred a wait and see attitude for BPI, even with the increase in major injuries suffered from the Second World War. If patients presented with avulsion of the surgical roots was suspected, or chronic nerve injuries, observation would be favored. Procedures such as Steindler's elbow flexorplasty (1918) [18] were more popular for their immediate effect and predictable results, which led to the development of other palliative techniques: pectoralis major muscle transfer by Clark (1946) [19] and Seddon (1949) [20, 21] or amputations for concomitant neurovascular injuries of the brachial plexus [22]. However, the Second World War brought back renewed interest in brachial plexus injuries with major BPI. With the increased prevalence of open, penetrating injuries from bullet and stab wounds, Davis (1947) [23] published a series of open and closed injuries to the brachial plexus. The authors recommended early exploration, neurolysis to free nerves from adjacent scars, and nerve grafts when end-to-end stump reapproximation was not possible. It is interesting to see the current principles of nerve repair/reconstruction recognized at such an early time [24]. In this period, the fundamentals of the modern science of nerve surgery appeared from two major contributors: Seddon and Sunderland's classification of the degree of nerve injury. The revolution in peripheral nerve surgery was initiated by Dr. Herbert Seddon (1943) [25], a British orthopedic surgeon, famed for his description of the three levels of nerve injury: neuropraxia (disruption injury of the endoneurium), axonotmesis (disruption injury of the mesoneurium), and neurotmesis (disruption injury of the epineurium). Dr. Sydney Sunderland (1968) [26], an Australian surgical anatomist, classified nerve injuries into five degrees. Sunderland expanded Seddon's axonotmesis concept into two separate degrees of injury (Sunderland 2 and 3, which means partial and incomplete injury) and also expanded neurotmesis into two more degrees (Sunderland 4 and 5, lesion in continuity and complete nerve division). The classification of nerve injury gave a rationale for the timing of nerve reconstruction. Meanwhile, notable tools such as cervical myelography [27], electromyography [28], and histamine test [29] were used to differentiate preganglionic from postganglionic injuries and improved preoperative diagnosis and planning. Seddon's experience in peripheral nerve injuries expanded from direct nerve repair to the use of autogenous nerve grafting (1947–1961) [30–33], and he cited unfavorable outcomes in BPI. At that time, discouraging results were reported by Barnes (1949) [34], Nulsen and Slade (1956) [35], Tracy and Brannon (1958) [36], and Bonney (1959) [24]. At the Paris meeting of the International Society for Orthopedic Surgery and Traumatology in1966, they concluded that surgical repair of brachial plexus lesions could not guarantee effective and predictable results [37]. This was a dismal time to become a brachial plexus surgeon.

"Period of Improvement (I)" by Microscopy Application (1964–1999)

The introduction of microscopy was in 1964. Seddon's speech in 1963 [32] at the Royal College of Surgeons argued against the mentality of always trying to primarily repair nerve gaps by mobilizing the nerve ends and keeping joint flexed, sometimes even beyond the "critical resection length" of the nerve leading to excessive tension. Millesi (1967–1988) [38–41] applied microsurgical technique to nerve dissection and interfascicular nerve grafting to improve outcomes. In his works, he particularly advocated for (1) differentiation of normal and pathological tissue with intraneural neurolysis, (2) interfascicular nerve graft for fascicular approximation (fascicular repair) with minimal manipulation, and (3) tensionless repair (Fig. 1.1). Millesi recognized that the poor establishment of circulation in the large graft can result from ischemic change in the center of the graft. Narakas (1969) [43] confirmed Millesi's work on interfascicular nerve grafting as his clinical outcomes *were* found satisfying even when dealing with extensive soft tissue loss. Rather than using a single thick nerve graft at the nerve root level of the brachial plexus, several nerve grafts (cable grafts) were needed to extend each fascicle of the root to the targets. Deburge (1967) [44], Lusskin and Campbell (1973) [45], Allieu (1977) [46], Narakas (1981) [47], Alnot (1987) [48], Millesi (1988) [49], and Terzis (1999) [50] published their large series of brachial plexus injury patients reconstructed with neurolysis, nerve transfer, nerve grafting, and

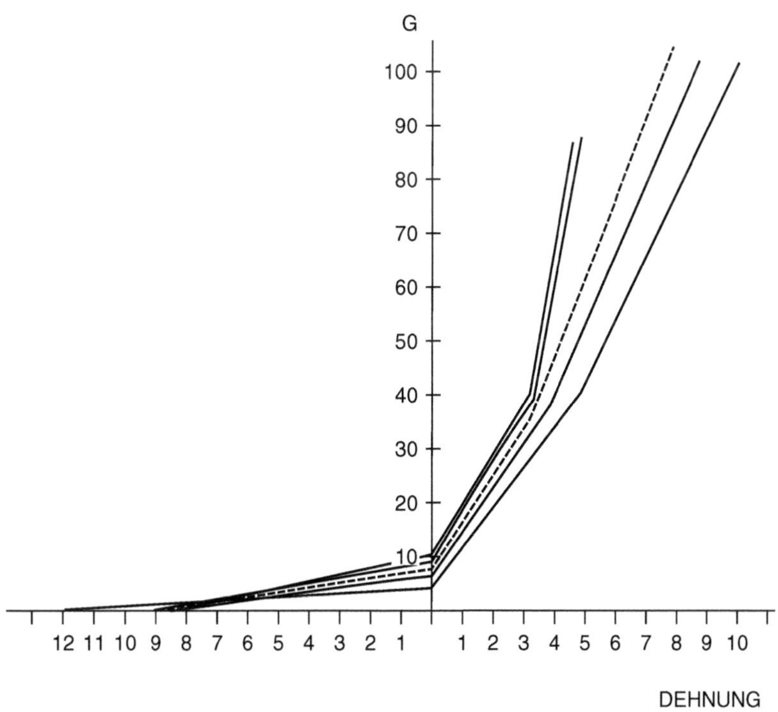

Fig. 1.1 Tension at the suture line increases with 2–3% gap of the whole length of the injured nerve. (From Berger and Millesi [42])

muscle transfers all with the employment of modern microsurgical techniques. Satisfactory results were reported in cases with penetrating or lacerating injuries. Improvement in nerve grafting was attributed to the blood supply in the grafts. By use of cabled grafts, vascular ingrowth was possible with the smaller individual strands in comparison to a single large diameter graft. When the recipient bed has inadequate blood supply, or the nerve gap is large, pedicled [51] and free vascularized nerve grafts [52] were introduced. In addition, when the proximal root was avulsed, or when the lower cervical roots were involved, nerve transfer using extraplexus or intraplexus donors became the next popular trend [53–55].

The introduction of microscopy in microneurosurgical and microvascular techniques, increased knowledge of brachial plexus anatomy (macro- and microanatomy) [56–59], advance of imaging and electrodiagnostic studies, improved techniques in nerve grafting, more donor nerves available for nerve transfer, introduction of functioning free muscle transplantation, advancements in palliative reconstruction, and increased understanding of rehabilitation and long-term follow-up have significantly improved the outcomes of brachial plexus reconstruction and brought forth unforeseen optimism.

"Period of Improvement (II)" by Nerve Transfer and Free Functioning Muscle Transplantation Application, 2000–Till Now

Neurotization is a surgical technique by transferring healthy and functional nerves to reinnervate denervated sensory or motor nerves or target of skin or muscle in the central or peripheral nerve lesions. Narakas (1988) [55] described five possible types of neurotization: cutaneocutaneous neurotization (healthy skin reinnervates the neighboring denervated skin), musculomuscular neurotization (healthy muscle reinnervates the neighboring denervated muscle), neuromuscular neurotization (functional nerve implants to a denervated muscle), neurocutaneous neurotization (functional nerve implants to the dermis of the skin), and neuroneural (motor or sensory nerve coaptation) neurotization. When "nerve transfer" is termed, it is actually a neuroneural neurotization, a procedure requiring division of a healthy donor nerve and coaptation to a denervated recipient nerve.

Revolution in Nerve Transfer

Credit should be given to Harris and Low (1903) [60], who first proposed suturing the distal stump of the damaged spinal nerve to healthy contiguous nerve (Fig. 1.2). This concept laid the foundation for the technique of nerve transfer, where adjacent healthy nerves can be sacrificed to serve as donors for injured stumps of more important recipient nerves. In a patient with avulsed 5th and 6th cervical nerves, Tuttle (1913) [61] used the anterior terminal branch of the 4th cervical nerve and sutured the donor to half of the distal stump of the upper trunk. Elbow flexion was shown to improve, although with little shoulder recovery. Vulpius and Stoffel (1920) [62] rerouted branches to the pectoralis muscle for transfer to ruptured musculocutaneous nerve and axillary nerves. The German surgeon Foerster (1929) [63], who operated on many war-related brachial plexus injuries, described transferring nerves of the

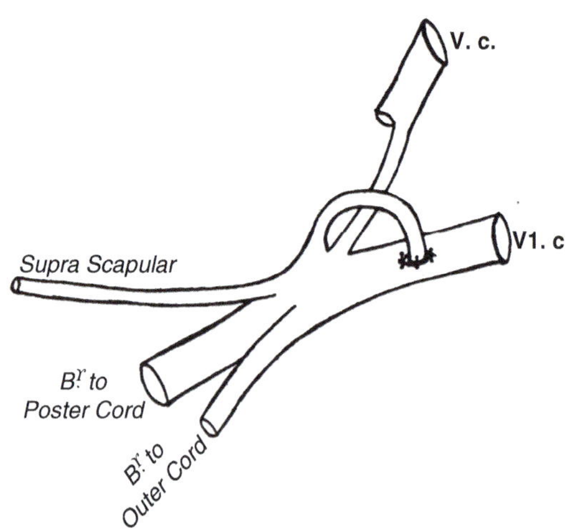

Fig. 1.2 The earliest description of nerve transfer. (From Harris and Low [60])

latissimus dorsi or subscapularis to ruptured axillary nerve and nerve of serratus anterior to the musculocutaneous nerve. Chiasserini (1934) [64] initiated the use of intercostal nerve transfer in paraplegics. Lurje (1948) [65] applied nerve transfer to upper division of the upper trunk in effort to restore deltoid and biceps function. With information gathered from 100 cadavers, he cited phrenic nerve, long thoracic nerve, medial pectoral nerve, lateral pectoral nerve, anterior rami of radial nerve, and subscapularis nerve as common donor nerves for nerve transfer. This was the first paper to describe transfer of branch to the triceps to the axillary nerve.

With increasing success on the management of brachial plexus injury, the recognition that upper roots are more prone to rupture and lower roots are more likely to be avulsed further ascended the popularity of nerve transfer. At that time, popular donor nerves in nerve transfer included intercostal nerve [66–69], spinal accessory nerve [70], phrenic nerve [71], and contralateral C7 [72]. Target nerves would be the suprascapular nerve, the musculocutaneous nerve, axillary nerve, median or ulnar nerves, even at more proximal level the upper trunk, the posterior cord, and occasionally the lateral or medial cords. Even with complete limb paralysis, contemporary techniques and experiences brought forth progress, which was never seen before.

Gu (1991) [72] was the first to present the use of the contralateral C7 (CC7) root (spinal nerve) as a rich source of axons to innervate the affected side nerve(s). The surgery proposed used a two-staged pedicled vascularized ulnar graft application to avoid central necrosis in a non-vascularized trunk graft. Gilbert (1992) [73] used the contralateral medial pectoral nerve of the healthy side as a donor nerve to innervate the musculocutaneous nerve on the affected side using a sural nerve graft as a bridge. Chuang (1993) [74] modified the CC7 technique by using a one-stage free vascularized ulnar nerve graft to bridge the gap between the contralateral C7 and the median nerve of the affected side as a one-stage procedure, or followed with functioning free muscle

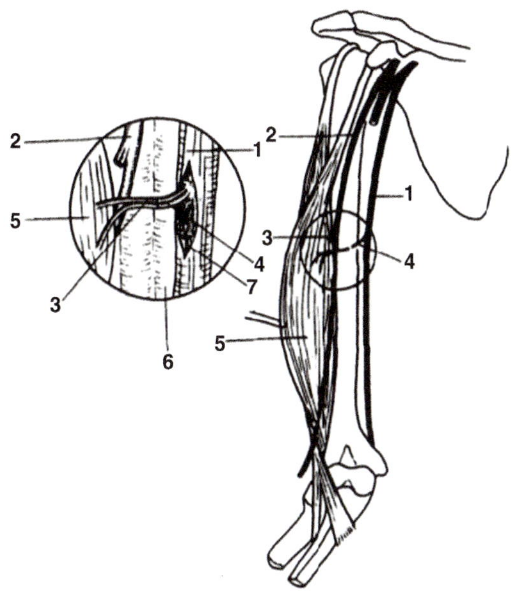

Fig. 1.3 Distal nerve transfer of a branch of the ulnar nerve to biceps branch of the musculocutaneous nerve for elbow flexion. (From Oberlin et al. [76])

transplantation as a two-stage procedure for total root avulsion reconstruction.

Narakas (1988) [75] recognized that distal nerve transfer would only be of benefit if the site of reconstruction was closer to the target muscle. Oberlin (1994) [76] (Fig. 1.3) described transferring 10% of the ulnar nerve at the upper arm to the motor nerve of the biceps for elbow flexion. In four cases, he reported no significant impairment of the hand. Using a similar technique but applying a nerve stimulator to preserve fascicles to the intrinsics of the hand, Leechavengvongs (1998) [77] reconfirmed the technique with high success rate and reliability: 31 of 32 patients with biceps muscle power of M3 or more and no subjective deficit in sensation or grip strength. In order to maximize elbow flexion recovery, Mackinnon et al. (2000–2008) [78–80] specifically delineated the expendable fascicles that innervated the flexor carpi radialis, flexor digitorum superficialis, palmaris longus of the median nerve, and the FCU of the ulnar nerve as possible donors in double fascicular transfer for elbow flexion (Fig. 1.4). Applying the same concept would be the transfer of the branch to the long

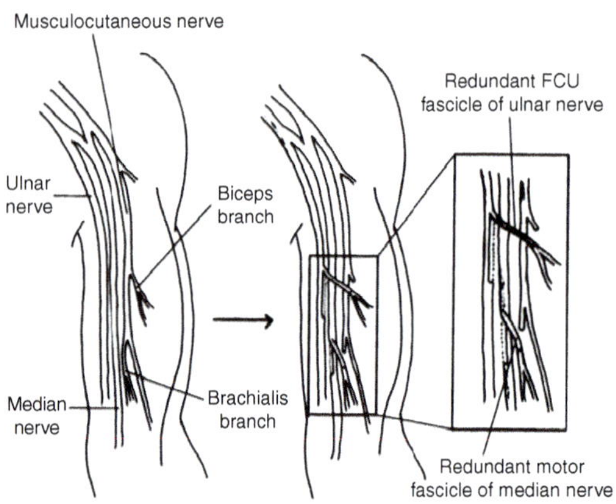

Fig. 1.4 Double fascicular transfer to the musculocutaneous nerve for elbow flexion. (From Mackinnon et al. [79])

head of the triceps [81], or the medial head of the triceps to the target axillary nerve for deltoid reinnervation [82]and the anterior interosseous nerve to the deep motor branch of the ulnar nerve for hand intrinsics reinnervation [82].

Functioning Free Muscle Transplantation (FFMT)

The management of total brachial plexus palsy underwent drastic changes over the past (twentieth) century. Seddon (1961) [33] abandoned reconstructive operations in favor of amputation and arthrodesis in such circumstances. Meanwhile, Narakas (1978) [53] laid out the functional priorities of the upper limb where (1) elbow joint control was upmost priority, followed by (2) wrist and finger flexion with median nerve sensation, (3) shoulder function, (4) wrist and finger extension, and (5) intrinsic hand and ulnar sensation. While elbow and shoulder function were reconstructed with extraplexus nerve transfer, the goals of restoring wrist and finger flexion and hand sensation were often abandoned. With the advancement of microsurgery, nerve transfer, and FFMT (Manktelow 1978 [83], Ikuta 1979 [84], Doi 1991 [85], Chuang 1996 [86]), attention shifted to restoring finger movement and hand sensation in total root avulsion patients. Nerve transfer and FFMT became the most reliable options.

FFMT is the transfer of a fresh muscle utilizing microvascular anastomoses for revascularization and subsequent microneural coaptation to the recipient motor nerve for muscle reinnervation. The use of FFMT in brachial plexus reconstruction is actually an example of the application of nerve transfer technique, and it has been shown to be effective and thus gained increased popularity.

Doi (1991) [85] described using free or pedicled latissimus dorsi muscle transfer to obtain elbow and finger flexion simultaneously, so-called one muscle for two functions. He would later publish the double FFMT technique that they have established as a protocol for complete root avulsions (1995) [87] (Fig. 1.5). He further added additional procedures such as nerve transfer for shoulder function, elbow extension, and hand sensation to improve the results (2000) [88].

Gracilis myocutaneous FFMT is the most frequently used donor muscle in brachial plexus reconstruction, in which the overlying skin flap is used for monitoring. The commonly used extraplexus donor nerves include the spinal accessory nerve, intercostal nerves, phrenic nerve with nerve graft elongation, and contralateral C7 with vascularized ulnar nerve graft elongation. The intraplexus donor nerves include part of the ulnar, part of the median nerve, or more proximally the infraclavicular or suprascapular nerve which requires nerve elongation in a two-stage procedure [89, 90].

At the end of the twentieth century and beginning of the twenty-first century, we saw the advances in three fields that changed the paradigms in brachial plexus injury: (1) intra- and extraplexus nerve transfers, or called proximal nerve transfers by using intraplexus nearby nerves or extraplexus donor nerves such as phrenic nerve, deep cervical motor branches, hypoglossal nerve, spinal accessory nerve, intercostal nerves, and contralateral C7 spinal nerve; (2) distal nerve transfers by using ulnar, median, or radial nerves as donor nerves; and (3) free functioning muscle transplantation. Attempts to reconstruct hand function in total root avulsions of the brachial plexus become more available and effective. In early or acute BPI, people recognized

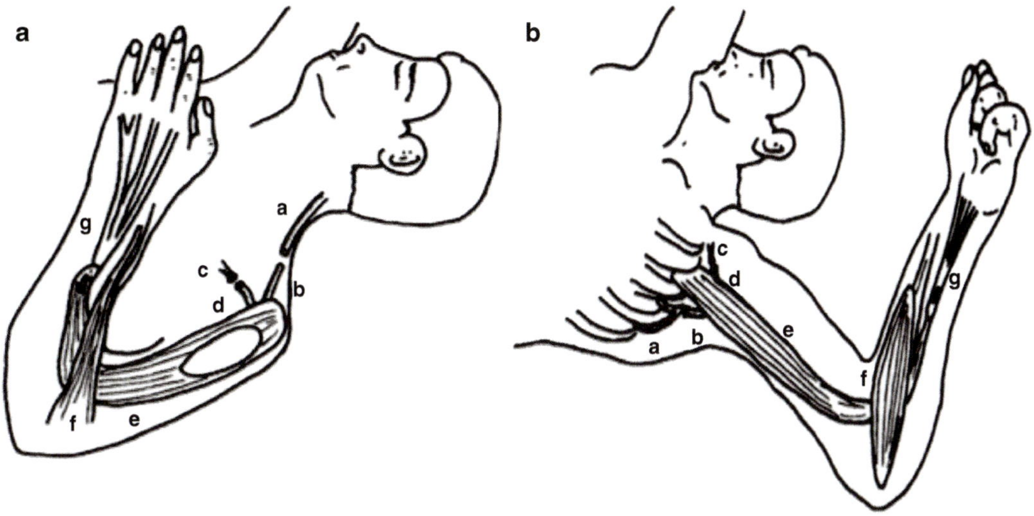

Fig. 1.5 Double muscle transplantation for total root avulsion reconstruction. (**a**) FFMT to restore elbow flexion and finger extension innervated by accesory nerve. (**b**) FFMT to restore finger flexion innervated by intercostal nerves. (From Doi et al. [87])

that timing of nerve transfer is a crucial factor in achieving successful results. In chronic BPI, nerve elongation first, followed by FFMT, is also an effective strategy for reconstruction.

Important milestones in the development of brachial plexus management are listed in Table 1.1.

Perspectives on the Future of BPI Reconstructive Microsurgery

The senior author, Chuang, had been trained by Terzis in 1984, Millesi in 1987, Narakas in 1987, and Kondo (Tsuyama group) in 1988 for peripheral nerve reconstruction. Till now he himself has performed more than 2000 cases of adult and pediatric brachial plexus exploration and reconstruction and more than 1000 cases of FFMT for different purposes. The senior author was continuously selected as the chapter author to edit the title of "Brachial Plexus Injuries" in the Textbook of "Plastic Surgery" (2nd edition 2006 [95], 3rd edition 2013 [96], and 4th edition 2018 [97]). The authors would like to make the following one proposal and few comments for the future of BPI reconstruction.

Table 1.1 Important milestones in the development of brachial plexus management

Main author	Period	Ref. No.	Message
Erb	1876	[8]	Recognition of C5/C6 root injuries for shoulder and elbow palsies
Klumpke	1885	[9]	Recognition of lower trunk or C8/T1 root injuries
Thorborne	1900	[14]	First to publish in detail the results of a surgically repaired brachial plexus lesion in a patient
Harris & Low	1903	[60]	First reported nerve transfer concept at root level for brachial plexus injury
Tuttle	1913	[61]	Transfer of nerves from cervical plexus to distal 5th, 6th roots
Seddon	1943	[25]	Classification of the three levels of peripheral nerve injuries
Seddon	1947	[30]	Description of autogenous grafts in nerve gaps
Sunderland	1951	[26]	Expanded the classification of nerve injury to 5 degrees
Millesi	1967	[40]	Introduction of microsurgery to nerve grafting

(continued)

Table 1.1 (continued)

Main author	Period	Ref. No.	Message
Berger & Millesi	1978	[91]	Emphasis on tension in nerve repair and the need for nerve grafting
Ikuta	1979	[84]	Use of free muscle graft for brachial plexus injury
Narakas	1985	[92, 104]	Neuroneural intraplexus transfer at root level
Terzis	1987	[52]	Vascularized nerve grafts
Gu	1989	[72]	Use of contralateral healthy C7 root for nerve transfer
Oberlin	1994	[76]	Distal nerve transfer of a branch of the ulnar nerve to biceps branch of the musculocutaneous nerve for elbow flexion
Doi	1995	[87]	Double FFMT transfer in total root avulsion
Bertelli	2011	[93]	T1 hand concept
Mackinnon	2005	[79]	Double fascicular transfer for elbow flexion
Chuang	2012	[94]	Multiple nerve transfers for total root avulsion as a one-stage reconstruction

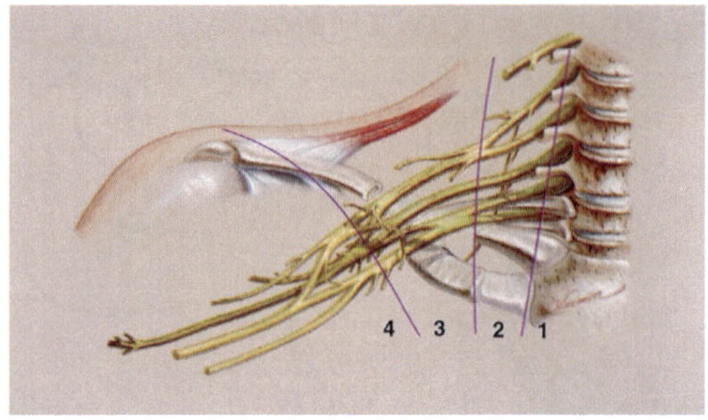

Fig. 1.6 New classification of level of brachial plexus injury: Level I, lesions inside the bone; Level II, lesions inside the muscle; Level III, lesions pre- and retroclavicular; Level IV, lesions infraclavicular. (From Chuang [97])

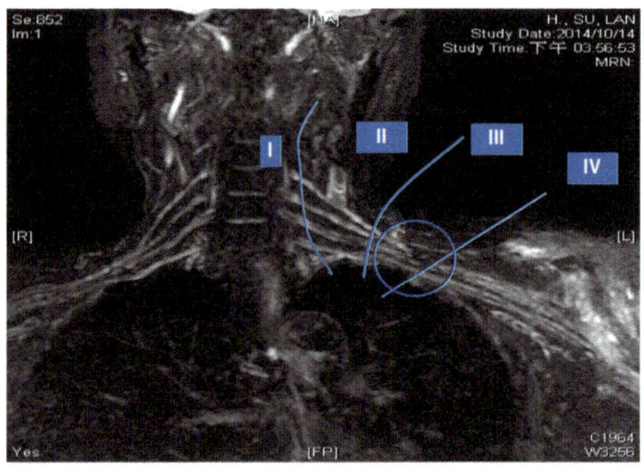

Fig. 1.7 New classification of level of brachial plexus injury in MRI. The MRI shows that the lesion is located in level III

One Proposal

Level of Brachial Plexus Injury

Various classifications of the level of BPI have been proposed without general consensus for unification [93, 96, 97]. The senior author has proposed that the classification is better expressed with the numbers, "Levels I to IV," rather than word descriptions [96, 97] (Figs. 1.6 and 1.7). The new classification is based on intraoperative findings and procedures, easily and quickly being understood:

- Level I: Injury inside the bone (vertebral bone), similar to the term preganglionic root injury which includes spinal cord, rootlet, and root injuries. Laminectomy and bone removal should be performed if the surgeon wants to visualize the underlying nerve structures.
- Level II: Injury inside the muscle (scalene anterior muscle), similar to the term postganglionic spinal nerve injury. Segmental resection of the scalene anterior muscle should be performed if the surgeon wants to visualize the underlying spinal nerves.
- Level III: Injury located pre- and retroclavicularly, including trunk and division injury. Osteotomy of the clavicle or elevation of the clavicle by connection of the supra- and infraclavicular fossa should be performed to facilitate nerve exploration and reconstruction.
- Level IV: The injury is infraclavicular, including cords and terminal branches. It usually encounters difficult dissection and requires long nerve grafts in closed BPI.

The new classification is simple and can facilitate the communication.

Comments on Two Major Debates

"Once debates, always debates" seems quite often in science researches. In the past three decades, there exist two major debates in the management of early and primary adult BPI. Which is the first choice for surgical treatment: (1) in total root avulsion, multiple nerve transfers vs. FFMTs? and (2) in incomplete BPI, proximal nerve grafts/transfers vs. distal nerve transfers?

In Total Root Avulsion BPI, Which Is the Treatment of Choice: Multiple Nerve Transfers or Free Functioning Muscle Transplantations?

Doi's (1991–2013) [85, 87, 88, 98] double FFMT across the elbow with a below-elbow pulley for hand reconstruction illustrates the "distal to proximal" in reconstruction priority, which means hand first and then elbow and shoulder. This is different from the traditional "proximal to distal" in reconstruction priority, in which elbow and shoulder are first and the hand is the last. The senior author (2012–2018) [89, 90, 94–97] advocates the use of multiple incisions for multiple nerve transfers (Fig. 1.8). In total root avulsion injury, Chuang advocates (1) CC7 transfer to the median nerve for finger and wrist flexion and finger sensation, (2) intercostal nerve transfer to the musculocutaneous nerve for elbow flexion, (3) phrenic nerve/deep cervical motor branch/hypoglossal nerve transfer to the distal C5 for shoulder function, and (4) preservation of the spinal accessory nerve for secondary enhancement. If the injury is C5 rupture and C6-T1 four root avulsion, then the C5, if the stump is healthy, will replace CC7 to the median nerve. If there is associated rib fracture with suspicious intercostal nerve injury, CC7 transfer contralaterally or healthy C5 ipsilaterally will transfer to musculocutaneous and median nerve two nerves together. FFMT is used predominantly as an adjuvant palliative reconstruction to enhance results in the later stage.

Advantages and disadvantages of multiple nerve transfers vs. FFMT in the acute BPI are shown in Table 1.2. Traditional strategy with multiple nerve transfers to obtain shoulder, elbow, and hand function is preferred by the authors.

In Incomplete Root Avulsion BPI, Which Is the Treatment of Choice: Proximal Nerve Grafts/Transfers or Distal Nerve Transfers?

Nerve transfer can be broadly separated into two categories: proximal nerve grafts and/or transfers and distal nerve transfers [99]. Definition of proximal and distal nerve transfers is based on (1) distance (from the nerve coaptation site to the neuromuscular junction), (2) scar encountered in dissection, and (3) whether or not the recipient nerve has nerve branching out distally [100] (Table 1.3).

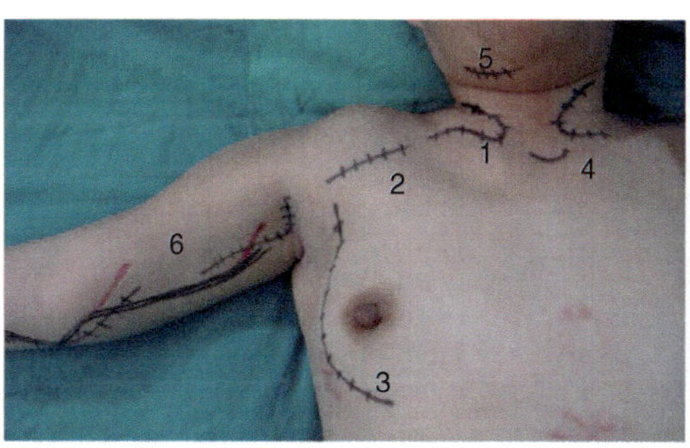

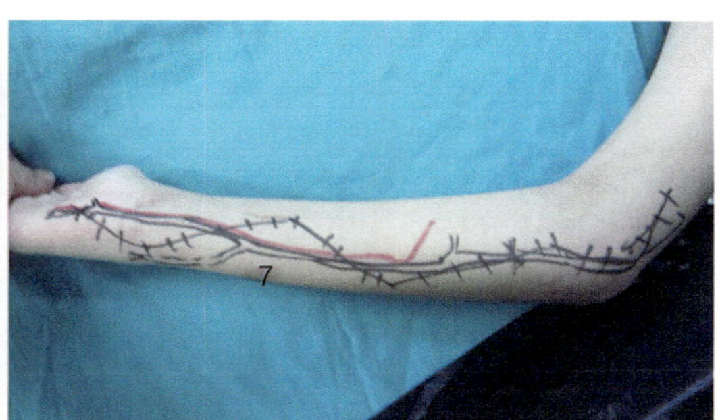

Fig. 1.8 Multiple incision lines for different purposes: (1) for supraclavicular brachial plexus exploration; (2) for infraclavicular brachial plexus exploration; (3) for intercostal nerve dissection; (4) for contralateral C7 dissection; (5) for hypoglossal nerve dissection; (6) for Oberlin or Mackinnon method of nerve transfer; (7) for vascularized ulnar nerve harvest

Table 1.2 Advantages and disadvantages of multiple nerve transfers vs. FFMTs in the acute BPI

	Multiple nerve transfers	FFMTs
Philosophy	Traditional strategy Proximal-to-distal in reconstruction priority	New strategy Distal-to-proximal in reconstruction priority
Reconstructive strategy	Multiple nerve transfers as a one-stage procedure FFMT, an adjuvant procedure to back up the results	Two FFMTs are essential Nerve transfers are adjuvant for shoulder and elbow extension and shoulder stability
Brachial plexus exploration	Yes	Maybe not
Nerve reconstruction		
For shoulder	Yes (by NT) for shoulder elevation	Shoulder fusion (or adjuvant by nerve transfer)
For elbow	Yes (by NT) for elbow flexion	Need FFMT for elbow flexion (adjuvant by nerve transfer for elbow extension)
For finger	Yes (by NT) for finger flexion	Need FFMTs for finger flexion and extension
Stage requirement for full reconstruction	Can be one stage	Always multiple stages
Rehabilitation period	Longer (at least 4 years)	2 years
Patient selection	Should be highly motivated, patient, and intelligent patient	Can be less intelligent and impatient patient
Predict outcomes		
Shoulder elevation	Better (≥60°)	Shoulder fusion (10–30°)
Elbow flexion	Usually better (M4)	M3–4
Finger flexion	M2–4	M2–4
Finger extension (EDC)	M0	M2–3
Finger sensation	Finger-like sensation, except 5th finger	Bizarre sensation (by ICN transfer)

NT nerve transfer, *FFMT* free functioning muscle transplantation, *ICN* intercostal nerve

Table 1.3 Advantages and disadvantages of proximal nerve grafts/transfers vs. distal nerve transfer in adult acute BPI

	Proximal nerve grafts/transfers	Distal nerve transfers
Philosophy	Traditional strategy	New strategy
Donor nerve	Intraplexus nerves, extraplexus (nearby) nerves Far from the target muscles	The donor nerve close to the target muscle
Definition	*Proximal nerve transfer*	*Distal nerve transfer*
Distance[a]	Longer (usually >10 cm)	Shorter (usually <5 cm)
Scar encountered	Yes	No
Target nerve with branching	Yes	No (direct to the muscle without branching)
Nerve graft required	Usually yes	No
Advantages	Diagnosis and treatment Mother nerves, more axons and power Nerve cut, less functional deficits Avoid unnecessary distal nerve transfer Check C5C6C7 stumps (especially C5) More options for shoulder reconstruction	Dissection in the healthy tissue, no scars, easy dissection Nerve-cut stump: healthy Direct nerve coaptation without nerve graft Shorter operation time Short rehabilitation time, faster recovery
Disadvantages	Operative site: more scars, difficult dissection, easy bleeding May have stump unhealthy, unpredictable Usually require nerve grafts Longer operation time Longer rehabilitation period, need patience	No diagnosis Risk to have iatrogenic injury, miss the powerful proximal nerve sources Risk of donor nerve cut causing some sequelae May need multiple incisions
Indication	All kinds of avulsion/rupture injury of brachial plexus injury	Not global BPI Intrinsic palsy of the hand

[a]Distance from the nerve coaptation to the neuromuscular junction

Proximal nerve graft/transfer is a traditional way that requires brachial plexus exploration to confirm the diagnosis. Diagnostic exploration is essential and especially true for ruptured C5 roots mistakenly presumed as root avulsion. Distal nerve transfer is a new strategy of reconstruction; it may or may not involve exploration of the brachial plexus. The superiority and which strategy is the best are yet to be investigated. However, in the last three decades, a major shift away from the traditional proximal nerve grafts/transfers to the more popular distal nerve transfers has occurred. Distal nerve transfer surgery has become part of the standard armamentarium offered to the BPI or high-level peripheral nerve injuries.

The senior author would like to make comments for this debate: (1) Proximal nerve grafts/transfers are still the main reconstructive procedure based on the principle of "no diagnosis, no treatment." Proximal nerve grafts/transfers allow intraoperative diagnosis as well as surgical intervention. This is especially true on C5, which is ruptured but the preoperative impression of avulsion (2). Distal nerve transfer provides only surgical intervention. It should not be applied in situations when proximal nerve graft/transfer is indicated. This is true in any peripheral nerve injury and reconstruction [101] (3). Proximal nerve graft/transfer requires less brain plasticity and allows easy spontaneous recovery without specific induction of exercise training (4). Proximal nerve transfer can avoid iatrogenic injury to the powerful proximal nerves (5). Proximal nerve graft/transfer can be applied in both complete and incomplete BPI.

However, disadvantages of proximal nerve graft/transfer include as follows: (1) Dense scars with difficult dissection will be encountered. Oozing and bleeding will be very often which requires diathermy carefully (2). Longer operation time is always required (3). The health of proximal ruptured stump is sometimes unpredictable, even when accessed microscopically (4). Interposition of nerve grafts is always required, which can jeopardize functional recovery (5). Longer rehabilitation time is necessary.

As such, the authors would like to make the following comments: Proximal nerve graft/transfer offers more accurate diagnosis and proper treatment to restore shoulder and elbow functions simultaneously. Distal nerve transfers can offer more efficient elbow flexion. Combining both strategies in primary nerve reconstruction when there is no healthy or insufficient donor nerve available is the authors' preferred choice.

Advantages and disadvantages of proximal nerve graft/transfer vs. distal nerve transfer for the incomplete BPI in the acute stage is shown in Table 1.3.

Uncertainty and Questions with Need of Future Investigation

The following subjects are still full of uncertainty with no universal acceptance in clinical application, although they have been proposed in the past:

1. Tissue engineering of nerve conduit (nerve tube) for the nerve gap
2. Nerve allograft with immunosuppressant medication
3. New nerve growth factor or stem cell application to improve regeneration
4. End-to-side neurorrhaphy [91, 102]
5. Spinal cord implantation of avulsed ventral roots [92]
6. Spinal cord injury and reconstruction
7. Sympathetic trunk injury and reconstruction
8. Intractable nerve shooting pain treatment (by encouraging medication or surgical approach?)
9. Others such as: How to differentiate motor/sensory fascicles in a mixed nerve intraoperatively? How to improve motor function of a FFMT? Will sensory axon input or motor axon input on the long nerve graft enhance the outcomes? Will supermicrosurgery or nanosurgery new technology improve the future nerve reconstruction?

Further investigation from research is warranted for clinical realization. These uncertainties may be resolved by new materials, new device, or new instruments, better researches, and innovative ideas in the future. As we have witnessed from the history of brachial plexus injury and reconstruction, change comes for optimism and the striving for better outcomes. Anything is possible.

Conclusion

Philosophy of Bunnell [103] "for a patient who has nothing, a little is a lot" should be always kept in mind when approaching brachial plexus injuries. Reconstruction of a completely paralyzed limb is no longer impossible, but achievable.

References

1. Robotti E, Longhi P, Verna G, Bocchiotti G. Brachial plexus surgery. An historical perspective. Hand Clin. 1995;11(4):517–33.
2. McHenry LC. Garrison's history of neurology. Springfield: Charles C. Thomas; 1969.
3. Smellie W. Collection of cases and observations in mid-wifery. 21768.
4. Flaubert A. Mémoire sur plusiers cas de luxations dans les efforts pour la réduction ont été suivis d'accidents graves. Répertoire générale d'anatomie et de physiologie pathologique. 1827;3:55–79.
5. Duplay SR. Trattato di Chirurgia. Torino Unione Tipografico-Editrice. 1895;8:142–3.
6. Delbert PCA. Les paralysies dans les luxation de l'epaule. Rev Chir. 1910;41:327–52.
7. Duchenne GB. De l'Electrisation Local- isee et de Son Application a la Pathologie et a la Therapeutique. 3rd ed. Paris. 1872.
8. Erb W. Diseases of the peripheral cerebrospinal nerves. In: von Ziemssen HW, editor. Cyclopaedia of the practice of medicine. New York: Wm. Wood & Co.; 1876.
9. Klumpke A. Contribution à l'étude des paralysies radiculaires du plexus brachial. Rev Med (Paris). 1885;5:591–790.
10. Duval P, Guillain G. Pathogénie des accidents nerveux consécutifs aux luxations et traumatismes de l'épaule. Arch Gén Méd. 1898;2:143–91.
11. Laugier M. Note sur la suture du nerf médian. Comptes rendus. 1864;1864:1139–43.
12. Phillipeaux J, Vulpian A. Note sur les essais de greffe d'un troncon de nerf lingual entre les deux bouts de l'hypoglosse. Arch Physiol Norm Path. 1870;3:618.
13. Albert E. Einige operationen an nerven. Wien Med Presse. 1885;26:1285–8.
14. Thorburn W. A clinical lecture on secondary suture of the brachial plexus. Br Med J. 1900;1(2053):1073–5.
15. Kennedy R. Suture of the brachial plexus in birth paralysis of the upper extremity. Br Med J. 1903;1(2197):298.
16. Taylor AS. Brachial birth palsy and injuries of similar type in adults. Surg Gynecol Obstet. 1920;30(5):494–502.
17. Sever JW. Obstetric paralysis: report of eleven hundred cases. J Am Med Assoc. 1925;85(24):1862–5.
18. Steindler A. A muscle plasty for the relief of flail elbow in infantile paralysis. Interstate Med J. 1918;35:235–41.
19. Clark JM. Reconstruction of biceps brachii by pectoral muscle transplantation. Br J Surg. 1946;34(134):180–1.
20. Brooks DM, Seddon HJ. Pectoral transplantation for paralysis of the flexors of the elbow; a new technique. J Bone Joint Surg Br. 1959;41-B(1):36–43.
21. Seddon HJ. Transplantation of pectoralis major for paralysis of the flexors of the elbow. Proc R Soc Med. 1949;42(10):837.
22. DeBakey ME, Simeone FA. Battle injuries of the arteries in World War II: an analysis of 2,471 cases. Ann Surg. 1946;123(4):534.
23. Davis L, Martin J, Perret G. The treatment of injuries of the brachial plexus. Ann Surg. 1947;125(5):647–57.
24. Bonney G. Prognosis in traction lesions of the brachial plexus. J Bone Joint Surg Br. 1959;41-B(1):4–35.
25. Seddon HJ. Peripheral nerve injuries. Glasgow Med J. 1943;139(3):61–75.
26. Sunderland S. A classification of peripheral nerve injuries producing loss of function. Brain. 1951;74(4):491–516.
27. Murphey L. Myelographic demonstration of avulsing injury of the brachial plexus. Am J Roentgenol Radium Ther. 1947;58:102–5.
28. Hodes R, Larrabee M, German W. The human electromyogram in response to nerve stimulation and the conduction velocity of motor axons: studies on normal and on injured peripheral nerves. Arch Neurol Psychiatr. 1948;60(4):340–65.
29. Bonney G. The value of axon responses in determining the site of lesion in traction injuries of the brachial plexus. Brain. 1954;77(4):588–609.
30. Seddon HJ. The use of autogenous grafts for the repair of large gaps in peripheral nerves. Br J Surg. 1947;35(138):151–67.
31. Seddon HJ. The practical value of peripheral nerve repair. Proc R Soc Med. 1949;42(6):427–36.
32. Seddon HJ. Nerve grafting. J Bone Joint Surg Br. 1963;45:447–61.
33. Yeoman PM, Seddon HJ. Brachial plexus injuries: treatment of the flail arm. J Bone Joint Surg Br. 1961;43(3):493–500.
34. Barnes R. Traction injuries of the brachial plexus in adults. J Bone Joint Surg Br. 1949;31B(1):10–6.

35. Nulsen F, Slade W. Recovery following injury to the brachial plexus. In: Peripheral nerve regeneration: a follow-up study of 3656 world war II injuries. Washington, DC: The National Academies Press; 1956. p. 389–408.
36. Tracy JF, Brannon EW. Management of brachial-plexus injuries (traction type). JBJS. 1958;40(5):1031–42.
37. Birch R. Brachial plexus injuries. J Bone Joint Surg. 1996;78(6):986–92.
38. Millesi H. Zum Problem der überbrückung von Defekten peripherer Nerven. Wien Med Wochenschr. 1968;118:182–7.
39. Millesi H. Surgical management of brachial plexus injuries. J Hand Surg Am. 1977;2(5):367–78.
40. Millesi H, Ganglberger J, Berger A. Erfahrungen mit der Mikrochirurgie peripherer Nerven. In: Chirurgia plastica et Reconstructiva: Springer; 1967. p. 47–55.
41. Millesi H, Meissl G, Katzer H. Zur Behandlung der Verletzungen des Plexus brachialis. Vorschlag einer integrierten Therapie. Bruns Beitr Klin Chir. 1973;220:429.
42. Berger A, Millesi H. Nerve grafting. ClinOrthopRelat Res. 1978;133:49–55.
43. Narakas A, Verdan C. Nerve grafts. Zeitschrift fur Unfallmedizin und Berufskrankheiten Revue de medecine des accidents et des maladies professionelles. 1969;62(3):137–52.
44. Deburge A, Merle D. Aubigné R: Etiologie, évolution et pronostic des paralysies traumatiques du plexus brachial. Rev Chir Orthop. 1967;53(1):23–42.
45. Lusskin R, Campbell JB, Thompson WA. Post-traumatic lesions of the brachial plexus: treatment by transclavicular exploration and neurolysis or autograft reconstruction. J Bone Joint Surg Am. 1973;55(6):1159–76.
46. Allieu Y. Exploration and direct treatment of neural lesions in traumatic paralysis caused by stretching of the brachial plexus in the adult. Revue de chirurgie orthopedique et reparatrice de l'appareil moteur. 1977;63(1):107–22.
47. Narakas A. Brachial plexus surgery. Orthop Clin North Am. 1981;12(2):303–23.
48. Alnot JY. Traumatic paralysis of the brachial plexus: preoperative problems and therapeutic indications. Philadelphia: WB Saunders; 1987.
49. Millesi H. Brachial plexus lesions: classification and operative technique. Philadelphia: WB Saunders; 1988.
50. Terzis JK, Vekris MD, Soucacos PN. Outcomes of brachial plexus reconstruction in 204 patients with devastating paralysis. Plast Reconstr Surg. 1999;104(5):1221–40.
51. Strange FSC. An operation for nerve pedicle grafting. Preliminary communication. Br J Surg. 1947;34(136):423–5.
52. Terzis JKBW. The anatomy of free vascularized nerve grafts. Philadelphia: Saunders; 1987.
53. Narakas A. Surgical treatment of traction injuries of the brachial plexus. Clin Orthop Relat Res. 1978;133:71–90.
54. Narakas A. Neurotization or nerve transfer for brachial plexus lesions. Ann Chir Main. 1982;1(2):101–18.
55. Narakas A. Neurotization or nerve transfer in traumatic brachial plexus lesions. Philadelphia: WB Saunders; 1987.
56. Bonnel F. Microscopic anatomy of the adult human brachial plexus: an anatomical and histological basis for microsurgery. Microsurgery. 1984;5(3):107–17.
57. Bonnel F, Allieu Y, Bruner P, Gilbert A, Rabischong P. Anatomical and surgical principles of the brachial plexus in newborn children. Int J Microsurg. 1980;2(1):12–5.
58. Leffert RD. The anatomy of the brachial plexus. New York: Churchill Livingstone; 1985.
59. Slingluff CLT, K J, Edgerton MT. The quantitative microanatomy of the brachial plexus in man. Reconstructive relevance. Philadelphia: WB Saunders; 1987.
60. Harris W, Low VW. On the importance of accurate muscular analysis in lesions of the brachial plexus; and the treatment of Erb's palsy and infantile paralysis of the upper extremity by cross-union of the nerve roots. Br Med J. 1903;2:1035–8.
61. Tuttle HK. Exposure of the brachial plexus with nerve transplantation. J Am Med Assoc. 1913;61(1):15–7.
62. Vulpius O, Stoffel A. Muskel-und Sehnentransplantation. Überpflanzungen an der oberen Extremität. Orthopädische Operationslehre 2nd ed. Part A Transplantation am Oberarm Stuttgart: Ferdinand Enke. 1920;266–271.
63. Foerster O. Die therapie der Schussverletzungen der peripheren Nerven, resultate der plexus operationen. Handbuch der neurologie von lewandowski. 1929;2:1676–91.
64. Chiasserini A. Tentativi di cura in casi di paraplegia da lesione de midollo lombare consecutiva a frattura vertebrale (anastomosi radiculo-intercostale). Il Policlinico. 1934;12:603–7.
65. Lurje A. Concerning surgical treatment of traumatic injury of the upper division of the brachial plexus (Erb's-type). Ann Surg. 1948;127(2):317–26.
66. Fantis A, Slezák Z. On the possibility of reinnervation in total lesions of the brachial plexus by intercosto-plexural anastomosis. Ceskoslovenska neurologie. 1965;28(6):412–8.
67. Kotani T. Trial surgical procedures of nerve transfer to avulsion injuries of plexus brachialis. Orthopaed Surg Traumatol. 1972:348–50.
68. Tsuyama N. Intercostal nerve transfer in the treatment of brachial plexus injury of root avulsion type. Paper presented at: Proceeding of the 12th congress of the international society of orthopaedic surgery and traumatology. 19721972.
69. Chuang DC, Yeh MC, Wei FC. Intercostal nerve transfer of the musculocutaneous nerve in avulsed

brachial plexus injuries: evaluation of 66 patients. J Hand Surg Am. 1992;17(5):822–8.
70. Allieu Y, Privat J, Bonnel F. Neurotization with the spinal nerve (nervus accessorius) in avulsions of roots of the brachial plexus. Neuro-Chirurgie. 1982;28(2):115.
71. Gu YD, Wu MM, Zhen YL, et al. Phrenic nerve transfer for brachial plexus motor neurotization. Microsurgery. 1989;10(4):287–9.
72. Gu Y, Zhang G, Chen D, et al. Cervical nerve root transfer from contralateral normal side for treatment of brachial plexus root avulsions. Chin Med J. 1991;104(3):208–11.
73. Gilbert A. Neurotization by contralateral pectoral nerve. Paper presented at: 10th symposium on the brachial plexus, Lausanne, Switzerland. 1992.
74. Chuang DC, Wei FC, Noordhoff MS. Cross-chest C7 nerve grafting followed by free muscle transplantations for the treatment of total avulsed brachial plexus injuries: a preliminary report. Plast Reconstr Surg. 1993;92(4):717–25. discussion 726-717
75. Narakas AO, Hentz VR. Neurotization in brachial plexus injuries. Indication and results. Clin Orthop Relat Res. 1988;237:43–56.
76. Oberlin C, Beal D, Leechavengvongs S, Salon A, Dauge M, Sarcy J. Nerve transfer to biceps muscle using a part of ulnar nerve for C5–C6 avulsion of the brachial plexus: anatomical study and report of four cases. J Hand Surg Am. 1994;19(2):232–7.
77. Leechavengvongs S, Witoonchart K, Uerpairojkit C, Thuvasethakul P, Ketmalasiri W. Nerve transfer to biceps muscle using a part of the ulnar nerve in brachial plexus injury (upper arm type): a report of 32 cases. J Hand Surg Am. 1998;23(4):711–6.
78. Tung TH, Novak CB, Mackinnon SE. Nerve transfers to the biceps and brachialis branches to improve elbow flexion strength after brachial plexus injuries. J Neurosurg. 2003;98(2):313–8.
79. Mackinnon SE, Novak CB, Myckatyn TM, Tung TH. Results of reinnervation of the biceps and brachialis muscles with a double fascicular transfer for elbow flexion. J Hand Surg Am. 2005;30(5):978–85.
80. Colbert SH, Mackinnon SE. Nerve transfers for brachial plexus reconstruction. Hand Clin. 2008;24(4):341–61.
81. Leechavengvongs S, Witoonchart K, Uerpairojkit C, Thuvasethakul P. Nerve transfer to deltoid muscle using the nerve to the long head of the triceps, part II: a report of 7 cases. J Hand Surg Am. 2003;28(4):633–8.
82. Novak CB, Mackinnon SE. Distal anterior interosseous nerve transfer to the deep motor branch of the ulnar nerve for reconstruction of high ulnar nerve injuries. J Reconstr Microsurg. 2002;18(6):459–64.
83. Manktelow RT, McKee NH. Free muscle transplantation to provide active finger flexion. J Hand Surg Am. 1978;3(5):416–26.
84. Ikuta Y, Yoshioka K, Tsuge K. Free muscle graft as applied to brachial plexus injury-case report and experimental study. Ann Acad Med Singap. 1979;8(4):454–8.
85. Doi K, Sakai K, Kuwata N, Ihara K, Kawai S. Reconstruction of finger and elbow function after complete avulsion of the brachial plexus. J Hand Surg Am. 1991;16(5):796–803.
86. Chuang DC. Functioning free muscle transplantation. In: Peimer CA, editor. Surgery of the hand and upper extremity. New York: McGraw-Hill; 1996. chapter 84. p. 1901–10.
87. Doi K, Sakai K, Kuwata N, Ihara K, Kawai S. Double free-muscle transfer to restore prehension following complete brachial plexus avulsion. J Hand Surg Am. 1995;20(3):408–14.
88. Doi K, Muramatsu K, Hattori Y, et al. Restoration of prehension with the double free muscle technique following complete avulsion of the brachial plexus: Indications and long-term results. JBJS. 2000;82(5):652.
89. Chuang DC. Neurotization and free muscle transfer for brachial plexus avulsion injury. Hand Clin. 2007;23(1):91–104.
90. Chuang DCC. Nerve transfer with functioning free muscle transplantation. Hand Clin. 2008;24(4):377–88.
91. Lundborg G, Kanje QZM, Danielsen N, Kerns JM. Can sensory and motor collateral sprouting be induced from intact peripheral nerve by end-to-side anastomosis. J Hand Surg (Br). 1994;19:277.
92. Hallin RG, Carlstedt T, Risling INRM. Spinal cord implantation of avulsed ventral roots in primates; correction between restored motor function and morphology. Exp Brain Res. 1999;124:304–10.
93. Bertelli JA, Ghizoni MF. Results and current approach for brachial plexus reconstruction. J Brachial Plex Peripher Nerve Inj. 2011;6:2–8.
94. Chuang DC, Hernon C. Minimum 4-year follow-up on contralateral C7 nerve transfers for brachial plexus injuries. J Hand Surg Am. 2012;37(2):270–6.
95. Chuang DCC. Adult brachial plexus injuries. In: Mathes S, Hentz VR, editors. Plastic surgery. 2nd ed. Philadelphia: Saunders Elsevier Inc., Vol VII, chapter 182; 2006. p. 515–38.
96. Chuang DCC. Brachial plexus injuries: adult and pediatric. In: Neligan PC, Chang J, editors. Plastic Surgery, vol. VI. 3rd ed. Philadelphia: Saunders Elsevier Inc; 2013. p. 789–816.
97. Chuang DCC. Brachial plexus injuries: adult and pediatric. In: Neligan PC, Chang J, editors. Plastic surgery, vol. VI. 4th ed. Philadelphia: Saunders Elsevier Inc; 2018. p. 812–44.
98. Doi K, Hattori Y, Sakamoto S, Dodakundi C, Satbhai NG, Montales T. Current procedure of double free muscle transfer for traumatic total brachial plexus palsy. JBJS Essent Surg Tech. 2014;3(3):e16.
99. Hu CH, Chang TN, Lu JCY, Laurence VG, Chuang DCC. Comparison of surgical strategies between proximal nerve graft and/or nerve transfer and dis-

tal nerve transfer based on functional restoration of elbow flexion: a retrospective review of 147 patients. Plast Reconstr Surg. 2018;141(1):68e–79e.
100. Chuang DCC. Distal nerve transfers: a perspective on the future of reconstructive microsurgery. J Reconstr Microsurg. 2018;34(09):669–71.
101. Pan CH, Chuang DCC, Rodríguez-Lorenzo A. Outcomes of nerve reconstruction for radial nerve injuries based on the level of injury in 244 operative cases. J Hand Surg Eur Vol. 2010;35(5):385–91.
102. Viterbo F, Trindada JC, Hoshino K, Mazzoni NA. End-to-side neurorrhaphy with removal of the epineurial sheath: an experimental study in rats. Plast Reconstr Surg. 1994;94:1038.
103. Boyes JH. Bunnell's surgery of the hand. 4th ed. Philadelphia: Lippincott; 1964.
104. Narakas A, Herzberg G. Neuro-neural intraplexal transfers in traumatic radicular avulsions of the brachial plexus. Report on fifteen cases. Ann Chir Main 1985;4:211–8.

Part I

Surgical Anatomy

Surgical Anatomy of the Brachial Plexus

2

Manuel Llusá, M. Rosa Morro, Joaquin Casañas, and Amy M. Moore

Supraclavicular Brachial Plexus and Collateral Branches

Surgical Anatomy

The brachial plexus contains between 85,000 and 160,000 nerve fibers (average of 120,000) that are distributed through the upper limb. The motor fibers represent one third of these and sensory fibers the other two thirds. According to Bonnel data, 40% of these motor fibers are intended for innervation of the shoulder girdle [1]. The brachial plexus, according to the classical form, consists of the ventral primary ramus of the last four cervical nerves (C5-C6-C7-C8) and the first thoracic (T1) [2–4] (Fig. 2.1). The roots of the C5 to C7 nerves emerge above the vertebral bodies of the same number, while C8 and T1 leave below the vertebral bodies C7 and T1.

M. Llusá
Hospital Vall d'Hebron, Brachial Plexus and Peripheral Nerve, Barcelona, Spain

M. R. Morro
Department of Human Anatomy and Embriology, Faculty of Medicine, University of Barcelona, Barcelona, Spain

J. Casañas
Department of Traumaunit, Brachial Plexus and Peripheral Nerve, Hospital Teknon, Barcelona, Spain

A. M. Moore (✉)
Department of Plastic and Reconstructive Surgery, The Ohio State University, Columbus, OH, USA

A. Y. Shin, N. Pulos (eds.), *Operative Brachial Plexus Surgery*,
https://doi.org/10.1007/978-3-030-69517-0_2

From their origin in the ventral rami of C5, C6, C7, C8, and T1 nerves, they mix to form the upper trunk (C5–C6), the middle trunk (C7), and lower trunk (C8 and T1). Each trunk gives rise to two divisions, anterior and posterior. The three posterior divisions form the posterior cord, the anterior division of the upper and middle trunks forms the lateral cord, and the anterior division of the lower trunk forms, itself, the medial cord. The lateral cord branches into the musculocutaneous nerve and lateral root of the median nerve; the medial cord divides into the medial root of the median nerve and the ulnar nerve. The posterior cord bifurcates into the axillary and radial nerves.

Roots, Spinal Nerve, and Branches

The spinal nerves have their origin from the spinal cord, leave the vertebral canal through the intervertebral foramen or neural foramen, and are distributed by specific sensory and motor territories. They have well-differentiated areas:

- The roots connect to the spinal nerve with the spinal cord. The dorsal root, i.e., sensory, emanates from the posterolateral sulcus of the spinal cord, originating from the posterior horn; it is larger (4–10 rootlets) and has an ovoid ganglion, the spinal ganglion or dorsal root ganglion, that is located in the middle area of the intervertebral foramen, containing

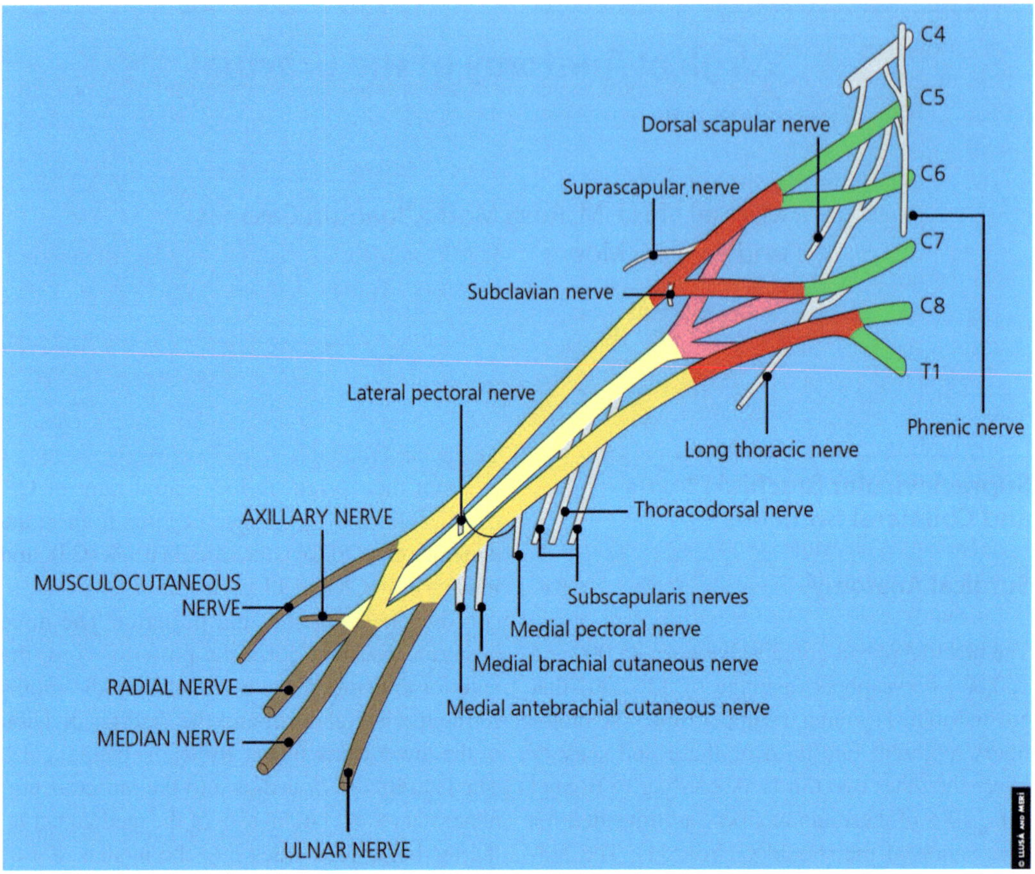

Fig. 2.1 Scheme of the brachial plexus and its collateral and terminal branches. Green: ventral ramus of the spinal nerve C5 to T1 and upper, middle and lower trunk. Red: anterior divisions of the trunks. Pink: posterior divisions of the trunks. Yellow: lateral and medial cords. Cream: posterior cord. Brown: terminal branches. White: collateral branches. [With permissions from Editorial Medica Panamericana]

the cell bodies of the sensory neurons. The ventral motor root is smaller (4–8 rootlets) and leaves the anterolateral sulcus of the spinal cord where its cellular body is located in the anterior horn (Fig. 2.2) [4].

- The spinal nerve is mixed containing motor and sensory fibers. It is formed by the union of four to eight ventral and dorsal rootlets that converge in the infundibulum of the dural sac; this takes place at the level of the midportion of neural foramen (see Fig. 2.2). The common trunk of the nerve is very short and rests in the costotransverse process between the ventral and dorsal tubercles of the cervical vertebrae [5]. The spinal nerve almost immediately divides into as follows:

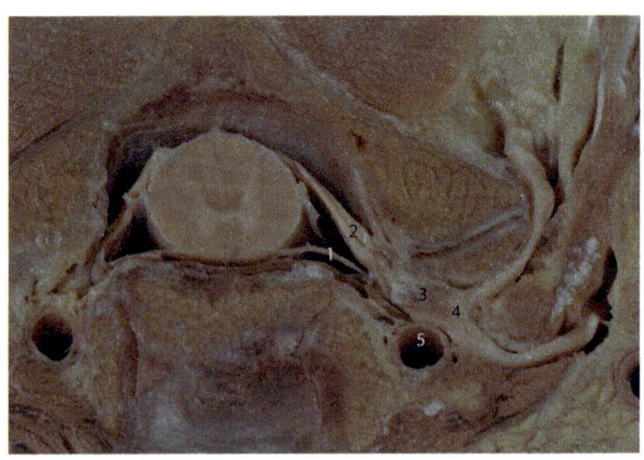

Fig. 2.2 Transverse section of the spinal cord and the roots that form the spinal nerve. 1 anterior rootlets, 2 posterior rootlets, 3 nerve ganglion, 4 spinal nerve, 5 vertebral artery. [With permissions from Editorial Medica Panamericana]

- The dorsal branch of the spinal nerve, i.e., dorsal primary ramus, runs posteriorly to innervate the paraspinal muscles and the skin of the back of the trunk (see Fig. 2.2). It is of dorsal embryological origin.
- The ventral branch of the spinal nerve, i.e., ventral primary ramus, retains the segmental character at the level of the thoracic region, but the fibers from the rest of the trunk intersect, divide, and interconnect to form the plexuses in the cervical and lumbosacral region. As the spinal nerves pass through the intervertebral foramen, their enveloping dura gradually turns into epineurium [6].
- Before the development of the plexuses, the ventral branches of C8 and T1 give two small nerve twigs: the white communicating branch, which joins it to the sympathetic ganglia, and the sinuvertebral nerve that, at the expense of a recurrent path, is reintroduced into the vertebral canal, innervating the meninges, vertebrae, and intervertebral discs (meningeal branches) [7].

From these origins, the axons of the roots of the plexus intersect, divide, and rejoin to give us the classic structure of the brachial plexus (see Fig. 2.1). The fibers that constitute the plexus are successively referred to as trunks (lower, middle, and upper), divisions (anterior and posterior), cords (lateral, medial, and posterior), terminal nerves, and collateral branches [8].

Trunks and Divisions

The trunks are named in the craniocaudal order as upper, middle, and lower trunks. According to the classic description, the upper trunk is formed by the "anastomosis" or union [1] of the anterior branches of C5 and C6, the middle trunk is constituted by C7, and the inferior one is formed by the union of the anterior branches of C8 and T1 (Fig. 2.3). These trunks will be subsequently split into an anterior and a posterior division (Fig. 2.4) [9], which has functional importance. They represent the separation of the fibers destined to innervate the ventral flexor muscles and those destined to innervate the extensor dorsal muscles. The union of the mentioned branches of the divisions will give rise to the cords.

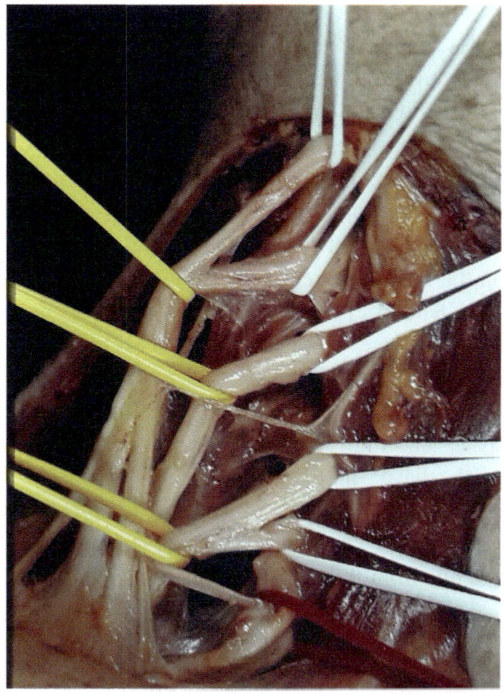

Fig. 2.3 Supraclavicular brachial plexus. White: anterior branches of the spinal nerve C5, C6, C7, C8 and T1. Yellow: upper, middle and lower trunk. Red: subclavian artery and posterior scapular artery

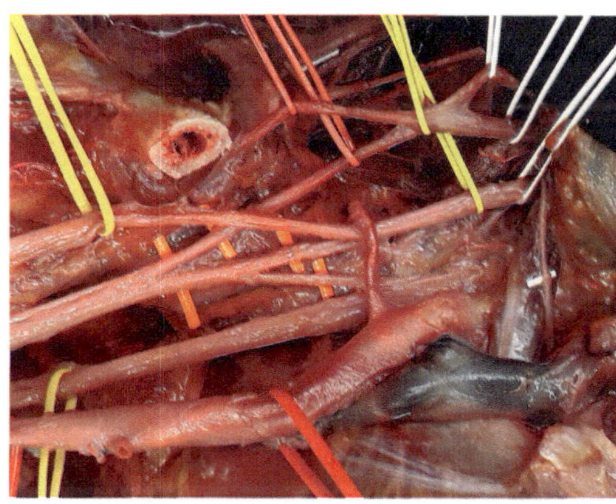

Fig. 2.4 Lateral view of a right supraclavicular brachial plexus. White: anterior branches of the spinal nerves C5, C6, C7, C8 and T1. Yellow: upper, middle and lower trunks. Orange: posterior divisions of the trunks and formation of the posterior cord. Red: axillary artery. Left yellow Lateral and medial cords

The direction of the spinal nerves C5 and C6 is descending, forming the upper trunk just at the outer edge of the interscalenic hiatus, at "Erb point" (Figs. 2.5 and 2.6) [10], about 3 cm above the clavicle. The direction of the spinal nerve C7 is horizontal, and it is located just at the medial edge of the anterior scalene. It will continue imperceptibly forming the middle trunk, located on the lateral border of the middle scalene muscle. C8 and T1 have an upward direction to join at the inner edge of the costal neck, just behind the insertion of the anterior scalene, forming the lower trunk, before leaving the interscalenic space (see Fig. 2.3). These roots and the lower trunk have more complicated relationships behind the subclavian artery and the pulmonary vertex, just above the Sibson fascia (which extends from the transverse process of C7 to the apex of the pleural dome) [11]. This detail helps us understand the reason for the posterior approach to the brachial plexus in cases of lesions or tumors of the lower roots. From the morpho-functional point of view, it is interesting to recognize that the C7 and C8 roots are the ones with the greatest size, C5 and T1 the smallest, and C6 in an intermediate situation; C7 is the root that carries the largest motor fiber quota. Of the trunks, the medial one has the lowest caliber since it is only formed by C7. The lower trunk mainly has fibers that will go to the anterior division, which will lead to the innervation of the intrinsic muscles of the hand. Its contribution to the posterior division is very small [12].

The trunks are located in the omoclavicular triangle, covered by the middle fascia of the neck

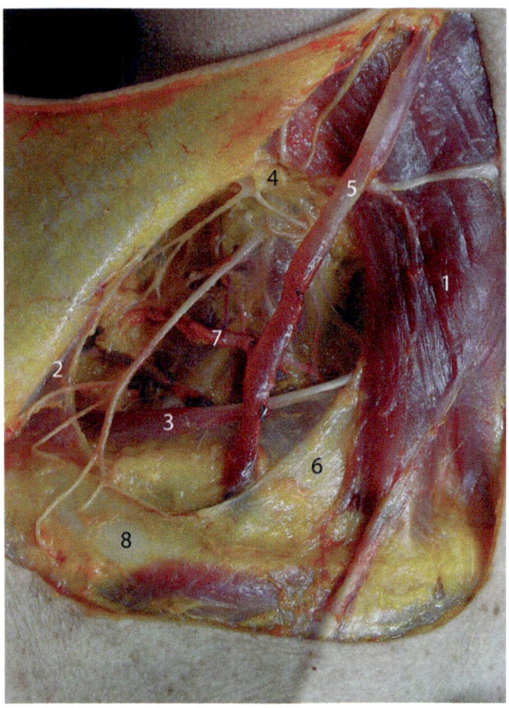

Fig. 2.5 Posterior cervical triangle and supraclavicular triangle (omoclavicular triangle) with their superficial anatomical structures and relationships. 1 ECLM, 2 trapezius, 3 omohyoid, 4 Erb´s neural point and superficial cervical plexus, 5 external jugular vein, 6 omohyoid fascia or middle cervical fascia, 7 superficial transverse cervical vessels, 8 clavicle. [With permissions from Editorial Medica Panamericana]

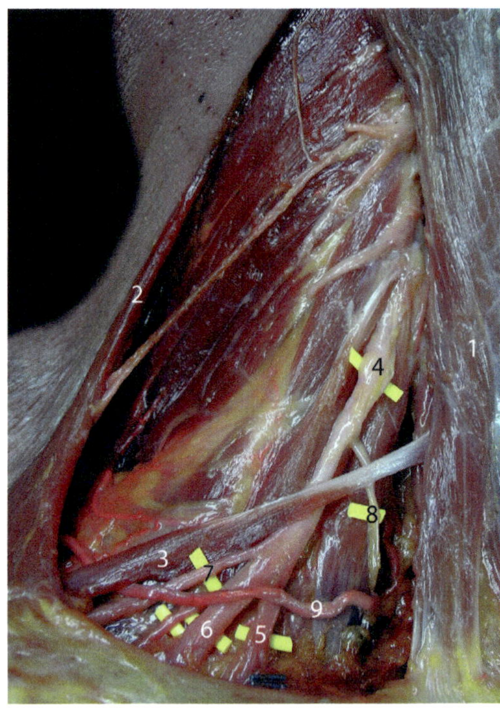

Fig. 2.6 Posterior cervical triangle and supraclavicular triangle (omoclavicular triangle) with their deep anatomical structures and relationships. 1 ECLM, 2 trapezius 3 omohyoid muscle, 4 upper trunk of brachial plexus, 5 anterior division of upper trunk, 6 posterior division of upper trunk, 7 suprascapular nerve, 8 communicating branch of upper trunk to the phrenic nerve, 9 superficial transverse cervical artery. [With permissions from Editorial Medica Panamericana]

that goes from the lower belly of the omohyoid to the clavicle [13]. At this level they are crossed by the supraclavicular nerves of the superficial cervical plexus. The external jugular vein runs in this same plane obliquely from the sternocleidomastoid to end at the lower angle between this muscle and the clavicle, where a fibrous reinforcement is formed around it called the falciform fold (see Fig. 2.5). The superficial transverse cervical artery and veins cross over the upper and middle trunks to supply the external area of the trapezius muscle, where it is located closely with the underlying spinal accessory nerve (XI cranial nerve), helping with its identification as a reference point (or hindering it in case of bleeding) (see Fig. 2.6). It is possible to confuse this artery with another one, of greater size, located more deeply called the posterior scapular artery or also known as the deep transverse cervical artery. This artery travels between the middle and upper trunk, or between the middle and lower trunk, and surrounds the edge of the middle and dorsal scalenes to branch along the dorsum of the scapula. It is also necessary to mention small muscular branches to the scalenous, which, although inconsistent in presence, is important to keep in mind when dissecting in this narrow area. Injury can cause bleeding due to avulsion from the main arterial trunk, especially when there is associated fibrosis or scarring. This artery is found ascending just behind the posterior aspect of the anterior scalene muscle, primarily supplying the middle and anterior scalene.

The three trunks descend to converge in the costoclavicular space where they branch into their divisions. At the point proximal to the concavity of the clavicle, the suprascapular artery crosses the divisions. The divisions will be located on the first muscular division of the anterior serratus muscle forming the cords [12].

Cords and Terminal Branches

The cords are named according to the relationship they present with the axillary artery, behind the pectoralis minor muscle. The *lateral cord* is formed by the union of the anterior divisions of the upper and middle trunks. The *medial cord* is formed by the anterior division of the lower trunk. The *posterior cord* is formed by the union of the posterior divisions of the three primary trunks (Figs. 2.7 and 2.8). The terminal branches emerge from the cords; from the lateral cord are the musculocutaneous nerve and the lateral root

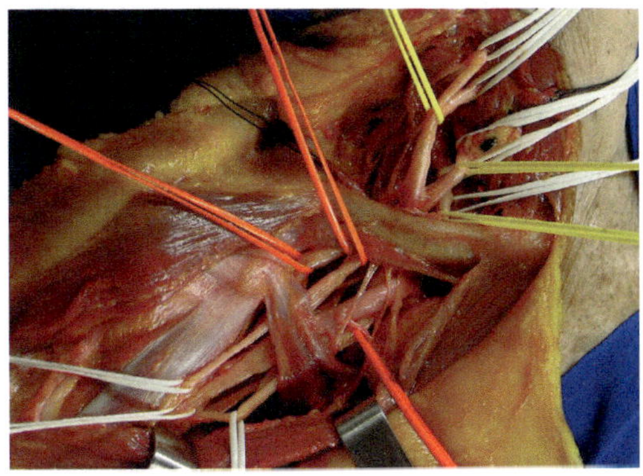

Fig. 2.7 General view of the supraclavicular and infraclavicular brachial plexus. Anatomical landmarks: omohyoid muscle, sectioned and retracted posteriorly, in the supraclavicular area; and pectoralis minor muscle and its tendon insertion in the coracoid process, in the infraclavicular area. [With permissions from Editorial Medica Panamericana]

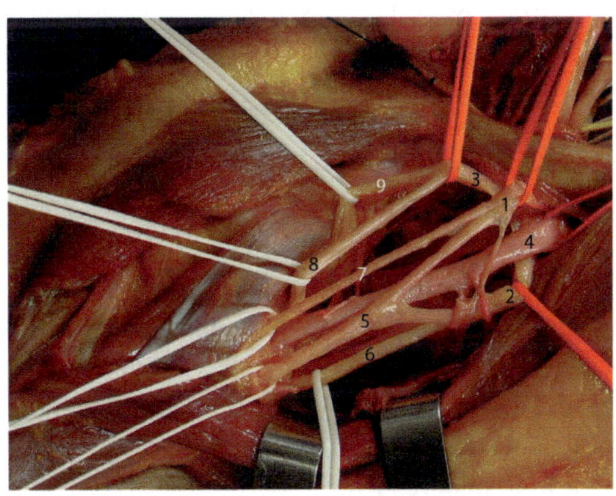

Fig. 2.8 Dissection of the infraclavicular brachial plexus. Pectoralis minor tendon sectioned and retracted distally to show the cords (orange vessel loops) and the terminal branches (white vessel loops). Axillary artery in red vessel loop. 1 lateral cord, 2 medial cord, 3 posterior cord, 4 axillary artery, 5 median nerve, 6 ulnar nerve, 7 musculocutaneous nerve, 8 radial nerve, 9 axillary nerve

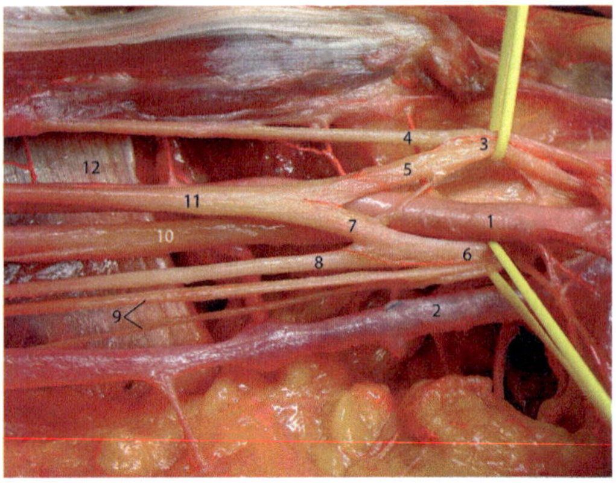

Fig. 2.9 Lateral and medial cords and their terminal branches, at the lateral border of the pectoralis minor muscle. 1 axillary artery, 2 axillary vein, 3 lateral cord, 4 musculocutaneous nerve, 5 lateral root of median nerve, 6 medial cord, 7 medial root of the median nerve , 8 ulnar nerve, 9 medial cutaneous nerve of the arm and medial cutaneous nerve of the forearm, 10 radial nerve, 11 median nerve, 12 tendon of insertion of the latissimus dorsi muscle

or lateral cord contribution to the median nerve. The medial cord gives rise to the medial root or medial cord contribution to the median nerve, the ulnar nerve, and the medial cutaneous nerve of the arm and medial cutaneous nerve of the forearm. The division of the lateral and medial cord into their terminal branches forms a figure of "M" over the axillary artery (Fig. 2.9). The posterior cord gives rise to the radial and axillary nerves [14].

Collateral Branches

Within the structural variability of the brachial plexus, the terminal and collateral branches are consistent. The terminal branches are intended to innervate the free part of the upper limb and the collaterals to innervate the scapular and periscapular musculature [13].

The collateral branches of the supraclavicular brachial plexus intended to innervate the muscles of the shoulder girdle or proximal part of the upper extremity are nerves for the deep musculature of the neck, subclavian nerve, suprascapular nerve, dorsal nerve of the scapula, and long thoracic nerve.

Types of Brachial Plexus

While the mapping of the posterior plane is generally simple and constant, that of the anterior plane is variable and complex because of the presence of a transition root (C7), whose contingent is distributed variably in the lateral and medial cords. According to Seddon [15] and Bonnel [16], among others, three types of plexuses are distinguished according to this transitional root.

Type A (classic) is found in 66% of cases. It is one in which all of the previous quota of C7 is destined to the lateral cord. In this case, the ulnar nerve cannot receive fibers from this root.

In type B, 24% of the cases observed, the C7 quota is destined for the medial cord, the ulnar nerve receiving part of these fibers.

In type C, 10% of the cases, the quota of C7 converges both in the lateral and medial cords, being able to distinguish two subtypes: C1, in which the point of union with the medial cord is above the origin of the ulnar nerve and, therefore, C7 participates in its constitution, and the subtype C2 in which the fusion occurs below such origin and, therefore, the ulnar nerve will not receive input from C7.

An unusual anatomical variation consists in the formation of the lateral and medial cord directly from the anterior divisions of the nerve trunks C5, C6, C7, C8, and T1, without prior formation of the upper, middle, and lower trunk.

The posterior cord, which is formed by the posterior divisions of the upper, middle, and lower trunks, presents variations in which frequently the posterior division of the upper and middle trunk forms a common cord that will then join with the posterior division of the lower trunk. Less frequently is the opposite: first the posterior division of the middle and lower trunk is joined and then that common cord with the posterior division of the upper trunk. The confluence of the three divisions at the same point is infrequent, even though it is usually described in all the textbooks [17–20]. The posterior divisions of the upper and middle trunks are larger than the previous divisions. In 10% of cases, there may be no posterior division of the lower trunk.

The existence of these multiple forms shows us the theoretical value of a unique anatomical description, although it is essential to perform it as a reference point for a subsequent clinical and surgical approach to the brachial plexus [21]. The introduction of perioperative electrodiagnostic records currently provides a great help in the knowledge of the nervous distribution in each particular patient [22], and maybe in the future, high-definition MRI or ultrasonography could also be useful [23].

Seddon [15] has defined two limit varieties of plexuses, based on the participation of the adjacent roots that constitute it (C4 and T2):

- The *pre-fixed plexus*, which is formed from the roots C4-C5-C6-C7-C8 and T1. It can exist in 60% of cases and coexist with the presence of a cervical rib or a hypertrophic transverse process. The posterior divisions of the upper and middle trunk have a similar diameter, but that of the lower trunk is smaller because it receives little or no T1 fiber.
- The *post-fixed plexus*, formed by C5-C6-C7-C8-T1-T2. It can exist in 15% of cases. In this case the contribution of C5 is smaller, with fewer fibers.

After the division of the primary trunks, the separation of the plexus into two planes is always constant:

- An anterior plane, formed by the two lateral and medial cords and their terminal branches, essentially intended for the flexor muscles of the upper limb.
- A posterior plane, formed by the posterior cord, which will give rise to the terminal branches that will innervate the extensor muscles.

The most frequent variations are found at the level of the cords, from small changes in their constitution to great anatomical variations as medial and lateral cords united in a single trunk. Kerr referenced 6% of anomalies in the formation of the entire path of the brachial plexus [24].

Morphology and Anatomical Relationships

From a morphological point of view, it should be noted that the plexus has a triangular shape with a broad origin, in a line that extends from the upper edge of the fifth cervical vertebra to the lower edge of the first thoracic. The apex of this triangular sheet ends in a very narrow area, the costoclavicular space, where the cords give rise to the terminal branches, already in the infraclavicular region.

In a general view, its shape is similar to a triangle, extending from the paravertebral line to the bottom of the axillary cavity (Fig. 2.10), or two triangles connected by their vertices at the costoclavicular space [12].

Inside this triangular area, the ventral primary ramus and trunks have a different obliqueness; the upper cervical branches have a descendent direction, the last cervical branch is almost horizontal, while the first thoracic branch is oblique upward.

These nervous structures have relationships with the anatomical regions to which they belong and that we can categorize into three areas: at the level of the intervertebral foramina and vertebral canal, at the level of the neck or supraclavicular region, and in the axilla or infraclavicular area [12].

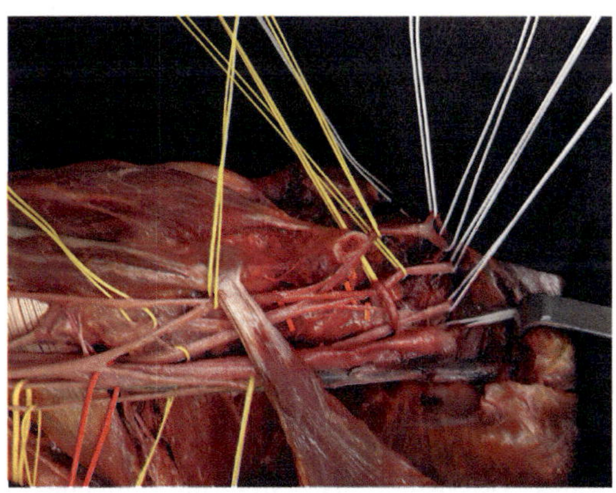

Fig. 2.10 General view of the supraclavicular and infraclavicular brachial plexus after clavicle resection. White: anterior branches of the spinal nerves C5, C6, C7, C8 and T1. Yellow: upper, middle and lower trunk. Orange: posterior divisions and posterior cord. Left yellow: terminal branches. Pectotalis minor muscles

Inside the intervertebral foramen and resting on the transverse process, we find the roots. Each root exits the canal on the upper face of the cervical transverse process or corresponding transverse canal, running between the short intervertebral muscles and in relation to the vertebral artery [25]. This is located inside the costovertebral foramen and from the sixth cervical vertebra to the axis. The vertebral artery is outside this foramen in front of the seventh cervical vertebra. The lower ventral primary rami (C8 and T1) are supported, at the exit of the intervertebral foramen, on and under the neck of the first rib, respectively. They do not have a direct relationship with the vertebral artery, which is located anterior to them. It is necessary to highlight the ventral tubercle of the C6 costotransverse process that is very prominent, being palpable under the pulse of the common carotid artery, known as the *Chassaignac carotid tubercle*. This is because the ventral tuber of C7 is almost non-existent, since no muscle is inserted in it and thus C6 appears as more bulky. This is a deep and difficult area of dissection, highlighting the vulnerability of important vascular structures, especially the subclavian and vertebral arteries. Even smaller branches such as the supreme thoracic artery, which is localized between C8 and T1 over the neck of the first rib, can present very worrisome bleeding due to its proximity to the subclavian trunk (the same thing happens with the scapular thyrocervical trunk). The cervicothoracic ganglion is located medially and posterior to the vertebral artery, near its origin in the subclavian artery.

The relationship of the anterior branches of C8 and T1 with the cervical sympathetic chain explain the clinical sign of Claude Bernard-Horner's syndrome (Fig. 2.11) (myosis, enophthalmos, ptosis, and anhidrosis). These connections with the sympathetic nervous system include both gray and white rami. The gray ramus brings postsynaptic fibers from the sympathetic ganglia to the spinal nerve, destined for sweat glands and vasoconstriction. The white ramus carries preganglionic fibers from spinal cord to sympathetic ganglia and is the base for the mentioned Horner's syndrome (interruption of the ciliary reflex travelling through the sympathetic chain) [14].

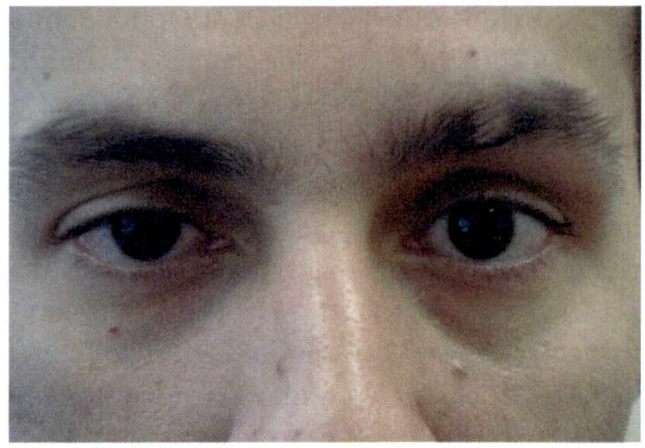

Fig. 2.11 Claude Bernard-Horner's syndrome: Enophthalmus, ptosis and myosis. [With permissions from Editorial Medica Panamericana]

Herzberg [26] describes in detail the anatomy of the area of the intervertebral foramen and costotransverse canal. He finds that there are reinforcements of dense connective tissue between the costotransverse processes and the epineurium of the underlying nerve, calling them the transverse root ligament. This ligament is just outside the intervertebral foramen where the inferior aspect of the spinal nerve is attached to the bone through connective tissue, protecting the weak intradural rootlets from traction injury that may cause avulsion from the spinal cord. These structures have greater consistency in the fifth, sixth, and seventh cervical nerves, being very thin or not existing in the eighth cervical and first thoracic nerves. This would explain the higher incidence of low root avulsions in contrast to those of C5–C6 and C7 due to the protective effect of the ligament. This ligament is located in the angle formed by the anterior and posterior division branches of the corresponding peripheral nerve. It also describes the relations of the subradicular arteries accompanying the roots C5, C6, and C7 from the ascending cervical artery.

In the neck, the brachial plexus is located within the lower part of the greater supraclavicular triangle, defined by the sternocleidomastoid anteriorly, the trapezius posteriorly, and the clavicle inferiorly, more precisely in the omoclavicular triangle (see Fig. 2.5), between the posterior belly of the omohyoid, the clavicle, and the spine [18]. At this level, we find the upper, middle, and lower trunks which are in close relationship with the scalene muscles. The origin of the scalene muscles is at cervical transverse processes and they direct to the first rib (anterior and middle scalene), inserting in front and behind the groove of the subclavian artery, and the second rib (posterior scalene).

The major interscalenic triangle or hiatus of the scalenes is found between the anterior and middle scalene. At this point the brachial plexus runs along with the subclavian artery, which is located below the upper and middle trunks but in front of the lower trunk [13] (see Fig. 2.3). The lower trunk can be separated, if present, by muscle *scalenus minimus*, or more frequently by their remaining form of a fibrous thickening. The aponeurosis that covers the scalene muscles comes from prevertebral aponeurosis and extends laterally forming a closed space constituting what is known in anesthesiology as a *sheath of the brachial plexus*. This sheath is the anatomical foundation of regional blocks at this level [27]. As mentioned, in this space we can inconstantly find the interscalenic artery that must be kept in mind to avoid its injury and consequent hemorrhage that can be difficult to stop due to the complexity of the area.

Within this regional anatomy, it should be remembered that the subclavian artery and its branches are divided into three segments with respect to its relationship with the anterior scalene muscle (Fig. 2.12) [18]: in the *pre- or intrascalenic portion,* we will find the subclavian artery supported on the pleural dome, adjacent with the vagus nerve (and recurrent nerve on the right side that surrounds it from below and behind), the ansa of Vieussens, and the phrenic nerve in front, in addition to its vertebral collateral branches, internal mammary, costocervical trunk (upper intercostal and deep cervical), and thyrocervical trunk (lower thyroid, ascending cervical, superficial transverse cervical, and suprascapular). The *interscalenic portion* rests on the upper face of the first rib, just behind the Lisfranc tubercle (insertion of the anterior scalene muscle). The *post- or extrascalenic* portion is found at the first muscular digitation of the anterior serratus muscle and gives rise to the posterior scapular artery. The artery is of considerable thickness, originating from its posterior face; this artery can pass between the primary trunks of the brachial plexus (between the upper and middle (see Fig. 2.3) or less frequently, between the middle and lower) to go to the upper angle of the scapula after surrounding the middle and posterior scalene muscles. It should be noted that sometimes its origin is located in the interscalene hiatus, with the risk that this entails during surgery in this area, and even in the intrascalenic portion, then running behind the tendon of the anterior scalene, and in front of the trunks of the plexus to pass between them (between the upper and middle or between the middle and lower) [13].

In front of the anterior scalene, the subclavian vein, and the phrenic nerve follows the anterior

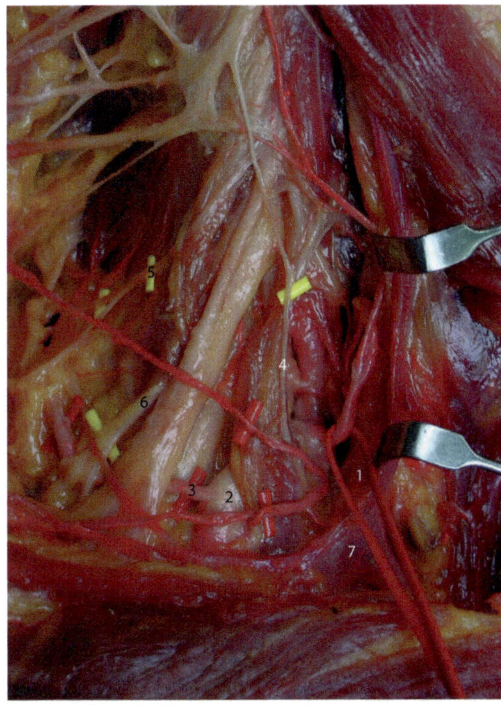

Fig. 2.12 Relationships of the anterior scalenus muscle. Subclavian artery (1) and its collateral branches in relation to the anterior scalenus muscles, prescalenic (internal thoracic artery, vertebral artery, costocervical trunk, and thyrocervical trunk-2), interscalenic, and postscalenic portions (posterior scapular artery-3). Anterior relation with the phrenic nerve-4, and posterior relation with the dorsal scapular nerve-5, and long thoracic nerve-6. Subclavian vein-7. [With permissions from Editorial Medica Panamericana]

edge of the muscle running from lateral to medial to enter into the thorax [28] (Fig. 2.13). At this level, we found the thyrocervical arterial trunk medial to the tendon; at this place emits its branches on the anterior scalene.

Dorsal to this area, between the middle and posterior scalene, another space is formed, the minor interscalenic triangle. This is narrow and difficult to visualize, through which the dorsal nerve of the scapula and the long thoracic nerve or Charles Bell, collateral branches of the brachial plexus (see Fig. 2.12), go. Usually the dorsal scapular nerve pierces the middle scalenes [29].

The omohyoid muscle crosses superficially to these structures, which as a whole are covered by the superficial cervical aponeurosis with the external jugular vein as already mentioned (see Fig. 2.5), and the platysma muscle in the subdermal layer.

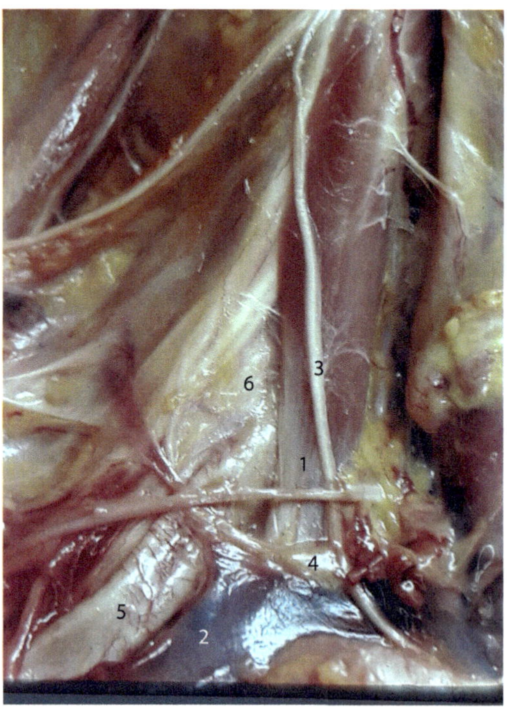

Fig. 2.13 Superficial relations of the anterior scalenus muscle. In front of the tendon of insertion-1, subclavian vein-2, phrenic nerve-3 and superficial transverse cervical artery and suprascapular artery-4 coming from the thyrocervical trunk. Behind the tendon and muscle, subclavian artery-5 (and lower trunk posterior to it) and middle and upper trunks-6 in the interscalenic space, inside the scalenic sheath

Finally, the separation of the trunks will occur in anterior and posterior divisions corresponding to the retroclavicular area, and the constitution of the lateral, medial, and posterior cords and their terminal branches (musculocutaneous, median, ulnar, cutaneous medial of the arm and cutaneous medial of the forearm, radial and axillary) that belong to the infraclavicular brachial plexus [28, 29].

The relationships of the cords with the axillary artery vary along its path [30]. Just below the clavicle, the posterior cord is located laterally to the axillary artery, the middle cord behind it, and the lateral cord in front. The nomenclature does not correspond in this area to the anatomical relationship. It is under the tendon of the pectoralis minor when the cords adopt the position appropriate to their nomenclature (see Fig. 2.8). Miller [31] described variations of the axillary artery with respect to the nerve cords in 2% of cases, the most frequent being the presence of the axillary artery in front of the three cords, keeping the median nerve behind it.

Regarding the appearance of the nerves of each of the cords, it should be mentioned that the branches of the posterior cord are usually constant in their sequence of appearance: first the upper subscapular nerve, the thoracodorsal, the lower subscapular, and finally the axillary nerve. The branches of the medial cord in order are medial pectoral nerve, medial cutaneous nerve of the arm, medial cutaneous nerve of the forearm, medial root or medial cord contribution (MCC) to the median nerve, and finally the ulnar nerve [13] (see Fig. 2.9). The branches of the lateral cord are more variable. In 10% of cases, the musculocutaneous nerve originates more distal than usual from the lateral cord, or even directly from the median nerve. On other occasions the external root of the median nerve can appear as two or three branches to finally continue with the main trunk, or more rarely this root has its origin directly from the musculocutaneous nerve itself at different heights. Nerve variations make it difficult to dissect and identify the components of the plexus [32].

Intraneural Anatomy

In peripheral nerve microsurgery, the fascicle with its perineurium is considered as the basic unit. Therefore it is important to know, when feasible, the quadratic location of the fascicles inside the nerve; this is what is known as intraneural pattern and topography. The longitudinal anatomy of the nerve trunk can be studied as advocated by Sunderland [33]. The fascicles are not individualized and in a constant position, but are divided and intermingled in a plexiform way along the nerve path, changing the number and size of the fascicles in short segments, especially in the proximal areas of the upper extremity.

The fascicular pattern indicates the number, size, and location of the fascicles at a given level. Sunderland established that, in general, every 1.5 cm the fascicular pattern could change. Since then, the fascicular arrangement maps of the motor and sensory fibers at different levels of the nerve length serve as a guide in the transverse topography to achieve a correct axial orientation of the fascicles during surgery. These maps are especially useful in the distal areas of the extremities, since then the variation of the fascicular pattern is smaller, being able to find long segments that maintain the same intraneural pattern in the distal part of the forearm, wrist, and hand (nerve disgregation or segregation) [20, 34, 35].This fact has been confirmed with stimulation and intraoperative nerve studies [20, 36].

In the intervertebral foramen, at the middle level of the nerve trunks, just after the union of the ventral and dorsal roots, a monofascicular arrangement of the nerve fibers is seen, in which the motor and sensory fibers are observed to intermingle. This occurs in the transition zone of the infundibulum when the epineurium continues. In the middle area of the ventral branch of the nerve trunk (or primary rami), after the dorsal branch (or primary rami) has been detached, an arrangement of the nerve fibers will be observed with an oligofascicular pattern, between 3 and 9 fascicular groups and with a mean of four to five groups. In the lateral zone of this branch, these fascicles will be separated into an anterior and a posterior group with a multifascicular pattern [17].

When the upper, middle, and lower trunks of the brachial plexus have been formed, the latter arrangement continues to be maintained in a ventral and dorsal plane in polyfascicular groups, a logical fact since they will originate the corresponding anterior and posterior divisions of the brachial plexus. The number of fascicles in each group is increasing progressively, while their size decreases as an expression of their separation [17]. This fact highlights the embryological and functional aspect of the anterior divisions with a flexopronator function and the posterior ones with an extensosupinator function of the upper limb.

In clinical practice, various schemes disseminated by the main authors in this area on the intraneural distribution and course of fascicular groups along their path from the origin of the plexus to the peripheral and collateral peripheral nerves are used. In our centers we mainly use the scheme of Narakas [11].

At present, a very good correlation between the histological studies of the intraneural topography and the studies with high-resolution ultrasound of Kubiena [23] has been demonstrated, corroborating the data reflected in the literature and checking dynamically the changes of fascicles and groups of fascicles along the entire path of the brachial plexus to its terminal branches. Thus, by ultrasound it has been shown, for example, how the anterior divisions, posterior divisions, and separation of the suprascapular nerve are located in the upper trunk with ultrasound images that are almost "histological" because of their ability to differentiate fascicular groups. The fascicles for the suprascapular nerve can be located in the cranial area, the fascicles for the musculocutaneous nerve in the anterior area, and those of the axillary nerve in the posterior area.

There are studies that have accounted for approximately the number of fibers for roots and terminal nerves (Bonnel [1] if you are going to mention studies). It is mentioned that C5 contains 16,000–23,000 nerve fibers, C6 about 26,000–27,500 fibers, C7 about 23,700–31,500, C8 24,000–30,600, and T1 about 19,700–22,000. In the terminal trunks, 15,900–18,000 fibers have been counted for the median nerve, for the musculocutaneous nerve 5000–6000, for the ulnar

14,000–16,000, for the radial 15,900–20,000, and for the axillary 6000–7000 fibers [12].

Collateral Terminal Branches and Motor Points

The collateral branches of the supraclavicular brachial plexus are:

- *Ventral collateral branches:* nerves for deep neck muscles, subclavian nerve, suprascapular nerve, and phrenic nerve.
- *Dorsal collateral branches:* dorsal nerve of the scapula and long thoracic nerve.

Nerves for Deep Neck Musculature (C2–C8)

Almost immediately after exiting the nerves C2 to C8, the branches that innervate the muscles of the long neck and anterior, middle, and posterior scalenes originate. They are cited for the diagnostic importance in electroneurophysiological tests [37] to determine pre- or postganglionic lesions due to the proximity of their origin to the spinal ganglion of roots C2 to C8 (T1 does not contribute to the innervation of this musculature). In clinical examination it is usually not a musculature that is studied specifically.

C2 to C4 form the cervical plexus, which in turn is divided into superficial (sensory) and deep (motor). From the superficial, sensory plexus originates the supra-acromial, supraclavicular, and suprasternal, transverse cervical, greater auricular, and lesser occipital nerves (see Fig. 2.5) radiating from the "neural point" located in the posterior edge of the sternocleidomastoid muscle (at the union of its upper third and middle third). From the deep cervical plexus, several cervical loops (between C2, C3, C4, and C5) are made up from which originates motor fibers for the sternocleidomastoid muscle, nerve for the rhomboid muscle and for the levator scapulae muscle known as the dorsal scapular nerve, and cervical fibers for the trapezius. Fibers will come out of the third cervical loop for the strap muscles of the neck, which, through the descending branch of the hypoglossal, will innervate the strap or hyoid muscles (see Fig. 2.12). Brunelli has studied this topic in detail and describes that the number of motor fibers from the deep cervical plexus contains about 3400–4100 myelinic fibers and the superficial cervical plexus about 2000 fibers [12, 38].

Phrenic Nerve (C3–C4)

The main component of the phrenic nerve originates from C4. Although it does not really belong to the brachial plexus, it is commented on the intimate relationship it has with it and the frequency with which a branch of the fifth cervical nerve contributes to its formation directly (accessory phrenic nerve) or through the subclavian nerve. It has a long path inside the aponeurosis of the anterior scalene muscle (see Figs. 2.6, 2.12, and 2.13), running along its anterior surface, close to its insertion, surrounding it medially running between the subclavian artery and vein. It enters the thoracic cavity and travels to its final destination innervating the corresponding hemidiaphragm, the main and automatic breathing muscle. It has been calculated that the number of myelinic fibers of this nerve is about 800 according to D. Chuang [39, 40].

Unilateral diaphragm paralysis is tolerated if there is no underlying respiratory pathology that results in a disorder of the ventilatory function, and that is why it should be systematically explored when there is a suspected suspicion of the brachial plexus. In addition, when it originates in the proximal area of the ventral nerve branches, it has a prognostic factor because it will indicate a possible preganglionic lesion.

The clinical examination of this nerve evaluates its function during breathing by auscultation and performing an x-ray in maximum inspiration and expiration to identify position of the diaphragm.

Subclavian Nerve (C5–C6)

It is a very thin nerve that originates from the anterior aspect of the upper trunk or, less frequently, directly from C5 or C6. It runs distally, above the plexus and in front of the subclavian artery and vein to innervate the subclavian muscle through its posterior face, at the level of the middle third, where its motor point is located.

Suprascapular Nerve (C5–C6)

The suprascapular nerve is a big collateral branch and with clinical and surgical importance not only for its function but also for serving as a reference point. It originates from the cranial border of the upper trunk or directly from C5, although in reality at this point a nerve trifurcation (Fig. 2.14) corresponding to the suprascapular nerve, and the posterior and anterior division of the upper trunk, arranged in this order. The suprascapular nerve runs parallel to the plexus and follows the lower belly of the omohyoid muscle to pass through the upper notch of the scapula and innervate the supraspinatus and infraspinatus muscles. It has proprioceptive fibers that are distributed through the shoulder joint, and skin sensory fibers have been described, being the only ones of the brachial plexus that originate above the clavicle.

The suprascapular nerve contains 3000 to 4000 myelinic fibers with a large component of afferent proprioceptive muscle fibers, and only

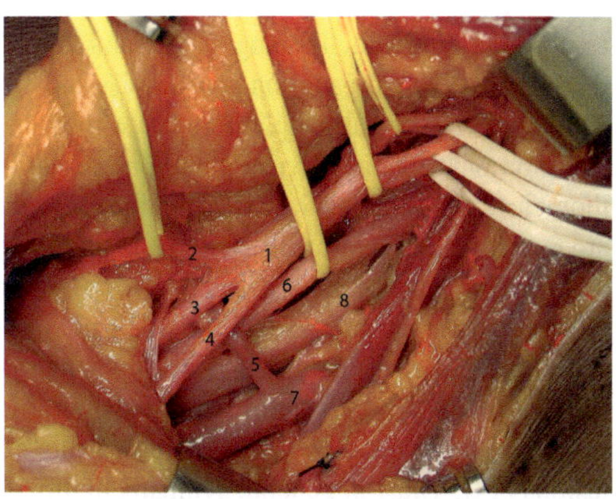

Fig. 2.14 Dissection of a supraclavicular brachial plexus. Upper trunk trifurcation (1) in suprascapular nerve (2), posterior division (3) and anterior division (4). Vascular relations of the posterior scapular artery (5) between the upper and middle trunks (6), and the subclavian artery (7) just posterior to the scalenus anterior and in front the lower trunk (8)

recently there are authors who have found sensory fibers of cutaneous distribution in a very limited area [41].

Dorsal Scapular Nerve (C4–C5)

It originates from the posterior aspect of the ventral primary rami of C5 and often from C4 and C6, near the intervertebral foramen. It penetrates the middle scalene muscle to go down and back in search of the vertebral edge of the scapula (Fig. 2.15). At this level it joins the posterior scapular artery or deep transverse cervical artery of the neck to descend under levator scapulae muscle to which it innervates in its middle area (motor point) and, subsequently, to run over the deep face of the major and minor rhomboid muscles. It innervates these muscles through their motor point located in the upper area of these muscles [13]. Note that C5 gives the component for this nerve within the intervertebral foramen while C6 makes it a bit more lateral, before the upper trunk is formed. The levator scapulae muscle is also innervated by direct cervical fibers of C3 and C4.

Long Thoracic Nerve (C5-C6-C7)

It has 1600 to 1800 myelinic fibers (Chuang [39], Narakas [42]). It originates from the posterior aspect of the ventral branches of C5, C6 (main component) and sometimes C7 (40% of cases), near the intervertebral foramen. They cross the middle scalene muscle, and when there is a component of C7, it usually joins the main component just above the middle scalene. At the exit of the muscular mass of the middle scalene muscle, it is directed vertically downward, behind the brachial plexus and the axillary vessels to be located near the angle that is formed between it and the subscapular muscle (see Fig. 2.15). It lies on the external face of the anterior serratus muscle while releasing nerve branches for the innervation of each of its muscular digitations (Fig. 2.16). The upper portion of the anterior serratus muscle is innervated by fibers of C5, the middle portion by fibers of C6, and the lower portion by fibers of C7. The long thoracic nerve at the level of the first

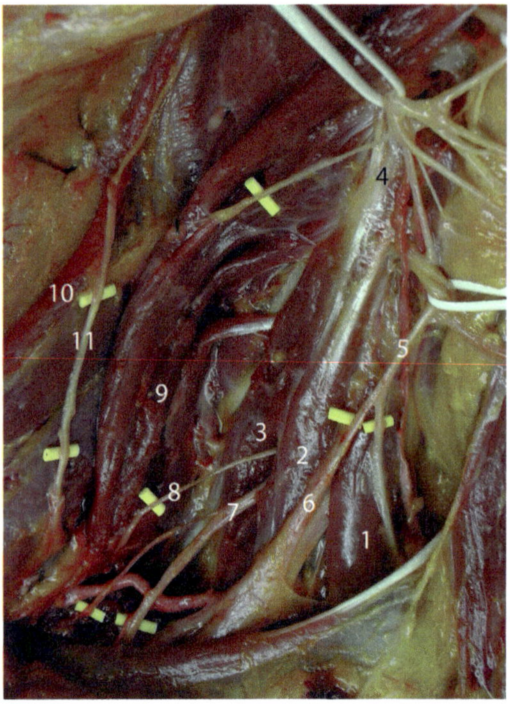

Fig. 2.15 Anterior, middle and posterior scalenus muscles and their neural relationships. 1 anterior scalenus, 2 middle scalenus, 3 posterior scalenus, 4 deep cervical plexus, 5 phrenic nerve, 6 upper trunk, 7 long thoracic nerve, 8 dorsal scapular nerve, 9 levator scapulae muscle, 10 trapezius muscle and 11 accessory or spinal nerve. [With permissions from Editorial Medica Panamericana]

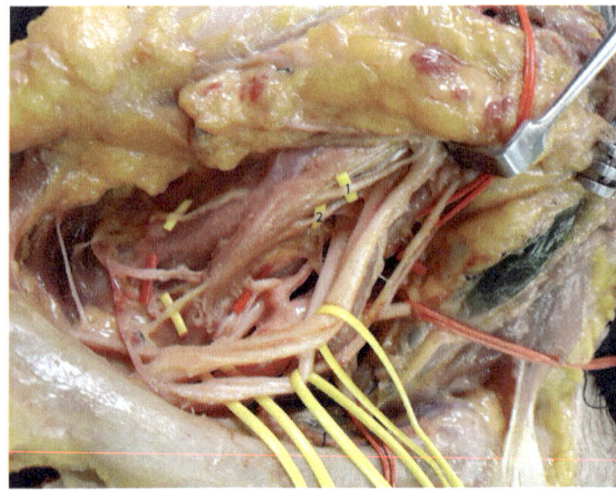

Fig. 2.16 Posterolateral view of a right brachial plexus. Observe the origin of the long thoracic nerve (1) and dorsal scapular nerve (2) in the dorsal part of C5 and C6, and their course

intercostal space is covered by aponeurotic fibers on the first muscular digitation that can produce a nerve compression (iatrogenic lesion at this level is feasible when performing a cervical rib removal by axillary route).

Sensory and Sympathetic Aspect

The spinal nerves, being mixed nerves, carry motor, sensory, and sympathetic fibers. The sensory fibers regroup to form cutaneous nerves during the course from the roots to the collateral and terminal nerves, to innervate a skin area of specific sensitivity [4]. In general, it is necessary to explore the sensitivity from the metameric point of view to study the spinoradicular lesions and the trunk sensitivity to study the lesions of the peripheral nerves.

The white communicating branches, which carry preganglionic fibers from the spinal cord to the sympathetic ganglia, run first through the ventral roots and then follow the nerve trunk and scale into the sympathetic ganglion. Following these sympathetic ganglia, gray communicating branches will emerge that will join the corresponding spinal nerves, to follow their peripheral path, to be distributed through their territory of specific vegetative innervation. The spinal nerves receive gray communicating branches of the corresponding sympathetic ganglia: C5 and C6 of the middle cervical ganglion and C7, C8 and T1 of the lower cervical ganglion and first thoracic ganglion or stellated cervical ganglion (cervicothoracic) [12, 13] (Fig. 2.17). Sympathetic fibers are responsible for vasoconstriction and the stimulation of sweat glands.

The sympathetic fibers of C8 and T1 are part of the ciliary reflex that explains the appearance of a Horner's syndrome (ptosis, enophthalmos, myosis, and anhidrosis) in the low brachial plexus lesions [14]. Thus, in general, sympathetic fibers determine vasomotor control, sweating, and pilomotor reflex.

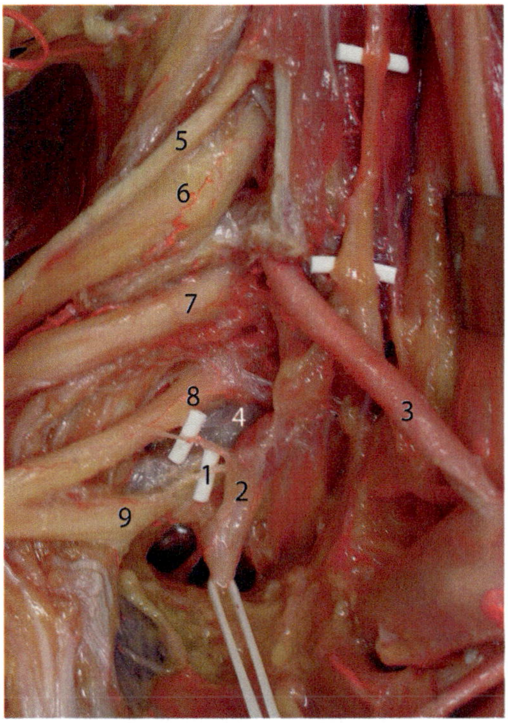

Fig. 2.17 Sympathetic chain communications (1) between the lower or stellated cervical ramus (2) and the anterior ramus of C8 and T1. The vertebral artery (3) is retracted medially to expose this deep area. Neck of the first rib (4). C5 (5), C6 (6), C7 (7), C8 (8), and T1 (9) anterior ramus of the brachial plexus. Observe the different thickness and obliquity of the nerves. [With permissions from Editorial Medica Panamericana]

Infraclavicular Brachial Plexus: Collateral and Terminal Branches

Surgical Anatomy and Relationships of the Terminal Branches

The divisions of the trunks are located resting in the muscular digitation of the anterior serratus muscle and at the level of the subscapular muscle, behind the subclavian muscle, in the two internal thirds of the clavicle [43].

The most distal part of the cords and the terminal branches of the plexus form at the level of the axilla.

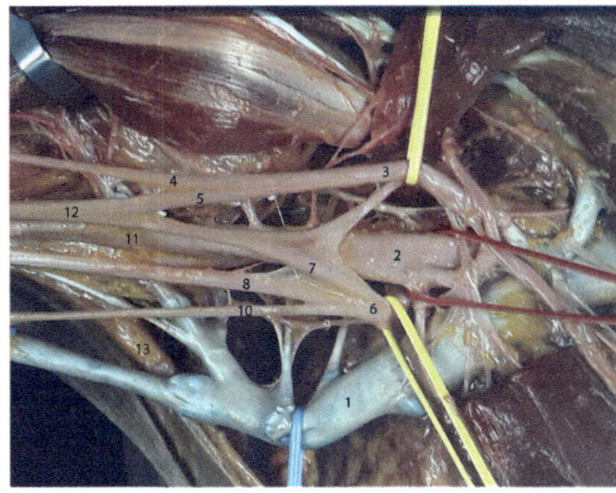

Fig. 2.18 General view of the infraclavicular brachial plexus. Retraction of the axillary vein to show the axillary artery and its relation with the lateral and medial cords and their terminal branches. 1 axillary vein, 2 axillary artery, 3 lateral cord, 4 musculocutaneous nerve, 5 lateral root of the median nerve, 6 medial cord, 7 medial root of the median nerve, 8 ulnar nerve, 9 medial cutaneous nerve of the arm, 10 medial cutaneous nerve of the forearm, 11 radial nerve, 12 median nerve, 13 tendon of insertion of latissimus dorsi muscle. [With permissions from Editorial Medica Panamericana]

The axillary cavity is shaped like a truncated triangular pyramid, limited in front by the subclavian, pectoral minor, Richet clavicoracoaxillary aponeurosis, pectoralis major, and its aponeurosis. Dorsally, it is limited by the subscapular, teres major, and latissimus dorsi muscles and, medially, by the ribs and anterior serratus muscle [12].

Inside the axillary cavity, the terminal branches of the brachial plexus and cords are closely related to the axillary artery and vein, its branches, and the lymphatic ganglia groups of the area. Neurovascular structures are involved in the axillary sheath, continuation of the aponeurosis of the scalenes, which continues to converge distally to pass through the retroclavicular space and finally diverge from the narrow costoclavicular to the upper limb [12, 28, 43].

The key point to be oriented in this area is the tendon of the pectoralis minor, inserting into the medial face of the coracoid process (Fig. 2.18). Behind it, the axillary artery is divided into three parts: pre-, retro-, and postpectoral segment (see Figs. 2.7 and 2.8) [43]. The nomenclature of the cords of the brachial plexus is according to their relationship with the second part or retropectoral part of the axillary artery since at this level they are outside (lateral cord), inside (medial cord), or behind (posterior cord) of the artery. Immediately distal to the clavicle, the relationships of the cords in the first part or prepectoral portion change substantially with the lateral cord separated and above the axillary artery, the middle cord completely behind, and the posterior cord located laterally to it [30]. This can be confusing in relation to the nomenclature; in the second portion, this nomenclature is classified as described; in the third part or postpectoral portion, the cords are arranged so that the lateral one is placed in front of the artery before dividing and forming the median and musculocutaneous nerve and the medial cord is arranged below it hidden between the artery and the vein axillary located in front, while the posterior cord remains in position (see Fig. 2.18) [43]. It is also interesting to know the division of the axillary artery in the three described segments and the collateral branches in each of them: upper thoracic artery in the prepectoral segment, acromiothoracic artery and lateral thoracic artery in the retropectoral segment, and the subscapular arteries and humeral circumflexes anterior and posterior in the postpectoral segment.

Sometimes it is possible to find an accessory muscle that extends from the lateral edge of the *latissimus dorsi* muscle to the posteroinferior border of the tendon of insertion of the pectoralis major or its vicinity, known as the axillopectoral muscle or the axillary arch of Langer. Knowledge of this accessory muscle is important in order to continue to be oriented correctly in the area and to correctly identify the neurovascular structures.

The lateral cord when reaching the lateral edge of the pectoralis minor muscle will divide originating laterally to the musculocutaneous nerve and medially its major component will form the lateral root or lateral cord contribution of the median nerve (which will provide innervation for the flexor carpi radialis muscle and sensory innervation of volar thumb, index, long, and annular fingers) (see Figs. 2.9 and 2.18). This contribution will carry fibers from C5 to C7, specifically to innervate the extrinsic musculature hand dependent on the median nerve and sensory territory in the skin [44]. The lateral cord will join the medial root or medial cord contribution to median nerve, which will carry C8 and T1 fibers to innervate the intrinsic musculature of the hand dependent on the median nerve (i.e. APB, opponens, FPB). All of this is placed in front of the third part of the axillary artery. In this area, anatomical variations of greater or lesser extent (double lateral root (see Fig. 2.18), union behind the artery, musculocutaneous fascicles transfer through the nerve to innervate biceps and brachialis at midarm level) may occur frequently. Despite being anatomical variations, its functional representation is usually not significant.

The medial cord appears between the axillary artery and vein, carrying C8 and T1 fibers, occasionally T2 and rarely C7. It runs along the medial side of the artery and, from its border, the medial cutaneous nerve of the arm and medial cutaneous nerve of the forearm, in this order (see Fig. 2.9) [45]. All of this happens distal to the minor pectoral muscle lateral border. At this level the medial cord divides giving rise to the ulnar nerve, which is its continuation, and laterally to the internal root of the median nerve for intrinsic muscles (APB, opponens, and FPB of the thenar eminence) already described above. From the anterior aspect of the medial cord, the medial pectoral nerve, hidden under the axillary artery, will branch and then curve between the artery and the vein, forming the so-called pectoral loop or ansa pectoralis along with the lateral pectoral nerve from the lateral cord (Fig. 2.19). The medial pectoral nerve penetrates the deep side of the pectoralis minor muscle to innervate it, with some of its branches that pass through it to innervate the sternocostal portion of the pectoralis major muscle (C8-T1). Clavipectoral aponeurosis of the anterior wall of the axillary cavity will be perforated by the lateral pectoral nerve (C5–C7) and the accompanying anterior thoracic vessels that will penetrate the deep side of the clavicular cord of the pectoralis major muscle to innervate it. From the pectoral loop, small nerve branches innervate the pectoralis major muscle

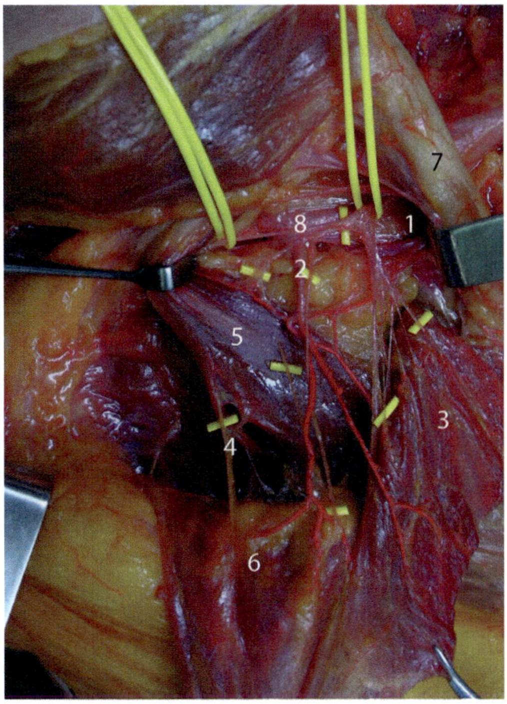

Fig. 2.19 The coracoclavipectoral fascia is perforated by branches of the lateral pectoral nerve (yellow vessel loop) originating from the lateral cord (1), and arterial branches of the thoracoacromial artery (2) that supply the clavicular part of the pectoralis major muscle (3). Observe the branches of the medial pectoral nerve (4) perforating the pectoralis minor muscle (5) to innervate the sternocostal part of the pectoralis major muscle (6). Clavicle (7). Axillary artery (8). [With permissions from Editorial Medica Panamericana]

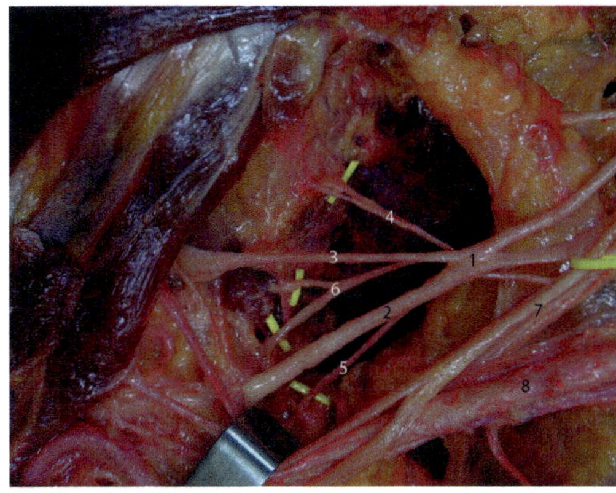

Fig. 2.20 Superior view of a right brachial plexus. Lateral and medial cords, and axillary artery are retracted anteriorly to show the posterior cord, and its terminal and collateral branches. 1 Posterior cord, 2 radial nerve, 3 axillary nerve, 4 upper subscapular nerve, 5 thoracodorsal nerve, 6 lower subscapular nerve. 7 lateral and medial cords. 8 axillary artery

and the pectoralis minor muscle. Many authors describe, instead of two nerves for the pectoral muscles, the existence of three or more nerve branches [46].

The posterior cord carries basically C5, C6, C7, and C8 fibers, the contribution of T1 being very small. It is formed by the union of the posterior divisions of the upper (C5–C6), middle (C7), and lower (C8-T1) trunks, at the level of the first muscular digitation or fascicles of the anterior serratus muscle (see Figs. 2.4 and 2.10). As an anatomical variation, the posterior cord may be absent, and then the radial and axillary nerve originates independently from the posterior divisions. The contribution of C5 and C6 is the main one for the axillary nerve. The contribution of C7 is distributed mainly by the radial nerve, the contribution of C8 and T1 being smaller. The upper subscapular nerve, thoracodorsal nerve, and inferior subscapular nerve in this order branch from it. Finally it gives rise to the axillary and radial nerves (Fig. 2.20). The axillary nerve originates in 80% of cases of the posterior cord, but can also originate from the posterior divisions of the upper and middle trunk. Likewise, the radial nerve originates in 80% of the cases of the posterior cord or the posterior divisions of the three trunks. Normally the radial nerve separates from the axillary nerve in the retropectoral area, running behind the third part of the axillary artery (see Figs. 2.8, 2.10, and 2.20) [21, 43].

In the inner wall of the axilla, we can see how the long thoracic nerve runs, all along the anterior serratus muscle covered by its aponeurosis and in the distal thorax in relation to the thoracic lateral artery (locate parallel to it), but in the line of insertion of their muscular digitations or fascicles in the ribs (see Fig. 2.16) [12, 21, 43, 44].

All this complex anatomy can be even more confusing due to the existence of arterial vascular variations, which occur in 10% of cases, and even more frequent venous variations. The most frequent arterial variation is the location of an axillary artery with a superficial situation in the median nerve [31], which can be disconcerting. The rest of the variations refer to the collateral branches of the three parts of the axillary artery, highlighting those of the acromiothoracic artery (second portion) and the subscapular artery (third portion).

Intraneural Anatomy

At the infraclavicular level, the intraneural distribution of the fascicles is more complicated because there are a greater number of them, although with small diameter, as an expression of the branching of the nerve to reach their final targets. This makes it difficult to recognize quadratic patterns in this area. However, Kubiena [23] shows with high-resolution ultrasound how the median nerve is formed through the internal and external roots from homonymous cords; despite this, the arrangement of fascicular groups is not specified.

Collateral Branches and Motor Points

The collateral branches of the infraclavicular brachial plexus that innervate the muscles of the shoulder girdle are:

- *Anterior collateral branches:* lateral pectoral nerve and medial pectoral nerve.
- *Posterior collateral branches:* superior subscapular nerve, thoracodorsal nerve, and inferior subscapular nerve.

Lateral Pectoral Nerve (C5–C7)

The lateral pectoral nerve originates from the anterior aspect of the lateral cord (Fig. 2.21), either as a single root or by the confluence of two or three rootlets. It can also originate from the anterior divisions of the upper and middle trunk. It leaves the lateral cord outside the first portion of the axillary artery, giving an upper branch of the pectoralis major that pierces the clavipectoral fascia to penetrate the deep aspect of the clavicular part of the pectoralis major muscle and innervate it (C5, C6, and C7) and a lower branch to join the medial pectoral branch that forms a loop (*ansa pectoralis*) contributing to the innervation of the sternocostal part of the pectoralis major muscle [46] (see Fig. 2.19).

Medial Pectoral Nerve (C8-T1)

The medial pectoral nerve originates from the anterior aspect of the medial cord at the level of the first portion of the axillary artery, that is, when it is located behind it (therefore dissection and visualization are difficult) (see Fig. 2.21). It curves around the artery, passing between it and the axillary vein, to form together with the lateral pectoral nerve, the so-called pectoral loop or ansa pectoralis (see Figs. 2.19 and 2.21), in front of the second portion of the axillary artery, just outside the acromiothoracic arterial trunk (anatomical landmark). All of this is located under the pectoralis minor muscle. Branches of the medial pectoral nerve that will penetrate the pectoralis minor muscle through its deep face will be detached from the pectoral loop, some of which will pass through it to innervate the sternocostal head of the pectoralis major muscle.

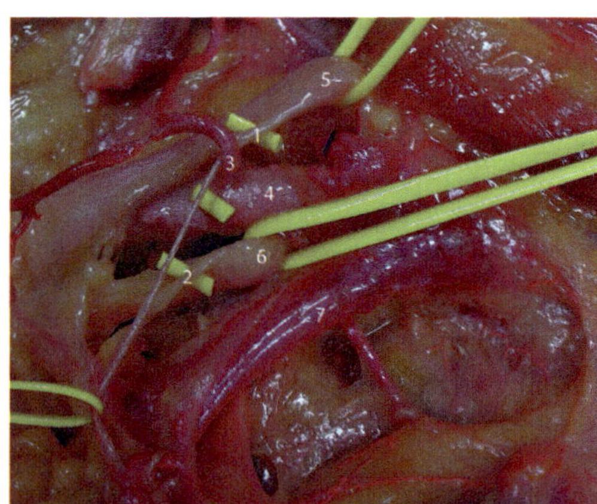

Fig. 2.21 Ansa pectoralis or pectoral loop formed by the lateral pectoral nerve (1) and the medial pectoral nerve (2) just distal to the origin of the thoracoacromial branch (3) of the axillary artery (4), under the pectoralis minor muscle. Lateral cord (5) and medial cord (6). Axillary vein (7) covering the medial cord and complicating the access to this structure. [With permissions from Editorial Medica Panamericana]

The number of myelinic fibers has been calculated at 400 to 600 according to the works of Chuang [39], Narakas [42], Oberlin [47], and Bertelli [48].

It should be noted that despite the medial and lateral nomenclature, this is done according to the cord from which these nerves originate and not to their anatomical location since the medial pectoral nerve is located "lateral" with respect to the lateral pectoral nerve, located more "medially" [43, 46].

The pectoralis major muscle consists of two heads, clavicular (innervated by the lateral pectoral nerve) and sternocostal (innervated by the medial pectoral nerve), with significant morphofunctional differences and function, but with a common insertion.

Upper Subscapular Nerve (C5-C6)

The upper subscapular nerve originates from the posterior cord carrying C5 and C6 fibers. It is directed to the subscapularis muscle to innervate its middle and upper portion. This branch is smaller than that of the inferior subscapular nerve [21, 30, 49] (Fig. 2.22).

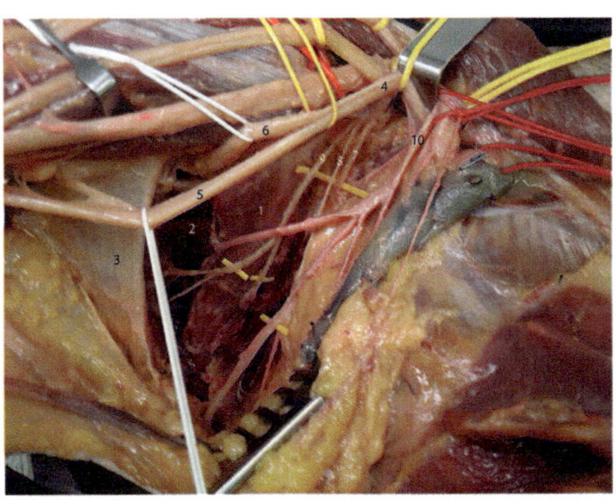

Fig. 2.22 View of the posterior wall of the axilla. 1 Subscapular muscle, 2 teres major muscle, 3 latissimus dorsi muscle. Elevating all the infraclavicular plexus we gain access to the posterior cord and its terminal an collateral branches: 4 posterior cord, 5 radial nerve, 6 axillary nerve, 7 upper subscapular nerve, 8 thoracodorsal nerve, 9 lower subscapular nerve. 10 axillary artery

Thoracodorsal Nerve (C6–C8)

The thoracodorsal nerve originates from the posterior cord between the upper and lower subscapular nerves (see Fig. 2.22). It carries mainly C7 but also C6 and C8 fibers. It can originate directly from the radial, axillary, or subscapular nerve. It is placed behind the subscapular artery and after its division into the superior scapular circumflex artery and thoracodorsal artery follows this last branch to penetrate the *latissimus dorsi* muscle with it. This is about 8–12 cm from its insertion tendon and about 2 cm from its leading edge [12, 21, 30, 43].

Lower Subscapular Nerve (C5–C6)

Although classically described as originating from the posterior cord, it can be detached independently from the axillary nerve. It is directed to the lower edge of the subscapular muscle, behind the subscapular vessels where it is divided into two branches, one to innervate the lower portion of the subscapular muscle and another to innervate the teres major muscle (see Fig. 2.22) [12, 21, 30, 43].

Sensory and Sympathetic Aspect

They will correspond to the specific sensory and sympathetic aspects of each of the nerves that compose it, and that we will see individually, or the sum of some of them according to the affected cord.

The collateral branches of the infraclavicular plexus have no cutaneous sensory but proprioceptive representation, which may explain the existence of pain when they are injured [4].

References

1. Bonnel F, Rabischong P. Anatomy and systematization of the brachial plexus in the adult. Anat Clin. 1981;2:289–98.
2. Shin AY, Spinner RJ. Clinically relevant surgical anatomy and exposures of the brachial plexus. Hand Clin. 2005;21(1):1–11.
3. Llusa M, Meri A, Ruano D. Surgical atlas of the musculoskeletal system. Rosemont: American Academy of Orthopaedic Surgeons; 2008.

4. Lazorthes G. Sistema nervioso periférico: descripción, sistematización y exploración. Barcelona: Toray-Masson; 1976.
5. Mumenthaler M, Schliack H. Peripheral nerve lesions. Diagnosis and therapy. New York: Thieme Medical; 1991.
6. Alnot JY, Narakas A. editores. Les Paralysies du Plexus Brachial. 2 ed. Monographie de la Société Française de Chirurgie de la Main. Paris: Expansion Scientifique Française; 1995.
7. Llusá M, Palazzi S, Carrera A, Forcada P. Anatomía quirúrgica del plexo braquial y nervios periféricos. Barcelona: Publicacions i Edicions de la Universitat de Barcelona; 2007.
8. Millesi H, Terzis JK. Nomenclature in peripheral nerve surgery. Committee report of the International Society of Reconstructive Microsurgery. Clin Plast Surg. 1984;11(1):3–8.
9. Tubiana R, McCullough CJ, Masquelet AC. An atlas of surgical exposures of the upper extremity. London: Martin Dunitz; 1990.
10. Shin AY, Spinner RJ, Steinmann SP, Bishop AT. Adult traumàtic brachial plexus injuries. J Am Acad Orthop Surg. 2005;13:382–96.
11. Alnot JY, Narakas A. Traumatic brachial plexus injuries. Paris: Expansion Scientifique Française; 1996.
12. Gilbert A, editor. Brachial plexus injuries. London: Martin Dunitz; 2001.
13. Socolovsky M, Rasulic L, Midha R, Garozzo D. Manual of peripheral nerve surgery. Stuttgart: Thieme; 2018.
14. Birch R, Bonney G. Wynn CB y parry, editores. Surgical disorders of the peripheral nerves. Edimburgo: Churchill Livingstone; 1998.
15. Seddon HJ. Surgical disorders of the peripheral nerves. Edinburgh and London: Churchill Livingstone; 1972.
16. Bonnel F. Microscopic anatomy of the adult human brachial plexus: an anatomical and histological basis for microsurgery. Microsurgery. 1984;5(3):107–17.
17. Yu HL, Chase RA, Strauch B. Atlas of hand anatomy and clinical implications. China: Mosby; 2004.
18. Doyle JR, Botte MJ. Surgical anatomy of the hand and upper extremity. Philadelphia: Lippincott Williams & Wilkins; 2003.
19. Bruce J, Walmsley R, Ross JA. Manual of surgical anatomy. E & S Livingstone: Edinburgh; 1964.
20. Omer JE, Spinner M, Van Beek AL. Management of peripheral nerve problems. 2nd ed. Nueva York: WB Saunders; 1998.
21. Mackinnon SE. Nerve surgery. New York: Thieme Medical Publishers, Inc.; 2015.
22. Kline DG, Hudson AR, Kim DH. Atlas of peripheral nerve surgery. Philadelphia: W.B. Saunders Company; 2001.
23. Kubiena H, Hormann M, Michlits W, Tschabitscher M, Groszschimdt K, Frey M. Intraoperative imaging of the brachial plexus by high-resolution ultrasound. J Reconst Microsurg. 2005;21(7):429–33.
24. Kerr AT. The brachial plexus of nerves in man, the variations in its formation and branches. Am J Anat. 1918;23(2):285–95.
25. Hollinshead WH. Anatomy for surgeons. 2nd ed. New York: Harper and Row Publishers, Inc.; 1968.
26. Herzberg G, Narakas A, Comtet JJ, Bouchet A, Carret JP. Microsurgical relations of the roots of the brachial plexus. Practical applications. Ann Chir Main. 1985;4(2):120–33.
27. Bollini CA, Urmey WF, Vascello L, Cacheiro F. Relationship between evoked motor response and sensory paresthesia in interscalene brachial plexus block. Reg Anesth Pain Med. 2003;28:384–8.
28. Rusell SM. Examination of the peripheral nerves injuries. An anatomical approach. New York: Thieme Medical Publishers, Inc; 2006.
29. Slutsky DJ, Hentz VR. Peripheral nerve surgery. Practical applications in the upper extremity. Philadelphia: Churchill Livingstone-Elsevier; 2006.
30. Chung KC, Yang LJ-S, JE MG, editors. Practical management of pediatric and adult brachial plexus palsies. New York: Elsevier Saunders; 2012.
31. Miller RA. Observations upon the arrangement of the axillary artery and brachial plexus. Am J Anat. 1939;64(1):143–63.
32. Alnot JY, Chammas M. Lésions traumatiques des nerf périphériques. Cahiers d'enseignement de la SOFCOT. Paris: Elsevier Masson; 2007.
33. Sunderland S. Nerves and nerve injuries. London: Churchill Livingston; 1972.
34. Jabaley ME, Wallace WH, Heckler FR. Internal topography of major nerves of the forearm and hand: a current view. J Hand Surg. 1980;5(1):1–18.
35. Watchmaker GP, Lee G, Mackinnon SE. Intraneural topography of the ulnar nerve in the cubital tunnel facilitates anterior transposition. J Hand Surg Am. 1994 Nov;19(6):915–22.
36. Gaul JS. Electrical fascicle identification as an adjunct to nerve repair. Hand Clin. 1986;2(4):709–22.
37. Kimura J, editor. Electrodiagnosis in diseases of nerve and muscle: principles and practice. Philadelphia: FA Davis Company; 1989.
38. Brunelli G, Monini L. Neurotization of avulsed roots of brachial plexus by means of anterior nerves of cervical plexus. Clin Plast Surg. 1984;11(1):149–52.
39. Chuang DC. Neurotization procedures for brachial plexus injuries. Hand Clin. 1995;11:633–45.
40. Chuang DC. Nerve transfers in adult brachial plexus injuries: my methods. Hand Clin. 2005;21:71–82.
41. Horiguchi M. The cutaneous branch of some human suprascapular nerves. J Anat. 1980;130(1):191–5.
42. Narakas AO. Thoughts on neurotization or nerve transfers in irreparable nerve lesions. Clin Plast Surg. 1984;11:153–9.
43. Llusa M, Palazzi S, Valer A. Anatomía quirúrgica del plexo braquial y los nerviós periféricos de la extremidad superior. Buenos Aires: Editorial Médica Panamericana S.A.; 2013.

44. Gelberman RH. Operative nerve repair and reconstruction. Philadelphia: JB Lippincott; 1991.
45. Palazzi S, Cáceres JP, Palazzi JL. Actualización y estrategia de tratamiento de las lesiones supraclaviculares del plexo braquial del adulto. Patología del Plexo Braquial. Madrid: Momento Médico Iberoamericano; 2004.
46. Aszmann OC, Rab M, Kamolz L, Frey M. The anatomy of the pectoral nerves and their significance in brachial plexus reconstruction. J Hand Surg Am. 2000 Sep;25(5):942–7.
47. Oberlin C, Belkheyar Z, Durand S. Paralysies traumatiques du plexu brachial de l'adulte par lésions radiculaires. En: Enciclopedie du Appareil locomoteur. Paris: Elsevier Masson SAS; 2007.
48. Bertelli JA, Ghizoni MF. Results and current approach for brachial plexus reconstruction. J Brachial Plex Peripher Nerve Inj. 2011;6:1–8.
49. Tubbs RS, Loukas M, Shahid K, Judge T, Pinyard J, Shoja MM, et al. Anatomy and quantitation of the subscapular nerves. Clin Anat. 2007 Aug;20(6):656–9.

Mechanisms of Injury

3

Kitty Wu, Peter Chang, and Christopher J. Dy

Introduction

The first description of traumatic brachial plexus injury dates to Homer's Iliad when "[Hector] hit [Teucer] just where the collar-bone divides the neck from the chest, a very deadly place, and broke the sinew of his arm so that his wrist was less, and the bow dropped from his hand" [1]. Nearly 3000 years later, trauma remains the leading cause of brachial plexus injuries (BPIs).

In his classic 1985 study of 1068 BPI patients, Narakas described the "rule of 7 x 70" summarized as follows: [1] more than 70% of BPI are caused by traffic accidents, [2] 70% of traffic accidents are a result of motorcycle or bicycle, [3] 70% of these patients suffered polytrauma, [4] 70% had infraclavicular lesion, [5] 70% had at least one root avulsion, [6] 70% of root avulsions affected the lower trunk, and [7] 70% of patients with root avulsions injuries suffered chronic pain. Other than the proportion of infraclavicular lesions being only 10%, Narakas' other observations have largely withstood the test of time [2, 3].

K. Wu
Department of Plastic and Reconstructive Surgery, Western University, London, ON, Canada
e-mail: kwu92@uwo.ca

P. Chang · C. J. Dy (✉)
Department of Orthopedic Surgery, Washington University School of Medicine, St. Louis, MO, USA
e-mail: peter.chang@wustl.edu; dyc@wustl.edu

From Homer to Narakas to the present day, this chapter summarizes the main mechanisms of adult brachial plexus injuries.

Closed Trauma

The most common cause of adult brachial plexus injury is a closed traction injury resulting from a high-velocity motor vehicle collision [4–8]. Motorcycle crashes are the most prevalent, accounting for 62% of operative BPI cases, followed by automobile collisions which account for an additional 13% of operative cases [4]. Other traumatic causes include snowmobile accidents, fall from a height, bicycle or pedestrian accidents, and workplace injuries [4, 9, 10]. In a North American study of 4538 multi-trauma patients, the overall incidence of BPI was 1.2%, with 29% resulting from automobile collisions, 22% from motorcycle accidents, and 4.8% from snowmobile accidents [11]. Although the proportion of closed BPI resulting from motorcycle collisions was slightly lower than those in automobile accidents, motorcycle driving is overall a higher-risk activity. Less than 1% of those involved in automobile accidents resulted in BPI, compared to 4.2% of those injured in a motorcycle accident and 4.8% of those injured in a snowmobile accident [11].

In motorcycle collisions, brachial plexus injury results from a direct, forceful vertical

A. Y. Shin, N. Pulos (eds.), *Operative Brachial Plexus Surgery*,
https://doi.org/10.1007/978-3-030-69517-0_3

impact to the shoulder from striking another immobile object such as another vehicle, the ground, a tree, or a utility pole [5]. The average motorcycle speed at the time of impact ranged from 47 km/h in India to 88 km/h in the United States [12, 13]. Motorcycle and snowmobile drivers are unprotected by a vehicular frame and are more frequently ejected from the vehicle, resulting in a high rate of associated polytrauma and higher injury severity scores [14].

Supraclavicular Injury

Ninety percent of traumatic BPI patients sustain supraclavicular injuries, and of these, 70% of injuries involve the avulsion of at least one root, and 12% involve avulsion of all five roots [4–6, 15]. Within all traumatic supraclavicular injuries, 50% of patients have complete C5-T1 pan-plexus involvement, followed by 39% with upper plexus lesions [4]. The prevalence of partial upper plexus lesions was further described by Bertelli in a series of 565 patients of which 23% had isolated C5–C6 injuries, 19% had C5–C7 injuries, and interestingly 52% had C5–C8 injuries [15], emphasizing the variability in injury patterns. The incidence of isolated lower plexus injuries is much less common and occurs in 2–6% of patients [3, 4, 10, 15, 16].

Upper plexus injuries are caused by a forceful widening of the shoulder-neck angle with a downward vertical force on the shoulder and traction on the neck while the shoulder is in an adducted position (Fig. 3.1a) [5, 6]. In contrast, lower plexus injuries occur from a widened scapulohumeral angle with the shoulder forced into hyper-abduction (Fig. 3.1b) [5, 6]. This finding is supported by biomechanical three-dimensional finite element studies of the brachial plexus. Strain to the upper plexus is evident with neck extension beyond 33° and neck flexion beyond 23.5° from the ipsilateral shoulder. Strain to the lower plexus occurs with shoulder abduction starting at 30° [7]. Upper plexus injuries occur more frequently in motorcycle and bicycle accidents, while lower plexus injuries were more common in those involved in car accidents [17]. Pan-plexus injuries result from increased severity of the transmitted forces or a combination of differential forces during the collision [11]. Motorcyclists not wearing helmets had a higher incidence of pan-plexus lesions [18].

The impact of seatbelts on the pattern of injury has been controversial. In a study of 43 surgically treated BPIs secondary to automobile accidents, Kaiser reported that all belted patients sustained upper plexus injuries on the side of the seatbelt crossing the shoulder [19]. In the same series, 86% of patients not wearing seatbelts suffered pan-plexus injuries. In contrast, Soldado reported on 11 patients with C7-T1 lesions on the side of the seatbelt crossing the shoulder and described a different mechanism for lower plexus injuries resulting from severe retropulsion of the shoulder as the body is projected forward and the shoulder

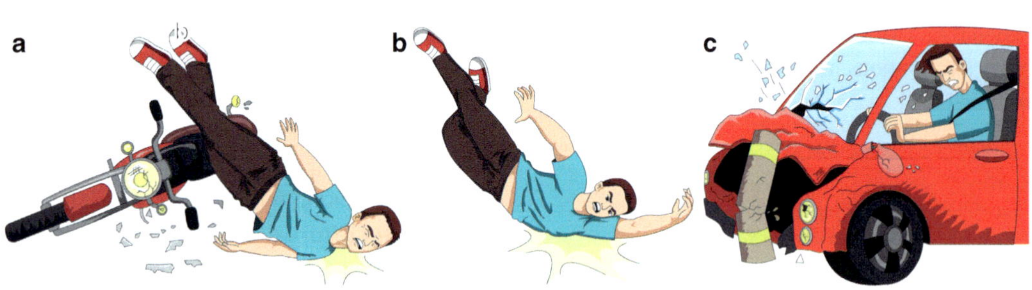

Fig. 3.1 *Mechanisms of supraclavicular injury.* Upper plexus injuries are caused by a forceful widening of the shoulder-neck angle with a downward vertical force on the shoulder and traction on the neck while the shoulder is in an adducted position (**a**). Lower plexus injuries occur from a widened scapulohumeral angle with the shoulder forced into hyper-abduction (**b**). Direct anterior shoulder compression, for example, from a seatbelt, predisposes intermediate-level injuries with C7 root involvement (**c**). (Image modified from Soldado et al. [5])

is kept immobilized by the seatbelt [5]. Brunelli theorized that direct anterior compression of the shoulder results in "intermediate BPI" with C7 root pathology and variable C5–C6 and C7-T1 involvement (Fig. 3.1c) [20]. The exact injury pattern may be determined by the direction and force of the impact in addition to the position of neck and shoulder. Furthermore, the retrospective nature of these studies involves interviewing patients regarding events at the time of a traumatic event and is subject to recall bias.

The upper brachial plexus is more susceptible to nerve rupture and the lower plexus to nerve avulsion. The C5–C6 nerve roots are suspended by the superior vertebral ligament and protected by dural sleeves and the tendinous portion of the anterior and middle scalene muscles as it exits from the intervertebral foramina [21, 22]. The C8-T1 roots are not supported by these structures and are more likely to avulse. Furthermore, nerves are more likely to rupture at branch points, where the adjacent soft tissues act as tethering points [23]. The supraclavicular branches of the upper plexus predispose rupture, whereas the C8-T1 roots do not have branch points and thus more likely to avulse [24].

Infraclavicular Injury

Infraclavicular injuries in motor vehicle collisions are less common, accounting for only 10–12% of traumatic cases overall, but are often just as severe with a high incidence of concomitant injury [3, 16, 25]. Twenty-three percent of patients have associated vascular injury, including axillary artery rupture or segmental occlusion, and 64% have concomitant fractures or dislocations of the humerus, clavicle, scapula, and shoulder. The presence of associated shoulder girdle trauma was predictive of increased severity of BPI and axonotmetic or neurotmetic lesions [3, 11].

Seventy-six percent of lesions are at the cord-terminal branch region and 24% at the division-cord level [3]. Internal rotation at the time of injury predisposed injury to the posterior cord, axillary, and radial nerve, and external rotation causes increased tension and likely injury to the musculocutaneous nerve [26]. Infraclavicular injuries are likely underreported as larger case series focus on operative BPI, and infraclavicular traction injuries are more often neurapraxic with a higher propensity for recovery without surgical intervention [11].

Combined Injuries

More extensive injuries include "skip-level" lesions, which can span both supra- and infraclavicular lesions along with the same level or include involvement of non-contiguous levels [27]. A horizontal "skip" lesion describes an injury to the same root at two different levels, for example, combined supraclavicular and infraclavicular lesions spanning an intact segment in between. A longitudinal "skip" lesion can involve, for example, avulsion of C5 and C7 but with the C6 root being spared [27]. Although rare, awareness of the possibility of such lesions is important both for prognostication and planning surgical reconstruction.

Open Trauma

Gunshot Wounds

Presently, the incidence of BPI with ballistic trauma is low, comprising of 3–12% of all operative BPI [5, 6]. The prevalence of civilian gunshot wounds (GSW) is the highest in the United States, ranging from 9.8 to 19.9% and lowest in India, Canada, and Germany, ranging from 0% to 11% [8, 11, 13, 28–30]. The extent of the injury is related to the type and caliber of the weapon, firing velocity, and presence of shrapnel [29, 31]. Larger caliber weapons achieve higher kinetic energy and cause more extensive damage to the surrounding tissues.

Nerve injury results from both the direct impact of the projectile and the secondary effects (heat, shock waves, and cavitation) [6, 32]. There is a high incidence of concomitant vascular, orthopedic, and soft tissue injuries, with 30% of patients requiring emergent operative intervention [6]. Vascular injuries include axillary artery pseudoaneurysms, arteriovenous fistulas, and expanding hematomas, which can lead to the continued progression or the delayed presentation of BPI [29, 33].

In contrast to traction injuries, 90% of GSW affect the infraclavicular plexus at the level of the cord or terminal branches [4, 29, 34]. Injuries at the cord level were most commonly to the medial cord (52%), followed by the lateral cord (26%) and posterior cords (22%) [35]. Injuries caused by shrapnel were more extensive, with a greater number of injured neural elements compared to bullet wounds [35]. The majority of lesions had some level of continuity; however, the zone of injury can be multi-leveled longitudinal or horizontal "skip-lesions" with a variable combination of in-continuity lesions and complete transection. Only 8% of lesions with complete loss of function on preoperative physical examination was found to be completely transected at the time of surgical exploration [10]. Lower-velocity injuries were more often neurapraxic or axonotmetic injuries with the propensity for recovery, while high-velocity missile injuries tend to be neurotmetic [31, 35]. The ballistic nature of the nerve injury makes it difficult to determine the zone of injury to the nerve and the extent of injury to the nerve. Both of these considerations make predicting prognosis challenging for peripheral nerve surgeons. While many patients may experience partial spontaneous recovery, there is a benefit to surgical exploration if neurologic recovery has plateaued.

Lacerations

Lacerating injuries to the brachial plexus are rare, with an incidence of 3–7% of all operative BPI [4, 10, 36]. Mechanisms include both sharp injuries from knife or glass and blunt injuries with engine motor blades, metal, and animal bites [4, 10]. Injuries are predominantly to the infraclavicular plexus. There are case reports of lacerating supraclavicular BPI from chainsaw kickback; however, these are often fatal from irreparable vascular injury and airway compromise and thus not represented in the operative BPI literature [37]. With sharp lacerations, the zone of injury is immediately discernible. Early exploration and repair are recommended to minimize the need for nerve grafts and optimize the chances of timely neural regeneration [36].

Sports-Related

The most common brachial plexus injury in athletes is the "burner" or "stinger," in which the athlete experiences burning or stinging pain from the neck, radiating down the arm that lasts for seconds to several minutes. It is most frequently encountered in contact sport athletes, particularly those playing American football and rugby [38, 39]. Forty-nine to 65 percent of American college football players experience this syndrome during their career [38]. Underlying cervical stenosis is a risk factor for the development of burners or stingers [40–42].

There are three different proposed mechanisms for stinger-type BPI. It can occur through brachial plexus traction injury, brachial plexus root compression in the neural foramen, or direct impact to the brachial plexus [43]. Traction injury can occur when the shoulder is depressed and the neck is laterally flexed contralateral to the affected extremity [43]. Traction injuries tend to occur in younger athletes without a history of any cervical pathology or trauma [44]. Brachial plexus root compression is caused by hyperextension and lateral flexion of the neck combined with a direct axial load that compresses the nerve root at the level of the neural foramen [45]. Direct impact to the brachial plexus can cause injury to the brachial plexus from shoulder pad compression of the plexus at Erb's point [45]. A recommendation to change the tackling technique from "leading with the head" to "shoulder tackling" is thought to contribute to an increase in BPI among American football players. In addition to BPI, cervical radiculopathy, cervical spondylosis, and spinal cord injury should be included in the differential diagnosis of peripheral neurologic deficits among athletes [38].

In addition to burners and stingers, more severe BPI can occur in athletes. Daly et al. described three patients who suffered permanent brachial plexus injuries related to football [46]. All patients underwent nerve transfers. Two out of the three patients were able to regain functional use of their arm; however, one patient was not able to regain any significant function. BPI can occur in non-contact athletes as well. In another large series of peripheral nerve injury, it was found that out of 16 BPI, 15 occurred in mountain climbers [47]. This occurred due to "backpack paralysis" where compression of the brachial plexus occurred due to the straps of the backpack carried by these climbers.

Glenohumeral Dislocation

BPI can occur in conjunction with glenohumeral (GH) dislocation or as a result of attempted reduction maneuvers. The incidence of neurologic injury and shoulder dislocation varies widely, with reported frequencies ranging from 5.4% to 55% [48–51]. In the largest series of associated injuries following a traumatic anterior GH dislocation, the incidence of associated neurological injury was 13.5% [52]. The likelihood of a neurologic injury was significantly greater in GH dislocation with a rotator cuff tear or greater tuberosity fracture. There are two primary groups of patients who suffer neurologic injury with GH dislocations: (A) young patients after high-energy trauma and (B) older patients who sustain low-energy same-level falls [52–55]. In addition to the GH dislocation and BPI, there are typically other injuries to the shoulder girdle and chest wall, such as fractures of the scapula, proximal humerus, clavicle, and first rib.

As the humeral head dislocates from the glenoid, the brachial plexus and peripheral nerves may be injured by traction and stretching or direct impact and compression. Stevens suggested that during GH dislocation, the axillary nerve is stretched across the surgical neck of the humerus as the arm is abducted and externally rotated [56]. The axillary nerve may also be injured from direct compression between the humeral head and the axillary border of the scapula [57]. The suprascapular nerve is also at risk due to its short distance from the posterior glenoid rim and the potential for tethering at the scapular and spinoglenoid notches [58]. Furthermore, concomitant vascular injury to the axillary artery or vein may result in a hematoma or pseudoaneurysm [53, 59, 60]. The axillary artery and brachial plexus travel in the same fascial sheath as they course through the axilla; thus, any swelling from arterial injury can result in compression on elements of the brachial plexus [61]. The subsequent scar tissue can lead to further constriction of the nerves [51]. Lastly, damage to the vasa nervorum during GH dislocation predisposes ischemic injury, leading to demyelination, mesoneurial disruption, and nerve infarction [61].

Joint reduction attempts, specifically with maneuvers that apply traction to the dislocated upper limb and countertraction in the axilla, can worsen neurovascular insult from the initial dislocation event or cause new injury [62]. In general, reduction maneuvers should be carried out with adequate sedation and full muscle relaxation to allow the reduction to be performed without excessive force.

BPI from GH dislocation most commonly affects the infraclavicular of the plexus at the level of the cords and branches [63–65]. While the axillary nerve is often considered most at risk in GH dislocation [52], several studies have demonstrated that injury to multiple nerves is more common than mononeuropathy [54, 59, 66–69]. Although the most commonly injured cord is the posterior cord, the medial cord is at a particular risk when the elbow and wrist are extended during the trauma. Given the lengthy distance from the site of injury to the intrinsic muscles of the hand, injury to the medial cord after GH dislocation is especially devastating to patients.

Iatrogenic Injury

Patient Positioning

Brachial plexus injuries due to improper patient positioning occur in 0.05% of surgical cases [70]. Fifteen percent of all closed medicolegal claims from the American Association of Anesthesiologists are due to peripheral nerve injuries with brachial plexus and ulnar nerve injuries being the most common [71, 72]. The use of muscle paralysis further diminishes intrinsic muscle tone and predisposes nonphysiologic positions. Patients placed in prone positioning are at increased risk, especially when the shoulders are abducted greater than 90° and externally rotated [70]. This places the brachial plexus under traction and compression between the clavicle and first rib. Lateral neck flexion towards the same side further compounds these compressive forces. Patients in lateral decubitus are at risk of compression if the dependent arm is placed underneath the thorax and compressed against the operating Table. A roll between under the chest can offload direct pressure to the axilla. Careful patient positioning, appropriate padding of all bony prominences, and avoidance of nonphysiologic positioning are crucial to preventing injury.

Regional Anesthesia

Regional nerve blocks can provide long-lasting analgesia and the avoidance of a general anesthetic; however, it is associated with a 2.84% risk of nerve injury [73]. The use of ultrasound guidance and nerve stimulators during regional blocks can help increase the accuracy of blocks and prevent intraneural injection. Nerve injury results from direct mechanical injury to the myelin sheath with intraneural needle insertion, chemical injury from the local anesthetic, and pressure exerted by the volume of administered local anesthetic [74]. Intrafascicular injections with greater than 12 psi result in persistent neurologic deficits [75].

The use of long-tapered needles for injection produces fewer transected axons compared to beveled needles, as the tapered end is thought to push the axons away [76]. Blunt short-bevel needles are less likely to penetrate the perineurium; however, when injuries occur, they are more severe [77].

The degree of injury also varies depending on the location of the block (interscalene, infraclavicular, axillary). The median nerve was most frequently affected with axillary regional blocks due to its superficial position, followed by combined median and ulnar neuropathies. Permanent upper trunk injuries have been reported following interscalene blocks [78] with periscapular atrophy developing within 10 days after surgery [78]. While the majority of regional anesthetic-related BPI recover spontaneously, the use of adjunctive modalities and prevention of intraneural injection are paramount.

Laparoscopic Surgery

There is a 0.16–1% incidence of brachial plexus injury with laparoscopic and robotic surgery, with increased risk associated with longer operative times and steep Trendelenburg positioning [79–81]. Shoulder braces and wrist restraints are often used to prevent patients from sliding from the operating table during steep Trendelenburg positioning. Both can predispose BPI as shoulder braces exert direct pressure over the acromion and clavicle and wrist restraints cause traction on the neck and shoulder [82]. Proper positioning and tucking arms by the patients' side rather than in an abducted position and limiting Trendelenburg less than 30 degrees are protective against BPI [83].

Cardiac Surgery

Intraoperative BPI is estimated at 0.2–10.6% in coronary artery bypass procedures [84–86]. Injury results from mechanical traction from sternotomy retractors and most commonly presents as either sensory disturbance in the lower C8-T1 roots or motor deficit in the upper or middle plexus [84]. The use of asymmetrically opening retractors for unilateral internal mammary artery harvest, cephalad retractor placement, wider retractor opening, and prolonged operative time increased the risk of BPI [86, 87]. Prolonged deep hypothermia for cardiopulmonary bypass has also been proposed as causative of ischemic nerve injury [88].

Shoulder Arthroplasty

The incidence of BPI during shoulder arthroplasty is estimated at 1% [89]. Shoulder abduction and external rotation combined with elbow extension place increased strain on the brachial plexus. Inferior capsular release increases risk to the axillary nerve. The brachial plexus can be injured during placement of retractors, from prolonged compression from retractors, during the bony work for implant preparation and insertion, and during implant reduction. In reverse total shoulder arthroplasty (TSA), positioning of the humerus in greater than 45° of extension increased strain on all nerves except for the axillary and ulnar nerve [90]. Glenoid exposure increased strain on all nerves except the median and ulnar nerve [90]. Supporting the arm from beneath the elbow and avoidance of prolonged external rotation can decrease tension on the brachial plexus and peripheral nerves, particularly during maneuvers to manipulate the proximal humerus [91, 92]. Excessive limb lengthening in reverse TSA (particularly >2 cm) may be associated with an increase in subclinical nerve injury compared to anatomic total shoulder arthroplasties [93, 94]. The reliance of the reverse TSA on deltoid strength makes avoidance of axillary nerve injury ever more important.

Oncologic Etiology

Primary Lesions

Primary brachial plexus tumors are very rare. Peripheral nerve sheath tumors, either neurofibromas (62%) or schwannomas (38%), are typically benign [95, 96]. Neurofibromas were more often isolated lesions, not associated with neurofibromatosis. Malignant lesions include peripheral nerve sheath, granular cell, synovial sarcoma, neurogenic sarcoma, and peripheral primitive neuroectodermal tumors [95]. The trunks were most commonly involved (48%), followed by the nerve roots (33%), cords or branches (15%), and multilevel involvement (4%) [95]. The most common clinical presentation was a palpable mass, paresthesia, or pain, with only 8% of patients presenting with motor deficits [95]. Treatment is dependent on the pathological diagnosis and includes both adjuvant radiotherapy and chemotherapy in addition to surgical resection; however, the 3-year survival is dismal at only 50% [96].

Metastatic Lesions

Metastasis to the brachial plexus is exceedingly rare but has been reported with non-melanoma skin cancer and breast cancer. Patients present with shoulder pain, decreased range of motion, and malignant lymphedema. Supraclavicular metastasis is more common with predominantly upper trunk involvement [97].

Radiation

Radiation-induced BPI is a sequela of breast, lung, head and neck, and nasopharyngeal cancer treatment [98, 99]. Standard fractionated radiation doses, higher overall dose, and shortened treatment times are risk factors for BPI [100]. Radiation-induced BPI is a manifestation of late toxicity and can present months or years following treatment [101]. Nerve injury occurs due to perineural fibrosis and demyelination [102]. With lung and breast cancer treatment, the infraclavicular plexus is more susceptible to injury being closer to the focus of treatment. The suggested total maximum dose to the brachial plexus is less than 60 Gy [103].

Neuralgic Amyotrophy

Neuralgic amyotrophy, also known as Parsonage-Turner syndrome and brachial neuritis, is characterized by the acute onset of painful neuropathy and is presumed to be autoimmune in origin [104]. Involvement is variable and can be limited to a terminal branch or involve multiple roots, although upper plexus involvement is more common [104]. In 90% of cases, acute pain is the first clinical symptom before the onset of weakness. In up to 50% of cases, a precipitation factor such as bacterial or viral infection, trauma, strenuous exercise, or surgery was identified occurring within 1 week to 1 month of onset [105]. Nerve injury results from focal inflammation-causing axonal damage and an hourglass-like constriction within the affected nerve [106, 107]. Generally, outcomes with nonoperative intervention are favorable, and 36% of patients recovering within 1 year, 75% within 2 years, and 89% in 3 years [105].

References

1. Aydn A, Tumerdem B, Yazar M, Erer M. Three-thousand-year-old written reference to a description of what might be the earliest brachial plexus injuries in the Iliad of Homer. Plast Reconstr Surg. 2004;114(5):1352–3.
2. Narakas AO. The treatment of brachial plexus injuries. Int Orthop. 1985;9(1):29–36.
3. Kim DH, Murovic JA, Tiel RL, Kline DG. Infraclavicular brachial plexus stretch injury. Neurosurg Focus. 2004;16(5):E4.
4. Kaiser R, Waldauf P, Ullas G, Krajcová A. Epidemiology, etiology, and types of severe adult brachial plexus injuries requiring surgical repair: systematic review and meta-analysis. Neurosurg Rev. 2018;1:1–10.
5. Soldado F, Ghizoni MF, Bertelli J. Injury mechanisms in supraclavicular stretch injuries of the brachial plexus. Hand Surg Rehabil. 2016;35(1):51–4.
6. Kim DH, Murovic JA, Tiel RL, Kline DG. Mechanisms of injury in operative brachial plexus lesions. Neurosurg Focus. 2004;16(5):E2.
7. Mihara A, Kanchiku T, Nishida N, Tagawa H, Ohgi J, Suzuki H, et al. Biomechanical analysis of brachial plexus injury: availability of three-dimensional finite element model of the brachial plexus. Exp Ther Med. 2018 Feb;15(2):1989–93.
8. Li GY, Xue MQ, Wang JW, Zeng XY, Qin J, Sha K. Traumatic brachial plexus injury: a study of 510 surgical cases from multicenter services in Guangxi, China. Acta Neurochir. 2019;161(5):899–906.
9. Faglioni W, Siqueira MG, Martins RS, Heise CO, Foroni L. The epidemiology of adult traumatic brachial plexus lesions in a large metropolis. Acta Neurochir. 2014;156(5):1025–8.
10. Kim DH, Cho YJ, Tiel RL, Kline DG. Outcomes of surgery in 1019 brachial plexus lesions treated at Louisiana State University Health Sciences Center. J Neurosurg. 2003;98(5):1005–16.
11. Midha R. Epidemiology of brachial plexus injuries in a multitrauma population. Neurosurgery. 1997;40(6):1182–8.
12. Terzis JK, Vekris MD, Soucacos PN. Outcomes of brachial plexus reconstruction in 204 patients with devastating paralysis. Plast Reconstr Surg. 1999;104(5):1221–40.
13. Jain DK, Bhardwaj P, Venkataramani H, Sabapathy SR. An epidemiological study of traumatic brachial plexus injury patients treated at an Indian Centre. Indian J Plast Surg. 2012;45(3):498–503.
14. Kaiser R, Mencl L, Haninec P. Injuries associated with serious brachial plexus involvement in polytrauma among patients requiring surgical repair. Injury. 2014;45(1):223–6.
15. Bertelli JA, Ghizoni MF, Soldado F. Patterns of brachial plexus stretch palsy in a prospective series of 565 surgically treated patients. J Hand Surg Am. 2017;42(6):443–446.e2.
16. Barman A, Chatterjee A, Prakash H, Viswanathan A, Tharion G, Thomas R. Traumatic brachial plexus injury: electrodiagnostic findings from 111 patients in a tertiary care hospital in India. Injury. 2012;43(11):1943–8.
17. Kaiser R, Waldauf P, Haninec P. Types and severity of operated supraclavicular brachial plexus injuries caused by traffic accidents. Acta Neurochir. 2012 Jul;154(7):1293–7.
18. Socolovsky M, Antoniadis G, Lovaglio A, Durner G, Bonilla G, Schmidhammer M, et al. A comparison of patients from Argentina and Germany to assess factors impacting brachial plexus and brain injury. J Brachial Plex Peripher Nerve Inj. 2019;14(01):e39–46.
19. Kaiser R, Haninec P. The influence of seatbelts on the types of operated brachial plexus lesions caused by car accidents. J Hand Surg Am. 2012;37(8):1657–9.
20. Brunelli GA, Brunelli GR. A fourth type of brachial plexus lesion: the intermediate (C7) palsy. J Hand Surg Br. 1991;16(5):492–4.
21. Zhong LY, Wang AP, Hong L, Chen SH, Wang XQ, Lv YC, et al. Microanatomy of the brachial plexus roots and its clinical significance. Surg Radiol Anat. 2017;39(6):601–10.
22. Sunderland S. Mechanisms of cervical nerve root avulsion in injuries of the neck and shoulder. J Neurosurg. 1974;41(6):705–14.

23. Mahan MA, Yeoh S, Monson K, Light A. Rapid stretch injury to peripheral nerves: biomechanical results. Neurosurgery. 2019;85(1):E137–44.
24. Yeoh S, Mahan MA. Brachial plexus stretch injury needs anatomical context. J Neurosurg Spine. 2019;14:1–2.
25. Lam WL, Fufa D, Chang NJ, Chuang DC. Management of infraclavicular (Chuang level IV) brachial plexus injuries: a single surgeon experience with 75 cases. J Hand Surg Eur Vol. 2015;40(6):573–82.
26. Milton GW. The circumflex nerve and dislocation of the shoulder. Br J Phys Med. 1954;17(6):136–8.
27. Chuang DC. Brachial plexus injuries: adult and pediatric. In: Chang J, editor. Plastic surgery. 3rd ed. Elsevier; 2013. p. 789–816.
28. Chambers JA, Hiles CL, Keene BP. Brachial plexus injury management in military casualties : who , what , when , why , and how. Mil Med. 2014;179(6):640–4.
29. Kim DH, Murovic JA, Tiel RL, Kline DG. Penetrating injuries due to gunshot wounds involving the brachial plexus. Neurosurg Focus. 2004;16(5):E3.
30. Ahmed-Labib M, Golan JD, Jacques L. Functional outcome of brachial plexus reconstruction after trauma. Neurosurgery. 2007;61(5):1016–22.
31. Samardzic MM, Rasulic LG, Grujicic DM. Gunshot injuries to the brachial plexus. J Trauma. 1997;43(4):645–9.
32. Kline DG. Civilian gunshot wounds to the brachial plexus. J Neurosurg. 1989;70(2):166–74.
33. Chen L, Peng F, Wang T, Chen D, Yang J. Traumatic pseudoaneurysm of axillary artery combined with brachial plexus injury. PLoS One. 2014;9(11):e113099.
34. Secer HI, Daneyemez M, Tehli O, Gonul E, Izci Y. The clinical, electrophysiologic, and surgical characteristics of peripheral nerve injuries caused by gunshot wounds in adults : a 40-year experience. Surg Neurol. 2008;69(2):143–52.
35. Secer HI, Solmaz I, Anik I, Izci Y, Duz B, Daneyemez MK, et al. Surgical outcomes of the brachial plexus lesions caused by gunshot wounds in adults. J Brachial Plex Peripher Nerve Inj. 2009;4:11.
36. Kim DH, Murovic JA, Tiel RL, Kline DG. Lacerations to the brachial plexus: surgical techniques and outcomes. J Reconstr Microsurg. 2005;21(7):435–40.
37. Kaiser R, Ullas G. Acutely reconstructed isolated supraclavicular brachial plexus injury caused by a chainsaw. Plast Surg Case Studies. 2016;2(1):7–8.
38. Levitz CL, Reilly PJ, Torg JS. The pathomechanics of chronic, recurrent cervical nerve root neuropraxia. The chronic burner syndrome. Am J Sport Med. 1997;25(1):73–6.
39. Bohu Y, Klouche S, Lefevre N, Peyrin JC, Dusfour B, Hager JP, et al. The epidemiology of 1345 shoulder dislocations and subluxations in French Rugby union players: a five-season prospective study from 2008 to 2013. Br J Sport Med. 2015;49(23):1535–40.
40. Kelly JD, Clancy M, Marchetto PA, Moyer RA. The relationship of transient upper extremity paresthesias and cervical stenosis. Orthop Trans. 1992;16:732.
41. Meyer SA, Schulte KR, Callaghan JJ, Albrigt JP, Powell JW, Crowley ET, et al. Cervical spinal stenosis and stingers in collegiate football players. Am J Sport Med. 1994;22(2):158–66.
42. Castro FP Jr, Ricciardi J, Brunet ME, Busch MT, Whitecloud TS 3rd. Stingers, the Torg ratio, and the cervical spine. Am J Sport Med. 1997;25(5):603–8.
43. Aval SM, Durand P Jr, Shankwiler JA. Neurovascular injuries to the Athlete's shoulder: part I. J Am Acad Orthop Surg. 2007;15(4):249–56.
44. Shannon B, Klimkiewicz JJ. Cervical burners in the athlete. Clin Sport Med. 2002;21(1):29–35.
45. Rihn J, Anderson DT, Lamb K, Deluca PF, Bata A, Marchetto PA, et al. Cervical spine injuries in American football. Sport Med. 2009;39(9):697–708.
46. Daly C, Payne SH, Seiler JG. Severe brachial plexus injuries in American football. Orthopedics. 2016;39(6):e1188–92.
47. Hirasawa Y, Sakakida K. Sports and peripheral nerve injury. Am J Sport Med. 1983;11(6):420–6.
48. Visser CP, Coene LN, Brand R, Tavy DL. The incidence of nerve injury in anterior dislocation of the shoulder and its influence on functional recovery. A prospective clinical and EMG study. J Bone Joint Surg Br. 1999;81(4):679–85.
49. DePalma AF. Surgery of the shoulder. Philadelphia: Lippincott; 1951.
50. Watson-Jones R. Fractures and joint injuries. Edinburgh: E&S Livingstone Ltd; 1952.
51. Gutkowska O, Martynkiewicz J, Urban M, Gosk J. Brachial plexus injury after shoulder dislocation: a literature review. Neurosurg Rev 2018 [Epub ahead of print].
52. Robinson CM, Shur N, Sharpe T, Ray A, Murray IR. Injuries associated with traumatic anterior glenohumeral dislocations. J Bone Joint Surg Am. 2012;94(1):18–26.
53. Travlos J, Goldberg I, Boome RS. Brachial plexus lesions associated with dislocated shoulders. J Bone Joint Surg Br. 1990;72(1):68–71.
54. Liveson JA. Nerve lesions associated with shoulder dislocation; an electrodiagnostic study of 11 cases. J Neurol Neurosurg Psychiatry. 1984;47(7):742–4.
55. Kosiyatrakul A, Jitprapaikulsarn S, Durand S, Oberlin C. Recovery of brachial plexus injury after shoulder dislocation. Injury. 2009;40(12):1327–9.
56. Stevens JH. Brachial plexus paralysis. In: Kreiger, editor. The shoulder: rupture of the supraspinatus tendon and other lesions in or about the subacromial bursa. Melbourne. 1934.
57. McGregor AL. A synopsis of surgical anatomy. Baltimore: William Wood & Company; 1942.
58. Zoltan JD. Injury to the suprascapular nerve associated with anterior dislocation of the shoulder: case report and review of the literature. J Trauma. 1979;19(3):203–6.

59. Wehbe J, Maalouf G, Habanbo J, Chidiac RM, Braun E, Merle M. Surgical treatment of traumatic lesions of the axillary nerve. A retrospective study of 33 cases. Acta Orthop Belg. 2004;70(1):11–8.
60. Razif MA, Rajasingam V. Anterior shoulder dislocation with axillary artery and nerve injury. Med J Malaysia. 2002;57(4):496–8.
61. Stenning M, Drew S, Birch R. Low-energy arterial injury at the shoulder with progressive or delayed nerve palsy. J Bone Joint Surg Br. 2005;87(8):1102–6.
62. Regauer M, Polzer H, Mutschler W. Neurovascular complications due to the Hippocrates method for reducing anterior shoulder dislocations. World J Orthop. 2014;5(1):57–61.
63. de Laat EA, Visser CP, Coene LN, Pahplatz PV, Tavy DL. Nerve lesions in primary shoulder dislocations and humeral neck fractures. A prospective clinical and EMG study. J Bone Joint Surg Br. 1994;76(3):381–3.
64. Martinoli C, Bianchi S, Santacroce E, Pugliese F, Graif M, Derchi LE. Brachial plexus sonography: a technique for assessing the root level. AJR Am J Roentgenol. 2002;179(3):699–702.
65. Takase F, Inui A, Mifune Y, Muto T, Harada Y, Kokubu T, et al. Concurrent rotator cuff tear and axillary nerve palsy associated with anterior dislocation of the shoulder and large glenoid rim fracture: a "terrible tetrad". Case Rep Orthop. 2014;312968
66. Yeap JS, Lee DJ, Fazir M, Kareem BA, Yeap JK. Nerve injuries in anterior shoulder dislocations. Med J Malaysia. 2004;59(4):450–4.
67. Visser CP, Tavy DL, Coene LN, Brand R. Electromyographic findings in shoulder dislocations and fractures of the proximal humerus: comparison with clinical neurological examination. Clin Neurol Neurosurg. 1999;101(2):86–91.
68. Gutkowska O, Martynkiewicz J, Stępniewski M, Gosk J. Analysis of patient-dependent and trauma-dependent risk factors for persistent brachial plexus injury after shoulder dislocation. Biomed Red Int. 2018;2018:14512137.
69. Fox M, Lambert S, Birch R. The terrible triad of the shoulder. J Bone Joint Surg. 2009;91-B(Suppl 1):13–20.
70. Uribe JS, Kolla J, Omar H, Dakwar E, Abel N, Mangar D, et al. Brachial plexus injury following spinal surgery. J Neurosurg Spine. 2010;13(4):552–8.
71. Duffy BJ, Tubog TD. The prevention and recognition of ulnar nerve and brachial plexus injuries. J Perianesthesia Nurs. 2017;32(6):636–49.
72. Grant I, Brovman EY, Kang D, Greenberg P, Saba R, Urman RD. A medicolegal analysis of positioning-related perioperative peripheral nerve injuries occurring between 1996 and 2015. J Clin Anesth. 2019;58:84–90.
73. Brull R, McCartney CJ, Chan VW, El-Beheiry H. Neurological complications after regional anesthesia: contemporary estimates of risk. Anesth Analg. 2007;104(4):965–74.
74. Vlassakov K, Lirk P, Rathmell JP. Intraneural injection: is the jury still out? Anesthesiology. 2018;129(2):221–4.
75. Kapur E, Vuckovic I, Dilberovic F, Zaciragic A, Cosovic E, Divanovic KA, et al. Neurologic and histologic outcome after intraneural injections of lidocaine in canine sciatic nerves. Acta Anaesthesiol Scand. 2007;51(1):101–7.
76. Maruyama M. Long-tapered double needle used to reduce needle stick nerve injury. Reg Anesth. 1997;22(2):157–60.
77. Jeng CL, Rosenblatt M. Intraneural injections and regional anesthesia: the known and the unknown. Minerva Anestesiol. 2011;77(1):54–48.
78. Avellanet M, Sala-Blanch X, Gonzalez-Viejo MA. Permanent upper trunk plexopathy after interscalene brachial plexus block. J Clin Monit Comput. 2016;30(1):51–4.
79. Romanowski L, Reich H, McGlynn F, Adelson MD, Taylor PJ. Brachial plexus neuropathies after advanced laparoscopic surgery. Fertil Steril. 1993;60(4):729–32.
80. Shveiky D, Aseff JN, Iglesia CB. Brachial plexus injury after laparoscopic and robotic surgery. J Minim Invasive Gynecol. 2010;17(4):414–20.
81. Eteuati J, Hiscock R, Hastie I, Hayes I, Jones I. Brachial plexopathy in laparoscopic-assisted rectal surgery: a case series. Tech Coloproctol. 2013;17(3):293–7.
82. Gagnon J, Poulin EC. Beware of the Trendelenburg position during prolonged laparoscopic procedures. Can J Surg. 1993;36(6):505–6.
83. Abdalmageed OS, Bedaiwy MA, Falcone T. Nerve injuries in gynecologic laparoscopy. J Minim Invasive Gynecol. 2017;24(1):16–27.
84. Unlu Y, Beliogu U, Hikmet K, Becit N, Ceviz M. Brachial plexus injury following median sternotomy. Interact Cardiovasc Thorac Surg. 2007;6:235–7.
85. Vahl CF, Carl I, Muller-Vahl H, Struck E. Brachial plexus injury after cardiac surgery. The role of internal mammary artery preparation: a prospective study on 1000 consecutive patients. J Thorac Cardiovasc Surg. 1991;102(5):724–9.
86. Healey S, O'Neill B, Bilal H, Waterworth P. Does retraction of the sternum during median sternotomy result in brachial plexus injuries ? Interact Cardiovasc Thorac Surg. 2013;17(1):151–7.
87. Chauhan A, Jacobs B, Andoga A, Baratz ME. Extensor tendon injuries in athletes. Sports Med Arthrosc Rev. 2014;22(1):45–55.
88. Lederman RJ, Breuer AC, Hanson MR, Furlan AJ, Loop FD, Cosgrove DM, et al. Peripheral nervous complications of coronary artery bypass graft surgery. Ann Neurol. 1982;12(3):297–301.
89. Bohsali KI, Wirth MA, Rockwood CA Jr. Complications of total shoulder arthroplasty. J Bone Joint Surg Am. 2006;88(10):2279–92.
90. Lenoir H, Dagneaux L, Canovas F, Waitzenegger T, Pham TT, Chammas M. Nerve stress during reverse

total shoulder arthroplasty: a cadaveric study. J Shoulder Elb Surg. 2017;26(2):323–30.
91. Kam AW, Lam PH, Haen PSWA, Tan M, Shamsudin A, Murrell GAC. Preventing brachial plexus injury during shoulder surgery: a real-time cadaveric study. J Shoulder Elb Surg. 2018;27(5):912–22.
92. Nagda SH, Rogers KJ, Sestokas AK, Getz CL, Ramsey ML, Glaser DL, et al. Peripheral nerve function during shoulder arthroplasty using intra-operative nerve monitoring. J Shoulder Elb Surg. 2007;16(3 Suppl):S2–8.
93. Ladermann A, Lubbeke A, Melis B, Stern R, Christofilopoulos P, Bacle G, et al. Prevalence of neurologic lesions after total shoulder arthroplasty. J Bone Joint Surg Am. 2011;93(14):1288–93.
94. Ladermann A, Williams MD, Melis B, Hoffmeyer P, Walch G. Objective evaluation of lengthening in reverse shoulder arthroplasty. J Shoulder Elb Surg. 2009;18(4):588–95.
95. Jia X, Yang J, Chen L, Yu C, Kondo T. Primary brachial plexus tumors: clinical experiences of 143 cases. Clin Neurol Neurosurg. 2016;148:91–5.
96. Kim DH, Murovic JA, Tiel RL, Moes G, Kline DG. A series of 146 peripheral non-neural sheath nerve tumors: 30-year experience at Louisiana State University Health Sciences Center. J Neurosurg. 2005;102(2):256–66.
97. Kim J, Jeon JY, Choi YJ, Choi JK, Kim SB, Jung KH, et al. Characteristics of metastatic brachial plexopathy in patients with breast cancer. Support Care Cancer. 2019:2–7.
98. Cai Z, Li Y, Hu Z, Fu R, Rong X, Wu R, et al. Radiation-induced brachial plexopathy in patients with nasopharyngeal carcinoma: a retrospective study. Oncotarget. 2016;7(14):18887–95.
99. Yan M, Kong W, Kerr A, Brundage M. The radiation dose tolerance of the brachial plexus: a systematic review and meta-analysis. Clin Transl Radiat Oncol. 2019;18:23–31.
100. Lindberg K, Grozman V, Lindberg S, Onjukka E, Lax I, Lewensohn R, et al. Radiation-induced brachial plexus toxicity after SBRT of apically located lung lesions. Acta Oncol. 2019;58(8):1178–86.
101. Johansson S, Svensson H, Denekamp J. Timescale of evolution of late radiation injury after postoperative radiotherapy of breast cancer patients. Int J Radiat Oncol Biol Phys. 2000;48(3):745–50.
102. Stoll BA, Andrew JT. Radiation-induced peripheral neuropathy. Br Med J. 1966;1(5491):834–7.
103. Jia Y, Gou W, Geng L, Wang Y, Chen J. Anatomic proximity of the peroneal nerve to the posterolateral corner of the knee determined by MR imaging. Knee. 2012;19(6):766–8.
104. Seror P. Neuralgic amyotrophy. An update. Joint Bone Spine. 2017;84(2):153–8.
105. Tsairis P, Dyck PJ, Mulder DW. Natural history of brachial plexus neuropathy. Report on 99 patients. Arch Neurol. 1972;27(2):109–17.
106. Suarez GA, Giannini C, Bosch EP, Barohn RJ, Wodak J, Ebeling P, et al. Immune brachial plexus neuropathy: suggestive evidence for an inflammatory-immune pathogenesis. Neurology. 1996;46(2):559–61.
107. Pan YW, Wang S, Tian G, Li C, Tian W, Tian M. Typical brachial neuritis (Parsonage-Turner Syndrome) with hourglass-like constrictions in the affected nerves. J Hand Surg Am. 2011;36(7):1197–203.

Biology of Nerve Injury

4

Jonathan E. Isaacs and Sarah M. Lamont

Nerve Injury

Like any biological tissue, the local nerve response to trauma depends on the intensity and mechanism of injury. However, more specific to nerve tissue, the physiological responses proximal to the injury, distal to the injury, and within the target organs all must be considered in understanding the implications towards healing and functional recovery. To further complicate the process, this healing response and potential is time dependent and degrades drastically with time.

The brachial plexus is vulnerable to a spectrum of injurious mechanisms. Blunt trauma directly to the supra- or infraclavicular region can result in acute nerve compression, while shoulder depression or distraction, shoulder hyperabduction or flexion, and cervical deviation can stretch the plexus or tear, rupture, or avulse plexus elements. Lacerations and sharp puncture wounds may have a tearing component but tend to have more focal nerve tissue disruption. Finally, gunshot wounds may combine shock wave-induced compression and rupture with mechanical transection from the bullet itself and are particularly hard to conceptualize.

Depending on the level of intensity, focal trauma disrupts connective tissue layers and blood vessels and results in both acute and delayed local cellular responses. However, understanding the more "nerve-specific" biological responses requires an appreciation of the unique nerve anatomy and normal physiology (Fig. 4.1).

The anatomically distinct "peripheral nerve" is a bundle of cellular extensions (axons) packaged in layers of connective tissue. The neural cell bodies from which these axons originate are in either the anterior horn of the spinal cord gray matter (motor neurons) or the proximate, but extra-spinal, dorsal root ganglions for sensory.

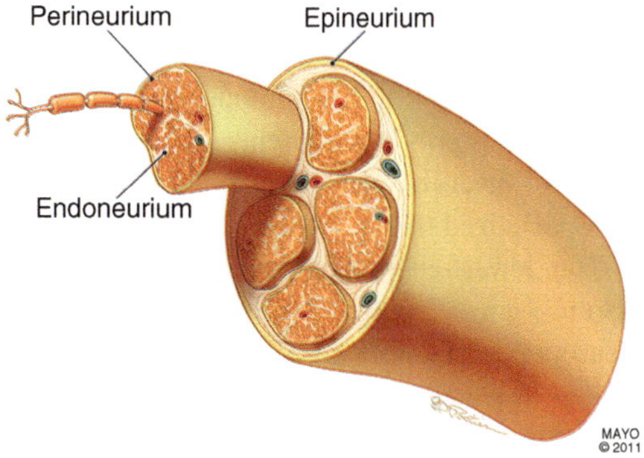

Fig. 4.1 The anatomy of a peripheral nerve. Myelin-wrapped axons run within endoneurial tubes grouped together within fascicles (encased with perineurium). The fascicles are packaged within the inner epineurium, and the outermost layer of the nerve is the outer epineurium. Blood vessels are seen running in all layers of the nerve

J. E. Isaacs (✉) · S. M. Lamont
Division of Hand Surgery, Department of Orthopedic Surgery, Virginia Commonwealth University Health System, Richmond, VA, USA
e-mail: jonathan.isaacs@vcuhealth.org

A. Y. Shin, N. Pulos (eds.), *Operative Brachial Plexus Surgery*,
https://doi.org/10.1007/978-3-030-69517-0_4

Each axon runs within an endoneurial sheath, and multiple endoneurial sheaths are packed together in fascicles contained by the toughest layer known as the perineurium. Fascicles are packaged within loose intraneural connective tissue (inner epineurium), and, finally, the outer layer of the nerve is the outer epineurium. Each motor axon innervates many muscle fibers via specialized connections known as endplates though there is only one mature functional endplate per muscle fiber. Sensory axons can innervate a variety of sensory organelles including Meissner and Pacinian corpuscles (fast-adapting receptors) and Merkel cells (slow-adapting receptors).

Many axons are insulated by a lipid-rich layer of myelin created and maintained by encircling Schwann cells (SCs). These and other SCs provide an essential supportive role to sustain normal nerve physiology. Between each segment of myelin, an uninsulated gap, known as a Node of Ranvier, exposes the intramembrane voltage-gated ion channels responsible for generating action potentials from shifting electrical gradients. Under the insulating myelin, these action potentials are not generated so that when a signal travels down a myelinated nerve, the combination of very fast passive conduction (under the insulated nerve segments) and the slower but self-propagating action potentials (known as saltatory conduction) allows the remarkably rapid transmission of signals over long nerve segments essential for normal sensory and musculoskeletal function. Finally, a rich intraneural plexus of blood vessels provides nutrients and oxygen necessary to meet the heavy metabolic demands of this specialized tissue.

The lowest-energy closed injuries may not disrupt any specific anatomic structure. Neuropraxic injuries involve either loss of homeostasis within the intraneural tissue or focal loss of myelin. Increased interstitial fluid (tissue edema or bleeding) from disrupted or permeable capillaries (depending on injury severity) may offset the delicately balanced electrical membrane gradient, affect the ability to propagate action potentials, or impede the delivery of nutrients and oxygen. Schwann cells become metabolically stressed (either due to the direct injury or to the altered microenvironment), and local myelination is lost. The net effect is conduction block and nerve dysfunction.

As the trauma intensity increases, the most anatomically vulnerable structure is the axon. With more tissue disturbance, damaged blood vessels produce visible ecchymosis, and the remaining blood vessels become permeable, allowing inflammatory cells and interstitial fluid accumulation. An influx of calcium releases membrane-bound vesicles which bridge across and seal off the disrupted axon ends to prevent the outflow of axoplasm [1], and the neuron shifts into "damage control" mode. The axon represents a substantial portion of the neuron, and axonotmesis triggers a cellular response marked by marginalization of the nucleus and dissolution of the Nissl bodies known as chromatolysis [2]. Many neurons (especially sensory and related to the level of the injury) do not survive this insult, and some animal reports demonstrate a 20 to 50% neuron loss from the dorsal root ganglia [3]. Endogenous neuroprotectants such as heat-shock protein-27 (HSP27) are upregulated and promote neuron survival [4] possibly in relation to SC-derived neurotrophic factors such as neurotrophic growth factor and brain-derived growth factors [5, 6]. Within hours of the trauma, damaged axons and their myelin sheaths on either side of the discontinuity begin a well-described degenerative process known as Wallerian degeneration (Fig. 4.2).

While the entire distal segment is affected, the process is more limited proximally and typically extends only to the first undamaged Node of Ranvier but can extend all the way to the cell body in more extreme cases [7]. An influx of extracellular ions such as Ca + trigger a cascade of events in which microtubules depolymerize, the cytoskeleton breaks down, and the axolemma (axon membrane) loses integrity resulting in cellular fragmentation and leaving disorganized cellular debris in place of the axon [8, 9]. The myelin sheath degrades within a few days as well. Endoneurial tubes swell for several weeks in response to the increased cellular activity though physiologic axonal continuity is lost within as little as 48 to 96 hours [7].

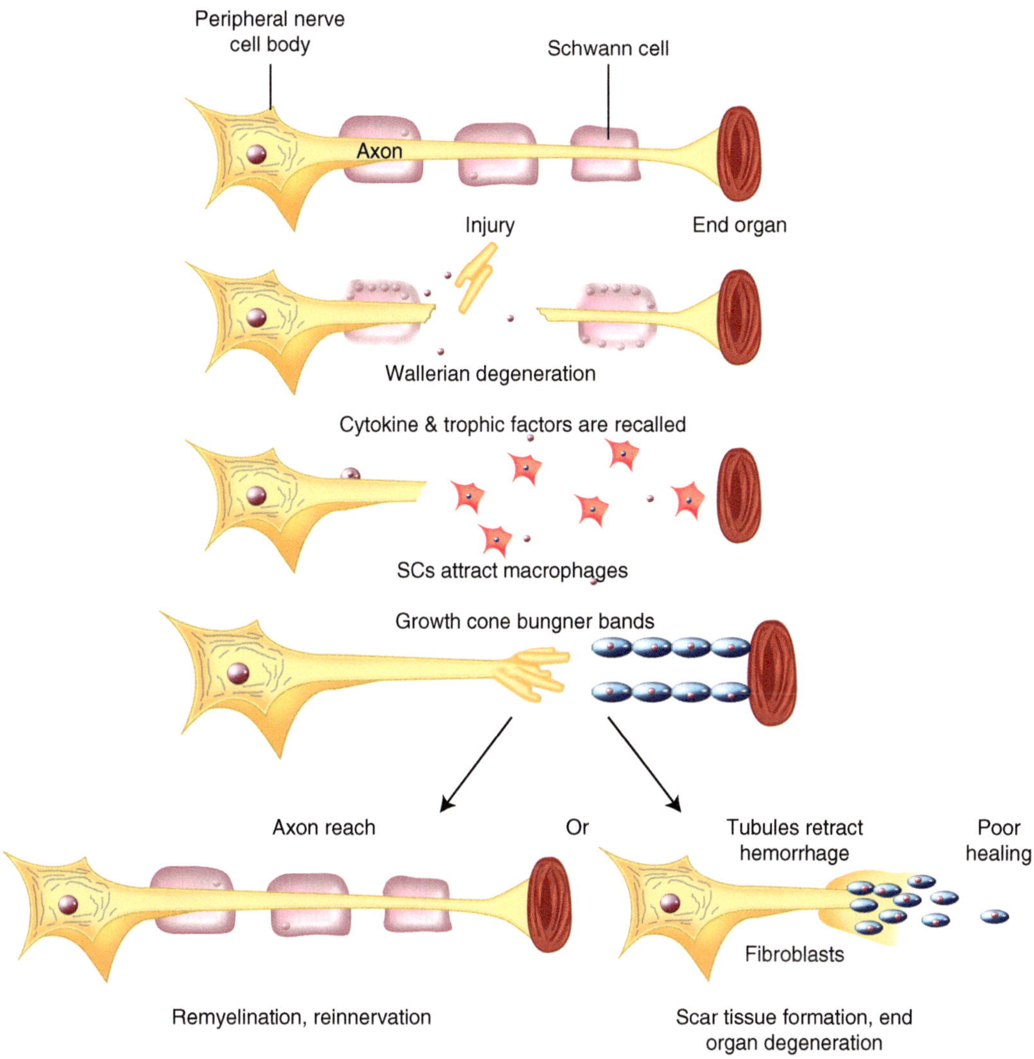

Fig. 4.2 Peripheral nerve injury consequences. After disruption of the nerve by injury, Wallerian degeneration begins, clearing the distal and (some of) the proximal axon through SCs and macrophages that are attracted by cytokines and trophic factors. The axon regeneration occurs through the formation of a growth cone. Growth cones unable to enter an endoneurial tube do not progress towards an end target and form a bulbous and often painful mass of scar tissue and swirling nerve fibers known as a neuroma

In response to cellular stress, factors released by damaged axons, or loss of trophic support from intact axons, SCs experience a rapid phenotype transformation into a very different cellular role orchestrating the clean-up and damage repair [10]. As the SCs enlarge and proliferate to shift towards a phagocytic state, released cytokines, interleukins, and chemotactic proteins attract circulating macrophages [11]. Histamine and serotonin released by incited endoneurial mast cells increase capillary wall permeability providing an avenue for macrophage migration into the zone of injury and along the degenerating axons [7]. The macrophages further promote SC activity by releasing additional communicative molecules [12]. Both SCs and macrophages phagocytize the cellular debris [13, 14] as the process clears the endoneurial tubes to accept regeneration axons. At the end of Wallerian degeneration, which may take several weeks, macrophages may remain for a longer period, die, or migrate to the lymphatic system [15, 16].

Greater levels of trauma disrupt deeper connective tissue layers including the endoneurium and even the perineurium. These layers have some elasticity and retract to create essentially an internal rupture, and the intraneural gap fills with hemorrhage and edema. The ensuing profound inflammatory response attracts infiltrating fibroblasts which proliferate and generate dense scar tissue [17]. The abundant bridging scar tissue creates a bulbous appearance to the nerve and is termed a neuroma-in-continuity. The inflammatory response extends beyond the nerve trunk resulting in gross perineural scarring as well. The more trauma, the more extensive the internal injury, tissue disruption, and fibrous response. The most severe insults stretch the last intact layer (the outer epineurium) to failure, tearing the nerve into two separate pieces though the tissue trauma still extends many centimeters from the point of failure often resulting in a large zone of injury. In these types of neurotemetic injuries, internal derangement, hemorrhage, and fibroblast-induced scarring can render large areas incapable of supporting axon regeneration.

Nerve Recovery

Neuropraxic injuries can recover within minutes to months depending on the damage. Local metabolic disruption can recover as soon as the insult is removed or as soon as intraneural swelling and ecchymosis resolve. Demyelination also can spontaneously resolve, and once SC function has stabilized, myelinating SCs will segmentally entubulate and wrap axons to restore physiological insulation and saltatory conduction. Reformed myelin sheaths have an immature quality with thinner and shorter segments (more Nodes of Ranvier per unit length) so that conduction velocity typically does not quite return to normal [18]. Within minutes of transection and well before the completion of Wallerian degeneration, neurons start downregulating maintenance genes (neurotransmitter production decreases, neurofilaments necessary to sustain axonal diameter decrease) and upregulating pro-regenerative genes [19]. Production of proteins (such as tubulin and actin) and lipids increases in preparation for cell repair [20]. This neuron phenotype shift is in part stimulated by withdrawal of end target-derived trophic factors (normally retrograde transported to the neuron cell body) [21] as well as SC and macrophage-derived neurotrophic factors and cytokines and is marked by the formation of a growth cone. The growth cone may be stimulated by the calcium influx seen immediately after injury and is formed by newly generated cytoskeleton and microtubules that fill the advancing cone. Stable microtubules aligned in parallel bundles serve as tracks for organelle transport (laminins or extracellular matrix proteins) to support the growing axon. This essential supply chain carrying building materials from the neuron cell body to the elongating tip is one reason for the clinically slow regeneration rates in human patients [22].

SCs shift from a phagocytic to a regenerative support role and, in addition to releasing neuron-stimulating neurotrophic factors, form longitudinal columns within the endoneurial space. These rows of SCs, referred to as Bands of Büngner, deposit channels of basal lamina inset with adhesion molecules such as (but not limited to) laminin that forms the essential guidance tracts for regenerating axons [23, 24]. Laminin is a glycoprotein attached to type IV collagen, proteoglycans, and entactin within the basal lamina. As the basal lamina becomes thicker, the endoneurial lumen becomes more narrow [25], and late in the Wallerian process, many endoneurial tubes appear to have collapsed [7].

Drawn by the neurotrophic factors, multiple small finger-like filopodia project from the growth cone to search the local microenvironment for these guidance cues within the basal lamina [26, 27]. Each axon tip still generates multiple exploratory axon branches though as these branches reach significant interference or enter tracts lacking neurotrophic support, they prune back. The remaining branches progress, and the narrowed endoneurial tubes expand to allow their passage [7]. Coincident neovascularization of the injury site is stimulated by vascular endothelial growth factor (VEGF) [28] and is necessary to rebuild the damaged circulatory network and meet the metabolic demands of the regenerating tissue.

For pure axonotmetic injuries in which the majority of endoneurial tubes are intact, the stimuli for axonal elongation are enough and the axons merely follow the intact pathways towards appropriate targets. Not all axons need to regenerate for normal or near normal recovery as regenerating axons can reinnervate (at least in animal models) up to five times the original number of muscle fibers [29]. With increasing levels of trauma, however, internal guidance is lost, and relative to the injury, axonal impeding scar tissue will have formed. Though SCs and growth cones release proteases and plasminogen activators and can grow through some scar tissue [30, 31], this effect is limited, and the interruption of defined pathways necessitates some level of neuron guidance if the axons are to reach any, and even more challenging – the correct, target. The greater the disruption, the more obstacles to accurate axonal regeneration and the slower and less likely meaningful end target reinnervation. Patient-specific differences (such as age) and the distance from the nerve cell body are also factors affecting nerve regeneration rates (proximal injuries regenerate faster than distal injuries).

Axonal guidance is one of the more controversial topics of nerve regeneration and may be best appreciated by differentiating neurotrophism (or nerve growth stimulation) from neurotropism (or nerve growth guidance) and from end-organ specificity (the tendency for a neuron type to grow towards the appropriately matched target) (Fig. 4.3).

Neurons are stimulated to form growth cones and to elongate by neurotrophic factors. Axons are directed and encouraged to elongate along a specific course by guidance cues such as the laminin and fibronectin within the SC basal lamina (neurotropism). At the same time, aberrant axonal growth is discouraged with growth inhibitors such as chondroitin sulfate proteoglycans [32]. SCs may also be target or end-organ specific – motor axons are supported by motor SCs and sensory axons are supported by sensory SCs (though experimental manipulation of this relationship has confirmed the ability of SCs to adapt their phenotypes to either axon source) [33]. Differences in SC generated guidance cues, and neurotrophic factors may direct axons towards specific targets. This theory is supported by the

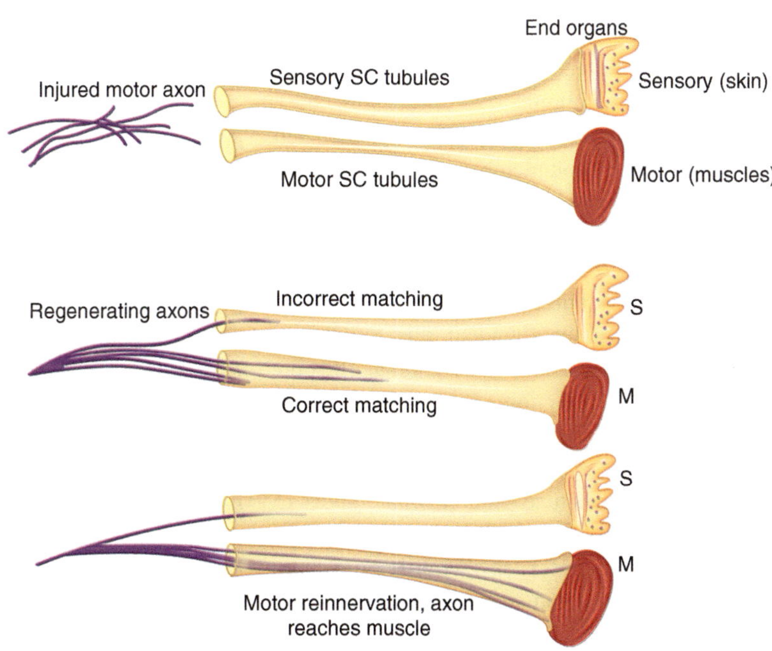

Fig. 4.3 The axonal guidance process. Branches of regenerating motor axons seem to have a preference for motor endoneurial tubes but can enter correct (motor) and incorrect (sensory) endoneurial tubes. Once correct end target contact is established, misdirected branches prune back

observation that sensory and motor neurons express distinct receptors [34] and end-organ-specific proteins have been demonstrated in motor versus sensory nerve basal lamina [35]. However, mismatching grafts (sensory nerve graft for motor regeneration) do not affect regeneration, somewhat diminishing the clinical importance of these biological distinctions [36].

Some researchers believe that motor neurons demonstrate more innate end-organ specificity than sensory nerve fibers [37]. This effect, termed preferential motor regeneration, has been demonstrated in animal studies. In a rodent model in which corresponding dorsal root ganglia were excised (eliminating any competing regenerating sensory axons), more motor axons regenerated down motor nerve paths than sensory nerve paths. Additionally, the axons regenerating into sensory pathways had greater collateralization suggesting an exploratory effort – as if the axons detected that they were on the wrong path and were trying to identify the correct path. The number of collaterals decreased, however, once correct end target contact was established (but not with "incorrect" contact and not when contact was prevented by transecting distal nerve tracts) [38]. This suggests that there are two phases to preferential motor reinnervation. Initially, pathway interactions draw more motor axons into motor tracts, and later, muscle contact must provide a retrograde feedback signal to promote further motor regeneration.

If enough intraneural disruption has occurred or if the nerve has completely ruptured, no meaningful spontaneous axonal regeneration can occur. Untreated, the undirected axons swirl around themselves and become entangled in the scar tissue in a bulbous neuroma. The distal stump also generates abundant scar tissue but, lacking axons, is referred to as a glioma. The purpose of surgical resection of damaged, scarred, and neuromatous tissue and surgical nerve repair is to remove the obstacles to axonal elongation and present opportune endoneurial tubes to receive and guide elongating axons. One key factor to functional recovery is obviously how many axons traverse the remaining (intraneural) gap and enter target matched tubes.

Reinnervation

Once meaningful contact is achieved with a motor target or sensory organelle, the neuron and SCs both go through another transition. The neurotrophins are downregulated (unnecessary axon branches are resorbed) though contact with an appropriate end target is not adequate for functional recovery, and the axon and its myelination must go through a maturation process of varying temporal length. The axon thickens, and myelinating SCs wrap around the axons to entubulate and form segments of myelin initially indicative of immature myelination. The SCs enter a maintenance state to support normal nerve function. Sensory organelle reinnervation seems to be more specific than motor reinnervation [37], and, while it is difficult to tell if a sensory organelle has been innervated by the wrong sensory axon, cortical remodeling will typically allow reestablishment of muscle function regardless of initial motor neuron-muscle circuitry.

Temporal Degradation of the Healing Process

Inadequate axonal guidance and other impedances to regeneration aside, time is the most significant factor in realizing functional sensory or motor reinnervation. Several researchers have offered convincing evidence that there is a temporal waning of axonal regeneration from the proximal stump, a loss of neurotrophic support within the distal nerve stump, and a loss of reinnervation potential in both chronically denervated muscle and sensory organelles. In rodent models, the number of regenerating axons begins to decrease after a 2-month repair delay with a precipitous drop by 6 months [39]. With chronic denervation of the distal stump, endoneurial tubes contract and suffer an accumulation of axon-inhibiting chondroitin sulfate proteoglycans [40]. Neurotrophic levels drop [41], and guidance cues degenerate until eventually, the bands of Büngner disappear [22, 42] possibly most likely in response to a degradation of SC function. With prolonged loss of axon contact, SCs enter a senescent state of inactivity. In this permanent state, SCs fail to proliferate and cease expressing pro-regenerative cytokines and neurotrophic factors [43] – they do not support axon regeneration. However, the mechanism of failed motor recovery is more complex, and in chronic denervation models, axons may regenerate to the muscle fibers but not form synapses [44].

Denervated muscles undergo a rapid and progressive atrophic process marked by loss of muscle mass, muscle fiber cross-sectional area (CSA), force generation, and stamina. Depending on the muscle and species, this loss of muscle mass (40% at 3 months [45], 50% at 1 month [46], 66% at 5 weeks [47]) and fiber CSA (76% at 5 weeks [47], 75% at 4 weeks [46]) can be quite substantial. A corollary loss of contraction strength is well recognized, and stimuli only produce 25% or less normal muscle contraction force within 3 months of denervation in small animal models [46, 48]. Human muscle experiences an approximately 50% loss of muscle fiber CSA within 2 to 3 months [49] though maximal contraction force of human denervated muscles has not been measured.

Muscle fibers function as a syncytium of fused nucleated cells [50]. With "denervation atrophy" these multinucleated muscle fibers lose size, nuclei, and contractile proteins [29, 51, 52]. Initially, a pool of reparative myoblast-like satellite cells (residing beneath the muscle basal lamina) are upregulated – proliferating, fusing into, and bolstering the shrinking muscle fibers [53–57]. While these mechanisms can temporarily maintain recovery potential, negative muscle changes become more pronounced with time, and consequently the longer a muscle takes to reinnervate, the poorer the final motor recovery [53, 58]. Though a complete physiologic explanation as to why this preservation process degrades with time is lacking, theories include irreversible changes to intracellular proteins and an eventual exhaustion of the satellite cell pool [29, 53, 58]. With "end-stage" denervation atrophy, the muscle fibers necrose and fragment, and the muscle tissue is completely replaced with fibrotic adipose tissue. The relative role of loss of neural stimulation versus the loss of trophic factors (from axonal interaction) in reaching this stage remains controversial [59].

Unlike muscle, sensory organelles such as the Meissner corpuscle can persist for years or degenerate and blend with surrounding dermal tissue. For instance, 40 percent of corpuscles remained after toe transplantation compared to normal toe pulp [60]. In general, sensory reinnervation is more difficult to analyze, and histologic findings do not necessarily correlate with exam findings [61].

Summary

The inconsistent and generally suboptimal clinical outcomes following major peripheral nerve and brachial plexus injuries are reflective of the biological challenges of axon regeneration. When axon regeneration is not necessary (as in neuropraxia), results are favorable, and when controlled axonal regeneration (axonotometic injuries with intact endoneurial tubes) is possible, at least some functional recovery can be expected. As the severity of the intraneural connective tissue disruption increases, however, fibroblast-induced scarring, endoneurial tube separation, and lack of intact guidance channels all compromise nerve recovery. Neurotrophic stimulation typically evokes a strong healing attempt. However, though well described, the innate ability of the body to direct axon elongation towards an appropriate (and correct) target is more limited. This mismatch between neuron regeneration and the ability of axons to traverse the zone of injury often results in neuromatous changes along the nerve or at the end of nerve stumps associated with full-thickness nerve rupture. Compounded by temporal related degradation of the robustness of axonal regeneration, the ability of distal nerve stumps to support regeneration, and the resilience of target end organs, the obstacles to functional recovery are often not overcome and certainly not without surgical intervention.

References

1. Spaeth CS, Boydston EA, Figard LR, Zuzek A, Bittner GD. A model for sealing plasmalemmal damage in neurons and other eukaryotic cells. J Neurosci. 2010;30(47):15790–800.
2. Watson WE. Observations on the nucleolar and total cell body nucleic acid of injured nerve cells. J Physiol. 1968;196(3):655–76.
3. Lundborg G. A 25-year perspective of peripheral nerve surgery: evolving neuroscientific concepts and clinical significance. J Hand Surg Am. 2000;25(3):391–414.
4. Dodge ME, Wang J, Guy C, Rankin S, Rahimtula M, Mearow KM. Stress-induced heat shock protein 27 expression and its role in dorsal root ganglion neuronal survival. Brain Res. 2006;1068(1):34–48.
5. Yan Q, Elliott J, Snider WD. Brain-derived neurotrophic factor rescues spinal motor neurons from axotomy-induced cell death. Nature. 1992;360(6406):753–5.
6. Yin Q, Kemp GJ, Frostick SP. Neurotrophins, neurones and peripheral nerve regeneration. J Hand Surg Br. 1998;23(4):433–7.
7. Burnett MG, Zager EL. Pathophysiology of peripheral nerve injury: a brief review. Neurosurg Focus. 2004;16(5):E1.
8. George EB, Glass JD, Griffin JW. Axotomy-induced axonal degeneration is mediated by calcium influx through ion-specific channels. J Neurosci. 1995;15(10):6445–52.
9. Adalbert R, Morreale G, Paizs M, Conforti L, Walker SA, Roderick HL, et al. Intra-axonal calcium changes after axotomy in wild-type and slow Wallerian degeneration axons. Neuroscience. 2012;225:44–54.
10. Scheib J, Hoke A. Advances in peripheral nerve regeneration. Nat Rev Neurol. 2013;9(12):668–76.
11. Mirsky R, Woodhoo A, Parkinson DB, Arthur-Farraj P, Bhaskaran A, Jessen KR. Novel signals controlling embryonic Schwann cell development, myelination and dedifferentiation. J Peripher Nerv Syst. 2008;13(2):122–35.
12. Shamash S, Reichert F, Rotshenker S. The cytokine network of Wallerian degeneration: tumor necrosis factor-alpha, interleukin-1alpha, and interleukin-1beta. J Neurosci. 2002;22(8):3052–60.
13. Goodrum JF, Earnhardt T, Goines N, Bouldin TW. Fate of myelin lipids during degeneration and regeneration of peripheral nerve: an autoradiographic study. J Neurosci. 1994;14(1):357–67.
14. Stoll G, Griffin JW, Li CY, Trapp BD. Wallerian degeneration in the peripheral nervous system: participation of both Schwann cells and macrophages in myelin degradation. J Neurocytol. 1989;18(5):671–83.
15. Gaudet AD, Popovich PG, Ramer MS. Wallerian degeneration: gaining perspective on inflammatory events after peripheral nerve injury. J Neuroinflammation. 2011;8:110.
16. Kuhlmann T, Bitsch A, Stadelmann C, Siebert H, Bruck W. Macrophages are eliminated from the injured peripheral nerve via local apoptosis and circulation to regional lymph nodes and the spleen. J Neurosci. 2001;21(10):3401–8.
17. Richard L, Topilko P, Magy L, Decouvelaere AV, Charnay P, Funalot B, et al. Endoneurial fibroblast-like cells. J Neuropathol Exp Neurol. 2012;71(11):938–47.
18. Schroder JM. Altered ratio between axon diameter and myelin sheath thickness in regenerated nerve fibers. Brain Res. 1972;45(1):49–65.
19. Holahan MRA. Shift from a pivotal to supporting role for the growth-associated protein (GAP-43) in the coordination of axonal structural and functional plasticity. Front Cell Neurosci. 2017;11:266.
20. Tetzlaff W, Alexander SW, Miller FD, Bisby MA. Response of facial and rubrospinal neurons to axotomy: changes in mRNA expression for cytoskeletal proteins and GAP-43. J Neurosci. 1991;11(8):2528–44.
21. Slack JR, Hopkins WG, Pockett S. Evidence for a motor nerve growth factor. Muscle Nerve. 1983;6(4):243–52.
22. Hoke A. Mechanisms of disease: what factors limit the success of peripheral nerve regeneration in humans? Nat Clin Pract Neurol. 2006;2(8):448–54.
23. Araki T, Milbrandt J. Ninjurin, a novel adhesion molecule, is induced by nerve injury and promotes axonal growth. Neuron. 1996;17(2):353–61.
24. Bunge RP, Bunge MB, Eldridge CF. Linkage between axonal ensheathment and basal lamina production by Schwann cells. Annu Rev Neurosci. 1986;9:305–28.
25. Sunderland S, Bradley KC. Endoneurial tube shrinkage in the distal segment of a severed nerve. J Comp Neurol. 1950;93(3):411–20.
26. Dodd J, Jessell TM. Axon guidance and the patterning of neuronal projections in vertebrates. Science. 1988;242(4879):692–9.
27. Gundersen RW, Barrett JN. Characterization of the turning response of dorsal root neurites toward nerve growth factor. J Cell Biol. 1980;87(3 Pt 1):546–54.
28. Hobson MI, Green CJ, Terenghi G. VEGF enhances intraneural angiogenesis and improves nerve regeneration after axotomy. J Anat. 2000;197(Pt 4):591–605.
29. Fu SY, Gordon T. Contributing factors to poor functional recovery after delayed nerve repair: prolonged denervation. J Neurosci. 1995;15(5 Pt 2):3886–95.
30. Akassoglou K, Kombrinck KW, Degen JL, Strickland S. Tissue plasminogen activator-mediated fibrinolysis protects against axonal degeneration and demyelination after sciatic nerve injury. J Cell Biol. 2000;149(5):1157–66.
31. Pittman RN. Release of plasminogen activator and a calcium-dependent metalloprotease from cultured sympathetic and sensory neurons. Dev Biol. 1985;110(1):91–101.
32. Joshi AR, Bobylev I, Zhang G, Sheikh KA, Lehmann HC. Inhibition of rho-kinase differentially affects axon regeneration of peripheral motor and sensory nerves. Exp Neurol. 2015;263:28–38.
33. Hoke A, Redett R, Hameed H, Jari R, Zhou C, Li ZB, et al. Schwann cells express motor and sensory phe-

notypes that regulate axon regeneration. J Neurosci. 2006;26(38):9646–55.
34. Boyd JG, Gordon T. Neurotrophic factors and their receptors in axonal regeneration and functional recovery after peripheral nerve injury. Mol Neurobiol. 2003;27(3):277–324.
35. Nichols CM, Brenner MJ, Fox IK, Tung TH, Hunter DA, Rickman SR, et al. Effects of motor versus sensory nerve grafts on peripheral nerve regeneration. Exp Neurol. 2004;190(2):347–55.
36. Kawamura DH, Johnson PJ, Moore AM, Magill CK, Hunter DA, Ray WZ, et al. Matching of motor-sensory modality in the rodent femoral nerve model shows no enhanced effect on peripheral nerve regeneration. Exp Neurol. 2010;223(2):496–504.
37. Brushart TM. Motor axons preferentially reinnervate motor pathways. J Neurosci. 1993;13(6):2730–8.
38. Redett R, Jari R, Crawford T, Chen YG, Rohde C, Brushart TM. Peripheral pathways regulate motoneuron collateral dynamics. J Neurosci. 2005;25(41):9406–12.
39. Sulaiman OA, Gordon T. Effects of short- and long-term Schwann cell denervation on peripheral nerve regeneration, myelination, and size. Glia. 2000;32(3):234–46.
40. Zuo J, Hernandez YJ, Muir D. Chondroitin sulfate proteoglycan with neurite-inhibiting activity is up-regulated following peripheral nerve injury. J Neurobiol. 1998;34(1):41–54.
41. Hoke A, Gordon T, Zochodne DW, Sulaiman OA. A decline in glial cell-line-derived neurotrophic factor expression is associated with impaired regeneration after long-term Schwann cell denervation. Exp Neurol. 2002;173(1):77–85.
42. Ide C. Peripheral nerve regeneration. Neurosci Res. 1996;25(2):101–21.
43. Saheb-Al-Zamani M, Yan Y, Farber SJ, Hunter DA, Newton P, Wood MD, et al. Limited regeneration in long acellular nerve allografts is associated with increased Schwann cell senescence. Exp Neurol. 2013;247C:165–77.
44. Ma CH, Omura T, Cobos EJ, Latremoliere A, Ghasemlou N, Brenner GJ, et al. Accelerating axonal growth promotes motor recovery after peripheral nerve injury in mice. J Clin Invest. 2011;121(11):4332–47.
45. Ashley Z, Sutherland H, Lanmuller H, Russold MF, Unger E, Bijak M, et al. Atrophy, but not necrosis, in rabbit skeletal muscle denervated for periods up to one year. Am J Physiol Cell Physiol. 2007;292(1):C440–51.
46. Willand MP, Lopez JP, de Bruin H, Fahnestock M, Holmes M, New System BJRA. Paradigm for chronic stimulation of Denervated rat muscle. J Med Biol Eng. 2011;31(2):87–92.
47. Dow DE, Cederna PS, Hassett CA, Kostrominova TY, Faulkner JA, Dennis RG. Number of contractions to maintain mass and force of a denervated rat muscle. Muscle Nerve. 2004;30(1):77–86.
48. Ashley Z, Salmons S, Boncompagni S, Protasi F, Russold M, Lanmuller H, et al. Effects of chronic electrical stimulation on long-term denervated muscles of the rabbit hind limb. J Muscle Res Cell Motil. 2007;28(4–5):203–17.
49. Aird RB, Naffziger HC. The pathology of human striated muscle following denervation. J Neurosurg. 1953;10(3):216–27.
50. Wozniak AC, Kong J, Bock E, Pilipowicz O, Anderson JE. Signaling satellite-cell activation in skeletal muscle: markers, models, stretch, and potential alternate pathways. Muscle Nerve. 2005;31(3):283–300.
51. Lien SC, Cederna PS, Kuzon WM Jr. Optimizing skeletal muscle reinnervation with nerve transfer. Hand Clin. 2008;24(4):445–54. vii
52. Cederna PS, Youssef MK, Asato H, Urbanchek MG, Kuzon WM Jr. Skeletal muscle reinnervation by reduced axonal numbers results in whole muscle force deficits. Plast Reconstr Surg. 2000;105(6):2003–9. discussion 10-1
53. Anzil AP, Wernig A. Muscle fibre loss and reinnervation after long-term denervation. J Neurocytol. 1989;18(6):833–45.
54. Ontell M. Muscle satellite cells: a validated technique for light microscopic identification and a quantitative study of changes in their population following denervation. Anat Rec. 1974;178(2):211–27.
55. Schultz E. Changes in the satellite cells of growing muscle following denervation. Anat Rec. 1978;190(2):299–311.
56. Moss F, LeBlond C. Satellite cells as a source of nuclei in muscles of growing rats. Anat Rec. 1971;170:421–36.
57. Hill M, Wernig A, Goldspink G. Muscle satellite (stem) cell activation during local tissue injury and repair. J Anat. 2003;203(1):89–99.
58. Kobayashi J, Mackinnon SE, Watanabe O, Ball DJ, Gu XM, Hunter DA, et al. The effect of duration of muscle denervation on functional recovery in the rat model. Muscle Nerve. 1997;20(7):858–66.
59. Gulati AK. Restoration of denervated skeletal muscle transplants after reinnervation in rats. Restor Neurol Neurosci. 1990;2(1):23–9.
60. Wei FC, Carver N, Lee YH, Chuang DC, Cheng SL. Sensory recovery and Meissner corpuscle number after toe-to-hand transplantation. Plast Reconstr Surg. 2000;105(7):2405–11.
61. Jabaley ME, Burns JE, Orcutt BS, Bryant M. Comparison of histologic and functional recovery after peripheral nerve repair. J Hand Surg Am. 1976;1(2):119–30.

Epidemiology of Adult Traumatic Brachial Plexus Injuries

5

Juan Manuel Breyer, Pamela Vergara, and Alfonso Perez

Adult traumatic brachial plexus injuries (BPI) are devastating lesions. These injuries both significantly affect function and daily living activities and also have a substantial social, economic, and psychological impact, creating lifelong disabilities. Epidemiological studies of traumatic BPI are critical for addressing the magnitude of the problem, determining the characteristics of the affected individuals in order to create prevention plans, and adequately allocating healthcare resources to treat and rehabilitate BPI patients. Unfortunately, there is a lack of epidemiological studies in this area, and the few studies are mainly focused on treatment and prognosis.

Although the true incidence of traumatic BPI is uncertain [1–3], there is concern that these complex injuries are increasing in frequency. This is partially due to high-speed motor vehicle accidents being more commonly observed, especially in urban areas. Fortunately, traumatic BPI are still uncommon. Even though the available literature about incidence is based on estimates, they are as uncommon as complex neurologic injuries. For example, BPI are 9 times less frequent than spinal cord injuries and almost 30 times less frequent than brain injuries [3]. The varying rates of BPI incidence in the general population have been described, based on the country or area studied. The estimated annual incidence of BPI in the general population lies between 0.17/100,000/year in Japan [4] and 1.6/100,000/year in the United States [5], with intermediate rates being reported worldwide: for example, Switzerland, 0.3–0.75 [6]; Czech Republic, 0.2 [7]; United Kingdom, 0.2 [8]; Serbia, 1.0 [9]; and Brazil, 1.5 [10].

When specific groups are studied, traumatic BPI have a significant relevance, representing 4.2–5% of injuries in the multitrauma setting. Snowmobiling and other high-risk and high-speed sports (i.e., skiing or snowboarding) account for 3–4.8% of injuries [3].

It is unquestionable that traumatic BPI represents a significant economic burden for patients and for health systems. Compared to other peripheral nerve injuries (PNI), traumatic BPI are the most care-consuming peripheral nerve injuries of the upper extremity [11], with higher direct treatment costs and inpatient lengths of stay. Furthermore, the costs of hospital treatment for upper extremity PNI and BPI have dramatically increased in the United States between 1993 and 2013 [1, 2]. The average nominal cost of

J. M. Breyer (✉)
Orthopedic Surgery – Hand Surgery Unit, Hospital del Trabajador, Santiago, RM, Chile

Orthopedic Surgery – Hand Surgery Unit, Clinica Alemana de Santiago, Santiago, RM, Chile

P. Vergara · A. Perez
Orthopedic Surgery – Hand Surgery Unit, Hospital del Trabajador, Santiago, RM, Chile

Orthopedic Surgery – Hand Surgery Unit, Clinica Las Condes, Santiago, RM, Chile

A. Y. Shin, N. Pulos (eds.), *Operative Brachial Plexus Surgery*,
https://doi.org/10.1007/978-3-030-69517-0_5

treatment for PNI and BPI increased from $10,000 to $15,000 per case to $20,000 to $30,000 per case, respectively [1].

There is limited information about the indirect cost from the patients' perspectives; however, Hong et al. estimated the indirect cost (sum of short-term and long-term wage losses plus disability payments). Given that the majority of patients in the United States with BPI are young, male, manual workers (mean 26 years, with a mean annual wage of $36,590 for year 2018), they estimated a median indirect cost of $801,723 during productive lifetime [12].

Patients

Narakas, in his seminal 1985 paper, described the demographics and etiology of traumatic BPI. As he noted, these injuries occur predominantly in young male patients in the context of road traffic accidents [6]. The male predominance was consistently repeated in subsequent studies [13–16]. A recent systematic review and meta-analysis by Kaiser et al. included ten studies conducted in eight countries (3032 patients) which described a pooled male prevalence of 93% with a male/female ratio of 13.3:1 [4]. The same meta-analysis showed traumatic BPI affecting mainly young patients, with a pooled mean age of 28.9 years (studies ranging from 23 to 34 years). Jain et al. studied 304 surgically treated patients in India, finding a mean age of 24, with nearly 45% of patients between 21 and 30 years old and 25% between 31 and 40 years old [17]. Another large case series of 406 surgically treated BPI in Brazil reported an average age of 28.4 years (range 9–67) [13]. These observations are comparable to the results of Li et al. in China (mean age 29, range 1–73) [16] and Songcharoen et al. in Thailand (mean age 23, range 2–53) [14].

There is no information explaining the marked tendency of BPI occurrence in younger male patients; however, it is likely due to increased exposure to risky behaviors culminating in road traffic accidents. In contrast, female patients are less frequently involved in both road traffic accidents in general and motorcycle accidents specifically [18]. In the latter, females show a more consistent helmet use, and alcohol intoxication is less common than in male patients [19]. All of these contexts provide additional explanations for the gender and age differences.

Associated Injuries

Traumatic BPI frequently occurs in polytraumatic contexts; thus they have a high frequency of associated injuries, ranging from 54% to 70% of patients [3, 17, 20]. Closed head injuries are the most common associated injuries (25–70%), ranging from minor concussions to coma (up to 19%). Concomitant spine fractures have been described for 5–68% of BPI patients, with cervical spine fractures being the most common. Combined traumatic BPI and spine cord injuries have been documented in 2–12.5% [3, 21] of patients. Upper limb fractures are frequently reported (17–55%), as well as lower limb fractures (19–33%). Other important associated injuries include thoracic cavity injury (pneumothorax, pulmonary contusions, and rib fractures) in 36–52% of patients, shoulder girdle injury (10–52%), and upper extremity vascular injuries (5–19%) [3, 17, 20, 21].

Psychosocial Impact of Brachial Plexus Injuries

Despite significant advances in the surgical treatment of traumatic BPI over the past two decades, this type of injury can lead to a severe and permanent upper extremity dysfunction. These patients report significantly worse outcomes in quality of life and related outcomes than the normal population, across physical, psychological, social, and environmental domains of quality of life questionnaires [22].

Pain is a common and debilitating problem for patients with traumatic BPI. Ciaramitaro et al. reported 77% of BPI patients with high levels of pain, with 90% of them describing neuropathic pain. This correlated with higher depression levels (Beck depression inventory) and low quality of life (Short form-36) [23]. These devastating injuries also affect patients in terms of financial status, employment, independence with daily living, body image, and psychological distress [24]. As a result, patients have high prevalence of post-traumatic stress disorder (19%) and depression (19%). Significantly, one-third of patients have experienced suicidal ideation [25].

Etiology

Closed Injuries

The leading cause of BPI is closed trauma in more than 90% of cases [4, 6, 26], with reports ranging from 72.9% [15] to 99.3% [17]. This variability in the reported prevalence of closed BPI can be explained by the studied populations, their geographical conditions, the center where patients were treated, or series, including operative and non-operative treated patients. For example, Kim et al. in their series of 1019 surgically treated patients (30-year period) in Louisiana, USA, described the lower rate of 72.9% of closed BPI, probably due to the high rate of gunshot wounds (GSW) found in this series (16.9%) [15], an uncommon finding compared to other series [4].

The main etiology of closed BPI is road traffic accidents. Already in 1985, Narakas (Switzerland) described in his series of 1068 patients a 70% of BPI related to road traffic accidents, with 70% of them as a result of motorcycle or bicycle accidents [6] (Table 5.1). Even though Narakas's classic work and his 70s rules are still considered valid today, newer studies suggest that the proportion of closed BPI related to road traffic accidents might be increasing. Kaiser's meta-analysis reported 81% of BPI cases as related to road traffic accidents (67% motorcycles, 14% cars) [4], with most of studies ranging from 60% to 91% [7, 9, 14, 17]. Mirroring this meta-analysis, motorcycles are the main cause involved among road traffic accidents, ranging from 46% to 82% [13, 14, 16]. It is important to note that a low rate of 22% of BPI has been described related to motorcycle accidents (Midha et al., Canada). This low rate is likely due to characteristics of the studied population, those of the Multitrauma Center, and the relatively low number of motorcycles in Toronto [3].

Table 5.1 Law of the Seven Seventies of Narakas [6]

70% of brachial plexus injuries are caused by traffic accidents
70% of traffic accidents are associated with motorcycles or bicycles
70% of these patients have multiple lesions
70% have supraclavicular injuries
70% of these cases will have at least one avulsion
70% of patients with avulsions will have commitment to the lower trunk
70% of avulsion patients will have persistent pain

Other less common causes (less than 10%) include fall from a height, pedestrians versus motor vehicle accidents, sports-related injury, traction by machinery, and fall of heavy object on shoulder [7, 14, 17]. Sports-related BPI have been described in contact sports (i.e., American football or rugby) and during recreational activities like snowmobiling. A specific brachial plexus injury has been described during these activities, termed "stingers" or "burners." These injuries are supposed to be a type of neuropraxia of the cervical roots or a transient brachial plexopathy. Among football players, the incidence of stingers during one season is estimated to be 26% [27] with a prevalence of 62%. There is a wide spectrum of presentations, and it is probably underestimated, considering that only 59% of the episodes of stingers are reported [27], because most of them (63.8%) have spontaneous and full recovery in less than 24 hours [28]. Similarly, the incidence of stingers among rugby players during one season has been reported as high as 20.9%, with a prevalence of history of a previous stinger of 33.9% [29].

Another source of BPI comes from snowmobiling, which has become a popular winter sport in North America, and along with the more frequent use of snowmobiles are increases of related injuries. Each year, in North America, snowmobile accidents are responsible for approximately 200 deaths and 14,000 injuries [30]. BPI represent 3% of snowmobile-related injuries [31], causing 3 to 4.8% of all brachial plexus injuries in North America [3].

Open Injuries

Brachial plexus lacerations, gunshot wounds (GSW), or iatrogenic injuries are less commonly associated with BPI and represent only 3% of patients undergoing surgical repair, according to the meta-analysis of Kaiser et al. [4]. GSW rates show significant variability between series from different countries, which can be explained by cultural, historical, and geopolitical circumstances. GSW rates as low as 0.7%, 1%, and 2.7% have been reported in India [17], China [16], and Thailand [14], respectively, compared with rates of 11–25% reported in the USA [15], Canada [3], and Brazil [10].

Work-Related Injuries

There is limited information in the literature about the mechanism of work-related injury related to BPI. Our institution, Hospital del Trabajador (a worker's compensation hospital), Santiago, Chile, focuses on worker accidents and diseases, and more than 90% of our BPI are worker compensation-related cases. During a 10-year period (2009–2018), 145 BPI cases were treated, and after excluding road traffic accidents (62% of patients), the most frequent causes were traction injuries with machinery at 22% (belt line, rollers), falls at ground level at 20%, direct blows at 15% (falling construction materials, tree trunks, machine pistons, etc.), and falls from height at 18% (construction scaffolds, stairs).

Type of Injury

When considering the anatomic location, the most frequent traumatic BPI are supraclavicular. Although Narakas described 70% of BPI being supraclavicular injuries [6], more recent studies have shown an increase in this type of injury, with rates closer to 90% (range 78–98%) [4]. Infraclavicular injuries are both less frequent (10%) and also have a more favorable prognosis, with lower rates of patients requiring surgery [32–34].

With regard to the cervical roots of each type of injury, supraclavicular BPI usually have two types of pattern: partial or complete. Partial injuries usually affect the C5 and C6 or the C5, C6, and C7 roots; partial injuries affecting only C8 and/or T1 are rare. Complete refers to injuries affecting all five roots. Complete supraclavicular BPI lesions are the most complex injuries to treat, frequently with incomplete functional recovery of the upper extremity and associated with poor outcomes [6, 33, 35]. Injuries involving all five roots are unfortunately frequent; the meta-analysis of Kaiser et al. described supraclavicular lesions in 53% of BPI (reports ranged from 43% to 64%) [4, 14, 16].

Regarding incomplete supraclavicular BPI (45%), upper-middle trunk (C5, C6, and C7) involvement is seen in 86.7% of incomplete lesions. Isolated lower trunk is only present in 13.3% [4]. Li et al. detail 511 operatively treated BPI, with 78% involving the upper and middle trunk (34% upper trunk exclusively) and 22% involving the middle and lower trunk (6% isolated LT) [16].

Root avulsion represents the most severe type of injury, and since repair or grafting is impossible, the only alternative to restore distal nerve function is nerve transfer. The frequency of avulsed roots is difficult to establish, based on diagnostic method (i.e., CT myelography, MRI) or operative findings. Narakas described 70% of patients having at least one root avulsion (70% of avulsions were lower trunk). Later studies have found ranges between 66% and 89% [14, 17]. The predilection of avulsions for lower trunk could be explained by the frail connective tissue attachments of the lower roots to the transverse process, as compared to upper and middle trunk roots. Cases with all five roots avulsed represents the worst possible scenario for BPI patients, because there is no possible spontaneous recovery and there are only few available therapeutic options. This condition, according to the previously cited meta-analysis from Kaiser et al., was present in 26% of the patients with traumatic BPI [4].

Conclusion

Traumatic brachial plexus injuries occur more frequently in young male patients. Most are closed lesions caused by road traffic accidents (motorcycles) involving the supraclavicular plexus. Open lacerations and gunshot wounds are less common among civilian populations.

As BPI represent a significant burden for patients and health systems, more epidemiological studies are required to fully comprehend the characteristics of the affected patients in order to create prevention policies and to adequately assign healthcare resources.

References

1. Lad SP, Nathan JK, Schubert RD, Boakye M. Trends in median, ulnar, radial, and brachioplexus nerve injuries in the United States. Neurosurgery. 2010;66(5):953–60.
2. Karsy M, Watkins R, Jensen MR, Guan J, Brock AA, Mahan MA. Trends and cost analysis of upper extremity nerve injury using the national (Nationwide) inpatient sample. World Neurosurg. 2019;123:e488–500.
3. Midha R. Epidemiology of brachial plexus injuries in a multitrauma population. Neurosurgery. 1997;4(6):1182–9.
4. Kaiser R, Waldauf P, Ullas G, Krajcová A. Epidemiology, etiology, and types of severe adult brachial plexus injuries requiring surgical repair: systematic review and meta-analysis. Neurosurg Rev. 2018;1:1–10.
5. Tapp M, Wenzinger E, Tarabishy S, Ricci J, Herrera FA. The Epidemiology of Upper Extremity Nerve Injuries and Associated Cost in the US Emergency Departments. Ann Plast Surg. 2019;83(6):676–80.
6. Narakas AO. The treatment of brachial plexus injuries. Int Orthop. 1985;9(1):29–36.
7. Kaiser R, Waldauf P, Haninec P. Types and severity of operated supraclavicular brachial plexus injuries caused by traffic accidents. Acta Neurochir. 2012;154(7):1293–7.
8. Macdonald BK, Cockerell OC, Sander JWAS, Shorvon SD, Macdonald CBK, Registrar S. The incidence and lifetime prevalence of neurological disorders in a prospective community- based study in the UK. Brain. 2000;123(4):665–76.
9. Rasulić L, Simić V, Savić A, Lepić M, Kovačević V, Puzović V, et al. Management of brachial plexus missile injuries. Acta Clin Croat. 2018;57(3):487–96.
10. Flores LP. Estudo epidemiológico das lesões traumáticas de plexo braquial em adultos. Arq Neuropsiquiatr. 2006;64(1):88–94.
11. Asplund M, Nilsson M, Jacobsson A, Von Holst H. Incidence of traumatic peripheral nerve injuries and amputations in Sweden between 1998 and 2006. Neuroepidemiology. 2009;32(3):217–28.
12. Hong TS, Tian A, Sachar R, Ray WZ, Brogan DM, Dy CJ. Indirect cost of traumatic brachial plexus injuries in the United States. J Bone Jt Surg. 2019;101(16):e80.
13. Faglioni W, Siqueira MG, Martins RS, Heise CO, Foroni L. The epidemiology of adult traumatic brachial plexus lesions in a large metropolis. Acta Neurochir. 2014;156(5):1025–8.
14. Songcharoen P. Brachial plexus injury in thailand: a report of 520 cases. Microsurgery. 1995;16(1):35–9.
15. Kim DH, Cho Y-J, Tiel R, Kine D. Outcomes of surgery in 1019 brachial plexus lesions treated at Louisiana State University Health Sciences Center. J Neurosurg. 2003;98(5):1005–16.
16. Li G, Xue M, Wang J, Zeng X, Qin J, Sha K. Traumatic brachial plexus injury : a study of 510 surgical cases from multicenter services in Guangxi, China. Acta Neurochir (Wien). 2019;161:899–906.
17. Jain DKA, Bhardwaj P, Venkataramani H, Sabapathy SR. An epidemiological study of traumatic brachial plexus injury patients treated at an Indian Centre. Indian J Plast Surg. 2012;45(3):498–503.
18. Boughton O, Jones GG, Lavy CBD, Grimes CE. Young, male, road traffic victims : a systematic review of the published trauma registry literature from low and middle income countries. SICOT J. 2015;1:10.
19. Hsieh C, Hsu S, Hsieh H, Chen Y. Differences between the sexes in motorcycle-related injuries and fatalities at a Taiwanese level I trauma center. Biom J. 2017;40(2):113–20.
20. Kaiser R, Mencl L, Haninec P. Injuries associated with serious brachial plexus involvement in polytrauma among patients requiring surgical repair. Injury. 2014;45(1):223–6.
21. Rhee PC, Pirola E, Hebert-Blouin MN, Kircher MF, Spinner RJ, Bishop AT, et al. Concomitant traumatic spinal cord and brachial plexus injuries in adult patients. J Bone Jt Surg – Ser A. 2011;93(24):2271–7.
22. Shen J, Wang Z. The level and influencing factors of quality of life in patients with brachial plexus injury. Int J Nurs Sci. 2014;1(2):171–5.
23. Ciaramitaro P, Mondelli M, Logullo F, Grimaldi S, Battiston B, Sard A, et al. Traumatic peripheral nerve injuries: epidemiological findings, neuropathic pain and quality of life in 158 patients. J Peripher Nerv Syst. 2010;15(2):120–7.
24. Franzblau L, Chung KC. Psychosocial outcomes and coping after complete avulsion traumatic brachial plexus injury. Disabil Rehabil. 2015;37(2):135–43.
25. Landers ZA, Jethanandani R, Lee SK, Mancuso CA, Seehaus M, Wolfe SW. The Psychological Impact of Adult Traumatic Brachial Plexus Injury. J Hand Surg Am. 2018;43(10):950.e1–6.

26. Terzis JK, Papakonstantinou KC. Surgical treatment of brachial plexus injuries in adults. Plast Reconstr Surg. 2000;106(5):1097–122.
27. Charbonneau RME, Mcveigh SA, Thompson K. Brachial neuropraxia in canadian atlantic university sport football players: what is the incidence of " stingers "? Clin J Sport Med. 2012;22:472–7.
28. Green J, Zuckerman SL, Dalton SL, Djoko A, Folger D, Kerr ZY. A 6-year surveillance study of "Stingers" in NCAA American Football. Res Sport Med. 2017;25(1):26–36.
29. Kawasaki T, Ota C, Yoneda T, Maki N, Urayama S, Nagao M, et al. Incidence of stingers in young rugby players. Am J Sports Med. 2015;43(11):2809–15.
30. Pierz JJ. Snowmobile injuries in North America. Clin Orthop Relat Res. 2003;409:29–36.
31. Plog BA, Pierre CA, Srinivasan V, Srinivasan K, Petraglia AL, Huang JH. Neurologic injury in snowmobiling. Surg Neurol Int. 2014;5:87.
32. Hems TEJ, Mahmood F. Injuries of the terminal branches of the infraclavicular brachial plexus: patterns of injury, management and outcome. J Bone Jt Surg – Ser B. 2012;94 B(6):799–804.
33. Kline DG, Tiel RL. Direct plexus repair by grafts supplemented by nerve transfers. Hand Clin. 2005;21(1):55–69.
34. Bertelli JA, Ghizoni MF, Soldado F. Patterns of brachial plexus stretch palsy in. J Hand Surg Am. 2017;42(6):443–6.
35. Mazurek MT, Shin AY. Upper extremity peripheral nerve anatomy: current concepts and applications. Clin Orthop Relat Res. 2001;383:7–20.

Brachial Plexus-Associated Injuries

6

Lauren Dutton and Nicholas Pulos

Introduction

The majority of patients with brachial plexus injuries suffer multiple trauma [1–4]. The high-energy mechanisms of injury frequently lead to concomitant trauma to vascular and musculoskeletal structures. Traumatic brain injury (TBI), chest wall trauma, spine fractures and spinal cord trauma, damage to potential extraplexal nerves and full-thickness rotator cuff tears wall have all been described [5–9].

Surgeons must be knowledgeable about concomitant injuries for two reasons. First, in the acute period, heightened suspicion for and accurate diagnosis of associated injuries can improve the initial treatment and potentially save life or limb. Further, distracting injuries can make diagnosing a brachial plexus lesion difficult and lead to delays in treatment. Second, when time to plan for brachial plexus reconstruction arrives, failure to recognize associated injuries may interfere with the planned procedure or lead to difficulties with rehabilitation. This chapter reviews the available literature on trauma associated with brachial plexus injuries from a reconstructive surgeon's point of view.

L. Dutton
Naval Hospital Jacksonville, Jacksonville, FL, USA

N. Pulos (✉)
Department of Orthopedic Surgery, Mayo Clinic, Rochester, MN, USA
e-mail: Pulos.Nicholas@mayo.edu

Vascular Injury

The incidence of major vascular injury in patients with brachial plexus injuries has been reported to be between 10% and 28% [1, 2, 10, 11]. The incidence of these combined injuries depends on what the authors report as the primary insult or denominator. Subclavian or axillary vascular injuries occur in approximately 56% of patients with a brachial plexus injuries, while brachial plexus injuries occur in approximately 43% of patients with a subclavian or axillary vascular injury [12, 13]. While injury to the subclavian or axillary vessels is most common, other injured vessels include the internal carotid artery and brachial, radial and ulnar arteries. Combined injuries of the brachial plexus and major vasculature may occur either as a result of direct injury to both structures or compression of the brachial plexus by an expanding haematoma secondary to the vascular injury [14]. Prolonged ischemia of the limb can also cause permanent neurologic as well as muscular damage, so an early accurate diagnosis of concomitant vascular injury is paramount.

A distal pulse on physical exam does not preclude the presence of a concurrent vascular injury. The axillary artery has six branches, which may provide collateral circulation to the upper extremity. Therefore, a low threshold for conventional angiography should exist in patients with suspected vascular trauma. Later, MR

A. Y. Shin, N. Pulos (eds.), *Operative Brachial Plexus Surgery*,
https://doi.org/10.1007/978-3-030-69517-0_6

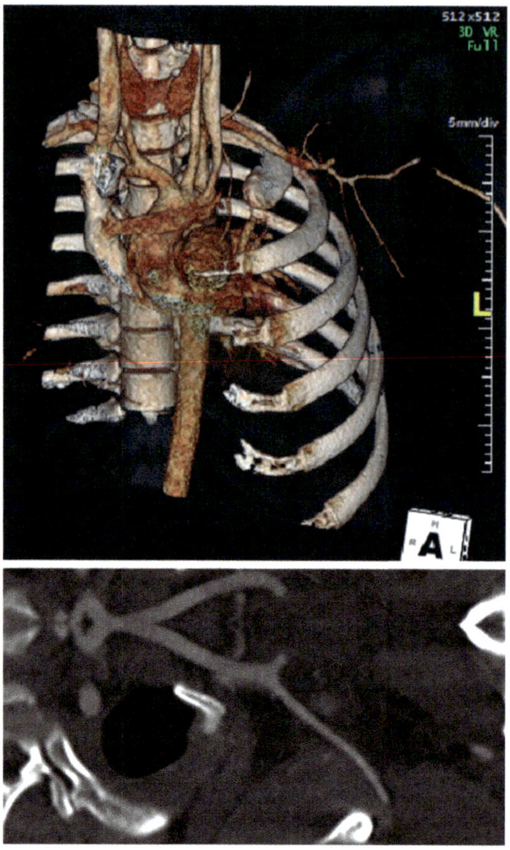

Fig. 6.1 Vascular injury. CT angiogram demonstrating occlusion of the distal segment of the left subclavian and proximal axillary artery at the level of the lateral edge of the second rib as well as multiple rib fractures in a 15-year-old patient who sustained a concomitant brachial plexus injury after a sledding accident. In addition to spinal accessory nerve transfer to the musculocutaneous nerve via sural nerve grafting, the patient also underwent reconstruction of the axillary artery

angiography or CT angiography may provide beneficial information regarding the patency of the subclavian artery, axillary artery and collateral circulation (Fig. 6.1). For patients undergoing reconstruction with a free functioning muscle, patency of the thoracoacromial trunk is assessed preoperatively with angiography to determine its suitability as a donor vessel [15, 16].

During the initial resuscitation, consultation with a vascular surgeon should be obtained to prevent prolonged ischemia time. Combined vascular and brachial plexus injuries may occur in the presence or absence of concomitant osseous injury. Following blunt trauma, many of these injuries have been associated with glenohumeral dislocations and proximal humerus fractures [17]. This may necessitate temporary shunting and fracture stabilization prior to definitive vascular repair. While the indications for acute brachial plexus exploration are few, open treatment of concomitant vascular injuries may allow the brachial plexus surgeon an opportunity to visualize the injury, repair (if cleanly lacerated) or tag any nerve structures for later identification. The primary concern in the acute setting, however, is limb reperfusion with or without skeletal stabilization.

Huang et al. compared the functional outcomes of patients with brachial plexus injury with and without concomitant vascular injury. Patients with an associated vascular injury were more likely to have suffered a pan-plexus lesion and other upper extremity injuries. The vascular injury group was more likely to require nerve grafting, whereas the control group was more often treated with nerve transfers. At final follow-up, only 43% of patients with a combined brachial plexus and vascular injury achieved antigravity biceps function compared to 73% of the patients who suffered a brachial plexus injury alone [18].

Spine and Spinal Cord Trauma

Spine fractures and spinal cord trauma make up the second most common concomitant injury in brachial plexus patients [19]. The frequency of brachial plexus injury in patients with known spinal cord trauma is reported to be between 0.6% and 1.8% [9]. There is less data, however, detailing the prevalence of spinal cord trauma in patients with a known brachial plexus injury [20]. Rhee et al. reviewed 255 adult patients who were evaluated for a traumatic brachial plexus injury, and 31 (12.2%) were found to have a concomitant injury of the spinal cord itself [9].

An accurate diagnosis of a brachial plexus or spinal cord injury can often be delayed following polytrauma, and the neurologic deficits imparted by each of these injuries may obscure the prompt and accurate diagnosis of the other [9]. Spine radiographs may reveal cervical fractures which put the spinal cord at risk or transverse process which is associated with root avulsions. Most commonly, the brachial plexus injury is initially unrecognized, while attention is focused on the spinal cord injury [21]. Unfortunately, the difficulty in identifying the concomitant brachial plexus injury frequently leads to a delay in diagnosis. Grundy and Silver reported that a diagnosis of a brachial plexus injury was delayed in 55% of patients, and Rhee et al. reported a mean time from injury to consultation at a brachial plexus clinic to be 9.1 months [9, 22].

Like the brachial plexus injury population in general, combined injuries are frequently seen in younger individuals, with the most common mechanism of injury being a high-speed motorized accident involving a motorcycle, automobile or other motorized vehicles (Fig. 6.2) [8, 9, 22–24]. In a large series of patients with combined injuries of the brachial plexus and spinal cord, 40–71% of these injuries were caused by motorcycle crashes [22, 23]. When the vehicle involved is an automobile, frequently the patient was not wearing a seatbelt at the time of the incident.

The classic brachial plexus injury mechanism of forcible separation of the head and neck from the shoulder via lateral flexion of the cervical spine may simultaneously result in a fracture of the thoracic spine and ribs (Fig. 6.3) [22]. The injury to the spinal cord itself may occur with lateral flexion injuries, as noted in one small case series [10], or hyperextension [9]. The exact mechanism of injury and forces that can lead to concurrent injuries to the brachial plexus and spinal cord are not fully understood.

Narakas reported in his series of cases with concomitant cervical spine trauma and brachial plexus injury that root avulsions were present 83% of the time, with nearly half of these patients having three or more roots avulsed from the spinal cord [23]. Some authors have hypothesized that an injury which primarily results in a traumatic root avulsion may secondarily cause an injury to the spinal cord itself. Flannery and Birch [25] lend support to this hypothesis by citing the four cases of incomplete Brown-Sequard syndrome reported by Narakas [23] that were attributed to haematoma formation within the canal. In their own two patients, the authors observed spinal cord lesions that were due to compression of the cord by a combination of CSF and haematoma. Both patients had appreciable return of function of the spinal cord but incomplete recovery of the brachial plexus lesions.

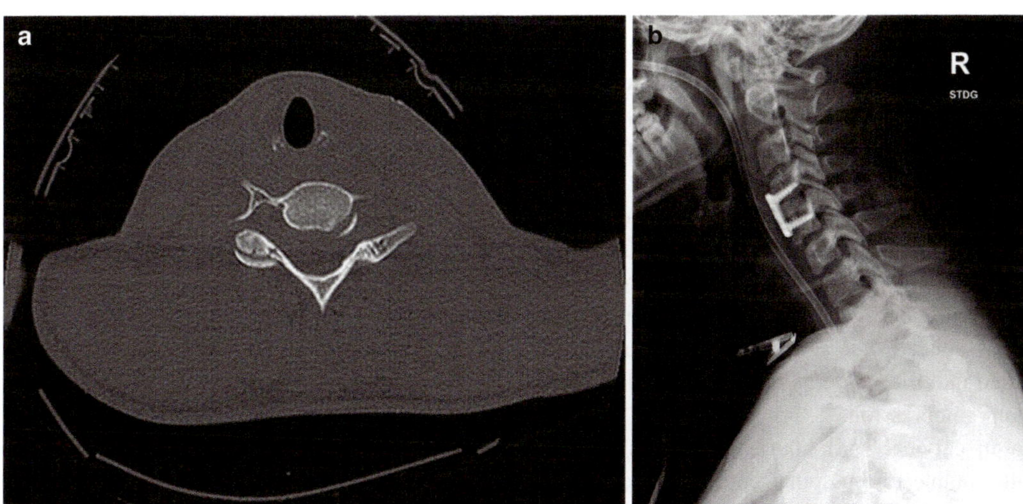

Fig. 6.2 Cervical spine injury. CT scan demonstrating a right-sided facet fracture at C6–C7 in a 15-year-old boy who was the passenger in a high-speed motor vehicle accident for which he underwent ACDF. The patient also had a contralateral brachial plexus injury

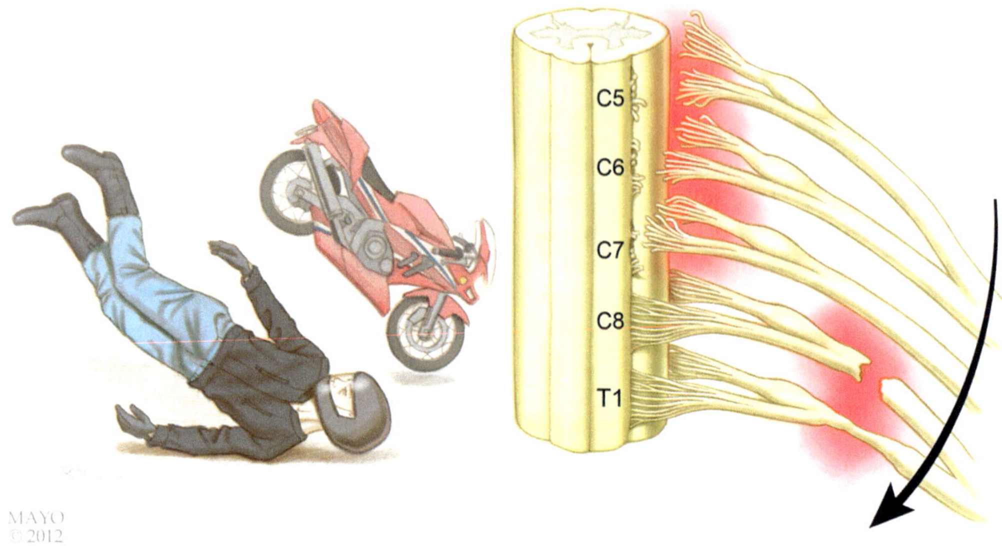

Fig. 6.3 Mechanism of brachial plexus injury. The classic brachial plexus injury mechanism of forcible separation of the head and neck from the shoulder via lateral flexion of the cervical spine may simultaneously result in a fracture of the thoracic spine and ribs

Nordin and Sinisi [12] reported on three patients presenting with preganglionic injuries of the brachial plexus that led to a partial Brown-Sequard syndrome. They described two distinct preganglionic injuries. In a peripheral intradural preganglionic rupture, the lesion occurs in the intradural course of the nerve root leaving central stumps. In a central preganglionic avulsion, the roots tear directly from the cord with central nervous tissue attached to the avulsed root leaving a resultant defect in the cord. The latter represents an injury to the central nervous system because it results in scarring within the spinal cord and has been estimated to cause a partial Brown-Sequard syndrome in 2–5% of patients with brachial plexus injuries. Russell and Mangan [26] presented a single case of brachial plexus avulsion injury and an associated subarachnoid haematoma that ruptured into the subdural space, ultimately causing cord compression.

In cervical cord injuries, paralysis is easily attributable to the spinal cord, and the brachial plexus injury may be masked by a co-existing tetraplegia [27]. Among patients who become paraplegic following combined injuries to the brachial plexus and spinal cord, as many as one in three may not achieve their expected level of independence due to the upper extremity paralysis attributable to the brachial plexus injury [22]. The consequences of missing or delaying the identification of a brachial plexus injury in the setting of spinal cord injury may be significant as many of the treatment options to maximize upper extremity function are time dependent [15].

A thorough physical examination, including evaluation of the upper and lower extremity reflexes, should be performed to rule out a concomitant upper motor neuron injury in presumed brachial plexus injuries [15]. Failure to properly account for a concomitant spinal cord injury in the setting of brachial plexus injury can lead to poor results, and the spasticity arising from the upper motor neuron lesion may compromise target sensorimotor function [9].

The use of intraplexal and extraplexal nerve transfers, tendon transfers, and free functioning muscles has been described for these patients to achieve enough strength for self-transfers and activities of daily living. Results of these interventions may be inferior to those seen in patients without associated spinal cord injuries, and expectations should be tempered [28].

Chest Wall Trauma

Injury to the chest including pneumothorax, hemothorax and lung contusions is of immediate concern in patients who present with blunt trauma. The principles of Advanced Trauma Life Support provide an algorithm to avoid missing these potentially life-threatening injuries. Ipsilateral rib fractures occur in approximately one-third of patients with brachial plexus injuries, and intraparenchymal lung injuries are reported in a similar number of patients (Fig. 6.4) [2, 3, 8, 29].

In addition to the life-threatening nature of chest wall trauma, critical evaluation of the chest is critical for the brachial plexus surgeon planning reconstruction. Injuries to the intercostal (ICN) and phrenic nerves have been reported to occur in conjunction with brachial plexus injuries [8, 22]. One study of 153 patients undergoing brachial plexus reconstruction reported a 10% incidence of phrenic nerve palsy [8]. The most common mechanism of injury for these patients with combined brachial plexus and chest wall injury was motorcycle accidents.

Inspiration and expiration chest radiographs or fluoroscopy of the diaphragm can evaluate the function of the phrenic nerve. However, diaphragm paralysis may also be seen with preganglionic injuries to the C5 nerve root. High-quality posteroanterior chest radiographs as well as dedicated rib films may identify rib fractures. Nevertheless, Kovachevich et al. found that nerve transfer using intercostal nerves was successful in 92% of patients despite concomitant chest wall trauma. Concurrent rib fractures were not found to be a risk factor for the overall rate of complications after intercostal nerve transfers for treatment of the brachial plexus injury, although rib fractures were found to be associated with a decreased likelihood of nerve viability [8]. This was in contrast to previous studies that had identified chest wall trauma, including ipsilateral rib fractures and phrenic nerve palsy, as a contraindication to ICN transfers [30, 31].

Injury to the spinal accessory nerve in the setting of brachial plexus palsy imparts added functional limitations to the patient, but may also render the nerve unable to be used for brachial plexus reconstruction [5]. In one study of 357 patients with stretch injuries of the brachial plexus, accessory nerve palsy was diagnosed in 6% of these patients with upper or complete brachial plexus palsy [5]. There were no patients with concurrent injuries of the lower brachial plexus and accessory nerve, and nearly one-third of patients with an accessory nerve injury also sustained a clavicle fracture. Complete recovery of the accessory nerve was seen in all seven patients who demonstrated contraction of the upper trapezius muscle with intraoperative electrical stimulation.

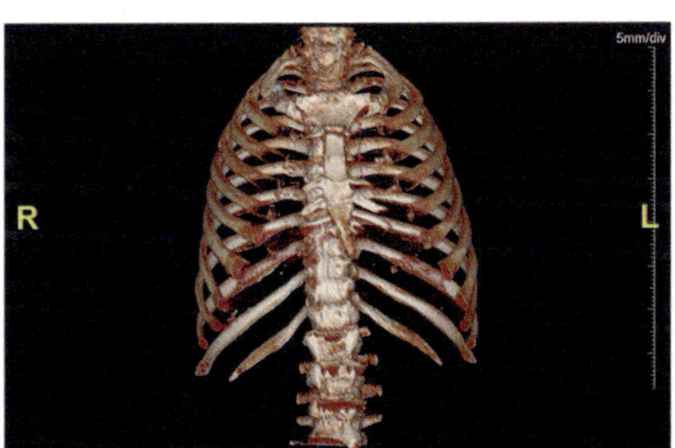

Fig. 6.4 Chest wall trauma. 3D reconstruction of a chest wall CT in this 74-year-old patient who sustained a brachial plexus palsy as well as right first through sixth rib fractures, left first through fifth rib fractures, a right clavicle fracture, and multiple spine fractures following a motorcycle injury

Scapulothoracic Dissociation

Scapulothoracic dissociation involves a laterally displaced scapula with separation of the acromioclavicular joint, sternoclavicular joint or clavicle fracture [32–34]. Motorcycle and motor vehicle accidents are the most common mechanism of injury followed by falls from heights and industrial accidents [35].

This junctional injury is essentially an internal forequarter amputation with intact skin, with disruption of osseous, muscular, vascular and neurologic structures [36]. Physical examination is often notable for asymmetric shoulder swelling and palpable shoulder girdle injuries. The limb is pulseless in nearly all cases with only 10% of patients having been reported to have limb-threatening ischemia [37, 38]. A thorough neurologic examination should be documented in patients who are able to cooperate.

This high-energy distraction injury may be initially diagnosed on an anteroposterior chest radiograph. The degree of scapular lateralization is measured by comparing the distance from a thoracic spinous process to the medial border of both scapulae. An increased displacement of greater than 1 cm or an increased ratio of the affected to the normal side (greater than 1.29) is concerning for scapulothoracic dissociation [38, 39]. Dedicated radiographs of the clavicle or AC and SC joints should also be obtained to aid in the radiographic diagnosis (Figs. 6.5 and 6.6) [40].

In the acute setting, consultation with a vascular surgeon will aid in the need for angiography or other imaging modalities. Again, an open vascular repair permits the brachial plexus surgeon the opportunity to evaluate the extent of the neurologic injury. Compared to axillary or brachial artery injuries, patients with subclavian artery disruption are significantly more likely to suffer

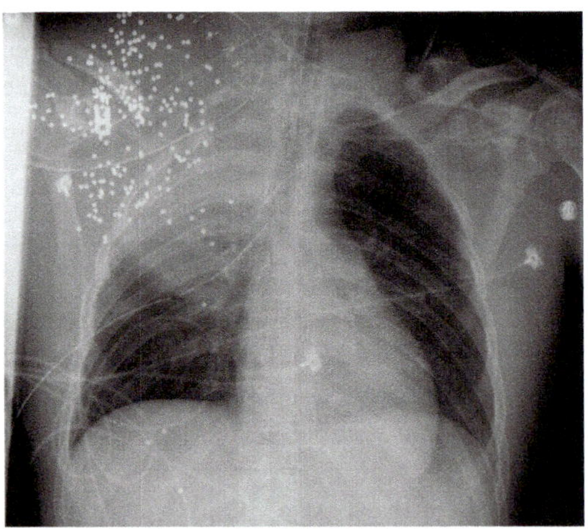

Fig. 6.5 Scapula and Clavicle Fractures. Chest x-ray of a 24-year-old man who sustained a gunshot wound to the right neck for which he sustained multiple injuries including disruption of the subclavian artery and fractures of the scapular body, clavicle, transverse process of C7 and first and second ribs. He underwent free functioning muscle transfer for treatment of the concurrent brachial plexus injury

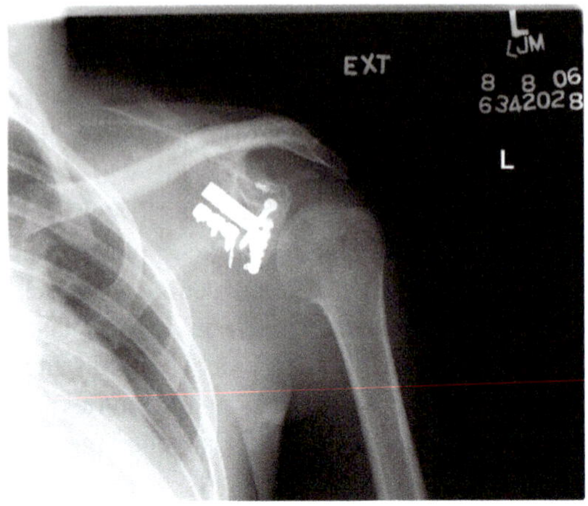

Fig. 6.6 Scapula fracture. Left shoulder x-ray of a 19-year-old man who sustained a brachial pan-plexopathy as well as a left scapula fracture for which he underwent surgical fixation

preganglionic nerve injuries [41]. Osseous stabilization not only protects any vascular repair or reconstruction and minimizes further trauma to soft tissues and neurovascular structures but also provides a stable shoulder girdle to support a cosmetic or functional prosthesis should the patient undergo amputation in the future. Ipsilateral fractures of the humerus, radius, ulna and/or hand occur in more than 40% of patients [37].

Historically, patients with a scapulothoracic dissociation and preganglionic nerve injuries were treated with transhumeral amputation and shoulder arthrodesis [40]. Advances in nerve surgery have changed the algorithm, and once the emergent needs of a patient with scapulothoracic dissociation are addressed, management of the neurologic injury is similar to other injuries of the brachial plexus.

Functional outcomes in following scapulothoracic dissociation are worse than those following isolated brachial plexus injuries alone [18, 42]. Zelle et al. followed 25 patients for an average of 12.6 years following scapulothoracic dissociation. During their initial hospital stay, three patients died from their injuries and six patients required an above the elbow amputation. Of the patients who underwent brachial plexus reconstruction, approximately half had suffered a pan-plexus injury. These patients were more likely to have worse physical and mental component summary scores on the Short Form-36 as well as poorer subjective shoulder function compared to those with partial brachial plexus lesions. The authors conclude that the functional outcome of patients with scapulothoracic dissociation depends primarily on the extent of the neurologic injury [38].

Other Musculoskeletal Injuries

Overall, fractures and dislocations are the most common associated pathology in patients with brachial plexus injury [2, 11, 29]. Conversely, peripheral nerve injuries are rare following extremity trauma and occur in less than 2% of patients. Crush injuries, dislocations and scapula fractures are more likely to be associated with a concomitant nerve injury [19, 43, 44]. In the setting of a brachial plexus injury, fractures to the scapula and clavicle occur with similar frequency to other long bone fractures in the ipsilateral extremity [2].

When treating concomitant long bone fractures, the effect of the brachial plexus injury should be taken into consideration. Brien et al. followed 21 patients with brachial plexus injuries and ipsilateral humeral shaft fractures. Of the 11 fractures treated non-surgically, there were 5 nonunions, 2 delayed unions and 2 malunions. In contrast, all three fractures that were treated with compression plating united [45]. Non-surgical treatment with functional bracing of isolated humeral shaft fractures remains a popular treatment with a low complication rate, but higher non-union and malunion rate than surgery [46–49]. However, in addition to soft tissue compression and gravity, fracture bracing relies on active muscle contraction to maintain alignment, which is often limited in patients with brachial plexus injuries. Another advantage of compression plating of humeral shaft fracture is that it maintains length and allows for early range of motion to keep shoulder and elbow joints supple while awaiting reinnervation or reconstruction.

Restoration of shoulder abduction and external rotation is considered the second priority in brachial plexus reconstruction (see previous chapter). One study identified that nearly one in ten patients with a traumatic brachial plexus injury sustained a concomitant tear of the rotator cuff [6]. Among these patients, those with infraclavicular brachial plexus injuries had a significantly higher rate of full-thickness tears of the rotator cuff. Obviously, failure to identify and address rotator cuff pathology can lead to suboptimal shoulder function regardless of reinnervation. Surgeons should have a low threshold to assess for each of these conditions with a thorough history, physical examination and appropriate imaging when formulating a treatment plan [50]. Open or arthroscopic rotator cuff repair is appropriate in these patients to maximize strength and functional outcomes [51]. However, a multidisciplinary team should consider the rehabilitation for each procedure so as not to interfere with healing of either the rotator cuff or brachial plexus reconstruction.

Traumatic Brain Injury

At the time of injury, the majority of patients will experience a brief loss of consciousness [3]. Up to one-third of patients with brachial plexus injuries will suffer more serious concomitant head trauma or coma [2, 11, 19, 29]. Coma and head trauma are associated with an increased risk of avulsion injuries and complete brachial plexus lesions [19].

One study identified a peripheral nerve injury in over one-third of traumatic brain injury (TBI) patients and a brachial plexus injury in 10 percent of patients. Alarmingly, no patient complained of neuropathy or weakness to clue the physician into the diagnosis [52]. Obtaining electrodiagnostic studies in coma patients is of little utility as it is unlikely that a brachial plexus reconstruction would be performed until the patient is able to comprehend his or her injury. However, for polytrauma patients who have awaken from coma, a thorough neurologic exam of the upper extremities is imperative to identify a brachial plexus injury in a timely fashion.

To date, no groups have reported their outcomes following brachial plexus reconstruction in patients who suffer TBI specifically. Anecdotally, TBI patients have severe difficulty understanding and comprehending the potentially complex reconstructions or non-anatomic nerve transfers to activate function. The diagnosis of TBI is broad and encompasses a spectrum of disability. Similarly, brachial plexus injuries are heterogenous, and it is difficult to make any meaningful comparisons between TBI patients and those who suffer brachial plexus injuries in the absence of head trauma. Importantly, the brachial plexus surgeon should be aware of the high incidence of head trauma in these patients and consult with physical medicine and rehabilitation colleagues as well as physical and occupational therapists if there is any concern that a patient may not be able to sufficiently participate in rehabilitation prior to commencing a complex reconstruction.

Conclusion

Brachial plexus injuries occur in 4 to 5 per cent of polytrauma patients depending on the mechanism of injury [19]. Motorcycle, motor vehicle and winter sports accidents should heighten the suspicion of trauma teams to a concomitant brachial plexus injury in polytrauma patients, especially in the setting of shoulder girdle fractures. Distracting injuries frequently delay the accurate diagnosis of a brachial plexus lesion.

For the brachial plexus surgeon, associated injuries may affect a planned brachial plexus reconstruction or lead to difficulties with rehabilitation following treatment. The most common concomitant injuries are long bone and shoulder girdle fractures, but vascular injuries, spinal cord lesions and traumatic brain injuries can negatively affect the prognosis following reconstruction and lead to long-term disability.

References

1. Terzis JK, Vekris MD, Soucacos PN. Outcomes of brachial plexus reconstruction in 204 patients with devastating paralysis. Plast Reconstr Surg. 1999;104:1221–40.
2. Rasulić L, Savić A, Lepić M, et al. Epidemiological characteristics of surgically treated civilian traumatic brachial plexus injuries in Serbia. Acta Neurochir. 2018;160:1837–45.
3. Midha R. Epidemiology of brachial plexus injuries in a multitrauma population. Neurosurgery. 1997;40:1182–8; discussion 1188-1189.
4. Noble J, Munro CA, Prasad VS, Midha R. Analysis of upper and lower extremity peripheral nerve injuries in a population of patients with multiple injuries. J Trauma. 1998;45:116–22.
5. Bertelli JA, Ghizoni MF. Combined injury of the accessory nerve and brachial plexus. Neurosurgery. 2011;68:390–5; discussion 396.
6. Brogan DM, Carofino BC, Kircher MF, et al. Prevalence of rotator cuff tears in adults with traumatic brachial plexus injuries. J Bone Joint Surg Am. 2014;96:e139.
7. Dubuisson AS, Kline DG. Brachial plexus injury: a survey of 100 consecutive cases from a single service. Neurosurgery. 2002;51:673–82; discussion 682-673.
8. Kovachevich R, Kircher MF, Wood CM, Spinner RJ, Bishop AT, Shin AY. Complications of intercostal nerve transfer for brachial plexus reconstruction. J Hand Surg Am. 2010;35:1995–2000.
9. Rhee PC, Pirola E, Hébert-Blouin MN, et al. Concomitant traumatic spinal cord and brachial plexus injuries in adult patients. J Bone Joint Surg Am. 2011;93:2271–7.
10. Robert R. Lateral flexion injuries of the cervical spine. J Bone Joint Surg. 1963;45-B:36–8.
11. Li GY, Xue MQ, Wang JW, Zeng XY, Qin J, Sha K. Traumatic brachial plexus injury: a study of 510 surgical cases from multicenter services in Guangxi, China. Acta Neurochir. 2019;161:899–906.
12. Nordin L, Sinisi M. Brachial plexus-avulsion causing Brown-Sequard syndrome: a report of three cases. J Bone Joint Surg Br. 2009;91:88–90.
13. Bucci G, Lucar-Lopez G, Sanchez-Gonzalez J, Malagelada F, Palencia Lopez J, Guevara-Noriega KA. Axillary artery injury and brachial plexus palsy as a complication of proximal humerus fractures. J Orthop. 2017;14:340–1.
14. McCready RA, Procter CD, Hyde GL. Subclavian-axillary vascular trauma. J Vasc Surg. 1986;3:24–31.
15. Noland SS, Krauss EM, Felder JM, Mackinnon SE. Surgical and clinical decision making in isolated long thoracic nerve palsy. Hand (N Y). 2018;13:689–94.
16. Maldonado AA, Romero-Brufau S, Kircher MF, Spinner RJ, Bishop AT, Shin AY. Free functioning gracilis muscle transfer for elbow flexion

reconstruction after traumatic adult brachial pan-plexus injury: where is the optimal distal tendon attachment for elbow flexion? Plast Reconstr Surg. 2017;139:128–36.
17. Brown FW, Navigato WJ. Rupture of the axillary artery and brachial plexus palsy associated with anterior dislocation of the shoulder. Report of a case with successful vascular repair. Clin Orthop Relat Res. 1968;60:195–9.
18. Huang AE, Noland SS, Spinner RJ, Bishop AT, Shin AY. Outcomes of reconstructive surgery in traumatic brachial plexus injury with concomitant vascular injury. World Neurosurg. 2020;135:e350–7.
19. Kaiser R, Mencl L, Haninec P. Injuries associated with serious brachial plexus involvement in polytrauma among patients requiring surgical repair. Injury. 2014;45:223–6.
20. Webb JC, Munshi P, Saifuddin A, Birch R. The prevalence of spinal trauma associated with brachial plexus injuries. Injury. 2002;33:587–90.
21. Grundy DJ, Silver JR. Problems in the management of combined brachial plexus and spinal cord injuries. Int Rehabil Med. 1981;3:57–70.
22. Grundy DJ, Silver JR. Combined brachial plexus and spinal cord trauma. Injury. 1983;15:57–61.
23. Narakas AO. Injuries of the brachial plexus and neighboring peripheral nerves in vertebral fractures and other trauma of the cervical spine. Der Orthopade. 1987;16:81–6.
24. Sturm JT, Perry JF Jr. Brachial plexus injuries from blunt trauma--a harbinger of vascular and thoracic injury. Ann Emerg Med. 1987;16:404–6.
25. Flannery MC, Birch R. Acute compression of the cervical spinal cord: a complication of preganglionic injury to the brachial plexus. Injury. 1990;21:247–8.
26. Russell NA, Mangan MA. Acute spinal cord compression by subarachnoid and subdural hematoma occurring in association with brachial plexus avulsion. Case report. J Neurosurg. 1980;52:410–3.
27. Akita S, Murase T, Yonenobu K, Shimada K, Masada K, Yoshikawa H. Long-term results of surgery for forearm deformities in patients with multiple cartilaginous exostoses. J Bone Joint Surg Am. 2007;89:1993–9.
28. Paul AW, Spinner RJ, Bishop AT, Shin AY, Rhee PC. two cases of traumatic brachial plexus injury with complete spinal cord injury. Hand (N Y). 2018;13:Np27–np31.
29. Faglioni W Jr, Siqueira MG, Martins RS, Heise CO, Foroni L. The epidemiology of adult traumatic brachial plexus lesions in a large metropolis. Acta Neurochir. 2014;156:1025–8.
30. Ruch DS, Friedman A, Nunley JA. The restoration of elbow flexion with intercostal nerve transfers. Clin Orthop Relat Res. 1995;314:95–103.
31. Wahegaonkar AL, Doi K, Hattori Y, Addosooki AI. Technique of intercostal nerve harvest and transfer for various neurotization procedures in brachial plexus injuries. Tech Hand Up Extrem Surg. 2007;11:184–94.
32. Oreck SL, Burgess A, Levine AM. Traumatic lateral displacement of the scapula: a radiographic sign of neurovascular disruption. J Bone Joint Surg Am. 1984;66:758–63.
33. Rubenstein JD, Ebraheim NA, Kellam JF. Traumatic scapulothoracic dissociation. Radiology. 1985;157:297–8.
34. Ebraheim NA, Pearlstein SR, Savolaine ER, Gordon SL, Jackson WT, Corray T. Scapulothoracic dissociation (closed avulsion of the scapula, subclavian artery, and brachial plexus): a newly recognized variant, a new classification, and a review of the literature and treatment options. J Orthop Trauma. 1987;1:18–23.
35. Damschen DD, Cogbill TH, Siegel MJ. Scapulothoracic dissociation caused by blunt trauma. J Trauma. 1997;42:537–40.
36. Covey CDC, Schwartz AK. Orthopaedic junctional injuries. J Bone Joint Surg Am. 2019;101:1783–92.
37. Lee L, Miller TT, Schultz E, Toledano B. Scapulothoracic dissociation. Am J Orthop (Belle Mead, NJ). 1998;27:699–702.
38. Zelle BA, Pape HC, Gerich TG, Garapati R, Ceylan B, Krettek C. Functional outcome following scapulothoracic dissociation. J Bone Joint Surg Am. 2004;86:2–8.
39. Lange RH, Noel SH. Traumatic lateral scapular displacement: an expanded spectrum of associated neurovascular injury. J Orthop Trauma. 1993;7:361–6.
40. Choo AM, Schottel PC, Burgess AR. Scapulothoracic dissociation: evaluation and management. J Am Acad Orthop Surg. 2017;25:339–47.
41. Sen RK, Prasad G, Aggarwal S. Scapulothoracic dissociation: level of vascular insult, an indirect prognostic indicator for the final outcome? Acta Orthop Belg. 2009;75:14–8.
42. Riess KP, Cogbill TH, Patel NY, Lambert PJ, Mathiason MA. Brachial plexus injury: long-term functional outcome is determined by associated scapulothoracic dissociation. J Trauma. 2007;63:1021–5.
43. Taylor CA, Braza D, Rice JB, Dillingham T. The incidence of peripheral nerve injury in extremity trauma. Am J Phys Med Rehabil. 2008;87:381–5.
44. Chamata E, Mahabir R, Jupiter D, Weber RA. Prevalence of brachial plexus injuries in patients with scapular fractures: a National Trauma Data Bank review. Plast Surg (Oakville, Ont). 2014;22:246–8.
45. Brien WW, Gellman H, Becker V, Garland DE, Waters RL, Wiss DA. Management of fractures of the humerus in patients who have an injury of the ipsilateral brachial plexus. J Bone Joint Surg Am. 1990;72:1208–10.
46. Ilyas AM, Mangan JJ, Graham J. Radial nerve palsy recovery with fractures of the humerus: an updated systematic review. J Am Acad Orthop Surg. 2020;28:e263–9.

47. Updegrove GF, Mourad W, Abboud JA. Humeral shaft fractures. J Shoulder Elb Surg. 2018;27:e87–97.
48. Denard A Jr, Richards JE, Obremskey WT, Tucker MC, Floyd M, Herzog GA. Outcome of nonoperative vs operative treatment of humeral shaft fractures: a retrospective study of 213 patients. Orthopedics. 2010;33(8). https://doi.org/10.3928/01477447-20100625-16. PMID: 20704103.
49. Sarmiento A, Zagorski JB, Zych GA, Latta LL, Capps CA. Functional bracing for the treatment of fractures of the humeral diaphysis. J Bone Joint Surg Am. 2000;82:478–86.
50. Güven O, Akbar Z, Yalçin S, Gündeş H. Concomitant rotator cuff tear and brachial plexus injury in association with anterior shoulder dislocation: unhappy triad of the shoulder. J Orthop Trauma. 1994;8:429–30.
51. Qi C, Cai Y, Yu T, Chen B, Meng Q. Diagnosis and treatment of rotator cuff tear and brachial plexus injury. Zhongguo Xiu Fu Chong Jian Wai Ke Za Zhi. 2014;28:802–5.
52. Stone L, Keenan MA. Peripheral nerve injuries in the adult with traumatic brain injury. Clin Orthop Relat Res. 1988;233:136–44.

Part II

Evaluation

Examination of the Adult Brachial Plexus Patient

7

Brittany N. Garcia, Angela A. Wang, and Alexander Y. Shin

Examination of the patient with a brachial plexus injury (BPI) is the foundation for early diagnosis as well as determining the outcome of surgical intervention(s) [1–3]. Examination needs to be performed in a standardized method that is detailed and complete. The goal of clinical examination of a new brachial plexus patient is to ascertain the location of the nerve injury (preganglionic vs postganglionic, and if postganglionic – trunk, division, cord, or terminal branches) and the severity of the injury (partial or complete). Examination of the patient should be done as soon as feasible to ascertain a baseline exam for comparison in the future to determine if there is spontaneous recovery. Ideally, the exam is performed by the same examiner each time to allow for consistency in exam styles. A global neurological exam of the upper and lower extremity is necessary to rule out spinal cord lesions [4].

Careful systematic motor and sensory exam should be performed and recorded. To facilitate record keeping, variations of Merle d'Aubigne's data sheet have been used [5] (Fig. 7.1). Our preference is to use the Mayo Clinic Brachial Plexus Exam Record [6] (Fig. 7.2). The tabular form allows easy comparison of prior examinations and a systematic exam to be recorded. Serial examinations over the first several months after injury can assist in determining if there is ongoing recovery and the prognosis for spontaneous functional recovery.

The British Medical Research Council (BMRC) muscle grading system and its many variations have been used for decades in the evaluation of muscle strength [6–9] (Table 7.1). The BMRC grading has received quite a bit of criticism, and its modifications have resulted in difficulties in comparing outcome studies. While there are many inherent limitations of the BMRC grading, it remains an easy-to-use system that has not been able to be replaced. There are important limitations that need to be understood about the BMRC grading system, however. In a study comparing BMRC grade to normalized torque measurements for elbow flexion or extension in brachial plexus injury patients, Shahgholi et al. demonstrated that patients who had been graded by experienced examiners as having BMRC 5 actually had less than 42% of the normal strength fulfilled [10]. In order to make the BMRC grading more precise, it has been our convention that a greater grade cannot be obtained unless the criteria of the lesser grade are obtained [11]. For example, in order to be a grade 3, active motion must be equal to passive motion. A grade 4 cannot

B. N. Garcia · A. A. Wang
University of Utah, Department of Orthopaedic Surgery, Salt Lake City, UT, USA
e-mail: Brittany.Garcia@hsc.utah.edu; Angela.Wang@hsc.utah.edu

A. Y. Shin (✉)
Department of Orthopedic Surgery, Mayo Clinic, Rochester, MN, USA
e-mail: shin.alexander@mayo.edu

A. Y. Shin, N. Pulos (eds.), *Operative Brachial Plexus Surgery*,
https://doi.org/10.1007/978-3-030-69517-0_7

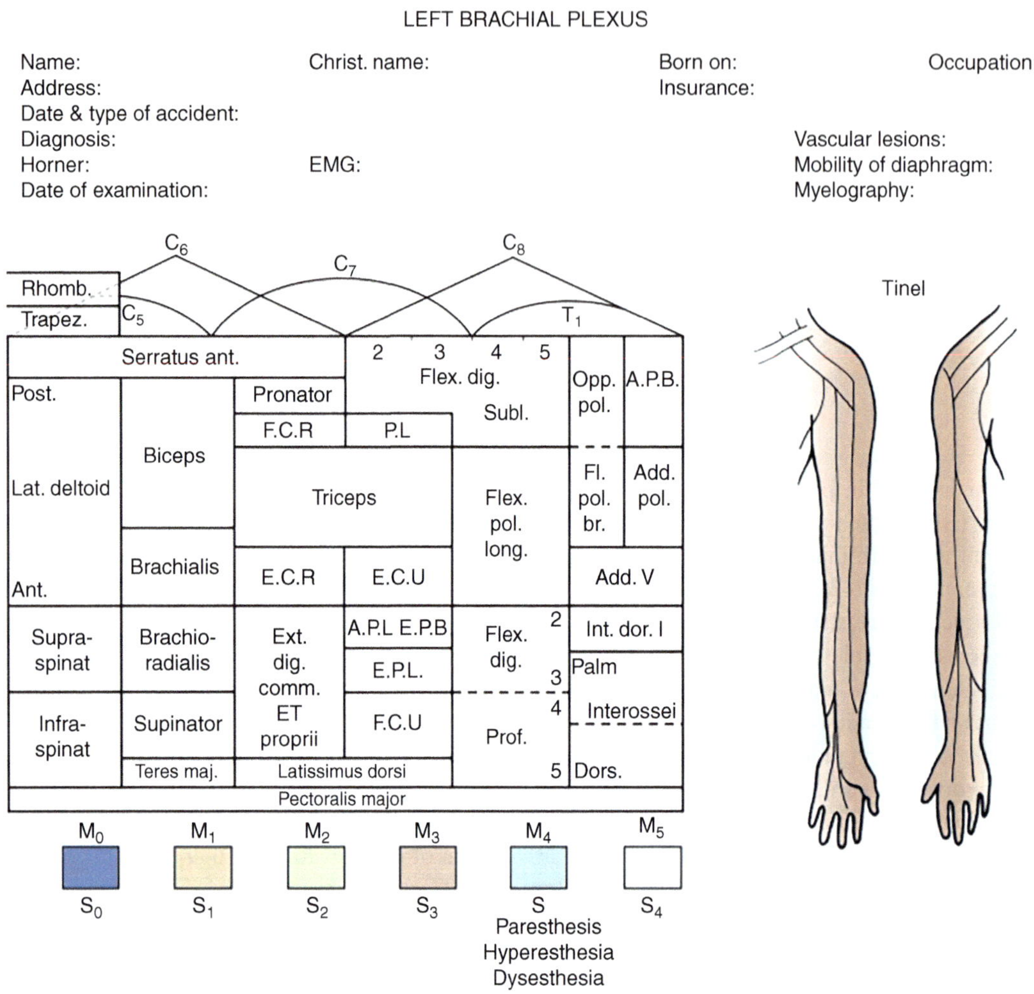

Fig. 7.1 The findings of clinical exam need to be accurately documented. The d'Aubigne Brachial Plexus Data Sheet is one example of motor and sensory documentation [5]

be assigned unless there is full active range of motion equal to passive range of motion and there is resistance strength. Addition of a + or – is assigned to further qualify the strength as a weak grade 4 or a strong grade 4. Manual muscle testing of every muscle of the upper extremity can be performed easily in about 6–10 minutes and recorded. It is important that the examiner be consistent in grading strength no matter what modification is used. When reporting motor strength, the conventions used should be accurately detailed to avoid confusion.

Clinical Exam

Clinical exam commences as soon as the surgeon meets the patient. The patient's gait and stance should be noted (for spinal cord injury). While obtaining the patient's history, the surgeon should observe the face, the ipsilateral eyelid, and pupils (for Horner's sign), the manner in which the patient holds his head (traumatic torticollis), as well as the manner of speech and how alert and oriented the patient is (closed head injury).

Brachial Plexus Nerve Muscle Record

Page 2 of 4

Provider: Pager:

Brachial Plexus | **Currently involved ☐ Left (L) ☐ Right (R) ☐ Both (B)**

Tinel's in Neck	
Horner's Sign	
Diaphragm	
EMG	
Pain	

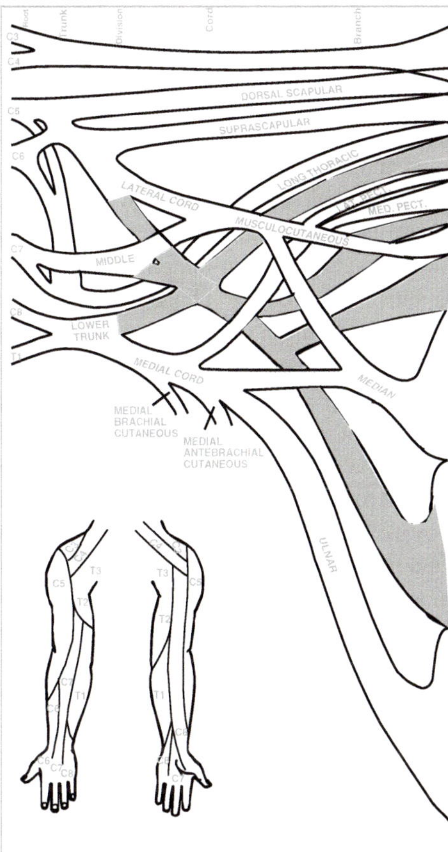

DATE	
	Side Involved
	Examiner
C3, C4, XI	Upper trapezius
C3, C4, XI	Middle trapezius
C3, C4, XI	Lower trapezius
C(3), C(4), C5	Levator scapulae
C4, C(5)	Rhomboids
C(5), C6	Supraspinatus
C(5), C6	Infraspinatus
C(5), C(6), C(7)	Serratus anterior
C5, C6	Teres major
C5, C6	Subscapularis
C5, C(6), C7	Clav. pect. major
C6, C(7), C(8), T1	Stern. pect. major
C6, C7, C8, T1	Pect. minor
C6, C(7), C8	Latissimus dorsi
C(5), C6	Biceps & Brachialis
C5, C6, C7	Coracobrachialis
C(5), C6	Deltoid anterior
C(5), C6	Deltoid middle
C(5), C6	Deltoid posterior
C5, C6	Teres minor
C7, C(8), T1	Pronator quadratus
C(6), C(7)	Pronator teres
C(6), C(7)	Flex. carpi rad.
C7, C(8), T1	Flex. dig. prof. II, III
C7, C(8), T1	Flex. dig. sup.
C7, C(8), T1	Palmaris longus
C7, C(8), T1	Flex. pol. long
C6, C7, C(8), T1	Flex. pol. brev. (long)
C6, C7, C(8), T1	Abd. pol. brev.
C(8), T(1)	Opponens pollicis
C8, T1	Lumbricales, 1, 2
C6, C(7), C8	Triceps
C(5), C6	Supinator
C(5), C6	Brachioradialis
C(6), C(7)	Ext. carpi rad. long.
C6, C7, C8	Ext. carpi rad. brev.
C(7), C8	Ext. carpi ulnaris
C(7), C8	Ext. dig. com.
C(7), C8	Ext. dig. minimi
C(7), C8	Ext. ind. prop.
C(7), C8	Ext. pol. longus
C6, C(7)	Ext. pol. brev
C6, C(7)	Abd. pol. long.
C7, C(8), T1	Flex. carpi uln.
C7, C(8), T1	Flex. dig. prof. IV, V
C8, T(1)	Abd. dig. minimi
C(8), T(1)	Add. pol.
C8, T(1)	Opp. dig. minimi
C(8), T(1)	1 Dorsal interosseous
C(8), T(1)	2 Dorsal interosseous
C(8), T(1)	3 Dorsal interosseous
C(8), T(1)	4 Dorsal interosseous
C8, T1	1 Palmar interosseous
C8, T1	2 Palmar interosseous
C8, T1	3 Palmar interosseous
C8, T1	Lumbricales 3,4
C8, T(1)	Flex. pol. brev. (short)
Others	

Grade	Degree of Muscle Strength	Descriptive Term
0 = Zero	No palpable contraction	Nothing
1 = Trace	Muscle contracts, but part does not move	Trace
2 = Poor	Partial movement of part with gravity eliminated	With gravity eliminated
3 = Fair	Muscle moves the part through full range of motion against gravity	Against gravity
4 = Good	Full range of motion against gravity plus added resistance	Near normal
5 = Excellent	Normal strength	Normal

Key Note on Roots	Legend bar for draw tool
	X = Avulsion O = Rupture == = Stretch

JOINT	Active	Passive
Shoulder		
flex		
ext		
abduct		
ext. rot		
int. rot		
Elbow		
flex		
ext		

Preoperative Findings

	Date	Exam / Study	Findings	Name / Initial
☐				
☐				
☐				
☐				
☐				

Preoperative Electrophysiologic Findings

Fig. 7.2 Mayo Clinic Brachial Plexus Nerve Muscle Record is another example of a data sheet that allows for evaluation over time. (With permission of the Mayo Foundation)

Table 7.1 The British Medical Research council system of grading muscles

Grade	Original description [9]	Commonly used description [8]
M0	No contraction	No contraction
M1	Return of perceptible contraction in proximal muscles	Very minimal or trace contraction, no motion of part
M2	Return of perceptible contraction in both proximal and distal muscles	Joint moves with gravity eliminated
M3	All important muscles against resistance	Joint moves against gravity
M4	All synergistic and independent movements are possible	Joint moves against resistance
M5	Complete recovery	Normal

There are two main components to the exam: sensory and motor (which includes active and passive range of motion).

Sensory Exam

Though subjective, the sensory examination is an important component of evaluating patients with brachial plexus injuries. In combination with an accurate motor exam, a comprehensive sensory exam assists the clinician with identifying the affected nerve roots and level of injury in brachial plexus patients and allows for evaluation of recovery over time. Sequential sensory exams should be performed and systematically recorded at each visit using tools such as the Merle d'Aubigne data sheet or Mayo Clinic Brachial Plexus Nerve Muscle Record (Figs. 7.1 and 7.2).

Different types of peripheral sensory receptors exist and relay somatosensory information such as light touch, pain, temperature, proprioception, and pressure to the sensory cortex. The most common way to evaluate sensory function in BPIs is to test the patient's ability to detect light touch. This is done with the patient's eyes closed and applying a stimulus directly to the skin – typically by the pad of the examiner's finger or with a light brush or cotton swab. If desired, pin prick can be used to evaluate sharp and dull sensation as well as ability to sense pain [12]. Intact or absent sensation can be compared to that of the contralateral limb. Patients may be asked to scale the amount of intact sensation using numbers 0–10 or percentages in order to compare examinations over time. Several types of sensory symptoms may be experienced by patients such as paresthesia, anesthesia, hyperesthesia, and dysesthesia. The quality of sensory symptoms should be noted and documented.

Given anatomic variability and overlapping of peripheral nerve distributions, the most accurate way to evaluate sensation (autonomic function) in patients with brachial plexus injuries is to examine the specific "autonomous zones." Nerve roots supply specific dermatomes; however, sensation to a single dermatome can have overlap from adjacent nerve roots [13]. Autonomous zones are small, distinct areas of skin where there is minimal to no overlapping of sensory innervation by a specific nerve root. Evaluating the affected limb in these particular zones allows for the most accurate clinical evaluation of intact vs insensate sensory function [13, 14]. The autonomous zones of the upper extremity used for evaluation are illustrated in Fig. 7.2.

Tinel's Sign

Determining the presence of Tinel's sign is a very important physical exam maneuver in brachial plexus patients. This exam maneuver has been validated in patients with supraclavicular, closed traction injuries and should be performed both at the time of initial injury and then during each subsequent follow-up visit [1, 15, 16]. It can be useful for detecting acute nerve lesions and later used to follow regeneration. In the acute setting, a strongly positive Tinel's sign at the location of an expected lesion can indicate that axons are ruptured rather than avulsed. In this setting the examiner can lightly tap over the posterior triangle of the neck. A positive Tinel's sign will elicit pain down to the level of the elbow in the case of C5 nerve lesions, the radial forearm and thumb in C6 lesions, and dorsal hand in C7 nerve lesions [16]. In the case of a neuropraxia or a conduction block, Tinel's sign will be absent, and in the setting of axonotmesis or neurotmesis, Tinel's sign will be present. Tinel's sign can assist with prediction of the clinical course of brachial plexus injuries. The examiner should lightly tap in a distal to proximal direction over the course of the affected nerve. The site at which the patient experiences paresthesias, such as pins and needles over the nerve, corresponds to the level of regeneration of axons. When compared to nerves that are repaired, the sign will progress at a quicker rate than in the setting of axonotmesis [16].

Sensory Outcomes and Monitoring Recovery

In addition to determining and recording the quality of pain, the visual analogue scale (VAS) can be used to monitor a patient's pain over time. Patients may rate their pain on a scale of 0–10 quantifying the severity. Patients may also be administered the Disability of the Arm, Shoulder, and Hand (DASH) questionnaire to better evaluate the disability experienced secondary to pain symptoms. Higher DASH scores are associated with greater levels of disability and poorer outcomes [17].

When evaluating sensory recovery in patients treated for brachial plexus injuries, several grading systems exist. The Medical Research Council from the work of Highet and Seddon developed a more widely used system for determining sensory recovery [15, 16]. This system focuses on pain and tactile sensibility and grades sensory recovery from S0 (absence of sensation in the respective autonomous zone) to S4 (total recovery of sensation in the involved zone) (Table 7.2). More subtle findings include evaluation of vasomotor and sudomotor (response of the sweat glands) fiber function in the recovering limb. Observation of the color, texture, and temperature of the palms of the hands can provide information to the surgeon regarding recovery of these functions. Sensory exam findings should be correlated with nerve conduction findings to determine if they are consistent with preganglionic or postganglionic injuries.

Table 7.2 The modified highet classification [15, 16]

Sensory recovery outcome	Highet	s2PD	m2PD	Recovery of sensibility
Failure	S0	–	–	No recovery of sensibility in the autonomous zone of the nerve
Poor	S1	–	–	Recovery of deep cutaneous pain sensibility with the autonomous zone of the nerve
	S1+	–	–	Recovery of superficial pain sensibility
	S2	–	–	Recovery of superficial pain and some touch sensibility
	S2+	–	–	As in S2, but with overresponse
	S3	>15 mm	>7 mm	Recovery of pain and touch sensibility with disappearance of overresponse
Good	S3+	7–15 mm	4–7 mm	As in S3, but with good localization of the stimulus and imperfect recovery of 2PD
Excellent	S4	2–6 mm	2–3 mm	Complete sensory recovery

Sensory recovery outcome (failure, poor, good, excellent); Highet classification (S0–S4), static two-point discrimination (s2PD), moving two-point discrimination (m2PD), and sensibility recovery. Source: Mackinnon and Dellon

Motor Exam

There are three parts to the motor exam: (1) observation of muscle atrophy, (2) measurement of passive and active range of motion (shoulder, elbow, wrist, thumb, and fingers), and (3) manual motor testing of the muscles of the upper extremity.

Observation of the patient's face, eyelids, shoulder girdle (trapezius, rhomboids, scapula), and upper extremity is done relatively rapidly. Asymmetries in eyelids may be consistent for Horner's syndrome which is associated with T1 preganglionic injuries (Fig. 7.3). Observation of the injured side can demonstrate atrophy of the trapezius (spinal accessory nerve injury) (Fig. 7.4), sternocleidomastoid (high spinal accessory nerve injury), and rhomboid (C4, C5 avulsion), scapular malposition (long thoracic nerve injury, scapulothoracic dissociation), or torticollis (severe paraspinal muscle injury) (Fig. 7.4). Observation of gait abnormalities or difficulties standing or balancing can be indicative of spinal cord injury that would require further evaluation.

After observation, active and passive range of motion of the shoulder, elbow, forearm, wrist, and fingers is performed. Conventions for measurement of motion have been previously described by the American Association of Orthopedic Surgeons (AAOS) [18]. Typically motion of the shoulder is evaluated first. Passive range of motion for forward flexion, abduction, extension, and external and internal rotation is performed and recorded. While measurement of shoulder forward flexion and abduction is fairly simple to perform, there are some inconsistencies in the literature regarding external and internal rotation measurement. External shoulder motion in the brachial plexus exam is measured with the upper arm adducted to the body, elbow flexed 90 degrees, and hand directly in front of the body. This is the neutral rotation position. External rotation is measured with the elbow at 90 degree flexion both actively and passively. If the patient does not have active elbow flexion, the examiner maintains elbow flexion at 90 degrees for the patient. Internal rotation is controversial as it has been measured by which vertebrae the patient can touch on his back or a degree from the neutral rotation position. The body blocks internal rotation measurements between 45 and 120 degrees when trying to use the convention of the elbow flexed to 90 degrees; thus, estimation of internal rotation is performed. If the patient allows his arm to be placed on the small of his back, internal rotation is approximately 110–120 degrees. While internal rotation is not often a motion restored by reconstructive surgeries, it should be measured.

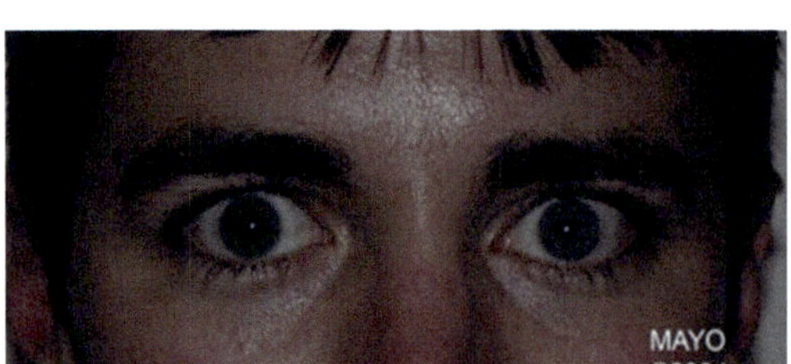

Fig. 7.3 Horner's sign of the left eye demonstrating ptosis and meiosis. (Copyright Mayo Foundation 2004)

Elbow range of motion of flexion and extension is fairly consistent and easy to obtain. Forearm rotation is measured with convention that neutral rotation is when the elbow is flexed 90 degrees and the thumb is pointed to the ceiling. It is important to measure the distal radius and ulna in pronation and supination and not the hand, as there are intercarpal pronation and supination which can overestimate the motion of the forearm. Wrist flexion, extension, and digital motion should be recorded as defined by the AAOS guidelines [18]. Any limitations of motion should be noted and evaluated appropriately (i.e., radiographs to evaluate for heterotopic bone, fractures, malunions, hardware issues, dislocations, etc.).

Once motion is recorded, a detailed and systematic clinical examination of a majority of the muscles in the upper extremity is performed. The patients should be undressed from the waist up (for females have a sports bra/tank top) to allow visualization and palpation of the muscle tested. It is important for the examiner to be cognizant of trick motions that patients often use and learn to compensate for paralyzed muscle [19]. Even for

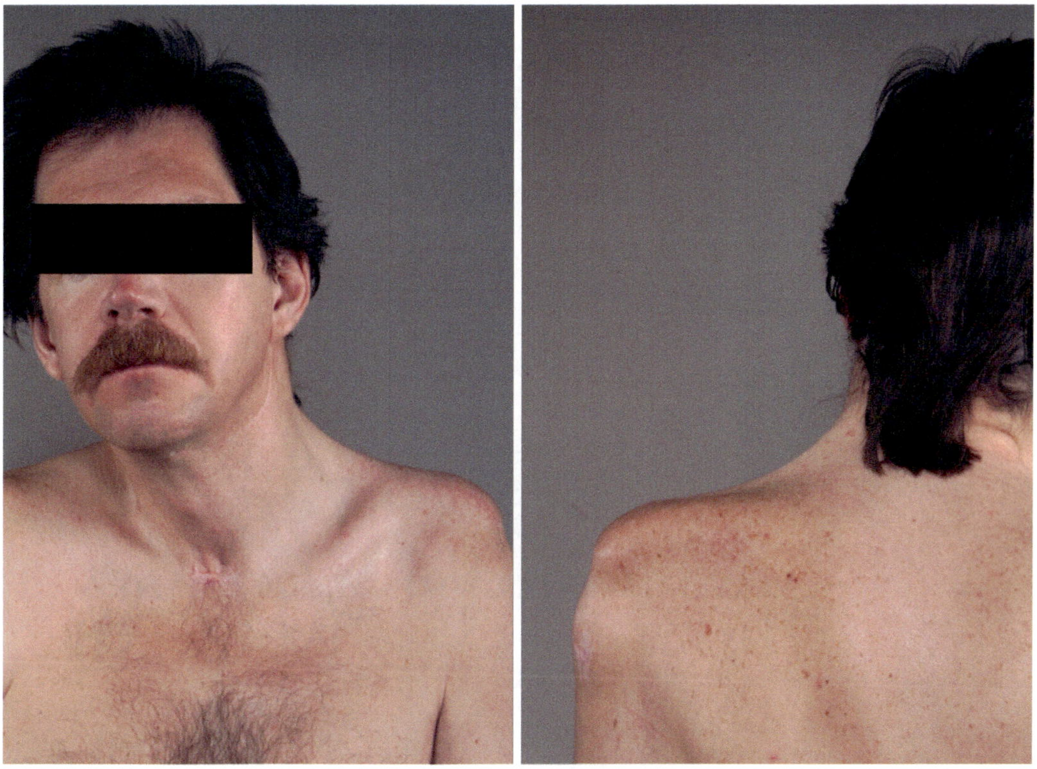

Fig. 7.4 Patient with severe brachial plexus injury with trapezius weakness from spinal accessory nerve injury with torticollis secondary to trauma to paracervical muscles

the expert surgeon, use of an exam template is recommended, to ensure there are not any missed muscle groups or exam parts. It is our preference to use the Mayo Clinic Brachial Plexus Nerve Muscle Record sheet (Fig. 7.2), which systematically lists muscle groups by nerve innervation and allows for easy serial exam referencing and recording. Some muscles are difficult to grade or examine consistently (i.e., serratus anterior, teres major) or cannot be readily examined (pectoralis minor, coracobrachialis) or have other muscle groups that perform the same function and are difficult to isolate (infraspinatus, supraspinatus, deltoid). This makes it even more imperative to have a consistent examiner and method of examination.

Exam is performed by examination of muscles in order of innervation from lowest cervical root to the first thoracic root. Thus, shoulder, chest, back, elbow flexors, wrist flexors, elbow extensors, wrist extensors, and hand function are examined sequentially. This nicely follows the Mayo Clinic Brachial Plexus Nerve Muscle Record.

Trapezius function (cranial nerve XI, spinal accessory nerve) is evaluated with a shoulder shrug, observing from both anterior and posterior sides (Fig. 7.5). Symmetry is evaluated as well as the strength of cephalad motion. The superior, middle, and lower trapezius function is recorded. Levator scapulae (dorsal scapular nerve) are not often examined; however, when it is examined, the head is rotated away from the injured side and flexed. The patient is then asked to position his head in neutral rotation and flexion. Weakness is consistent with dorsal scapular injury. Rhomboids (dorsal scapular nerve) are tested by having the patient attempt to touch his shoulder blades together, and symmetry is observed. While subtle, rhomboid paralysis can lead to a slight tilting of the head toward the injured side.

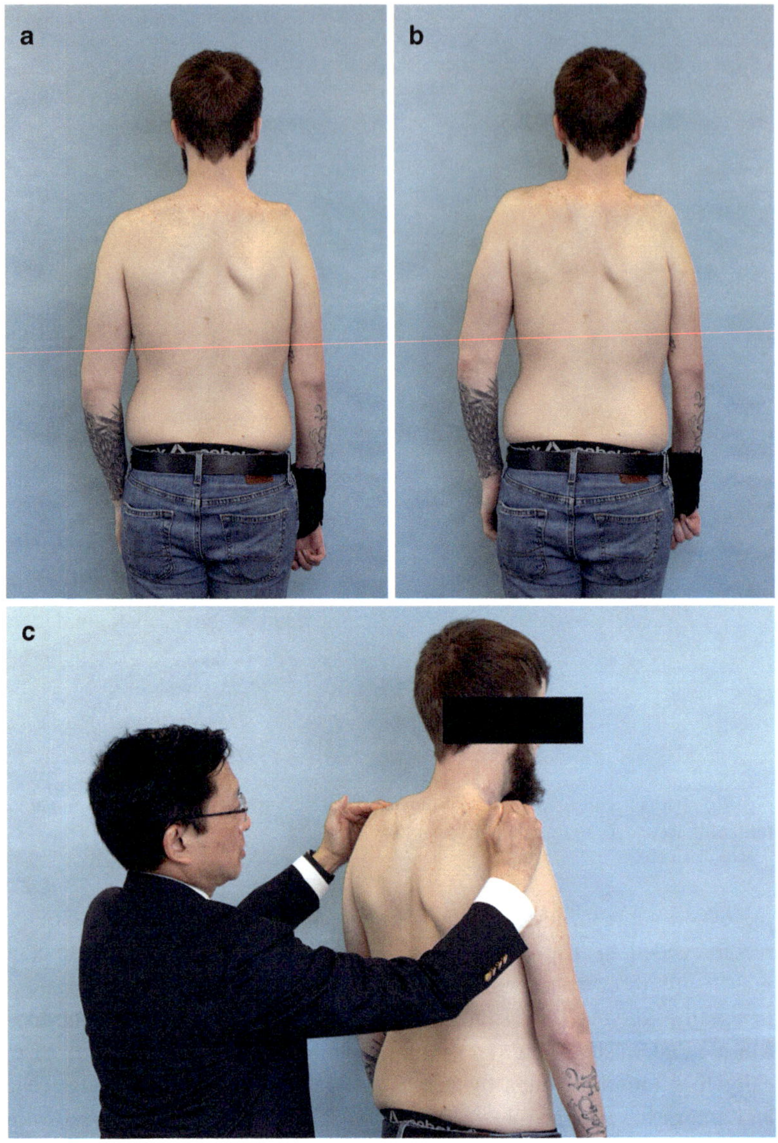

Fig. 7.5 The trapezius is examined by having the patient shrug his shoulders (**a**, **b**). As well as with resistance (**c**)

The shoulder is one of the most complicated joints to examine secondary to the numerous muscles about the shoulder with often similar functions. This needs to be considered when trying to isolate specific muscles. The supraspinatus (suprascapular nerve) is evaluated by forward flexing and/or abduction of the shoulder typically below 90 degrees of forward flexion or abduction. Occasionally, the supraspinatus is powerful enough to give the patient full shoulder forward flexion and abduction. The infraspinatus (suprascapular nerve) is evaluated by holding the arm adducted to the body with the elbow flexed 90 degrees and asking the patient to externally rotate his shoulder (Fig. 7.6). The serratus anterior muscle (long thoracic nerve) is a complicated muscle to examine. Its purpose is to stabilize the scapula against the posterior thorax when the arm is forward flexed or abducted. Isolated serratus anterior palsy is relatively easy to examine, as the scapula wings when the patient loads the forward flexed arm (exam is performed by asking patient to do a push-up against the wall) (Fig. 7.7). However, as part of a brachial plexus injury, this

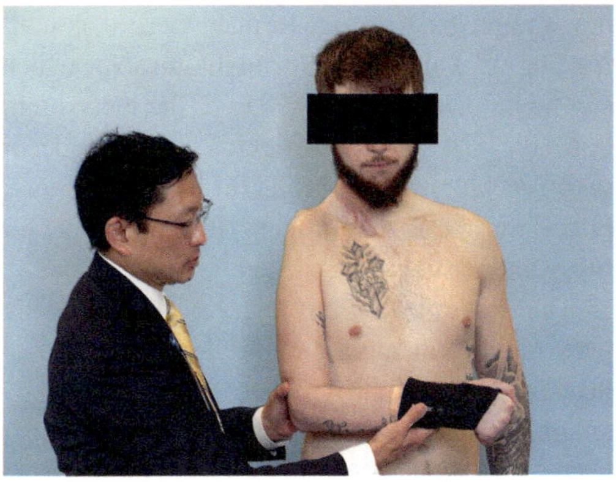

Fig. 7.6 Infraspinatus is examined by adducting the upper arm to the side of the body and placing the forearm against the abdomen. The patient is asked to externally rotate the arm off the abdomen

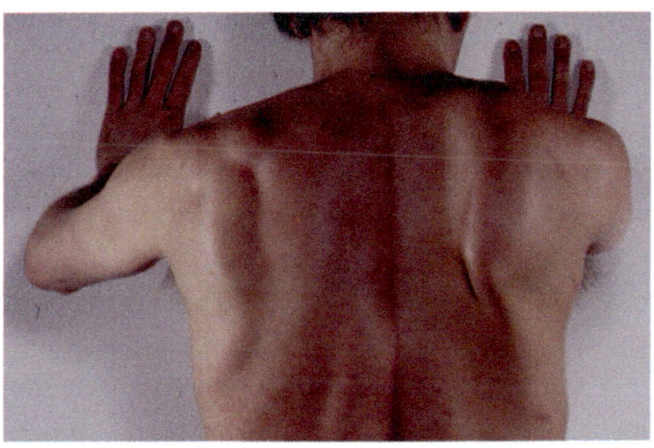

Fig. 7.7 In isolated serratus anterior weakness, pushing on a wall in a push-up-type position results in the scapula winging

exam finding can be subtle. The inferior corner of the scapula is palpated, and the examiner's fingers are held over it. The examiner's other hand pushes the shoulder posteriorly (Fig. 7.8). If the serratus anterior has function, the inferior corner and scapula are felt to stabilize against the thorax. If the serratus does not function, the inferior corner and scapula are pushed posteriorly.

The subscapularis muscle (upper and lower subscapular nerves) is an internal rotator of the shoulder along with the teres major and latissimus dorsi. To isolate the subscapularis muscle, the palm of the hand is placed on the abdomen, the elbow is brought anterior (to neutralize the latissimus dorsi and teres major), and the patient is asked to push his hand into his abdomen while the examiner resists this maneuver (Fig. 7.9). The teres major (lower subscapular nerve) is difficult to isolate and is an internal rotator and adductor of the shoulder and is typically examined along with the latissimus dorsi muscle (long thoracic nerve). The pectoralis muscles are next examined. The clavicular (upper) head of the pectoralis muscle is innervated by the lateral pectoral nerve, while the sternal (lower) head is innervated by the medial pectoral nerve. The pectoral muscles are adductors of the arm. To test the pectoralis muscles, the patient is asked to push his hands together with the elbows extended. The upper and lower portions of the muscle are pal-

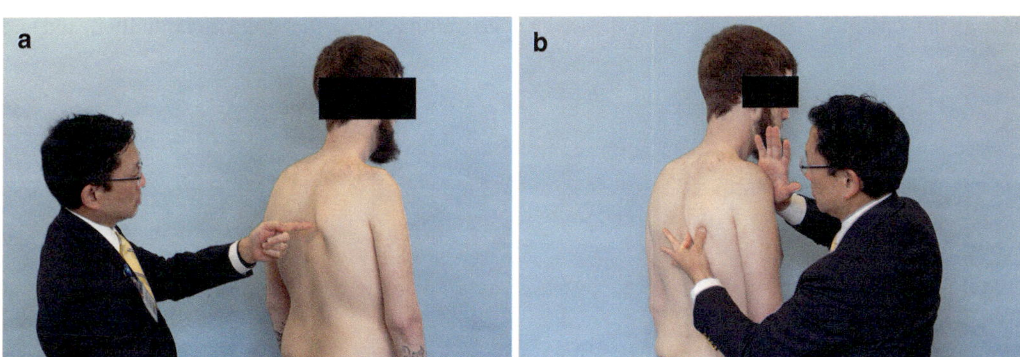

Fig. 7.8 In global brachial plexus injury, or C5–C7 injury, the serratus anterior exam is more subtle and difficult. In a thin patient, the scapula can be seen winging (**a**). The inferior corner of the scapula is palpated, and a posterior directed force is applied to the anterior shoulder, which forces the scapula posteriorly. If the serratus anterior fires, the scapula is forced to the rib cage. If the serratus is weak or paralyzed, the scapula is translated posteriorly with this maneuver (**b**)

pated and tested (Fig. 7.10). The latissimus dorsi presence can be quickly ascertained by the cough test (Fig. 7.11a). The cough test is performed by the examiner placing both hands under the posterior fold of the arm and asking the patient to cough. There will be an involuntary contraction of the latissimus dorsi muscles if they are functioning. To grade the strength, the arm is extended and the patient asked to hold his hand against the gluteal region (Fig. 7.11b). The examiner abducts the arm to evaluate the latissimus dorsi strength.

The biceps and brachialis (musculocutaneous nerve) are elbow flexors, with the biceps also being a supinator of the forearm. The biceps tendon should be palpated to make sure it is contracting as well as the brachialis muscle, which can be palpated on either side of the biceps tendon (Fig. 7.12). Elbow flexion can also occur with brachioradialis or forearm flexor (Steindler effect) muscle activation; thus, it is imperative for the examiner not to be tricked.

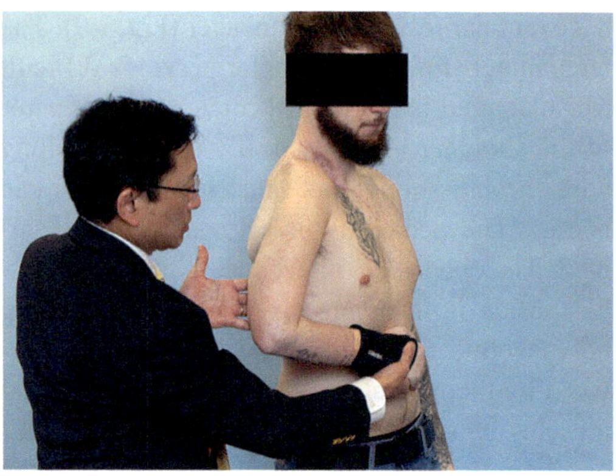

Fig. 7.9 The subscapularis muscle is examined by placing the patient's hand on his abdomen, bringing his elbow forward and having the patient push in against his abdomen. Alternatively, the hand can be placed on the small of the back, and the patient is asked to elevate his hand off the small of his back

The deltoid (axillary nerve) is classically divided into an anterior, middle, and posterior head. Function of the deltoid can be mimicked by an intact supraspinatus, and thus the examiner needs to make sure the muscle is actually firing and activating with motion. The bulk and tone of the muscle should be evaluated. Forward flexion, abduction, and extension are examined. For weak or reinnervating axillary nerve injuries, the arm is placed by the patient's side and the patient is asked to abduct or forward flex while the examiner's thumb and index fingers are placed around the deltoid to feel for contraction (Fig. 7.13a). A sensitive test for posterior deltoid function is the swallowtail test described by Nishijima et al. [20]. In this test the patient leans forward and extends the shoulders (Fig. 7.13b). A lag in extension is a sign for posterior deltoid weakness.

Exam of the median nerve motor function includes exam of the pronator quadratus, pronator teres, flexor carpi radialis, flexor digitorum profundus of index/middle, flexor digitorum superficialis, flexor pollicis longus and brevis, abductor pollicis brevis, opponens, and index and middle finger lumbricals. The pronator quadratus is examined with the elbow maximally flexed and

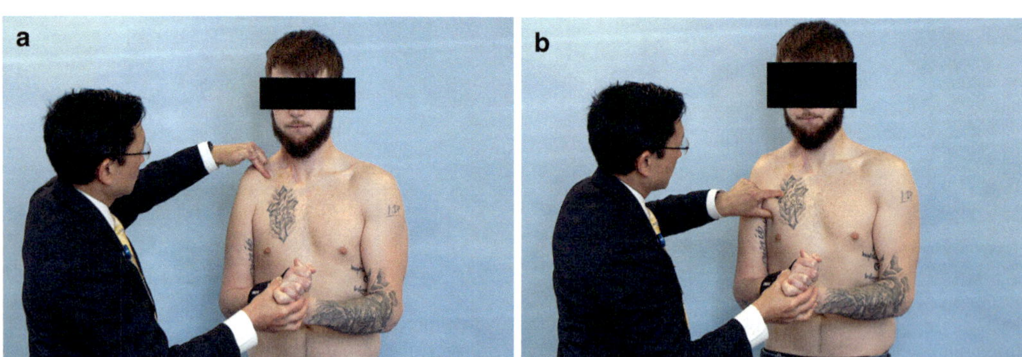

Fig. 7.10 The pectoralis muscles (clavicular (**a**) and sternal (**b**)) are examined by having the patient adduct his arm to his side while the examiner palpates both heads of the muscle

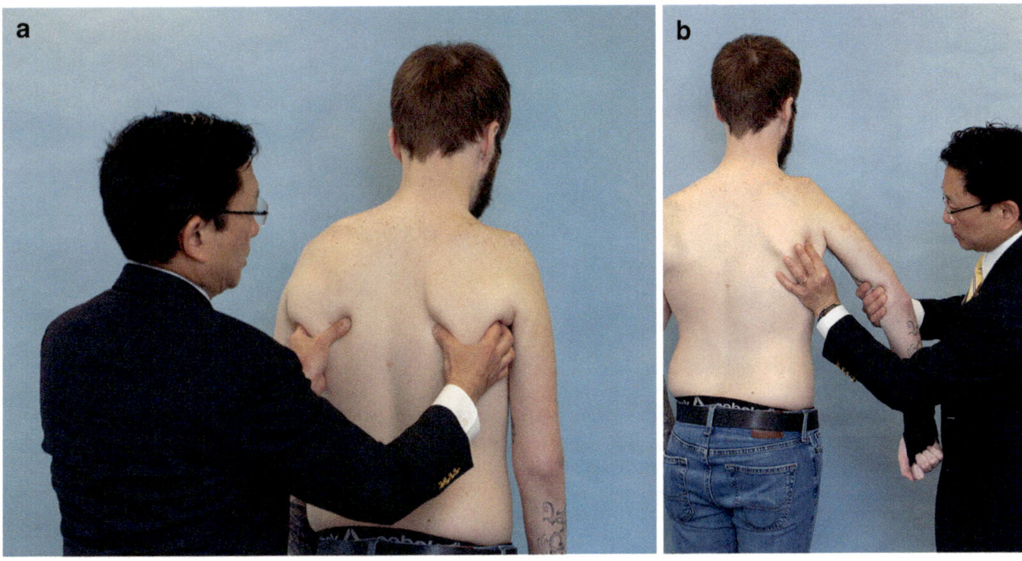

Fig. 7.11 (**a**). A quick screening test of the function of bilateral latissimus dorsi muscles is the cough test (**a**). The examiner holds the latissimus muscles from behind and asks the patient to cough. The cough results in an involuntary contraction of the muscle which is palpated. To grade the strength of the muscle, the hand is placed on the gluteal region with the elbow extended, and the patient is asked to maintain this position while the examiner abducts the arm (**b**)

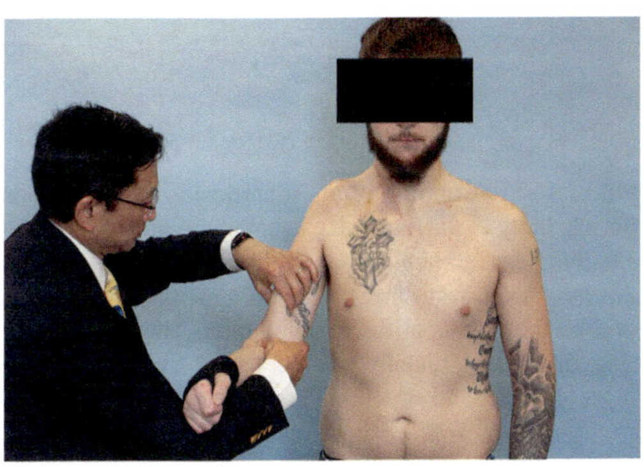

Fig. 7.12 The biceps tendon is palpated to ensure it is firing and elbow flexion not occurring through the brachioradialis. The brachialis muscle can be palpated on either side of the biceps tendon

the forearm in supination. The patient pronates his forearm while the examiner resists this motion (if possible). Pronator teres is examined with the elbow extended in a similar fashion. The flexor carpi radialis is the radial wrist flexor. It is tested by resisted wrist flexion. The fingers should be kept extended, and tendon of the flexor carpi radialis should be palpated to ensure that the wrist flexion is not occurring through another wrist flexor (palmaris longus or flexor carpi ulnaris) (Fig. 7.14). The flexor digitorum profundus of the index and middle finger is isolated by holding the proximal interphalangeal joints of the fingers extended while the patient flexes the distal interphalangeal joints (Fig. 7.15). The flexor digitorum superficialis has a common muscle belly and flexes the fingers at the proximal interphalangeal joint. To isolate the superficialis, the index, ring, and small fingers are kept fully extended and the patient is asked to flex the middle finger (Fig. 7.16). The palmaris longus is just ulnar to the flexor carpi radialis muscle and can be absent in up to 16% of individuals. The easiest way to identify it is to have the patient flex the wrist while touching his thumb to the small finger (Fig. 7.17). The flexor pollicis longus is the only flexor of the interphalangeal joint of the thumb. It is isolated and examined by stabilizing the proximal phalanx of the thumb and while the patient attempts to flex the distal joint of the thumb (Fig. 7.18). The flexor pollicis brevis is one of three thenar muscles, and it has a deep and super-

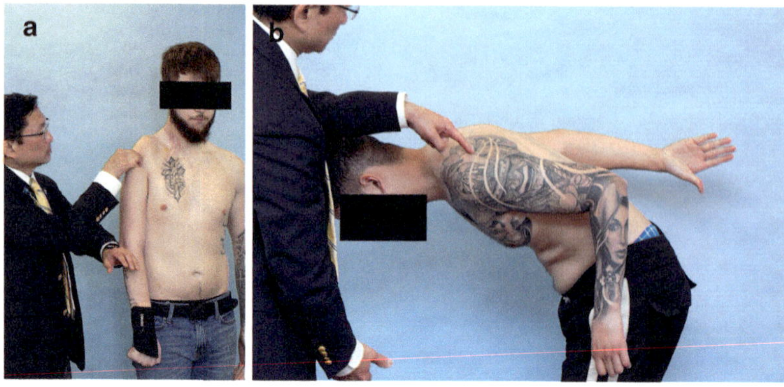

Fig. 7.13 (**a**). The deltoid is palpated with two fingers, and the patient asked to abduct or forward flex the arm. The contraction of the deltoid can be felt. (**b**). To examine posterior deltoid function, the swallowtail test is performed. The patient leans forward and extends his shoulders. If there is weakness or no function, this test demonstrates an asymmetry to the normal side

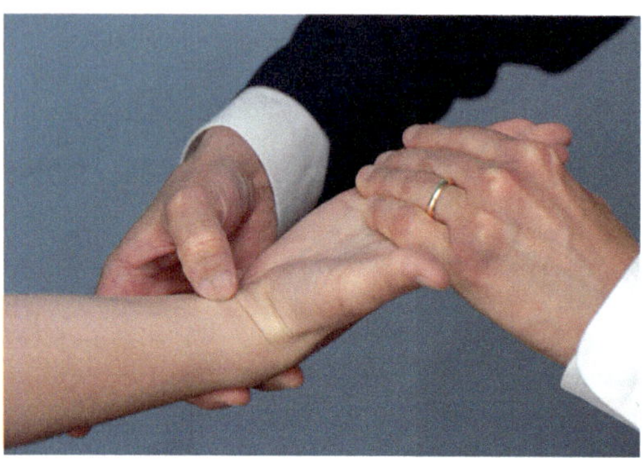

Fig. 7.14 The flexor carpi radialis is palpated with resisted wrist flexion while the patient (if able) keeps his fingers extended (to eliminate wrist flexion from finger flexors)

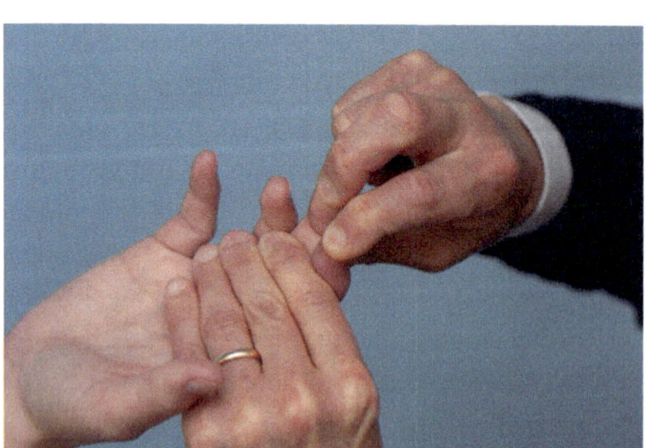

Fig. 7.15 The median nerve-innervated flexor digitorum profundus of the index and middle fingers is tested by blocking the metacarpophalangeal joint and proximal interphalangeal joint in extension while the patient flexes the index and middle finger. The ulnar-innervated profundus tendons are tested similarly

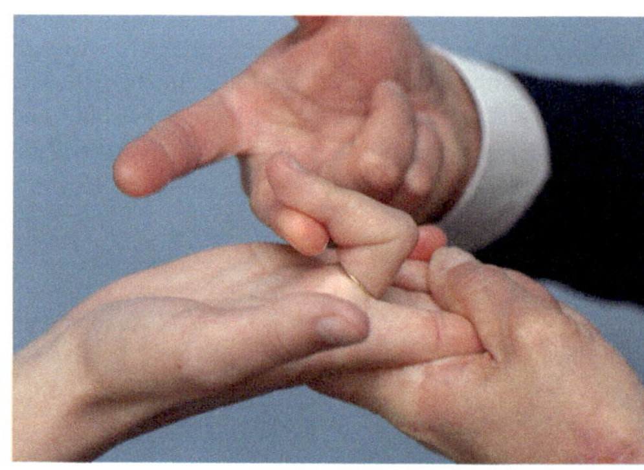

Fig. 7.16 Flexor digitorum superficialis is a common muscle belly to the digits. By keeping the index, ring, and small fingers fully extended, the flexor digitorum profundus is blocked from flexing the digits with the exception of the superficialis of the middle finger. Alternatively, the ring finger superficialis can be tested by blocking the index, middle, and small finger in full extension

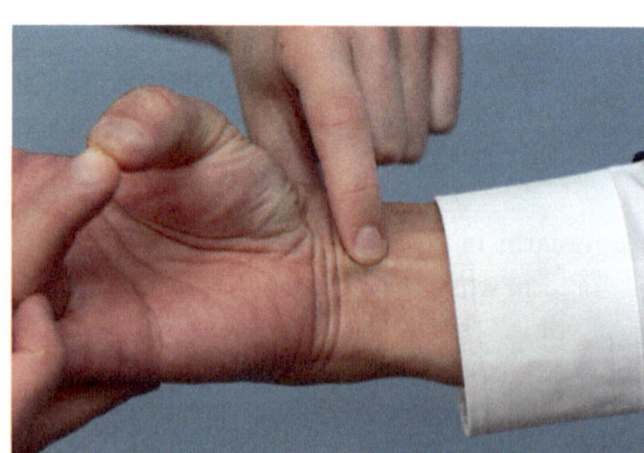

Fig. 7.17 The palmaris longus is best tested with wrist flexion while the patient opposes the thumb to the small finger if possible

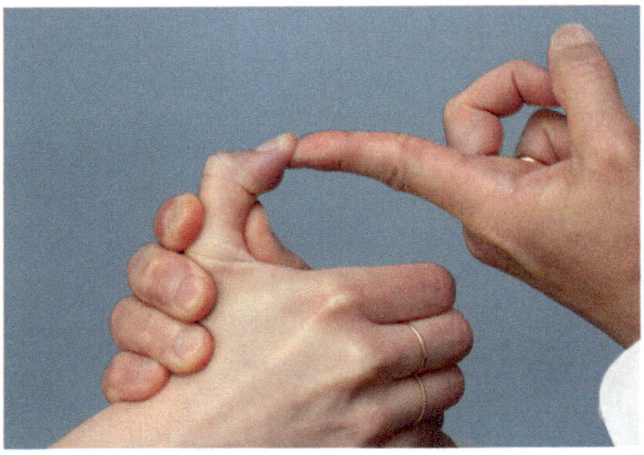

Fig. 7.18 The flexor pollicis longus is tested by blocking the thumb at the metacarpophalangeal joint and having the patient flex the thumb tip

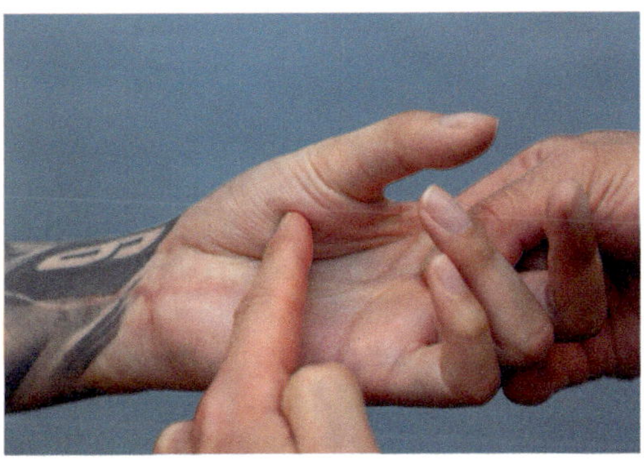

Fig. 7.19 Thenar muscles include the flexor pollicis brevis, opponens, and abductor pollicis brevis. The flexor pollicis brevis has median and ulnar nerve innervation that is difficult to separate. The three muscles are often examined as a unit. The hand is supinated on the table and the patient asked to point the tip of his thumb to the ceiling. The thenar muscles are palpated, and resistance is applied to push the thumb tip radially and toward the table

ficial head. The superficial head is innervated by the median nerve, while the deep head is innervated by the ulnar nerve; it flexes the thumb at the metacarpophalangeal joint and assists in opposition of the thumb as well. It is difficult to distinguish which head is firing clinically. The opponens pollicis produces opposition of the thumb and works with the other thenar muscles. The abductor pollicis brevis is the third thenar muscle. The flexor pollicis brevis, opponens, and abductor pollicis brevis are typically tested as a group by flexion of the thumb at the metacarpophalangeal joint, palmar abduction, and opposition to the small finger (Fig. 7.19). The last median nerve-innervated muscle to be tested is the lumbricals of the index and middle finger, also known as the first and second lumbrical. The lumbrical flexes the metacarpophalangeal joint and extends the interphalangeal joint. They are tested by having the patient flex the metacarpophalangeal joint 90 degrees while extending the interphalangeal joint fully (Fig. 7.20).

The terminal branches of the radial nerve are next tested and include the triceps, supinator, brachioradialis, extensor carpi radialis longus and brevis, extensor carpi ulnaris, extensor digitorum communis, extensor digitorum minimi, extensor digitorum proprius, extensor pollicis longus and brevis, and abductor pollicis longus. The triceps should be tested for antigravity strength by abducting/forward flexing the shoulder above horizontal and asking the patient to extend his elbow (Fig. 7.21). If unable to overcome gravity,

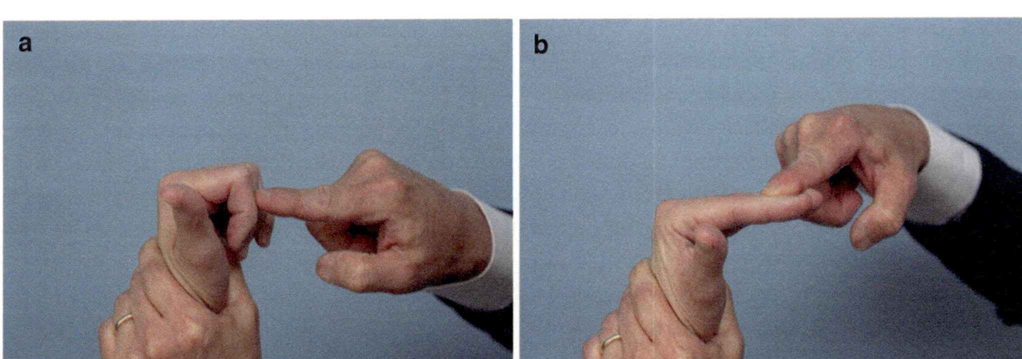

Fig. 7.20 The lumbricals are tested by having the patient hold his metacarpophalangeal joints at 90 degrees with the proximal interphalangeal joints fully flexed (**a**), and then the patient is asked to extend the proximal interphalangeal joint. Palmarly directed force is applied to the middle phalanx to test the strength of the lumbricals (**b**)

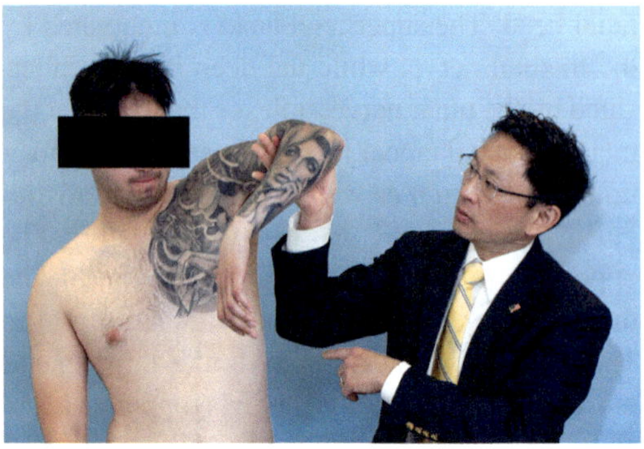

Fig. 7.21 Triceps are examined by placing the arm overhead and asking the patient to extend his elbow. If the patient cannot do this secondary to limitation of shoulder motion, an antigravity position is chosen (patient leaning to one side). Strength is tested by flexing the elbow to 90 degrees and having the patient extend while resistance is applied

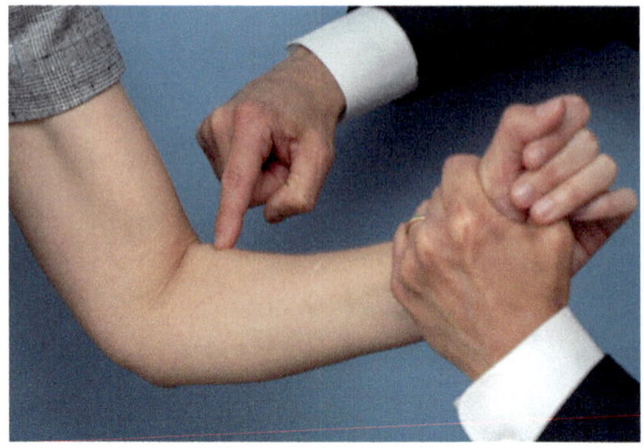

Fig. 7.22 Brachioradialis is tested by having the patient isometrically contract the elbow at 90 degrees. The muscle of the brachioradialis can been seen and palpated. The brachioradialis typically fires concomitantly with the triceps, so if there is no triceps function, the examiner needs to stabilize the forearm for the brachioradialis to fire

the upper arm is placed parallel to the ground and the patient asked to extend with gravity eliminated. When testing a strong triceps, it should be tested starting at less than 90 degrees of flexion, asking the patient to fully extend with the examiner resisting the extension. A locked elbow in extension may falsely give the examiner the impression the triceps is much stronger than it really is. Supinator function is tested with the elbow extended (to eliminate biceps from supinating the forearm), forearm fully pronated, and the patient asked to supinate the forearm. Brachioradialis is tested by resisting elbow flexion at 90 degrees of flexion (Fig. 7.22). Wrist extensors are examined by having the patient extend and radially deviate the wrist (extensor carpi radialis longus) and extending the wrist in neutral (extensor carpi radialis brevis). When the patient can only extend and radially deviate the wrist, the extensor carpi radialis brevis is not firing. The base of the second (insertion of extensor carpi radialis longus) and third metacarpals (insertion of extensor carpi radialis brevis) can be palpated to feel tendon tension if it is uncertain which of the wrist extensors is firing. Extensor digitorum communis is examined by having the patient extend his lesser digits. The extensor indicis proprius is examined by having the patient make a fist and only extending the index finger. Similarly, the extensor digiti minimi is examined by having the patient make a fist and extending the small finger. The extensor pollicis longus is examined by placing the hand flat on the table and having the patient lift the thumb off the table (Fig. 7.23). Alternatively, the examiner can block the metacarpophalangeal joint in extension and have the patient extend the interphalangeal joint of the thumb. Extensor pollicis brevis and the abductor pollicis longus extend and abduct the thumb metacarpal and the carpometacarpal joint, respectively.

The last part of the motor exam is examination of the ulnar nerve-mediated muscles of the forearm and hand which include the flexor carpi ulnaris, flexor digitorum of the ring and small finger, abductor digiti minimi, adductor pollicis, the dorsal and palmar interossei, the third and fourth lumbricals, and the flexor pollicis brevis. The flexor carpi ulnaris is tested by wrist flexion with ulnar deviation. If there is difficulty ascertaining if the flexor carpi ulnaris is actually firing, the tendon of the muscle just proximal to the pisiform can be palpated to confirm its activation (Fig. 7.24). Abductor digiti minimi is tested by having the patient abduct the small finger with the digit fully

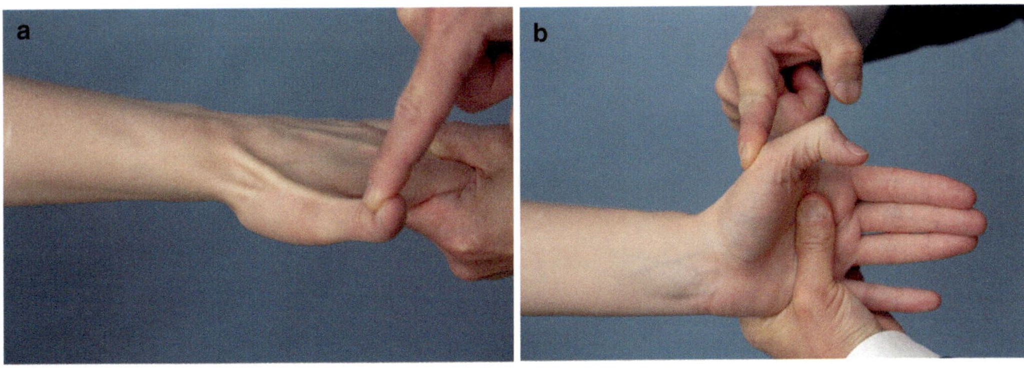

Fig. 7.23 The extensor pollicis longus is the only muscle than can lift the thumb off the table when the hand is placed palm side down (**a**). Alternatively, the thumb axis can be stabilized, and the patient is asked to extend the interphalangeal joint. The abductor pollicis longus and extensor pollicis brevis are examined by asking the patient to abduct and extend the metacarpophalangeal joint of the thumb (**b**)

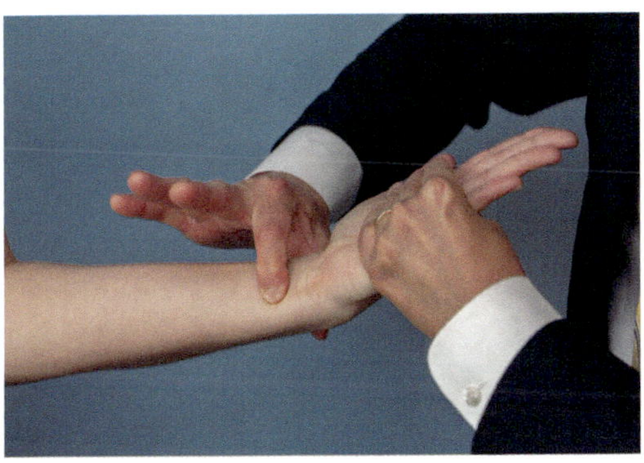

Fig. 7.24 The flexor carpi ulnaris is examined by having the wrist flexed with fingers extended while palpating the tendon at the level of the pisiform

extended. The adductor pollicis is one of three muscles that adducts the thumb. The opponens and flexor pollicis brevis also adduct the thumb, thus making examination of the adductor pollicis difficult to isolate (Fig. 7.24). The first dorsal interosseous abducts the index finger and can be tested by having the patient extend and radially abduct the index finger (Fig. 7.25). Adduction and abduction of the fingers in extension test the palmar and dorsal interossei, respectively. The lumbricals flex the metacarpophalangeal joint and extend the interphalangeal joint (Fig. 7.26). They are tested by having the patient flex the metacarpophalangeal joint 90 degrees while extending the interphalangeal joint fully (Fig. 7.20).

Vascular Exam

As severity of BPI increases, so does the risk of associated vascular injuries [21]. The association of vascular injuries has been shown to be relatively high with closed, blunt injury in BP patients, and concomitant BPI and vascular injury correlate with worse long-term disability, morbidity, and mortality [22, 23]. The incidence of a major vascular injury associated with a BPI has been shown to be between 13% and 23% [4, 22, 24]. The vascular structures typically affected include the subclavian and axillary arteries and veins [13, 23, 24].

Surgeons should have a high index of suspicion of vascular injury when evaluating patients with BPI as 5–15% of patients with upper extremity trauma and concurrent vascular injuries can present with an initially normal pulse examination [22]. Unrecognized vascular injury can potentially cause irreversible limb ischemia, loss of limb, and a worse prognosis. There are "hard" signs that can alert the examiner to the increased risk of vascular injury in upper extremity trauma,

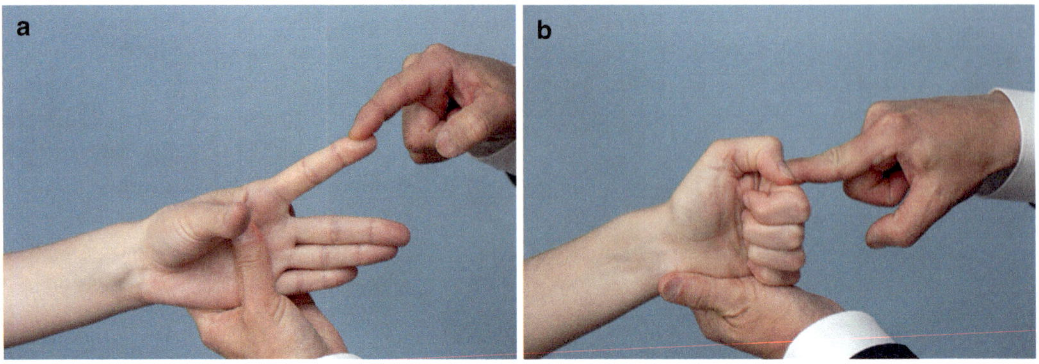

Fig. 7.25 First dorsal interosseous is examined by having the index finger radially abducted (**a**). It can also be palpated. The adductor can be tested with a key pinch maneuver, where the patient makes a fist and uses the thumb to pinch against the radial aspect of the index finger. Weakness is demonstrated by a Froment's sign (**b**) (flexion of the interphalangeal joint and supination of the thumb)

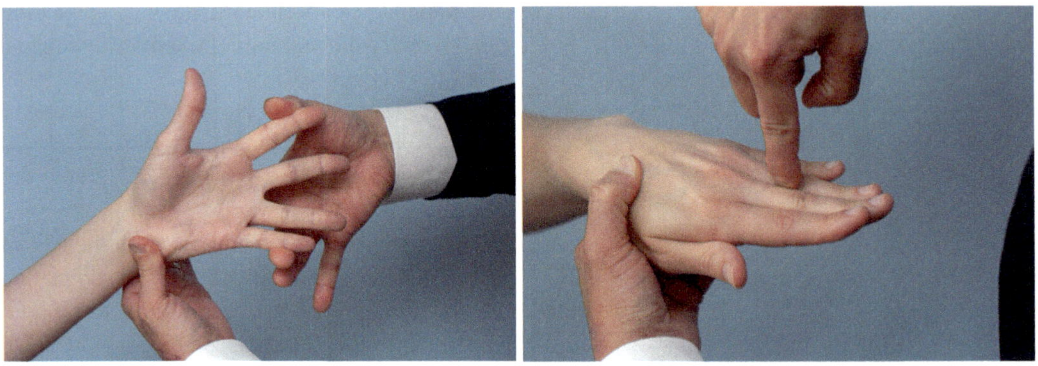

Fig. 7.26 Palmar interossei adduct the digits, and the dorsal interossei abduct the digits. With the hand flat on a table, the patient is asked to abduct and adduct the digits. Strength can be tested by having the patient hold the digits adducted while the examiner tries to push his finger between the patient's fingers

including findings such as pulselessness, rapidly expanding hematomas in the supra- or infraclavicular fossae, obvious acute bleeding, and pallor. Unfortunately in the setting of a BPI, signs such as paresthesias, pain, and paralysis can occur due to nerve or vascular injury and may not reliably indicate one or the other, but should be considered when evaluating for either injury.

The vascular exam in BP patients should begin with palpation of the ulnar and radial pulses in addition to evaluation of capillary refill. If pulses are unable to be palpated, Doppler ultrasonography should be utilized. Auscultation of the supraclavicular and infraclavicular fossae may also be performed to assess for thrills or bruits which can be indicative of major vascular injury [3, 22]. Another noninvasive tool that can be used in evaluation is the arterial pressure index (API), which is the ratio of the systolic blood pressure in the injured limb to that of the systolic pressure of the uninjured limb. An API of greater than 0.90 is considered normal. Ratios below this threshold should prompt further workup. If a vascular injury is highly suspected and/or the patient has a concerning exam, or API <0.90, angiography, though more invasive, is the gold standard diagnostic study of choice for evaluating vascular injuries of the affected extremity. This can be done with a conventional computed tomography angiography (CTA), digital subtraction angiography (DSA), or magnetic resonance (MR) angiography [13, 22]. A CTA is fast, is commonly utilized, and has high sensitivity and specificity for detecting vascular injury. CTA is a good first choice diagnostic treatment modality; however, should the study be inconclusive despite a high index of suspicion, or if vascular intervention is necessary, a DSA may be a more preferable choice given it can provide both diagnostic and therapeutic utility. Vascular injury should initiate a prompt consultation with vascular surgery colleagues. If the patient is taken to the operating room for emergent exploration or repair of vascular structures, it may be appropriate to proceed with an initial brachial plexus exploration after vascular status is addressed and if the patient is stable. Finally, angiography studies are also helpful when planning for long-term reconstructive options. In such cases, the success of free functioning muscle transfer depends on adequate patency of recipient vasculature, such as the thoracoacromial trunk of the injured limb [2].

Deafferentation Pain

Attention to the development of neuropathic type pain is key as this can significantly affect the patient's quality of life, and recognition of this pain is an integral part of the patient's care. Patients with BPIs can experience severe, unremitting pain following nerve root avulsions, known as deafferentation pain, or pain in the deafferented extremity [25, 26]. The quality of pain experienced due to deafferentation in BP patients is commonly characterized as burning or crushing and is constant with intermittent paroxysms of sharper, shooting pain as well. The pain occurs at night and throughout the day and has been shown to worsen in cases of increased emotional or psychologic stress or tension; patients may grasp their arm or massage it to help improve the pain [15, 25, 27]. These paroxysms of more abrupt, lightning-type pain can have some consistency in quality and location and may occur frequently such as every few minutes, or infrequently such as every few days. Neuropathic pain is more frequent than causalgia pain and occurs more commonly in patients with root avulsion injuries [27]. Cold sensitivity has also been described in BP patients. Deafferentation pain can occur in a paralytic limb, is different than phantom limb pain, and may be extremely limiting for patients and cause significant prevention or delay of return to work and hobbies. It should be treated in conjunction with a pain clinic to provide coordinated efforts from different subspecialties to best address this difficult and debilitating problem.

Spinal Cord Injury

Ruling out compromise of the spinal cord is important; suspicion arises if the lower extremities are affected. Though rare, and often difficult to diagnose, patients with brachial plexus injuries may have concomitant injuries of the spinal cord. Spinal cord injuries can present with symptoms consistent with complete cord transections, anterior cord syndrome, Brown-Sequard syndrome, or mixed lesions [4]. Evaluation of motor function, sensory, and reflexes in the lower extremities is imperative in patients with BPIs. Upper motor neuron signs such as hyperreflexia can assist with diagnosis of these dual injury patterns. Brown-Sequard syndrome is associated with root avulsion-type injuries and will present with signs and symptoms consistent with hemitransection of the cord. This typically manifests with weakness in motor function and deficits in proprioception and vibratory sensation on the ipsilateral side of the injury. This is due to injury to the corticospinal tract and dorsal columns. On the contralateral side of the injury, the patient may experience hypoesthesia with deficits in pain and temperature sensation below the level of the injury due to insult to the spinothalamic tract. Depending on the severity of cord injury endured, these deficits may be permanent or transient [4, 28, 29]. If there is suspicion for spinal cord injury, prompt consultation with Neurology should be instituted.

References

1. Haymaker W, Woodhall B. Peripheral nerve injuries: principles of diagnosis. Philadelphia: W. B. Saunders Company; 1945.
2. Noland SS, et al. Adult Traumatic Brachial Plexus Injuries. J Am Acad Orthop Surg. 2019;27(19):705–16.
3. Spinner RJ, et al. In: Wolfe SW, et al., editors. Traumatic brachial plexus injury, in green's operative hand surgery. Philadelphia: Elsevier; 2017.
4. Rhee PC, et al. Concomitant traumatic spinal cord and brachial plexus injuries in adult patients. J Bone Joint Surg Am. 2011;93(24):2271–7.
5. D'Aubigne M, Deburge A. Etiology, development and prognosis of traumatic paralysis of the brachial plexus. Rev Chir Orthop Reparatrice Appar Mot. 1967;53(1):23–42.
6. Shin AY, et al. Adult traumatic brachial plexus injuries. J Am Acad Orthop Surg. 2005;13(6):382–96.
7. James MA. Use of the Medical Research Council muscle strength grading system in the upper extremity. J Hand Surg Am. 2007;32(2):154–6.
8. MacAvoy MC, Green DP. Critical reappraisal of Medical Research Council muscle testing for elbow flexion. J Hand Surg Am. 2007;32(2):149–53.
9. Seddon HJ. In: Seddon HJ, editor. Peripheral Nerve Injuries. Medical Research Council Special Report Series, No. 282. London: Her Majesty's Stationary Office; 1954.
10. Shahgholi L, et al. A comparison of manual and quantitative elbow strength testing. Am J Phys Med Rehabil. 2012;91(10):856–62.
11. Maldonado AA, et al. Free functioning gracilis muscle transfer versus intercostal nerve transfer to musculocutaneous nerve for restoration of elbow flexion after traumatic adult brachial pan-plexus injury. Plast Reconstr Surg. 2016;138(3):483e–8e.
12. Htut M, et al. Pain phenomena and sensory recovery following brachial plexus avulsion injury and surgical repairs. J Hand Surg Br. 2006;31(6):596–605.
13. Limthongthang R, et al. Adult brachial plexus injury: evaluation and management. Orthop Clin North Am. 2013;44(4):591–603.
14. Maffi TR, et al. Enhanced survival using the distally based sural artery interpolation flap. Ann Plast Surg. 2005;54(3):302–5.
15. Birch R, Bonney G, Wynn Parry CB. Surgical disorders of the peripheral nerves. London: Churchill Livingstone; 1998.
16. Birch R, Quick T. In: Wolfe SW, et al., editors. Nerve injury and repair, in green's operative hand surgery. Philadelphia: Elsevier; 2017.
17. Gummesson C, Atroshi I, Ekdahl C. The disabilities of the arm, shoulder and hand (DASH) outcome questionnaire: longitudinal construct validity and measuring self-rated health change after surgery. BMC Musculoskelet Disord. 2003;4:11.
18. Heck CV, Hendryson IE, Rowe CR. Joint motion – method of measuring and recording. Chicago: American Academy of Orthopaedic Surgeons; 1965.
19. Suh N, et al. Trick elbow motions in patients with brachial plexus injuries. J Hand Surg Am. 2014;39(11):2312–4.
20. Nishijma N, et al. The swallow-tail sign: a test of deltoid function. J Bone Joint Surg Br. 1995;77(1):152–3.
21. Huang AE, et al. Outcomes of reconstructive surgery in traumatic brachial plexus injury with concomitant vascular injury. World Neurosurg. 2020;135:e350–7.
22. Lebowitz C, Matzon JL. Arterial injury in the upper extremity: evaluation, strategies, and anticoagulation management. Hand Clin. 2018;34(1):85–95.
23. Johnson SF, et al. Brachial plexus injury: association with subclavian and axillary vascular trauma. J Trauma. 1991;31(11):1546–50.
24. Narakas AO. The treatment of brachial plexus injuries. Int Orthop. 1985;9(1):29–36.
25. Thomas DG. Brachial plexus injury: deafferentation pain and dorsal root entry zone (DREZ) coagulation. Clin Neurol Neurosurg. 1993;95(Suppl):S48–9.
26. Parry CB. Pain in avulsion lesions of the brachial plexus. Pain. 1980;9(1):41–53.
27. Zhou Y, et al. The clinical characteristics of neuropathic pain in patients with total brachial plexus avulsion: a 30-case study. Injury. 2016;47(8):1719–24.
28. Chechick A, et al. Brown-Sequard syndrome associated with brachial plexus injury in neck trauma. J Trauma. 1982;22(5):430–1.
29. Oller DW, Boone S. Blunt cervical spine Brown-Sequard injury. A report of three cases. Am Surg. 1991;57(6):361–5.

Adult Brachial Plexus Injuries: Neurodiagnostic Evaluation

8

Brian A. Crum

Introduction

Nerve conduction studies (NCSs) and needle electromyography (EMG) should be considered extensions of the neurologic history and examination of the peripheral sensory and motor systems. NCSs assess large, myelinated sensory and motor nerve fibers. EMG assesses primarily type 1 muscle fibers. Both studies are critical to understanding the distribution and severity of brachial plexus injuries and assist in the surgical teams' approach to intervention [1, 2].

The main reasons to perform NCSs and EMG are to obtain objective evidence of disease within the peripheral nervous system and to assist with localization of the problem. NCSs and EMG can aid in answering several clinical questions: Is the problem focal, multifocal, or diffuse? Does it involve peripheral nerve, neuromuscular junction, or muscle? For conditions affecting the nerve, one can try to assess where along the course of the nerve is the disease (e.g., root, plexus, nerve) and how much of the pathophysiologic mechanism is axonal or demyelinating (or neurapractic). The natural evolution of abnormalities found on EMG can be helpful in determining the timing of a neurologic process and assisting in prognostication (e.g., is there reinnervation occurring?).

B. A. Crum (✉)
Mayo Clinic, Rochester, MN, USA
e-mail: crum.brian@mayo.edu

Anatomy

The main motor neuroanatomical structures that are important in NCSs and EMG are the anterior horn cell in the ventral spinal cord, the motor root and axon of the peripheral nerves, the neuromuscular junction, and the muscle fiber. In the sensory system, the dorsal root ganglion and its peripheral axon to a sensory receptor can be assessed with NCSs. The location of the dorsal root ganglion is an important feature in interpretation of NCSs because preganglionic sensory lesions (e.g., radiculopathy, nerve root avulsion, or a central nervous system process) will not show NCS abnormalities, but postganglionic lesions (e.g., plexopathy or peripheral neuropathy) will show abnormalities on sensory NCSs.

Nerve Conduction Studies

Basic Concepts

NCSs are performed by percutaneously stimulating a peripheral nerve and then recording a response over nerve or muscle. In motor studies the response is recorded over muscle, whereas in sensory studies, the response is recorded at

A. Y. Shin, N. Pulos (eds.), *Operative Brachial Plexus Surgery*,
https://doi.org/10.1007/978-3-030-69517-0_8

another point on the nerve. Various factors are measured in the resulting response, including the amplitude (height) of the response, the conduction velocity, and the distal latency (time from stimulus to onset of response). Attention is also paid to changes in the morphologic pattern of the resulting waveforms with different points of stimulation along the course of the nerve.

Stimulation is performed with a negatively charged stimulator (cathode) applied percutaneously to the nerve being studied. Because the inside of the axon is negatively charged, this stimulation depolarizes the axon and leads to an action potential generated at that point on the nerve. Large, myelinated axons have lower stimulation thresholds. Approximately 2 cm proximal to the cathode on the stimulator is an anode that hyperpolarizes the axon at that point on the nerve; this hyperpolarization can yield a theoretical anodal block. Thus, any component of the initiated action potential that is heading proximally may be blocked.

With increasing stimulus intensity (typically measured in milliamperes), the amplitude (height) of the resulting response increases because of excitation of more and more axons within the nerve up to a point at which a further increase in the stimulus intensity does not lead to an increase in the amplitude of the response. This level of stimulus intensity is called *supramaximal stimulation* and must be attained at each point of stimulation along the nerve to ensure that all axons in the nerve that can be stimulated have been stimulated.

In motor NCSs, the active recording electrode (G1) is placed over the motor end plate of the muscle, which is typically halfway along the course of the muscle. The reference recording electrode (G2) is placed distally over the corresponding tendon. This arrangement allows acquisition of a compound muscle action potential (CMAP) (Fig. 8.1). In sensory NCSs, the recording electrode is placed over the nerve, and the referential electrode is also placed on the nerve, typically 3–4 cm farther away from the recording electrode. The resulting sensory nerve action potential (SNAP) often has a triphasic waveform with an initial downward (positive) deflection (Fig. 8.2). Sensory NCSs can be done *orthodromically* (stimulating distally, recording proximally) or *antidromically* (stimulating proximally, recording distally). A ground electrode is used in all NCSs and EMG and is usually placed at a point between the cathode stimulus and G1.

The CMAP amplitude is generally measured in millivolts. At both proximal and distal sites of stimulation, the CMAP morphologic pattern stays essentially the same without any considerable change or decrease in amplitude. A CMAP response is a measure not only of the motor axon

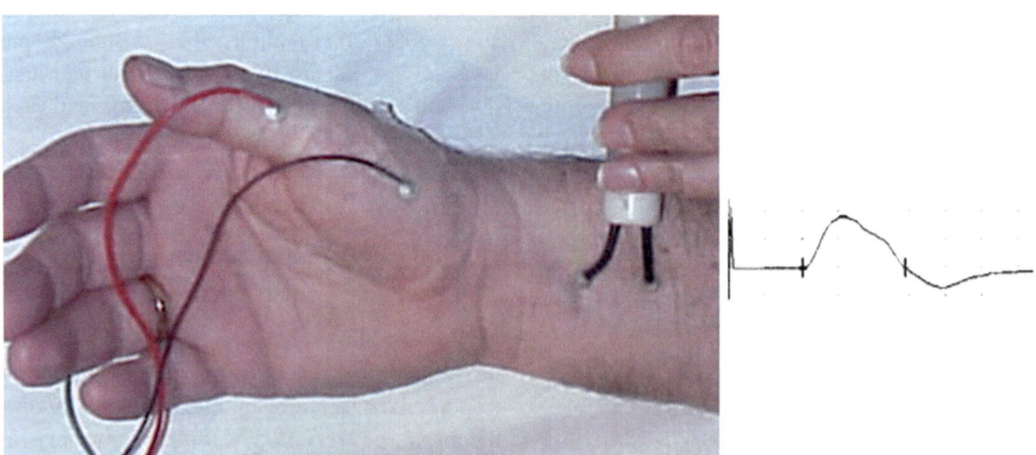

Fig. 8.1 Median motor NCS. Left: Stimulation of median nerve, recording abductor pollicis brevis. Right: Resulting compound muscle action potential (CMAP) waveform

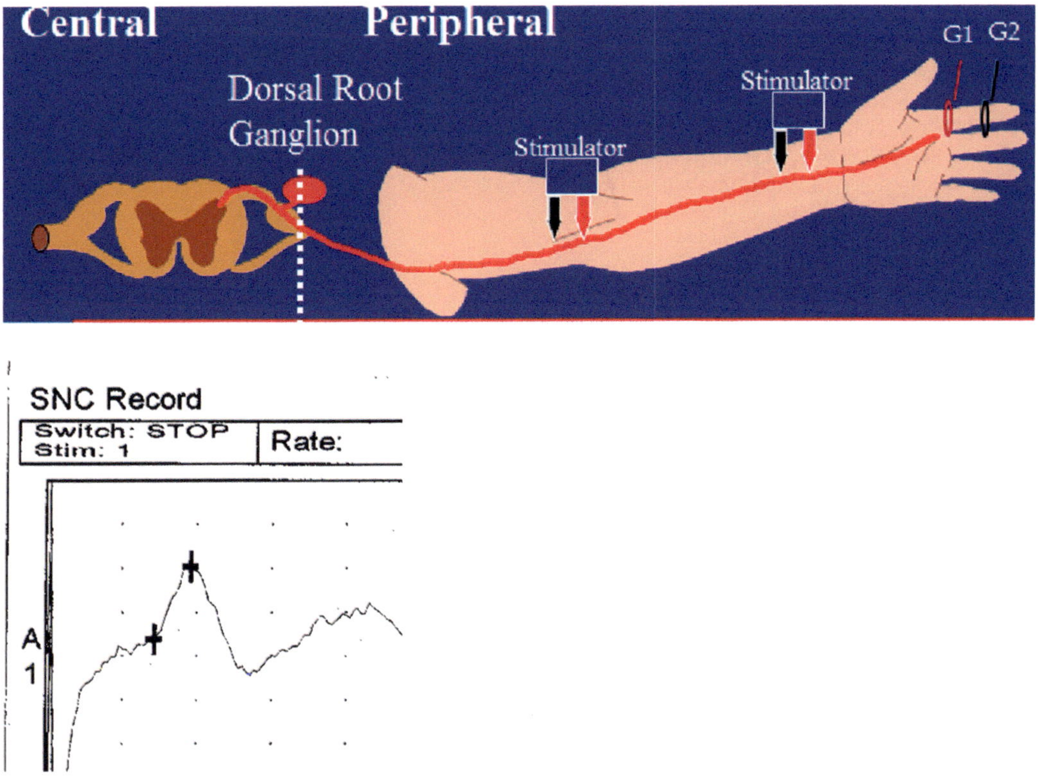

Fig. 8.2 Top, schema for an antidromic sensory NCS of the median nerve showing stimulation at the wrist and elbow and recording from the second digit. Bottom, sensory nerve action potential (SNAP) waveform with wrist stimulation

but also of the neuromuscular junction and the muscle itself.

For sensory NCSs, a nerve-generated potential is recorded, so the amplitude is much smaller (generally on the order of microvolts). As a result, the signal-to-noise ratio is less favorable than with motor studies, and several stimuli may have to be averaged to ensure a high-quality SNAP. In normal sensory NCSs, the morphologic pattern of the waveform changes (decreased amplitude and prolonged duration) between proximal and distal sites because of phase cancellation of the traveling wave.

Measurements

Several parameters are measured in NCSs. These include the amplitude, distal latency, and, at times, the conduction velocity. The *amplitude* of the CMAP or SNAP is the height of the response. *Distal latency* is the time between the stimulation and the onset of the waveform when the most distal site is stimulated (usually at the ankle or wrist). *Conduction velocity* is calculated by measuring the distance between points of stimulation and dividing by the difference in latencies between the two stimulation sites. These values are compared to normal controls and, at times, to the contralateral limb if asymptomatic (especially in sensory NCSs) (Fig. 8.3).

In motor studies, the duration and area of the CMAP are also marked and may be important in certain clinical conditions. If the morphology of the waveform is different between the distal and proximal sites of stimulation, temporal dispersion or conduction block may be present. As mentioned above, the CMAP should be almost identical in amplitude, duration, and overall morphologic findings along all sites of stimulation in a motor nerve. Considerable loss of amplitude at the proximal site compared with the distal

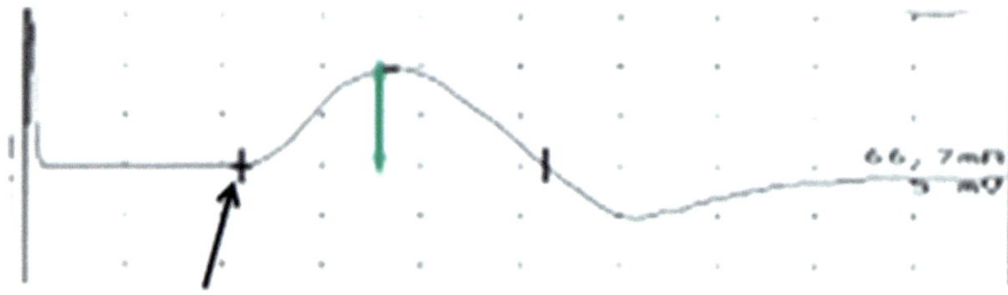

Fig. 8.3 CMAP waveform with latency (arrow) and amplitude (double arrow) highlighted

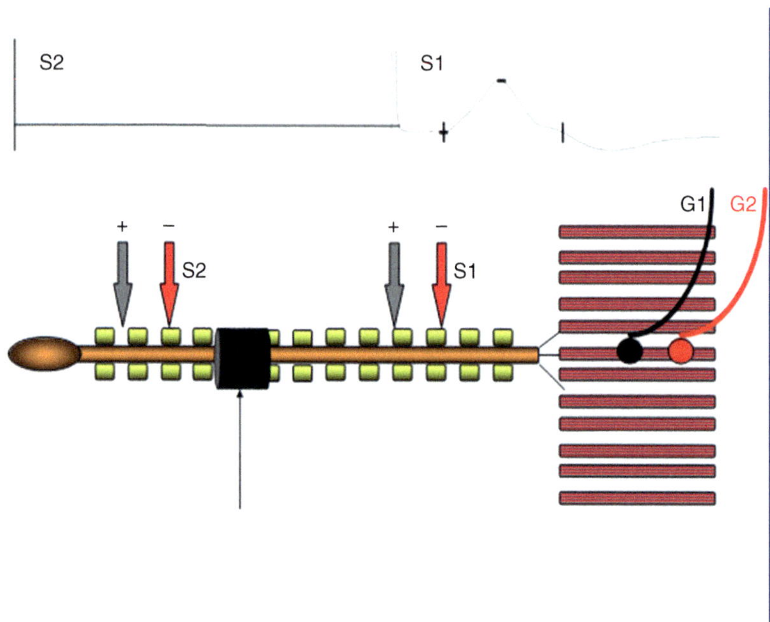

Fig. 8.4 Conduction block (at bottom arrow). Stimulation proximal (S2) and distal (S1) to a lesion showing normal response with distal stimulation and lack of response with proximal stimulation

site suggests a conduction block, and prolonged duration at the proximal site compared with the distal site suggests temporal dispersion. In general, a 20% decrease in CMAP amplitude is consistent with conduction block (Fig. 8.4), and an increase in duration of the CMAP waveform of more than 30% is consistent with temporal dispersion (Fig. 8.5). Both findings generally indicate some degree of underlying demyelination, or neuroapraxia, between the points of stimulation. Stimulation at Erb's point can thus reveal focal abnormalities in brachial plexus or proximal nerve lesions. In sensory studies, amplitudes normally decrease as a function of distance so that proximal amplitudes are smaller than distal amplitudes. Due to this, assessment for conduction block and temporal dispersion is not helpful.

Late Responses

The motor and sensory NCSs described above are relatively direct measures of the integrity of the more distal segments of nerves. In proximal segments of nerves, NCSs have technical limitations for direct assessment of nerves because of difficulty in isolated stimulation of nerves and isolated recording from nerves or muscle. Although direct measures are not reliable, indirect measures of the proximal segments of nerves are possible with F wave assessment (Fig. 8.6).

In elicitation of an F wave, the nerve is stimulated as usual for the distal CMAP, but the anode is rotated off the nerve to allow the action potential generated at the point of stimulation at the distal stimulation site to travel proximally. This action potential travels exclusively up the motor

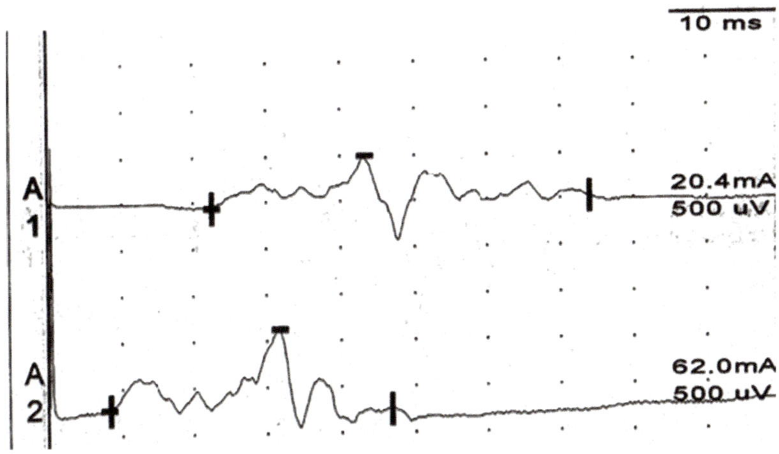

Fig. 8.5 Ulnar motor NCS showing very long duration, polyphasic CMAP at both proximal (top waveform) and distal (bottom waveform) sites of simulation with more prominent dispersion with proximal stimulation

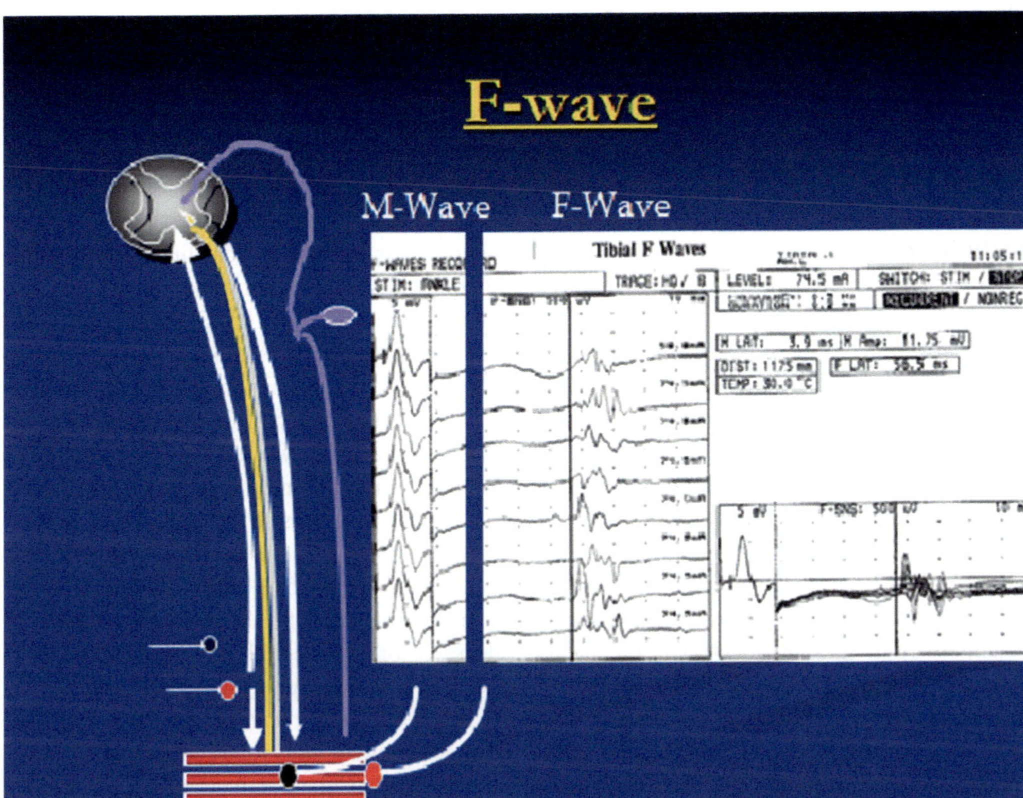

Fig. 8.6 F waves: Stimulation distally with proximal volley of the evoked action potential proximally to anterior horn cells and resulting distal volley to the muscle to generate F wave. Recording (right) showing the CMAP waveform (M wave) followed by the F wave

axon to the anterior horn cell and causes depolarization of a small pool of anterior horn cells. These anterior horn cells, in turn, send an action potential back down the motor nerve to the muscle, where the small evoked responses can be recorded, representing the F wave. Because each stimulus excites a different pool of anterior horn cells, the elicited F waves vary in configuration, amplitude, and, to a lesser extent, latency. The F wave represents a signal that has traversed the entire peripheral segment of the motor nerve proximally and then back distally. The F wave therefore serves as an indirect way to assess proximal motor nerve segments (plexus and root).

The F latency is typically measured as the time between stimuli at the distal site on the motor nerve and the appearance of the first two F waves. The resulting F latency can be compared to normal values or to an estimate that takes into consideration the nerve conduction velocity and the distance of the pathway traveled to the spinal cord. An F latency that is longer than the F estimate suggests that conduction was slowed proximally, which is consistent with an underlying pathophysiologic mechanism of acquired demyelination or neuroapraxia in this proximal nerve segment.

Needle EMG

Technique

Needle EMG assesses electrical activity of the muscle fibers themselves. Because needle EMG includes analysis of electrical activity with the muscle at rest and assessment with mild levels of voluntary contraction, this technique is typically performed on an awake patient who can both relax a muscle and voluntarily contract it with mild force. The test can be mildly to moderately painful to the patient. It is done by inserting a small needle into a muscle to record the electrical potentials from muscle fibers near the needle electrode (Fig. 8.7). There are few contraindications to needle EMG. For patients on anticoagulants, the test can be done after INR testing, if appropriate, and a discussion with the patient regarding the small risk of bleeding and bruising. Patients with pacemakers or spinal cord stimulators can be tested safely. Areas of active skin infection are avoided with the needle insertion.

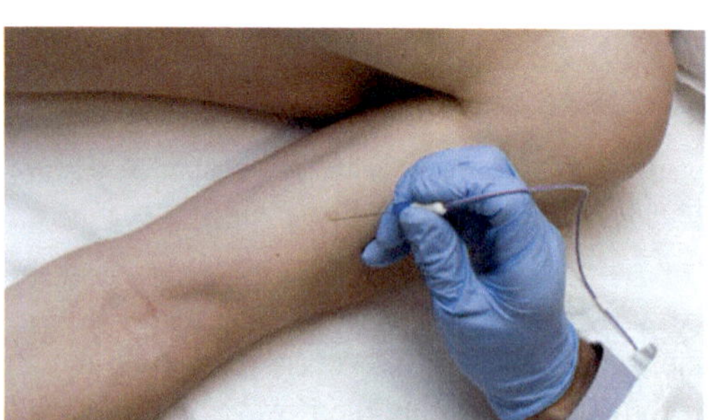

Fig. 8.7 Needle EMG of biceps demonstrated

Spontaneous Activity

Spontaneous activity is assessed with the muscle at rest. A needle is inserted through the skin into the muscle, and spontaneous activity is assessed (with minimal movement of the needle) in several areas of the muscle. Insertional activity occurs with each tiny movement of the needle. At rest, a normal muscle usually has no spontaneous activity, but several abnormalities in spontaneous activity may be detected and indicate certain disease processes.

Fibrillation potentials, which indicate denervation of individual muscle fibers, are regular, rhythmic discharges of muscle fibers and can be heard or seen only with EMG. They are not visible clinically. Positive sharp waves have a pathophysiologic meaning similar to that of fibrillation potentials but a different morphologic pattern in that they have a downward (positive) deflection rather than upward (negative) deflection. Fibrillation potentials or positive sharp waves can be seen as early as 2 weeks after injury to a nerve and almost always by 3 weeks. With reinnervation of muscle, fibrillation potentials may decrease or resolve. Fibrillation potentials can occur in any neurogenic process.

Fasciculation potentials are irregular discharges of motor units (one anterior horn cell and all the muscle fibers it innervates); as a result, they are larger than fibrillation potentials and can be seen clinically under the skin. Unlike fibrillation potentials, which indicate a pathologic process, fasciculations can be seen in normal persons but are also seen as part of disorders involving anterior horn cells, motor roots, or motor nerves.

Myotonic discharges are another spontaneous discharge characterized by waxing and waning frequency and amplitude with a sound resembling that of a dive-bomber. They occur in various disorders affecting muscle, including several channelopathies, and they are not seen with the naked eye. These discharges can also be seen in neurogenic processes. Patients who have electrical myotonia may not always have clinical myotonia (delayed relaxation of a contracted muscle, like relaxing a clenched fist).

Myokymic potentials are most commonly due to radiation damage to nerves. They are regularly occurring bursts of motor units that fire spontaneously, giving rise to a sound resembling that of marching soldiers. Not usually visible to the naked eye, myokymic potentials are occasionally found in demyelinating neuropathies and in mononeuropathies. When occurring in the face, they are often associated with brainstem disorders such as multiple sclerosis or glioma. They are most highly associated with radiation damage to nerves, especially in brachial plexopathy due to radiation therapy [3].

Voluntary Activation

Voluntary motor units are assessed during muscle contraction. Several parameters are assessed, the most important of which is the motor unit potential duration. The morphologic pattern of the waveform is also analyzed for polyphasia or complexity. With reinnervation, the size of each motor unit increases and so does the degree of polyphasia or complexity. This can be from terminal axonal reinnervating muscle fibers or from more axonal growth through an area of nerve injury. Early regenerating motor units can appear very complex and small and are termed "nascent" motor units (Fig. 8.8). Motor units that are immature or in the process of reinnervating can also display a characteristic called "variability" or "instability" which reflects variation of the moment to moment motor unit potential seen with activation of the muscle. This is a result of the immaturity of the nerve terminal that is newly reinnervating with inconsistent transmission across the neuromuscular junction.

Recruitment of motor unit potentials refers to the number of motor unit potentials firing at a given force. As a muscle is contracted more forcefully, more and more motor units are recruited to supply the force needed. In a neurogenic process, fewer motor units are available, so despite a stronger contraction, fewer motor units are present to supply that force, and recruitment is reduced (e.g., a small number of motor unit potentials fire at inappropriately high frequencies). In severe neurogenic disease, there may be only one or two motor units that can be activated, often called "discrete" recruitment.

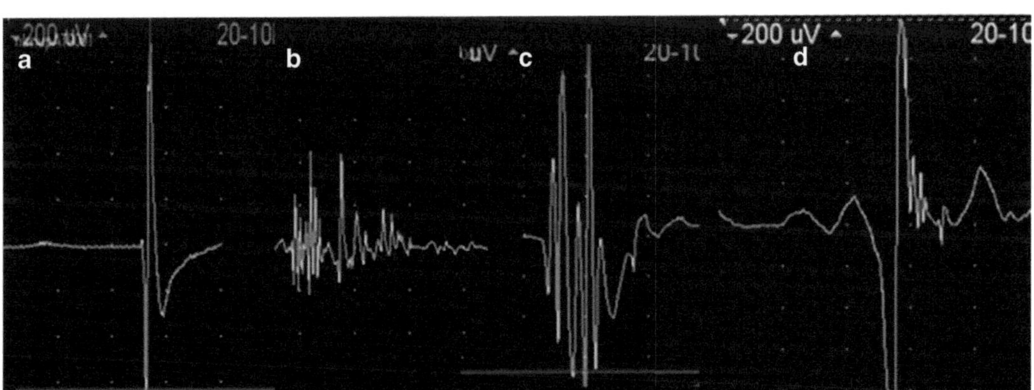

Fig. 8.8 Voluntary motor unit morphology and size. (**a**) Normal motor unit. (**b**). Nascent motor unit. (**c**). Complex, polyphasic motor unit. (**d**) A large, less complex, motor unit. (**b–d**) represent the typical evolution after reinnervation of a muscle

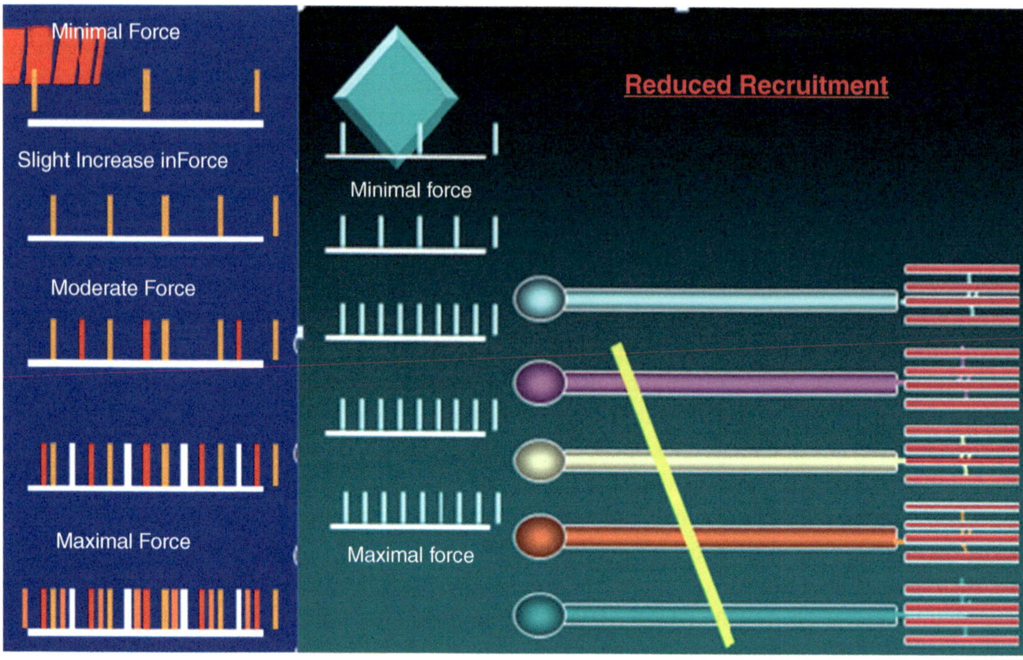

Fig. 8.9 Left, normal recruitment of motor units (shown as different colored lines). Right, reduced/discrete recruitment showing extreme example of only one motor unit firing with maximal voluntary activation

In summary, in neurogenic disorders, the typical EMG pattern includes fibrillation potentials, fasciculation potentials, and large, occasionally complex, motor units firing with reduced recruitment (Fig. 8.9).

Application to Brachial Plexus Assessment

Motor NCSs reflect the functioning of motor axons; the reduction or absence of the CMAP amplitude is reflective of damage to motor axons. In very acute injuries or in the setting of neuroapraxia, conduction block may be seen in incomplete or complete injuries. Sensory NCSs measure primarily the postganglionic pathway, and their normalcy when testing an area of sensory loss is evidence for a preganglionic lesion. The reduction in the amplitude or even loss of the response will indicate postganglionic injury, though some degree of preganglionic injury cannot be excluded in those circumstances.

The distribution of the needle EMG abnormalities is important to localize the lesion(s) after brachial plexus injury. In upper extremity processes, this can be approached by a distal to proximal and a rostral to caudal analysis. The electromyographer will examine muscles innervated by C5-T1 nerve roots and different nerves to attempt to understand the anatomic localization (e.g., upper trunk vs lateral cord vs axillary or suprascapular nerve). In addition, assessment will be made of nerve root vs peripheral injury by assessing the paraspinal muscles and very proximal muscles like rhomboid, which is innerved just at the C5 root level. It is important to realize that the paraspinals are innervated by multiple roots, so abnormality here implies preganglionic injury, but the precise root localization is not possible.

The goal of the EMG is to guide the referring clinician to the most likely sites of injury. Often there is a combination of sites as in upper trunk AND axillary nerve or C5/6 root *and* brachial plexus. And, at times, precise localization is simply not possible with EMG when there are multiple sites involved and one can imply likelihood but not definitive conclusions. It is important to consider the technical ability of the electromyographer to adequately perform NCSs and EMG which can be negatively affected by patient factors like previous injuries, surgeries, scars, tolerance for the examination, body habitus, muscle atrophy after injury, and use of anticoagulants.

Evolution and Timing of EMG Abnormalities

After an initial nerve injury, needle EMG shows an immediate decrease in the recruitment of motor units because of the loss of action potentials firing through the point of injury. In severe injury, no motor units are seen. At this early juncture, both conduction block/neuroapraxia and axonal damage can produce this picture; very early needle EMG therefore can indicate a problem, but not confirm the pathophysiology. Fibrillation potentials begin to appear in the first 2 weeks. Increased size and/or polyphasia or complexity of voluntary motor units may take 1 to 2 months to appear if coming from reinnervation in terminal axons and 3 months or more if coming from axonal regrowth (dependent on the distance from the injury to the muscle). The early nascent motor units are often the first sign of reinnervation, even occurring before there is demonstrable muscle activation or limb movement.

On NCSs, conduction block can be identified with stimulation above and below the injury site. Within the initial 10 days, NCSs can be used to identify the presence of a conduction block and the location of a lesion but not the pathophysiologic process, similar to needle EMG. When a focal process affects axons (*axonotmesis*), Wallerian degeneration occurs, and NCSs performed 2 to 4 weeks later yield low-amplitude CMAPs stimulating at both proximal and distal sites. In this situation, localization is not possible, but pathophysiologic findings are consistent with an axonal lesion. Stimulation above the brachial plexus is technically challenging and requires either stimulation at Erb's point or at the spinal nerve level. In both approaches, there can be difficulty obtaining supramaximal stimulation on the nerve of interest. Recording in these cases is usually distally in the hand from ulnar or median-innervated muscles assessing mainly lower trunk function.

In summary, soon after axonal injury, needle EMG reveals fibrillation potentials and reduced recruitment. A conduction block, if able to be assessed, can be found. However, with a focal demyelinating process (*neuroapraxia*), a focal conduction block will still be seen with stimulation both proximal and distal to the lesion at 4 weeks and beyond. The EMG will again show reduced recruitment, but fibrillation potentials will be absent or very mild.

Brachial Plexopathy Neurodiagnostic Assessment

The EMG approach includes taking a focused history and doing a limited neurological examination to assist in the planning of the full EMG study. Special attention is paid not only to the peripheral nerve examination but also to central nervous system examination findings such as hyperreflexia, spasticity, and Babinski signs which may further add to the weakness or impaired function of the patient. A Horner's sign (ptosis and miosis) often suggests nerve root avulsion of C8/T1. Combining their own focused evaluation and the clinical notes from the surgical team, the electromyographer should then plan the EMG study to answer the most important questions of the clinicians; often this is around distribution and severity of abnormalities and intactness of the nerve roots. The EMG study is tailored to the clinical questions at hand. Timing of the initial EMG is best at least 4 weeks after injury as some electrophysiological findings (fibrillation potentials) may only appear after this time. At this point, conduction block, if found, is more suggestive of a neurapraxic lesion as enough time has passed to allow for Wallerian degeneration.

NCSs are done initially to evaluate median and ulnar function (motor and sensory NCSs), and further studies are guided by the clinical scenario. Radial motor and sensory studies can be done to assess radial nerve and also upper trunk/

posterior cord integrity. Medial and lateral antebrachial cutaneous sensory NCSs are key tools to assess lower and upper trunk (and medial and lateral cord) localizations, respectively. More proximal nerve studies are uncommonly done, mainly used for more focal neuropathies (axillary, musculocutaneous, suprascapular). Spinal accessory NCSs can be done to assess for injury to that nerve and also to test integrity for possible use in brachial plexus reconstructive surgery. Sensory NCSs are vital to suggesting a preganglionic component to the injury; preserved responses in the setting of clear sensory loss in that nerve distribution indicate preganglionic damage/root avulsion. Absent or reduced sensory NCSs indicate at least postganglionic damage, though cannot exclude concomitant preganglionic damage. An important technical note for most sensory NCSs, comparison with the contralateral side (if unaffected) is important as normal values are not as consistent in some of these studies (especially the antebrachial cutaneous studies). Also, in otherwise healthy younger individuals, the amplitudes of sensory NCSs can be very high, and comparison with the opposite side may reveal a relative loss of amplitude even when a normal amplitude is found on the symptomatic side. A side-to-side difference of >50% on sensory NCSs is usually significant to imply neurogenic involvement on the affected side.

As mentioned above, the needle EMG is used to help localize more precisely, and a number of muscles are usually assessed. First dorsal interosseous, extensor indicis proprius, pronator teres, triceps, biceps, deltoid, infraspinatus, rhomboid, and paraspinals are commonly done (Table 8.1). More detailed assessment can be undertaken of specific distributions based on findings in these muscles as well as the clinical scenario. Needle EMG of trapezius, intercostals, and even diaphragm can be done to assist in surgical planning.

Figure 8.10 shows the EMG study on a patient seen 4 months after a brachial plexus injury. The ulnar and median motor responses were absent, indicating significant axonal damage in the C8/T1, lower trunk, or medial cord pathways. The sensory responses being absent or low amplitude indicate a large degree of postganglionic (e.g., plexus) damage. The fact that the median sensory response is present, though low, could indicate some preganglionic/root involvement at C6. The needle examination revealed fibrillation potentials in most limb muscles with no voluntary motor units, going along with severe axonal damage with no reinnervation occurring. Lower cervical paraspinals showed fibrillation potentials, but no abnormalities were noted in mid-cervical paraspinals or in rhomboid. This suggests nerve root involvement at C8/T1 but intact C5 root. Involvement of the C7 root is difficult to judge from this study. As is the case with many EMG studies in post-traumatic brachial plexopathy, there appears to be a mixture of pre- and postganglionic damage, though clearly no signs of active reinnervation in this diffuse process.

The presence of multiple voluntary motor units with voluntary contraction suggests reasonable chance for meaningful outcome; and no motor units seen usually predicts lack of recovery spontaneously. In patients followed with upper trunk traumatic brachial plexopathy, the lack of any motor units by needle EMG assured poor functional outcome (0/29 patients reaching at least MRC 4/5 strength after 2 years), and the presence of even discrete recruitment was associated with a small (25%) chance of at least MRC 4/5 strength outcome [4].

Table 8.1 NCS and needle EMG and corresponding root and trunk distributions

Root	Trunk	Motor NCS	Sensory NCS	Needle EMG
C5C6	Upper	Suprascapular, axillary, musculocutaneous	Lateral ABCRadialMedian Digit I/II	Rhomboid (C5) Spinati, deltoid, biceps, pronator teres (C6)
C7	Middle	Radial (EDC)	Median digit II/III	Triceps, EDC, pronator teres (some C7)
C8T1	Lower	MedianUlnar	UlnarMedial ABC	EIP (C8)FDI, APB, FDB

ABC antebrachial cutaneous, *EDC* extensor digitorum communis, *EIP* extensor indices proprius, *FDI* first dorsal interosseous, *APB* abductor pollicis brevis, *FDP* flexor digitorum profundus

NERVE CONDUCTIONS

* = Repetitive Stim. NR = No Response.

Stimulate	(Record)	AMPLITUDE (milli/micro) volts right	left	normal	VELOCITY meters/sec. right	left	normal	DISTAL LATENCY milliseconds right	left	normal	F-WAVE LATENCY milliseconds right	left
Median, motor	(Abductor pollicis br)	–	0.0	(>4.0)	–		(>48)	–	NR	(<4.5)	–	
Median, sensory	(Index)	–	7	(>15)	–	52	(>56)	–	3.0	(<3.6)	–	
Radial, sensory	(Dorsal hand)	–	0	(>20)	–		(>49)	–	NR	(<2.9)	–	
Ulnar, motor	(Abductor digiti mini)	–	0.0	(>6.0)	–		(>51)	–	NR	(<3.6)	–	
Lateral antebrachial, sensory	(Forearm)	11 –	0		–			2.7 –	NR		–	

VOLUNTARY MOTRO UNIT POTENTIALS

MUSCLE	INSERT. ACTIVITY	SPONTANEOUS Fib.	Fasc.	MUP NORMAL	RECRUITMENT Act.	Reduced	Rapid	DURATION LONG	SHORT	AMPLITUDE HIGH	LOW	PHASES %	TURNS
L. Biceps brachii	Decreased	0	0		None								
	Comment:	Dense fibrosis,	no muscle										
L. Deltoid	Increased	+++	0		None								
L. First dorsal interosseous	Increased	+++	0		None								
L. Infraspinatus	Increased	+++	0		None								
L. Pronator teres	Increased	+++	0		None								
L. Rhomboid major	Normal	0	0	Normal									
L. Triceps brachii	Increased	+++	0		None								
L. Paraspinal, cervical (lower)	Normal	++	0	----									
L. Paraspinal, cervical (mid)	Normal	0	0	Normal									

Fig. 8.10 Initial EMG done in a patient with brachial plexus injury

Neurodiagnostics to Assist in Selection of Nerve Donor for Transfer

When selecting a potential donor nerve for transfer surgery, preoperative needle EMG can be useful by assessing the activity in the innervated muscle(s). A study of recruitment in donor nerve-innervated muscles found that in those muscles with normal or mildly abnormal recruitment, these nerves when transferred produced a better outcome measured by motor strength and active range of motion compared to donor nerves displaying very reduced recruitment on pre-transfer needle EMG [5]. Another study similarly found correlation between the number of motor units in a donor nerve and the eventual muscle strength after nerve transfer surgery [6].

Follow-Up Neurodiagnostic Evaluations

In follow-up of patients who have undergone brachial plexus reconstructive surgery or being considered for such, repeat neurodiagnostic testing provides information on interval reinnervation. The electromyographer should understand the details of any reconstructive surgery, if done, to direct the electrophysiological assessment. After reconstructive nerve surgery, needle EMG is done in the downstream muscles to compare to previous or preoperative needle EMG studies. Improvement may take months to appear given rate of axonal growth and reinnervation. Close communication between the surgical team and the electromyographer is critical to help assess and answer the key clinical questions as a routine EMG study done without this information may not be as helpful to surgical team. Re-emergence of motor units has been shown to correlate to the measurements of force in downstream muscles, including after nerve/muscle transfer as in gracilis muscle transfer [7]. While fibrillation potentials may or may not persist, the emergence of motor units in muscles that previously did not have motor units or the improvement in recruitment abnormalities (which indicates more motor units functioning) is a positive electrophysiological sign. Improvement in the CMAP amplitude is also a positive sign indicating more functioning motor units.

Summary

Neurodiagnostic evaluation of brachial plexus injuries is vital to understand the distribution, severity, and evolution of the neurogenic picture in each patient. Using NCSs and needle EMG at the initial evaluation will provide the surgical team important information to guide subsequent treatment or testing. Those performing neurodiagnostic studies should be experienced in testing less common NCSs and needle EMG studies and should have clear direction from the surgical team regarding the most important clinical questions to address with testing. Follow-up neurodiagnostic testing can assist in tracking re-innervation (or lack thereof). Close communication between the surgical team and the neurodiagnostician is key to ensure adequate testing and interpretation of findings for maximal clinical assistance to the patient and surgical team caring for the patient.

References

1. O'Shea K, Feinberg JH, Wolfe SW. Imaging and electrodiagnostic work-up of acute adult brachial plexus injuries. J Hand Surg Eur. 2011;36(9):747–59.
2. Ferrante MA. Electrodiagnostic assessment of the brachial plexus. Neurol Clin. 2012;30(2:551–80.
3. Harper CM Jr, Thomas JE, Cascino TL, Litchy WJ. Distinction between neoplastic and radiation-induced brachial plexopathy, with emphasis on the role of EMG. Neurology. 1989;39(4):502–6.
4. Impastato DM, Impastato KA, Dabestani P, Ko JH, Bunnell AE. Prognostic value of needle electromyography in traumatic brachial plexus injury. Muscle Nerve. 2019;60(5):595–7.
5. Schreiber JJ, Feinberg JH, Byun DJ, Lee SK, Wolfe SW. Preoperative donor nerve electromyography as a predictor of nerve transfer outcomes. J Hand Surg Am. 2014;39(1):42–9.
6. Mandeville RM, Brown JM, Sheean JL. Semi-quantitative electromyography as a predictor of nerve transfer outcome. Clin Neurophysiol. 2019;130(5):701–6.
7. Kazamel M, Sorenson E. Electromyographic findings in gracilis muscle grafts used to augment elbow flexion in traumatic brachial plexopathy. J Clin Neurophysiol. 2016;33(6):549–53.

Intraoperative Brachial Plexus Neurophysiological Monitoring

9

Brian A. Crum and Jeff Strommen

Introduction

The assessment of brachial plexus and cervical and upper thoracic nerve roots is an important function of intraoperative monitoring (IOM) in the setting of reconstructive brachial plexus surgery. Whether a particular nerve root is functionally connected to the spinal cord is vital information in the surgical decision-making process as the presence or absence of this functional connection will often dictate between different, often quite disparate, procedures. In addition, the functional integrity of elements of the brachial plexus is important in this decision-making process. To help make these determinations, intraoperative electrophysiological testing is necessary. This requires the use of nerve conduction studies (NCSs) and somatosensory and motor evoked potentials (SEPs and MEPs). With close attention to potential technical problems, this vital information can be quickly and accurately obtained.

Once it is decided to undergo surgical exploration and reconstruction, the preoperative EMG study is used to provide guidance regarding the distribution and severity of the injury (see previous Neurodiagnostic Evaluation section). Localization is supplemented by advanced imaging, but it is important to note that myelography and MRI may not be able to clearly identify root avulsion [1, 2]. In one study, the preoperative judgment of nerve root continuity (with EMG and imaging studies) was compared to nerve root assessment during IOM. In 25% of cases of suspected nerve root avulsion preoperatively, continuity was found during IOM [3]. Intraoperatively, anatomic continuity of the nerve root can generally be visually determined although, if an avulsed root remains intradural or, as is frequently the case, is very scarred, anatomic continuity cannot be determined by visual inspection alone. Additionally, even with full exposure (with laminectomy), nerve roots in anatomic continuity may not conduct electrically [4, 5]. In this setting, IOM is the only reliable means to determine functional continuity of axons in order to ensure a maximally effective reconstructive surgical procedure.

This chapter will provide background on the equipment and techniques used for IOM of the brachial plexus and the interpretation of the findings thereby. It will include the use of NCS, EMG, and evoked potentials (EPs). For the purpose of this review, the term "peripheral nerve" will apply to nerve distal to the spinal cord and also distal to the intervertebral foramen (spinal root/nerve, plexus, peripheral nerve). The application of these electrodiagnostic techniques will be described for specific clinical scenarios.

B. A. Crum (✉)
Mayo Clinic, Rochester, MN, USA
e-mail: crum.brian@mayo.edu

J. Strommen
Abbott Northwester Hospital, Allina Health, Minneapolis, MN, USA
e-mail: Jeffrey.Strommen@allina.com

A. Y. Shin, N. Pulos (eds.), *Operative Brachial Plexus Surgery*,
https://doi.org/10.1007/978-3-030-69517-0_9

IOM Techniques

Somatosensory Evoked Potentials

Responses from stimulation of peripheral nerves can be recorded from the spinal cord and cerebral cortex as somatosensory evoked potentials (SEPs). Intraoperative stimulation of peripheral nerve directly will depolarize both motor and sensory axons; however, selective orthodromic recording from central sensory pathways ensures that only the large fiber/dorsal column pathway is assessed, just as it does with percutaneous stimulation in routine SEPs. Since the primary goal for intraoperative SEPs in brachial plexus injury is to assess nerve root integrity, stimulation is performed as close to the intervertebral foramen as possible. (Fig. 9.1) Bipolar handheld stimulation probes are usually used by the surgeon with the cathode (red electrode) directed proximally. Monopolar stimulators with the return electrode near the wound may be used in some settings but have the disadvantage of providing a non-focal stimulation which may lead to spread to other nerve structures. Recording is performed from the cervical spine level via either a nasopharyngeal electrode or from a needle electrode placed directly on the lamina in the cervical spine. These responses are small in amplitude, so many stimuli must be averaged, typically at least 20–50, stimulating at 1.1-1.9 Hertz. It is very important to ensure that the individual holding the stimulator on the nerve maintain their position until the stimulation is finished. Stimulus intensity is typically between 10–20 mA. (Fig. 9.2a, b)

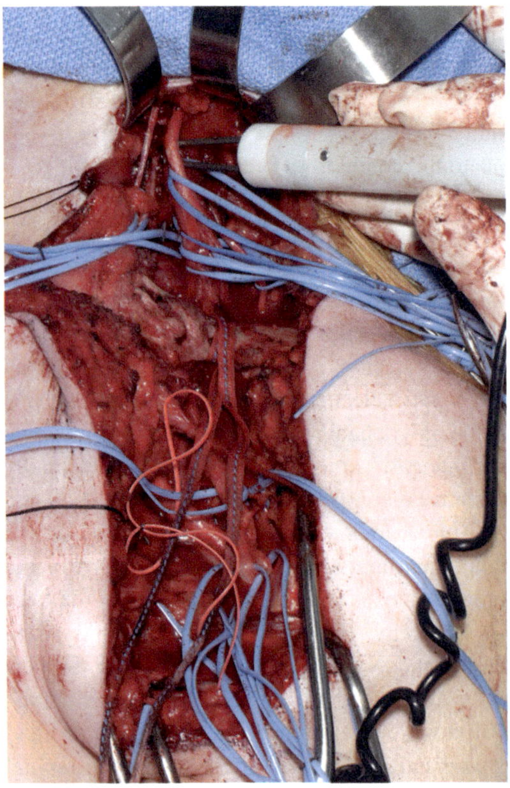

Fig. 9.1 Bipolar stimulator held by surgeon on C6 spinal nerve just outside exit from intervertebral foramen (top center)

Motor Evoked Potentials

Motor evoked potentials (MEPs) are most commonly obtained with transcranial electrical stimulation, recorded directly on the nerve at the intervertebral foramen, the same location as stimulation for SEPs. Similar to SEPs, the goal of MEP is to assess nerve root continuity (Fig. 9.2c–e). Anodal stimulation is utilized with a short duration (0.05 msec), rapid rise time stimulus using subcutaneously placed EEG electrodes placed over the motor cortex. Several [2–5] stimuli with an interstimulus interval of 2–4 msec are given with intensity of 200–600 Volts [4]. Direct nerve recording is performed with bipolar hook electrodes (Fig. 9.3), usually placed onto the spinal nerve as close to the exit from the intervertebral foramen as possible (Fig. 9.1).

Nerve Action Potentials

Recording of a nerve action potential (NAP) is performed with direct nerve stimulation and recording using bipolar electrodes as shown in Fig. 9.3. A variety of commercial electrodes are available for this purpose. The electrodes are

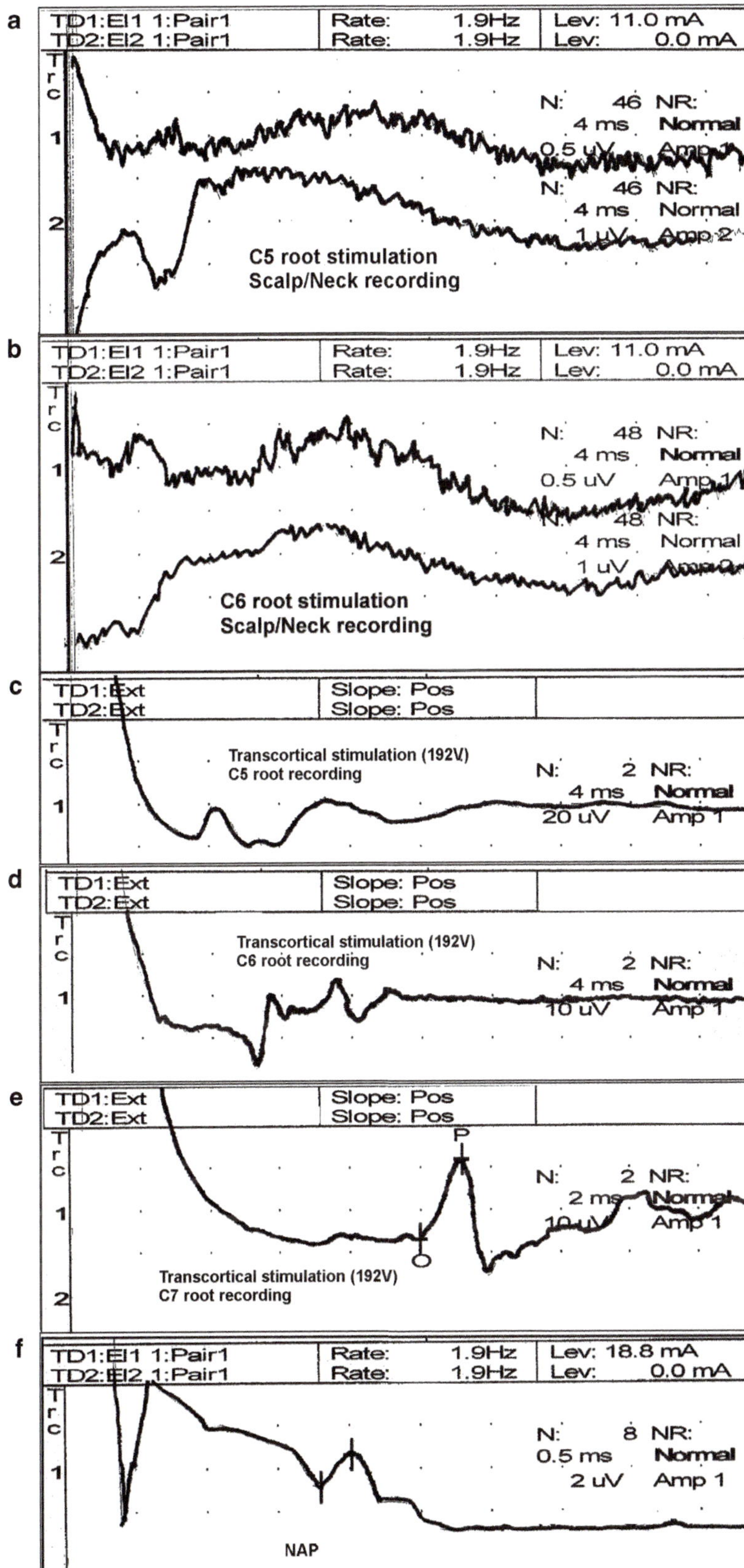

Fig. 9.2 Bipolar electrodes. Left, pointed tip electrodes often used for stimulation Right, hook electrodes often used for recording

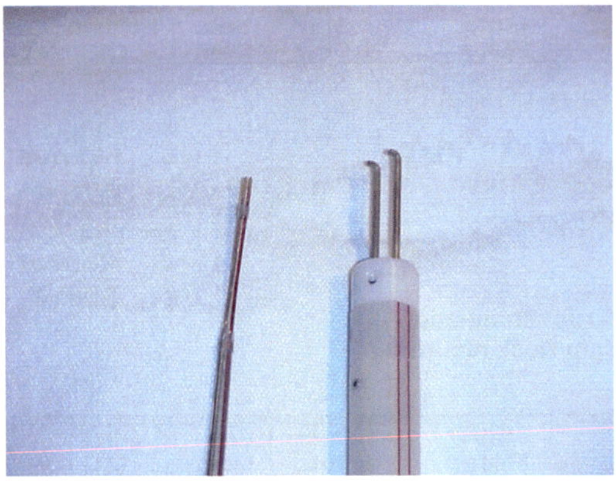

Fig. 9.3 Intraoperative recordings during brachial plexus exploration and reconstruction
(**a**) SEP recording over the scalp and neck, respectively, with direct intraoperative C5 root stimulation. The presence of the response supporting C5 sensory root integrity.
(**b**) SEP recording over the scalp and neck, respectively, with direct intraoperative C6 root stimulation. The presence of the response supporting C6 sensory root integrity.
(**c**) Transcortical electrical stimulation with direct MEP recording over the C5 root supporting integrity of C5 motor fibers.
(**d**) Transcortical electrical stimulation with direct MEP recording over the C6 root supporting integrity of C6 motor fibers.
(**e**) Transcortical electrical stimulation with direct MEP recording over the C7 root supporting integrity of C7 motor fibers.
Nerve action potential with stimulation distal and recording proximal to the lesion. No reproducible response could be recorded across the lesion

separated by at least 4 cm, and the nerve is held out of the surgical field if possible to avoid current shunting due to surrounding fluid. Stimulation is typically performed at the distal site with recording proximally across the lesion (Figs. 9.3f and 9.4). Stimulus intensities of only a few milliamperes are required, though if no NAP is obtained with low stimulus intensity, we often increase the intensity to 20–25 milliamperes to ensure sufficient intensity to depolarize even damaged axons. The presence of a NAP across a lesion assures functional continuity of at least 4000 axons in which it has been shown that this degree of axonal continuity translates into functional end-organ reinnervation [6]. Conversely, when no NAP response is recorded across a lesion, it is unlikely functional reinnervation will occur.

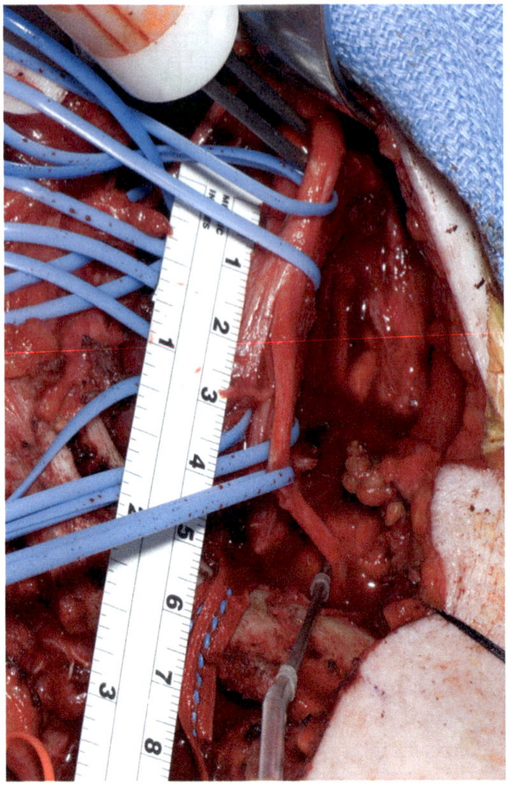

Fig. 9.4 Intraoperative NAP recording with bipolar stimulation electrodes (bottom) and recording electrodes (top)

Triggered EMG

To assess for nerve continuity, direct nerve stimulation can be performed proximal to the lesion with recording a distal muscle innervated by that nerve. A response will confirm continuity of that nerve and imply at least some continuity of at least one nerve root supplying that nerve. It can also help identify anomalous innervation in confusing cases. A few limitations should be considered. The size of the muscle recording in this situation may have more to do with the distance between any depolarizing muscle fibers and the recording electrodes than with the actual number of functioning axons. While a response does indicate some continuity or reinnervation to the target end-organ muscle, it cannot prove the continuity of individual roots as all muscles have multiple root innervation. Due to the amplification of the motor response when recording from muscle, quantification of the number of functional axons is difficult but does provide evidence of at least some continuity or reinnervation. The lack of a muscle response with triggered EMG, however, does not indicate a lesion without continuity as the axons may be regenerating through the lesion but have not yet reached the target muscle. In this setting, the continuity can only be assessed with NAP across the peripheral nerve lesion or MEP and SEP across the root segment. An absent muscle response cannot distinguish between a pre- or post-ganglionic lesion. For all of these reasons, recording MEPs over the spinal nerve, not with direct nerve stimulation, is ideal when assessing nerve root integrity.

Technical Issues

Muscle artifact from neck and proximal arm muscles is a major technical challenge in MEP studies. With transcranial stimulation there is activation of motor neurons diffusely which can be recorded directly over the muscle but will also be detected from a distant electrode (volume conduction). This may lead to a recorded response in the target muscles which actually arises from a different nerve/muscle element, leading to a false-positive result. When there is concern about a false-positive MEP response, recording of a spinal nerve from a known avulsed ventral root is helpful; a response there confirms a likely false-positive response due to volume conduction. If this is not possible, neuromuscular blocking agents can also be used to make this distinction. If the waveform in question disappears or decreases in size, a volume-conducted response is most likely as spinal root-recorded MEP would not be affected by neuromuscular blockade. The cervical SEP potential from nerve root stimulation is also subject to this artifact with a similar troubleshooting approach. NAP recordings can also be distorted by volume-conducted muscle artifact, and the use of a neuromuscular blocking agent is useful to enhance interpretation.

Excessive stimulus artifact can also hamper recordings, particularly given the short distance between stimulating and recording electrodes. Occasionally one must move the recording (for MEP) or stimulating (for SEP) electrodes distally onto brachial plexus elements to obviate this problem. The polarity of the MEP stimulus can also be alternated and several stimuli averaged in an attempt to reduce the stimulus artifact by phase cancellation. Stimulus artifact is a problem in NAP recordings as the recording electrode will "see" the electrical shock given to depolarize the nerve. If the distance is short between the stimulating and recording electrodes, then this stimulus artifact may obscure the NAP. A distance of no less than 4 cm, therefore, and preferably longer must be used. Additionally, in all these settings, the surgical bed should be dry or the nerve gently retracted out of the fluid to improve the recording.

Anesthesia can have a major detrimental impact on IOM, especially the use of inhalational agents that suppress cortical excitability. For SEPs, this negatively impacts scalp recordings more than cervical spine or nasopharyngeal recordings. Inhalational anesthetic agents reduce the effectiveness of transcranial electrical stimulation in initiating a MEP. NAP recordings, however, are not affected by anesthesia. Neuromuscular blocking agents may be desirable for SEP, MEP, or NAP studies in which muscle artifact must be eliminated, though they are not used (or sparingly used) when recording responses from muscle. Our preferred anesthetic regimen is total intravenous anesthesia (TIVA) with narcotic and propofol and use of short-acting neuromuscular blocking agents only as necessary. Once the monitoring is completed, low-level halogenated agents can then be added as determined by the anesthesia team.

Accurate communication with the surgical team is vital. The IOM physician and technicians cannot always see the operative field during the NAP, SEP, or MEP studies. Before beginning the stimuli, it must be confirmed that the surgeon is holding the electrodes in the proper place with the proper orientation and that they continue to hold their position until the stimuli are finished. In the hectic environment of the operating room, often with multiple surgeons and surgical team members, this can be a challenge but is critical for optimal decision-making. Communication with the anesthesia team is also important, especially as it relates to the use of inhalational agents or neuromuscular blocking agents during the procedure.

Interpretation

The presence of a central SEP response (scalp or cervical spine) after spinal nerve stimulation indicates the continuity of the dorsal root in cases where avulsion is questioned [5, 7]. Although it does not directly test the ventral root, its separate continuity is often assumed when a SEP response is obtained [5]. Lack of a response argues for dorsal nerve root avulsion or disruption, especially when NAPs can be recorded from the corresponding spinal nerve or plexus element distal to the foramen. In a pure preganglionic lesion affecting the dorsal roots, the cell body and peripheral axon are still intact, and a peripheral NAP would be expected. A MEP response indicates continuity of the ventral root, while absence suggests avulsion [1]. It is important to realize that the integrity of the dorsal root does not guarantee integrity of the ventral root and vice versa [5]. In addition, the loss of SEP responses occurs with less apparent root damage as judged by visual inspection and is more likely to be absent when there is anatomic continuity [5]. A mismatch (partially avulsed dorsal or ventral roots) was noted in 11% of roots studied by laminectomy [1]. In most of these instances, the ventral root was avulsed with an intact dorsal root. A combination of these two IOM techniques (SEP and MEP), therefore, is ideal [8, 9]. From the surgical reconstruction perspective, the continuity of the ventral roots is the most functionally important to determine, as a functioning ventral root can be utilized as the proximal stump for nerve grafting. The loss of the ventral roots as a grafting vehicle will necessitate other transposition procedures utilizing nerve and/or nerve-muscle transfers from other territories [10, 11].

Application to Brachial Plexus Reconstruction

The following case represents the use of these IOM techniques. A 42-year-old man presented with a flail left arm after a snowmobile accident. Six months after the injury, complete loss of motor and sensory function persisted in the arm. On clinical examination voluntary contraction was possible only in the rhomboid, trapezius, and serratus anterior muscles, and diffuse sensory loss was present throughout the limb. Muscle stretch reflexes were absent. A Tinel's sign was present in the supraclavicular region radiating to the thumb. There was no evidence of a Horner syndrome. Routine NCSs of the left arm revealed absent median and ulnar motor responses and a low-amplitude median SNAP. The lateral antebrachial sensory response was absent. Needle examination showed dense fibrillation potentials with no motor unit potentials activated in all left upper limb muscles plus infraspinatus. Rhomboids were normal as were the mid-cervical paraspinals. Prominent fibrillation potentials were noted in low cervical paraspinals. These findings were consistent with a very severe left pan-brachial plexopathy with mixed preganglionic and postganglionic injury and probable complete root avulsion affecting the lower segments (C8, T1, and possibly C7). There was likely at least partial preservation of the C5 root although this was difficult to predict with absolute certainty as in some cases the rhomboids may be innervated by C4. A CT myelogram was consistent with left C8 and T1 nerve root avulsions. It was felt that he likely had intact nerve roots at C5 and C6. The continuity of C7 was uncertain, but given the serratus anterior activation, this was likely to be intact. Reconstructive surgery was indicated with IOM to determine root continuity and assist with surgical decision-making.

After surgical exposure, visual inspection suggested that the C5, C6, and C7 roots were intact with probably significant postganglionic injury. The C8 and T1 roots were visibly avulsed. Intraoperative SEP testing with stimulation of the C5 and C6 roots showed reproducible responses

(Fig. 9.2a, b). Motor evoked potentials were also present on C5, C6, and C7 roots while under a short-acting paralytic agent (Fig. 9.2c–e). This confirmed that there was both motor and sensory root continuity of C5 and C6 and at least motor root integrity of C7. Attention then turned to determining whether there was continuity across the injured brachial plexus. No reproducible NAP could be recorded across the upper or middle trunk segments, but a NAP was present stimulating and recording proximal to this level (Fig. 9.2f). Based on these findings, the following grafting procedures were performed: C5 to axillary nerve, C6 to musculocutaneous nerve, and C7 to radial nerve. In this particular case, IOM confirmed continuity of the C5–C7 roots which were then used as grafting vehicles. It also helped to define the proximal extent of the nerve injury.

Figure 9.5 shows examples of various injuries with the expected IOM findings. Fig. 9.5a and b

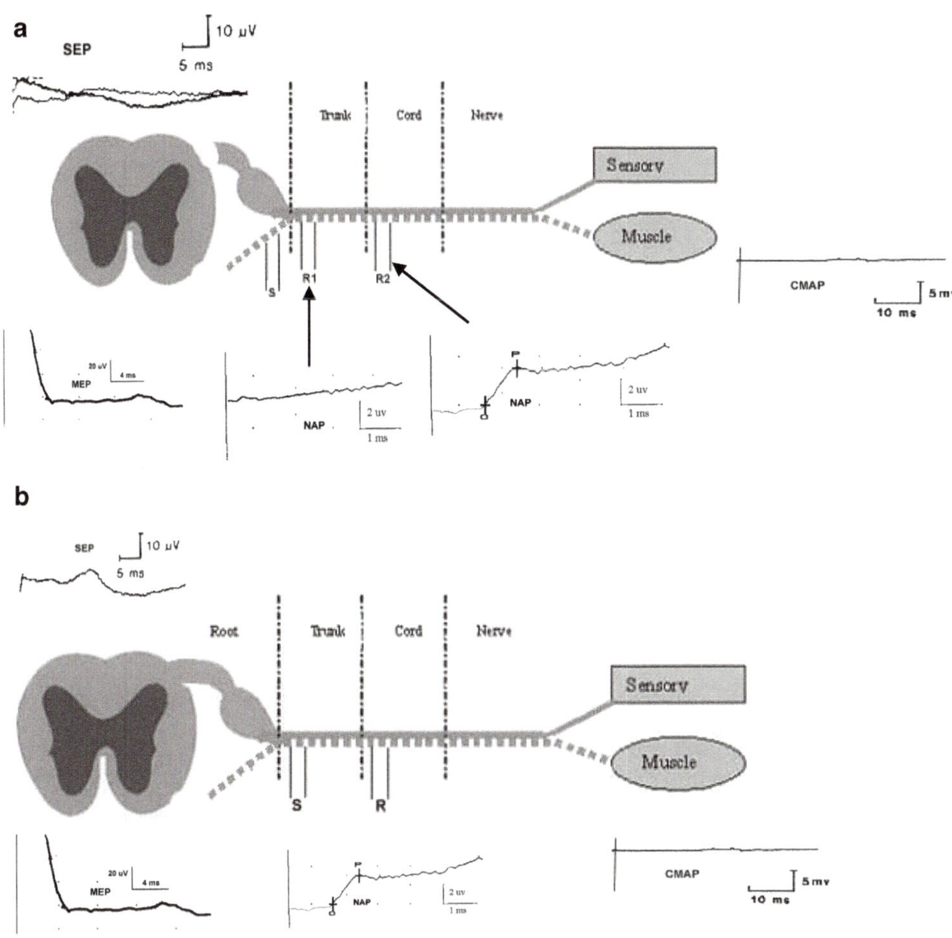

Fig. 9.5 Expected intraoperative recording with various lesions of the roots or plexus. (**a**) Complete ventral and dorsal avulsion. Preservation of NAP due to intact sensory fibers, MEP and SEP absent. (**b**) Ventral root disruption with preservation of dorsal root. Preservation of NAP and SEP with root stimulation but MEP absent. (**c**) Complete postganglionic lesion. Preservation of SEP, MEP, and NAP proximal to lesion. No NAP recorded across the lesion indicating no evidence of functional axons across the lesion. (**d**) Severe postganglionic lesion but with some regeneration through the injured segment. Note presence of all responses with the exception of the compound muscle action potential amplitude given there has not yet been end-organ reinnervation. (**e**) Mixed preganglionic and postganglionic lesions with no recordable SEP or NAP, but a positive MEP response

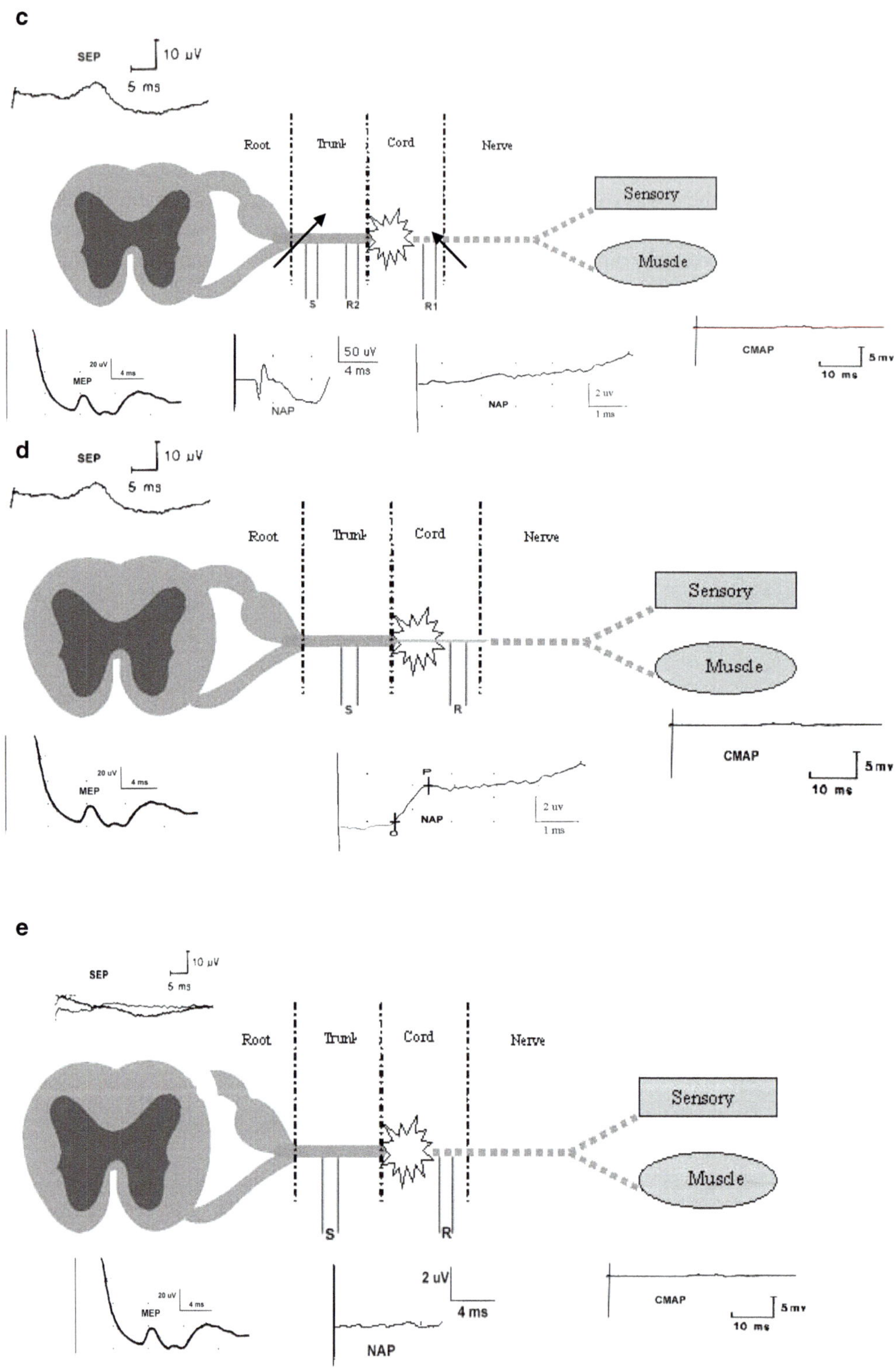

Fig. 9.5 (continued)

both show ventral root avulsion, eliminating a grafting procedure, even with the presence of a SEP in Fig. 9.5b. A complete postganglionic injury is depicted in Fig. 9.5c. The SEP and MEP are present, whereas a NAP across the plexus is not present. Stimulation and recording in the proximal plexus yield a NAP, identifying the proximal extent of the lesion. In this setting, nerve grafting/transfers or end-to-end anastomosis could be appropriate. If a NAP is present across elements of the brachial plexus (Fig. 9.5d), only neurolysis of that segment would be performed. A mixed lesion with sensory root avulsion and severe postganglionic injury is shown in Fig. 9.5e. In this case, the utility of performing both MEP and SEP studies is demonstrated, as absence of a SEP without testing of a MEP would have been interpreted as a low likelihood of a successful grafting procedure when, in reality, that was likely to be most beneficial.

Summary

Performing IOM for brachial plexus reconstructive operations requires the use of multiple modalities (SEP, MEP, and NAP) and is crucial in providing vital information to the surgical team to assist in reconstructive surgical decision-making. This data is especially indispensable in the timely assessment of the functional continuity of nerve roots. There are, however, many technical challenges that must be realized and overcome in order to acquire reliable electrophysiological data which require constant, accurate communication between the IOM, surgical, and anesthesiology teams.

References

1. Carvalho GA, Nikkhah G, Matthies C, Penkert G, Samii M. Diagnosis of root avulsions in traumatic brachial plexus injuries: value of computerized tomography, myelography and magnetic resonance imaging. J Neurosurg. 1997;86:69–76.
2. Oberle J, Antoniadis G, Rath SA, Seitz K, Schneider O, Braun V, Kahamba JF, Richter HP. Radiological investigations and intra-operative evoked potentials for the diagnosis of nerve root avulsion: evaluation of oth modalities by intradural root inspection. Acta Neurochir. 1998;140(6):527–31.
3. Clarkson JH, Ozyurekoglu T, Mujadzic M, Iyer V, Breidenbach WC. An evaluation of the information gained from the use of intraoperative nerve recording in the management of suspected brachial plexus root avulsion. Plast Reconstr Surg. 2011;127(3):1237–43.
4. Turkof E, Millesi H, Turkof R, Pfundner P, Mayr N. Intraoperative electroneurodiagnostics (transcranial electrical motor evoked potentials) to evaluate the functional status of anterior spinal roots and spinal nerves during brachial plexus surgery. Plast Reconstr Surg. 1997;99:1632–41.
5. Oberle J, Antoniadis G, Kast E, Richter HP. Evaluation of traumatic cervical nerve root injuries by intraoperative evoked potentials. Neurosurgery. 2002;51:1182–90.
6. Kline DG, Hackett ER, May PR. Evaluation of nerve injuries by evoked potentials and electromyography. J Neurosurg. 1969;31:128–36.
7. Hashimoto T, Mitomo M, Hirabuki N, Miura T, Kawai R, Nakamura H, Kawai H, Ono K, Kozuka T. Nerve root avulsion of birth palsy: comparison of myelography with CT myelography and somatosensory evoked potential. Radiology. 1999;178:841–5.
8. Burkholder LM, Houlden DA, Midha R, Weiss E, Vennettilli M. Neurogenic motor evoked potentials: role in brachial plexus surgery. Case Report Neurosurg. 2003;98:607–10.
9. Harper CM. Preoperative and intraoperative electrophysiologic assessment of brachial plexus injuries. Hand Clin. 2005;21:39–46.
10. Shin AY, Spinner RJ, Steinmann SP, Bishop AT. Adult traumatic brachial plexus injuries. J Am Acad Orthop Surg. 2005;13:382–96.
11. Spinner RJ, Kline DG. Surgery for peripheral nerve and brachial plexus injuries or other nerve lesions. Muscle Nerve. 2000;23:680–95.

10 Adult Brachial Plexus Injuries: Evaluation: Radiologic Evaluation

Felix E. Diehn, John C. Benson, and Dong Kun Kim

Introduction

Imaging is critical in the evaluation of preganglionic brachial plexus injury (BPI). The identification of nerve root avulsions is a vital component of prognostication and surgical decision-making. The principal modalities used to assess injuries proximal to the dorsal root ganglia are conventional myelography, computed tomography myelography (CTM), and magnetic resonance imaging (MRI), including myelography-type MRI sequences. Additional radiological evaluation in the setting of traumatic injury to the neck and/or shoulder girdle (including the postganglionic brachial plexus, bones, soft tissues and vasculature) is beyond the scope of this chapter; prior review articles discussing such imaging are available for the interested reader [1–4]. In this chapter, the imaging modalities, normal imaging anatomy, and imaging findings of *preganglionic* BPI in adult non-penetrating trauma will be considered.

Conventional Myelography

Through the 1980s, prior to the advent and refinement of advanced imaging (CT and MRI), conventional myelography was the gold standard for evaluation of the thecal sac and root sleeves of the brachial plexus nerve roots. However, this fluoroscopic/radiographic modality had major limitations compared to the advanced imaging available today: it relied on planar rather than cross-sectional imaging, was unable to evaluate the ventral and dorsal nerve roots separately, and lacked sensitivity for partial root avulsion. Conventional myelography continues to be utilized as the initial part of CTM (technical details to follow) when intrathecal contrast is injected in the fluoroscopy suite prior to transfer of the patient to the CT scanner. Since CTM can suffer from artifacts in the lower cervical and upper thoracic regions, the plain radiographic images obtained during conventional myelography prior to CTM may be complementary to the CT images.

Conventional myelography is performed by injecting iodinated contrast intrathecally, usually via lumbar puncture. Using a tiltable table, the contrast is observed flowing cephalad to the craniovertebral junction under fluoroscopy. Spot radiographic images are obtained, typically including anteroposterior (AP), oblique, and lateral projections.

F. E. Diehn (✉) · J. C. Benson · D. K. Kim
Department of Radiology, Division of Neuroradiology, Mayo Clinic, Rochester, MN, USA
e-mail: diehn.felix@mayo.edu

A. Y. Shin, N. Pulos (eds.), *Operative Brachial Plexus Surgery*,
https://doi.org/10.1007/978-3-030-69517-0_10

CT Myelography

CTM begins with conventional myelography. The patient is rolled several times to allow for optimal distribution of contrast throughout the thecal sac and transferred to the CT scanner for high spatial resolution cross-sectional imaging.

The current state-of-the-art multidetector row CT scanner allows for sub-millimeter resolution of approximately 0.5 mm, allowing for visualization of cervical rootlets which measure approximately 1 mm in thickness. The technology enables imaging with isotropic voxels (volumetric, three-dimensional pixels), such that high-resolution multiplanar reformats can be achieved. Such reformatted images are typically created in the sagittal, coronal, and oblique planes. Examples include oblique sagittal at the level of the foramina, oblique axial parallel to the disc spaces, and curved coronal aligned with the spinal canal.

CTM does have a few inherent limitations. In order for the contrast injected in the lumbar thecal sac to ascend to the craniocervical junction, the patient cannot have a flow-limiting stenosis in the cervical, thoracic, or upper lumbar spine. Extremely large body habitus can diminish visualization of normal anatomy and contrast material. The shoulders can similarly attenuate the imaging, particularly at the cervicothoracic junction. In an acute or hyperacute setting, blood products within the spinal canal, especially if intrathecal, can prevent contrast from adequately outlining the spinal canal. For this reason, and because pseudomeningocele formation does not occur immediately after injury, a CTM (or MRI) should not be performed immediately, but rather at least 1 week if not 3–4 weeks after the traumatic event [1–3, 5]. Careful evaluation of the intrathecal contents is required to distinguish nerve root mimics, such as normal vessels and scar tissue/adhesions [4].

MRI

Both conventional and myelographic-type MR sequences are typically performed to assess for preganglionic BPI; conventional (e.g., spin echo) sequences alone do not adequately depict intradural nerve roots. Specifically, conventional sequences often have CSF flow artifact within the intrathecal compartment that can obscure intradural nerve roots. Such artifact is mitigated on conventional gradient recalled echo (GRE) sequences, which allow for better definition of nerve roots but have inherently lower image quality due to reduced signal to noise ratio and resolution.

Advancements in MRI sequence technology have yielded iterative improvements in these aspects. Myelographic-type pulse sequences rely on heavy T2- or T2-like weighting, i.e., imaging sequences in which fluid is hyperintense (bright). On modern scanners, such sequences are three-dimensional, with submillimeter resolution and good signal to noise ratio. CSF flow artifacts are mitigated on such imaging, and individual ventral and dorsal rootlets can be distinguished similar to CTM. Trade names for such sequences from vendors used at our institution include Cube and fast imaging employing steady-state acquisition (FIESTA) on General Electric magnets and sampling perfection with application-optimized contrasts using different flip angle evolution (SPACE) and constructive interference in steady state (CISS) on Siemens machines. Cube and SPACE sequences are three-dimensional fast spin echo sequences optimized for isotropic imaging and using T2-weighting for MR myelography, while FIESTA and CISS are heavily T2-weighted (T2/T1) three-dimensional gradient echo sequences with very high contrast to noise ratio and fewer flow artifacts. These three-dimensional sequences can be performed in the axial, coronal, or sagittal plane, and relevant two-dimensional reformatted images can be made in any plane from the acquired data. As FIESTA and CISS are heavily T2-weighted but not purely T2-weighted, the signal intensity of tissues such as the spinal cord and bone marrow is best evaluated on conventional T2- and T1-weighted images.

CTM vs MRI

On MRI, the quality of preganglionic BPI imaging with the aforementioned high-resolution sequences is often excellent. MRI inherently affords greater soft tissue contrast resolution, so structures like the spinal cord can be better evaluated. In addition to evaluation of the spinal cord, MRI enables complementary assessment of other anatomic and physiologic changes, such as those involving nerve roots and paraspinal muscles (refer to subsequent sections on imaging findings). Postganglionic injuries involving the brachial plexus can be evaluated with MRI but not CTM. MRI is noninvasive, compared to the minimally invasive nature of CTM, and does not require intrathecal contrast material. In addition, MRI does not utilize ionizing radiation, unlike CT. However, despite progressive improvement in MRI technology, MRI may still suffer from artifacts. For example, large pseudomeningoceles can make visualization of nerve roots challenging, and CSF pulsation artifacts remain problematic. Furthermore, CT imaging has wider availability and has greater patient acceptance due to inherently faster imaging and fewer issues with claustrophobia. CT is also less subject to motion artifact, including that which stems from patient motion due to a variety of sources (e.g., tremor/patient movement, swallowing, respiratory, cardiac) and from CSF pulsation. Moreover, CT has fewer contraindications compared to MRI. For instance, patients with certain implanted devices may not be MRI candidates.

Several studies have assessed and compared the diagnostic accuracy of CTM and MRI for preganglionic BPI [6–8]. Generally, CTM has been shown to be at least equivalent if not able to outperform MRI [6–11]. CTM still affords slightly higher spatial resolution and slightly better visualization of nerve roots [12]. Historically, the reported diagnostic accuracy of MRI for nerve root avulsions has been quite variable; Tagliafico et al. cited literature in which its accuracy ranged between 52% and 88% [13]. Some studies have shown promising results for MRI. In a study of the accuracy of MRI compared to surgical results for brachial plexus lesions of various etiologies, traumatic injuries (both pre- and postganglionic lesions combined) were detected with a sensitivity and specificity of 84% and 91%, respectively [13]. Given such results and the inherent advantages of MRI over CTM, some centers prefer MRI over CTM as the primary modality to evaluate for preganglionic injuries [14–18].

Nevertheless, we believe CTM currently remains the clinical practice gold standard for nonoperative visualization of nerve root avulsions in adults. A recent systematic review was inconclusive with respect to the diagnostic accuracy of MRI compared to CTM for traumatic BPI [19]. Another current systematic review and meta-analysis found the accuracy of MRI for nerve root avulsion to be modest, with a sensitivity of 93% and a specificity of 72% compared to surgical exploration [20]. This review included a recent study that showed the accuracy of MRI for detecting nerve root avulsions to be 79% [21]. In our practice and in other high-volume centers [3, 22], CTM remains the imaging modality of choice for preganglionic BPI in adults, although the two modalities are often used complementary to one another [22]. We concur with authors who suggest that no single imaging modality has been definitively demonstrated to be superior in this realm [3]. A survey of experienced peripheral nerve surgeons for BPI management demonstrated that 94% use CTM or MRI and 41% use both [23]. This probably reflects the practice at many centers. If MRI is performed as the initial study, CTM can be especially useful when the MRI is discordant with clinical/electromyographic data or when the MRI is of poor quality [6]. The setting of partial nerve root avulsion identified on MRI is also one in which CTM may be particularly valuable [7]. Ultimately, modality choice depends on institution-specific factors such as physicians' preferences and available imaging equipment, as well on individual patient-specific factors. It is worth noting that some authors view CTM and MRI merely as supplemental investigations, with surgical exploration being the diagnostic reference standard [20, 21].

Normal Imaging Anatomy

Both CTM and MRI depict the normal anatomy of the cervical spinal canal in fine detail (Figs. 10.1 and 10.2). Normally, the spinal cord is

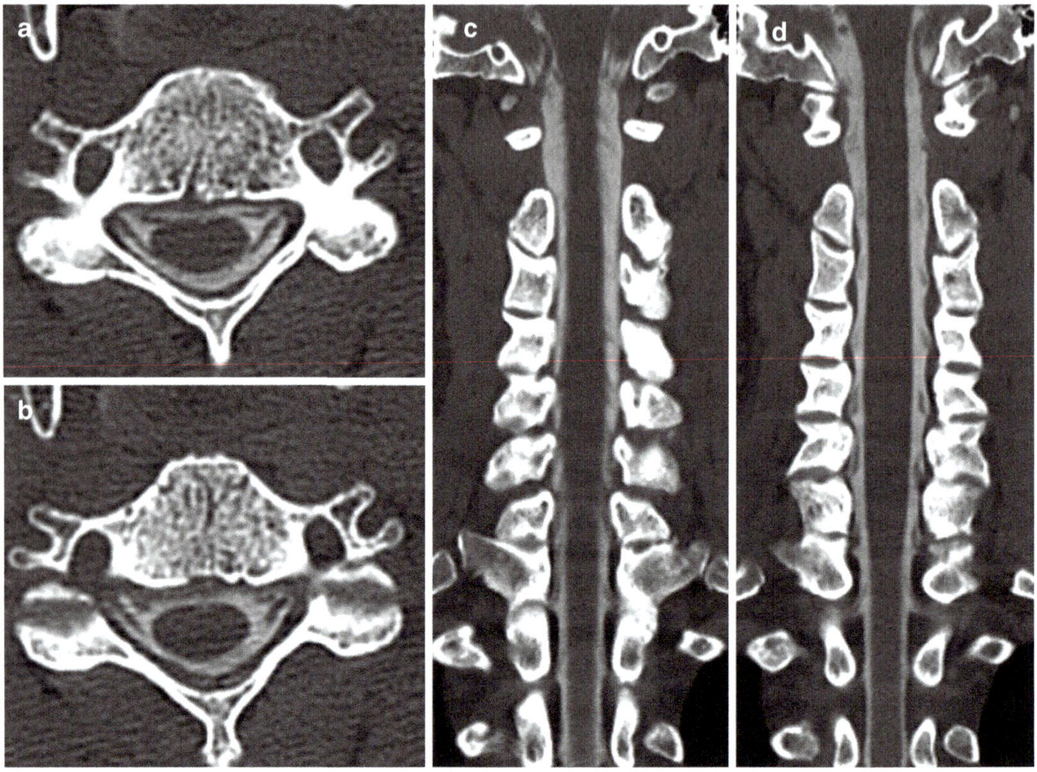

Fig. 10.1 Normal anatomy on axial (**a**, **b**) and coronal (**c**, **d**) CTM images. At the C5–6 level (**a**, **b**), the spinal cord is situated in the middle of the thecal sac. The bilateral ventral and dorsal nerve roots course laterally from the spinal cord (**a**) toward the neural foramina (**b**). The nerve roots are continuous on contiguous slices and of regular caliber. The dorsal nerve roots are slightly more prominent than the ventral counterparts. On coronal images, the dorsal rootlets at several levels are demonstrated as they coalesce into roots and course from the spinal cord (**c**) ventrolaterally toward the neural foramina (**d**)

situated in the middle of the thecal sac. The ventral and dorsal nerve rootlets and roots can be resolved individually as they course anteriorly, laterally, and inferiorly toward their neural foramina and coalesce into the spinal nerve at the level of the root sleeve. The nerve rootlets enter or exit the spinal cord approximately one vertebral level above their foramen. These nerve rootlets and the roots they coalesce into are symmetric in number, location, and caliber. CTM and MRI often more clearly delineate the dorsal compared to ventral roots, as the former are comprised of more rootlets and therefore thicker than the latter [9, 24].

Primary Imaging Findings of Preganglionic BPI

The two classic imaging findings of a preganglionic BPI are avulsion of the nerve root and pseudomeningocele formation, spanning from C5 to T1 (in some anatomically variant cases, also C4 and/or T2). Nerve root avulsion is the direct sign of injury and can be complete or partial; partial avulsions involve at least one but not all of the rootlets or roots. Although avulsion typically occurs at the level of the spinal cord, preganglionic injuries also encompass injuries located slightly more distally within the spinal canal or

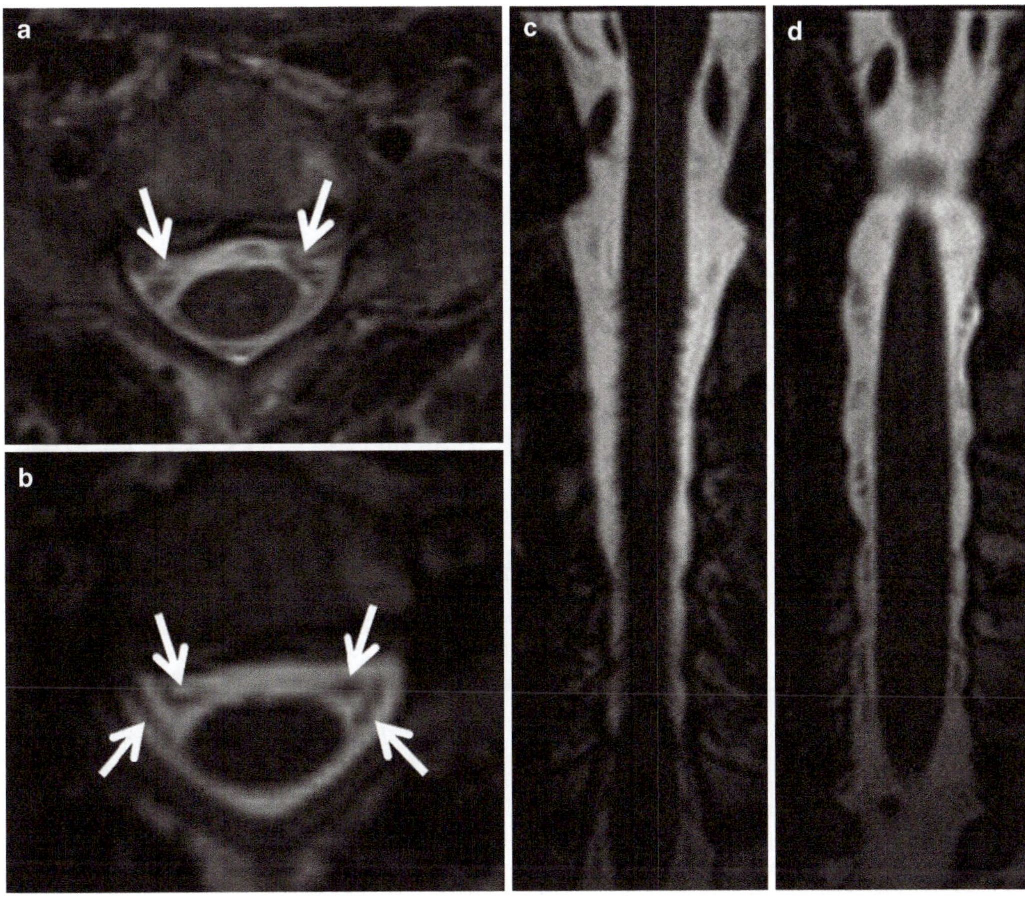

Fig. 10.2 Normal anatomy on axial (**a**, **b**) and coronal (**c**, **d**) MR images. On a conventional axial T2-weighted image at the C5–6 level (**a**), the spinal cord is located in the middle of the thecal sac. The nerve roots are not well visualized, in part due to their inherent low resolution and in part due to CSF flow artifact (arrows). At the same level on a high-resolution T2-weighted axial reformatted image (**b**; SPACE sequence, Siemens, acquired in the sagittal plane), the CSF flow artifact is mitigated, and the ventral and dorsal nerve roots can be identified as hypointense linear/curvilinear structures within the hyperintense CSF as they course laterally from the spinal cord to their neural foramina (arrows). A coronal reformatted image of this same sequence demonstrates the dorsal rootlets at several levels as they coalesce into roots and course from the spinal cord (**c**) ventrolaterally toward the neural foramina (**d**)

within the neural foramen, proximal to the dorsal root ganglion. A completely avulsed nerve root can be diagnosed by complete absence or lack of complete continuity of the nerve root within the spinal canal (Figs. 10.3, 10.4, 10.5, and 10.6). MRI may demonstrate displacement of the cord contralaterally (Figs. 10.5 and 10.6) and/or focal abnormal T2 signal (usually hyperintense edema) in the adjacent spinal cord at the root avulsion site. A partially avulsed nerve root may be missing either its ventral or dorsal roots (Fig. 10.4a) or one or more of its rootlets, or one or more of its roots/rootlets may be thinned or irregular but partially visible. Avulsion of ventral roots with preservation of the dorsal roots is the most common pattern of partial avulsion [9]. An asymmetrically abnormal course of the nerve root is an additional finding compatible with at least partial avulsion [25]. Occasionally, blood products can be identified in the injured nerve

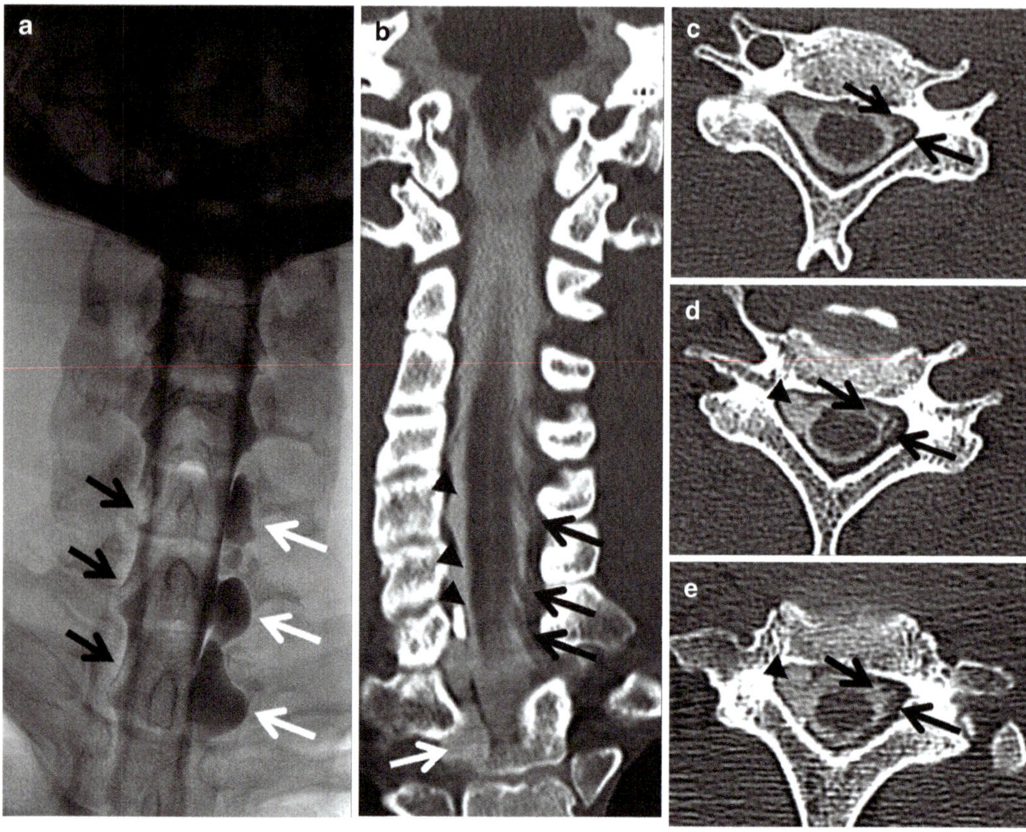

Fig. 10.3 Complete nerve root avulsions and pseudomeningoceles. Conventional frontal myelographic image in a prone patient (**a**), coronal reformatted CTM image (**b**), and axial CTM images (**c, d, e**). The frontal myelographic image (**a**) demonstrates multiple right-sided pseudomeningoceles (white arrows), from C6–7 through T1–2. The normal filling defects of nerve roots within contrast-opacified CSF (black arrows) are present on the right side but absent on the affected left side. The coronal reformatted CTM image (**b**) shows absence of the right C6, C7, and C8 nerve rootlets (arrowheads) compared to the normal left side (arrows), as well as multilevel pseudomeningoceles at C6–7 through T1–2 (e.g., T1–2, white arrow). On selected axial images, at C5–6 (**c**), C6–7 (**d**), and C7–T1 (**e**), the right C6, C7, and C8 ventral and dorsal nerve roots are not visualized, respectively, consistent with complete avulsions; note the normal left-sided nerve roots (arrows). Pseudomeningoceles (arrowheads in **d**, **e**) are present at C6–7 and C7-T1, but not at C5–6 (**c**)

root [26], characteristically manifesting as T2* hypointensity (increased susceptibility artifact) on hemosiderin-sensitive sequences such as GRE. One potential pitfall of nerve root avulsion diagnosis exists in the subacute phase, when perineural scarring at the site of an avulsed nerve root can mimic a partially intact neural element [4, 27].

A pseudomeningocele is the primary indirect, though imperfect, sign of preganglionic BPI. This is caused by injury of the dura surrounding the nerve roots and manifests as a laterally positioned well-defined but unencapsulated CSF-containing outpouching of the dural sac, without neural elements (Figs. 10.3, 10.4, and 10.6). Extradural collections represent a healing response of the injured dura and are best visualized in the days and weeks after injury rather than in the hyperacute phase. The presence of a pseudomeningocele is common with, but does not imply, nerve root avulsion, as the former can exist in the latter's absence. Similarly, nerve root avulsions can occur without pseudomeningocele formation

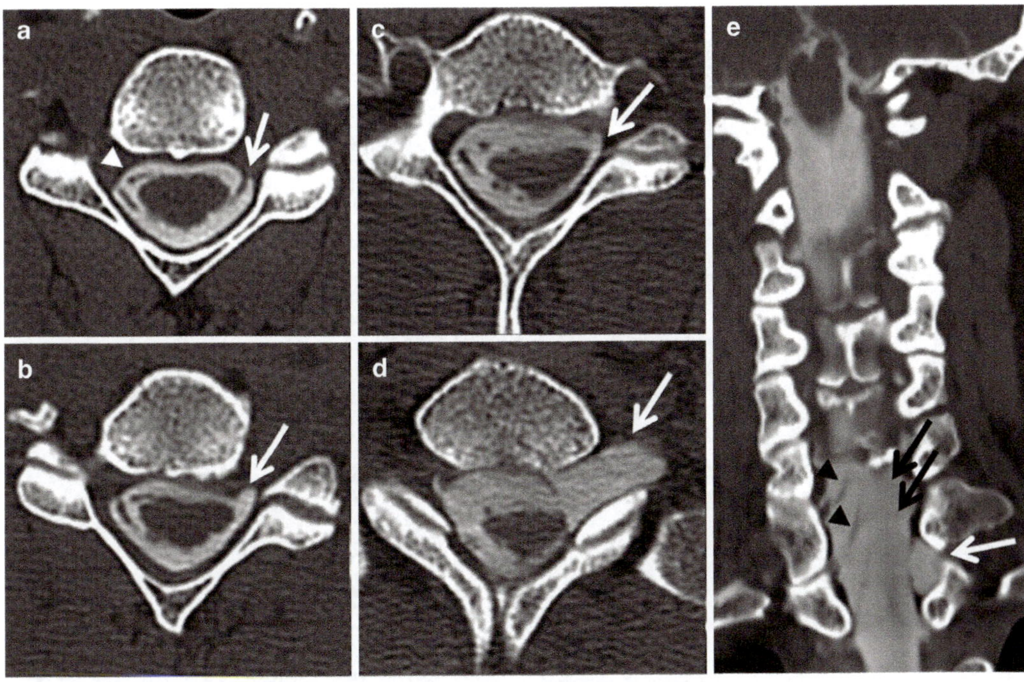

Fig. 10.4 Partial and complete nerve root avulsions and a pseudomeningocele. Axial (**a–d**) and coronal (**e**) CT myelography images. At C4–5 (**a**), a partial left C5 nerve root avulsion is present, with nonvisualization of the left ventral nerve root (compared to normal right (arrowhead)); the left dorsal root is intact (arrow). At C5–6 (**b**) and C6–7 (**c**), complete left C6 and C7 nerve root avulsions are demonstrated, respectively, with nonvisualization of both the ventral and dorsal nerve roots (arrows) and no pseudomeningocele. At C7-T1 (**d**), a complete left T1 nerve root avulsion is evident, with nonvisualization of either ventral or dorsal nerve roots and a large lateral spinal canal through extraforaminal pseudomeningocele (arrow). A coronal reformatted image at a ventral level (**e**) also demonstrates the absent left nerve rootlets at C6–7 and C7-T1 (black arrows), compared to the normal right side (arrowheads), and the left pseudomeningocele at C7-T1 (white arrow)

(Figs. 10.3, 10.4, and 10.5) [21, 28–32]. Pseudomeningoceles can range in size and conspicuity from large and obvious to small and subtle. They can be located within the spinal canal, neural foramina, and/or extraforaminal zones (Figs. 10.3, 10.4, and 10.6). When nerve root avulsions are concurrent, thinned or discontinuous nerve roots may be seen in or immediately distal to the pseudomeningoceles, and retracted neural tissue may be present distally [22]. While CTM generally relies on communication with the thecal sac for pseudomeningocele visualization, MRI can demonstrate such lesions even when they do not communicate with the intrathecal compartment [6, 22, 33]. In some cases, small necks and/or adjacent epidural scar may prevent such communication [6, 33].

Associated Imaging Findings of Preganglionic BPI

Associated findings of preganglionic BPI are generally better visualized on MRI than on CTM [32, 34–37]. Specifically, spinal cord injuries may be seen in association with preganglionic BPI, and MRI is especially better suited to diagnosing such cord injuries. In a 2011 study of 255 patients, clinical and/or imaging findings of spinal cord injury were present in ~15% of BPI patients [38]. Additional imaging findings in the acute phase include cord displacement (typically contralateral due to lack of normal traction from nerve roots (Fig. 10.6)), a divot at the neural avulsion site, cord parenchymal edema (T2 hyperintensity) and/or hemorrhage (often T2 hypointensity but variable depending

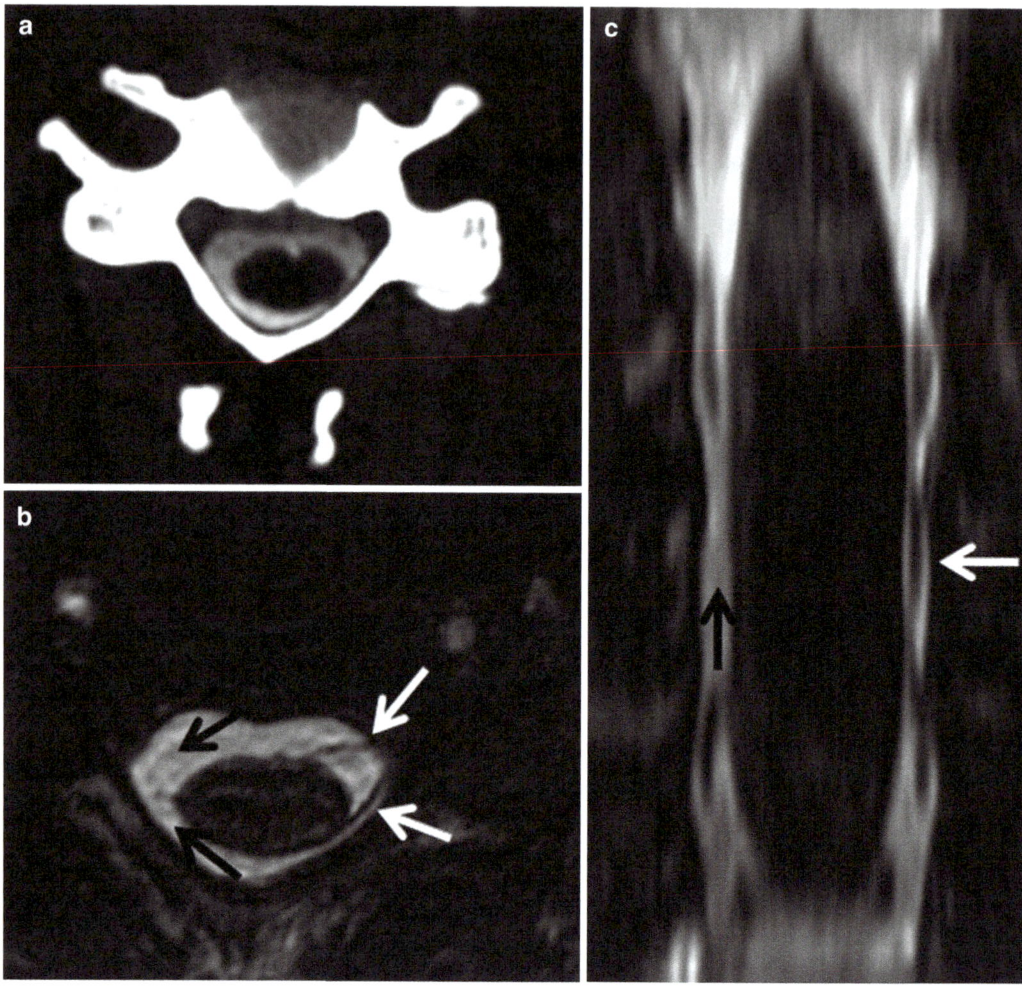

Fig. 10.5 Complete nerve root avulsion; CTM and MRI can be complementary. Axial CT myelographic image (**a**) and heavily T2-weighted axial (**b**) and reformatted oblique coronal (**c**) MR images, FIESTA sequence (GE). The CTM (**a**) does not convincingly demonstrate nerve roots at the level of interest on the right. However, the left nerve roots on the asymptomatic side are also not well seen. On the MRI (**b**, **c**), the right-sided nerve rootlets and roots are convincingly absent (black arrows), consistent with complete avulsion, compared to the definitely present and normal left-sided counterparts (white arrows). Note that a pseudomeningocele is not present

on age/type of blood products, with susceptibility artifact on hemosiderin-sensitive sequences), or mass effect on the cord from space-occupying lesions such as epi- or subdural hematomas. Frank cord transection is a rare presentation, as is transdural cord herniation. In the subacute to chronic phases, myelomalacia (abnormal T2 hyperintensity and volume loss) and syringomyelia (fluid-bright T2 signal) may be observed [12, 33, 39, 40].

Unlike CT, MRI can also depict the physiologic effects of trauma. Though uncommon, MRIs performed with intravenous gadolinium (not routinely done for BPI in our practice) may demonstrate pathologic enhancement of a nerve root, stump, or nerve root exit zone if these struc-

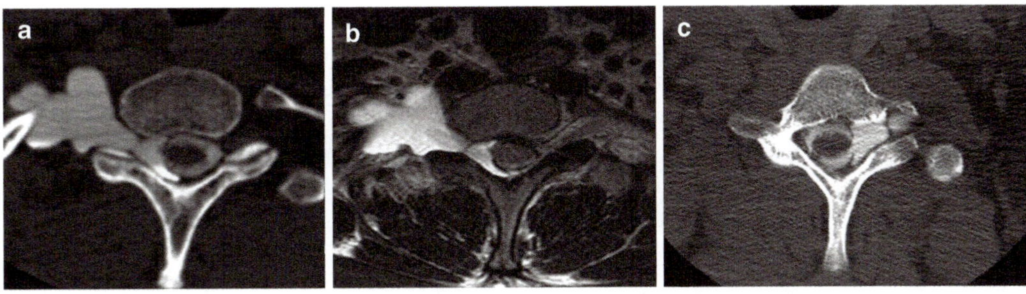

Fig. 10.6 Pseudomeningoceles in two different patients. Axial CTM (**a**) and axial conventional T2-weighted MR (**b**) images in the same patient demonstrate a large intraspinal through extraforaminal pseudomeningocele on the right, with lack of visualization of the right ventral and dorsal nerve roots at this level. Both examinations demonstrate these findings equally well. Axial CTM (**c**) in a different patient demonstrates a smaller left-sided pseudomeningocele. In both patients, the spinal cord is deviated contralaterally

tures have functional impairment [33, 34]. Such enhancement implies breakdown of the blood-nerve barrier, even in the presence of anatomic continuity [33]. Associated denervation changes in the posterior cervical paraspinal muscles and more distal innervated muscles may also be seen on MRI. These changes are easiest to see post-gadolinium and may be present even in the acute/early subacute phase after injury. Denervation changes can be diagnosed by the presence of edema-type signal abnormality (hyperintensity on T2, hypointensity on T1) and enhancement of the muscles [33, 35, 41]. Such changes occurring in the multifidus muscle are most specific for preganglionic BPI, given its single root rather than multisegmental innervation [33, 35].

Uncommonly observed findings associated with preganglionic BPI in typically the subacute to chronic phases include CSF leak and superficial siderosis. In a 2013 study of 145 patients with traumatic BPI, 15% of patients described new-onset headache, and in 5% these were classic postural headaches likely due to post-traumatic CSF leak [42]. Preganglionic BPI is one of many potential causes of superficial siderosis [43], which is due to chronic repetitive bleeding in the subarachnoid space. Typically this entity presents clinically decades after the traumatic event (Fig. 10.7).

Summary

Advanced imaging with either CTM or MRI plays a critical role in the evaluation of adult preganglionic BPI. Although CTM is considered the imaging gold standard and probably the first choice for advanced imaging in adults at most centers, MRI also offers excellent diagnostic performance. Due to their differing strengths and weaknesses, the two modalities are considered complementary at many institutions. Both modalities can detect the hallmark primary findings of preganglionic BPI: nerve root avulsions (complete or partial) and pseudomeningocele formation. The presence of one of these findings does not definitely imply the other. Secondary findings of preganglionic BPI may also be observed, typically better on MRI. These findings include injury of the spinal cord, physiologic findings such as nerve root enhancement or denervation changes in the paraspinal muscles,

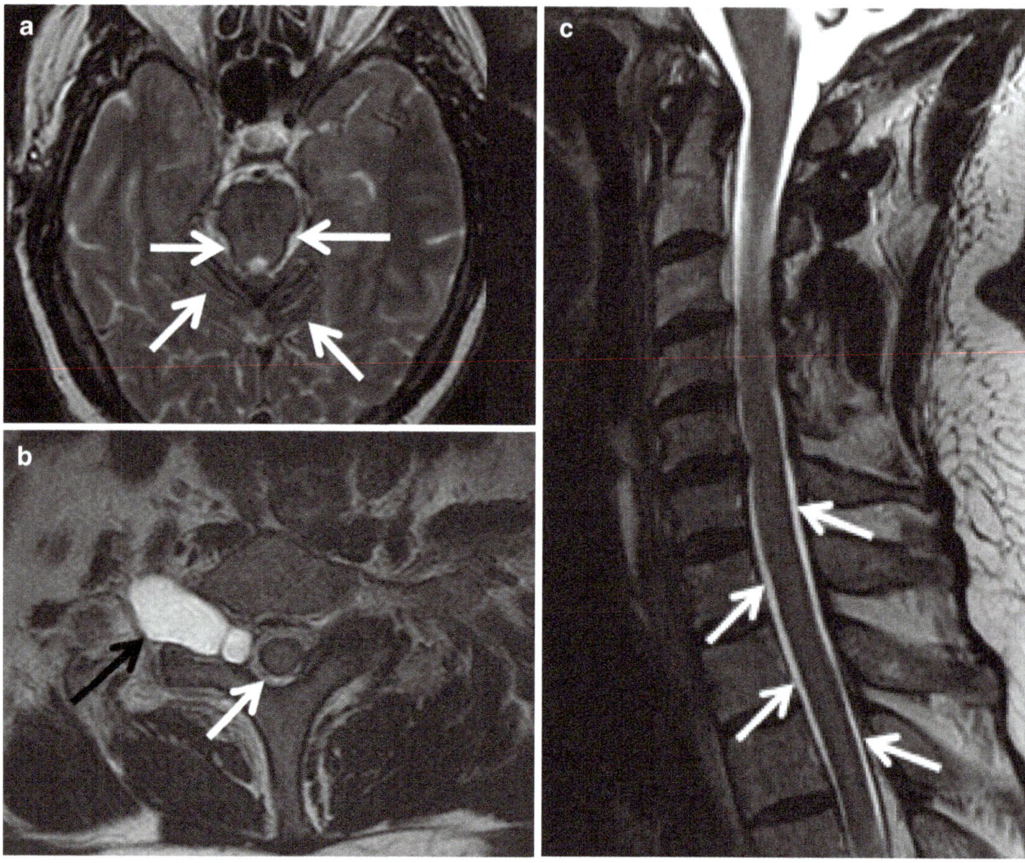

Fig. 10.7 Superficial siderosis as a chronic phase complication of traumatic preganglionic brachial plexus injury. T2-weighted axial brain (**a**) and axial (**b**) and sagittal (**c**) cervical spine MR images obtained 40 years after trauma. The pial surface of the brain and spinal cord is diffusely lined with T2 hypointense material (white arrows). A low cervical right-sided traumatic pseudomeningocele (black arrow) related to the remote trauma extends from the spinal canal through the foramen into the extraforaminal zone (**b**)

and, uncommonly, CSF leak or superficial siderosis.

References

1. Shin AY, Spinner RJ, Steinmann SP, Bishop AT. Adult traumatic brachial plexus injuries. J Am Acad Orthop Surg. 2005;13(6):382–96.
2. Sakellariou VI, Badilas NK, Mazis GA, Stavropoulos NA, Kotoulas HK, Kyriakopoulos S, et al. Brachial plexus injuries in adults: evaluation and diagnostic approach. ISRN Orthop. 2014;2014:726103.
3. O'Shea K, Feinberg JH, Wolfe SW. Imaging and electrodiagnostic work-up of acute adult brachial plexus injuries. J Hand Surg Eur Vol. 2011;36(9):747–59.
4. Amrami KK, Port JD. Imaging the brachial plexus. Hand Clin. 2005;21(1):25–37.
5. Vargas MI, Gariani J, Delattre BA, Dietemann JL, Lovblad K, Becker M. Three-dimensional MR imaging of the brachial plexus. Semin Musculoskelet Radiol. 2015;19(2):137–48.
6. Gasparotti R, Ferraresi S, Pinelli L, Crispino M, Pavia M, Bonetti M, et al. Three-dimensional MR myelography of traumatic injuries of the brachial plexus. AJNR Am J Neuroradiol. 1997;18(9):1733–42.
7. Doi K, Otsuka K, Okamoto Y, Fujii H, Hattori Y, Baliarsing AS. Cervical nerve root avulsion in brachial plexus injuries: magnetic resonance imaging classification and comparison with myelography and computerized tomography myelography. J Neurosurg. 2002;96(3 Suppl):277–84.
8. Nakamura T, Yabe Y, Horiuchi Y, Takayama S. Magnetic resonance myelography in brachial plexus injury. J Bone Joint Surg Br. 1997;79(5):764–9.
9. Carvalho GA, Nikkhah G, Matthies C, Penkert G, Samii M. Diagnosis of root avulsions in traumatic brachial plexus injuries: value of computerized tomogra-

phy myelography and magnetic resonance imaging. J Neurosurg. 1997;86(1):69–76.
10. van Es HW. MRI of the brachial plexus. Eur Radiol. 2001;11(2):325–36.
11. Castillo M. Imaging the anatomy of the brachial plexus: review and self-assessment module. AJR Am J Roentgenol. 2005;185(6 Suppl):S196–204.
12. Caranci F, Briganti F, La Porta M, Antinolfi G, Cesarano E, Fonio P, et al. Magnetic resonance imaging in brachial plexus injury. Musculoskelet Surg. 2013;97(Suppl 2):S181–90.
13. Tagliafico A, Succio G, Serafini G, Martinoli C. Diagnostic accuracy of MRI in adults with suspect brachial plexus lesions: a multicentre retrospective study with surgical findings and clinical follow-up as reference standard. Eur J Radiol. 2012;81(10):2666–72.
14. Rankine JJ. Adult traumatic brachial plexus injury. Clin Radiol. 2004;59(9):767–74.
15. Singer AD, Meals C, Kesner V, Boulis N. F MG, Umpierrez M, et al. the multidisciplinary approach to the diagnosis and management of nonobstetric traumatic brachial plexus injuries. AJR Am J Roentgenol. 2018;211(6):1319–31.
16. Tharin BD, Kini JA, York GE, Ritter JL. Brachial plexopathy: a review of traumatic and non-traumatic causes. AJR Am J Roentgenol. 2014;202(1):W67–75.
17. Mallouhi A, Marik W, Prayer D, Kainberger F, Bodner G, Kasprian G. 3T MR tomography of the brachial plexus: structural and microstructural evaluation. Eur J Radiol. 2012;81(9):2231–45.
18. Tsai PY, Chuang TY, Cheng H, Wu HM, Chang YC, Wang CP. Concordance and discrepancy between electrodiagnosis and magnetic resonance imaging in cervical root avulsion injuries. J Neurotrauma. 2006;23(8):1274–81.
19. Fuzari HKB. Dornelas de Andrade a, Vilar CF, Sayao LB, Diniz PRB, Souza FH, et al. diagnostic accuracy of magnetic resonance imaging in post-traumatic brachial plexus injuries: a systematic review. Clin Neurol Neurosurg. 2018;164:5–10.
20. Wade RG, Takwoingi Y, Wormald JCR, Ridgway JP, Tanner S, Rankine JJ, et al. MRI for detecting root avulsions in traumatic adult brachial plexus injuries: a systematic review and meta-analysis of diagnostic accuracy. Radiology. 2019;293(1):125–33.
21. Wade RG, Itte V, Rankine JJ, Ridgway JP, Bourke G. The diagnostic accuracy of 1.5T magnetic resonance imaging for detecting root avulsions in traumatic adult brachial plexus injuries. J Hand Surg Eur Vol. 2018;43(3):250–8.
22. Aralasmak A, Karaali K, Cevikol C, Uysal H, Senol U. MR imaging findings in brachial plexopathy with thoracic outlet syndrome. AJNR Am J Neuroradiol. 2010;31(3):410–7.
23. Belzberg AJ, Dorsi MJ, Storm PB, Moriarity JL. Surgical repair of brachial plexus injury: a multinational survey of experienced peripheral nerve surgeons. J Neurosurg. 2004;101(3):365–76.
24. Silbermann-Hoffman O, Teboul F. Post-traumatic brachial plexus MRI in practice. Diagn Interv Imaging. 2013;94(10):925–43.
25. Wade RG, Takwoingi Y, Wormald JCR, Ridgway JP, Tanner S, Rankine JJ, et al. Magnetic resonance imaging for detecting root avulsions in traumatic adult brachial plexus injuries: protocol for a systematic review of diagnostic accuracy. Syst Rev. 2018;7(1):76.
26. Fan YL, Othman MI, Dubey N, Peh WC. Magnetic resonance imaging of traumatic and non-traumatic brachial plexopathies. Singap Med J. 2016;57(10):552–60.
27. Chhabra A, Thawait GK, Soldatos T, Thakkar RS, Del Grande F, Chalian M, et al. High-resolution 3T MR neurography of the brachial plexus and its branches, with emphasis on 3D imaging. AJNR Am J Neuroradiol. 2013;34(3):486–97.
28. van Es HW, Bollen TL, van Heesewijk HP. MRI of the brachial plexus: a pictorial review. Eur J Radiol. 2010;74(2):391–402.
29. Nagano A, Ochiai N, Sugioka H, Hara T, Tsuyama N. Usefulness of myelography in brachial plexus injuries. J Hand Surg Br. 1989;14(1):59–64.
30. Walker AT, Chaloupka JC, de Lotbiniere AC, Wolfe SW, Goldman R, Kier EL. Detection of nerve rootlet avulsion on CT myelography in patients with birth palsy and brachial plexus injury after trauma. AJR Am J Roentgenol. 1996;167(5):1283–7.
31. Ochi M, Ikuta Y, Watanabe M, Kimori K, Itoh K. The diagnostic value of MRI in traumatic brachial plexus injury. J Hand Surg Br. 1994;19(1):55–9.
32. Volle E, Assheuer J, Hedde JP, Gustorf-Aeckerle R. Radicular avulsion resulting from spinal injury: assessment of diagnostic modalities. Neuroradiology. 1992;34(3):235–40.
33. Yoshikawa T, Hayashi N, Yamamoto S, Tajiri Y, Yoshioka N, Masumoto T, et al. Brachial plexus injury: clinical manifestations, conventional imaging findings, and the latest imaging techniques. Radiographics. 2006;26(Suppl 1):S133–43.
34. Hayashi N, Yamamoto S, Okubo T, Yoshioka N, Shirouzu I, Abe O, et al. Avulsion injury of cervical nerve roots: enhanced intradural nerve roots at MR imaging. Radiology. 1998;206(3):817–22.
35. Hayashi N, Masumoto T, Abe O, Aoki S, Ohtomo K, Tajiri Y. Accuracy of abnormal paraspinal muscle findings on contrast-enhanced MR images as indirect signs of unilateral cervical root-avulsion injury. Radiology. 2002;223(2):397–402.
36. Gupta RK, Mehta VS, Banerji AK, Jain RK. MR evaluation of brachial plexus injuries. Neuroradiology. 1989;31(5):377–81.
37. Hems TE, Birch R, Carlstedt T. The role of magnetic resonance imaging in the management of traction injuries to the adult brachial plexus. J Hand Surg Br. 1999;24(5):550–5.
38. Rhee PC, Pirola E, Hebert-Blouin MN, Kircher MF, Spinner RJ, Bishop AT, et al. Concomitant traumatic spinal cord and brachial plexus inju-

ries in adult patients. J Bone Joint Surg Am. 2011;93(24):2271–7.
39. Rehman I, Chokshi FH, Khosa F. MR imaging of the brachial plexus. Clin Neuroradiol. 2014;24(3):207–16.
40. Bowen BC, Pattany PM, Saraf-Lavi E, Maravilla KR. The brachial plexus: normal anatomy, pathology, and MR imaging. Neuroimaging Clin N Am. 2004;14(1):59–85. vii-viii
41. Uetani M, Hayashi K, Hashmi R, Nakahara N, Aso N, Ito N. Traction injuries of the brachial plexus: signal intensity changes of the posterior cervical paraspinal muscles on MRI. J Comput Assist Tomogr. 1997;21(5):790–5.
42. Hebert-Blouin MN, Mokri B, Shin AY, Bishop AT, Spinner RJ. Cerebrospinal fluid volume-depletion headaches in patients with traumatic brachial plexus injury. J Neurosurg. 2013;118(1):149–54.
43. Cohen-Gadol AA, Krauss WE, Spinner RJ. Delayed central nervous system superficial siderosis following brachial plexus avulsion injury. Report of three cases. Neurosurg Focus. 2004;16(5):E10.

11 Adult Brachial Plexus Injuries: Determinants of Treatment (Timing, Injury Type, Injury Pattern)

Robla Costales and M. Socolovsky

Traumatic brachial plexus lesions are devastating injuries in adults. Brachial plexus lesions may have a profound, lifelong social and economic impact on patients, because most will face severe residual morbidity. Great efforts should therefore be made to optimize the treatment of these patients. Recent years have witnessed tremendous progress in surgical techniques for brachial plexus repair [1, 2].

With the progress achieved in recent decades, there is currently a surgical indication in the vast majority of cases. The only absolute contraindication to performing nerve repair surgery for a brachial plexus injury is when too much time has elapsed since the injury occurred, such that the muscular atrophy associated with the disappearance of motor endplates has eliminated any potential for muscle reinnervation. More relative contraindications include a patient's poor general condition, joint stiffness, and the inability to adhere to an adequate postoperative rehabilitation program [3].

R. Costales
Department of Neurosurgery. Hospital HM Regla / HM San Francisco, León, Spain

M. Socolovsky (✉)
Peripheral Nerve & Brachial Plexus Surgery Program, Department of Neurosurgery, University of Buenos Aires School of Medicine, Buenos Aires, Argentina

There are many determinants to consider in the treatment of brachial plexus injuries. The most important determinants are surgical timing and injury type.

Injury Type

Traumatic brachial plexus injuries can be classified into open injuries and closed injuries that result from stretching. The latter are much more frequent and generally caused by high-speed vehicle accidents, especially involving motorcycles [3, 4]. The plexus may be affected at its origin in the spinal cord (root avulsion), in the supraclavicular region (root or trunk injury), or in the infraclavicular region (cord or terminal nerve injury). On many occasions, various combinations of the afore-mentioned injury types occur.

The classification system proposed by Seddon and Sunderland allows for establishing the degree of peripheral nerve lesion severity and the potential for spontaneous recovery [5, 6]. While these classifications are useful for understanding and establishing the management of these lesions, in reality, there is generally a combination of several degrees of injury in the same patient. This is especially true in the case of brachial plexus lesions [1, 3].

Regarding location, brachial plexus lesions can be classified in two ways: pertaining to

A. Y. Shin, N. Pulos (eds.), *Operative Brachial Plexus Surgery*,
https://doi.org/10.1007/978-3-030-69517-0_11

their position relative to the dorsal root ganglion and their position relative to the clavicle.

Preganglionic Versus Postganglionic Injury

Whether a brachial plexus lesion is preganglionic, postganglionic, or mixed is of paramount importance for therapeutic planning and prognosis determination [1].

Proximal ganglion lesions, called preganglionic lesions, are more severe and are usually associated with root avulsions, while lesions distal to the ganglion, called postganglionic lesions, are generally less severe, have the potential for some degree of spontaneous recovery, and have more options for surgical reconstruction. For this reason, no kind of spontaneous recovery should be expected with preganglionic injuries, and early nerve transfer surgery is indicated [1, 7, 8].

Differentiating between these types of lesion must be made with the data provided by the clinical evaluation, imaging tests, and electrophysiological studies. With the exception of direct inspection at the site of the lesion, which in general is not performed, the findings obtained via the complementary studies are suggestive, but do not irrefutably verify the diagnosis [3].

During the clinical evaluation, some information may be useful for determining the lesion's location. Intense pain, located mainly in the forearm and hand, described by the patient as a severe burning or compression sensation, indicates some degree of deafferentation and is strongly suggestive of root avulsion, which ultimately is identified in roughly 90% of cases [9], mainly involving inferior elements of the plexus [10]. In about half of patients, the pain becomes manifest immediately after the injury and, when associated with Claude Bernard-Horner syndrome, is highly suggestive of avulsion of C8 and T1 [3, 11].

Tinel's sign, elucidated by percussing the posterior triangle of the neck in the supraclavicular region, may be useful for differentiating between rupture and root avulsion [12]. When the sign is positive, there is a high probability that there is a neuroma and, therefore, at least part of the lesion is postganglionic, which means that the surgeon will probably have root stumps available for grafting. The sign is formed by radiation of painful paresthesia in the lateral region of the shoulder and arm (C5 root) and the lateral surface of the forearm, with extension to the thumb and index finger (C6 root) after supraclavicular percussion [11]. Eventually, this radiation can be directed towards the chest, indicating possible injury to the superficial cervical plexus. Paresthesia originating with a C7 root lesion is not well defined [3]. The search for Tinel's sign can be repeated in subsequent evaluations, and, when it progresses distally, axonal regeneration is presumed. A negative sign suggests root avulsion [3].

Functional loss of muscles innervated by nerve branches originating directly from the cervical roots is highly suggestive of a preganglionic root rupture.

With complete paralysis of the brachial plexus, the classically described maneuver to show a winged scapula to signify a long thoracic nerve injury is infeasible, due to paralysis of the musculature of the entire limb, so that a more suitable test in such patients is shoulder antepulsion in the supine position [3]. The long thoracic nerve originates in spinal nerves C5, C6, and C7 in the interscalenic space and innervates the serratus anterior muscle. The fibers coming from the C5 root that participate in formation of the nerve are responsible for the shoulder antepulsion [13]. Rhomboid muscle paralysis, caused by dorsal scapular nerve injury, is also considered a sign of C5 avulsion [3]. These muscles are responsible for adducting the scapula, aided by the trapezius muscle [14].

Electroneuromyography evaluation can provide important clues when attempting to locate the lesion in the dorsal root ganglion; these clues include identifying denervation of the paravertebral muscles and rhomboid and serratus anterior muscles and the determination of sensory conduction velocity. Imaging can also reveal findings indicative of root avulsion.

Supraclavicular, Retroclavicular, and Infraclavicular

Relative to the clavicle, brachial plexus injuries are classified as supraclavicular, retroclavicular, and infraclavicular. Supraclavicular injuries include a high incidence of preganglionic root rupture [3].

Retroclavicular lesions are uncommon and generally associated with another site of injury above or below the clavicle.

Infraclavicular brachial plexus injuries are complex and variable, with cord and terminal nerve injuries, and, in about 20% of cases, associated with a preganglionic lesion involving the inferior roots of the plexus [15]. Many times, there is an associated vascular injury, given the adjacency of the large axillary vessels with plexus structures at this level [16]. Associated supra- and infraclavicular lesions occur in about 10% of patients [3].

Injury Pattern

The brachial plexus supplies the whole upper extremity, except for a small strip of skin on the inner side of the upper arm, which receives sensory fibers from T2 [17].

Brachial plexus injuries include a broad spectrum of patterns. At one extreme, complete injury to the brachial plexus leads to a flail arm, which has no function and also entails additional problems like pain. The other extreme is a partial lesion involving only one root, with minimal loss of function because the vast majority of the muscles receive nerve fibers from at least two roots. The best example is an isolated lesion of C7. If two or three neighboring roots are involved, a characteristic paralysis pattern develops [1, 3, 17].

C5–C6 Root Injury

Patients with a C5–C6 root injury present with a palsy of shoulder abduction and external rotation, elbow flexion, and forearm supination. The coracobrachialis remains innervated. The flexor carpi radialis and pronator teres are functional, but weak. Wrist flexion is usually preserved, because the palmaris longus and the flexor carpi ulnaris are unaffected. Hand grasp and pinch strength and wrist extension and elbow extension strength are diminished compared to the normal strength values in the unaffected arm [2, 17].

C5–C7 Root Injury

The clinical picture of a C5–C7 root injury is similar to that observed with C5–C6 injuries. Wrist, finger, and elbow extension are also usually preserved, but with greater loss of strength than in C5–C6 patients. The flexor carpi radialis and pronator teres are paralyzed, as well as the latissimus dorsi muscle in roughly half of patients. Hand grasp and pinch strength and wrist extension and elbow extension strength are significantly weaker than in those with a C5–C6 injury.

There is usually a reduction of sensation in all fingers, especially in the thumb, but hand protective sensation is preserved. There is a longitudinal area of anesthesia along the lateral aspect of the forearm and arm and over the deltoid chevron [2, 17].

C5–C8 Root Injury

In addition to shoulder and elbow flexion palsy, the teres major, latissimus dorsi, pectoralis major, and triceps are paralyzed. Wrist extension is paralyzed, but some patients can extend the wrist with the help of thumb and finger extensors. Wrist flexion is possible, thanks to the palmaris longus, and pronation is possible because the pronator quadratus is still functional. Hand grasp and pinch strength are less than in C5–C6 and C5–C7 patterns [2].

There is a continuous longitudinal zone of lost protective sensation over the lateral forearm, lower arm, and deltoid chevron, as in the C5–C7 group, but wider. Unlike the previous group, the dorsal aspect of the hand is affected. With respect to the fingers, there is no particular pattern of sensory disturbance. Some patients present with thumb anesthesia, but in no instance is there complete anesthesia of all fingers. Horner's sign is absent [2].

C5-T1 Root Injury with Partially Preserved Finger Flexion and Horner's Sign

In these patients, the shoulder is completely paralyzed. Adduction is not possible, because the pectoralis major is totally paralyzed, and there is also palsy of finger and wrist extension. Wrist flexion is weak, but preserved in some patients because the palmaris longus remains functional. Finger flexion is possible, but incomplete in excursion and not functional for all fingers. Grasping and pinch are extremely weak and, thereby, nonfunctional. Thumb anesthesia is frequent. The dorsal aspect of the hand is completely anesthetized. The lateral longitudinal area of anesthesia over the forearm and arm is wider than in C5–C8 patients, comprising 2/3 of the limb circumference. There is still a zone of normal sensation over the ulnar border. The findings observed in this group of patients may be due to a partial root injury of T1 or, more likely, to a post-fixated brachial plexus [2, 3, 17].

C8-T1 Root Injury

In these patients, shoulder function and elbow flexion are normal. Wrist and finger extension are preserved. The flexor carpi radialis is preserved, but the flexor carpi ulnaris and palmaris longus are paralyzed. The pronator teres is also preserved. Intrinsic muscles of the hand are partially preserved. The flexor pollicis longus is paralyzed. Wrist extension is weaker than in the normal wrist [2, 3].

Sensory disturbances compromise the ulnar aspect of the hand and forearm. Horner's sign is always present [2, 17].

C7-T1 Root Injury

In C7-T1 patients, shoulder and elbow range of motion are normal, but strength is markedly reduced relative to the patient's normal side and to the affected limb in C8-T1 patients [16].

Wrist extension is weak, roughly half the strength of the normal side, and with radial deviation due to extensor carpi ulnaris palsy [2, 16].

Sensory disturbance is present along the ulnar aspect of the hand, forearm, and arm. As opposed to C8-T1 patients, decreased sensation also is present in the third finger [2].

C8-T1 Root Injury

Triceps paralysis and weak wrist extension are the main differences in this group compared to the previous group of patients. Shoulder motion and elbow flexion are almost normal [2].

C5-T1 Palsy

In these patients, the clinical picture is a flail limb. All patients present with a Horner's sign. The sensory deficit includes the entire limb, except for the inner aspect of the arm [2, 3, 17].

Timing of Surgery

Deciding on the right time to operate on a traumatic brachial plexus injury must be done following a thorough analysis of each case.

Patients with total palsy of the brachial plexus following the causal trauma have almost no chance of spontaneous recovery, so early surgery is usually indicated, even more so if root avulsions are diagnosed [2].

Conversely, with partial injuries some spontaneous improvement might occur. The best time to operate on such patients is after the third month, but before the sixth month after injury. Good results can be achieved after the seventh month, but the rate of good results decreases drastically, especially after 9 months [2, 3, 17].

One year since the trauma that caused the brachial plexus injury is the maximum time generally accepted to perform primary repair surgery expecting good results [3].

Other Determinants of Treatment

As mentioned previously, it is well established that certain factors play an important role in the outcomes experienced by patients who undergo brachial plexus reconstructive surgery. Among these factors, the time from trauma to surgery and the extent of the primary lesion seem to be the most important [18].

Recently, other factors like compliance with postoperative rehabilitation [19, 20], the patient's age [18], and the patient's body mass index [21–23] have been considered, though they seem to be less major determinants.

Body Mass Index

Body mass index (BMI), which reflects a patient's weight relative to height, has only recently been reported as another prognostic factor, with its influence appearing not to be as strong as the timing of surgery [22, 24].

Data published in the literature seem to favor lower BMI as a predictor of enhanced outcome, with an inverse relationship between mean BMI and clinical results [23–25].

Socolovsky et al. analyzed the influence of BMI on the outcomes for abduction following spinal accessory to suprascapular nerve transfers, and a high BMI was found to predict a poorer outcome, measured as the degrees of shoulder abduction achieved after a minimum 24 months of follow-up [22].

Lee et al. identified BMI as one of the factors affecting deltoid strength after triceps motor branch transfer for axillary nerve reinnervation. Patients with a higher BMI do not necessarily have larger deltoid muscles and need more deltoid strength to elevate their heavier arms [25].

Proximal muscle reinnervation is more dependent upon BMI than distal muscle reinnervation, because proximal muscles must support more of the limb's weight [23].

Patient Age

It has long been known that the pediatric nervous system has greater plasticity and regenerative potential than the adult's, and it is common experience that younger adults recover faster and more robustly than older adults.

Data also suggest that age is linked to the outcomes of brachial plexus surgery. A number of case series have demonstrated poorer outcomes for nerve repair and reconstruction in older patients [23]. It has been suggested that this trend may be related to a decreased capacity for nerve regeneration in older patients [26].

In one analysis of 194 musculocutaneous nerve reconstructions in the context of brachial plexus injuries, patients younger than 20 demonstrated significantly superior biceps/brachialis power than those older than 40 [27].

In 2009, Terzis et al. analyzed axillary nerve reconstructions in posttraumatic plexopathy patients and found that people younger than 20 years old obtained superior deltoid power (mean = M3.18) than those older than 20 years (mean = M2.70) [28].

Poor outcomes have also been observed in older patients specifically receiving nerve transfers. Lee et al. found that deltoid strength after a triceps to axillary nerve transfer correlated inversely with the patient's age [28].

A recent study found that increasing age adversely affects outcomes with respect to elbow flexion, but could not demonstrate it for shoulder abduction [18].

It appears that increasing age is associated with steadily worsening elbow flexion and shoulder abduction outcomes, perhaps indicating a need for earlier surgery and/or more aggressive repairs in older patients.

There is very little published data available to evaluate the outcomes of nerve transfers in patients older than 70 [25]. As described earlier, although age has been identified as an independent risk factor in the literature, there are other more important determinants, like the duration of time from injury to surgery [2, 26, 28]. The current literature on brachial plexus surgery in elderly patients questions the dogma that older patients who receive nerve transfers fare poorly [23].

Rehabilitation

The influence of an intense and prolonged rehabilitation program on the final result in patients with a brachial plexus injury is well-known among peripheral nerve surgeons.

Outcomes related to compliance with postoperative rehabilitation have recently been analyzed [19, 20, 29], with statistically superior outcomes achieved in patients who followed a specialized neuro-rehabilitation program than in those who either failed to follow a rehabilitation program or were deficient in their compliance.

References

1. Siqueira MG, Malessy MJA. Traumatic brachial plexus lesions: clinical and surgical aspects. In: Treatment of peripheral nerve lesions: Prism Books; 2011. p. 93–110.
2. Bertelli JA, Ghizoni MF. Results and current approach for Brachial Plexus reconstruction. J Brachial Plex Peripher Nerve Inj. 2011;6:2.
3. Siquiera MG, Martins R, Heisse O, Socolovsky M (2010) Lesiones traumáticas del plexo braquial e adultos: Parte 1. Mecanismos de lesión, métodos diagnósticos e indicaciones del tratamiento quirúrgico. In: Neurocirugía, Aspectos Clínicos y Quirurgícos, 1st Ed. Corpus.
4. Jones SJ, Parry CB, Landi A. Diagnosis of brachial plexus traction lesions by sensory nerve action potentials and somatosensory evoked potentials. Injury. 1981;12:376–82.
5. Seddon HJ. A classification of nerve injuries. Br Med J. 1942;2:237–9.
6. Sunderland S. A classification of peripheral nerve injuries producing loss of function. Brain. 1951;74:491–516.
7. Terzis JK, Papakonstantinou KC. The surgical treatment of brachial plexus injuries in adults. Plast Reconstr Surg. 2000;106:1097–122. quiz 1123–1124
8. Midha R. Nerve transfers for severe brachial plexus injuries: a review. Neurosurg Focus. 2004;16:E5.
9. Parry CB. Pain in avulsion lesions of the brachial plexus. Pain. 1980;9:41–53.
10. Narakas AO. Lesions found when operating traction injuries of the brachial plexus. Clin Neurol Neurosurg. 1993;95(Suppl):S56–64.
11. Bertelli JA, Ghizoni MF. Use of clinical signs and computed tomography myelography findings in detecting and excluding nerve root avulsion in complete brachial plexus palsy. J Neurosurg. 2006;105:835–42.
12. Landi A, Copeland S. Value of the Tinel sign in brachial plexus lesions. Ann R Coll Surg Engl. 1979;61:470–1.
13. Bertelli JA, Ghizoni MF. Long thoracic nerve: anatomy and functional assessment. J Bone Joint Surg Am. 2005;87:993–8.
14. Smith J, Padgett DJ, Kaufman KR, et al. Rhomboid muscle electromyography activity during 3 different manual muscle tests. Arch Phys Med Rehabil. 2004;85:987–92.
15. Birch R. Injuries to the brachial plexus: controversies and possibilities. Neurosurg Clin N Am. 2001;12:285–94.
16. Birch R. Infraclavicular lesions. In: Boome RB, editor. The hand and upper extremity: the brachial plexus. Edinburgh and New York: Churchill Livingstone; 1997. p. 79–88.
17. Millesi H. Update on the treatment of adult brachial plexus injuries. In: Brachial plexus injuries. Martin Dunitz Ltd. 2001.
18. Socolovsky M, di Masi G, Bonilla G, et al. Age as a predictor of long-term results in patients with brachial plexus palsies undergoing surgical repair. Oper Neurosurg (Hagerstown). 2018;15:15–24.
19. Socolovsky M, Di Masi G, Battaglia D. Use of long autologous nerve grafts in brachial plexus reconstruction: factors that affect the outcome. Acta Neurochir. 2011;153:2231–40.
20. Socolovsky M, di Masi G, Bonilla G, et al. The phrenic nerve as a donor for brachial plexus injuries: is it safe and effective? Case series and literature analysis. Acta Neurochir. 2015;157:1077–86; discussion 1086.
21. Elhassan B, Bishop AT, Hartzler RU, et al. Tendon transfer options about the shoulder in patients with brachial plexus injury. J Bone Joint Surg Am. 2012;94:1391–8.
22. Socolovsky M, Di Masi G, Bonilla G, Malessy M. Spinal to accessory nerve transfer in traumatic brachial plexus palsy: is body mass index a predictor of outcome? Acta Neurochir. 2014;156:159–63.
23. Socolovsky M, Martins RS, Di Masi G, et al. Influence of body mass index on the outcome of brachial plexus surgery: are there any differences between elbow and shoulder results? Acta Neurochir. 2014;156:2337–44.

24. Socolovsky M, Paez MD. A literature review of intercostal-to-musculocutaneous-nerve transfers in brachial plexus injury patients: does body mass index influence results in Eastern versus Western countries? Surg Neurol Int. 2013;4:152.
25. Lee J-Y, Kircher MF, Spinner RJ, et al. Factors affecting outcome of triceps motor branch transfer for isolated axillary nerve injury. J Hand Surg Am. 2012;37:2350–6.
26. Johnsen PH, Wolfe SW. Successful nerve transfers for traumatic brachial plexus palsy in a septuagenarian: a case report. Hand (N Y). 2016;11:NP30–3.
27. Bonnard C, Anastakis DJ, van Melle G, Narakas AO. Isolated and combined lesions of the axillary nerve. A review of 146 cases. J Bone Joint Surg Br. 1999;81:212–7.
28. Terzis JK, Barbitsioti A. Primary restoration of elbow flexion in adult post-traumatic plexopathy patients. J Plast Reconstr Aesthet Surg. 2012;65:72–84.
29. Terzis JK, Barmpitsioti A. Axillary nerve reconstruction in 176 posttraumatic plexopathy patients. Plast Reconstr Surg. 2010;125:233–47.

12 Priorities of Treatment and Rationale in Adult Brachial Plexus Injuries

Allen T. Bishop

Goals of Chapter: To Provide a Framework for the Initial Neurosurgical Management of Adult BPI

Planning the initial treatment of brachial plexus injuries in adult patients is a complex process, requiring acquisition of information from the medical history, physical examination, imaging, preoperative and intraoperative electrophysiologic studies, as well as anatomical findings at surgery.

The goal of initial management is to restore as much function as possible to the limb, at the earliest appropriate time following injury. Immediate intervention of closed injury has its advocates, but is generally chosen primarily for penetrating or iatrogenic injuries when primary nerve repair is possible. Exploration and identification of stretched or ruptured plexal elements at the time of vascular or fracture surgery also have value, with a plan for later reconstruction to bridge areas of scar. Tagging of nerves at physiologic length at initial inspection is to be recommended in these instances, expecting the need to further resect scarred nerve stumps.

Suspected nerve root avulsions warrant early intervention due to the poor prognosis for spontaneous recovery. Intradural injury may be inferred by a detailed examination of proximally innervated motors, absence of a Tinel's sign in the posterior cervical triangle, associated injury to phrenic or spinal accessory nerves, deviation of the head and neck towards the opposite side, and/or presence of an ipsilateral Horner's syndrome. In addition, myelographic abnormalities and electrophysiologic studies demonstrating preservation of sensory nerve conduction in insensate areas provide additional evidence. If other medical factors permit, intervention in the first 1–3 months is encouraged.

Surgery should be delayed in incomplete injuries, or complete injuries without evidence of avulsion until after 3 months, as there is currently no method to differentiate a neuropraxic conduction block from a more severe axonotmetic or neurotmetic injury. Most surgeons would plan for this period of observation, with careful serial exams and EMG to document any observed improvement. Absence of improvement in one or more segments of the plexus provides the indication for surgery. Delay beyond 6 months, however, will result in generally poorer outcomes [1].

Why Set Priorities?

Every patient understandably desires restoration of normal limb function. Unfortunately,

A. T. Bishop (✉)
Department of Orthopedic Surgery, Mayo Clinic, Rochester, MN, USA
e-mail: bishop.allen@mayo.edu

A. Y. Shin, N. Pulos (eds.), *Operative Brachial Plexus Surgery*,
https://doi.org/10.1007/978-3-030-69517-0_12

recovery from most adult brachial plexus injuries generally precludes full recovery. It is necessary to plan to reconstruct what is *achievable* rather than what is *desired or desirable* for this reason. Multiple factors affect recovery from plexal injury. The most important of these are discussed below:

High-Energy Mechanism of Injury

Most injuries in adults result from motor vehicle accidents or falls. These closed injuries frequently produce both irreparable nerve root avulsions and extensive longitudinal axonotmetic damage. Separation of ventral and dorsal rootlets from the spinal cord, termed a "root avulsion," is not practically reparable. If not avulsed, there is commonly an extensive damage to plexal elements extradurally, with axonotmesis and extensive scarring and/or rupture resulting in large nerve gaps.

Limited Sources of Autologous Nerve Graft

Sources of expendable nerves are generally limited to small diameter sensory nerves, occasionally combined with vascularized ulnar nerve grafts when both C8 and T1 are avulsed [2, 3]. The amount of available material may fall short of what is needed to satisfy all available proximal nerves. One or both sural nerves are among the most expendable and useful sources. Sensory nerves from an insensate area of the paralyzed arm may also be used, commonly including the radial sensory nerve and lateral antebrachial cutaneous nerves.

Problems with Autograft Alternatives: Nerve Conduits and Allograft

Results of motor recovery, when using engineered conduits or allogeneic nerve material are generally poorer than those with autograft nerve [4–6]. Although engineered nerve conduits are readily available, they are generally contraindicated for defects other than short gaps in sensory nerves. Fresh and less-immunogenic processed nerve allografts have been extensively studied for major mixed nerve reconstruction. Reports of processed allogeneic nerves used to reconstruct brachial plexus injury are largely anecdotal [7, 8], and experimental studies demonstrate poorer functional outcomes [4, 9]. Fresh allografts require prolonged immunosuppressive treatment to facilitate axon regrowth, risk late rejection, and carry some risk of disease transmission [7, 10–13].

Decellularized or processed allografts provide results intermediate to conduits and autograft [4, 13]. Efforts are ongoing to improve allograft performance and hold future promise [11, 14–16].

At present, however, nerve autografts, either conventional or vascularized, remain the "gold standard" for mixed motor nerves and most especially for proximal locations such as the brachial plexus [9].

Limited Sources for Intra- or Extraplexal Nerve Transfer Donors

Nerve transfers provide an attractive alternative to grafting and often have proven superior when used to target specific needed functions. Transfers from expendable non-plexus nerves as well as intraplexal sources in incomplete injuries have greatly expanded options and improved results of these devastating injuries.

Time-Related Muscle Changes in Lower-Motor Neuron Injury

Elapsed time from injury to motor regeneration remains a critical problem in peripheral nerve surgery. The basic problem lies in the distance from the proximal nerve coaptation and the target muscle or sensory end organ. At the typical rate of 1–2 mm/day, nerve regeneration is a prolonged process. The importance of distance cannot be overemphasized, due to the current inability to mitigate the effects of lower motor neuron injuries on the muscles they supply. With loss of the lower motor neuron, involved muscles are completely denervated. A series of physical and metabolic changes occur as a result. These changes effect acetylcholine receptors, cellular metabolism as well as cytoskeletal and contractile proteins. Eventually, muscle may be replaced with scar and adipose tissue [17, 18]. Nerve regeneration time may be shortened by use of vascularized nerve grafts, direct nerve transfers closer to the desired muscle's point of innervation, or even skeletal shortening [19–22].

Slow and Imperfect Regeneration of Nerve Axons

While neuropraxic injury will generally recover, axonotmesis and neurotmesis disrupt not only the nerve fibers but also intraneural blood supply, connective tissue layers, and supporting cells.

Proximal Neuron Death

The distal axon, separated from its cell body, cannot be sustained. Depending upon the severity of the disruption, the ability of reparative mechanisms to permit axon regeneration will be variably compromised. The neuron itself has limited ability to regenerate and may at times not survive the axonal injury. This proximal dieback of neurons is more likely in sensory than motor neurons and more likely with disruption close to the cell body.

Associated Injury

Injury to adjacent soft tissue hampers nerve regeneration as well, due to exposure to the environment, vascular compromise, and/or infection. Vascular injury requiring stents or grafts in the subclavian or axillary vessels of the paralyzed limb is at the least a relative contraindication for free functioning muscle flap reconstruction. Ipsilateral fractures of ribs 3–7 carry a 10% risk/rib of intercostal nerve damage, limiting their use at times for extraplexal nerve damage. Phrenic nerve palsy is also associated with proximal plexus injury [23]. The use of intercostal nerves in the face of an ipsilateral phrenic nerve injury is a further clinical consideration, although generally found to be well tolerated. Similarly, damage to the spinal accessory nerve (eleventh cranial nerve) is common in conjunction with plexal injury. The resultant weak or paralyzed ipsilateral trapezius muscle eliminates another often important extraplexal nerve or tendon transfer source. Skeletal injury causing bone or joint instability, if left uncorrected, will also disturb the nerve recovery process.

Technical Factors

Technical factors also greatly affect nerve repair. These include accuracy of nerve alignment, tension at the repair site, number and location of sutures, as well as proper positioning of the nerve stumps without either excessive gapping or crowding/folding of fascicles.

In most cases, tension-free coaptation is not possible due to rupture with retraction and intraneural scarring. Nerve grafts to bridge such defects are required if direct reconnection of proximal nerve and distal targets is required. Regardless of the type of reconstruction, accuracy is facilitated by microsurgical technique [24]. Use of fibrin glue, nerve wrapping, and similar tools has improved or at least not adversely affected results [25–27].

Despite meticulous technique and the best available microsurgical equipment, nerve reconstruction remains grossly inaccurate at the scale of the nerve fiber. Axonal growth is often misdirected or blocked entirely, resulting in results that seldom meet the aspirations of surgeons and the expectations of their patients.

Brachial Plexus Injury Priorities

Priorities for neurosurgical reconstruction are based on assessment of what needed functions are both most important *and* likely to be successfully restored. There is general agreement regarding these priorities. The approach selected to achieve the desired function will vary depending upon the pattern of injury and surgeon experience, skill, and preferences, but should be largely based upon careful analysis of outcomes. From highest to lowest, the priorities for reconstruction are:

1. Elbow flexion
2. Shoulder stabilization and external rotation
3. Grasp and release function wrist extension/finger flexion and wrist flexion/finger extension

4. Hand sensation
5. Intrinsic hand function

Elbow Flexion

Elbow Flexion in Pan-plexal Injury

Global injuries generally are the result of motor vehicle accidents or similar high-energy insults. The result is a supraclavicular injury, most commonly causing avulsion of four or five nerve roots. In our experience, neither the C5 nor the C6 nerve root is usually available for nerve grafting, and extraplexal nerve options must usually be selected.

Grafting from a normal C5 or C6 root for elbow flexion when available would seem logical, to restore normal activation of elbow flexors. Reported results when performed within 6 months of injury have been somewhat disappointing. A study of 68 such grafts evaluated results by donor root (C5 or C6), time from injury to surgery, and length of nerve graft. Sixty-two percent of patients operated within 6 months of injury achieved MRC III or better function [28]. Forty-four percent of those operated between 7 and 12 months reached functional strength, and only 12.5% thereafter. Grafts longer than 12 cm produced a poorer result. There was no significant difference between C5 or C6 root donors. A larger series reported 53% good or excellent results with grafting from either C5 or C6 [29]. Efforts to improve results have focused primarily on extraplexal direct transfers from intercostal nerves as originally described by Tsuyama [30].

Nerve Transfers for Elbow Flexion

Nerve transfer from extraplexal nerves has become routine for reconstruction of elbow flexion. This is of course mandatory when all proximal roots are avulsed but also often preferred to intraplexal nerve grafts when roots are available by many surgeons. Many such transfers have been reported, using two or more intercostal nerves, the spinal accessory nerve with an interposed graft, phrenic nerve, and contralateral C7 with or without grafts. It should be intuitive that intraplexal transfers cannot be performed in global injury.

Intercostal nerve crossing, originally described by Tsuyama et al. [30], has been the "gold standard" procedure for reconstruction of elbow flexion in patients with complete avulsive injury. A later review of their experience demonstrated 82% at least MRC III recovery in adults younger than 40 treated within 7 months of injury [31]. Results have varied significantly in other reports, including a review of 19 studies and 635 cases reported in which 35% achieved at least MRC IV, and an additional 31%, MRC III [32].

Spinal accessory nerve transfer provided 72.5% MRC III or better in a large series of 216 patients [33] and 71% of another when surgery was performed by 6 months. Thereafter, results were much less satisfactory (55% at 7–12 months, and 0% when performed after 1 year) [28].

Phrenic nerve transfer has been controversial, given reasonable concern about pulmonary function after phrenic transection. A systematic review of 7 phrenic nerve transfer series including 124 patients was reported by de Mendonça [34]. 70.1% of patients achieved MRC III or greater strength, but with some initial impairment of pulmonary function. When transferred directly to anterolateral bundles of the anterior division, upper trunk, the phrenic nerve results did not differ statistically from intercostal nerve transfer [35]. Fifteen of 23 phrenic transfers achieved full elbow flexion (65%).

Functioning Free Muscle Transfer for Elbow Flexion

Functioning free muscle transfers can be performed for elbow flexion alone or combined with an additional, more distal function (e.g., combined with wrist or finger extension) [36] or finger flexion [37]. The use of a free muscle for combined elbow flexion and a hand or wrist function will weaken elbow flexion strength—a fact that must be weighed against the importance of the added function [38]. Additionally, distal function requires the ability to stabilize the elbow with triceps reinnervation, provided by another extraplexal nerve transfer [39]. Although other muscles have been used, the gracilis has been the most commonly selected donor, due to its favorable anatomy [40].

Free muscle flaps have the advantage of no period of denervation prior to the surgical procedure. When used for elbow flexion, the motor nerve may be placed in close proximity to the intercostal or spinal accessory nerve, also limiting the time period required for reinnervation, averaging 5 months in one series [38]. In 62 cases of pan-plexus injury, 68% of gracilis free flaps neurotized with intercostal nerves regained at least M3 function [41]. These results were superior to direct intercostal nerve transfer to biceps (42% M3 or greater). For this reason, we generally consider a free muscle flap in acute reconstruction to be our preferred method for global injuries. Significantly, the addition of direct nerve crossing to the biceps in addition did not significantly improve results [42].

Elbow Flexion in C5–6 or C5–7 Pattern

Injuries to the upper trunk, Erb-Duchenne palsy, produce paralysis of shoulder abduction and external rotation as well as loss of elbow flexion. The addition of C7 or middle trunk injury results in some variable additional weakness of elbow and/or wrist extension. Restoration of elbow flexion in these injuries is most successfully done by an intraplexal fascicular transfer to the biceps motor branch of the musculocutaneous nerve from the adjacent ulnar nerve [43]. Recovery of elbow flexion is rapid and reliable, particularly in purely upper trunk lesions.

The addition of brachialis reinnervation by addition of a second transfer from median nerve is a logical procedure to further improve strength [43–49]. We have not found this addition to result in statistically significant increased strength when compared to ulnar fascicular transfer alone and prefer to avoid risking further disturbance of wrist and hand motor and sensory function in most cases [47].

Shoulder Stability and External Rotation

Goals

Shoulder motion and dynamic stability depends upon innervation from the brachial plexus, primarily upper and middle trunks. The complex and coordinated interaction of multiple nerves and muscles required for positioning the arm and forearm is a challenge to restore with plexus injury. Paralysis of the shoulder results in subluxation of the humeral head due to the unopposed weight of the arm, which is frequently painful. Recovery of muscles crossing the joint will improve subluxation. Alternatively, glenohumeral arthrodesis will serve the same purpose.

Restoration of lost motion is also an important surgical goal. Although older papers have emphasized shoulder abduction in reporting successful outcomes, it is now recognized that external rotation is functionally the motion of greater importance [50]. External rotation allows active positioning of the hand in front of the body for better manipulation of the environment, while abduction allows motion only in the coronal plane.

Shoulder in Pan-Plexal Injury

In pan-plexal injury, the only shoulder girdle muscles reliably functioning are the trapezius, innervated by the spinal accessory nerve; rhomboid, variably through C4; and levator scapulae (C3–5). Severe injuries often damage more proximal cervical nerves as well as the spinal accessory nerve, weakening or paralyzing all remaining shoulder musculature. In such cases, particularly when all nerve roots are avulsed, options to restore active motion are limited.

A careful physical exam must be performed to assess potential treatment options, later confirmed by electrophysiologic studies and myelography.

Options to improve shoulder girdle symptoms in a global injury may include nerve grafts, nerve transfers, tendon transfer, and arthrodesis. The latter two are generally considered after the acute phase of treatment, but must be considered at the time of injury when resources are limited for other desired functions. Reconstructive procedures that stabilize the shoulder will improve more distal function, including strength of elbow flexion and extension. Improved positioning of the hand provided by shoulder positioning results in more functional grasp as well [51]. Shoulder reconstruction is generally directed to the axillary and suprascapular nerves.

Nerve Graft

Reconstruction of axillary and suprascapular nerve function by nerve graft from available plexal nerve roots or extraplexal transfer is desirable in global injury. The C5 nerve root, if available, should be routinely selected for shoulder reconstruction if available. Unfortunately, our experience has found most adult global palsies to have all five nerve roots avulsed, confirmed by evoked potential monitoring. In these cases, either nerve transfer or a later procedure (tendon transfer or arthrodesis) are the only possibilities for the shoulder.

Nerve Transfers

Intraplexal nerve transfer is, of course, not possible in global injuries. The most common extraplexal shoulder procedure is the direct spinal accessory to suprascapular nerve transfer. It targets the most desired function (external rotation) and requires no interposed graft. Other sources of nerve to the shoulder have included intercostal nerves, phrenic nerve, cervical plexus motor nerve, and the contralateral C7 procedure [51, 52, 53]. The desired result of shoulder external rotation by reinnervation of the infraspinatus muscle has proven to be less successful than abduction, particularly with pan-plexal injury.

Arthrodesis

When grasp is not attempted in global avulsive injury, reconstruction of elbow flexion as an initial intervention followed by later shoulder arthrodesis is a time-tested option [30, 54]. Results have generally been satisfactory in global palsy, resulting in improved shoulder girdle active motion at the scapulothoracic joint. At times, humeral rotational osteotomy may also be considered to improve external rotation position [55].

Tendon Transfer

The recognition of the importance of external rotation for function has led to the development of new methods to animate the shoulder. Unlike the Saha procedure, which moved the trapezius with the acromion to the deltoid tuberosity, transfers are now more commonly directed to the infraspinatus tendon, using the inferior third of the trapezius or (if ipsilateral distal muscle paralyzed by injury or spinal accessory transfer) contralateral lower trapezius [56, 57]. More conventional tendon transfers using latissimus dorsi or teres major are of course not possible due to paralysis in global palsy.

Shoulder in C5–6 or C5–7 Injury

The same options exist in incomplete plexus injury. Preservation of partial shoulder girdle function in some of these patients leads to predictably better range of motion by either nerve graft or nerve transfer [58].

Grasp and Release

Goals

Restoring grasp is a challenging undertaking, with results generally poor enough to make this desirable function at the bottom of the prioritized function list. A discussion of grasp should also include release. Grasp ideally requires active wrist extension and finger flexion as well as positioning of the thumb for key pinch against the radial border of the index finger. Release requires wrist flexion and finger and thumb extension. Finally, the proper pattern of finger flexion requires positioning of finger metacarpophalangeal (MP) joints in flexion prior to activation of long finger flexors. As intrinsic function is virtually never restored in proximal nerve injury, this requires a MP joint tenodesis or arthrodesis procedure in order to avoid an "intrinsic minus" or claw deformity. The ability to position the thumb for oppositional pinch similarly requires thenar motor recovery. As this is not practical, some form of thumb CMC positioning for key pinch by arthrodesis or tenodesis is needed, as well as stabilization of the IP joint to simplify the multiple-joint thumb axis.

Indications

Loss of wrist and hand function results from injury to the C8 and T1 nerve roots, generally occurring in complete or global plexus injury. In the majority of these injuries, the spinal nerves are avulsed. The irreparable nature of the injury and the long distance and time required for motor axon growth from proximal transfers to distal targets make meaningful recovery challenging without special techniques using free gracilis muscle flaps or contralateral C7 transfers. These procedures have demonstrated the ability to restore some useful (if rudimentary) grasp in some patients.

Contraindications

Stiff Hand

In order for useful grasp to occur, the hand and wrist must be sufficiently supple to allow the desired motion. In some patients with plexus injuries, the hands are dystrophic and stiff. In our experience, intensive physiotherapy with and without capsulotomy has generally not proven successful in obtaining the desired degree of tension-free movement of interphalangeal joints.

Vascular Injury

When functioning free muscle flaps are decided upon for hand function in brachial plexus injury, the absence of usable nerves in the arm requires both proximal fixation as well as proximal nerve and microvascular connections. Damage to the axillary or subclavian vessels in general is a contraindication to free muscle transfers, although collateral flow may at times allow a successful outcome [59].

Grasp and Release in Pan-plexal Injury

Contralateral C7

The use of the opposite limb (contralateral) C7 nerve root was pioneered by Yu-Dong Gu, applied to a variety of distal targets but most notably the median nerve for hand sensation and flexion [60]. The entire C7 nerve root may be used, with surprisingly little donor morbidity in most cases, although use of a portion is preferred by some [61]. When targeting the median nerve, a pedicled vascularized ulnar nerve graft from the paralyzed arm is used to optimize axon regrowth. Alternatively, direct C7 transfer retro-esophageally prolonged to include the middle trunk and its divisions avoids the use of any intervening graft and allows targeting a variety of additional functions, including elbow flexion and ulnar nerve motors [19, 20]. At times, direct transfer may also require shortening the humerus of the paralyzed arm, bringing the selected distal targets closer to the proximal nerve stumps. The size and age of the patient are factors influencing recovery, as is elapsed time from injury. We have abandoned the hemi-contralateral C7 procedure as originally described in adults due to poor outcomes [62], but find if of use in neonatal global palsy with complete avulsions.

Free Muscle for Grasp

Another approach to solving the grasp problem has been to use the gracilis muscle, whose anatomy is favorable for animating the hand. This is primarily due to the proximal location of its major vascular pedicle and adjacent obturator nerve supply, combined with its length [40]. These factors allow the pelvic origin of the muscle to be secured to the clavicle and acromion, with vascular repairs to available infraclavicular vessels (most commonly thoracoacromial trunk or thoracodorsal arteries and veins). Harvest of the entire muscle with its distal tendon of insertion at the pes anserinus allows it to reach distal to the elbow to connect with wrist or finger extrinsic tendons. Variations described have included transfer of one, two, or three muscles in an effort to obtain useful hand function.

Double Free Muscle Procedure

The ability to restore grasp in brachial plexus injury via functioning free muscle microsurgical flap transfer was described by Doi et al. [63], using one gracilis free muscle flap for combined elbow flexion and finger extension with spinal accessory nerve transfer, followed shortly thereafter with a second gracilis flap to provide finger flexion controlled by two intercostal motor nerves. Additionally, reinnervation of the triceps is required to position the hand in space. Triceps function is restored at the time of the second procedure with two additional intercostal nerves. Sensory intercostal nerves are generally transferred as well, to the median nerve or lateral cord contribution to median nerve.

Shoulder function has been restored using a C5 nerve root if available, or by a contralateral C7 procedure. Alternatively, arthrodesis or tendon transfer options may be considered. Shoulder function has been demonstrated to be important by some means in order for adequate grasp function [51]. Later thumb CMC fusion, tenolysis of one or both gracilis flaps, or shoulder fusion may be required to optimize function. Doi has reported 96% successful restoration of elbow flexion, and 65%, grasp with at least 30° of total active motion. In our experience, 75% of patients recovered M4 elbow flexion, and 65%, similar finger flexion obtaining at least M3 elbow flexion [38]. We prefer to transfer the first gracilis to wrist rather than finger extensors to augment the tenodesis effect for finger flexion, as adequate wrist extension was otherwise absent, or required activation of finger extensors crossing the wrist which adversely affected grasp.

Single Gracilis Muscle for Grasp

We have found patients reluctant to undergo the extensive commitment of two lengthy microsurgical procedures and in recent years have developed a single gracilis procedure that restores grasp, but not release. The procedure is described in detail in a subsequent chapter, but relies upon intercostal nerve transfer to both biceps and gracilis for elbow flexion and grasp and transfer of the spinal accessory nerve to the triceps long head motor branch. Sensory neurotization is performed with intercostal sensory nerves, and shoulder function by available C5 nerve root or later stabilization. A subsequent wrist fusion optimizes the mechanics of finger flexion, and the thumb repositioned for key pinch at the same time.

Triple Muscle Transfer for Grasp and Wrist Extension

Transfer of the adductor longus with the gracilis is occasionally possible with a single vascular pedicle with separate obturator nerve branches [64]. This enables a modification of the double free muscle procedure to include a separate motor for another purpose, such as wrist extension, combined with gracilis-provided finger flexion. The feasibility of this procedure has been published by Yuan-Kun Tu, but results as a triple transfer not reported in print.

Amputation and Prosthetic Fitting

Amputation remains an option, requested at times by patients troubled by painful shoulder subluxation or uncontrollable, insensate limbs [65]. Relief is provided for these bothersome problems with appropriate patient selection. Fitting with a passive cosmetic or limited-function prosthesis has proven to be of social or functional use in some of our patients.

Advances in prosthetics and prosthetic control using targeted reinnervation have revolutionized care of traumatic amputations and have opened the door for similar advances, just beginning to make inroads for brachial plexus injury patients [66–69]. Most such cases have been in incomplete injuries with substantial spontaneous or postsurgical recovery. The need to maximize return of proximal function including sufficient strength and motion to position a prosthesis for useful function will make the need for initial reconstructive surgery likely, rather than a "bionic arm" substitute without need for other interventions.

Outcome

Truly useful grasp requires the ability to position the wrist in extension with activation of finger flexors. Ideally, wrist extension is actively rather than passively positioned by arthrodesis. This is often challenging to accomplish, requiring double or even triple muscle transfers [38, 70] or modifications to the contralateral C7 procedure permitting direct transfer of multiple extraplexal transfers to provide a chance for useful recovery [19]. Whether reconstructed by contralateral C7 technique or by functioning free muscle transfer(s), useful function requires a number of anticipated steps to all be successful and to function together to be useful.

Release in a normally innervated extremity occurs with activation of wrist flexors and digit extensors. In a paralyzed hand, restoration of either motor may be useful. Active wrist flexion if present or reconstructed may enable later tenodesis of extensor digitorum and extensor pollicis longus tendons to the distal radius to provide better finger extension. Alternatively, active finger extension may achieve a similar result, although wrist extension will tend to occur simultaneously and may inhibit finger extension by tensioning the extrinsic flexor tendons. Given the problems with providing release function, many pan-plexus patients with some recovery of grasp place and remove objects to be manipulated with assistance from the opposite hand, making truly independent bimanual activity an unlikely outcome in even the most successful surgery.

Sensation

Goals

Recovery of at least protective sensation in brachial plexus injury is certainly desirable. Some form of sensorial feedback is required for grasp function. As Erik Moberg recognized in quadriplegic injury, "ocular" sensation, or observation of the hand visually during use, is one form of feedback not requiring cutaneous innervation of proven value [71]. Alternatively, nerve transfers are often utilized to provide critical sensibility.

Sensation in Pan-plexal Injury

Recovery of sensation in global injury may be provided in global injuries by extraplexal nerve transfer. Both intercostal nerve and contralateral C7 procedures have documented ability to restore sensation, although without cortical re-orientation [61, 72, 73].

Sensation in C5–6 or C5–7 Injury

The sensory deficit in upper brachial plexus injury chiefly affects index and thumb, extending to the middle finger with C7 involvement. Distal sensory transfers may allow recovery of critical sensory areas provided by the proper ulnar digital nerve of the thumb and proper radial digital nerve of the index finger. This may be accomplished by transfer of the common digital nerve to the fourth web, end to end with recovery of S2 or S3 function [74]. Sensory reeducation is mandatory in order to obtain a good result. The role of end-to-side neurorrhaphy performed in a similar fashion may potentially improve sensation without loss of donor area feeling. While appealing, considerable variability of reported outcomes in the literature makes this a less certain intervention.

Intrinsic Function

Lowest on the list, the complex functions provided by thenar, hypothenar, interosseous, and lumbrical muscles intrinsic to the hand provide the fine, coordinated control that many patients expect to recover with surgical intervention. Time and distance, limited available nerves for transfer, and changes to chronically denervated skeletal muscle in lower motor neuron injury make recovery of meaningful intrinsic function extremely unlikely. Patient education is required to lower expectations to realistic levels. In the (possibly near) future, powered orthoses or amputation with prosthetic fitting with "smart" or programmable terminal devices may enable a semblance of coordinated hand function to be obtainable. Efforts to overcome the muscular changes associated with lower motor neuron injury, to improve the rate and extent of axon regrowth, deficiencies in amount and performance of nerve grafts and their substitutes, as well as avulsive injury will continue to challenge the next generation of reconstructive surgeons.

Conclusions

Despite meticulous technique and the best available microsurgical equipment, nerve reconstruction remains grossly inaccurate at the scale of the nerve fiber. Axonal growth is often misdirected or blocked entirely, resulting in results that seldom meet the aspirations of surgeons and the expectations of their patients.

References

1. Akasaka Y, Hara T, Takahashi M. Free muscle transplantation combined with intercostal nerve crossing for reconstruction of elbow flexion and wrist extension in brachial plexus injuries. Microsurgery. 1991;12(5):346–51.
2. Bertelli JA, Ghizoni MF. Results of c5 root grafting to the musculocutaneous nerve using pedicled, vas-

cularized ulnar nerve grafts. J Hand Surg Am Vol. 2009;34(10):1821–6.
3. Birch R, et al. Experience with the free vascularized ulnar nerve graft in repair of supraclavicular lesions of the brachial plexus. Clin Orthop Relat Res. 1988;237:96–104.
4. Giusti G, et al. Return of motor function after segmental nerve loss in a rat model: comparison of autogenous nerve graft, collagen conduit, and processed allograft (AxoGen). J Bone Joint Surg (Am Vol). 2012;94(5):410–7.
5. Rbia N, Shin AY. The role of nerve graft substitutes in motor and mixed motor/sensory peripheral nerve injuries. J Hand Surg Am Vol. 2017;42(5):367–77.
6. Shin RH, et al. Treatment of a segmental nerve defect in the rat with use of bioabsorbable synthetic nerve conduits: a comparison of commercially available conduits. J Bone Joint Surg (Am Vol). 2009;91(9):2194–204.
7. Elkwood AI, et al. Nerve allograft transplantation for functional restoration of the upper extremity: case series. J Spinal Cord Med. 2011;34(2):241–7.
8. Squintani G, et al. Nerve regeneration across cryopreserved allografts from cadaveric donors: a novel approach for peripheral nerve reconstruction. J Neurosurg. 2013;119(4):907–13.
9. Sahakyants T, et al. Return of motor function after repair of a 3-cm gap in a rabbit peroneal nerve: a comparison of autograft, collagen conduit, and conduit filled with collagen-GAG matrix. J Bone Joint Surg (Am Vol). 2013;95(21):1952–8.
10. Larsen M, et al. Epstein-Barr virus infection as a complication of transplantation of a nerve allograft from a living related donor. Case report. J Neurosurg. 2007;106(5):924–8.
11. Kim JP, et al. The effect of full dose composite tissue allotransplantation immunosuppression on allograft motor nerve regeneration in a rat sciatic nerve model. Microsurgery. 2018;38(1):66–75.
12. Atchabahian A, et al. Regeneration through long nerve grafts in the swine model. Microsurgery. 1998;18(6):379–82.
13. Moore AM, et al. Acellular nerve allografts in peripheral nerve regeneration: a comparative study. Muscle Nerve. 2011;44(2):221–34.
14. Rbia N, et al. A simple dynamic strategy to deliver stem cells to decellularized nerve allografts. Plast Reconstr Surg. 2018;142(2):402–13.
15. Hundepool CA, et al. Comparable functional motor outcomes after repair of peripheral nerve injury with an elastase-processed allograft in a rat sciatic nerve model. Microsurgery. 2018;38(7):772–9.
16. Ray WZ, et al. Effect of cold nerve allograft preservation on antigen presentation and rejection. J Neurosurg. 2011;114(1):256–62.
17. Isaacs J. Major peripheral nerve injuries. Hand Clin. 2013;29(3):371–82.
18. Frostick SP. The physiological and metabolic consequences of muscle denervation. Int Angiol. 1995;14(3):278–87.
19. Wang L, et al. Contralateral C7 transfer to lower trunk via the prespinal route in the repair of brachial plexus injury: an experimental study in rats. J Plast Reconstr Aesthet Surg JPRAS. 2014;67(9):1282–7.
20. Wang SF, et al. Contralateral C7 nerve transfer with direct coaptation to restore lower trunk function after traumatic brachial plexus avulsion. J Bone Joint Surg (Am Vol). 2013;95(9):821–7. S1-2
21. Terzis JK, Skoulis TG, Soucacos PN. Vascularized nerve grafts. A review. [Review] [53 refs]. Int Angiol. 1995;14(3):264–77.
22. Kanaya F, et al. Functional results of vascularized versus nonvascularized nerve grafting. Plast Reconstr Surg. 1992;89(5):924–30.
23. Kovachevich R, et al. Complications of intercostal nerve transfer for brachial plexus reconstruction. J Hand Surg Am Vol. 2010;35(12):1995–2000.
24. Millesi H. Nerve grafting. [Review] [83 refs]. Clin Plast Surg. 1984;11(1):105–13.
25. Leite APS, et al. Heterologous fibrin sealant potentiates axonal regeneration after peripheral nerve injury with reduction in the number of suture points. Injury. 2019;50(4):834–47.
26. Sameem M, Wood TJ, Bain JR. A systematic review on the use of fibrin glue for peripheral nerve repair. Plast Reconstr Surg. 2011;127(6):2381–90.
27. Lee JY, et al. Does the addition of a nerve wrap to a motor nerve repair affect motor outcomes? Microsurgery. 2014;34(7):562–7.
28. Samii A, Carvalho GA, Samii M. Brachial plexus injury: factors affecting functional outcome in spinal accessory nerve transfer for the restoration of elbow flexion. J Neurosurg. 2003;98(2):307–12.
29. Nagano A, Ochiai N, Okinaga S. Restoration of elbow flexion in root lesions of brachial plexus injuries. J Hand Surg Am Vol. 1992;17(5):815–21.
30. Tsuyama N, et al. Intercostal nerve transfer for traumatic brachial nerve palsy. [Japanese]. Seikei Geka Orthop Surg. 1969;20(14):1527–9.
31. Nagano A, et al. Direct nerve crossing with the intercostal nerve to treat avulsion injuries of the brachial plexus. J Hand Surg Am Vol. 1989;14(6):980–5.
32. Kawai H. Intercostal nerve transfer. In: Kawai H, Kawabata H, editors. Brachial Plexus Palsy, vol. 161-236. Singapore: World Scientific; 2000.
33. Songcharoen P, Mahaisavariya B, Chotigavanich C. Spinal accessory neurotization for restoration of elbow flexion in avulsion injuries of the brachial plexus. J Hand Surg Am Vol. 1996;21(3):387–90.
34. de Mendonca Cardoso M, Gepp R, Correa JF. Outcome following phrenic nerve transfer to musculocutaneous nerve in patients with traumatic brachial palsy: a qualitative systematic review. Acta Neurochir. 2016;158(9):1793–800.
35. Liu Y, Lao J, Zhao X. Comparative study of phrenic and intercostal nerve transfers for elbow flexion after global brachial plexus injury. Injury. 2015;46(4):671–5.

36. Akasaka Y, Hara T, Takahashi M. Restoration of elbow flexion and wrist extension in brachial plexus paralyses by means of free muscle transplantation innervated by intercostal nerve. Annales de Chirurgie de la Main et du Membre Superieur. 1990;9(5):341–50.
37. Doi K, et al. Free muscle transfer can restore hand function after injuries of the lower brachial plexus. J Bone Joint Surg Br Vol. 1998;80(1):117–20.
38. Barrie KA, et al. Gracilis free muscle transfer for restoration of function after complete brachial plexus avulsion. Neurosurg Focus. 2004;16(5):E8.
39. Doi K, et al. Significance of elbow extension in reconstruction of prehension with reinnervated free-muscle transfer following complete brachial plexus avulsion. Plast Reconstr Surg. 1997;100(2):364–72; discussion 373-4.
40. Doi K, et al. Basic science behind functioning free muscle transplantation. [Review] [41 refs]. Clin Plast Surg. 2002;29(4):483–95, v-vi.
41. Maldonado AA, et al. Free functioning gracilis muscle transfer versus intercostal nerve transfer to musculocutaneous nerve for restoration of elbow flexion after traumatic adult brachial pan-plexus injury. Plast Reconstr Surg. 2016;138(3):483e–8e.
42. Maldonado AA, et al. Free Functioning Gracilis Muscle Transfer With and Without Simultaneous Intercostal Nerve Transfer to Musculocutaneous Nerve for Restoration of Elbow Flexion After Traumatic Adult Brachial Pan-Plexus Injury. J Hand Surg Am Vol. 2017;42(4):293.e1–7.
43. Oberlin C, et al. Nerve transfer to biceps muscle using a part of ulnar nerve for C5-C6 avulsion of the brachial plexus: anatomical study and report of four cases. J Hand Surg Am Vol. 1994;19(2):232–7.
44. Toussaint CP, Zager EL. The double fascicular nerve transfer for restoration of elbow flexion. Neurosurgery. 2011;68(1 Suppl Operative):64–7; discussion 67.
45. Sneiders D, et al. Outcomes of single versus double fascicular nerve transfers for restoration of elbow flexion in patients with brachial plexus injuries: a systematic review and meta-analysis. Plast Reconstr Surg. 2019;144(1):155–66.
46. Loy S, et al. Ulnar nerve fascicle transfer onto to the biceps muscle nerve in C5-C6 or C5-C6-C7 avulsions of the brachial plexus. Eighteen cases. [French]. Annales de Chirurgie de la Main et du Membre Superieur. 1997;16(4):275–84.
47. Carlsen BTMD, et al. Comparison of single versus double nerve transfers for elbow flexion after brachial plexus injury. Plast Reconstr Surg. 2011;127(1):269–76.
48. Mackinnon SE, et al. Results of reinnervation of the biceps and brachialis muscles with a double fascicular transfer for elbow flexion. J Hand Surg Am Vol. 2005;30(5):978–85.
49. Liverneaux PA, et al. Preliminary results of double nerve transfer to restore elbow flexion in upper type brachial plexus palsies. Plast Reconstr Surg. 2006;117(3):915–9.
50. Boe CC, Elhassan BT. Restoration of shoulder function. Hand Clin. 2016;32(3):303–10.
51. Doi K, et al. Significance of shoulder function in the reconstruction of prehension with double free-muscle transfer after complete paralysis of the brachial plexus. Plast Reconstr Surg. 2003;112(6):1596–603.
52. Chuang DC, et al. Restoration of shoulder abduction by nerve transfer in avulsed brachial plexus injury: evaluation of 99 patients with various nerve transfers. Plast Reconstr Surg. 1995;96(1):122–8.
53. El-Gammal TA, Fathi NA. Outcomes of surgical treatment of brachial plexus injuries using nerve grafting and nerve transfers. J Reconstr Microsurg. 2002;18(1):7–15.
54. Hara T, Tsuyama N. [Pectoral nerve transplantation in traumatic paralysis of the brachial plexus]. [Japanese]. Shujutsu–Oper. 1969;23(9):1087–96.
55. Alnot JY. Paralytic shoulder secondary to post-traumatic peripheral nerve lesions in the adult. [Review] [50 refs] [French]. Acta Orthop Belg. 1999;65(1):10–22.
56. Elhassan B, et al. Tendon transfer options about the shoulder in patients with brachial plexus injury. J Bone Joint Surg (Am Vol). 2012;94(15):1391–8.
57. Elhassan B, et al. Shoulder tendon transfer options for adult patients with brachial plexus injury. J Hand Surg Am Vol. 2010;35(7):1211–9.
58. Baltzer HL, et al. Evaluation of infraspinatus reinnervation and function following spinal accessory nerve to suprascapular nerve transfer in adult traumatic brachial plexus injuries. Microsurgery. 2017;37(5):365–70.
59. Hattori Y, et al. Complete avulsion of brachial plexus with associated vascular trauma: feasibility of reconstruction using the double free muscle technique. Plast Reconstr Surg. 2013;132(6):1504–12.
60. Gu YD, et al. Seventh cervical nerve root transfer from the contralateral healthy side for treatment of brachial plexus root avulsion. J Hand Surg. 1992;17B(5):518–21.
61. Songcharoen P, et al. Hemi-contralateral C7 transfer to median nerve in the treatment of root avulsion brachial plexus injury. J Hand Surg [Am]. 2001;26(6):1058–64.
62. Sammer DM, et al. Hemi-contralateral C7 transfer in traumatic brachial plexus injuries: outcomes and complications. J Bone Joint Surg (Am Vol). 2012;94(2):131–7.
63. Doi K, et al. Double free-muscle transfer to restore prehension following complete brachial plexus avulsion. J Hand Surg Am Vol. 1995;20(3):408–14.
64. Sananpanich K, et al. Anatomic variance in common vascular pedicle of the gracilis and adductor longus muscles: feasibility of double functioning free muscle transplantation with single pedicle anastomosis. J Reconstr Microsurg. 2008;24(4):231–8.
65. Maldonado AA, et al. The role of elective amputation in patients with traumatic brachial plexus injury. J Plast Reconstr Aesthet Surg JPRAS. 2016;69(3):311–7.

66. Aszmann OC, et al. Bionic reconstruction to restore hand function after brachial plexus injury: a case series of three patients. Lancet. 2015;385(9983):2183–9.
67. Nadi M, Midha R. Editorial. Myoelectric functional hand prosthesis for total brachial plexus injury. J Neurosurg. 2017;127(5):1160–2.
68. Resnik L, et al. Use of the DEKA Arm for amputees with brachial plexus injury: a case series. PLoS One [Electronic Resource]. 2017;**12**(6):e0178642.
69. Bueno RA Jr, et al. Targeted muscle reinnervation of a muscle-free flap for improved prosthetic control in a shoulder amputee: case report. J Hand Surg Am Vol. 2011;36(5):890–3.
70. Doi K, et al. Restoration of prehension with the double free muscle technique following complete avulsion of the brachial plexus. Indications and long-term results. J Bone Joint Surg. 2000;82A(5):652–66.
71. Moberg E. Surgical treatment for absent single-hand grip and elbow extension in quadriplegia. Principles and preliminary experience. J Bone Joint Surg (Am Vol). 1975;57(2):196–206.
72. Hattori Y, et al. Sensory recovery of the hand with intercostal nerve transfer following complete avulsion of the brachial plexus. Plast Reconstr Surg. 2009;123(1):276–83.
73. Gao K, et al. Outcome of contralateral C7 transfer to two recipient nerves in 22 patients with the total brachial plexus avulsion injury. Microsurgery. 2013;33(8):605–11.
74. Emamhadi M, Andalib S. Successful recovery of sensation loss in upper brachial plexus injuries. Acta Neurochir. 2018;160(10):2019–23.

Part III

Treatment Options in Adults

Root Grafting in Adult Brachial Plexus Injuries

13

Jayme Augusto Bertelli, Neehar Patel,
and Francisco Soldado

For decades, root nerve grafting has been the main standard of repair for brachial plexus injuries [1, 2]. However, the surgical exploration of root nerves is technically more demanding than nerve transfers. For example, most C6 stumps are retroscalenic in patients with a complete BPI, requiring a demanding and risky harvesting technique for which plexus surgeons must be comfortable to optimize functional and pain control outcomes [3].

Nerve transfers have become popular for surgeons without experience in surgical brachial plexus exploration, as they are performed in non-scarred areas with normal and reproducible anatomy [4]. The use of isolated nerve transfers has been justified because of certain theoretical advantages, relative to nerve grafting, like faster reinnervation and the avoidance of co-contractions. However, in a recent Systematic Review of Individual Participant Data on elbow flexion reconstruction for BPI, isolated nerve transfers only were superior to isolated nerve grafting for upper-type BPI. Nerve transfers failed to generate better results than nerve grafting in complete palsies, older patients, or late cases [5, 6]. The authors of this review hypothesized that nerve transfers "lose" their biological advantages when the donor nerve is not connected to a terminal muscle motor branch, very close to the target.

Current literature has focused on comparing nerve transfers and nerve grafting; but, in fact, it is the combination of these two techniques that optimizes BPI reconstruction results [5, 7]. Nerve grafting can be combined with nerve transfers, either because it is dictated by the availability of donors or to enhance and optimize reconstructive options. Benefits of the combination of nerve transfers and nerve grafting include the reinnervation of muscles other than those targeted by the nerve transfer, which in turn stabilizes the joint, thereby improving joint motion [7].

To conclude, mastering nerve root exploration and grafting techniques remains of paramount importance for BPI reconstruction. The clinical exam, imaging studies, and surgical exploration performed to determine nerve root availability and adequacy for grafting will be addressed in this chapter. We will also discuss our preferred nerve grafting strategies for each pattern of BPI.

J. A. Bertelli (✉)
Center of Biological and Health Sciences, Department of Neurosurgery, University of the South of Santa Catarina (Unisul), Tubarão, SC, Brazil

Department of Orthopedic Surgery, Governador Celso Ramos Hospital, Florianópolis, SC, Brazil

N. Patel
Bombay Hospital Institute of Medical Sciences, New Marine Lines, Mumbai, Maharashtra, India

F. Soldado
Pediatric Hand Surgery and Microsurgery Unit, Barcelona University Children's Hospital HM Nens, HM Hospitales, Barcelona, Spain

Pediatric Hand Surgery and Microsurgery Unit, Vall d'Hebron Barcelona Hospital Campus, Barcelona, Spain

A. Y. Shin, N. Pulos (eds.), *Operative Brachial Plexus Surgery*,
https://doi.org/10.1007/978-3-030-69517-0_13

Preoperative Judgment of Root Availability

Preoperative root availability evaluations, which combine clinical and radiological exams, are focused to ascertain the need for surgical exploration of the upper roots (C5 and C6) for potential nerve grafting. For lower roots (C7 to T1), surgical exploration is not indicated for two main reasons: first, in complete BPI or lower BPI, they are almost always avulsed; and second, middle and lower trunk reconstruction yields very poor results [3, 8].

For preoperative planning to verify C5-C6 availability post BPI, we recommend combining Tinel's sign, the protraction sign (in complete palsies), and a CT-myeloscan [3]. In one study, a preoperative clinical-radiological systematic evaluation that combined CT myelography and these signs was 96.8% accurate identifying graftable roots in patients with a complete BPI [3].

Although electrophysiological studies have also been used for preoperative planning in BPI, they are of limited value, and we do not rely on them for our clinical-radiological preoperative planning [9].

Clinical Examination and Root Availability in BPI (Tinel's Sign and Protraction Sign)

The most useful clinical signs to diagnose root rupture versus avulsions in patients with a total BPI are Tinel's sign and the protraction sign [3, 10, 11].

Tinel's sign is performed using gentle percussion over the supraclavicular region. Painful paresthesias radiating to the arm and eventually to the forearm (C5 root) or hand (C6 root) are considered a positive Tinel's sign. Approximately 90% of patients with a positive Tinel's sign have a C5+/-C6 root available for grafting [3].

The protraction sign is evaluated with the shoulder protraction test, which indicates postganglionary C5 injury, as the upper motor branch of the long thoracic nerve stems directly from C5, innervating the upper digitations of the serratus anterior muscle [3]. Forward motion of the shoulder girdle around the chest wall is evaluated with the patient in a supine position, separating the scapula from the bed. Motion is resisted by the examiner's hand placed over the anterior side of the shoulder, while concomitant shoulder elevation is avoided to prevent trapezius muscle participation. The sign is considered positive when protraction range of motion on the involved side is similar to that of the contralateral side and scores at least BMRC M4 in strength. Approximately 95% of patients with a complete BPI and a positive protraction sign have a C5 root available for grafting [3].

The presence of both a positive Tinel's and a positive protraction test, together with the absence of signs of avulsion on CT-myeloscan, is our indication for root nerve surgical exploration. However, according to Echalier, in total BPI with positive Tinel's and protraction tests, imaging studies might not be indicated, because their accuracy is 95%, with no false negatives [11].

Imaging Evaluation and Root Availability

Several studies have demonstrated an accuracy of CT myelography greater than 95% for detecting whether a nerve root is avulsed or ruptured [3, 12, 13]. Detractors of CT myelography argue that it is an invasive examination, but their opinion is based on isolated clinical reports of complications [14].

Magnetic resonance imaging (MRI) has also been used to assess root avulsion in BPI. However, the reported accuracy of 1.5 T MRI detecting root avulsions is far poorer than for CT-myeloscan, ranging between 52% and 79% [15, 16]. This said, Echalier has recently reported 89% diagnostic accuracy with this imaging modality [11]. Finally, MRI myelography has exhibited accuracy similar to CT myelography for the diagnosis of nerve root lesions [17].

Intraoperative Evaluation and Root Availability

Patients with a BPI and positive Tinel's sign or protraction test (total palsies) and myelo-CT that does not reveal avulsions of upper brachial plexus roots will undergo surgical root exploration. General anesthesia is used without muscle relaxants. The C5-C6 roots of the brachial plexus are explored through a vertical 6-cm incision centered over Chassaignac's tubercle, 1 cm anterior to the sternocleidomastoid muscle (Fig. 13.1). Roots are dissected medial to the phrenic nerve to check for continuity and to perform nerve trimming inside a healthy zone (Figs. 13.2 and 13.3).

Roots are stimulated electrically to confirm paralysis using an insulated 21-gauge needle (Contiplex D; B. Braun Melsungen AG, Melsungen, Germany) connected to a nerve stimulator (Stimuplex HNS 11; B. Braun Melsungen AG). Stimulation begins with 1 mA; and, if no muscle contraction is observed, stimulus intensity is progressively raised to 5 mA. The occurrence of muscle contraction following electrical stimulation indicates at least a partially preserved root. Any root lesion proximal to the point of nerve stimulation will preclude muscle contractions, because of inherent Wallerian degeneration of the entire segment of the nerve distal to the site of the lesion. A root stump also is considered graft-eligible if electrical stimulation of root branches produces muscle contraction of root-innervated muscles (e.g., of the serratus anterior muscle), if the root is uninterrupted from the

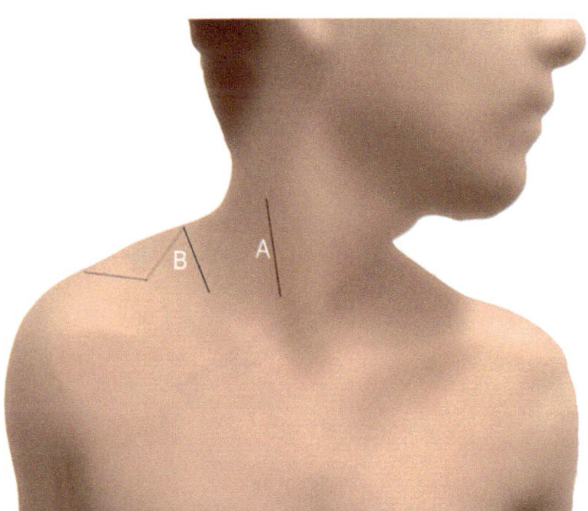

Fig. 13.1 C5-C6 graft-able roots are explored surgically through a vertical incision over Chassaignac's tubercle (A). The upper trunk divisions, SSN and SAN, are explored through a transversal incision over the supraclavicular region (B). "B" incision can be extended zig-zagged to detach the trapezius muscle allowing dissection of the suprascapular nerve distal to the suprascapular notch

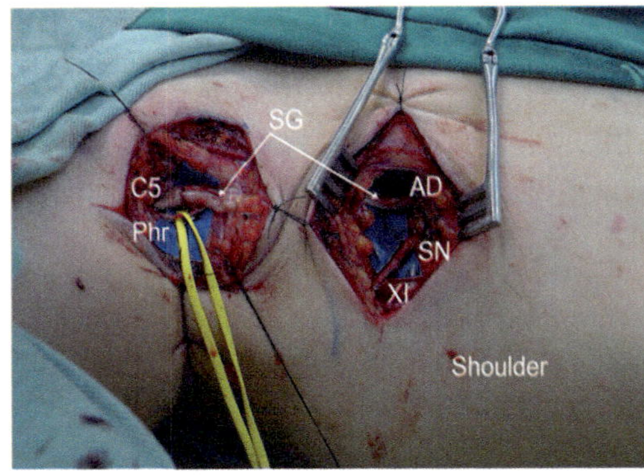

Fig. 13.2 Intraoperative view of the right neck depicting the C5 root grafted with two strands of sural nerve grafts (SG) to the anterior division of the upper trunk (AD). The healthy C5 root stump is medial to the phrenic nerve (Phr). The spinal accessory nerve (XI) is connected to the suprascapular nerve (SN)

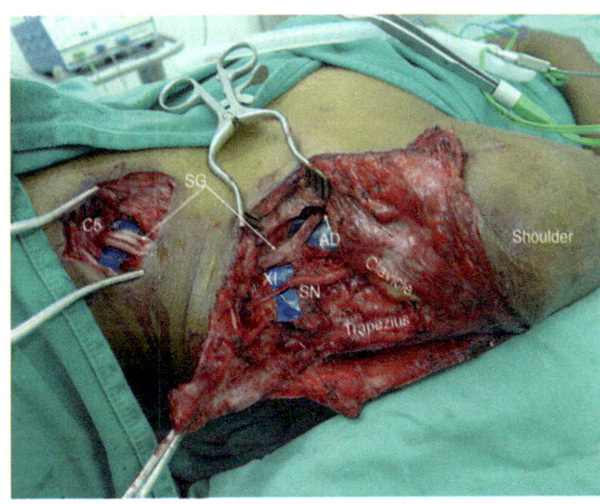

Fig. 13.3 Intraoperative view of the right neck depicting the C5 root grafted with three strands of sural nerve grafts (SG) to the anterior division of the upper trunk (AD). The trapezius muscle is detached from the clavicle allowing extended dissection of the suprascapular nerve (SS), till a healthy stump is available to be coapted with the spinal accessory nerve (XI)

supraclavicular or retro-scalenic region to the intervertebral foramen, and if a fascicular pattern and mushroom formation are observed after trimming. When a neuroma is present at the root stump, it always is considered a graft-eligible root.

We do not perform electrophysiological studies or histological studies to monitor root quality, because they are either unreliable or have not been proven effective [18–20].

Nerve Grafting Strategies in BPI

C5-C6+/-C7 BPI

Approximately 80% of patients with an upper-type BPI (C5-C6, C5-C7) present with a graft-able root. Our policy is that, even when we have two graft-able roots (C5+C6), we combine roots grafting to the upper trunk and triple nerve transfer (SAN to SSN, Oberlin and triceps to axillary) [7].

A supraclavicular vertical incision is made over the trapezius muscle and the distal third of the clavicle to allow for upper trunk anterior and posterior division dissection, as well as for a SAN to SSN transfer (Fig. 13.1).

When both C5 and C6 are available for grafting, one graft from the anterior part of each root (with neurons responsible for shoulder and elbow flexion) is connected to the anterior division of the upper trunk (ADUT), while one graft from the posterior part of each root (with neurons responsible for shoulder and elbow extension) is connected to the posterior division of the upper trunk (PDUT) (Fig. 13.4). When only C5 is available, two strands of a sural graft are interposed to the ADUT. This strategy provides better results than isolated nerve transfers, with a mean increase of 20° of shoulder abduction and elbow flexion strength [7, 21].

The benefits of combining nerve grafting and nerve transfer might be explained by the improvement in joint stability that results from the reinnervation of accessory agonist and antagonist muscles, which stabilizes joints [22]. Thus, shoulder outcome improvement is ascribed to reinnervation of accessory agonist and antagonist muscles that stabilize the shoulder joint: in particular, the clavicular portion of the pectoralis muscle and the coracobrachialis muscle, both of which actively participate in abduction beyond the horizontal position. When the C6 root is also available, grafting the PDUT provides reinnervation of the subscapular muscle, which contributes

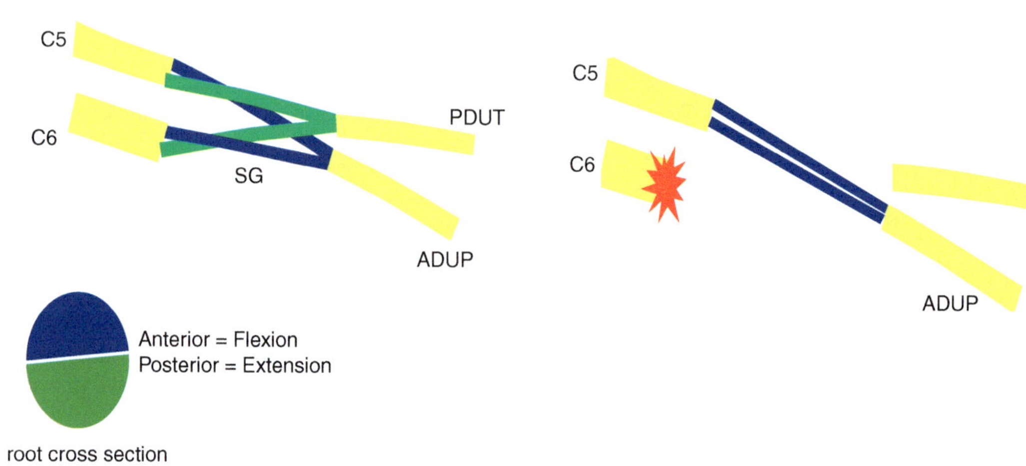

Fig. 13.4 Schematic representation of the surgical strategy for root grafting in upper-type paralysis of the brachial plexus. (SG) Sural nerve grafts, (ADUP) anterior division of the upper trunk, and (PDUT) posterior division of the upper trunk

to shoulder stabilization. Elbow flexion improvement owes to grafting the ADUT, which results in reinnervation of the brachialis, brachioradialis, and clavicular portion of the pectoralis muscle. Of these, the former two contribute directly to elbow flexion, and the latter to increased shoulder stability. In fact, in our patients, during maximal elbow flexion strength measurement, pectoralis major contractions are observed promptly.

C5-T8 BPI (T-1 Hand)

The most common pattern of upper-type BPI is the T-1 hand, which accounts for roughly 55% of these injuries [7, 8, 22]. When there is traction on the brachial plexus, in general C5 and C6 rupture because of the line of pull and the buttress provided by the transverse process. Meanwhile, C7 and C8 are avulsed because of fragile attachments to the bone. Conversely, T1 is more protected from injury under the first rib [23].

Nerve grafting is of paramount importance in these patients, owing to several functions that must be reconstructed (shoulder, elbow flexion, elbow extension, wrist extension, and finger extension in 50% of patients) relative to the scarce available donors [8]. The grafting strategy and surgical approach are similar to that of C5-C6+/-C7 injuries. However, when only a root is available for grafting, the recipient depends on pectoralis major function. If the pectoralis major is functional, grafts are connected to the PDUT. In these injuries, triceps branches are not available for nerve transfer, and deltoid functional recovery is dependent on root grafting.

Complete Paralysis

Complete paralysis accounts for 50% of all brachial plexus injuries [24]. In almost 90% of such patients, at least one graft-able root is available for grafting [24]. Identifying a graft-eligible root is important in patients with a pan-plexal BPI, due to three main potential benefits: neuropathic pain control, elbow flexion reanimation, and lateral forearm and hand protective sensory restoration.

The classic established reconstructive priorities for BPI are restoring elbow flexion, followed by reestablishing at least some degree of shoulder control [25]. On the other hand, we think that pain control should be the first priority in complete BPI, because 84% of patients with complete BPI suffer from neuropathic pain [26]. This highly disabling condition can be addressed in 50% of individuals in the days after root grafting, resulting in tremendously improved quality of life [26, 27]. We have postulated that pain in BPI originates from ruptured rather than avulsed roots, challenging classical beliefs which blame deafferentation as the origin of pain [27, 28]. In patients who have been grafted but pain persists, we have attributed pain to the growth of axons, because this process is associated with the extensive production of neurotrophic factors that produce pain [27, 29].

The second priority in complete BPI should be restoring elbow flexion. The results attained from reconstruction of these injuries when there is no graft-eligible root are clearly worse than when a root is available for grafting [30]. Currently, for complete BPI, we recommend exploring only the C5 or C6 roots, if available on CT scan in the setting of positive Tinel's and protraction tests. The C7 root is not explored, even when not avulsed, because grafting of C7 to the middle trunk leads to very poor results.

Our current reconstructive strategy for complete BPI employs one or two long grafts (>10 cm, mean 14 cm) connected to the infraclavicular structures (cords) (Fig. 13.5), because they provide better outcomes than when connected in the supraclavicular space (trunks or divisions) [31]. When either C5 or C6 is available for grafting, it is connected to the musculocutaneous nerve (MCN) in the infraclavicular region (Fig. 13.3). The MCN is also explored in the arm region before grafting to rule out a secondary lesion, which was identified in 18% of our cases, a situation that requires longer grafts (Fig. 13.6). When two roots are available, both are connected to the lateral cord, while the distal part of the long

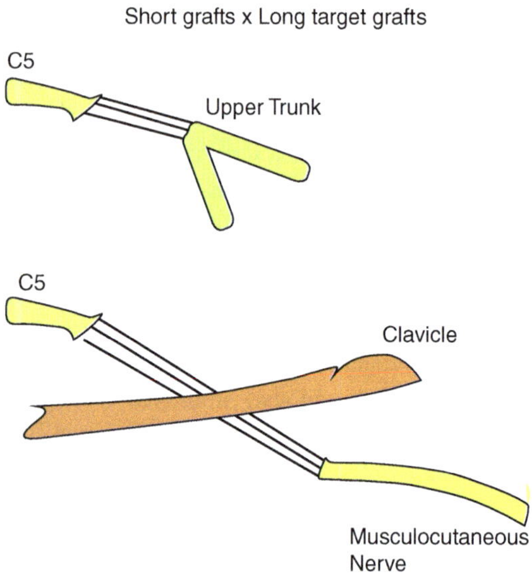

Fig. 13.5 Schematic representation of the surgical strategies for root grafting in complete paralysis of the brachial plexus using sural nerve grafts. Results of long grafts, around 14 cm in length, to the musculocutaneous nerve below clavicle are better than C5 root grafting to the anterior division of the upper trunk

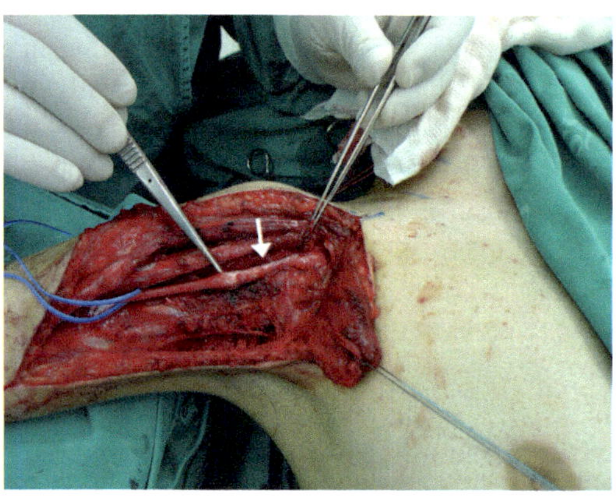

Fig. 13.6 Intraoperative view of a double lesion of the musculocutaneous nerve (arrow) at the level of the coracoid process

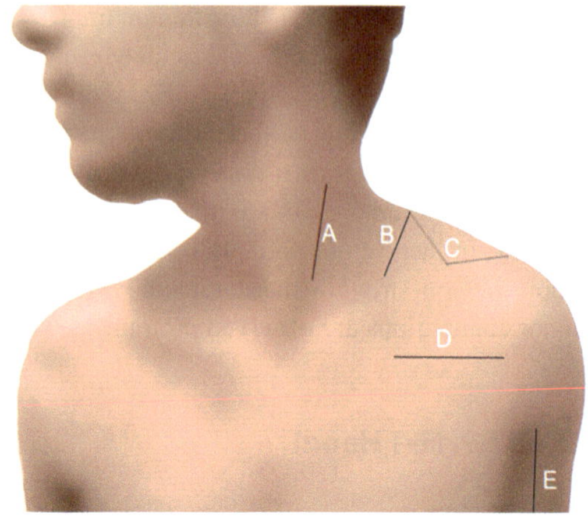

Fig. 13.7 Schematic representation of the surgical incisions for repairing a complete paralysis of the brachial plexus. Via incision A we explore C5 and C6 roots. Via incision B we connect the spinal accessory nerve to the suprascapular nerve. Via incision C, if needed, we extend "B" approach by detaching the trapezius from the clavicle to find a healthy distal stump of the suprascapular nerve. We then check the musculocutaneous nerve for double lesion by incision E. Finally, we approach the musculocutaneous nerve using incision "D." This is a transpectoral approach, which is faster than the deltopectoral approach and preserves the cephalic and thoracoacromial vessels in case a free gracilis muscle is needed in the future. After locating the musculocutaneous nerve through "E," it is tracked proximally as possible within the lateral cord to decrease the length of sural grafts

thoracic nerve is connected to the triceps long head motor branch. We do not connect C6 to the posterior cord, because it results in co-contractions between elbow flexors and extensor, leading to worse results. Incisions are represented in Fig. 13.7.

Using the C5 root to repair the MCN has been successful in 91% of our patients, generating at least grade M3 strength [31]. This is an enhanced success rate relative to our previous reconstructive strategy, with which we used short grafts to connect the C5 root to the anterior division of the upper trunk, resulting in antigravity elbow flexion in just 78% of patients [32]. The 22% failure rate that we observed with the previous strategy of grafting the ADUT could be related not only to poor root quality, despite continuity, but to other problems distal to the root itself, like disrupted nerve coaptation, double lesions involving the MCN, or a traumatized biceps. In addition, because of the character of longitudinal stretch of the BPI, micro-histologic alterations that remain undiagnosed on eye observation during trimming and repair might cause some failures [32].

We do not use intercostal nerves to restore elbow flexion as a first choice, saving them for backup surgery in case our initial reconstruction fails. The pectoralis major muscle has a high rate of spontaneous recovery, even when complete paralysis is demonstrated by CT scan; hence, it is not currently a target of our repair. Finally, we do not use grafts to reconstruct hand function. Excepting when two roots are available for grafting and are connected to the lateral cord. Neither do we use grafting in the supraclavicular region (short grafts) or very long grafts to the motor part of the median nerve at the elbow as this yields unpredictable results [31, 32]. Only 30% of supraclavicular grafting attain BMRC M3 level function for either wrist or finger flexion or extension [32]. In addition, spontaneous recovery of hand function occurs in roughly 10–15% of patients with complete paralysis, as a result of a post fixed brachial plexus [32]. We have abandoned the use of long vascularized ulnar nerve grafts because results can be worse than with sural grafts [33].

We have given up the use of contralateral roots, because of the procedure's risk and lack of convincing results [34]. Even when we have grafted the entire C7 root via a spinal cord approach, we attained no recovery of hand function. Patients who only experience M3 level finger flexion recovery, despite scientific enthusiasm for this, are largely dissatisfied, not only because of difficulties opening their hand and weakness but also because of poor control independent of the donor arm. The risk of the procedure, the potential for donor defects after nerve harvesting, and disappointing outcomes have made us abandon contralateral roots as donors. Using this same rationale — disappointing outcomes following sacrifice of a vital organ — we are biased against employing phrenic nerve transfers for elbow flexion [35].

Another benefit of root grafting in complete BPI is providing sensation to the limb. Grafting of the C5 root to the musculocutaneous nerve restores protective sensation over the lateral elbow, forearm, and hand [36]. All these patients recover thermo-algesic sensation in a variable territory that varies from just over the thenar eminence to the entire lateral forearm and hand, with 70% of patients capable of perceiving 2–0 monofilament pressure over the thenar eminence, palm, and dorsoradial aspect of the hand. This protective sensation is important in these anesthetic limbs to avoid inadvertent skin injuries. We do not recommend transferring other nerves, like the cervical plexus or intercostal nerves, to achieve sensory recovery, because the results are poor [32].

References

1. Narakas AO. The surgical treatment of traumatic brachial plexus lesions. Int Surg. 2019;65(6):521–7.
2. Hentz VR, Narakas A. The results of microneurosurgical reconstruction in complete brachial plexus palsy. Assessing outcome and predicting results. Orthop Clin North Am. 1988;19(1):107–14.
3. Bertelli JA, Ghizoni MF. Use of clinical signs and computed tomography myelography findings in detecting and excluding nerve root avulsion in complete brachial plexus palsy. J Neurosurg. 2006;105(6):835–42.
4. Oberlin C, Béal D, Leechavengvongs S, Salon A, Dauge MC, Sarcy JJ. Nerve transfer to biceps muscle using a part of ulnar nerve for C5-C6 avulsion of the brachial plexus: anatomical study and report of four cases. J Hand Surg Am. 1994;19(2):232–7.
5. Ayhan E, Soldado F, Fontecha CG, Bertelli JA, Leblebicioglu G. Elbow flexion reconstruction with nerve transfer or grafting in patients with brachial plexus injuries: a systematic review and comparison study. Microsurgery. 2019:40(7).
6. Soldado F, Ayhan E, Bertelli JA, Leblebicioglu G. Comparison of outcomes following nerve transfers versus nerve grafting. 491 A systematic review of individual participant data for restoration of elbow flexion after adult brachial plexus injuries. In: Giddins G, Leblebicioğlu G, editors. Evidence based data in hand surgery and therapy: Iris Publications; 2017.
7. Bertelli JA, Ghizoni MF. Nerve root grafting and distal nerve transfers for C5-C6 brachial plexus injuries. J Hand Surg Am. 2010 [cited 2019 Dec 8];35(5):769–75.
8. Bertelli JA, Ghizoni MF. C5–8 brachial plexus root injury: the "T-1 hand.". J Neurosurg. 2012;116(2):409–13.
9. Brunelli GA, Brunelli GR. Preoperative assessment of the adult plexus patient. Microsurgery. 1995 [cited 2019 Dec 8];16(1):17–21.
10. Tinel J. Le signe du « fourmillement » dans les lesions des nerfs peripheriques. Presse Med. 1915;23:388–9.
11. Echalier C, Teboul F, Dubois E, Chevrier B, Soumagne T, Goubier J-N. The value of preoperative examination and MRI for the diagnosis of graftable roots in total brachial plexus palsy. Hand Surg Rehabil [Internet]. 2019;38(4):246–50.
12. Walker AT, Chaloupka JC, de Lotbiniere AC, Wolfe SW, Goldman R, Kier EL. Detection of nerve rootlet avulsion on CT myelography in patients with birth

palsy and brachial plexus injury after trauma. AJR Am J Roentgenol. 1996;167(5):1283–7.
13. Yamazaki H, Doi K, Hattori Y, Sakamoto S. Computerized tomography myelography with coronal and oblique coronal view for diagnosis of nerve root avulsion in brachial plexus injury. J Brachial Plex Peripher Nerve Inj. 2007;2(01):16.
14. Romesburg J, Ragozzino M. Aseptic meningoencephalitis after iohexol CT myelography. AJNR Am J Neuroradiol [Internet]. 2009;30(5):1074–5.
15. Wade RG, Itte V, Rankine JJ, Ridgway JP, Bourke G. The diagnostic accuracy of 1.5T magnetic resonance imaging for detecting root avulsions in traumatic adult brachial plexus injuries. J Hand Surg Eur Vol. 2018;43(3):250–8.
16. Carvalho GA, Nikkhah G, Matthies C, Penkert G, Samii M. Diagnosis of root avulsions in traumatic brachial plexus injuries: value of computerized tomography myelography and magnetic resonance imaging. J Neurosurg. 1997;86(1):69–76.
17. Gasparotti R, Ferraresi S, Pinelli L, Crispino M, Pavia M, Bonetti M, et al. Three-dimensional MR myelography of traumatic injuries of the brachial plexus. AJNR Am J Neuroradiol. 1997;18(9):1733–42.
18. Oberle JW, Antoniadis G, Rath SA, Richter H-P. Value of nerve action potentials in the surgical management of traumatic nerve lesions. Neurosurgery. 1997;41(6):1337–43.
19. Murji A, Redett R, Hawkins C, Clarke H. The role of intraoperative frozen section histology in obstetrical brachial plexus reconstruction. J Reconstr Microsurg. 2008;24(3):203–9.
20. Malessy MJ, van Duinen SG, Feirabend HK, Thomeer RT. Correlation between histopathological findings in C-5 and C-6 nerve stumps and motor recovery following nerve grafting for repair of brachial plexus injury. J Neurosurg. 1999;91(4):636–44.
21. Bertelli JA, Ghizoni MF. Reconstruction of C5 and C6 brachial plexus avulsion injury by multiple nerve transfers: spinal accessory to suprascapular, ulnar fascicles to biceps branch, and triceps long or lateral head branch to axillary nerve. J Hand Surg Am. 2004;29(1):131–9.
22. Gribble PL, Ostry DJ. Independent coactivation of shoulder and elbow muscles. Exp Brain Res. 1998;123(3):355–60.
23. Metaizeau JP, Gayet C, Plenat F. [Brachial plexus birth injuries. An experimental study (author's transl)]. Chir Pediatr. 1979;20(3):159–63.
24. Bertelli JA, Ghizoni MF, Soldado F. Patterns of Brachial Plexus Stretch Palsy in a Prospective Series of 565 Surgically Treated Patients. J Hand Surg Am. 2017;42:443–6.
25. Alnot JY, Daunois O, Oberlin C, Bleton R. [Total paralysis of the brachial plexus caused by supraclavicular lesions]. Rev Chir Orthop Reparatrice Appar Mot. 1992;78(8):495–504.
26. Bertelli JA, Ghizoni MF, Loure Iro Chaves DP. Sensory disturbances and pain complaints after brachial plexus root injury: a prospective study involving 150 adult patients. Microsurgery. 2011;31(2):93–7.
27. Bertelli JA, Ghizoni MF. Pain after avulsion injuries and complete palsy of the brachial plexus: the possible role of nonavulsed roots in pain generation. Neurosurgery. 2008;62(5):1104–13.
28. Parry WCB. Pain in avulsion lesions of the brachial plexus. Pain. 1980;9(1):41–53.
29. Quintão NLM, Santos ARS, Campos MM, Calixto JB. The role of neurotrophic factors in genesis and maintenance of mechanical hypernociception after brachial plexus avulsion in mice. Pain. 2008;136(1–2):125–33.
30. Bertelli J. Results and current approach for Brachial Plexus reconstruction. 2016;(2011):1–8.
31. Bertelli JA, Ghizoni MF. Reconstruction of complete palsies of the adult brachial plexus by root grafting using long grafts and nerve transfers to target nerves. J Hand Surg Am. 2010;35(10):1640–6.
32. Bertelli JA, Ghizoni MF. Results of grafting the anterior and posterior divisions of the upper trunk in complete palsies of the brachial plexus. J Hand Surg Am. 2008;33(9):1529–40.
33. Bertelli JA, Ghizoni MF. Results of c5 root grafting to the musculocutaneous nerve using pedicled, vascularized ulnar nerve grafts. J Hand Surg Am. 2009;34:1821–6.
34. Wang S, Li P, Xue Y, Yiu H, Li Y-C, Wang H. Contralateral C7 nerve transfer with direct coaptation to restore lower trunk function after traumatic brachial plexus avulsion. J Bone Joint Surg Am. 2013;95(9):821–7, S1-2.
35. Siqueira MG, Martins RS. Phrenic nerve transfer in the restoration of elbow flexion in brachial plexus avulsion injuries: how effective and safe is it? Neurosurgery. 2009;65(4 Suppl):A125–31.
36. Bertelli JA, Ghizoni MF. Grafting the C5 root to the musculocutaneous nerve partially restores hand sensation in complete palsies of the brachial plexus. Neurosurgery. 2012;71(2):259–62; discussion 262–3.

Nerve Transfers to Shoulder and Elbow

14

Andrew L. O'Brien, Jana Dengler, and Amy M. Moore

Introduction

Nerve transfer surgery makes use of redundant and synergistic innervation of spared muscle groups to restore motor function, by the transfer of intact nerves or fascicles to injured nerves closer to the end target, shortening the distance (and time) to reinnervation. Following injury, nerve axons undergo Wallerian degeneration distal to the site of injury [1, 2]. Subsequent regeneration of nerve axons occurs at a rate of 1 mm per day, or 1 inch per month [3]. In the intervening time, the now denervated motor end plate and associated muscle are subject to potentially irrevocable fibrosis and atrophy if not reinnervated by the newly sprouting axon [4]. The timeframe in which this reinnervation must be completed to preserve muscle function is not completely elucidated; yet, general consensus states this time to be 12–18 months. Proximal nerve injuries, such as that seen in brachial plexus injuries, often exhibit too great of distances for nerve and axonal regeneration to overcome within this timeframe. As such, nerve transfers allow for early reinnervation of these target muscles through coaptation of more distal nerve donors.

As detailed in previous chapters, planning and performing nerve transfer surgery requires thorough knowledge of anatomy, function, internal nerve topography, and electrodiagnostic testing. In the setting of brachial plexus injuries, there is a hierarchy of importance of recovery. For adults, this is in decreasing order of importance: elbow flexion, external rotation, shoulder abduction, elbow extension, and finally, finger motion. Several nerve transfer techniques have been described to restore shoulder and elbow function in the setting of brachial plexus injuries. Here we present indications for nerve transfers, perioperative considerations, surgical techniques available to restore shoulder and elbow function, and outcomes of these transfers.

A. L. O'Brien · A. M. Moore (✉)
Department of Plastic and Reconstructive Surgery, The Ohio State University Wexner Medical Center, Columbus, OH, USA

J. Dengler
Division of Plastic and Reconstructive Surgery, Sunnybrook Health Sciences Centre, University of Toronto, Toronto, ON, Canada
e-mail: jana.dengler@mail.utoronto.ca

Indications for Nerve Transfers

Considerations for nerve transfers to restore elbow and shoulder function in the setting of brachial plexus injuries include (1) available donor(s) and (2) presentation within an appropriate timeframe.

A. Y. Shin, N. Pulos (eds.), *Operative Brachial Plexus Surgery*,
https://doi.org/10.1007/978-3-030-69517-0_14

Donor Selection

Appropriate donor selection is crucial for success of nerve transfer surgery. Donor nerves should provide redundant function (such that sacrifice of these nerve fascicles does not result in functional loss), be adequately free from injury (innervating muscles demonstrating at least MRC grade 4), provide synergistic function to recipient nerves (provides more intuitive motor reeducation), and be anatomically located near recipient nerve end targets. Electromyography (EMG) can be used to evaluate possible donor nerves by assessing motor unit recruitment and relative absence of positive sharp waves and fibrillations [5].

Timing

For successful reinnervation from nerve transfers, surgery must be performed before irreversible damage to motor end plates and fibrosis of recipient muscle occurs [6]. However, this must be balanced with allowing for native recovery of axons following brachial plexus injury in the setting of blunt injuries. We advocate for performing nerve transfer surgery prior to 9 months after injury. Serial exams during the first 12 weeks after injury will allow recovery from neuropraxic injuries. Electromyography (EMG) can provide evidence of recovery before functional improvement is seen. Ultimately, in the absence of palpable muscle contraction on physical exam or electrodiagnostic indication of reinnervation in the form of motor unit action potentials by 12–16 weeks on EMG, nerve transfers should be considered. Adult patients with presentation greater than 12 months from injury are no longer primary nerve transfer candidates, and tendon transfers and/or free functional muscle transfers are offered.

Perioperative Considerations

Several perioperative considerations can facilitate successful nerve transfer. To allow donor nerve evaluation intraoperatively, long-acting depolarizing paralytics should be avoided during induction of anesthesia. Similarly, local anesthetics such as lidocaine should not be administered until after all necessary electrical stimulation of nerves is complete. We recommend the use of intraoperative nerve stimulation to evaluate nerve function. Donor nerves should exhibit strong muscular contractions at 0.5 milliamps (mA), whereas recipient muscles should be devoid of contraction at 2.0 mA.

All nerve coaptations must be tension-free. Donor and recipient nerves should be divided such that adjacent joints can move through full range of motion without tension on the coaptation [7]. This is done by neurolyzing donor nerves as distally as possible and neurolyzing recipient nerves as proximally as possible ("donor distal, recipient proximal"). Intraneural dissection and coaptations are facilitated by use of an operating room microscope to ensure appropriate tissue handling and prevent inadvertent injury. Coaptations are performed with 9–0 nylon epineurial sutures making sure not to overtighten the repair and cause fascicular bunching.

Early post-operative care is directed at protecting the coaptation, controlling edema, and managing pain. For nerve transfers to restore elbow function, immobilization is used in the initial 21 days as the blood-brain barrier is restored within the nerve by this time indicating healing [8]. For nerve transfers to restore shoulder function, the shoulder is immobilized for up to 4 weeks to protect the pectoralis muscle tendon repair (if taken down during the nerve transfer surgery) [8]. As reinnervation of the recipient muscle occurs at the rate of rate of 1 mm per day or 1 inch per month, therapy should focus on range of motion, muscle strengthening and balancing, and remapping of the motor cortex [8]. Relearning is aided by voluntary contraction of the donor nerve distribution to illicit function of the target muscle, which is eventually not needed [9].

Nerve Transfers to Restore Shoulder Function

Recovery of shoulder function following brachial plexus injury is directed at restoring shoulder stability, external rotation, and abduction through reinnervation of the suprascapular and axillary nerves. The axillary nerve is reported to be the most common recipient target; however, dual-innervation of the axillary and suprascapular nerves has demonstrated superior shoulder function over single-nerve innervation [10–12]. Dual innervation should be attempted when donor nerve availability allows.

Spinal Accessory to Suprascapular Nerve Transfer

Indications To restore supraspinatus and infraspinatus muscle function: shoulder stabilization, initiation of shoulder abduction, and external rotation.

Contraindications This nerve transfer is contraindicated if the spinal accessory nerve (SAN) has been previously damaged or in the setting of a total plexus injury where the spinal accessory will serve as the donor nerve for an innervated free functional muscle tissue transfer.

Surgical Technique Both anterior or posterior supraclavicular approaches can be used for this nerve transfer.

In the *anterior approach*, the patient is placed in the supine position. A transverse incision is made 2 cm above the medial half of the clavicle. Dissection is carried down through the platysma muscle. The supraclavicular nerves are identified and protected. The fat pad is elevated cephalad. The external jugular vein and sternocleidomastoid muscle are mobilized and retracted medially, exposing the omohyoid. The omohyoid is then divided and retracted to reveal a fatty plane, through which the brachial plexus is exposed. The suprascapular nerve (SSN) is identified as the lateral-most branch of the upper trunk after the confluence of the C5 and C6 spinal nerves. If the brachial plexus injury involves C5/C6 root avulsions, the suprascapular nerve may be displaced inferiorly, deep to the clavicle, necessitating an infraclavicular approach for identification.

The spinal accessory nerve (SAN) is located on the undersurface of the trapezius muscle just deep to the fascia. It is identified by following the superior border of the trapezius muscle from lateral to medial along the clavicle. Identification of the SAN can use of intraoperative nerve stimulation. Once located, the SAN is dissected free from the surrounding tissues and followed distally. The nerve is then transected as distally as possible to transpose anteriorly toward the suprascapular nerve for coaptation.

In the *posterior approach*, the patient can be positioned prone, lateral, or in the semi-fowler (beach chair) position; the authors prefer prone positioning. In the prone position, key surface landmarks are identified and marked as follows: the acromion, the superior-medial border of the scapula, and the midline spinous processes (Fig. 14.1). The spinal accessory nerve is located approximately 40% of the distance from midline to the acromion, and the suprascapular nerve is found approximately half the distance from the acromion to the superior-medial border of the scapula [13, 14]. A transverse incision is made 2 fingerbreadths superior to the scapular spine. Dissection is carried though the trapezius by splitting the fibers as they run transversely. The SAN is found on the deep (i.e., anterior) surface of the trapezius with the help of intraoperative nerve stimulation.

The SSN is identified by dissecting the trapezius muscle laterally. The supraspinatus muscle

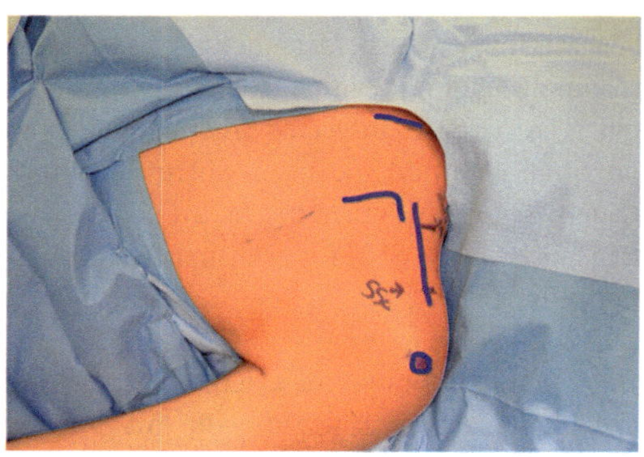

Fig. 14.1 Key surface landmarks for the spinal accessory nerve transfer (SAN) to suprascapular nerve (SSC) include the acromion laterally, the superior-medial border of the scapula, and the midline spinous processes. A transverse incision is made 2 fingerbreadths superior to the scapular spine

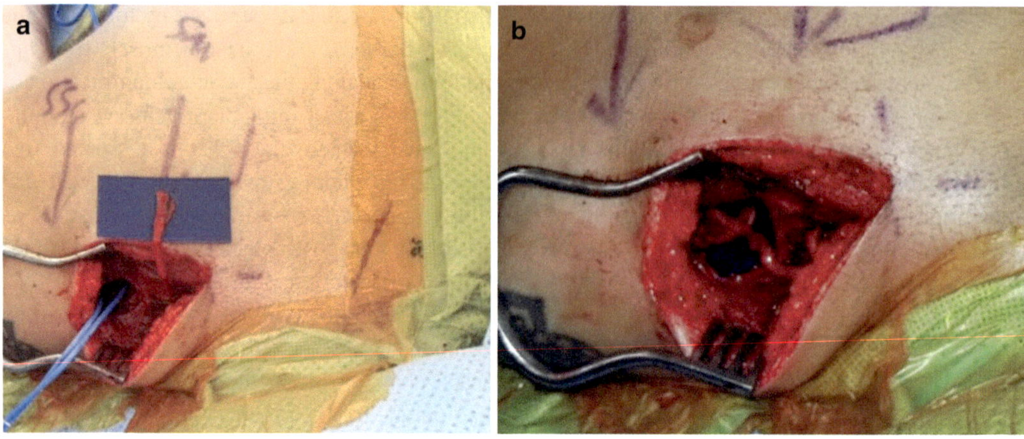

Fig. 14.2 Transfer of the spinal accessory nerve to the suprascapular nerve. (**a**) The spinal accessory nerve is identified and transected distally. (**b**) transfer of the spinal accessory nerve to the suprascapular nerve is achieved without tension

and fascia, which is often atrophied, is identified. The dissection proceeds superior to the supraspinatus muscle, which is retracted inferiorly, and directed deep toward the suprascapular notch. A combination of careful dissection and finger palpation is used to identify the anterior scapular edge. The suprascapular vessels are then visualized, typically overlying the notch and lateral to the SSN. The ligament lies either directly beneath or medial to the vessels. Using finger palpation and the assistance of a peanut, the suprascapular ligament is identified running in a superior to inferior direction, following the edge of the scapula. It is then carefully divided revealing the notch. The SSN is found directly beneath the ligament; if there is a history of a scapula fracture, it can be tethered to the scapula. The nerve is dissected free and followed proximally toward the neck where it is transected. The SAN is then transected distally and transposed to the SSN for a tension-free coaptation (Fig. 14.2).

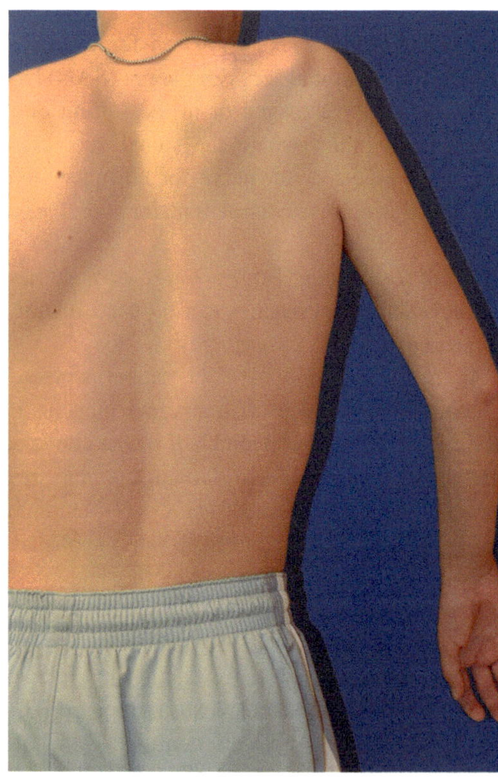

Fig. 14.3 Outcome demonstrating initiation of abduction and external rotation after spinal accessory to suprascapular nerve transfer

Outcomes Restoration of external rotation and abduction can be achieved with this transfer (Fig. 14.3). In a 22-patient series by Emamhadi et al. with an average follow-up time of 21.7 months [15], restoration of external rotation to MRC grade 4 was achieved in 63.6% of patients, and to MRC grade 3 in 13.6% of patients. The remaining 22.7% of patients recovered MRC grade 2 function. In a study by Manske et al., patients who underwent SAN to SSN nerve transfer following brachial plexus birth injury demonstrated improved external rotation compared to those who underwent nerve grafting from C5 and C6 nerve roots to SSN [16]. In this study, the nerve transfer group exhibited a mean Active Movement Scale (AMS) score of 3.21 versus 2.7 in the nerve grafting group. Furthermore, 24% of nerve transfer patients achieved an AMS of >5 compared to only 5% of graft patients. Bertelli and Ghizoni published a report of 30 patients who underwent SAN to SSN transfer [17]. Patients with C5-C6 injuries regained 122 degrees of shoulder abduction and 118 degrees of external rotation on average. In a follow-up study of 110 patients with complete brachial plexus palsy, mean recovery of shoulder abduction was 58.5° [18]. Notably, a subset of the patients ($n = 17$) required more extensive dissection and exposure due to the extent of their initial injury.

Triceps to Axillary Nerve Transfer

Indications Axillary nerve dysfunction from isolated axillary nerve injury or C5-C6 brachial plexus injuries. Must have triceps (C7) function intact.

Contraindications Poor triceps muscle function, as seen in C7 injuries.

Nerve transfers using each of the heads of triceps nerve branches have been described. We advocate for use of the medial branch to triceps; it has demonstrated predictable anatomy and adequate length [13, 19–21].

Surgical Technique This nerve transfer can be performed from an anterior [22, 23] or posterior approach [13, 24]. The authors prefer to perform this transfer from a posterior approach with the patient in prone positioning, as it is usually combined with the SAN to SSN transfer described above.

A 10 cm incision is made extending from the lateral border of the scapula, along the posterior border of the deltoid and down the lateral border of the long head of triceps (Fig. 14.4). When approaching the investing fascia between the deltoid and long head of triceps, it is important to look for the cutaneous branch of the axillary nerve. Identification of this nerve can serve as a guide to the axillary nerve. Dissection is carried toward to the quadrilateral space, bordered by teres major (inferiorly), teres minor (superiorly), long head of the triceps (medially), and humeral shaft (laterally). The axillary nerve is identified existing the quadrangular space. Lack of muscle contraction is confirmed with intraoperative stimulation of the nerve.

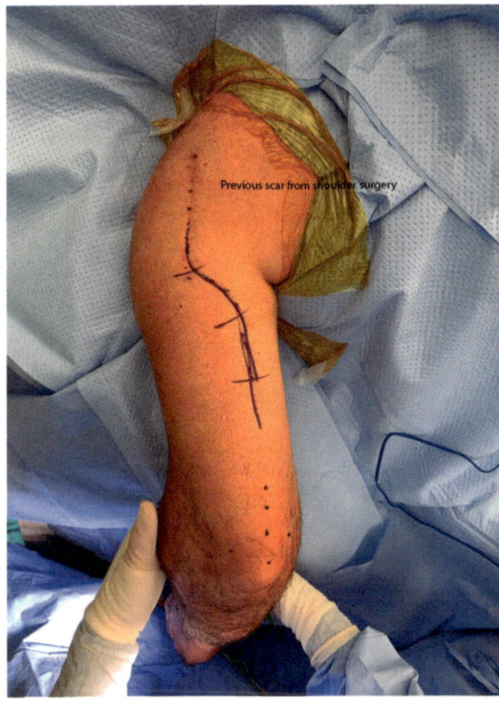

Fig. 14.4 Triceps to axillary nerve transfer. This image demonstrates a previous shoulder incision (dotted line) that was incorporated into the posterior arm incision for the triceps to axillary nerve transfer. Hanging the elbow off the table during the markings can assure a midline posterior approach to the triceps branches

The radial nerve is then identified between the long and lateral head of triceps in its characteristic fat pad. Discrete branches to each of the respective heads of the triceps are identified. The branch to the medial head runs anteriorly and distally and is tagged with a vessel loop or blue background (Fig. 14.5). The donor triceps nerve is transected as distally as possible and transposed 180° to meet the axillary nerve. The axillary nerve is transected proximally to ensure inclusion of the

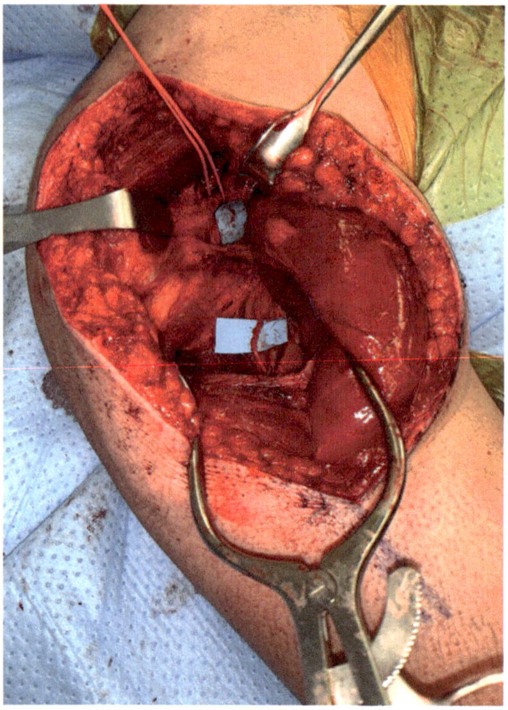

Fig. 14.5 The medial triceps branch is identified overlying the radial nerve proper (lying over the blue background) and the axillary nerve is surrounded by the vessel loop

branch to teres minor, an important contributor to external rotation. Coaptation of the triceps branch to the anterior and posterior branches of the axillary nerve is performed (Fig. 14.6).

Outcomes Restoration of shoulder abduction can be achieved with this transfer. In a case series by Desai et al., 27 patients underwent triceps to axillary nerve transfer, most commonly from the medial head (40%), followed by long head (27%) and lateral head (22%) [25]. In 15 patients (56%), single nerve transfer was performed, whereas the remainder had an additional transfer – other than the radial nerve – to the axillary nerve. At an average follow-up times of 22 months, 81% of patients recovered MRC grade 3 or above function with a mean shoulder abduction range of 110°. There was no significant down grade in donor nerve function.

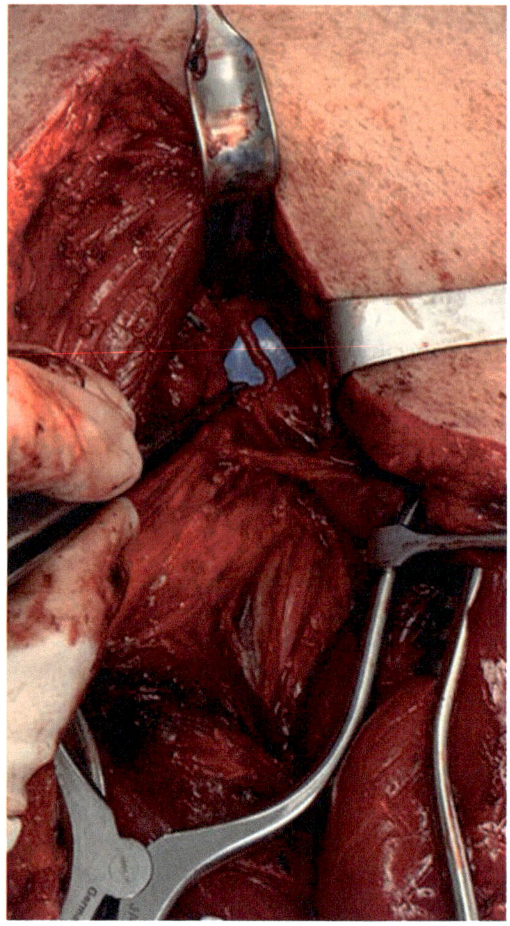

Fig. 14.6 The medial triceps branch is transferred to the axillary nerve without tension

The radial to axillary nerve transfer has also been shown to be an important adjunct to the SAN to SSN nerve transfer when performed concurrently, also known as dual nerve transfers. In a comparative study by Texakalidis et al., patients who underwent dual nerve transfers demonstrated a statistically significant increase in shoulder abduction (median range 90°) as compared to single nerve transfer (median range 42.5°) [26]. Additionally, 4 of 4 patients who underwent dual nerve transfer regained deltoid function of MRC grade 3, compared to 3 of 10 patients who underwent SAN to SSN transfer alone.

Medial Pectoral to Axillary Nerve Transfer

Indications Weak or absent triceps function (C5-C7 brachial plexus injuries). The medial pectoral nerve arises from the lower trunk (C8-T1) near the coracoid process and enter the pectoralis major on its deep aspect.

Contraindications Weak or absent pectoralis major function; or nerve to triceps available as a donor.

Surgical Technique An infraclavicular approach is used for this nerve transfer. An incision is made along the anterior deltopectoral groove extending onto the medial arm. Dissection is carried down to the deep fascia; the cephalic vein is identified and retracted superiorly with the deltoid muscle. At its insertion onto the humerus, the pectoralis major muscle is dissected circumferentially and disinserted, leaving a 1 cm cuff of tendon on the humerus for later repair. A Krackow locking stitch at the proximal end of the pectoralis major tendon is used to retract the muscle. The medial pectoral nerves are seen emerging from the underside of the pectoralis minor muscle. Function of nerve branches is confirmed with intra-operative stimulation. Three to four distal nerve branches are selected for nerve transfer; the more proximal branches can be left intact to preserve innervation to pectoralis major. The fascicles for transfer are followed distally to where they enter the muscle, and transected.

To expose the axillary nerve, the coracoid process and the subscapularis muscle are identified. As this muscle extends inferiolaterally toward the humeral head, the axillary nerve can be palpated as it runs toward the quadrilateral space. The axillary artery is dissected and mobilized to reveal the posterior circumflex humeral artery. Posterolateral to the posterior circumflex humeral artery lie the axillary and radial nerves. The axillary nerve is followed proximally to its division from the posterior cord. Direct coaptation between the medial pectoral nerve branches and the axillary nerve is possible (Fig. 14.7); however, in some instances short nerve grafts are required to maintain a tension-free coaptation [10, 27].

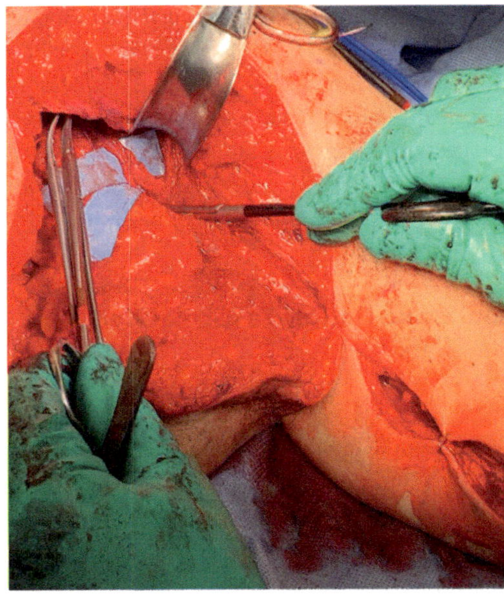

Fig. 14.7 Medial pectoral nerve transfer to the axillary nerve from an anterior approach

Outcomes In a series of eight patients with upper brachial plexus injuries, Ray et al. reported six patients recovered "deltoid function" $\geq$ MRC grade 4, and two patients did not [27]. In another series of 13 patients, 83.3% of patient recovered shoulder abduction, and 58.3% recovered external rotation to a level of MRC grade 3 or higher [28].

Nerve Transfers to Restore Elbow Flexion

Restoration of elbow flexion is prioritized in brachial plexus injuries [29]. The musculocutaneous nerve provides motor innervation to the biceps brachii and brachialis (in addition to the coracobrachialis) and is ultimately responsible for elbow flexion.

Numerous donors have been described for restoring elbow flexion, including nerve fascicle to flexor carpi ulnaris (FCU) (Oberlin) [30], FCU and flexor digitorum superficialis (FDS) (double fascicular transfer) [31, 32], median pectoral [33], thoracodorsal [34–36], spinal accessory [37], and intercostal nerves [38] – all of which are described below. Careful history, physical exam, and pre-operative electrodiagnostic studies guide the surgeon's choice of donor(s).

Single and Double Fascicular Nerve Transfers

Indications Fascicular transfers from the median and ulnar nerve are indicated when there is lack of elbow flexion, but intact hand and wrist function.

Contraindications Weak wrist flexion (indicates lack of redundancy and/or inadequate donor); weakness or absence of FDS.

Surgical Technique With the patient in the supine position and their affected arm stretched out on a hand table, an incision is made along the medial arm from the axilla to 3–4 cm proximal to the antecubital fossa (Fig. 14.8). The subcutaneous tissue is dissected with care to preserve branches of the medial antebrachial cutaneous (MABC) nerve. The median nerve is the first nerve to be encountered lateral to the basilic vein. Dissection of the median nerve is performed along the length of the incision. The ulnar nerve is found medial to the basilic vein and is also dissected along the length of the incision.

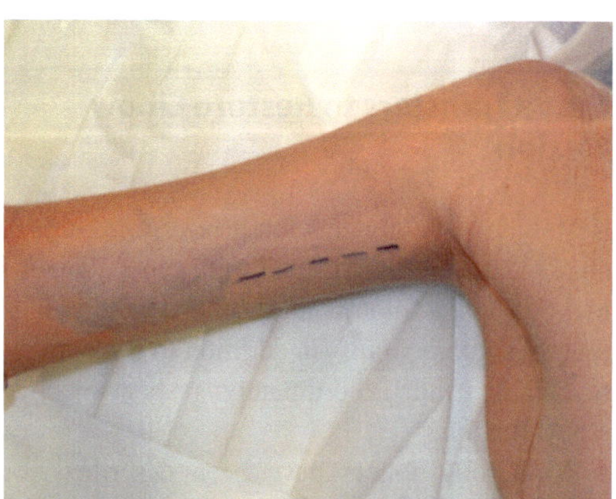

Fig. 14.8 Incision for performing a single or double fascicular nerve transfer to restore elbow flexion

The musculocutaneous (MC) nerve arises from the lateral cord, travels under the coracobrachialis, and is found on the medial surface of the biceps brachii muscle traveling over the brachialis muscle. Identifying the plane between the coracobrachialis and the biceps is helpful when identifying the nerve more proximally. At the junction of the mid-humerus, there is a group of vessels that enter the biceps muscle. It is at this point, that the nerve to the biceps can be found entering the muscle. There is often more than one nerve branch supplying the biceps muscle; inclusion of all branches in the nerve transfer is important. After giving off branches to biceps, the MC nerve then continues on to give off branches to brachialis in the mid- to distal-third of the arm and terminates as the lateral antebrachial cutaneous (LABC) nerve. The brachialis branch(es) dives deep into the brachialis muscle, whereas the LABC continues distally superficial to the muscle. Gentle traction on the LABC translates to the skin over its sensory distribution and can be seen as gentle tugging on the skin. It should be noted that the branch to the biceps innervates the muscle on its deep aspect, while the branch to brachialis innervates the muscle on its superficial aspect. Intraoperative stimulation confirms lack of muscle function. The branches to the biceps and brachialis are neurolyzed proximally to obtain length for transposition to the donor nerve(s).

Intra-fascicular dissection of the median and ulnar nerves is performed adjacent to where the brachialis and biceps branches reach to provide tension-free closure(s). Intraoperative nerve stimulation is used to identify donor fascicles in the ulnar and median nerves and ensure redundancy of function in what is left behind. Importantly, the median nerve topography is such that the sensory component fascicles are noted to be lateral, whereas the motor fascicles are medial. The redundant median nerve fascicles (FDS) typically lie medially in the nerve and lie between the fascicles to pronator teres and to the anterior interosseous nerve, both of which are not expendable. The FCU fascicles of the ulnar nerve typically lie in the posterolateral aspect of the ulnar nerve. The FDS and FCU donor fascicles are transected distally and coaptation is performed (Fig. 14.9).

Outcomes Single and fascicular nerve transfers can reliably restore strong elbow flexion (Fig. 14.10). Oberlin first described the ulnar fascicle to biceps nerve transfer in four patients [30]. He reported restoration of elbow flexion in all patients of MRC grade 3 or greater, without any impairment of hand function. He later published a cohort of 32 patients, where 75% regained MRC grade 3 or above elbow flexion [39]. In Mackinnon's initial 2005 series of six patients that underwent the double fascicular nerve transfer, mean elbow flexion strength of MRC grade 4 was noted at an average follow-up of 21 months [32]. Subsequently, Ray and Mackinnon reported a larger series of 29 patients, in which 23 regained MRC grade 4 or higher elbow flexion and four patients regained MRC grade 3 [40]. Liverneaux and Oberlin published a cohort of 15 patients in 2007 in which all 10 patients who had minimum 6 months follow-up demonstrated MRC grade 4 elbow flexion [31].

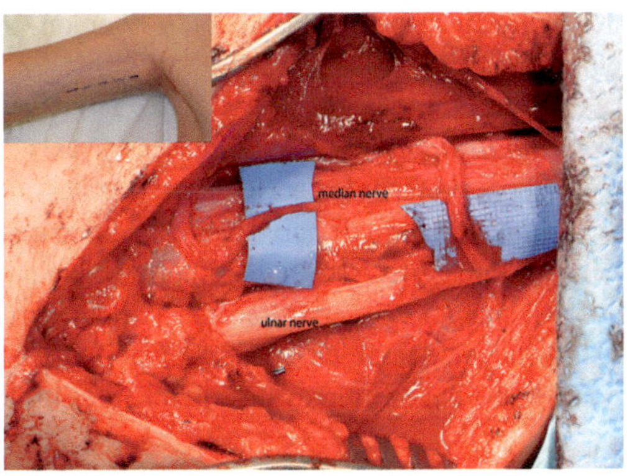

Fig. 14.9 Double fascicular transfer of the ulnar fascicle to the biceps branch and the median fascicle to the brachialis branch of the musculocutaneous nerve

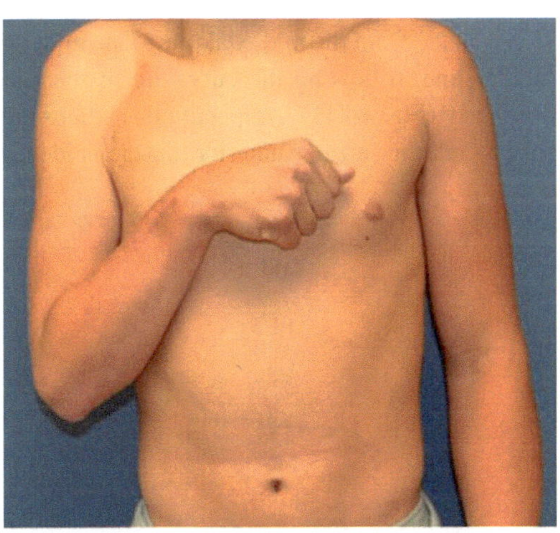

Fig. 14.10 Restoration of strong and full elbow flexion after double fascicular transfer

The superiority of the double fascicular transfer over the single fascicular transfer remains debated. A retrospective review performed by Carlsen et al. compared 23 patients who underwent single fascicular transfer to 32 patients that underwent double fascicular transfer, and they found that both groups demonstrated MRC grade 4 or greater elbow flexion without a statistically significant difference [41]. Of note, those who underwent single-fascicle transfers in this series were noted to have more severe injuries, precluding the availability of additional donors [41]. A prospective trial by Martins et al. was unable to identify significant differences in functional outcome between the single fascicular and double fascicular nerve transfers in 40 randomized patients [42]. A meta-analysis and subsequent quantitative analysis of 29 studies and 341 patients by Sneiders et al. concluded that there were no differences in elbow flexion strength between single fascicular and double fascicular nerve transfers, with most patients regaining MRC grade 3 elbow flexion [43]. However, a greater proportion of double fascicular nerve transfer patients demonstrated MRC grade 4 or greater elbow flexion strength if performed 6 months or less from the initial injury which was a statistically significant improvement over single fascicular transfers [43]. A meta-analysis of 176 cases by Donnelly et al. found double fascicular transfers superior to single fascicular transfers, with 83% of patients with double fascicular transfer regaining elbow flexion of MRC 4 or greater compared to only 63% of patients with single ulnar nerve fascicular nerve transfer [44].

Thoracodorsal to Musculocutaneous Nerve Transfer

Indications The thoracodorsal nerve is a viable donor for the recovery of elbow flexion when no other donors are available [34–36, 45–47]. The thoracodorsal nerve has been touted for its potential length and concentration of motor fascicles [36].

Contraindications Poor thoracodorsal nerve function, as evidenced by weakness or absence of latissimus dorsi contraction.

Surgical Technique With the patient in the supine position, an incision is made in the midbrachium to expose the musculocutaneous nerve (described in the previous sections). The dissection proceeds proximally to identify its takeoff from the lateral cord underneath the retracted pectoralis major muscle. The pectoralis major muscle does not need to be disinserted from the humerus to access the proximal MC nerve takeoff. However, if there is difficulty visualizing or dissecting the MC nerve due to scar or a high takeoff, there should be no hesitancy to release the pectoralis major muscle from its insertion on the humerus with plans to reinsert at the end of the case.

Once the MC nerve is carefully dissected, another incision is made on the chest in the midaxillary line just anterior to the palpable latissimus muscle. The authors often mark this with the patient awake in the preoperative holding area. Dissection through the subcutaneous tissue is performed down to the anterior surface to the latissimus muscle. The nerve lies on the anterior surface of the latissimus with the vascular pedicle. There are two branches of the thoracodorsal nerve which can be neurolyzed distally into the muscle. Intraoperative stimulation confirms strong contraction of the muscle. Both branches are transected distally, neurolyzed proximally, and brought into the axilla through a subcutaneous tunnel. The coaptation to the MC nerve is performed end-to-end without tension. The shoulder is placed through full range of motion to confirm lack of tension.

Outcomes An early report of the thoracodorsal to musculocutaneous nerve transfer by Novak et al. evaluated restoration of elbow flexion among ten patients with brachial plexus injuries secondary to trauma and oncologic interruption [34]. Nine of these patients regained MRC grade 4 or above elbow flexion. Samardzic similarly reported a series of 13 patients that all regained MRC grade 3 or above elbow flexion [28].

Intercostal to Musculocutaneous Nerve Transfer

Indications In the setting of a brachial plexus injury involving all nerve roots, intercostal (IC) nerve transfers are indicated for restoration of elbow flexion.

Contraindications While no consensus exists, the authors prefer to avoid IC nerve transfers in the setting of a phrenic nerve palsy. Additionally, while previous rib fractures are not an absolute contraindication to nerve transfer, an increased likelihood of compromised nerve viability was noted in patients with previous rib fractures [48].

Surgical Technique The patient is placed in the supine position with the arm extended on an arm board. The chest is prepped from the midline to the posterior axillary line, and from the shoulder to anterior superior iliac spine. A curvilinear incision is made from the midaxial line to the midclavicular line, following the curvature of the ribs anteriorly (Fig. 14.11). Adipocutaneous flaps are raised, and the serratus anterior muscle is identi-

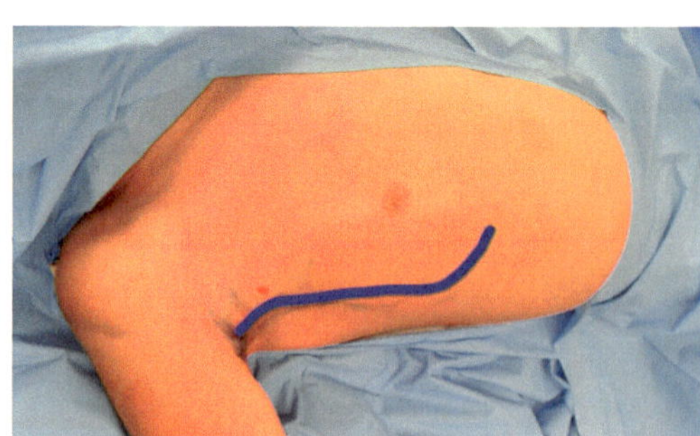

Fig. 14.11 Markings for intercostal nerve transfers

fied. Electrocautery is used to split the serratus anterior muscle and periosteum directly over each rib exposed (T2-T6). The sub-periosteal plane is developed with a periosteal elevator to expose the neurovascular bundle at the inferior aspect of each rib. The intercostal nerve is identified carefully and stimulated to confirm muscle function. It is then neurolyzed anteriorly and posteriorly from the surrounding muscle and vascular bundle using bipolar cautery. Dissection of the motor nerves extends from the costochondral junction to the midaxillary line. Given the small size of the intercostal nerves, they are not transected until all levels are exposed. The authors prefer to transfer four ICs to the musculocutaneous nerve with an end-to-end coaptation. For levels T5 or T6 it is common to need a short 2–3 cm nerve graft to avoid unnecessary tension. Sensory intercostal nerves or a branch of the MABC are great sources of nerve graft material if needed.

The musculocutaneous nerve dissection to its takeoff from the lateral cord proceeds in a similar fashion as previously mentioned. The IC nerves are transected distally and transposed into the axilla for coaptation with the MC nerve (Fig. 14.12). Dissection of the axillary fat can be performed to decrease the distance between nerves. Of note, the authors advocate using the intercostobrachial nerves to reinnervate the lateral cord contribution to the median nerve in order to restore sensation into the limb. For future free functional muscle innervation, the authors also bank on sural nerve graft powered by the nerves to the rectus abdominis muscles (Fig. 14.12). This long graft is coapted distally in the arm to the medial antebrachial cutaneous nerve for a distal vascular source to the graft.

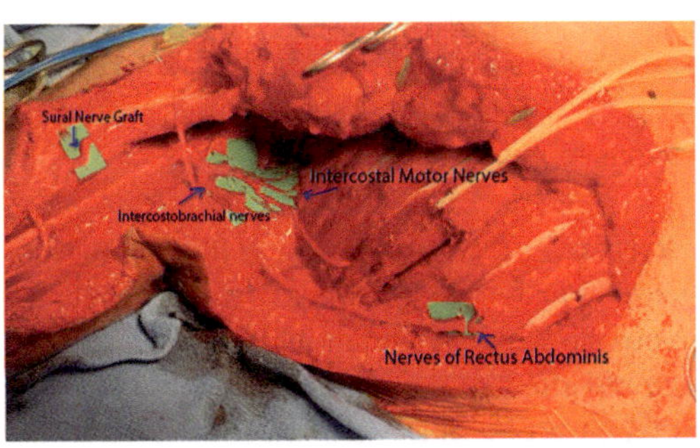

Fig. 14.12 Intraoperative exposure of the intercostal nerve transfers to restore elbow flexion. Four levels of intercostal nerves were transferred end-to-end to the musculocutaneous nerve. Two intercostobrachial nerves were transferred to the lateral cord contribution to the median nerve to restore hand sensation. Lastly, two rectus abdominis nerves were transferred to a 25 cm sural nerve graft. Distally the coaptation was to the medial antebrachial cutaneous nerve to re-establish a vascular supply for the long nerve graft. This graft can be used for future innervation of a free functional muscle to help restore finger flexion

Outcomes Strong elbow flexion can be achieved with intercostal nerve transfers (Fig. 14.13). A large cohort study of 112 patients who underwent intercostal to musculocutaneous nerve transfer demonstrated restoration of elbow flexion strength MRC grade 3 or above in 87% of patients [49]. A meta-analysis of 27 studies and 965 patients showed that 72% of patients recovered MRC grade 3 or greater elbow flexion without the use of an interpositional graft. Forty-seven percent of patients who required a nerve graft recovered elbow flexion of MRC grade 3 or above [50].

To determine the optimal number of intercostal donor nerves, Xiao et al. reviewed a cohort of 30 patients [38]. Elbow flexion was restored in 66.7%, 82.4%, and 75% of patients who underwent transfer with two, three, and four intercostal nerves, respectively. A systematic review by Leland et al. found no functional advantage of

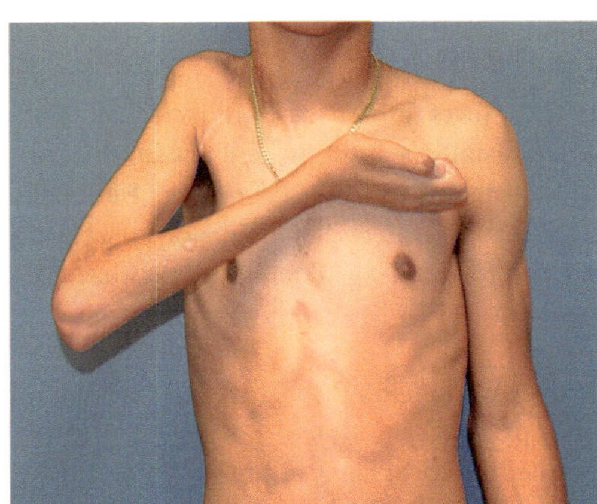

Fig. 14.13 One year outcome after intercostal nerve transfers to the musculocutaneous nerve to restore elbow flexion

transferring two, three, or four intercostal nerves, and thereby recommended the transfer of only two intercostal levels [51]. A study by Kovachevich et al. found a 2.49 increased odds of complication with each additional intercostal nerve harvested [48].

Medial Pectoral to Musculocutaneous Nerve Transfer

Indications If hand function is weak or if the patient refuses the use of redundant median and ulnar nerve fascicles to restore elbow flexion, the medial pectoral nerves are an option.

Contraindications Absent or weak medial pectoral nerve function; presence of redundant median or ulnar nerve fascicles for transfer.

Surgical Technique An incision is made longitudinally along the medial arm and crosses the axilla, avoiding the hair-bearing skin. The musculocutaneous nerve is identified in the upper arm as described in the previous section and neurolyzed proximally from the lateral cord. The medial pectoral nerves are identified by disinserting the pectoralis major muscle off its insertion on the humerus and reflecting it medially to expose its underside where the medial pectoral nerves can be seen emerging from the pectoralis minor. Often, the pectoralis minor is released from the coracoid and reflected to obtain adequate length on the nerves. Several branches are selected, transected distally, and transposed toward the musculocutaneous nerve for coaptation. Following neurorrhaphy, the pectoralis major is repaired, and the patient's shoulder is immobilized for 4 weeks.

Outcomes Samardzic et al. report a series of nine patients in which 90.5% of patients regained MRC grade 3 or above elbow flexion [28]. A study by Pondaag and Malessy reports return of elbow flexion with MRC >3 in 23 of 25 patients [52]. Blaauw and Slooff presented similar results in a cohort of 25 patients with obstetrical brachial plexus injuries. In their series, 88% of patients recovered elbow flexion MRC grade 3 or above [53].

Nerve Transfers to Restore Elbow Extension

After the restoration of elbow flexion and shoulder function, elbow extension can be regained through nerve transfers to nerve branches of triceps. While previously elbow extension function was not restored and left to be gravity dependent, recent studies have highlighted the importance of concurrent elbow extension and flexion to control hand position in space [54]. Similarly, patients who exhibit elbow flexion without extension report poor elbow and hand control and require the use of their contralateral extremity to hold their arm in extension [55, 56].

Ulnar Nerve Fascicle to Long Head of Triceps Nerve Transfer

Indications Upper plexus injury with C7 involved and hand function is intact.

Contraindications Absent or weak wrist flexion and intrinsic hand function are indicative of poor ulnar nerve function and should act as contraindications to this nerve transfer.

Surgical Technique The ulnar-to-triceps nerve transfer is performed from an anterior approach with the patient in the supine position and the affected arm on an arm board. Starting at the insertion of the pectoralis major, a 10 cm incision is made between the anterior and posterior compartments of the arm. Through this incision, the ulnar nerve is identified on the medial aspect to the brachial artery and found deep to the MABC. A longitudinal incision is made through the epineurium, and nerve stimulation is used to identify a motor fascicle that contributes largely to wrist flexion without innervation of intrinsic function to the hand; this is then transected distally for transfer.

At the interval between the ulnar nerve and the vascular structures in the upper arm, the branches to the triceps can be found. With dissection deep to the vessels, the radial nerve is identified. The branch to the long head of the triceps runs parallel between the radial and ulnar nerves. This branch is transected proximally, and a tension-free end-to-end coaptation is performed with the transected donor fascicle of the ulnar nerve.

Outcomes The original description of this nerve transfer by Flores presents two patients with C5-C6 traumatic brachial plexus injury [57]. Both patients recovered MRC grade 4 elbow extension following the ulnar nerve fascicle to long head of triceps nerve transfer. Importantly, each patient had additional available donors to restore elbow flexion and shoulder function (which were prioritized). A study by Goubier et al. reports a return of MRC 4 elbow extension 6–7 months after this nerve transfer in nine of ten patients; the remaining patient recovered MRC 3 elbow extension. Interestingly, eight patients required tendon transfers for subsequent wrist and finger palsies [58].

Thoracodorsal to Triceps Nerve Transfer

Indications The thoracodorsal nerve provides an excellent donor nerve for elbow extension, provided it is not required for restoration of elbow flexion.

Contraindications Poor thoracodorsal nerve function, as evidenced by weakness or absence of latissimus dorsi contraction; or unavailability of thoracodorsal nerve due to use in other nerve transfers.

Surgical Technique A medial arm incision is made to expose the radial nerve and associated triceps musculature. The branch to the long head of the triceps is identified running between the radial and ulnar nerves and can be seen innervating the long head of the triceps at the proximal third of the muscle. The branch is then followed proximally to the takeoff of the branch to the medial head of the triceps. The nerves to the medial and lateral triceps coalesce into a single nerve trunk near the border of the latissimus muscle, which is then transected as a single recipient nerve.

Through a separate incision on the chest in the midaxillary line, the thoracodorsal nerve is identified as previously described (see section "Thoracodorsal to Musculocutaneous Nerve Transfer"). The nerve is found lying on the anterior surface with the vascular pedicle. There are two branches of the thoracodorsal nerve which can be neurolyzed distally into the muscle. Intraoperative stimulation confirms strong contraction of the muscle. Both branches are transected distally, neurolyzed proximally, and brought into the axilla through a subcutaneous tunnel. The donor nerves are coapted to the previously dissected medial and long heads of the triceps nerve branches in an end-to-end fashion. The shoulder is put through a full range of motion.

Outcomes A single report of this transfer was initially published by Pet et al. as one of four patients with reinnervation of the triceps using different nerve transfers; the patient that underwent thoracodorsal to triceps nerve transfer ultimately recovered MRC grade 4 elbow extension [59]. In a larger series of eight patients by Soldado et al., all patients demonstrated return of elbow flexion within 12 months, and all but one patient recovered MRC 4 elbow extension [35].

Intercostal to Triceps Nerve Transfer

Indications Intercostal nerve transfers are indicated for restoration of elbow extension in the absence of other additional donors.

Contraindications The authors prefer to avoid IC nerve transfers in the setting of a phrenic nerve palsy.

Surgical Technique As previously described (see section "Intercostal to Musculocutaneous

Nerve Transfer"), the patient is placed in the supine position with the affected arm extended on an arm board. A curvilinear incision is made from the midaxial line to the midclavicular line, following the curvature of the ribs anteriorly. Adipocutaneous flaps are raised, and the serratus muscle is identified and split over each exposed rib. The sub-periosteal plane is developed to expose the neurovascular bundle at the inferior aspect of each rib. The intercostal nerve is identified carefully and stimulated to confirm muscle function. It is then neurolyzed anteriorly and posteriorly from the surrounding muscle and vascular bundle using bipolar cautery. Dissection of the motor nerves extends from the costochondral junction to the midaxillary line. Given the small size of the intercostal nerves, they are not transected until all levels are exposed.

The radial nerve and branch to the long head of triceps are again identified through a mid-brachial incision. The branch to the long head of triceps is dissected to its origin on the radial nerve and transected. The IC nerves are then coapted to the branch of the triceps.

Outcomes In a study by Goubier and Teboul, seven of ten patients who underwent this transfer recovered MRC 4 elbow extension. The average time for recovery of initial muscle contraction was 7 months, and the average time to extension against resistance was 15 months [60]. After long-term follow-up (average 24 months), nine of eleven patients recovered MRC 3 to MRC 4 elbow extension. Of three patients who regained less than MRC 3 function, two patients underwent transfer more than 6 months following their initial injury [61]. In a series of 25 patients with root avulsion brachial plexus injury by Gao et al., 56% of patients regained at least MRC grade 3 elbow [62].

Pediatric Implications

Obstetrical brachial plexus injury results from excessive traction on the head and/or neck during birth [63]. As many as 5400 cases of brachial plexus injuries occur annually in the United States, and global incidences are estimated to be between 0.13 and 5.1 per 1000 live births in industrialized countries [64–67]. These injuries are commonly organized into three groups with distinct distributions and functional deficits – upper plexus, lower plexus, and global injury [68]. Upper plexus injuries involve C5 and C6 nerve roots with occasional involvement of C7. This distribution of injuries results in internal rotation and adduction of the shoulder, extension of the elbow, pronation of the forearm, and flexion of the wrist; a presentation colloquially known as "Erb's Palsy." Lower never injury, or Klumpke palsy, includes C8 and T1 and primarily affects the hand. Global injury typically presents as flail arm and claw hand as a result of injury of all roots from C5 to C8.

Restoration of elbow flexion takes precedence to shoulder abduction in upper plexus injuries; however, hand reinnervation becomes priority in global plexus injuries [68–70]. Numerous donor nerves have been described in the pediatric population including suprascapular nerve, spinal accessory nerve, intercostal nerve, phrenic nerve, pectoral nerves, ulnar nerve fascicles, and median nerve fascicles [52, 53, 71–73]. Recently, nerve transfers for restoration of elbow flexion and shoulder abduction have shown to be as successful as direct repair in children with birth-related brachial plexus injuries [74].

Conclusion

Nerve transfers are an important tool for the restoration of upper extremity function following brachial plexus injury. The success of nerve transfers relies on an intimate understanding of upper extremity anatomy, a thorough evaluation of donors and recipients through history, exam, and electrodiagnostic studies, careful operative technique, and commitment to cortical re-education and postoperative hand therapy. Our understanding of nerve physiology and surgical outcomes continues to grow. Critical analysis and investigation will continue to define the role of nerve transfers in upper extremity reconstruction of shoulder and elbow function.

References

1. Waller A. Experiments on the section of the glossopharyngeal and hypoglossal nerves of the frog, and observations of the alterations produced thereby in the structure of their primitive fibres. Philos Trans R Soc Lond. 1850;140:423–9.
2. Coleman MP, Höke A. Programmed axon degeneration: from mouse to mechanism to medicine. Nat Rev Neurosci. 2020;21(4):183–96.
3. Seddon HJ, Medawar PB, Smith H. Rate of regeneration of peripheral nerves in man. J Physiol Lond. 1943;102(2):191–215.
4. Nath RK, Mackinnon SE. Nerve transfers in the upper extremity. Hand Clin. 2000;16(1):131–9, ix.
5. O'Shea K, Feinberg JH, Wolfe SW. Imaging and electrodiagnostic work-up of acute adult brachial plexus injuries. J Hand Surg Eur Vol. 2011;36(9):747–59.
6. Fu SY, Gordon T. Contributing factors to poor functional recovery after delayed nerve repair: prolonged denervation. J Neurosci. 1995;15(5 Pt 2):3886–95.
7. Boyd K, Nimigan A, Mackinnon S. Nerve reconstruction in the hand and upper extremity. Clin Plast Surg. 2011;38(4):643–60.
8. Moore AM, Novak CB. Advances in nerve transfer surgery. J Hand Ther. 2014;27(2):96–105.
9. Kahn LC, Moore AM. Donor activation focused rehabilitation approach: maximizing outcomes after nerve transfers. Hand Clin. 2016;32(2):263–77.
10. Mackinnon SE, Yee A, Ray WZ. Nerve transfers for the restoration of hand function after spinal cord injury. J Neurosurg. 2012;117(1):176–85.
11. Kostas-Agnantis I, Korompilias A, Vekris M, Lykissas M, Gkiatas I, Mitsionis G, et al. Shoulder abduction and external rotation restoration with nerve transfer. Injury. 2013;44(3):299–304.
12. Xiao F, Zhao X, Lao J. Comparative study of single and dual nerve transfers for repairing shoulder abduction. Acta Neurochir. 2019;161(4):673–8.
13. Leechavengvongs S, Witoonchart K, Uerpairojkit C, Thuvasethakul P. Nerve transfer to deltoid muscle using the nerve to the long head of the triceps, part II: a report of 7 cases. J Hand Surg Am. 2003;28(4):633–8.
14. Bahm J, Noaman H, Becker M. The dorsal approach to the suprascapular nerve in neuromuscular reanimation for obstetric brachial plexus lesions. Plast Reconstr Surg. 2005;115(1):240–4.
15. Emamhadi M, Alijani B, Andalib S. Long-term clinical outcomes of spinal accessory nerve transfer to the suprascapular nerve in patients with brachial plexus palsy. Acta Neurochir. 2016;158(9):1801–6.
16. Manske MC, Kalish LA, Cornwall R, Peljovich AE, Bauer AS. Reconstruction of the suprascapular nerve in brachial plexus birth injury: a comparison of nerve grafting and nerve transfers. JBJS. 2020;102(4):298–308.
17. Bertelli JA, Ghizoni MF. Transfer of the accessory nerve to the suprascapular nerve in brachial plexus reconstruction. J Hand Surg Am. 2007;32(7):989–98.
18. Bertelli JA, Ghizoni MF. Results of spinal accessory to suprascapular nerve transfer in 110 patients with complete palsy of the brachial plexus. J Neurosurg Spine. 2016;24(6):990–5.
19. Jerome JTJ. Anterior deltopectoral approach for axillary nerve neurotisation. J Orthop Surg (Hong Kong). 2012;20(1):66–70.
20. Bertelli JA, Ghizoni MF. Reconstruction of C5 and C6 brachial plexus avulsion injury by multiple nerve transfers: spinal accessory to suprascapular, ulnar fascicles to biceps branch, and triceps long or lateral head branch to axillary nerve. J Hand Surg Am. 2004;29(1):131–9.
21. Colbert SH, Mackinnon S. Posterior approach for double nerve transfer for restoration of shoulder function in upper brachial plexus palsy. Hand (N Y). 2006;1(2):71–7.
22. Bertelli JA, Kechele PR, Santos MA, Duarte H, Ghizoni MF. Axillary nerve repair by triceps motor branch transfer through an axillary access: anatomical basis and clinical results. J Neurosurg. 2007;107(2):370–7.
23. Bauer AS, Rabinovich RV, Waters PM. The anterior approach for transfer of radial nerve triceps fascicles to the axillary nerve. J Hand Surg Am. 2019;44(4):345.e1–6.
24. Witoonchart K, Leechavengvongs S, Uerpairojkit C, Thuvasethakul P, Wongnopsuwan V. Nerve transfer to deltoid muscle using the nerve to the long head of the triceps, part I: an anatomic feasibility study. J Hand Surg Am. 2003;28(4):628–32.
25. Desai MJ, Daly CA, Seiler JG, Wray WH, Ruch DS, Leversedge FJ. Radial to axillary nerve transfers: a combined case series. J Hand Surg Am. 2016;41(12):1128–34.
26. Texakalidis P, Tora MS, Lamanna JJ, Wetzel J, Boulis NM. Combined radial to axillary and spinal accessory nerve (SAN) to Suprascapular nerve (SSN) transfers may confer superior shoulder abduction compared with single SA to SSN transfer. World Neurosurg. 2019;126:e1251–6.
27. Ray WZ, Murphy RKJ, Santosa K, Johnson PJ, Mackinnon SE. Medial pectoral nerve to axillary nerve neurotization following traumatic brachial plexus injuries: indications and clinical outcomes. Hand (N Y). 2012;7(1):59–65.
28. Samardzic M, Rasulic LG, Grujicic DM, Bacetic DT, Milicic BR. Nerve transfers using collateral branches of the brachial plexus as donors in patients with upper palsy—thirty years' experience. Acta Neurochir. 2011;153(10):2009.
29. Belzberg AJ, Dorsi MJ, Storm PB, Moriarity JL. Surgical repair of brachial plexus injury: a multinational survey of experienced peripheral nerve surgeons. J Neurosurg. 2004;101(3):365–76.
30. Oberlin C, Béal D, Leechavengvongs S, Salon A, Dauge MC, Sarcy JJ. Nerve transfer to biceps muscle using a part of ulnar nerve for C5-C6 avulsion of the brachial plexus: anatomical study and report of four cases. J Hand Surg Am. 1994;19(2):232–7.

31. Liverneaux PA, Diaz LC, Beaulieu J-Y, Durand S, Oberlin C. Preliminary results of double nerve transfer to restore elbow flexion in upper type brachial plexus palsies. Plast Reconstr Surg. 2006;117(3):915–9.
32. Mackinnon SE, Novak CB, Myckatyn TM, Tung TH. Results of reinnervation of the biceps and brachialis muscles with a double fascicular transfer for elbow flexion. J Hand Surg Am. 2005;30(5):978–85.
33. Wellons JC, Tubbs RS, Pugh JA, Bradley NJ, Law CR, Grabb PA. Medial pectoral nerve to musculocutaneous nerve neurotization for the treatment of persistent birth-related brachial plexus palsy: an 11-year institutional experience. J Neurosurg Pediatr. 2009;3(5):348–53.
34. Novak CB, Mackinnon SE, Tung THH. Patient outcome following a thoracodorsal to musculocutaneous nerve transfer for reconstruction of elbow flexion. Br J Plast Surg. 2002;55(5):416–9.
35. Soldado F, Ghizoni MF, Bertelli J. Thoracodorsal nerve transfer for elbow flexion reconstruction in infraclavicular brachial plexus injuries. J Hand Surg Am. 2014;39(9):1766–70.
36. Dai S-Y, Lin D-X, Han Z, Zhoug S-Z. Transference of thoracodorsal nerve to musculocutaneous or axillary nerve in old traumatic injury. J Hand Surg Am. 1990;15(1):36–7.
37. Samii A, Carvalho GA, Samii M. Brachial plexus injury: factors affecting functional outcome in spinal accessory nerve transfer for the restoration of elbow flexion. J Neurosurg. 2003;98(2):307–12.
38. Xiao C, Lao J, Wang T, Zhao X, Liu J, Gu Y. Intercostal nerve transfer to neurotize the musculocutaneous nerve after traumatic brachial plexus avulsion: a comparison of two, three, and four nerve transfers. J Reconstr Microsurg. 2014;30(5):297–304.
39. Teboul F, Kakkar R, Ameur N, Beaulieu J-Y, Oberlin C. Transfer of fascicles from the ulnar nerve to the nerve to the biceps in the treatment of upper brachial plexus palsy. J Bone Joint Surg Am. 2004;86(7):1485–90.
40. Ray WZ, Pet MA, Yee A, Mackinnon SE. Double fascicular nerve transfer to the biceps and brachialis muscles after brachial plexus injury: clinical outcomes in a series of 29 cases. J Neurosurg. 2011;114(6):1520–8.
41. Carlsen BT, Kircher MF, Spinner RJ, Bishop AT, Shin AY. Comparison of single versus double nerve transfers for elbow flexion after brachial plexus injury. Plast Reconstr Surg. 2011;127(1):269–76.
42. Martins RS, Siqueira MG, Heise CO, Foroni L, Teixeira MJ. A prospective study comparing single and double fascicular transfer to restore elbow flexion after brachial plexus injury. Neurosurgery. 2013;72(5):709–14; discussion 714–715; quiz 715.
43. Sneiders D, Bulstra L, Hundepool C, Treling W, Hovius SE, Shin A. Outcomes of single versus double fascicular nerve transfers for restoration of elbow flexion in patients with brachial plexus injuries: a systematic review and meta-analysis. Plast Reconstr Surg. 2019;144(1):155–66.
44. Donnelly MR, Rezzadeh KT, Vieira D, Daar D, Hacquebord J. Is one nerve transfer enough? A systematic review and pooled analysis comparing ulnar fascicular nerve transfer and double ulnar and median fascicular nerve transfer for restoration of elbow flexion after traumatic brachial plexus injury. Microsurgery. 2020;40(3):361–9.
45. Schusterman MA, Jindal R, Unadkat JV, Spiess AM. Lateral branch of the thoracodorsal nerve (LaT branch) transfer for biceps reinnervation. Plast Reconstr Surg Glob Open. 2018;6(3):e1698.
46. Samardzic MM, Grujicic DM, Rasulic LG, Milicic BR. The use of thoracodorsal nerve transfer in restoration of irreparable C5 and C6 spinal nerve lesions. Br J Plast Surg. 2005;58(4):541–6.
47. Sulaiman OAR, Kim DD, Burkett C, Kline DG. Nerve transfer surgery for adult brachial plexus injury: a 10-year experience at Louisiana State University. Neurosurgery. 2009;65(suppl_4):A55–62.
48. Kovachevich R, Kircher MF, Wood CM, Spinner RJ, Bishop AT, Shin AY. Complications of intercostal nerve transfer for brachial plexus reconstruction. J Hand Surg Am. 2010;35(12):1995–2000.
49. Nagano A, Yamamoto S, Mikami Y. Intercostal nerve transfer to restore upper extremity functions after brachial plexus injury. Ann Acad Med Singap. 1995;24(4 Suppl):42–5.
50. Merrell GA, Barrie KA, Katz DL, Wolfe SW. Results of nerve transfer techniques for restoration of shoulder and elbow function in the context of a meta-analysis of the English literature. J Hand Surg Am. 2001;26(2):303–14.
51. Leland HA, Azadgoli B, Gould DJ, Seruya M. Investigation into the optimal number of intercostal nerve transfers for musculocutaneous nerve reinnervation: a systematic review. Hand (N Y). 2018;13(6):621–6.
52. Pondaag W, Malessy MJA. Intercostal and pectoral nerve transfers to re-innervate the biceps muscle in obstetric brachial plexus lesions. J Hand Surg Eur Vol. 2014;39(6):647–52.
53. Blaauw G, Slooff ACJ. Transfer of pectoral nerves to the musculocutaneous nerve in obstetric upper brachial plexus palsy. Neurosurgery. 2003;53(2):338–42.
54. Gribble PL, Mullin LI, Cothros N, Mattar A. Role of cocontraction in arm movement accuracy. J Neurophysiol. 2003;89(5):2396–405.
55. Bertelli JA. Lower trapezius muscle transfer for reconstruction of elbow extension in brachial plexus injuries. J Hand Surg Eur Vol. 2009;34(4):459–64.
56. Doi K, Shigetomi M, Kaneko K, Soo-Heong T, Hiura Y, Hattori Y, et al. Significance of elbow extension in reconstruction of prehension with reinnervated free-muscle transfer following complete brachial plexus avulsion. Plast Reconstr Surg. 1997;100(2):364–72; discussion 373–374.
57. Flores LP. Transfer of a motor fascicle from the ulnar nerve to the branch of the radial nerve destined to the long head of the triceps for restoration of elbow

extension in brachial plexus surgery: technical case report. Neurosurgery. 2012;70(2):E516–20; discussion E520.
58. Goubier J-N, Maillot C, Asmar G, Teboul F. Partial ulnar nerve transfer to the branch of the long head of the triceps to recover elbow extension in C5, C6 and C7 brachial plexus palsy. Injury. 2019;50 Suppl 5:S68–70.
59. Pet MA, Ray WZ, Yee A, Mackinnon SE. Nerve transfer to the triceps after brachial plexus injury: report of four cases. J Hand Surg Am. 2011;36(3):398–405.
60. Goubier J-N, Teboul F. Transfer of the intercostal nerves to the nerve of the long head of the triceps to recover elbow extension in brachial plexus palsy. Tech Hand Up Extrem Surg. 2007;11(2):139–41.
61. Goubier J-N, Teboul F, Khalifa H. Reanimation of elbow extension with intercostal nerves transfers in total brachial plexus palsies. Microsurgery. 2011;31(1):7–11.
62. Gao K, Lao J, Zhao X, Gu Y. Outcome after transfer of intercostal nerves to the nerve of triceps long head in 25 adult patients with total brachial plexus root avulsion injury. J Neurosurg. 2013;118(3):606–10.
63. Pollack RN, Buchman AS, Yaffe H, Divon MY. Obstetrical brachial palsy: pathogenesis, risk factors, and prevention. Clin Obstet Gynecol. 2000;43(2):236–46.
64. Benjamin KR. Part 1. Injuries to the brachial plexus: mechanisms of injury and identification of risk factors. [Miscellaneous Article]. Adv Neonatal Care. 2005;5(4):181–9.
65. Hoeksma AF, Wolf H, Oei SL. Obstetrical brachial plexus injuries: incidence, natural course and shoulder contracture. Clin Rehabil. 2000;14(5):523–6.
66. Gilbert WM, Nesbitt TS, Danielsen B. Associated factors in 1611 cases of brachial plexus injury. Obstet Gynecol. 1999;93(4):536–40.
67. Mollberg M, Hagberg H, Bager B, Lilja H, Ladfors L. High birthweight and shoulder dystocia: the strongest risk factors for obstetrical brachial plexus palsy in a Swedish population-based study. Acta Obstet Gynecol Scand. 2005;84(7):654–9.
68. Terzis JK, Kokkalis ZT. Pediatric brachial plexus reconstruction. Plast Reconstr Surg. 2009;124(6S):e370.
69. Marcus JR, Clarke HM. Management of obstetrical brachial plexus palsy evaluation, prognosis, and primary surgical treatment. Clin Plast Surg. 2003;30(2):289–306.
70. Haerle M, Gilbert A. Management of complete obstetric brachial plexus lesions. J Pediatr Orthop. 2004;24(2):194–200.
71. Ladak A, Morhart M, O'Grady K, Wong JN, Chan KM, Watt MJ, et al. Distal nerve transfers are effective in treating patients with upper trunk obstetrical brachial plexus injuries: an early experience. Plast Reconstr Surg. 2013;132(6):985e–92e.
72. O'Grady KM, Power HA, Olson JL, Morhart MJ, Harrop AR, Watt MJ, et al. Comparing the efficacy of triple nerve transfers with nerve graft reconstruction in upper trunk obstetric brachial plexus injury. Plast Reconstr Surg. 2017;140(4):747–56.
73. Goubier J-N, Teboul F, Papadogeorgou E. Nerve transfers in children with traumatic partial brachial plexus injuries. Microsurgery. 2008;28(2):117–20.
74. Chim H, Kircher MF, Spinner RJ, Bishop AT, Shin AY. Reconstruction of pediatric brachial plexus injuries with nerve grafts and nerve transfers. J Hand Surg Am. 2014;39(9):1771–8.

15 Free-Functioning Muscle Transfer

Andrés A. Maldonado and Louis H. Poppler

Introduction

A free-functioning muscle transfer or transplantation (FFMT) is when a muscle is detached to its origin with its nerve and vascular pedicle and transferred to another location for the purpose of restoring function. Use of a FFMT for brachial plexus reconstruction was first reported by Ikuta and colleagues, who used it to restore elbow flexion in a child seen with a chronic loss of elbow flexion [1]. With the improvement of strategy, techniques, and technology, especially with the advance in microsurgery, the indications of FFMT have been expanded.

FFMT has become an attractive option for many brachial plexus injuries in late presentations with absent function, due to delay in referral or failed prior nerve surgery. Typically, it has been recommended to restore elbow function, especially when the time from injury to surgery is greater than 9–12 months [2–4]. Another valuable role has been to restore grasp in acute cases [5, 6], or more recently, to restore elbow flexion in acute scenarios [7, 8]. Using a long muscle with a proximally located neurovascular pedicle, such as the gracilis FFMT, makes such reconstructions possible. A gracilis transfer, when fixed to the clavicle proximally and tunneled to the forearm, can animate the wrist or the hand. Because the motor point of the muscle is located at the shoulder, a nerve transfer to this area will reinnervate the muscle within 6 months or less [9].

This chapter will attempt to highlight our current FFMT strategies and techniques in acute and chronic brachial plexus injuries.

Prerequisites for Functioning Free Muscle Transfer

FFMT is possibly one of the most complex techniques in brachial plexus surgery. Before considering to perform this kind of reconstruction, the following general points should be analyzed [10]:

Preoperative Planning

1. Passive range of motion across the joint for the planned transfer. If stiffness is present, physical therapy should be first considered. Some patients with avulsion injury develop a stiff and edematous intrinsic-minus posture

A. A. Maldonado (✉)
Peripheral Nerve and Brachial Plexus Unit, Department of Plastic Surgery, University Hospital Getafe, Madrid, Spain

Department of Plastic, Hand and Reconstructive Surgery, BG Unfallklinik Frankfurt, Frankfurt, Germany
e-mail: mail@andresmaldonado.es

L. H. Poppler
Private Practice, Boise, ID, USA

A. Y. Shin, N. Pulos (eds.), *Operative Brachial Plexus Surgery*,
https://doi.org/10.1007/978-3-030-69517-0_15

with a flattened palm and fixed finger metacarpophalangeal joint extension. Success in these situations will require restoration of supple joints or later positioning of metacarpophalangeal joints in a flexed posture by tenodesis, capsulodesis, or arthrodesis.
2. Vascular assessment of the affected limb. A good artery is mandatory before the FFMT is performed. Generally, we use the thoracoacromial artery if the FFMT is transferred for elbow flexion reconstruction, and the brachial, radial, or ulnar artery for hand reconstruction. Vascular injuries are common in adult brachial plexus injury, occurring in 10% or more of patients [11]. The incidence is higher when the first rib is fractured. Avulsion of the subclavian or axillary vessels is generally considered a contraindication for free muscle transfer because patency of the thoracoacromial or thoracodorsal vessels is usually needed for FFMT to be successful. Concomitant vascular injury has been associated with worse functional outcome following reconstructive surgery of traumatic brachial plexus injury [12]. Computed tomography angiography (CTA) or digital subtraction angiography (DSA) can be useful to assess upper extremity vascularity and potential recipient vessels. Magnetic resonance angiography (MRA) can also be used but is contraindicated when there is metal artifact in the area of the vessels (i.e., prior orthopedic fracture fixation or vascular repair/clips).
3. Donor nerve: There must be an expendable motor nerve in the vicinity of the muscle neurovascular pedicle. In most brachial plexus injury cases, this will mean an extraplexal source (spinal accessory nerve or two to three intercostal motor nerves). Other nerves may be used as available, including regenerated contralateral C7 nerve transfer or elements of the brachial plexus in partial injuries (i.e., a fascicle of the ulnar nerve) [13]. Electromyography (EMG) could help to discard any previous nerve injury – i.e., EMG in the trapezius muscle if the spinal accessory is going to be used as donor nerve. Sometimes, intraoperative assessment by nerve stimulation may require a change in surgical plans and goals.
4. Adequate skin coverage, a stable and well-vascularized bed for tendon gliding.

Donor Muscle Selection

The gracilis, latissimus dorsi, adductor longus, and rectus femoris muscles have all been used as donor muscles for FFMT. The gracilis is maybe the most frequently used free-functioning muscle [9]. It is a strap muscle rather than a pennate muscle, with excellent fiber length, but it has considerably less cross-sectional area than the biceps that it is intended to replace. Thus, data suggest that it is poorly matched for strength but well matched for needed excursion. Experience has demonstrated that both the gracilis and the latissimus can provide useful function [14]. The gracilis generates sufficient force to flex the elbow against gravity in most cases and has other desirable qualities. Most importantly, the proximal position of its neurovascular pedicle permits rapid reinnervation from either the spinal accessory or intercostal motor nerves, whereas its length and shape facilitate its passage into the forearm to animate the wrist and hand [9].

Gracilis Harvest

The harvest of the gracilis muscle is described in detail in articles by Shin and colleagues [15] as well as in Chap. 11 in this textbook. We refer the reader to this detailed article for more technical information.

Based on the position of the recipient vessels, the contralateral gracilis is preferred for biceps and finger extensor reconstruction. Either contralateral or ipsilateral gracilis can be used for finger flexor reconstruction. Briefly, the steps for gracilis free functional muscle dissection are [16]:

1. The gracilis muscle can be topographically identified by drawing a line between the proximal pubic tubercle and the distal gracilis muscle tendinous insertion at the pes anserine.
2. The gracilis tendon at the pes anserine can be identified via a 3-cm longitudinal incision over the pes anserine and a 4-cm longitudi-

nal incision in the distal medial thigh. At the pes anserine, the gracilis tendon can be easily palpated as the most superior tendinous insertion. The inferior tendon at the pes anserine is the semitendinosus tendon (Fig. 15.1). Dissection is carried between the tendons until the medial collateral ligament of the knee is visualized. Umbilical tape is then placed around the superior, gracilis tendon, and the multiple soft tissue attachments to the gracilis tendon are divided (Fig. 15.2).

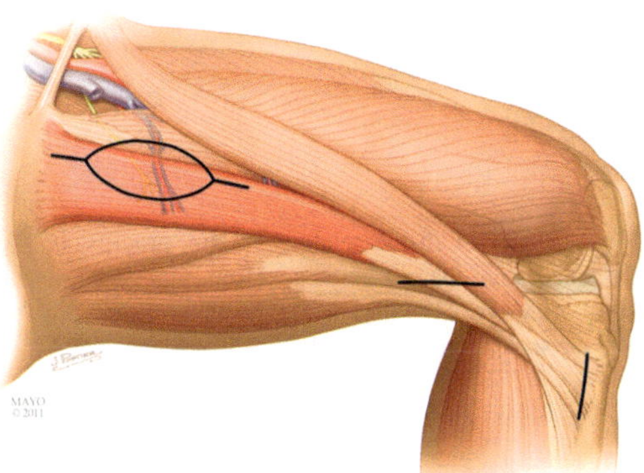

Fig. 15.1 Incisions performed for gracilis free functional muscle dissection. (Reproduced by permission of Mayo Foundation for Medical Education and Research. All rights reserved)

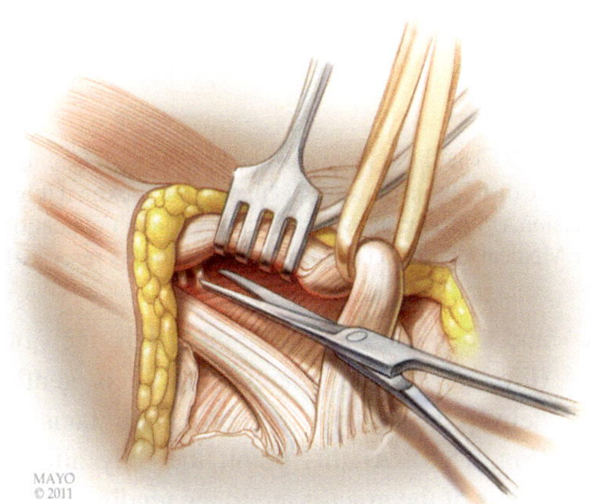

Fig. 15.2 Umbilical tape is placed around the gracilis tendon, and the multiple soft tissue attachments to the gracilis tendon are divided. (Reproduced by permission of Mayo Foundation for Medical Education and Research. All rights reserved)

3. A 4-cm incision is made over the distal medial thigh, where the myotendinous portion of the gracilis is identified. The gracilis is pulled to confirm the gracilis tendon previously identified inserting into the proximal tibia. All soft tissue attachments to the gracilis are divided between these two incisions.
4. Skin island is placed slightly anterior to the muscle. The dimensions may include the proximal two-thirds of the medial thigh skin with a maximum width of 8 cm to allow for primary closure (remember that the location of the dominant vascular pedicle into the medial muscle belly is around 10 cm from the pubic tubercle). A handheld, sterile Doppler device can be used to identify and mark skin perforators overlying the proximal gracilis muscle. An elliptically shaped incision is drawn slightly anterior to the anterior border of the gracilis muscle, centered about the identified skin perforators.
5. The proximal thigh incision is made along the anterior border of the skin paddle, and dissection is carried toward the adductor longus (Fig. 15.3).
6. In the interval between the adductor longus and gracilis muscles, the fascia of the adductor longus is gently retracted to expose the obturator nerve and the dominant proximal artery and venae comitantes (Fig. 15.4).
7. The adductor longus is retracted medially and superiorly while the vascular perforators

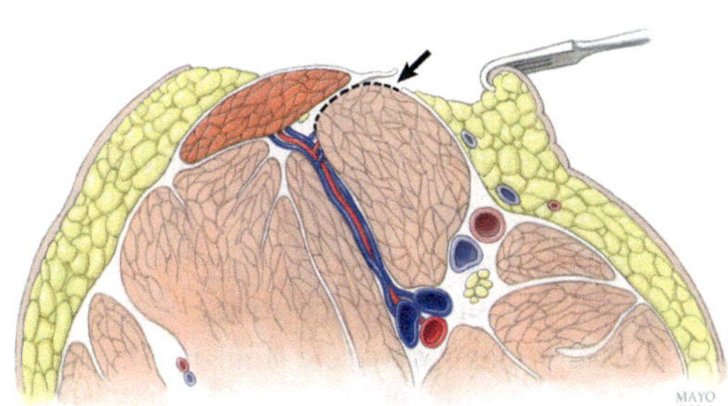

Fig. 15.3 The proximal thigh incision is made along the anterior border of the skin paddle, and dissection is carried toward the adductor longus (black arrow). (Reproduced by permission of Mayo Foundation for Medical Education and Research. All rights reserved)

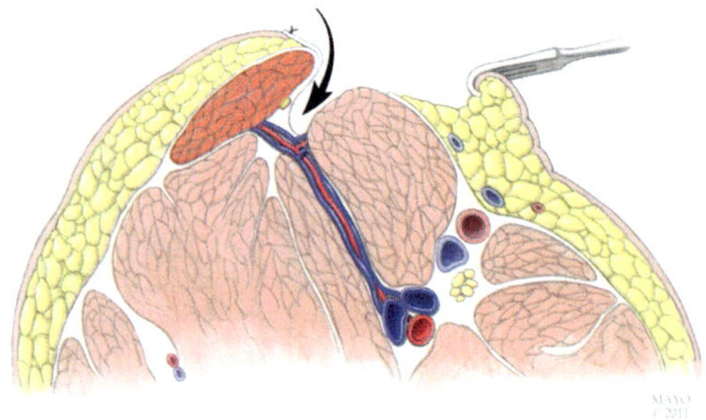

Fig. 15.4 The pedicle is found in the interval between the adductor longus and gracilis muscles. (Reproduced by permission of Mayo Foundation for Medical Education and Research. All rights reserved)

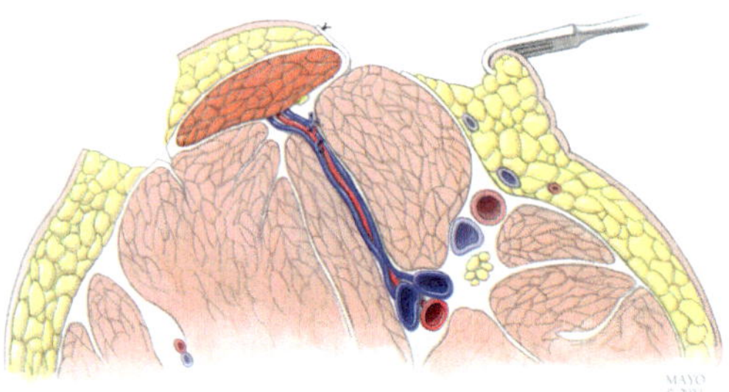

Fig. 15.5 The posterior skin paddle incision is made, and dissection is carried to the level of the adductor magnus muscle. (Reproduced by permission of Mayo Foundation for Medical Education and Research. All rights reserved)

to the adductor longus are carefully dissected and ligated, and the main pedicle is dissected to the profunda femoral artery and vein.

8. The obturator nerve is identified entering the deep surface of the gracilis obliquely to the vascular pedicle and stimulated with a disposable nerve stimulator to verify contraction. A vessel loop is placed around the nerve, and the dissection progresses as far proximal as possible.
9. The posterior skin paddle incision is made, and dissection is carried to the level of the adductor magnus muscle (Fig. 15.5).
10. Between the two thigh incisions, blunt finger dissection is performed in a subfascial plane. The secondary pedicle can often be felt or seen and is ligated.
11. The distal tendon of the gracilis is then detached from the pes anserine (Fig. 15.6) and passed first into the distal thigh incision and then to the proximal thigh incision (Fig. 15.7). The gracilis muscle is gently delivered out of the proximal incision (Fig. 15.8). At this point, the only attachments of the gracilis are to the tendinous origin at the pubic tubercle and the vascular pedicle.
12. The gracilis muscle is replaced back into its native bed, and the proximal attachment is addressed. The proximal attachment is tendinous laterally and more muscular

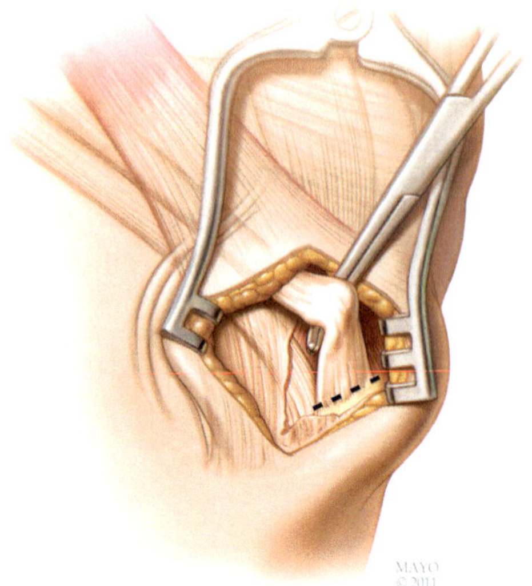

Fig. 15.6 The distal tendon of the gracilis is then detached from the pes anserine. (Reproduced by permission of Mayo Foundation for Medical Education and Research. All rights reserved)

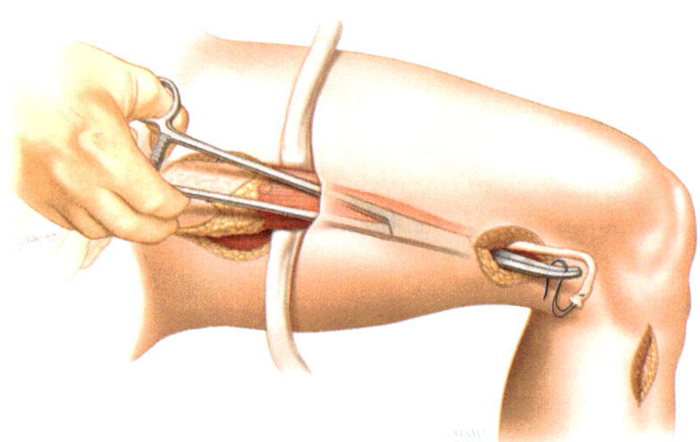

Fig. 15.7 The distal tendon of the gracilis is passed first into the distal thigh incision and then to the proximal thigh incision. (Reproduced by permission of Mayo Foundation for Medical Education and Research. All rights reserved)

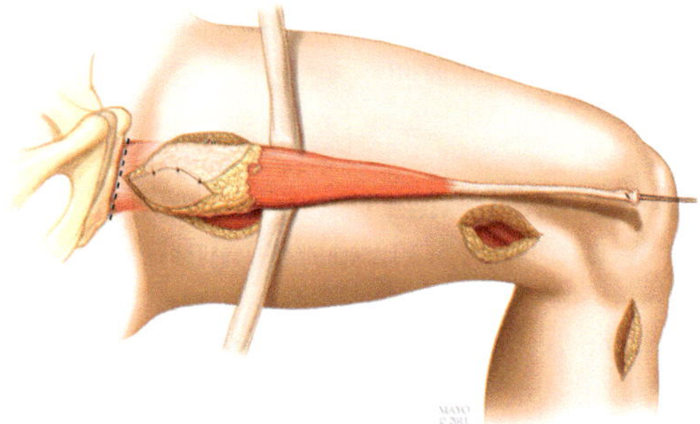

Fig. 15.8 The gracilis muscle is gently delivered out of the proximal incision. (Reproduced by permission of Mayo Foundation for Medical Education and Research. All rights reserved)

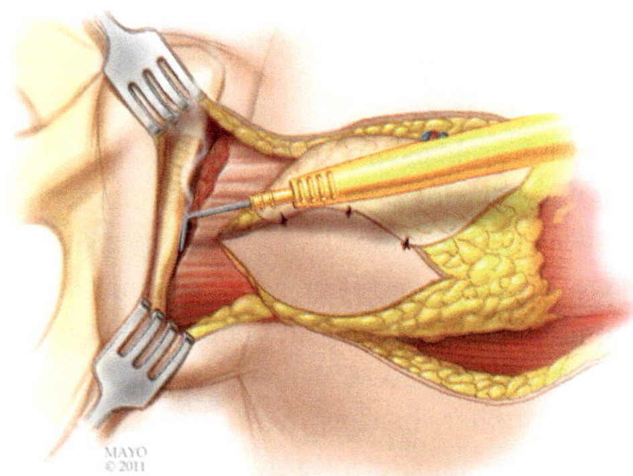

Fig. 15.9 The gracilis tendon is detached from the pubic rami. (Reproduced by permission of Mayo Foundation for Medical Education and Research. All rights reserved)

medially. The tendon is dissected off the adductor longus tendon and adductor magnus muscles, and using an angled electrocautery tip (bent by the surgeon), the gracilis tendon is detached from the pubic rami (Fig. 15.9).

13. The flap harvest is now complete, and the gracilis is perfusing only from its dominant pedicle. A papaverine-soaked sponge is placed over the vessels until the recipient site has been prepared. Once the recipient site is ready for the transfer, the pedicle of the gracilis is ligated (Fig. 15.10).

Once freed from the leg, the gracilis FFMT is brought immediately to the arm and positioned within the recipient site. The ideal goal is to

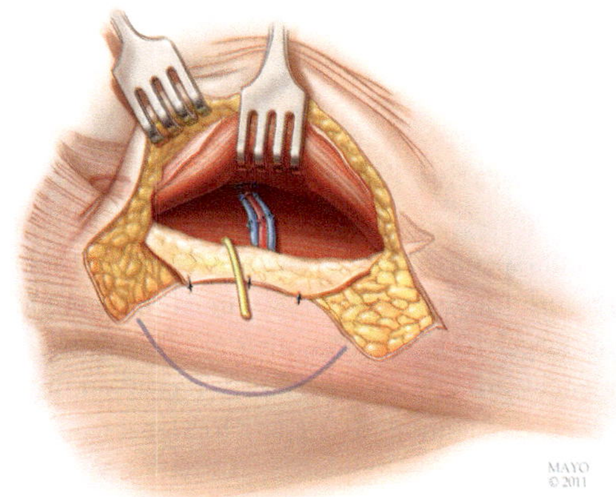

Fig. 15.10 The pedicle of the gracilis is ligated, once the recipient site is ready for the transfer. (Reproduced by permission of Mayo Foundation for Medical Education and Research. All rights reserved)

have the ischemic time of the muscle less than 60 minutes when possible, and no greater than 90 minutes.

Intraoperative Planning

To be more efficient, at least two teams should work simultaneously. Brachial plexus exploration or recipient vessel preparation and flap dissection with magnifying loupes are performed at the same time. During the FFMT insetting, the donor site is closed. Vein anastomoses are carried out with a coupler system (Synovis, Birmingham, USA), and arterial anastomosis is performed with 8/0 or 9/0 nylon using the microscope. Intravenous heparin (1000 I.U.) is used before flap reperfusion.

The gracilis is proximally attached to the clavicle and lateral acromion with suture anchors such that the vessels of the gracilis are at the same level of the donor vessel, which is typically the thoracoacromial trunk. The distal tendon is passed under the skin tunnel and temporarily clamped to prevent retraction. The arterial anastomosis is typically accomplished first, followed by venous anastomosis. The superior vein of the gracilis pedicle is the largest and is most frequently used. The inferior vein is ligated. Donor motor nerve coaption is performed, followed by distal gracilis tendon attachment.

Postoperative Planning

Patients spend the first 24 hours in our ICU. Blood pressure (target MAP 75–80 mmHg), hemoglobin (target 10 g/dL), and other electrolytical disbalances are controlled. Hourly flap monitoring is performed during the first 48 h. Signal from the Cook-Swartz Doppler (Cook Medical, Bloomington, Indiana, USA) probe connected to the artery, and clinical evaluation of the skin island are performed.

Patients must be willing and able to undergo a complex and lengthy microsurgical procedure and comply with a supervised postoperative rehabilitation protocol that minimizes problems associated with scar formation and strengthens and reeducates the neurotized muscle flap for the needed function. Our protocol has two stages. The first one is started after 3 weeks, once immobilization is completed. The new muscle origin and insertion need to be protected during this initial period (specially the first 8 weeks). Joint mobility and tendon gliding should be maintained as much as possible with passive range of motion exercises (at least 5 minutes per hour), always with attention to protection of the tenorrhaphy sites. The second stage is started after 6 weeks, but with a stronger focus when the first signs of reinnervation (clinically or in the EMG study) are appreciated. The time of onset of spontaneous contraction depends on the site of neurorrhaphy relative to the transferred FFMT, but typically begins between 3 and 6 months postoperatively. The role of the therapist is critical, guiding the patient in muscle contraction, initially using the previous muscle function of the recipient nerve to initiate the new muscle contraction.

In the German healthcare system, some patients (i.e., work-related injuries) have the opportunity to spend 3 weeks in our Department to undergo an intensive physical therapy program. We believe the time of onset of spontaneous contraction is the perfect time to guide, teach, and motivate the patient through a more intensive rehabilitation program.

Free-Functioning Muscle Transfer in Acute Brachial Plexus Injuries

As described by Doi and associates, the goal after a brachial plexus injury with avulsion of four or five nerve roots is to obtain voluntary elbow flexion and extension, hand sensation, and grasp and release function in patients [3, 5, 17]. One of the major advances in brachial plexus surgery has been the application of FFMT in the acute setting (during the first 9 months). There are two main reasons/advantages of using FFMT after an acute brachial plexus injury:

1. Restore prehension. After complete brachial plexus avulsion, several surgical approaches have been developed to restore prehension [18–21]. A powerful grip independent of the contralateral limb and the independent use of both hands would be the ideal reconstruction. Active rather than passive (tenodesis) finger flexion is imperative for a powerful grip. Release of grasp is another useful function in prehension. To achieve voluntary finger extension independent of elbow position, a second free muscle transfer is required. The complexity of this undertaking for the patient, the surgeons, and the therapist, as well as the need for all aspects of the procedure to function properly, makes this procedure among the most challenging and, when successful, most rewarding of the reconstructive options for a patient with a complete brachial plexus injury. The double free muscle transfer developed by Doi [17, 22] is based on two stages:
   - Stage I: during the first operation, the exploration of the brachial plexus and reconstruction of the proximal ruptured motor nerves is performed, if possible. Additionally, the contralateral gracilis (neurotized by the spinal accessory nerve) is used for elbow flexion and finger extension (see Fig. 15.11). The motor nerve of the transferred gracilis is passed

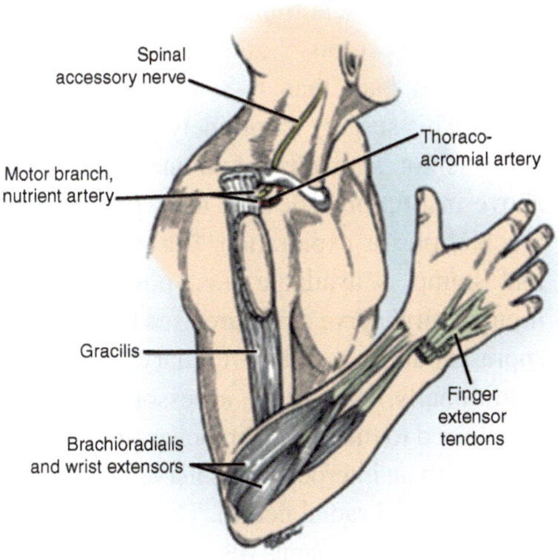

Fig. 15.11 Schematic representation of the stage I of Doi's double free muscle transfer for reconstruction of elbow flexion and prehension after complete brachial plexus avulsion. During the first operation, the exploration of the brachial plexus is performed, repaired if possible, and the gracilis FFMT (neurotized by the spinal accessory nerve) is used for elbow flexion and finger or wrist extension. (Reproduced by permission of Mayo Foundation for Medical Education and Research. All rights reserved)

behind the clavicle and coapted to the distal branch of the spinal accessory nerve in the supraclavicular area. Thoracoacromial artery and vein or the cephalic vein are used as recipient vessels. The FFMT is attached proximally to the acromion with non-absorbable sutures and placed on the anterolateral aspect of the arm and dorsal surface of the forearm. To prevent bowstringing, the free muscle is passed deep to the brachioradialis muscle. Correct muscle tension is critical for good postoperative function. Before detaching the muscle, the resting length of the muscle is reproduced, and silk sutures can be placed on the surface of the muscle at 5-cm intervals, as described by Manktelow and colleagues [23, 24]. The original muscle length is restored by stretching the muscle until the distance between the markers is once again 5 cm. Tension is adjusted with the shoulder in 60 degrees of abduction and 15 degrees of anterior flexion, the elbow in 150 degrees of flexion, the wrist in neutral, and the fingers in full extension. After adjusting the tension, the position of coaptation is marked over the tendon of the extensor digitorum and the donor muscle tendon. The elbow is flexed to 90°, and with the wrist in neutral and the fingers fully flexed, the tenorrhaphies between the donor muscle tendon and extensor digitorum tendon are completed.

- Stage II: during the second operation (2 or 3 months after the first one), a second gracilis FFMT (neurotized by the fifth and sixth intercostal nerves) is used for finger flexion. The thoracodorsal artery and vein are used as recipient vessels. The muscle is proximally attached to the second and third ribs and placed on the medial aspect of the upper part of the arm and forearm so that it does not act as an elbow flexor. The distal attachment of the gracilis tendon is passed deep to the flexor pronator origin, to the flexor digitorum profundus muscles and tendons. The flexor digitorum profundus tendons are first interconnected to provide a cascade of increasing flexion from the index finger to the small finger, and they are then joined with the gracilis tendon with a Pulvertaft weave; an additional flexor carpi radialis tendon graft is often required to prolong the gracilis. Muscle tension is determined as previously described.

  Additionally, the third and fourth intercostal nerves are used to neurotize the motor branch of the triceps brachii muscle for elbow extension and the intercostal sensory rami to the lateral cord contribution to the median nerve to restore sensibility of the hand (see Fig. 15.12). A third operation (1.5 years after stage I) is usually necessary to stabilize (arthrodesis) the CMC-thumb and wrist joints. Tenolysis of both FFMT may also be necessary.

Thirty of 36 patients undergoing double free muscle procedure reconstruction (with a mean follow-up of 40 months) were assessed for the long-term outcome of prehension,

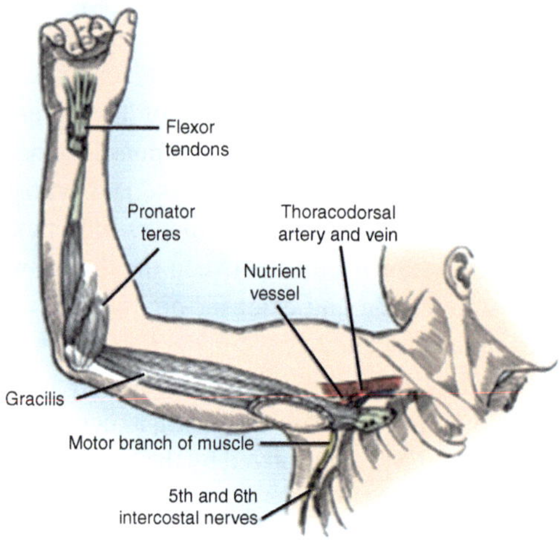

Fig. 15.12 Schematic representation of the stage II of Doi's double free muscle transfer for reconstruction of elbow flexion and prehension after complete brachial plexus avulsion. During the second operation, a second gracilis FFMT (neurotized by the fifth and sixth intercostal nerves) is used for finger flexion. (Reproduced by permission of Mayo Foundation for Medical Education and Research. All rights reserved)

including motion and stability of the shoulder and elbow, voluntary and independent motion of the fingers, sensibility, and performance of activities of daily living [5, 25]. The functional outcome of prehension according to the authors' classification was excellent in six patients (which implies restoration of more than 90 degrees of elbow flexion, dynamic stability of the elbow while moving the fingers, and more than 60° of total active motion of the fingers), good in 11 patients (same as excellent, except for total active motion of 30°–60°), fair in three patients (total active motion of less than 30°), and poor in ten patients. Satisfactory results (excellent and good) were achieved in 17 of 30 patients (57%).

A modification of the above technique is the single-stage FFMT for prehension developed by the Mayo Clinic group [9, 20]. This algorithm combines the reconstruction of the elbow flexion and hand prehension in one surgery, using only one gracilis muscle. The indications for this approach are the same as for a double free muscle transfer: avulsion of four or five nerve roots. Surgery should be performed no later than 6–8 months after the injury. This surgery is routinely performed by three senior surgeons simultaneously at the above institution. The first team perform the brachial plexus exploration. If a viable proximal stump is available (i.e., postganglionic injury), sural nerve grafts are used to target the suprascapular and axillary nerves. Additionally, the spinal accessory nerve is transferred to the triceps branches of the radial nerve with an interpositional nerve graft (often the superficial radial nerve). The second team prepares the recipient vessels (thoracoacromial artery and cephalic vein), two intercostal motor nerves (T3 and T4) for the gracilis muscle, and another pair (T5 and T6) for the biceps motor branch of the musculocutaneous nerve. Additionally, the four intercostal sensory rami are dissected for the lateral cord contribution to the median nerve to restore sensibility of the hand. Finally, the third team dissects the contralateral gracilis muscle. The gracilis is attached to the acromion and distal clavicle, and the distal tendon is woven into the flexor digitorum profundus and flexor pollicis longus to produce finger flexion and thumb pinch. An antecubital pulley must be used to avoid bowstringing. The intact lacertus fibrosus, reinforced if needed by weaving the flexor carpi ulnaris across the antecubital fossa to the lateral epicondyle and back, is generally used for this purpose. To balance the elbow flexion and hand prehension motion (the gracilis muscle is crossing two joints), triceps function is needed. Based on this, the spinal accessory nerve is transferred to the triceps branches as previously mentioned. Figure 15.13a, b summarize the whole single-stage concept. Arthrodesis of the CMC-thumb and wrist joints is performed 1.5 years after the main reconstruction, depending on the extent of recovery.

Some preliminary data from the Mayo Clinic group (in the process of being published) found that 20 out of 27 patients presented active pull-through finger flexion after

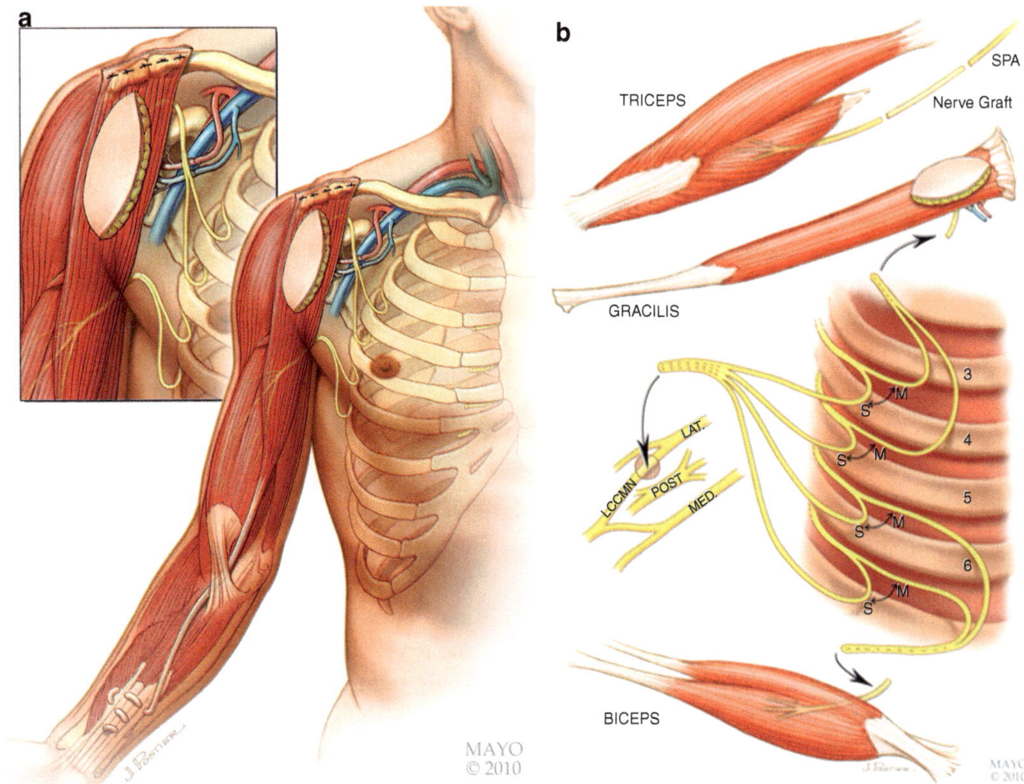

Fig. 15.13 Schematic representation of the single single-stage FFMT for prehension developed by the Mayo Clinic group. (**a**) The gracilis is attached to the acromion and distal clavicle, and the distal tendon is woven into the flexor digitorum profundus and flexor pollicis longus to produce finger flexion and thumb pinch. Note that two intercostal nerves (T5 and T6) are transferred to the biceps muscle and two (T3 and T4) to the gracilis muscle. (**b**) Overall representation of all the nerve transfer: spinal accessory for triceps muscle and intercostal nerves for biceps, gracilis muscle, and lateral cord contribution to the median nerve. LAT lateral cord, LCCMN lateral cord contribution to the median nerve, M,motor, MED medial cord, POST posterior cord, S sensory, SPA spinal accessory nerve. (Reproduced by permission of Mayo Foundation for Medical Education and Research. All rights reserved)

the single-stage FFMT technique for prehension previously described. However, only 6 (25%) patients considered their hand function as useful for daily activities. The DASH score pre- vs. post-reconstruction was 43.8 and 30.8, respectively. The mean follow-up of these 27 patients was 38 (range 24–132) months. Regarding the secondary procedures of this group of patients, 89% underwent wrist fusion, 78% thumb CMC fusion, and 74% thumb IP fusion. Further analysis is needed to determine how useful is this grade of finger flexion in daily activities.

Recently, a different application of the FFMT to restore prehension has been described. The combination of initial arm reconstruction and elective amputation with final prosthetics fitting (called "bionic reconstruction" developed by Aszmann and colleagues [26, 27]) has been published in the last few years with promising results. In this innovative concept, the FFMT has been performed before the elective amputation with the intent of restoring function in the actual wrist and hand, but in other cases, the FFMT was done a priori to create a signal site for future prosthetic control. We believe this is another potential application of FFMT in acute and chronic brachial plexus injuries. Further studies and more experience by other groups are needed to further establish this reconstruction strategy.

2. Restore elbow flexion. Elbow flexion is widely accepted as the most important function to restore after a pan-plexus injury [6]. Extraplexal nerve transfers have been widely used to reconstruct elbow flexion in acute scenarios (when the time from injury to surgery is less than 9–12 months). Intercostal (ICN) and spinal accessory (SAN) nerves are the most commonly used donors [2]. Many reports with different results have been published using ICN transfer for reconstruction of elbow flexion [28–44]. The outcomes have varied from 0% [44] to 78% [36] of patients recovering M4 elbow flexion after ICN transfer. These varied results make it difficult to educate patients as well as surgeons regarding the expected outcomes from this surgery.

A recent study by Maldonado et al. [8] has shown that gracilis FFMT reconstruction achieves better elbow flexion strength than ICN to MCN transfer for elbow flexion after pan-plexus injury. In this study, 62 patients after traumatic pan-plexus injury underwent gracilis FFMT reconstruction (gracilis group) or ICN to musculocutaneous nerve (MCN) transfer (MCN group) for elbow flexion reconstruction following a pan-plexus injury. The two groups were compared with respect to postoperative elbow flexion strength according to the British Medical Research Council grading system. In the FFMT group 67.7% patients achieved M3 or M4 elbow flexion. In the ICN to MCN group 41.9% patients achieved M3 or M4 elbow flexion. The difference was statistically significant (p-value <0.05). Based on this study, we believe the role of gracilis FFMT should be carefully considered in acute reconstruction. ICN transfer to the MCN is a technically simpler procedure compared to FFMT. This nerve transfer is used to reinnervate the biceps, which is a stronger muscle and has some biomechanical advantages for elbow flexion over the gracilis muscle [14]. However, the gracilis FFMT has the advantages of immediate muscle reinnervation (denervation time of the muscle is hours not months) and the possibility of being performed any time after the injury. Additionally, the varied results previously reported of the ICN to MCN transfer may be consequence of the secondary trauma at different levels (biceps muscle, neuromuscular plaque, biceps branch, etc.), which cannot be observed/detected during the macroscopically surgical exploration. Taking an uninjured gracilis muscle with a healthy motor nerve and vascular pedicle may improve the reliability of the reconstruction. Interestingly, a second study [7] was published in 65 patients after traumatic pan-plexus injury comparing the gracilis FFMT alone (gracilis group) vs. the combination of gracilis FFMT and ICN to MCN transfer (gracilis + MCN group). The use of ICN to MCN transfer associated with gracilis FFMT did not improve the elbow flexion BMRC grade. This second study reinforce the hypothesis of the important role of using/adding a FFMT in the reconstructive plan even in the acute scenario.

Functioning Free Muscle Transfer in Chronic Brachial Plexus Injuries

In the complete or upper type of brachial plexus injury, when the time from injury to surgery is greater than 9–12 months, a free-functioning muscle transfer (FFMT) in conjunction with an extraplexal or intraplexal (if available) motor nerve transfer to restore elbow function has been recommended [2, 4]. The above general principles are the same for chronic and acute scenarios: a free passive range of motion of the elbow joint, good skin coverage, available recipient vessels, and an uninjured donor nerve are needed for a successful FFMT.

Vascular injuries of the subclavian artery, specially the thoracoacromial trunk, are a relative contraindication. Dissection through dense scar tissue in proximity to a subclavian artery injury or arterial reconstruction is technically challenging. Surgical confirmation of adequate vessels to permit microvascular anastomoses to the free-functioning muscle is required before muscle harvest, and a vascular surgery team should be available in the operating room if needed. We perform preoperative a computed tomography angiography (CTA) or digital subtraction angiography (DSA) to evaluate potential recipient vessels.

Selection of the donor nerve depends on the availability of functioning nerves after the brachial plexus injury. After pan-plexus injuries, the spinal accessory nerve and the intercostal nerve are good potential candidates [20]. When these proximal intercostal nerves have already been used, more inferior intercostal nerves can be harvested. In upper type of brachial plexus injury, the ulnar or median nerves are excellent option as a donor motor nerve for innervated muscle transfer [45].

The two most commonly used muscles for upper extremity reconstruction are the gracilis muscle and the latissimus dorsi muscle. The rectus femoris is occasionally selected. For elbow flexion reconstruction, the muscle is attached to the acromion and distal clavicle, and the distal tendon is woven into the biceps tendon (Fig. 15.14) or into the flexor digitorum profundus and flexor pollicis longus (wrist arthrodesis is necessary, especially if the flexor digitorum profundus is used for the distal attachment). A recent study has shown biomechanically and clinically superior elbow flexion strength, if the gracilis muscle is distally attached to the flexor digitorum profundus compared to the biceps tendon [46]. The rest of the technique is previously discussed in this chapter.

Results are relatively predictable if an experienced microsurgical team is involved and the patient is a good candidate with high motivation. More than 90% of patients who have undergone FFMT for elbow flexion have recovered more than 90 degrees of elbow flexion after transfer of the spinal accessory nerve or intercostal nerves [5, 47]. Patients older than 40 years did not consistently recover comparable degrees of elbow flexion despite successful reinnervation to the transferred muscle. The final quantitative assessment of muscle strength showed 10% to 20% of the mean values of normal elbow flexion more than 2 years after surgery.

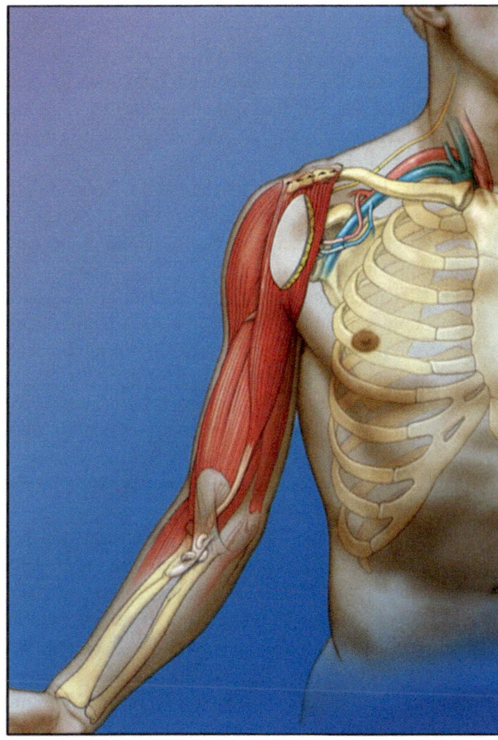

Fig. 15.14 Schematic representation of the gracilis free-functioning muscle transfer for elbow flexion reconstruction in a late brachial plexus injury. Note the spinal accessory nerve is transferred to the gracilis motor branch. Alternatively, intercostal nerves can be used. The thoracoacromial vessels are used as recipient vessels. (Reproduced by permission of Mayo Foundation for Medical Education and Research. All rights reserved)

Summary

Free-functioning muscle transfer is a powerful tool in upper extremity reconstruction when other options are not available. Patient selection, an experienced microsurgical team, and a dedicated postoperative rehabilitation program are key factors for success in these complex surgeries. Additionally, other reconstruction methods are usually required: selected joint arthrodesis, neurolysis, nerve grafting, nerve transfer, tendon transfer, etc. A multimodal and multidisciplinary reconstruction, including functional free muscle transfer, is essential for restoration of lost function and patient satisfaction.

References

1. Ikuta Y, Yoshioka K, Tsuge K. Free muscle graft as applied to brachial plexus injury-case report and experimental study. Ann Acad Med Singap. 1979;8(4):454–8.
2. Giuffre JL, Kakar S, Bishop AT, Spinner RJ, Shin AY. Current concepts of the treatment of adult brachial plexus injuries. J Hand Surg Am. 2010;35(4):678–88.
3. Doi K, Kuwata N, Muramatsu K, Hottori Y, Kawai S. Double muscle transfer for upper extremity reconstruction following complete avulsion of the brachial plexus. Hand Clin. 1999;15(4):757–67.
4. Akasaka Y, Hara T, Takahashi M. Restoration of elbow flexion and wrist extension in brachial plexus paralyses by means of free muscle transplantation innervated by intercostal nerve. Ann Chir Main Memb Super. 1990;9(5):341–50.
5. Doi K, Muramatsu K, Hattori Y, Otsuka K, Tan SH, Nanda V, et al. Restoration of prehension with the double free muscle technique following complete avulsion of the brachial plexus. Indications and long-term results. J Bone Joint Surg Am. 2000;82(5):652–66.
6. Shin AY, Spinner RJ, Steinmann SP, Bishop AT. Adult traumatic brachial plexus injuries. J Am Acad Orthop Surg. 2005;13(6):382–96.
7. Maldonado AA, Kircher MF, Spinner RJ, Bishop AT, Shin AY. Free functioning gracilis muscle transfer with and without simultaneous intercostal nerve transfer to musculocutaneous nerve for restoration of elbow flexion after traumatic adult brachial pan-plexus injury. J Hand Surg Am. 2017;42(4):293.e1–7.
8. Maldonado AA, Kircher MF, Spinner RJ, Bishop AT, Shin AY. Free functioning gracilis muscle transfer versus intercostal nerve transfer to musculocutaneous nerve for restoration of elbow flexion after traumatic adult brachial pan-plexus injury. Plast Reconstr Surg. 2016;138(3):483e–8e.
9. Spinner RJ, Shin AY, Elhassan BT, Bishop AT. Traumatic brachial plexus injury. In: Wolfe SW, Hotchkiss RN, Pederson WC, Scott H, Kozin MD, Cohen MS, editors. Green's operative hand surgery. Philadelphia: Elsevier; 2016. p. 1146–207.
10. Stevanovic M, Sharpe F. Functional free muscle transfer for upper extremity reconstruction. Plast Reconstr Surg. 2014;134(2):257e–74e.
11. Sturm JT, Perry JF. Brachial plexus injuries from blunt trauma – a harbinger of vascular and thoracic injury. Ann Emerg Med. 1987;16(4):404–6.
12. Huang AE, Noland SS, Spinner RJ, Bishop AT, Shin AY. Outcomes of reconstructive surgery in traumatic brachial plexus injury with concomitant vascular injury. World Neurosurg. 2020;135:e350–7.
13. Soldado F, Bertelli J. Free gracilis transfer reinnervated by the nerve to the supinator for the reconstruction of finger and thumb extension in longstanding C7-T1 brachial plexus root avulsion. J Hand Surg Am. 2013;38(5):941–6.
14. Doi K, Hattori Y, Tan S-H, Dhawan V. Basic science behind functioning free muscle transplantation. Clin Plast Surg. 2002;29(4):483–95.
15. Giuffre JL, Bishop AT, Shin AY. Harvest of an entire gracilis muscle and tendon for use in functional muscle transfer: a novel technique. J Reconstr Microsurg. 2012;28(5):349–58.
16. Maldonado AA, Spinner RJ, Elhassan BT, Bishop AT, Shin AY. Strategies for multimodal reconstruction of challenging injury patterns: combining nerve grafting and transfers, free functioning muscles and tendon transfers. In: Dy CJ, Isaacs JE, editors. Nerve reconstruction. Chicago: American Society for Surgery of the Hand. p. 177–86.
17. Doi K, Sakai K, Kuwata N, Ihara K, Kawai S. Double free-muscle transfer to restore prehension following complete brachial plexus avulsion. J Hand Surg Am. 1995;20(3):408–14.
18. Doi K. New reconstructive procedure for brachial plexus injury. Clin Plast Surg. 1997;24(1):75–85.
19. Xu WD, Lu JZ, Qiu YQ, Jiang S, Xu L, Xu JG, et al. Hand prehension recovery after brachial plexus avulsion injury by performing a full-length phrenic nerve transfer via endoscopic thoracic surgery. J Neurosurg. 2008;108(6):1215–9.
20. Barrie KA, Steinmann SP, Shin AY, Spinner RJ, Bishop AT. Gracilis free muscle transfer for restoration of function after complete brachial plexus avulsion. Neurosurg Focus. 2004;16(5):E8–9.
21. Wang SF, Li PC, Xue Y-H, Yiu H-W, Li YC, Wang HH. Contralateral C7 nerve transfer with direct coaptation to restore lower trunk function after traumatic brachial plexus avulsion. J Bone Joint Surg Am. 2013;95(9):821–7.
22. Doi K. Management of total paralysis of the brachial plexus by the double free-muscle transfer technique. J Hand Surg Eur Vol. 2008;33(3):240–51.
23. Manktelow RT, McKee NH. Free muscle transplantation to provide active finger flexion. J Hand Surg Am. 1978;3(5):416–26.
24. Manktelow RT, Zuker RM, McKee NH. Functioning free muscle transplantation. J Hand Surg Am. 1984;9A(1):32–9.
25. Doi K, Sakai K, Fuchigami Y, Kawai S. Reconstruction of irreparable brachial plexus injuries with reinnervated free-muscle transfer. Case report. J Neurosurg. 1996;85(1):174–7.
26. Hruby LA, Sturma A, Mayer JA, Pittermann A, Salminger S, Aszmann OC. Algorithm for bionic hand reconstruction in patients with global brachial plexopathies. J Neurosurg. 2017;127(5):1163–71.
27. Aszmann OC, Roche AD, Salminger S, Paternostro-Sluga T, Herceg M, Sturma A, et al. Bionic reconstruction to restore hand function after brachial plexus injury: a case series of three patients. Lancet. 2015;385(9983):2183–9.
28. Schreiber JJ, Byun DJ, Khair MM, Rosenblatt L, Lee SK, Wolfe SW. Optimal axon counts for brachial

plexus nerve transfers to restore elbow flexion. Plast Reconstr Surg. 2015;135(1):135e–41e.
29. Friedman AH, Nunley JA, Goldner RD, Oakes WJ, Goldner JL, Urbaniak JR. Nerve transposition for the restoration of elbow flexion following brachial plexus avulsion injuries. J Neurosurg. 1990;72(1):59.
30. El-Gammal TA, Fathi NA. Outcomes of surgical treatment of brachial plexus injuries using nerve grafting and nerve transfers. J Reconstr Microsurg. 2002;18(1):7–15.
31. Coulet B, Boretto JG, Lazerges C, Chammas M. A comparison of intercostal and partial ulnar nerve transfers in restoring elbow flexion following upper brachial plexus injury (C5-C6+/-C7). J Hand Surg Am. 2010;35(8):1297–303.
32. Bhandari PS, Sadhotra LP, Bhargava P, Bath AS, Mukherjee MK, Bhatti T, et al. Surgical outcomes following nerve transfers in upper brachial plexus injuries. Indian J Plast Surg. 2009;42(2):150–60.
33. Merrell GA, Barrie KA, Katz DL, Wolfe SW. Results of nerve transfer techniques for restoration of shoulder and elbow function in the context of a meta-analysis of the English literature. J Hand Surg Am. 2001;26(2):303.
34. Ruch DS, Friedman A, Nunley JA. The restoration of elbow flexion with intercostal nerve transfers. Clin Orthop Relat Res. 1995;314:95–103.
35. Okinaga S, Nagano A. Can vascularization improve the surgical outcome of the intercostal nerve transfer for traumatic brachial plexus palsy? A clinical comparison of vascularized and non-vascularized methods. Microsurgery. 1999;19(4):176–80.
36. Ogino T, Naito T. Intercostal nerve crossing to restore elbow flexion and sensibility of the hand for a root avulsion type of brachial plexus injury. Microsurgery. 1995;16(8):571–7.
37. Ochiai N, Mikami Y, Yamamoto S, Nakagawa T, Nagano A. A new technique for mismatched nerve suture in direct intercostal nerve transfers. J Hand Surg Br. 1993;18(3):318–9.
38. Nagano A, Ochiai N, Okinaga S. Restoration of elbow flexion in root lesions of brachial plexus injuries. J Hand Surg Am. 1992;17(5):815–21.
39. Malessy MJ, Thomeer RT. Evaluation of intercostal to musculocutaneous nerve transfer in reconstructive brachial plexus surgery. J Neurosurg. 1998;88(2).
40. Krakauer JD, Wood MB. Intercostal nerve transfer for brachial plexopathy. J Hand Surg Am. 1994;19(5):829–35.
41. Chuang DC, Yeh MC, Wei FC. Intercostal nerve transfer of the musculocutaneous nerve in avulsed brachial plexus injuries: evaluation of 66 patients. J Hand Surg Am. 1992;17(5):822–8.
42. Chalidapong P, Sananpanich K, Kraisarin J, Bumroongkit C. Pulmonary and biceps function after intercostal and phrenic nerve transfer for brachial plexus injuries. J Hand Surg Br. 2004;29(1):8–11.
43. Nagano A, Tsuyama N, Ochiai N, Hara T, Takahashi M. Direct nerve crossing with the intercostal nerve to treat avulsion injuries of the brachial plexus. J Hand Surg Am. 1989;14(6):980–5.
44. Sulaiman OAR, Kim DD, Burkett C, Kline DG. Nerve transfer surgery for adult brachial plexus injury: a 10-year experience at Louisiana State University. Neurosurgery. 2009;65:A55–62.
45. Hattori Y, Doi K, Baliarsing AS. A part of the ulnar nerve as an alternative donor nerve for functioning free muscle transfer: a case report. J Hand Surg Am. 2002;27(1):150–3.
46. Maldonado AA, Romero-Brufau S, Kircher MF, Spinner RJ, Bishop AT, Shin AY. Free functioning gracilis muscle transfer for elbow flexion reconstruction after traumatic adult brachial pan-plexus injury: where is the optimal distal tendon attachment for elbow flexion? Plast Reconstr Surg. 2017;139(1):128–36.
47. Chuang DC, Epstein MD, Yeh MC, Wei FC. Functional restoration of elbow flexion in brachial plexus injuries: results in 167 patients (excluding obstetric brachial plexus injury). J Hand Surg Am. 1993;18(2):285–91.

Tendon Transfers of the Shoulder, Elbow, Wrist, and Hand

16

Eric Richard Wagner, Bassem T. Elhassan, and Charles A. Daly

Tendon Transfers After Brachial Plexus Injury: Shoulder and Elbow

Peripheral nerve and brachial plexus injuries are life-altering events, given the extensive compromise in shoulder, arm, and hand function. When these injuries do not recover, or attempts at nerve reconstructions fail to restore various functions of the upper extremity, patients are often left quite limited in their daily lives. One of the most common areas not to recover is the shoulder, leading to a very limited overall function of the patient's upper extremity [1]. With variable or non-existent recovery of deltoid and rotator cuff function, patients are left with limited ability to raise their arm or rotate if away from their abdomen. Even in those patients that obtain a recovery of elbow flexion and some shoulder musculature, and thus shoulder stability, their arm is left internally rotated against their abdomen limiting their elbow flexion, without the ability to externally rotate to neutral [2, 3].

Nerve grafting and transfers are the preferred treatment for brachial plexus and peripheral nerve injuries involving the shoulder and elbow that do not recover within 6–9 months from the injury. However, either when the patient presents after 9–12 months, or when the reconstructions fail to recover, patients are left with limited options, including tendon and muscle transfers or shoulder fusions. The range of deficits can range across a wide spectrum, from lack of shoulder stability and no function, to limitations in certain motions. As mentioned above, the most common deficits often involve a lack of shoulder abduction and elevation, as well as shoulder external rotation [2, 3]. Thus, patients are unable to position their hand in space or reach their mouths with their hand.

Although one option to reconstruct the patient's shoulder involves a glenohumeral fusion, this should be reserved as a last resort for patients with no other options [4]. In the setting of a glenohumeral fusion, shoulder motion is dependent on scapulothoracic motion [4–6]. In patients with brachial plexus injuries, their scapulothoracic articulations are often involved and limited, thus, markedly compromising their ability to regain meaningful motion after glenohumeral arthrodesis and leading to a high rate of scapulothoracic pain [4, 7].

Shoulder and elbow tendon transfers represent viable options for patients in the late stages (>9–12 months) after brachial plexus and peripheral nerve injuries. The viability of these transfers is dependent on which muscles are spared by the injury, and thus expendable and available as viable donors. The trapezius muscle is innervated by

E. R. Wagner · C. A. Daly
Department of Orthopaedic Surgery, Emory University, Atlanta, GA, USA

B. T. Elhassan (✉)
Shoulder Fellowship at MGH, Boston, MA, USA
e-mail: belhassan@partners.org

A. Y. Shin, N. Pulos (eds.), *Operative Brachial Plexus Surgery*,
https://doi.org/10.1007/978-3-030-69517-0_16

the spinal accessory nerve (cranial nerve XI), and thus is a viable option in most adult injury patterns [8–12]. In upper trunk injuries, the latissimus dorsi, teres major, levator scapulae, and pectoralis major are often viable options.

When considering a tendon transfer, certain principles are critical in order to achieve an optimal outcome:

1. The recipient and transferred tendon must have similar musculo-tendinous excursion.
2. The recipient and transferred tendon should have similar lines of pull.
3. One tendon (the transferred) should be designed to replace one function (of the recipient).
4. The transferred tendon and muscle's function should be expendable without a significant donor site morbidity.
5. Strength of transferred muscle must be at least grade 4 or greater.

When considering these principles around the shoulder, it is important to keep in mind the distinct roles of the various musculature when driving shoulder motion. As described by Goldner, Herzberg, and others [9, 13–15], the deltoid drives most aspects of shoulder motion, while the rotator cuff functions both as a dynamic joint stabilizer and driver of internal/external rotation and abduction. These are complemented by the latissimus dorsi, teres major, and pectoralis major as secondary internal rotators and joint depressors, while the scapulohumeral rhythm is coordinated by the serratus anterior, trapezius, rhomboids, levator scapulae, and pectoralis minor. With regard to the rotator cuff, its function as a dynamic shoulder stabilizer involves the anterior-posterior force couple between the subscapularis and infraspinatus-teres minor. A paralysis of infraspinatus alone leads to a loss of ~50% abduction and ~70% external rotation strength, while a paralysis of supraspinatus and infraspinatus combined is associated with a loss of ~75% abduction and ~80% external rotation strength [16]. Furthermore, it is important to keep in mind the critical role of scapulothoracic motion and coordination of scapulohumeral rhythm that drives shoulder function. For example, isolated serratus anterior palsy leads to scapular winging and marked limitations in shoulder motion. Finally, the line of pull, muscle strengths, tensions, and excursions are critical to consider when attempting to reconstruct and rebalance a paralytic shoulder, as described by Herzberg et al. [15] (Fig. 16.1).

Keeping these considerations in mind, we will review various types of shoulder and elbow functional deficits and the various tendon transfer options to reconstruct each one. In addition to the principles of tendon transfers, it is important to remember that the joint must be passively supple and mobile prior to the transfer.

Upper Trunk: Shoulder Stability

Shoulder stability remains one of the most critical downstream consequences of brachial plexus injuries. In complete or severe upper trunk injuries, the shoulder subluxates inferiorly, markedly compromising function, while leading to pain and eventual glenohumeral dysplasia. If this stability is not restored either through nerve recovery or reconstructions, it is one of the first priorities when considering various tendon transfers to reconstruct the shoulder girdle. Fortunately, many upper trunk injuries have multiple available options to stabilize the shoulder.

The initial technique of the upper trapezius transfer first described by Hoffa (1891), Lewis (1910), and Lange (1911), with fascia lata prolongation from the tendon to the greater tuberosity, was associated with adhesions and poor outcomes [11, 17]. However, a modification by Bateman and later Saha [12] (whose name now is denoted with the surgery) in the 1960s to include the acromion insertion of the upper trapezius has shown promising results at restoring shoulder stability [8–11, 17, 18]. This transfer is performed via a mid-lateral incision, detaching the trapezius' lateral insertion on the acromion using an oscillating saw. The atrophied deltoid is then split, and the acromial insertion of the upper trapezius is transferred to the proximal humerus. The bony insertion is anchored to the proximal

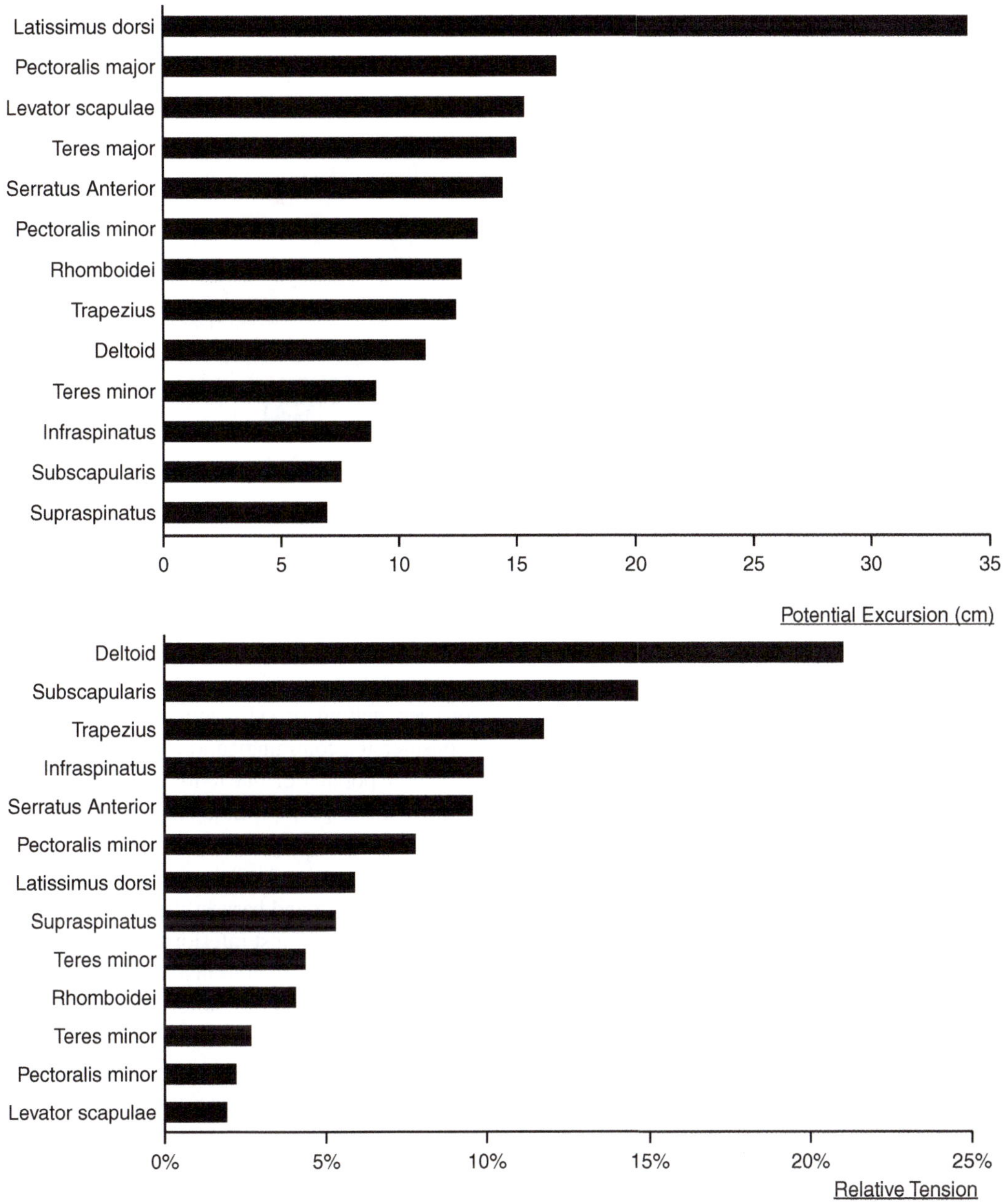

Fig. 16.1 Graphs representing the potential excursions and relative tensions of the various shoulder musculature. (Borrowed from: Herzberg et al. [15]. Copyright Elsevier 1999.)

humerus 2–5 cm distal to the lateral edge of the greater tuberosity with the shoulder in >65–75° of abduction, fixed with either screws alone or a plate and screws. The deltoid is then repaired either in placed or advanced proximally in maximal tension [17] (Fig. 16.2). Most studies show >80% reduction of glenohumeral subluxation with subtle improvements in joint function [8–11, 17, 18]. For example, Aziz et al. demonstrated a mean 40° in final abduction and elevation, with a reduction of shoulder subluxation in all patients that underwent the transfer [8]. Another example is seen in the series by Ruhmann et al., where patients with upper trunk injuries gained between

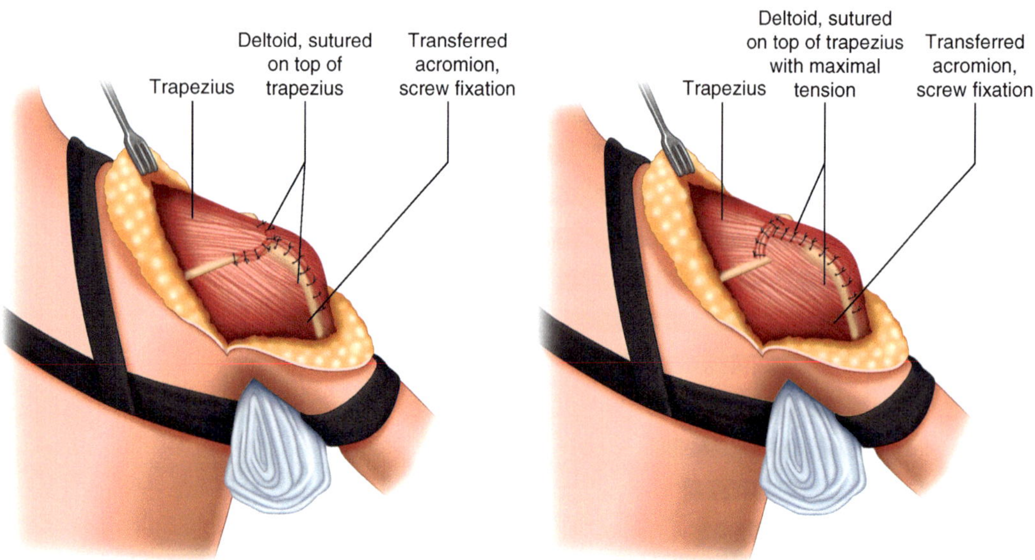

Fig. 16.2 Two variations of the upper trapezius transfer technique as described by Saha in 1967. (Borrowed from: Ruhmann et al. [17]. Original Article: Saha [12])

40° and 50° of flexion and abduction, while those with a complete injury gained between 20° and 30° of flexion and abduction [17].

Upper Trunk: External Rotation +/− Abduction

Although it was traditionally thought that shoulder abduction is the most critical function [9, 17–19], many patients with recovery of elbow flexion would argue that shoulder external rotation is actually the most critical function [2, 20]. In these patients, many of the shoulder's accessory internal rotators at least partially recover, including the latissimus dorsi, teres major, pectoralis major, and subscapularis. Therefore, the patient is left with an arm that is internally rotated against their abdomen, without the ability to position their hand in space and reach their mouth or top of their heads.

The traditional transfer to restore shoulder external rotation is the latissimus dorsi transfer to either the teres minor or infraspinatus insertions on the greater tuberosity. This has been reported extensively in patients with massive, irreparable rotator cuff injuries involving the supraspinatus and infraspinatus, with predictable restoration in shoulder abduction and external rotation [21–24]. However, deltoid or subscapularis insufficiency is considered a contraindication to this transfer in this patient population due to its role as a humeral head depressor [21, 24, 25]. The transfer is performed through either an anterior or posterior incision. Anteriorly, the deltopectoral interval is utilized to expose and harvest the latissimus tendon off its insertion just inferior to the subscapularis tendon. It is then transferred posteriorly around the humerus to the teres minor insertion [26]. Alternatively, a posterior incision along the posterior axillary fold is used to harvest the latissimus dorsi incision off its insertion, and then it is anchored into place either via an open deltoid split or arthroscopic approach onto the greater tuberosity [23] (Fig. 16.3). In patients with brachial plexus injuries, it has been demonstrated to lead to improvements in clinical external rotation and better positioning of the arm in space in the pediatric population [20, 27]. However, its use in the adult population has not been examined, likely because many adult brachial plexus injuries are associated with weak or paralyzed latissimus dorsi, deltoid, or subscapularis muscles.

Originally described by Elhassan et al. [28] in 2009, the transfer of the lower trapezius has been used successfully to restore shoulder external

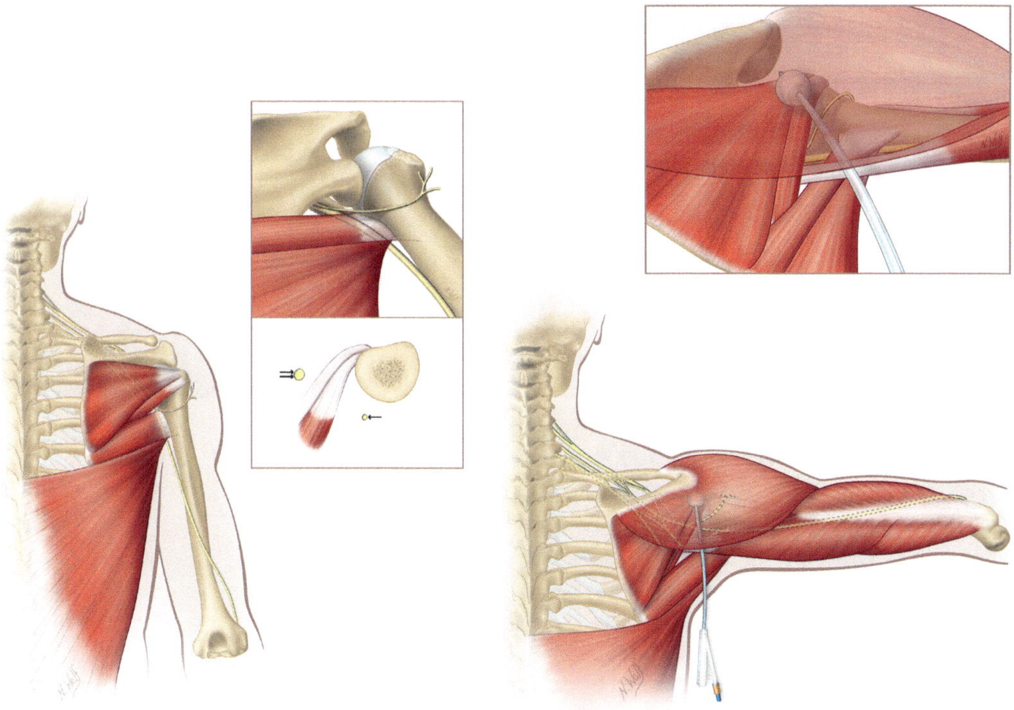

Fig. 16.3 Latissimus dorsi transfer. (The figure adapted from a technique article by Wagner et al. demonstrates the posterior and insertional anatomy of the latissimus dorsi, and the transfer interval posteriorly around the proximal humerus. Borrowed from: Wagner et al. [23])

rotation in patients with brachial plexus injuries [2, 28–30]. This is partly due to its "in-phase" contraction with the native shoulder external rotators and abductors [31], a similar excursion when compared to the infraspinatus [15], and "in-line" pull the simulates the infraspinatus line of pull. These potentially overcome some of the limitations of the latissimus dorsi transfer, including the humeral head depression and anterior translation in the setting of subscapularis insufficiency, as well as lack of synchronous contraction [32]. In patients with massive irreparable posterosuperior rotator cuff tears, this transfer has been shown to have very good results when performed via the open technique [33]. Recently this has been modified to the arthroscopic-assisted technique [23, 34]. This technique is performed by harvesting the lower trapezius off the medial scapular spine. The tendon is then either directly transferred to the infraspinatus tendon or is prolonged with an Achilles tendon allograft and anchored to the anterior aspect of the greater tuberosity (Fig. 16.4). The exposure of the greater tuberosity can either be done via an open deltoid split or trans-acromial approach, or via an arthroscopic-assisted approach. Finally, the contralateral lower trapezius can be utilized in the setting of a non-functional ipsilateral lower trapezius due to a prior spinal accessory nerve transfer [35, 36] (Fig. 16.5).

Posterior Cord: Axillary Nerve

In the setting of deltoid paralysis, patients are often quite limited in their shoulder flexion, abduction, and elevation. As the primary driver of shoulder motion, these patients lack much of their active shoulder motion. It is particularly disabling in the setting of a brachial plexus injury when other muscles around the shoulder are not optimally functioning. The treatment options for

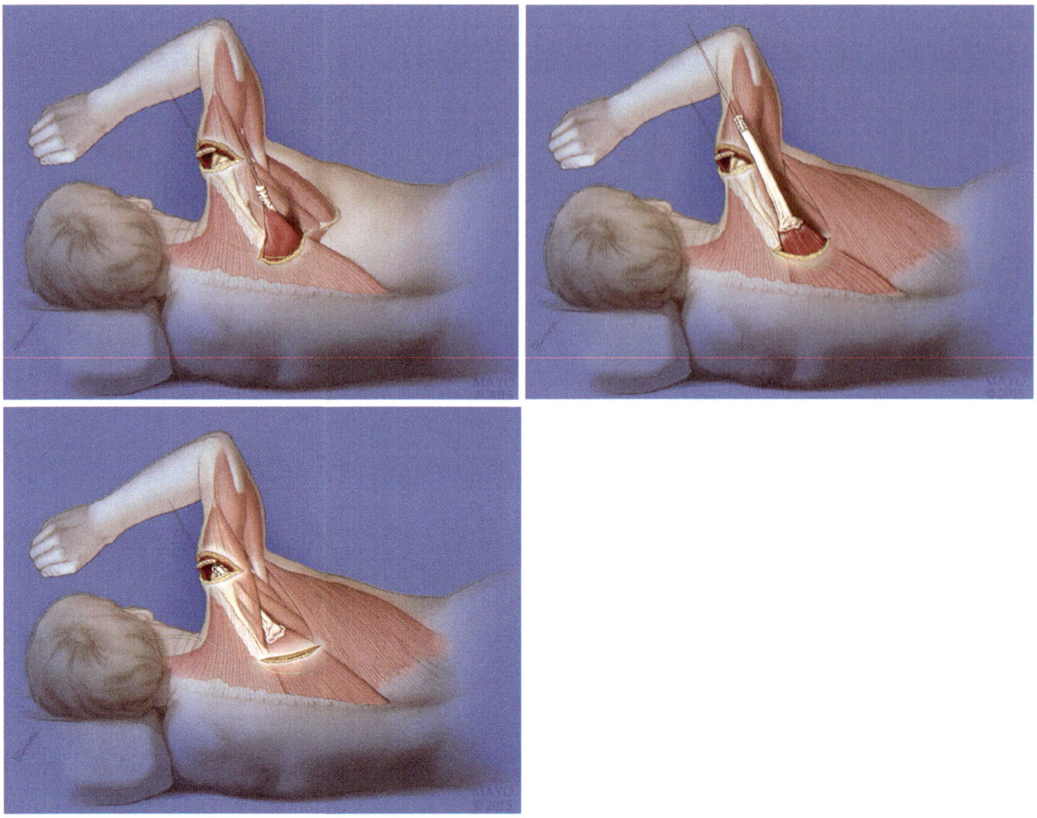

Fig. 16.4 Open lower trapezius transfer. The lower trapezius is harvested from the medial scapular spine, then transferred to the anterior aspect of the greater tuberosity. (Borrowed from: Elhassan et al. [33])

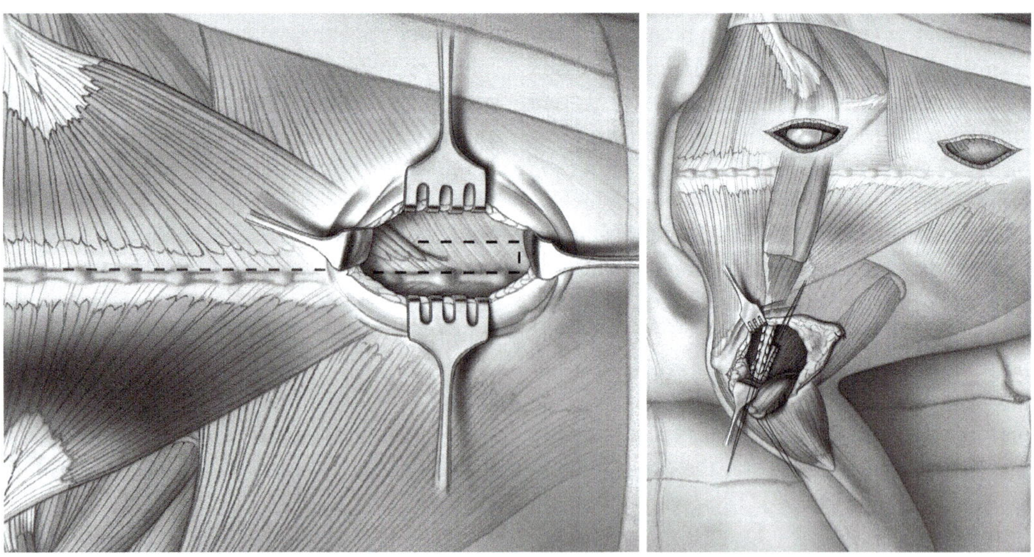

Fig. 16.5 Contralateral lower trapezius transfer. In the setting of a prior spinal accessory nerve transfer, the contralateral lower trapezius can be harvested (prolonged with lumbar fascia) and transferred to the greater tuberosity. (Borrowed from: Elhassan et al. [35])

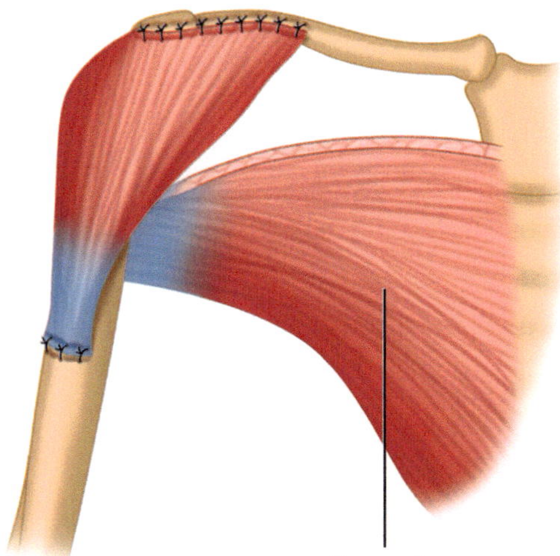

Fig. 16.6 Bipolar pedicled latissimus transfer. The latissimus dorsi is transferred to the anterior aspect of the shoulder, deep to the pectoralis major, and rotated 180° and inverted before securing to the anterior acromion and humeral shaft. (Borrowed from: Ferrier et al. [46])

deltoid paralysis involve nerve transfers [37–39], tendon transfers [2, 40, 41], or glenohumeral arthrodesis [42–44]. Most of the successful reported reconstructions have been in the setting of isolated deltoid paralysis, with a functional rotator cuff and other shoulder musculature. The two main tendon transfer options involve the latissimus dorsi or the pectoralis major.

The latissimus dorsi muscle was one of the original descriptions to reconstruct the anterior and middle deltoid in the setting of deltoid paralysis [45–47]. The bipolar pedicled latissimus dorsi transfer involves detaching the latissimus dorsi muscular origin and tendon insertion and isolating the neurovascular pedicle. The muscle is then transferred to the anterior aspect of the shoulder, deep to the pectoralis major, and rotated 180° and inverted before securing to the anterior acromion and humeral shaft (Fig. 16.6). This technique has been associated with improvements in shoulder function if performed in the setting of isolated deltoid paralysis [45–47]. For example, Itoh et al. demonstrated improvements in active shoulder flexion to at least 90° in 60%, with most regaining shoulder flexion strength of either M3 or M4.

The pectoralis major tendon transfer for isolated deltoid paralysis was first reported by Hou and Tai [40] in 1991 with promising results, which were later reinforced in 2009 by Lin et al. [41]. This reconstruction is based on the three parts of the pectoralis major muscle, the clavicular (origin on the clavicle), sternocostal (origin on the first to sixth sternocostal regions), and abdominal (origin on the lower sternocostal and rectus abdominis fascia). These converge to insert on the greater tuberosity of the humerus, supplied by different branches of the thoracoacromial artery and innervated by the lateral pectoral nerve (upper part) or the medial pectoral nerve (lower part). These separate blood supplies and innervation make this pedicled muscle transfer feasible. Pedicled transfer of the upper part of the pectoralis muscle involves harvesting the clavicular and upper sternal parts on their pedicle, then turned over 180° with the deep surface now superficial. The muscular origins are then attached in a transosseous fashion to the lateral clavicle and acromion, while the tendinous portion is anchored to a bony groove at or distal to the deltoid tuberosity [48] (Fig. 16.7). This can be done alone in the setting of isolated deltoid insufficiency, or can be combined with a reverse shoulder arthroplasty in the setting of an upper trunk brachial plexus injury or glenohumeral arthritis [48].

Hou and Tai [40] reported on the outcomes of this transfer either alone (4 patients) with improvements in abduction to 40° or combined with the upper trapezius transfer (3 patients) with improvements in abduction to 70°–90° and forward flexion was 60°–150°. Lin et al. [41] demonstrated a mean 74° abduction and 75° forward flexion postoperatively. Finally, Elhassan et al. reported on the largest series of patients with deltoid paralysis (n = 31) combined with arthritis, performing a pedicled pectoralis transfer with a reverse shoulder arthroplasty [48]. In this series, the mean shoulder flexion of 83° and external rotation of 15°, with reasonable postoperative SSV and DASH scores. This series demonstrates how the pedicled pectoralis functions in a similar fashion to the anterior deltoid; this tendon trans-

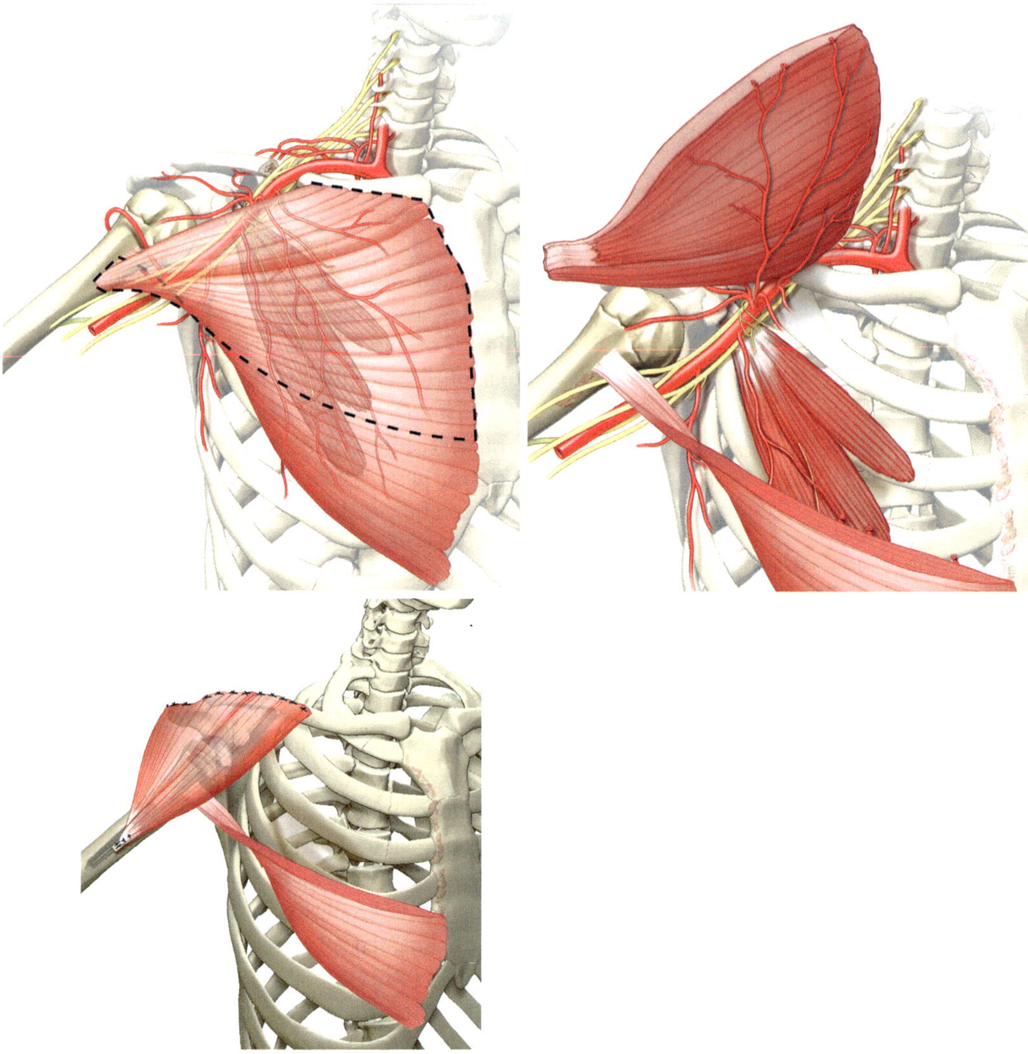

Fig. 16.7 Pedicled pectoralis transfer. The clavicular and upper sternal portion of the pectoralis major muscle is harvested and inverted, and its origin is anchored to the lateral clavicle and acromion while its insertion is anchored to the humeral shaft. (Borrowed from: Elhassan et al. [48])

fer provides similar biomechanical advantages when using the reverse prosthesis.

Long Thoracic Nerve

The serratus anterior represents one of the main stabilizers of the scapula and coordinators of scapulothoracic motion and subsequent scapulohumeral rhythm during shoulder elevation [49–53]. The scapular external rotation plays a key role in shoulder abduction and forward elevation. Therefore, serratus anterior paralysis leads to destabilization of the scapula and marked limitations of the shoulder function. In addition to limited motion, many patients experience fatigue, subjective instability, and pain, in part from the loss of the subacromial space secondary to the resultant limitations in scapular external rotation and humeral abduction [49–55]. In patients with penetrating injury, direct nerve repair or nerve transfer performed before the irreversible loss of the neuromuscular endplate units can lead to good recovery [56–58]. However, if it fails or the muscle does not recover, the patients have limited options. Traditionally, these patients were treated with scapulothoracic fusions or fascial slings. Fusions significantly limit patients' motion and are associated with a high rate of nonunion and pulmonary complications, while slings stretch and loosen with time [49, 59–61]. Therefore, we prefer to perform the pectoralis major tendon transfer.

Initially described by Tubby in 1904 and modified in the 1940s and 1950s, the pectoralis major transfer involves transfer of the sternal or clavicular heads to the inferior angle of the scapula [62–64]. This dynamic stabilization of the scapula restores its motion along the plane of the thorax, improving the patient's pain and shoulder function. Although initially prolonged with a tendon allograft, given the mixed results of these studies [49–55, 65–69], it is now preferred to perform a direct transfer without allograft prolongation [70]. Many recent studies have shown very predictable results with this direct transfer [51, 52, 54, 70], particularly when including its bony insertion [52, 71]. The transfer is performed by harvesting the pectoralis major, separating the clavicular and sternal heads from each other, and then transferring the sternal head to the inferior angle of the scapular. The bony insertion of the sternal head is anchored into the inferior angle of the scapula via multiple transosseous sutures, while the clavicular head is fixed back into the humerus (Fig. 16.8).

Spinal Accessory Nerve

Trapezius paralysis from spinal accessory nerve injury may result in significant dysfunction of the shoulder as a result of the loss of the support of the scapula on the chest wall, with drooping and loss of scapula external rotation [72–74]. This results in shoulder girdle instability from disruption of the dynamic of the scapulohumeral rhythm and resultant shoulder dysfunction [72–76]. Although most spinal accessory nerve injuries recover, those who do not are left with tendon transfers as their main option [72–74, 77–85]. Originally described by Eden in 1924, verified by Lange in the 1950s and modified by Bigliani [72], the Eden-Lange transfer entails transfer of the levator scapulae to the spine of the scapula and rhomboid minor and major to the mid body of the scapula [72–74, 76, 81]. However, this transfer was associated with variable outcomes [72–75, 81, 83, 86, 87], given it did not replicate the line of pull of the trapezius and did not produce a scapular external rotation force.

A modification of this technique, known as the triple tendon transfer or "T3," moved the levator scapulae to the lateral spine of the scapula, the rhomboid minor next to it on the scapular spine, and then the rhomboid major on the medial scapular spine [88, 89]. Thus, this technique almost perfectly recreates the upper and middle trapezius anatomy, producing a better scapular external rotation force and normal biomechanics of

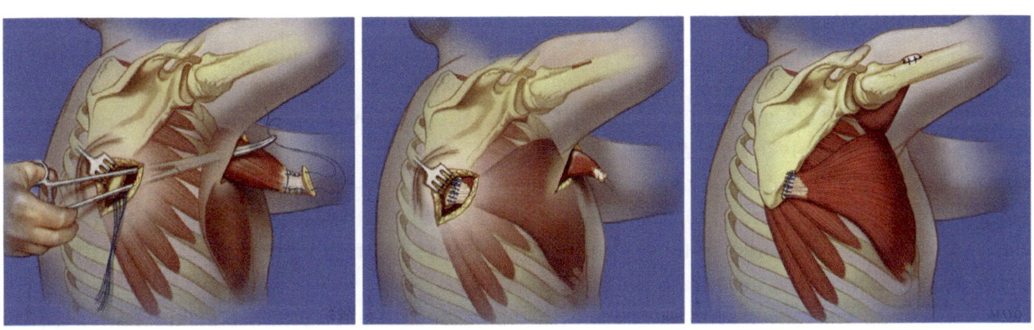

Fig. 16.8 Pectoralis major transfer. The sternal head of the pectoralis major is transferred to the inferior angle of the scapula, while the clavicular head is secured back into the humeral insertion. (Borrowed from: Elhassan and Wagner [71])

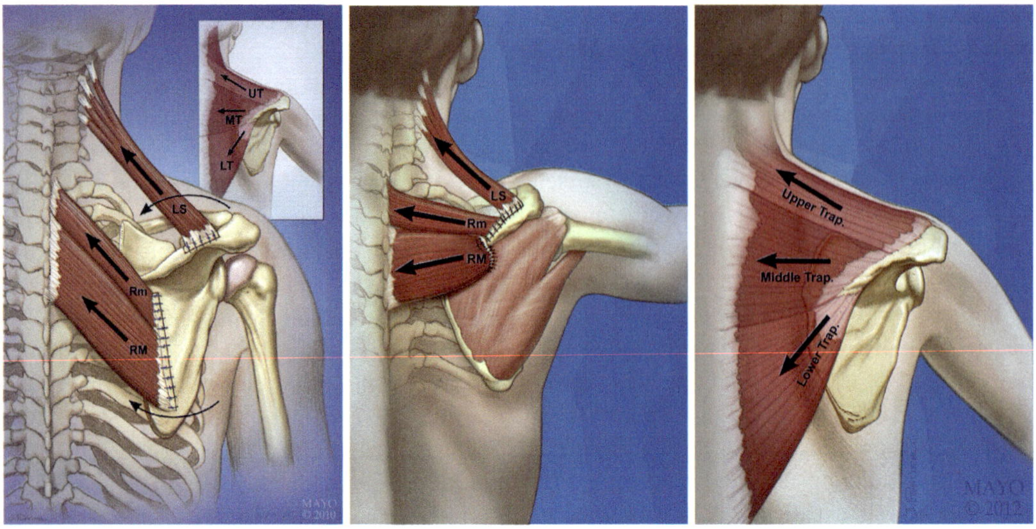

Fig. 16.9 Triple transfer. The Eden-Lange transfer (left) is compared to the modified technique, the T3 triple transfer (middle), with the normal trapezius as a reference on the right. (Borrowed from: Elhassan and Wagner [89])

the scapula [88]. In a clinical series of 22 patients at 35 months follow-up, the T3 transfer improved patients' abduction to 118° and forward flexion to 150°, with improvements in all clinical outcome measures [89]. The technique is performed via exposing and harvesting the rhomboid major, rhomboid minor, and levator scapulae along with the bony insertions. The levator scapulae is then transferred to the lateral scapular spine, while the rhomboid minor next to it and the rhomboid major on the medial scapular spine (Fig. 16.9).

Elbow: Upper Radial Nerve and Musculocutaneous Nerve

In the setting of elbow paralysis without a functional recovery, patients are often quite limited in many activities of daily living. Although nerve transfers and grafts are often quite predictable at reconstructing elbow function [90–92], in the setting of chronic nerve injuries or those that fail a nerve reconstruction, the use of a free functioning muscle transfer of the gracilis has been demonstrated to be quite effective [93–97]. See the chapter of free functioning muscle transfers for more details on this technique.

If the free functioning muscle transfer fails or is not an option, patients are left with very limited options. The bipolar latissimus dorsi transfer, performed in a similar fashion to the reconstruction of the anterior deltoid, represents a reasonable option for patients with preserved latissimus dorsi muscle function. Alternatively, a pedicle lower trapezius transfer can be used for elbow flexion or extension, similar to the contralateral lower trapezius transfer for shoulder external rotation [35]. Additionally, the triceps muscle can be transferred to the biceps in the setting of preserved elbow extension but no elbow flexion. Finally, many trick motions of the elbow can be utilized in patients with brachial plexus injuries, including the Steindler flexorplasty where the elbow flexor origins are moved proximally to facilitate elbow flexion [95, 98–101].

Tendon Transfers After Brachial Plexus Injury: Forearm and Hand

For treatment of brachial plexus palsy, tendon transfer in the hand and forearm has not been studied in the literature to the extent of transfers for treatment of shoulder and elbow pathology.

Tendon transfer following incomplete brachial plexus palsy is difficult and poorly described as a result of the heterogeneous characteristics of these lesions. Furthermore, loss of sensibility and proprioception is often more severe than that of single distal nerve palsies making reconstruction more complicated. Affected extremities often present with deficits that span typical distributions resulting in weakness in those muscle groups which may otherwise be suitable for transfer. Furthermore, extremities affected by brachial plexus palsy in which the hand and forearm are affected often have such profound involvement that there is a lack of noncritical but functional muscles available for transfer. For these reasons, free functional muscle is often chosen for reconstruction and discussed further in Chap. 15. Despite these challenges, tendon transfers in the hand and forearm can offer excellent results for secondary reconstruction when donor muscle-tendon units are available. For this purpose in particular, tendon transfers should be conceptualized as a tool to restore a hand function rather than replace a nonfunctional muscle.

As a result of the mixed deficits present, classic discussion of tendon transfers' myotomal distributions is not as applicable in the setting of the brachial plexus, and these are best viewed as individual motor deficits. These transfers must be individualized based on injury patterns and available donors, and the staging and timing of multiple procedures must be thought out such that only tendon transfer procedures which can be rehabilitated concomitantly are performed together.

Radial Nerve

Wrist Extension

PT to ECRB

The pronator teres to extensor carpi radialis brevis is the most common transfer for restoration of wrist extension. It can be utilized in as an internal splint and transferred in an end to side if recovery expected [102]. End to end transfer is ideal if recovery is not expected as has more direct line of pull.

Finger Extension

Finger extension can be restored by tenodesis or transferring the FCU, FCR, or an FDS tendon. FCU is thought to perform a more critical function than FCR as it allows for flexion and ulnar deviation, a critical component of the dart thrower's motion. If tendon transfer is performed, tenorrhaphy should occur proximal to the flexor retinaculum to prevent bowstringing [103].

Tenodesis of the finger extensor tendons can be performed either to the radius with transosseous sutures or sutured end to side to the FDS tendons through the interosseous membrane [104]. The tenodesis should be tensioned such that the metacarpophalangeal joints are in slight extension with the wrist in neutral position.

Thumb Extension

Many different transfer options are available to recreate thumb extension. Palmaris longus and ring finger FDS are the two most common transfers. PL as a transfer reroutes the line of pull volarly allowing for thumb abduction with extension [102]. FDS to the ring can be split and transferred to EIP and EPL producing composite thumb and index finger extension.

Median Nerve

Wrist Flexion

In incomplete brachial plexus injuries, complete loss of wrist flexion is fortunately rare. In injuries severe enough to completely impair wrist flexion, the chances of functional hand recovery are unfortunately small, and any functional donor units are likely going to be best utilized for other functions, as such wrist fusion is often considered rather than tendon transfer in these settings.

Thumb Flexion

Thumb IP flexion deficits often occur, and degree of hyperextensibility of the thumb IP joint and resting posture often dictate associated degree of disability. Thumb IP fusion in slight flexion can be considered, as well as tendon transfer. Tendon transfer motors can include BR, ECRL, and ECU, but unfortunately none of these transfers

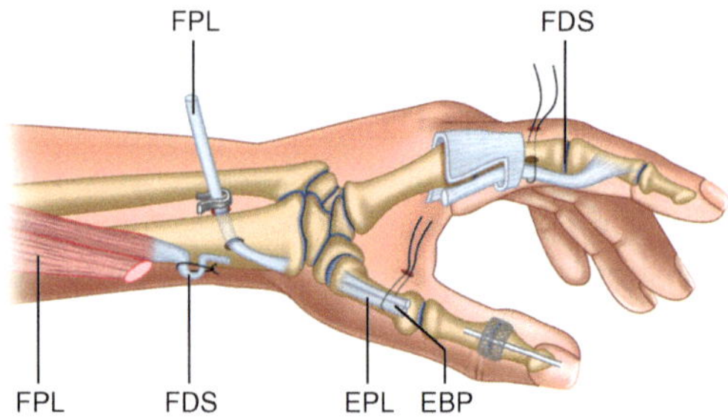

Fig. 16.10 Several modifications of the key grip procedure have helped to eliminate sources of prior patient satisfaction. The thumb IP joint is fused, and with a flexible MP joint, the EPL and EPB tenodesis is performed just proximal to the MP joint. Furthermore, FDS can be tenodesed to the proximal phalanx to help with thumb flexion if needed. (Borrowed from Hentz et al. [107])

offer an excursion that adequately recapitulates that of the native FPL. Fifteen patients with tetraplegia who had undergone BR to FPL transfer were described by Waters et al. [105] 15 of 16 thumbs demonstrated functional improvement, and 80% were able to perform at least 4 more ADLs than prior to surgery [105].

The Moberg procedure has been described for tetraplegia with only brachioradialis intact (Fig. 16.10). In this procedure, BR is transferred to ECRB, and the FPL is tenodesed to the ulnar aspect of the distal radius [106]. The IP joint of the thumb is stabilized to allow all motion to occur through the MP joint of the thumb allowing wrist extension to recapitulate lateral key pinch [107].

Finger Flexion

Tendon transfers for restoration of finger flexion depend on the degree of weakness. If possible, independent index finger function would be ideal. With incomplete loss of finger flexion, side-to-side transfer to tendons with intact FDP function can be considered. Alternatively, transfer of BR or ECRL to FDP of the index finger may be attempted (most commonly utilizing BR for FPL and ECRL for FDP to the index).

Bertelli and Ghizoni described transfer of the brachialis to finger flexors in six patients typically utilizing local tendon autograft. The improvement in finger flexion was moderate; those with complete preoperative absence of finger flexion obtained finger flexion to 1–2 cm from the palm [108]. In a separate study, grade 3 or better strength was obtained in 11 of 18 patients and grade 4 or better in 8 of 18 patients. In this study only about 56% of patients were satisfied postoperatively demonstrating the limitations inherent in this procedure and the utilizing of free functional muscle in many of these patients [109].

Thumb Opposition

Thumb opposition is a complex motion involving palmar abduction, pronation, and flexion of the thumb metacarpal and proximal phalanx. The ideal insertion for restoration of this function is the insertion of the abductor pollicis brevis with an ideal angle of pull from the trajectory of the pisiform to best recapitulate the pull of the abductor pollicis brevis.

Ring FDS

Most commonly the ring finger flexor digitorum superficialis opponensplasty utilizing the flexor carpi ulnaris tendon is utilized, but this transfer may not be available in brachial plexus palsy due to the concern for weak ring finger FDP function. It is typically transferred utilizing the FCU as a pulley.

PL

The palmaris longus has also been utilized for transfer to restore opposition, but similar to the ring finger FDS it is often not functional in lesions of the brachial plexus. It is transferred typically through a pulley utilizing the transverse carpal ligament as a pulley and requires harvesting a long slip of palmar fascia to gain the length necessary for transfer. Due to the line of pull, it mainly functions to restore palmar abduction of the thumb due to the line of pull [110].

EIP

The EIP opponensplasty can be utilized in high or low ulnar nerve palsy and is a good option in treatment of lesions of the brachial plexus as it may be available as a donor. The EIP is sectioned just prior to its expansion into the extensor hood and transferred ulnarly utilizing the ulna as a pulley. It is then routed across the palm and inserted into the APB [111]. Anderson noted good to excellent results following this transfer in 87.5% of 40 patients managed with this technique [112].

Huber

The Huber transfer utilizes the abductor digiti minimi and is mostly employed in cases of congenital absence or when EIP and FDS are not available. The ADM is released from its insertion and turned 180° to insert on the APB insertion. This transfer provides improved bulk improving the cosmetic result as compared to other transfers but palmar abduction not improved as significantly as pronation and flexion with this transfer.

Ulnar Nerve

Intrinsic Muscle Function

Bouvier's test in which the MP joints are passively flexed and the patient is asked to extend at the IP joints allows for determination of the requirement for dynamic vs static tendon transfer options to correct clawing. Multiple procedures have been described for treatment of this pathology. Volar metacarpophalangeal joint capsulodesis has been described although there is concern that results following this procedure will decrease with time as the volar plate laxity recurs. Brown reported on 44 cases with less than half having improvement in clawing and having 5 hands with near immediate failure of the ring and small fingers and 18 hands in which hyperextension recurred over the first year [113]. Static and dynamic tenodesis has been described as have a number of tendon transfer procedures. Tendon transfers can be powered by flexor digitorum superficialis or wrist motors.

Flexor digitorum superficialis transfers can include transfer into either only the ring and small finger or all four lesser digits. These tendon transfers can be inserted into the lateral band which may help to restore PIP extension, particularly in those with a suggestive Bouvier's test, but this also may cause PIP hyperextension particularly in lax individuals, due to the loss of the FDS and overpull of the lateral band. To combat PIP hyperextension, Burkhalter recommended insertion directly into the proximal phalanx [114]. Brandsma reported on 76 hands for which FDS was utilized for restoration of intrinsic function with variable insertions utilized with clawing fully corrected in 21% of patients and improvement in 57% [115]. Zancolli described a lasso whereby the FDS tendon is passed through the A1 pulley and sutured to itself to correct MP flexion which prevents PIP hyperextension [116].

Flexor digitorum superficialis tendon transfers unfortunately never improve and often weaken grip strength. Only tendon transfers for clawing which utilize wrist extensors and intercalary tendon graft are able to improve grip strength. Tendon transfers utilizing BR, ECRL, and ECRB have been described which utilize tendon graft split into two or four tails which are subsequently passed in the intermetacarpal spaces and may be inserted into the proximal phalanx, lateral band, or proximal pulley system. By preserving FDS, concern for PIP hyperextension is also diminished.

Key Pinch

ECRB and BR are good donors both requiring tendon graft to lengthen and are passed between the index and long finger metacarpals in the palm with second metacarpal used as a pulley and tendon inserted onto the adductor pollicis insertion. Hastings and Smith separately have described improvement of pinch strength up to 200% with this procedure [117, 118].

Ring or long finger FDS can also be utilized; the flexor digitorum superficialis is divided in the digit and passed deep to the flexor tendons and inserted on the adductor pollicis insertion, unfortunately not replicating the pull of adductor pollicis as well as ECRB or BR [119]. When FDS is utilized, it should be divided just proximal to Camper's chiasm between the A1 and A2 pulleys to prevent PIP hyperextension; furthermore the ring finger FDS should only be utilized in low ulnar nerve palsy as in high ulnar nerve palsy FDP to the ring finger may be the only functional finger flexor to that digit [111, 120].

Occasionally the thumb IP and MP flexors will overpower the thumb extensors resulting in

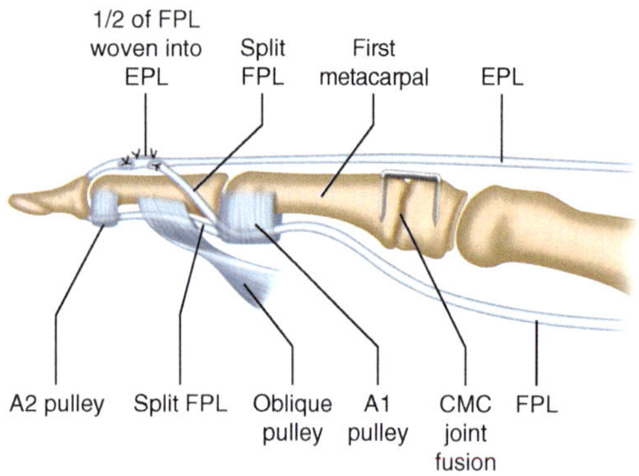

Fig. 16.11 The radial half of FPL tendon can be woven and sutured into the EPL with tensioning the appropriate pulp placement in key pinch position via a split FPL transfer. (Borrowed from Van Heest et al. [121])

a persistent Froment sign. Depending on patient demands, either fusion or split FPL transfer can be considered. Split FPL transfer involves a radial midaxial incision and detachment of the radial half of the FPL distally. It is extracted from between the oblique and annular pulley and passed radially deep to the neurovascular bundle and wrapped deep to and around the EPL tendon and sutured to itself in such tension as to make the tension equal between the two slips of FPL (Fig. 16.11). Van Heest described 12 cases in all of which the Froment sign was completely eliminated and IP joint flexion limited to 15–30° [121].

References

1. Doi K, Hattori Y, Ikeda K, Dhawan V. Significance of shoulder function in the reconstruction of prehension with double free-muscle transfer after complete paralysis of the brachial plexus. Plast Reconstr Surg. 2003;112(6):1596–603. Epub 2003/10/28.
2. Elhassan B, Bishop A, Shin A, Spinner R. Shoulder tendon transfer options for adult patients with brachial plexus injury. J Hand Surg Am. 2010;35(7):1211–9. Epub 2010/07/09.
3. Shin AY, Spinner RJ, Steinmann SP, Bishop AT. Adult traumatic brachial plexus injuries. J Am Acad Orthop Surg. 2005;13(6):382–96. Epub 2005/10/15.
4. Wagner ER, McLaughlin R, Sarfani S, Cofield RH, Sperling JW, Sanchez-Sotelo J, et al. Long-term outcomes of glenohumeral arthrodesis. J Bone Joint Surg Am. 2018;100(7):598–604. Epub 2018/04/04.
5. Cofield RH, Briggs BT. Glenohumeral arthrodesis. Operative and long-term functional results. J Bone Joint Surg Am. 1979;61(5):668–77. Epub 1979/07/01.
6. Hawkins RJ, Neer CS 2nd. A functional analysis of shoulder fusions. Clin Orthop Relat Res. 1987;223:65–76. Epub 1987/10/01.
7. Vastamaki M. Shoulder arthrodesis for paralysis and arthrosis. Acta Orthop Scand. 1987;58(5):549–53. Epub 1987/10/01.
8. Aziz W, Singer RM, Wolff TW. Transfer of the trapezius for flail shoulder after brachial plexus injury. J Bone Joint Surg. 1990;72(4):701–4. Epub 1990/07/01.
9. Goldner JL. Strengthening of the partially paralyzed shoulder girdle by multiple muscle-tendon transfers. Hand Clin. 1988;4(2):323–36. Epub 1988/05/01.
10. Karev A. Trapezius transfer for paralysis of the deltoid. J Hand Surg Br. 1986;11(1):81–3. Epub 1986/02/01.
11. Ruhmann O, Wirth CJ, Gosse F. Trapezius transfer in deltoid paralysis. Orthopade. 1997;26(7):634–42. Epub 1997/07/01.
12. Saha AK. Surgery of the paralysed and flail shoulder. Acta Orthop Scand. 1967;Suppl 97:5–0. Epub 1967/01/01.
13. Brand PW, Beach RB, Thompson DE. Relative tension and potential excursion of muscles in the forearm and hand. J Hand Surg Am. 1981;6(3):209–19. Epub 1981/05/01.
14. Comtet JJ, Herzberg G, Naasan IA. Biomechanical basis of transfers for shoulder paralysis. Hand Clin. 1989;5(1):1–14. Epub 1989/02/01.
15. Herzberg G, Urien JP, Dimnet J. Potential excursion and relative tension of muscles in the shoulder girdle: relevance to tendon transfers. J Shoulder Elb Surg. 1999;8(5):430–7. Epub 1999/10/30.
16. Gerber C, Blumenthal S, Curt A, Werner CM. Effect of selective experimental suprascapular nerve block on abduction and external rotation strength of the shoulder. J Shoulder Elb Surg. 2007;16(6):815–20. Epub 2007/10/13.
17. Ruhmann O, Schmolke S, Bohnsack M, Carls J, Wirth CJ. Trapezius transfer in brachial plexus palsy. Correlation of the outcome with muscle power and operative technique. J Bone Joint Surg. 2005;87(2):184–90. Epub 2005/03/02.
18. Monreal R, Paredes L, Diaz H, Leon P. Trapezius transfer to treat flail shoulder after brachial plexus palsy. J Brachial Plex Peripher Nerve Inj. 2007;2:2. Epub 2007/01/16.
19. Kotwal PP, Mittal R, Malhotra R. Trapezius transfer for deltoid paralysis. J Bone Joint Surg. 1998;80(1):114–6. Epub 1998/02/14.
20. Waters PM, Bae DS. The early effects of tendon transfers and open capsulorrhaphy on glenohumeral deformity in brachial plexus birth palsy. Surgical technique. J Bone Joint Surg Am. 2009;91 Suppl 2:213–22. Epub 2009/10/14.

21. Gerber C, Rahm SA, Catanzaro S, Farshad M, Moor BK. Latissimus dorsi tendon transfer for treatment of irreparable posterosuperior rotator cuff tears: long-term results at a minimum follow-up of ten years. J Bone Joint Surg Am. 2013;95(21):1920–6. Epub 2013/11/08.
22. Gerber C, Vinh TS, Hertel R, Hess CW. Latissimus dorsi transfer for the treatment of massive tears of the rotator cuff. A preliminary report. Clin Orthop Relat Res. 1988;232(232):51–61. Epub 1988/07/01.
23. Wagner ER, Woodmass JM, Welp KM, Chang MJ, Elhassan BT, Higgins LD, et al. Novel arthroscopic tendon transfers for posterosuperior rotator cuff tears: latissimus dorsi and lower trapezius transfers. JBJS Essent Surg Tech. 2018;8(2):e12. Epub 2018/09/21.
24. Warner JJ, Parsons IM. Latissimus dorsi tendon transfer: a comparative analysis of primary and salvage reconstruction of massive, irreparable rotator cuff tears. J Shoulder Elbow Surg/Am Shoulder Elbow Surg [et al]. 2001;10(6):514–21. Epub 2001/12/18.
25. Woodmass JM, Wagner ER, Chang MJ, Welp KM, Elhassan BT, Higgins LD, et al. Arthroscopic treatment of massive posterosuperior rotator cuff tears: a critical analysis review. JBJS Rev. 2018;6(9):e3. Epub 2018/09/12.
26. Boileau P, Chuinard C, Roussanne Y, Neyton L, Trojani C. Modified latissimus dorsi and teres major transfer through a single delto-pectoral approach for external rotation deficit of the shoulder: as an isolated procedure or with a reverse arthroplasty. J Shoulder Elb Surg. 2007;16(6):671–82. Epub 2007/12/07.
27. Waters PM. Update on management of pediatric brachial plexus palsy. J Pediatr Orthop B. 2005;14(4):233–44. Epub 2005/06/03.
28. Elhassan B, Bishop A, Shin A. Trapezius transfer to restore external rotation in a patient with a brachial plexus injury. A case report. J Bone Joint Surg Am. 2009;91(4):939–44. Epub 2009/04/03.
29. Elhassan B. Lower trapezius transfer for shoulder external rotation in patients with paralytic shoulder. J Hand Surg Am. 2014;39(3):556–62.
30. Elhassan B, Bishop AT, Hartzler RU, Shin AY, Spinner RJ. Tendon transfer options about the shoulder in patients with brachial plexus injury. J Bone Joint Surg Am. 2012;94(15):1391–8. Epub 2012/08/03.
31. Smith J, Padgett DJ, Dahm DL, Kaufman KR, Harrington SP, Morrow DA, et al. Electromyographic activity in the immobilized shoulder girdle musculature during contralateral upper limb movements. J Shoulder Elb Surg. 2004;13(6):583–8. Epub 2004/12/01.
32. Iannotti JP, Hennigan S, Herzog R, Kella S, Kelley M, Leggin B, et al. Latissimus dorsi tendon transfer for irreparable posterosuperior rotator cuff tears. Factors affecting outcome. J Bone Joint Surg Am. 2006;88(2):342–8. Epub 2006/02/03.
33. Elhassan BT, Wagner ER, Werthel JD. Outcome of lower trapezius transfer to reconstruct massive irreparable posterior-superior rotator cuff tear. J Shoulder Elbow Surg/Am Shoulder Elbow Surg [et al]. 2016;25(8):1346–53. Epub 2016/03/13.
34. Elhassan BT, Alentorn-Geli E, Assenmacher AT, Wagner ER. Arthroscopic-assisted lower trapezius tendon transfer for massive irreparable posterior-superior rotator cuff tears: surgical technique. Arthrosc Tech. 2016;5(5):e981–e8. Epub 2016/12/03.
35. Elhassan BT, Wagner ER, Spinner RJ, Bishop AT, Shin AY. Contralateral trapezius transfer to restore shoulder external rotation following adult brachial plexus injury. J Hand Surg Am. 2016;41(4):e45–51. Epub 2016/01/21.
36. Elhassan BT, Wagner ER, Bishop AT. Feasibility of contralateral trapezius transfer to restore shoulder external rotation: part I. J Shoulder Elb Surg. 2012;21(10):1363–9. Epub 2011/12/06.
37. Leechavengvongs S, Malungpaishorpe K, Uerpairojkit C, Ng CY, Witoonchart K. Nerve transfers to restore shoulder function. Hand Clin. 2016;32(2):153–64.
38. Leechavengvongs S, Witoonchart K, Uerpairojkit C, Thuvasethakul P. Nerve transfer to deltoid muscle using the nerve to the long head of the triceps, part II: a report of 7 cases. J Hand Surg Am. 2003;28(4):633–8.
39. Witoonchart K, Leechavengvongs S, Uerpairojkit C, Thuvasethakul P, Wongnopsuwan V. Nerve transfer to deltoid muscle using the nerve to the long head of the triceps, part I: an anatomic feasibility study. J Hand Surg Am. 2003;28(4):628–32.
40. Hou CL, Tai YH. Transfer of upper pectoralis major flap for functional reconstruction of deltoid muscle. Chin Med J. 1991;104(9):753–7.
41. Lin H, Hou C, Xu Z. Transfer of the superior portion of the pectoralis major flap for restoration of shoulder abduction. J Reconstr Microsurg. 2009;25(4):255–60. Epub 2008/12/09.
42. Atlan F, Durand S, Fox M, Levy P, Belkheyar Z, Oberlin C. Functional outcome of glenohumeral fusion in brachial plexus palsy: a report of 54 cases. J Hand Surg Am. 2012;37(4):683–8. Epub 2012/04/03.
43. Ruhmann O, Schmolke S, Bohnsack M, Flamme C, Wirth CJ. Shoulder arthrodesis: indications, technique, results, and complications. J Shoulder Elbow Surg/Am Shoulder Elbow Surg [et al]. 2005;14(1):38–50.
44. Safran O, Iannotti JP. Arthrodesis of the shoulder. J Am Acad Orthop Surg. 2006;14(3):145–53. Epub 2006/03/08.
45. De Smet L. The latissimus dorsi flap for reconstruction of a paralysed deltoid. Acta Chir Belg. 2004;104(3):328–9. Epub 2004/08/03.
46. Ferrier JA, Owens T, Singer DI. Functional reconstruction of the shoulder with a latissimus dorsi pedi-

cle flap and a hemiarthroplasty: a case report. J Hand Surg Am. 1995;20(2):284–7. Epub 1995/03/01.
47. Itoh Y, Sasaki T, Ishiguro T, Uchinishi K, Yabe Y, Fukuda H. Transfer of latissimus dorsi to replace a paralysed anterior deltoid. A new technique using an inverted pedicled graft. J Bone Joint Surg. 1987;69(4):647–51. Epub 1987/08/01.
48. Elhassan BT, Wagner ER, Werthel JD, Lehanneur M, Lee J. Outcome of reverse shoulder arthroplasty with pedicled pectoralis transfer in patients with deltoid paralysis. J Shoulder Elb Surg. 2018;27(1):96–103. Epub 2017/09/25.
49. Borges CS, Ruschel PH, Ferreira MT. Pectoralis major to scapula transfer for patients with serratus anterior palsy. Tech Hand Up Extrem Surg. 2011;15(3):135–7. Epub 2011/08/27.
50. Noerdlinger MA, Cole BJ, Stewart M, Post M. Results of pectoralis major transfer with fascia lata autograft augmentation for scapula winging. J Shoulder Elb Surg. 2002;11(4):345–50. Epub 2002/08/27.
51. Streit JJ, Lenarz CJ, Shishani Y, McCrum C, Wanner JP, Nowinski RJ, et al. Pectoralis major tendon transfer for the treatment of scapular winging due to long thoracic nerve palsy. J Shoulder Elb Surg. 2012;21(5):685–90. Epub 2011/07/05.
52. Tauber M, Moursy M, Koller H, Schwartz M, Resch H. Direct pectoralis major muscle transfer for dynamic stabilization of scapular winging. J Shoulder Elb Surg. 2008;17(1 Suppl):29S–34S. Epub 2008/02/08.
53. Warner JJ, Navarro RA. Serratus anterior dysfunction. Recognition and treatment. Clin Orthop Relat Res. 1998;349:139–48. Epub 1998/05/19.
54. Galano GJ, Bigliani LU, Ahmad CS, Levine WN. Surgical treatment of winged scapula. Clin Orthop Relat Res. 2008;466(3):652–60. Epub 2008/01/16.
55. Perlmutter GS, Leffert RD. Results of transfer of the pectoralis major tendon to treat paralysis of the serratus anterior muscle. J Bone Joint Surg Am. 1999;81(3):377–84. Epub 1999/04/13.
56. Novak CB, Mackinnon SE. Surgical treatment of a long thoracic nerve palsy. Ann Thorac Surg. 2002;73(5):1643–5. Epub 2002/05/23.
57. Schippert DW, Li Z. Supraclavicular long thoracic nerve decompression for traumatic scapular winging. J Surg Orthop Adv. 2013 Fall;22(3):219–23. Epub 2013/09/26.
58. Uerpairojkit C, Leechavengvongs S, Witoonchart K, Malungpaishorpe K, Raksakulkiat R. Nerve transfer to serratus anterior muscle using the thoracodorsal nerve for winged scapula in C5 and C6 brachial plexus root avulsions. J Hand Surg Am. 2009;34(1):74–8. Epub 2008/12/17.
59. Jakab E, Gledhill RB. Simplified technique for scapulocostal fusion in facioscapulohumeral dystrophy. J Pediatr Orthop. 1993;13(6):749–51. Epub 1993/11/01.
60. Howard R. Thoraco-scapular arthrodesis. J Bone Joint Surg. 1961;43-B:175.
61. Atasoy E, Majd M. Scapulothoracic stabilisation for winging of the scapula using strips of autogenous fascia lata. J Bone Joint Surg Br. 2000;82(6):813–7. Epub 2000/09/16.
62. Steindler A. The traumatic deformities and disabilities of the upper extremity. Springfield: Charles C Thomas; 1946. p. 162–3.
63. Tubby A. A case illustrating the operative treatment of paralysis of the serratus magnus by muscle grafting. Br Med J. 1904;2:1159–60.
64. Durman D. An operation for paralysis of the serratus anterior. J Bone Joint Surg. 1945;27:380–2.
65. Connor PM, Yamaguchi K, Manifold SG, Pollock RG, Flatow EL, Bigliani LU. Split pectoralis major transfer for serratus anterior palsy. Clin Orthop Relat Res. 1997;341:134–42. Epub 1997/08/01.
66. Gozna ER, Harris WR. Traumatic winging of the scapula. J Bone Joint Surg Am. 1979;61(8):1230–3. Epub 1979/12/01.
67. Iceton J, Harris WR. Treatment of winged scapula by pectoralis major transfer. J Bone Joint Surg Br. 1987;69(1):108–10. Epub 1987/01/01.
68. Steinmann SP, Wood MB. Pectoralis major transfer for serratus anterior paralysis. J Shoulder Elb Surg. 2003;12(6):555–60. Epub 2003/12/13.
69. Vastamaki M. Accessory nerve palsy and serratus palsy. Ann Chir Gynaecol. 1996;85(2):167–71. Epub 1996/01/01.
70. Povacz P, Resch H. Dynamic stabilization of winging scapula by direct split pectoralis major transfer: a technical note. J Shoulder Elb Surg. 2000;9(1):76–8. Epub 2000/03/16.
71. Elhassan BT, Wagner ER. Outcome of transfer of the sternal head of the pectoralis major with its bone insertion to the scapula to manage scapular winging. J Shoulder Elb Surg. 2015;24(5):733–40. Epub 2014/12/03.
72. Bigliani LU, Compito CA, Duralde XA, Wolfe IN. Transfer of the levator scapulae, rhomboid major, and rhomboid minor for paralysis of the trapezius. J Bone Joint Surg Am. 1996;78(10):1534–40. Epub 1996/10/01.
73. Bigliani LU, Perez-Sanz JR, Wolfe IN. Treatment of trapezius paralysis. J Bone Joint Surg Am. 1985;67(6):871–7. Epub 1985/07/01.
74. Kuhn JE, Plancher KD, Hawkins RJ. Scapular winging. J Am Acad Orthop Surg. 1995;3(6):319–25. Epub 1995/11/01.
75. Teboul F, Bizot P, Kakkar R, Sedel L. Surgical management of trapezius palsy. J Bone Joint Surg Am. 2005;87 Suppl 1(Pt 2):285–91. Epub 2005/09/06.
76. Lange M. [The operative treatment of irreparable trapezius paralysis]. Istanbul Tip Fak Mecmuasi. 1959;22:137–41. Epub 1959/01/01.
77. Anderson R, Flowers RS. Free grafts of the spinal accessory nerve during radical neck dissection. Am J Surg. 1969;118(5):796–9. Epub 1969/11/01.

78. Dunn AW. Trapezius paralysis after minor surgical procedures in the posterior cervical triangle. South Med J. 1974;67(3):312–5. Epub 1974/03/01.
79. Hoffman JC. Permanent paralysis of the accessory nerve after cannulation of the internal jugular vein. Anesthesiology. 1983;58(6):583–4. Epub 1983/06/01.
80. Olarte M, Adams D. Accessory nerve palsy. J Neurol Neurosurg Psychiatry. 1977;40(11):1113–6. Epub 1977/11/01.
81. Skedros JG, Kiser CJ. Modified Eden-Lange procedure for trapezius paralysis with ipsilateral rotator cuff-tear arthropathy: a case report. J Bone Joint Surg Am. 2011;93(22):e131(1–5). Epub 2012/01/21.
82. Tucker JA, Gee W, Nicholas GG, McDonald KM, Goodreau JJ. Accessory nerve injury during carotid endarterectomy. J Vasc Surg. 1987;5(3):440–4. Epub 1987/03/01.
83. Wiater JM, Bigliani LU. Spinal accessory nerve injury. Clin Orthop Relat Res. 1999;368:5–16. Epub 1999/12/29.
84. Woodhall B. Trapezius paralysis following minor surgical procedures in the posterior cervical triangle; results following cranial nerve suture. Ann Surg. 1952;136(3):375–80. Epub 1952/09/01.
85. Wright TA. Accessory spinal nerve injury. Clin Orthop Relat Res. 1975;108:15–8. Epub 1975/05/01.
86. Guettler JH, Basamania CJ. Muscle transfers involving the shoulder. J Surg Orthop Adv. 2006 Spring;15(1):27–37. Epub 2006/04/11.
87. Romero J, Gerber C. Levator scapulae and rhomboid transfer for paralysis of trapezius. The Eden-Lange procedure. J Bone Joint Surg Br. 2003;85(8):1141–5. Epub 2003/12/05.
88. Werthel JD, Wagner ER, Sperling JW, Elhassan B. Tendon transfer options for trapezius paralysis: a biomechanical study. J Am Acad Orthop Surg. 2019;27(5):e235–e41. Epub 2018/09/15.
89. Elhassan BT, Wagner ER. Outcome of triple-tendon transfer, an Eden-Lange variant, to reconstruct trapezius paralysis. J Shoulder Elb Surg. 2015;24(8):1307–13. Epub 2015/04/07.
90. Mackinnon SE, Novak CB, Myckatyn TM, Tung TH. Results of reinnervation of the biceps and brachialis muscles with a double fascicular transfer for elbow flexion. J Hand Surg Am. 2005;30(5):978–85.
91. Oberlin C, Beal D, Leechavengvongs S, Salon A, Dauge MC, Sarcy JJ. Nerve transfer to biceps muscle using a part of ulnar nerve for C5-C6 avulsion of the brachial plexus: anatomical study and report of four cases. J Hand Surg Am. 1994;19(2):232–7.
92. Oberlin C, Durand S, Belheyar Z, Shafi M, David E, Asfazadourian H. Nerve transfers in brachial plexus palsies. Chir Main. 2009;28(1):1–9.
93. Chim H, Kircher MF, Spinner RJ, Bishop AT, Shin AY. Free functioning gracilis transfer for traumatic brachial plexus injuries in children. J Hand Surg Am. 2014;39(10):1959–66.
94. Chuang DC. Functioning free muscle transplantation for brachial plexus injury. Clin Orthop Relat Res. 1995;314:104–11.
95. Giuffre JL, Kakar S, Bishop AT, Spinner RJ, Shin AY. Current concepts of the treatment of adult brachial plexus injuries. J Hand Surg Am. 2010;35(4):678–88; quiz 88. Epub 2010/04/01.
96. Shin AY, Spinner RJ. Clinically relevant surgical anatomy and exposures of the brachial plexus. Hand Clin. 2005;21(1):1–11.
97. Bishop AT. Functioning free-muscle transfer for brachial plexus injury. Hand Clin. 2005;21(1):91–102.
98. Suh N, Wagner ER, Spinner RJ, Bishop AT, Shin AY. Trick elbow motions in patients with brachial plexus injuries. J Hand Surg Am. 2014;39(11):2312–4. Epub 2014/06/09.
99. Al-Qattan MM. Elbow flexion reconstruction by Steindler flexorplasty in obstetric brachial plexus palsy. J Hand Surg Br. 2005;30(4):424–7. Epub 2005/06/07.
100. Brunelli GA, Vigasio A, Brunelli GR. Modified Steindler procedure for elbow flexion restoration. J Hand Surg Am. 1995;20(5):743–6. Epub 1995/09/01.
101. Goldfarb CA, Burke MS, Strecker WB, Manske PR. The Steindler flexorplasty for the arthrogrypotic elbow. J Hand Surg Am. 2004;29(3):462–9. Epub 2004/05/14.
102. Sammer DM, Chung KC. Tendon transfers: part I. Principles of transfer and transfers for radial nerve palsy. Plast Reconstr Surg. 2009;123(5):169e–77e.
103. Ratner JA, Peljovich A, Kozin SH. Update on tendon transfers for peripheral nerve injuries. J Hand Surg Am. 2010;35(8):1371–81.
104. Goubier J-N, Teboul F. Management of hand palsies in isolated C7 to T1 or C8, T1 root avulsions. Tech Hand Up Extrem Surg. 2008;12(3):156–60.
105. Waters R, Moore KR, Graboff SR, Paris K. Brachioradialis to flexor pollicis longus tendon transfer for active lateral pinch in the tetraplegic. J Hand Surg Am. 1985;10(3):385–91.
106. Bednar MS, Woodside JC. Management of upper extremities in tetraplegia: current concepts. J Am Acad Orthop Surg. 2018;26(16):e333–e41. Epub 2018/07/20.
107. Hentz VR, Brown M, Keoshian LA. Upper limb reconstruction in quadriplegia: functional assessment and proposed treatment modifications. J Hand Surg Am. 1983;8(2):119–31.
108. Bertelli JA, Ghizoni MF. Brachialis muscle transfer to reconstruct finger flexion or wrist extension in brachial plexus palsy. J Hand Surg Am. 2006;31(2):190–6.
109. DeGeorge BR Jr, Becker HA, Faryna JH, Spinner RJ, Bishop AT, Shin AY. Outcomes of muscle brachialis transfer to restore finger flexion in brachial plexus palsy. Plast Reconstr Surg. 2017;140(2):307e–17e. Epub 2017/07/27.

110. Braun RM. Palmaris longus tendon transfer for augmentation of the thenar musculature in low median palsy. J Hand Surg Am. 1978;3(5):488–91.
111. Sammer DM, Chung KC. Tendon transfers: part II. Transfers for ulnar nerve palsy and median nerve palsy. Plast Reconstr Surg. 2009;124(3):212e–21e.
112. Anderson GA, Lee V, Sundararaj GD. Extensor indicis proprius opponensplasty. J Hand Surg. 1991;16(3):334–8.
113. Brown PW. Zancolli capsulorrhaphy for ulnar claw hand. Appraisal of forty-four cases. J Bone Joint Surg Am. 1970;52(5):868–77. Epub 1970/07/01.
114. Burkhalter WE. Restoration of power grip in ulnar nerve paralysis. Orthop Clin North Am. 1974;5(2):289–303. Epub 1974/04/01.
115. Brandsma JW, Ottenhoff-De Jonge MW. Flexor digitorum superficialis tendon transfer for intrinsic replacement. Long-term results and the effect on donor fingers. J Hand Surg Br. 1992;17(6):625–8. Epub 1992/12/01.
116. Hastings H, McCollam SM. Flexor digitorum superficialis lasso tendon transfer in isolated ulnar nerve palsy: a functional evaluation. J Hand Surg Am. 1994;19(2):275–80.
117. Hastings H 2nd, Davidson S. Tendon transfers for ulnar nerve palsy. Evaluation of results and practical treatment considerations. Hand Clin. 1988;4(2):167–78. Epub 1988/05/01.
118. Smith RJ. Extensor carpi radialis brevis tendon transfer for thumb adduction—A study of power pinch. J Hand Surg Am. 1983;8(1):4–15.
119. Hamlin C, Littler JW. Restoration of power pinch. J Hand Surg Am. 1980;5(4):396–401. Epub 1980/07/01.
120. Lee DH, Rodriguez JA. Tendon transfers for restoring hand intrinsic muscle function: a biomechanical study. J Hand Surg Am. 1999;24(3):609–13.
121. Van Heest A, Hanson D, Lee J, Wentdorf F, House J. Split flexor pollicus longus tendon transfer for stabilization of the thumb interphalangeal joint: a cadaveric and clinical study. J Hand Surg Am. 1999;24(6):1303–10.

Glenohumeral Arthrodesis in Brachial Plexus Palsy

17

Idris S. Gharbaoui

Introduction

Fusion of any joint is often viewed by the orthopedic surgeon as a failure. This is particularly true when it applies to an articulation as complex and mobile as the shoulder. Glenohumeral arthrodesis, also known as shoulder fusion, has been recommended as a last resort procedure after failure of more accepted treatments such as nerve reconstruction, nerve transfers, or tendon transfers. Historically, indications for this procedure have included treatment of severe joint destruction resulting from infections and tuberculosis, neurologic deficits such as poliomyelitis, and different degenerative diseases. It has also occasionally been recommended for rheumatoid arthritis, irreparable injury of the rotator cuff, and severely comminuted fractures of the proximal aspect of the humerus. The development of shoulder arthroplasties has resulted in a significant reduction of the indications of glenohumeral arthrodesis, which are now mostly recommended for sequela of brachial plexus palsies [1], with secondary inefficiency of both deltoid and rotator cuff muscles. In these situations, a flail shoulder represents a considerable disability, often resulting in a painful inferior subluxation of the glenohumeral joint (Fig. 17.1) with inability to control the entire upper extremity and position the hand in space.

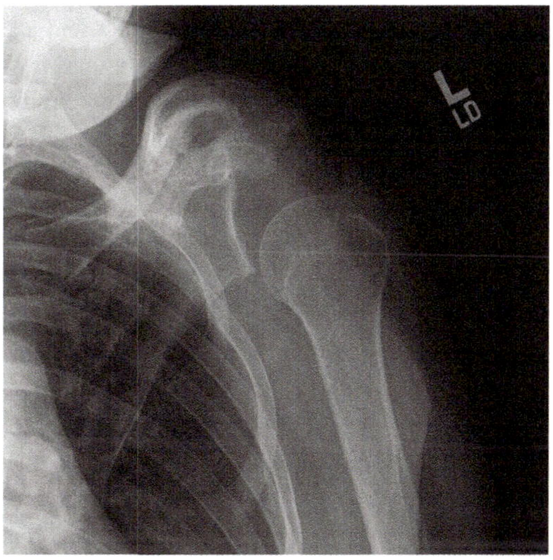

Fig. 17.1 Inferior subluxation of the glenohumeral joint

The best results of glenohumeral fusion are achieved with normal or near normal scapulothoracic muscles. The trapezius, levator scapulae, rhomboids, and serratus are all necessary to provide stable and strong scapular motion. In addition, the acromioclavicular and sternoclavicular joints will be stressed after fusion of the glenohumeral joint. The innervation of the trapezius and

Electronic Supplementary Material The online version of this chapter (https://doi.org/10.1007/978-3-030-69517-0_17) contains supplementary material, which is available to authorized users.

I. S. Gharbaoui (✉)
Texas Orthopedic Hospital, Houston, TX, USA

A. Y. Shin, N. Pulos (eds.), *Operative Brachial Plexus Surgery*,
https://doi.org/10.1007/978-3-030-69517-0_17

the levator scapulae is usually intact in brachial plexus palsy. Hence, when glenohumeral fusion is undertaken in this setting, it allows for both shoulder stability and a certain degree of motion through the scapulothoracic, as well as the acromioclavicular and sternoclavicular joints, particularly in abduction and rotation. The rhomboids are usually preserved, except in the situation of C5 avulsion. The serratus anterior however is more often weak. A functional serratus anterior allows a better forward flexion through scapular rotation. Ideally, glenohumeral fusions should allow patients to use the paralyzed upper extremity independently, as well as the ability to perform bimanual activities, reach their mouth, face, and head, their front pocket, perineum, and possibly back pocket. As at least half of the motion of the shoulder is eliminated, the position of the fusion must be extremely precise.

Stabilization of the glenohumeral joint has been historically recommended in selected patients to improve both shoulder pain and the function of the upper extremity. It has been typically recommended in patients with functional scapulothoracic muscles as well as with active elbow flexion and a functional and sensate hand. A high rate of complications has been associated with this procedure, as it creates a huge lever over the fusion site. Patients with severe brachial plexus injuries often have poor bone quality from severe osteoporosis and lack the normal muscular compressive forces that would help with the bone healing. The rate of reported complications in the literature is very high. In addition to the usual complications such as hematomas and infections, nonunions, fractures (usually at the distal end of the plate or rarely through the scapular neck), and skin breakdown over prominent hardware are common in these patients with severe muscle atrophy (Fig. 17.2). More recent studies have shown significant decreases in the number and severity of these complications with improvement of the surgical techniques and modern hardware.

The goal of this chapter is to incorporate a review of the literature with personal clinical experience and present the best surgical techniques, types of hardware, and position of the fusion and review surgical indications.

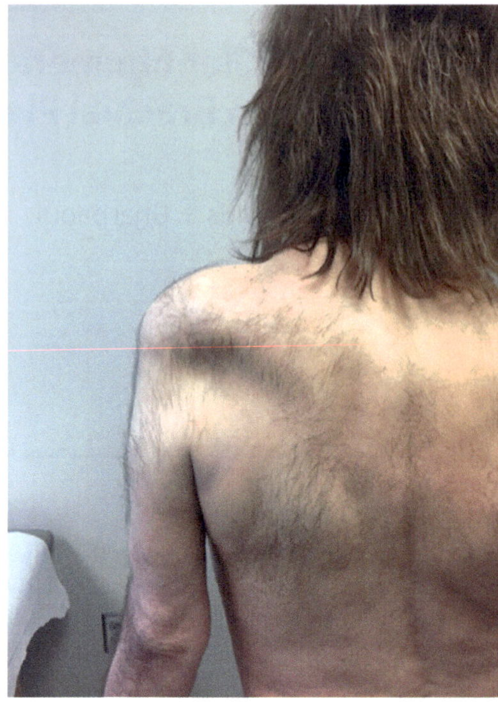

Fig. 17.2 Muscle atrophy, involving deltoid, supraspinatus, and infraspinatus

Operative Techniques

Patient position Glenohumeral fusions can be performed in the beach chair position (with wide exposure of the back of the shoulder), or more often, in the lateral decubitus position. The entire upper extremity and the chest, shoulder, and back are prepped and draped. The ideal position should allow complete exposure of the scapula, in order to control abduction, forward flexion, and rotation of the glenohumeral joint. Placement of temporary pins through the glenohumeral joint and mobilization of the extremity intraoperatively is highly advisable, to assess the amount of motion, the position of the hand, and the severity of the scapular winging. The lateral decubitus is preferred by most authors [2–11]. Others [12–15] prefer the beach chair position.

Surgical approach The surgical approach is usually very easy in these patients due to severe atrophy of the deltoid. The proximal part of the incision is usually performed along the spine of the scapula toward the lateral and anterior aspect of the acromion. Distally, three different approaches can be found in the literature: (1) Posterior approach [9], which can put at risk the axillary nerve and may result in some loss of sensation or dysesthesia in its distribution; (2) lateral approach [2–7, 10, 11, 14] through the deltoid; and (3) anterior approach [12, 13, 16] through the deltopectoral interval. A two-incision technique has also been described by Irlenbush [17], combining a deltopectoral approach with a second incision along the spine of the scapula. More recently, arthrodesis of the shoulder has been performed arthroscopically [15].

Intra, extra-articular fusion The contact surface between humerus and glenoid is very limited. The labrum has to be removed as well as the rotator cuff. Presence of one or multiple screws further diminishes this bony contact. For this reason, most contemporary authors (Table 17.1) recommend both an intra-articular (glenohumeral) and extra-articular (acromiohumeral) fusion. Some recommend bone grafting to increase the chances for healing (Table 17.1). Atlan [6] compared 2 series of patients, all with bone grafting: 26 of them had both intra- and extra-articular arthrodesis using massive tricortical bone graft, while 28 patients had a glenohumeral only fusion with cancellous bone graft. The rate of nonunion was 4% in the first group, versus 43% in the second group. In order to improve the bony contact between acromion and humeral head, some authors recommended an osteoclasis [9] of the acromion, osteotomy of the acromion distally [2], or near its junction with the scapular spine in addition to an osteotomy of the distal 2 cm of the clavicle [4], allowing the acromial arch to hinge downward for better apposition with the superior aspect of the humeral head.

Bone grafting Few authors have systematically used bone grafting (Table 17.1). In the previously mentioned article, Atlan [6] compared massive tricortical bone graft, placed in the glenohumeral and acromiohumeral spaces in 26 patients and reported 1 nonunion (4%), versus a 43% nonunion rate using cancellous bone graft only in the glenohumeral joint. He concluded that massive subacromial graft significantly reduced pseudarthrosis. Another difference between the two groups was the extent of the fusion, involving both glenohumeral and acromiohumeral spaces in the first group, versus glenohumeral joint only in the second group. The vast majority of authors (Table 17.1), however, have obtained a high rate of bone healing, without graft.

Bone fixation (Table 17.2) Methods of fixation have improved over time. In older articles, fixa-

Table 17.1 Type of arthrodesis (intra, extra-articular), bone grafting

Year	Cases	Author	Type of fusion	Bone grafting	Nonunions	Remarks
1988	11	Richards	IA + EA	No	0	
1991	13	Rouholamin	IA + EA	No	2	1 satisfactory fibrous union
1992	17	Pruitt	IA + EA	3	1	Pediatric population
1997	12	Emmelot	IA + EA	No	0	Paralyzed upper extremity
1998	18	El-Said	IA + EA	No	1	
1999	14	Ruhmann	IA + EA	No	1	
2004	27	Chammas	IA?	No	0	
2005	6	Wong	IA + EA	No	0	
2011	4	Lerch	IA + EA	No	0	
2011	11	Esenyel	IA + EA	Yes	No	
2012	26	Atlan	IA + EA	Yes	1	Massive tricortical graft
2012	28	Atlan	IA	Yes	12	Cancellous graft
2017	8	Lenoir	IA	No	0	Arthroscopic fusion + ex fix
2017	7	Thangarajah	IA + EA	5	1	Nonunion: lag screws only
2018	11	Irlenbush	IA + EA	Some	0	

IA (intra-articular) glenohumeral fusion, *EA* (extra-articular) acromiohumeral fusion

Table 17.2 Position of fusion and postoperative motion

			Position of fusion (degrees)			Results (degrees)			
Year	Author	Specificities	Abd	FF	IR	Abd	FF	IR	Findings/Recommendations
1988	Richards	*N* = 11, 1 total	30	30	30	65	75		All have mild winging
1991	Rouholamin	*N* = 13	30	20	20–30	56	50		
1992	Pruitt	*N* = 17, pediatric	50	25	20	63	64	40	Better in BP 74/75/55
1997	Gonzalez-Diaz	*N* = 13	30	30	45	65	75		
1997	Emmelot	*N* = 12, flail UE	30	20–30	20		80		
1999	Ruhmann	*N* = 14	20	30	40	59	51		More power/motion than trapezius transfer
2002	Rtaimate	*N* = 15	52	20	20	48	46	40	
2004	Chammas	*N* = 11 good hand *N* = 16 flail hand	24 31	21 27	14 28	59 63	61 62	42 45	
2011	Lerch	*N* = 4	20	30	40	60	40		
2011	Esenyel	*N* = 8	30	30	30	68	67		
2011	Sousa	*N* = 19	30	32	44				Abd > 35, FF > 30, IR < 45
2012	Atlan	22 upper, 32 total	30	30	30	59		48	
2017	Lenoir	*N* = 8	30	30	30	80	59		
2018	Belkheyar	*N* = 8 ad with OBPP	Allow HM, HP, 0 rot			67		−21	21 ext. rot
2018	Van Der Lingen	*N* = 12	31	20	22	48	60	32	IR < 40
2018	Irlenbush	*N* = 11	30	30	20	63	79	47	Abd = 25, FF = 20, IR = 30

Abd abduction, *FF* forward flexion, *Int rot* internal rotation, *Ext rot* external rotation, *HM* hand to mouth, *HP* hand to perineum, *0 rot* neutral rotation

tion has been performed using a smooth K-wire and Hagie pins [18], or a Rush pin augmented with a tension-band wiring from the acromion to the neck of the humerus [2]. Later, the need for compression through the arthrodesis was established, and multiple authors [3, 4, 19, 20] have recommended fixation using lag screws. All of these techniques required postoperative immobilization in a spica cast or a brace until complete healing of the fusion and were often associated with a high rate of nonunion. In addition, early physical therapy was not possible resulting in severe atrophy of the scapulothoracic muscles. More recently, stronger fixation methods have been advocated, using AO DCP (Arbeitsgemeinschaft für Osteosynthesefragen, Dynamic Compression Plate) plates [1, 6–10, 14, 16–18, 21] or pelvic reconstruction plates [11–13]. Both offer very strong fixation with no need for rigorous postoperative immobilization. The DCP plates are probably stronger than the pelvic reconstruction plates; however, they are very rigid and very hard to bend and even harder to twist and mold over this particular bony anatomy. Many patients experience painful prominent hardware, skin ulceration, and breakdown, necessitating removal of the hardware. In Rtaimate's [9] series, all 15 patients complained of painful and prominent hardware under the skin necessitating premature hardware removal. The reconstruction plates are narrow and less bulky. They are easier to bend, twist, mold, and apply directly against the bone, avoiding skin irritation. No failure of these plates has been reported in this review of the literature.

External fixators have also been recommended. Their main advantage is the possibility to correct the position of the fusion postoperatively, improving the final outcome. However, they have been associated with a high rate of nonunions. More recently, authors have recommended augmenting the external fixation with compressive lag screws. Both Emmelot [5] and Lenoir [15] used a combination of external fixation and lag screws, via open and arthroscopic techniques, respectively, with 100% bone healing.

Position of fusion In order to restore the best possible function, without painful excessive winging of the scapula, the position of fusion must be as precise as possible. Malposition represents the most critical complication of glenohumeral arthrodesis. There is no consensus in the literature, about the position of fusion of the glenohumeral joint. Large variations in multiple planes have been reported [22]: 10–80° abduction, 10–60° forward flexion, and from 60° of internal rotation to 45° of external rotation. The tendency, however, throughout the years has evolved, to favor less abduction and forward flexion and more internal rotation. The most frequently recommended position, within a 10° variation, is 30-30-30° of abduction, forward flexion, and internal rotation. The most important functional goals for the patient are the ability to reach the face, perineum, and pockets and achieve a position of the arm allowing for maximum strength for lifting, pushing, and pulling all while resting the shoulder in a comfortable position with the arm at the side of the body. Excessive abduction or forward flexion may force the scapula to rotate medially or posteriorly, resulting in winging when the shoulder is at rest. Excessive abduction does not improve the final range of motion but significantly increases postoperative pain (Table 17.2). Cofield and Briggs [23], in an earlier long-term review of 71 cases, did not correlate periscapular pain with fusions beyond 45° of abduction. They suggested that the final position of fusion in abduction and forward flexion has little effect on the results. Pruitt [18] reported unsatisfactory outcomes (pain, prominent scapular winging, and poor cosmetic appearance), in pediatric patients fused in 70° abduction. In one case the arthrodesis was revised, and the patient was re-fused in less than 45° abduction with a good final outcome. Table 17.2 summarizes the positions of fusion in our reviewed articles, as well as the final maximum motion in abduction, forward flexion, and internal rotation. Regarding internal rotation, Van Der Helm [22] analyzed loading of the shoulder girdle muscles after glenohumeral arthrodesis. He recommended, in order to achieve mobility area in the mid-sagittal plane, to fuse the shoulder at 60° of internal rotation with a little abduction and forward flexion. He also recommended external fixation, in order to be able to adjust fusion angles postoperatively. Sousa [11] suggested that exaggerated internal rotation >45° significantly correlates with inability of the hand to reach the mouth. Cofield and Briggs [23], as well as Hawkins and Neer [24, 25], found that the degree of internal rotation was the most important factor for functional success. Most recent articles recommend a position of fusion between 20° and 40° of internal rotation (Table 17.2).

Complications The main complications include nonunion, fractures at both ends of the plate, infections, hematomas, and most commonly malposition resulting in severe and painful scapular winging or poor function necessitating a revision. The rate of complications has significantly improved overtime, with better osteosynthesis techniques. Table 17.3 shows the rate of complications in our reviewed articles. Nonunions and infections have become less common with modern techniques. Reconstruction plates allow for a better apposition against the bone. Also, having a low profile, they are rarely responsible of prominent and painful hardware or skin breakdown in these patients with severe muscle atrophy. With the newer recommendations regarding the position of fusion, painful winging of the scapula has also been significantly reduced, and in some studies eliminated. Fractures are still common, particularly at the distal end of the plate. They can be treated conservatively, in a cast or a brace, or surgically in case of severe displacement. These fractures can be, in a sense, providential, as they may allow, when necessary, adjustments to the position of the upper extremity and improvement of the function.

Table 17.3 Complications

Year	Author	# cases	Nonunions	Fractures	Infections	Hardware	Malpositions
1988	Richards	11	0		0	0	0
1992	Pruitt	17	1			5	1
1998	El-Said	18	1	1	2	0	0
2002	Rtaimate	15	1	1		15	0
2004	Chammas	27	2	3	1	1	0
2011	Sousa	13	1	1			1
2011	Esenyel	8	0	1	1	0	0
2012	Atlan	54: 26 (IA + EA fusion)	1	4	2	1	0
		28 (IA fusion)	12				
2017	Thangarajah	7	1	0	0	0	0
2018	Belkheyar	8	0	0	0	0	0
2018	Ulrich	11	0	0	0	0	0

Results The quality of the results depends on multiple factors such as bone healing, complications, pain, and function. Satisfied patients are typically pain-free, with a good functional result and no or minimal painless winging. They should be able to maintain their arm against her body while at the same time being able to control their shoulder and position their hand in space. The happiest patients report a feeling of stability of the shoulder, improvement of the cosmetic appearance, and improvement with regard to dressing, personal hygiene, walking, running, and performing activities of daily living. The shoulder pain from the inferior subluxation is usually cured by the fusion. Neuropathic pain can also improve from reduced traction on the brachial plexus with less irritation on nerve endings. In recent studies, fusions in less abduction and forward flexion, with increased internal rotation, have helped achieve these goals. The results depend mostly on the final position of the fusion, but also on the strength of the elbow flexors, the functional quality of the forearm, wrist, and hand, and of course, the power and integrity of the scapulothoracic muscles. In the reviewed articles, most patients achieved 50 and 65° of abduction, 40–80° of forward flexion, and 32–47° of internal rotation (Table 17.2). It appears from these studies that a fusion in a high degree of abduction or forward flexion does not lead to a better range of motion postoperatively. It may however increase the risk of postoperative winging and pain. Patient satisfaction has been excellent in most series. The subjective assessment of satisfaction depends on the amount of any residual pain, the capability to maintain the arm against the body at rest, and the ability to reach the mouth [17]. Van Der Lingen [8] found that satisfaction was more dependent on shoulder function than residual pain. The most satisfied patients, with better DASH scores, showed better degrees of abduction and forward flexion. All reviewed articles reported a satisfaction rate above 80%. Many [2, 4, 5, 8, 12–14] achieved 100%.

Poor subjective outcomes were mainly related to residual pain, neuropathic in nature, or resulting from a malposition of the fusion, from excessive abduction or forward flexion, with painful scapular winging. Pruitt reported that all his patients were satisfied but one. The shoulder had been fused at more than 70° of abduction, resulting in pain and poor appearance. The arthrodesis was revised and re-fused in less abduction (45°). In El-Said's [2] article, 4 patients out of 18 complained of residual pain. All had been placed in more than 80° of abduction.

Author's Preferred Technique

The position of the fusion is without doubt one of the most important parameters of this procedure. The goal is to obtain the maximum amount of abduction and anterior flexion without creating any painful winging of the scapula when the arm lies against the body. Revision of the fusion would be very complicated after internal fixation. While the best position of the fusion usually falls around 20–30° of abduction, 20–30° of anterior flexion, and 30–40° of internal rotation, it varies from patient to patient, depending on the strength of the scapulothoracic muscles, the power of the elbow flexion and extension, the presence or not of active pronation and supination, the body mass, and the particular needs of the patient, based on his occupation or hobbies. This ideal position is difficult to predict with certainty from clinical assessment. In order to predict the best position of fusion, and allow a possible and simple adjustment, a percutaneous pinning of the glenohumeral joint can be performed a few days or weeks prior to the surgery (Fig. 17.3). Many of these patients also have absence of antigravity biceps, and the percutaneous pinning can be performed at the time of the flexorplasty (Fig. 17.4). Postoperatively, the elbow is usually immobilized in a long-arm cast, and the patient can enjoy and assess the benefits of a stable glenohumeral joint, as well as the newly recovered function, while assessing the impact from the loss of the passive motion. Adjustments to this position may then be planned, to improve function, at the time of the fusion. The infectious risk is minimal. However, these pins can create some damage to the articular surface when kept for long periods of time. A brace maintained part of the time can help minimize this damage.

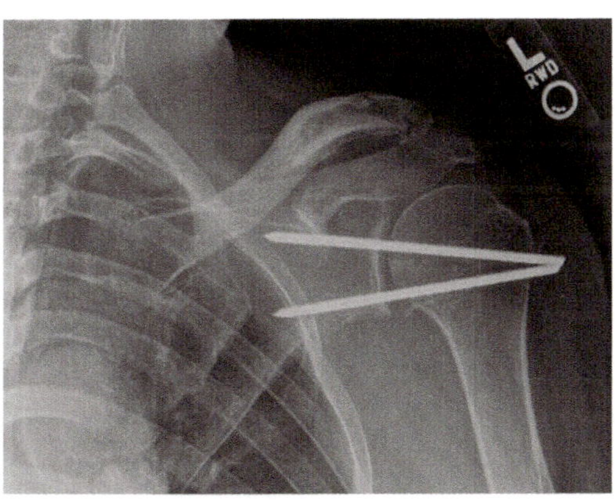

Fig. 17.3 Percutaneous pinning

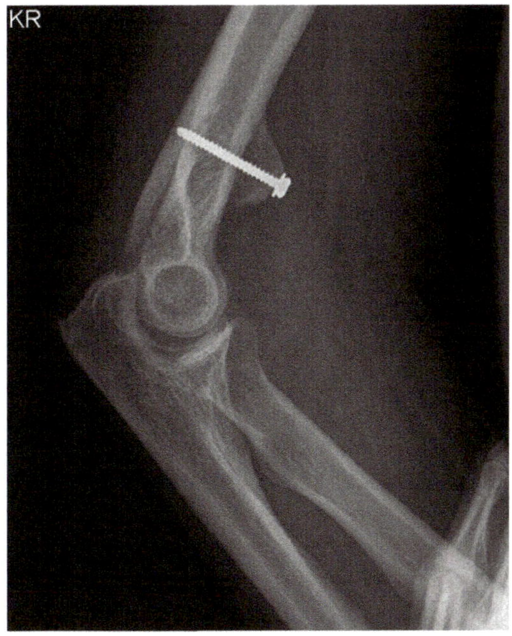

Fig. 17.4 The percutaneous pinning was performed as the same time as the Steindler procedure

The glenohumeral fusion is performed on a patient in the beach chair position or on the lateral position on the opposite site. The pelvis is perfectly immobilized. In order to preserve the anatomy and to provide coverage of most of the hardware, a deltopectoral approach is preferred, extended proximally to the back of the shoulder, over the acromion, then following the spine of the scapula. The proximal insertion of the deltoid is elevated to fully expose the glenohumeral joint. The labrum is excised, as well as the rotator cuff. When percutaneous pins had been previously inserted, a template is applied to the bones, following the spine of the scapula, the superior and lateral aspect of the acromion and the lateral aspect of the humerus. The pins are then removed, and a decortication of the humeral head, glenoid fossa, and undersurface of the acromion is performed. It is important to obtain a fusion in both glenohumeral joint and acromiohumeral space. The humeral head has to sit in tight contact with both glenoid and acromion. Temporary K-wires are then inserted to maintain the position. No osteotomy of the acromion is necessary, especially in sequela from obstetric palsies, where the acromion is deformed and down sloped. No bone graft is usually necessary, except in the rare cases with poor bony contact between the humeral head and the acromion. The bone fixation is then performed using a pelvic reconstruction plate, molded to match the template. All screws are inserted through the plate taking care to place at least two cancellous lag screws through the humeral head and the glenoid fossa and 1–2 more screws through the acromion and the neck of the scapula (Fig. 17.5). Additional cortical screws are inserted proximally in the spine of the scapula and distally in the humeral shaft. The wound is closed after reattachment of the proximal deltoid to the bone. Postoperatively, the patient is placed in a simple shoulder abduction pillow, maintaining the arm in mild abduction.

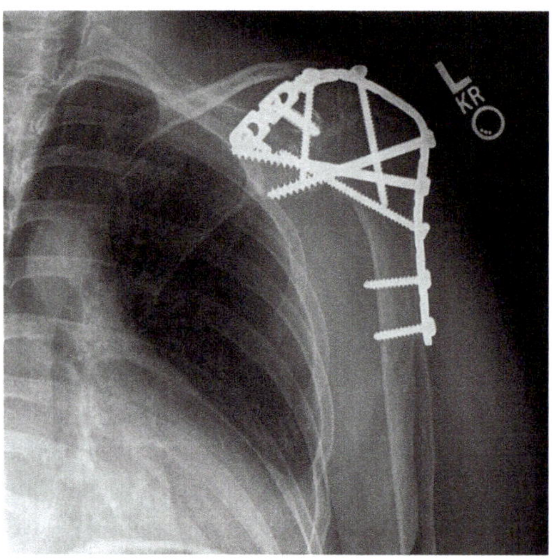

Fig. 17.5 Internal fixation using a reconstruction plate. Lag screws are inserted through the plate, across the glenohumeral joint and the acromiohumeral space

Discussion

Upper vs total, flail hand vs functional hand (Table 17.4) Prerequisites to a glenohumeral arthrodesis traditionally include active elbow flexion as well as a functional and sensate hand. Many patients with a total brachial plexus palsy, sometimes in spite of a surgical treatment, can have a weak hand, sometimes insensate. Many authors looked at the outcomes of shoulder arthrodesis in total brachial plexus palsy, versus upper brachial plexus palsy. Richards [12] reported on 11 adults, one of them with a total palsy that demonstrated a comparable range of motion as the rest of the group, and his shoulder pain was completely relieved. Rouholamin [4] reported on 13 patients, 6 of them having a total brachial plexus palsy. Similarly, his results found that total palsies were comparable to the upper palsies. Chammas [20] compared 2 groups of patients: 11 with upper palsy and a functional hand and 16 with a total palsy and a flail hand. All of them had active elbow flexion against resistance after nerve reconstruction, tendon transfers, or free muscle transfer. The position of fusion was different in the two groups with 24° and 21° of abduction and forward flexion, respectively, in the upper palsy and 31° and 27° in the total palsies. Postoperatively, active range of motion of 59°, 61°, and 42° of abduction, forward flexion, and internal rotation, respectively, was achieved in the upper palsy group versus 63°, 62°, and 45° in the total palsy group. In spite of increasing the position of fusion abduction, all patients except one, in the total palsy group, had recovered a strong brachiothoracic grasp, 7 could perform bimanual activities such as holding a tray, 14 could use the hand as a

Table 17.4 Results in total BPP

			Position			Results			
Year	Author	Specificities	Abd	FF	Int Rot	Abd	FF	Int Rot	Particularities
1988	Richards	$N = 1$	30	30	30	75	85		Poor hand function
1991	Rouholamin	$N = 6$	23	27	47	65	51		
2004	Chammas	$N = 16$	31	27	28	63	62	45	Flail hand
2012	Atlan	$N = 32$	30	30	30	57		46	
2017	Lenoir	$N = 3$	30	30	30	50	80		

Abd abduction, *FF* forward flexion, *Int Rot* internal rotation paperweight, and 8 of them could sleep on the fused upper extremity. Patients with upper palsy showed better strength in abduction, adduction, and internal and external rotation. Finally, he reported that the strength of the pectoralis major was a significant prognostic factor in terms of ultimate excursion of the hand and of shoulder strength. Atlan [6] looked retrospectively at 54 cases of glenohumeral fusion, 32 total palsies, and 22 partial palsies. All patients had prior recovery of active elbow flexion. The mean range of motion was 59° in abduction (57°, for complete, and 62° for partial palsy) and 48° in internal rotation (50° for complete and 46° for partial palsy). He concluded that there was no significant difference between the partial and total palsy groups. Lenoir [15] reported a series that included arthroscopic glenohumeral fusion in eight patients, three of them with a total palsy, and two of these also had a transfer of the inferior branch of the spinal accessory nerve to the suprascapular nerve. Their postoperative range of motion was 50° of abduction and 80° of forward flexion as opposed to 59° and 80° for the entire group. These authors agreed that active antigravity elbow flexion is absolutely necessary, as all their patients had recovered it. Emmelot [5] reported a series of 28 patients with total brachial plexus palsy and a flail shoulder, elbow, and a poorly functional hand. He performed a shoulder fusion in combination with an elbow stabilizing orthosis in 12 patients; 16 additional patients refused the operation and where used as a control group. He performed fusions at 30° of abduction, 20–30° of forward flexion, and 20° of internal rotation. Postoperatively, all patients said they benefited from the surgery, and none regretted undergoing the shoulder fusion. There was overall improvement in most cases with regard to dressing (100%), cosmetic appearance (91%), physical hygiene (91%), walking (83%), running (75%), and particularly feeling more stable (91%). There was a significant difference in functional activities between the group with glenohumeral arthrodesis and the group without.

Patients with previous spinal accessory nerve transfer It is admitted that the quality of the results correlates directly with the quality of the trapezius, rhomboids, serratus, and levator scapulae. In the primary treatment of brachial plexus palsies, many patients undergo nerve transfers, sometimes using the spinal accessory nerve, most often to the suprascapular nerve. The most proximal branches of the spinal accessory nerve to the upper trapezius are usually preserved maintaining some control over the scapula. The lower trapezius, however, is denervated. Few authors have specifically looked at the results. Thangarajah [16] reported on seven patients, two of them having had a spinal accessory to suprascapular nerve transfer. He analyzed his results, using the Oxford Shoulder Score (OSS) and Subjective Shoulder Value (SSV). The average OSS in his cases improved from 11 preoperatively to 27 postoperatively (range 16–40). This was accompanied by a significant increase in the mean SSV from 7 preoperatively (range 0–15) to 45 postoperatively (range 15–100). In the patients with previous spinal accessory nerve transfer, the OSS improved from 11 to 22 in one patient and from 15 to 26 in another, while the SSV improved from 10 to 30, and from 0 to 50. Chammas [20] reported on 27 patients, 11 of which had an upper palsy with a functional hand and 16 a total palsy with a flail hand. Eleven patients had undergone suprascapular nerve repair, which failed in all with a muscle power of MRC grade 2 or less. Seven other patients had a direct transfer of the terminal branch of the spinal accessory nerve, and four had nerve grafting to the suprascapular nerve. A total of 22/27 patients had a weak or nonfunctioning trapezius. He reported a postoperative range of motion of 59, 61, and 42°, respectively, for the abduction, forward flexion, and internal rotation in the patients with upper palsies, and 63, 62, and 45° for the patients with total palsy. Compared to other series, it did not appear that a partially or totally denervated trapezius hindered the outcome. Atlan [6] reported on 54 patients who had shoulder arthrodesis. All patients had preganglionic avulsions. A spinal accessory nerve transfer for elbow flexion was performed in seven cases. Their results showed slightly smaller abduction and rotational arc of motion in these patients, even though this trend was not significant.

While it would make sense that a healthy trapezius should be a prerequisite, there is no evidence that partial or even total denervation of the trapezius significantly hinders the outcome. Until a more detailed study is performed, one can safely assume that glenohumeral arthrodesis can be performed in patients with previous and failed spinal accessory nerve transfer, particularly, when the rest of the scapulothoracic muscles are functional. However, it would be highly advisable to avoid such transfers in patients with multiple root avulsions, who could become candidates for a glenohumeral joint fusion at a later time.

Weak serratus The serratus is a very important muscle for the stability of the scapula. It plays a major role in scapular protraction and upward rotation, resulting in forward flexion of the arm. It is both an antagonist to the rhomboids when pulling the scapula forward around the thorax and an agonist and synergistic by keeping the scapula pressed against the thorax when the superior and inferior parts fire together. In cases of weakness of the serratus, excessive position of the fusion in forward flexion would result in posterior winging of the scapula caused by the weight of the arm. It has therefore been recommended by Emmelot [5] to reduce the forward flexion angle to 10–15° in such cases.

Poor acromioclavicular joint A resection of the lateral end of the clavicle has been recommended by Cofield [23], in the setting of a painful, osteoarthritic AC joint. A fusion of the acromioclavicular joint, as recommended by Richards [12], is a less attractive option.

Pediatric patients The proximal growth plate of the humerus is responsible for 80% of the growth, and does not fuse before 17 years of age. Hence, concerns in children include severe shortening of the arm segment, decreased bone surface area in which to obtain a solid fusion, as well as loss of position over time, resulting in decreased abduction. For that reason, fusions have been recommended in as much as 90° of abduction. Pruitt [18] reported on 17 patients with 91% satisfactory results and recommended fusions to be performed in around 50° of abduction and after age 10. Mah and Hall [26] in their series of 10 patients with a follow-up between 5 and 27 years did not find any loss of abduction over time. They recommended fusion at 45° abduction and 25° flexion, and did not consider shortening to be functionally important, provided the patient could reach his mouth with his hand.

Indications

Indications for glenohumeral arthrodesis in brachial plexus palsies have been historically a salvage procedure, typically considered after failure of more accepted treatments, such as nerve reconstruction or tendon transfers. It would be however interesting to compare their outcomes. The functional results of direct nerve repairs to the shoulder are less predictable than those for the elbow [27, 28]. Modern nerve transfer techniques [29], including spinal accessory to suprascapular, combined with triceps long or lateral branch to the axillary nerve are usually very successful. When more roots than C5 and C6 are involved however, it is often impossible to use one of the triceps branches to neurotize the axillary nerve. Results of the isolated transfer of the spinal accessory to suprascapular, without reconstruction of the axillary nerve, have been disappointing [30], particularly for external rotation, for both amplitude and strength.

In cases with failure of the surgical nerve reconstruction or in the absence of surgery, persistent brachial plexus palsies with a flail shoulder are very difficult to treat. Tendon transfers have been reported to have only limited success owing to the complex biomechanics of shoulder girdle [31]. Ruhmann [10] compared the outcomes of two groups of patients with persistent brachial plexus palsy. Sixty-three patients underwent a trapezius transfer, and 14, a shoulder arthrodesis. In all cases, the trapezius transfer resulted in increased abduction from 6.1° to an average of 36.4° (20–80°) and forward flexion from 13.8° to an average of 31.9° (10–90°). The multidirectional shoulder instability was improved in 60 patients. Strength and functional improvement were, on average, greater following shoulder arthrodesis with an increased abduction from 9.6° to 59.3° (40–90°) and forward flexion from 11.4° to 50.7° (30–90°). The main advantage of the trapezius transfer was to maintain the passive motion, while the patients with the fusion obtained more strength and better function. He concluded that the shoulder fusion was more suitable for those patients who require the best possible extent of function and strength in the shoulder.

Le Hanneur [32] reported on a series of 45 consecutive patients with either C5-C6-C7 or C5-C6-C7-C8 brachial plexus palsy. Glenohumeral arthrodesis was performed in 24 patients with a flail shoulder, either primary, in avulsion injuries and late cases, or secondary, in cases of failure of the nerve surgery. Nerve surgery for reconstruction of the shoulder was performed in 14 patients. He reported 23/24 good results in the arthrodesis group, versus 6/14 in the nerve surgery group. Degeorge [33] compared two similar groups of adults with brachial plexus palsy. Twenty were managed by transfer of the spinal accessory nerve to the suprascapular nerve, and 38 by shoulder arthrodesis. After an average follow-up of 46 months, the DASH scores and the ranges of motion of the shoulder were comparable between the two groups; however, the strength was significantly greater in the arthrodesis group, in all directions of motion. In addition, the heterogeneity of the data suggested poor predictability and reliability of the nerve transfer, in contrast to the modest but predictable and uniform results of the shoulder arthrodesis. He concluded that arthrodesis should not be considered anymore as a salvage procedure, but rather, deserves to be viewed as a valid alternative to nerve transfer.

To summarize, the functional outcome of glenohumeral arthrodesis is superior to those of isolated spinal accessory to suprascapular nerve transfer and those of trapezius transfer. While the gold standard of surgical reconstruction of brachial plexus palsy should primarily involve nerve reconstruction, in cases with multiple root avulsions, when a nerve reconstruction of both suprascapular and axillary nerve is not possible, a shoulder arthrodesis should become part of the overall strategy, providing a better outcome for the shoulder. In these situations, no nerve donors should be wasted on the shoulder, and all available roots should then be directed to other functions allowing a higher axonal count with a superior outcome for the rest of the extremity. The shoulder fusion would then be planned as a secondary procedure which would be part of the overall strategy of treatment.

Contraindications

Poor postoperative satisfaction can be the result of lack of function or persistent pain [8, 17]. It can also be the result of unrealistic expectations. The quality of the results directly correlate with the strength and function of the scapulothoracic muscles. Even in case of complete (C5 to T1) avulsions, the spinal accessory nerve is usually preserved, allowing some degree of function and stability. An associated paralysis or weakness of the trapezius represents the only absolute contraindication. In case of extraforaminal rupture of the upper roots, the rhomboids, levator scapulae, and serratus function are usually preserved. More often, patients with C7 and/or C6 avulsions demonstrate additional weakness of the serratus. A thorough clinical examination, possibly augmented with a nerve conduction study, can help in the assessment of the level of denervation. In these situations, a meeting with comparable patients can be very helpful in establishing realistic expectations. Residual pain is also a significant source of patient unhappiness, especially when coupled with a limited function. While the shoulder pain from the inferior subluxation is usually eliminated by the fusion, no promise should be made regarding the neuropathic pain. In our practice, candidates for shoulder fusion with questionable indications are encouraged to meet with similar patients (with comparable extent of the palsy), having undergone it previously. In addition, a percutaneous pinning can also help the patient predict and assess his function, as well as the impact on his pain.

Conclusion

Glenohumeral arthrodesis is a safe, satisfactory, and reproducible procedure. Complications have become rare with modern techniques. Pelvic reconstruction plates are easier to mold and allow for a stable fixation with a high rate of union, without skin irritation. Bone grafting is not necessary. Malposition of the fusion, resulting in painful winging and/or suboptimal function, represents the most challenging complication. The most frequently recommended position is 30° of abduction, 30° of forward flexion, and 30° of internal rotation. The tendency has been, however, to reduce the amount of abduction and forward flexion and increase the amount of internal rotation. Preoperative placement of percutaneous pins across the glenohumeral joint can be very helpful in fine-tuning the position of the fusion at the time of surgery.

Shoulder fusions are beneficial in secondary settings, after failure of more conventional procedures. Their outcome is superior to that of trapezius transfer. They can also be indicated, in primary settings, as part of the overall strategy of treatment, in cases of multiple avulsions with limited available nerve material. When a reconstruction of both suprascapular and axillary nerves cannot be achieved, shoulder fusion provides a better outcome than isolated repair of the suprascapular. It can achieve a better outcome for the shoulder, but also the rest of the extremity (as no nerves would be wasted on the shoulder and more donor nerves would be directed to the elbow and hand). Total brachial plexus palsies do not represent a contraindication, as the final motion is comparable to that of upper palsy, although with slightly less strength. Active antigravity elbow flexion and a functional and sensate hand are usually prerequisites for this procedure. Patients without active elbow flexion and a functional hand can however still benefit from it, by combining it with an elbow orthosis (and possibly wrist orthosis or fusion). Recovery of a brachiothoracic pinch and complete resolution of the shoulder pain can lead to a high level of satisfaction. Even in patients with weak scapulothoracic muscles, shoulder fusions are still beneficial. Patients with a previous spinal accessory nerve transfer are also good candidates for this procedure. When the fusion is planned primarily, as part of the overall strategy, it is advisable to avoid using the spinal accessory nerve for any nerve transfer. Furthermore, it can finally be performed in adolescents, as close as possible to skeletal maturity.

Even though glenohumeral arthrodesis is an accepted procedure in brachial plexus palsies, it has remained mostly unpopular. Sacrifice of part of the passive range of motion can be a reasonable price to pay for patients in demand of stability, pain relief, and better function. The satisfaction rate is very high, but to avoid unrealistic expectations, it would be highly advisable to have the patients meet and talk to previous patients who underwent this procedure.

Number of complications: nonunions, fractures (above or below the plate), infections (deep or superficial), painful hardware (including skin irritation and ulceration)

Figures 17.6, 17.7, 17.8, 17.9, 17.10, 17.11, and 17.12: Results in an obstetric brachial plexus

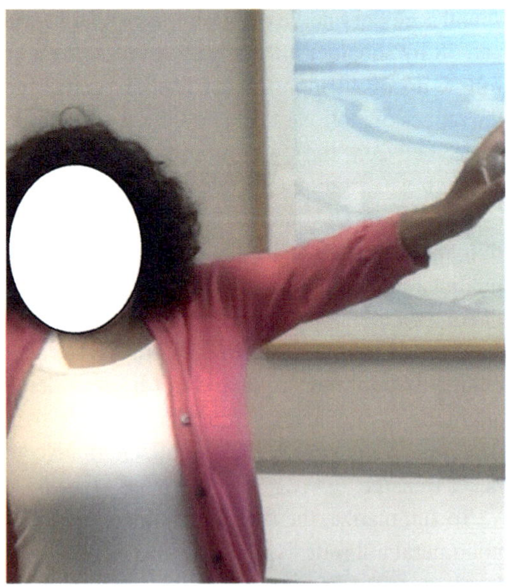

Fig. 17.6 Abduction

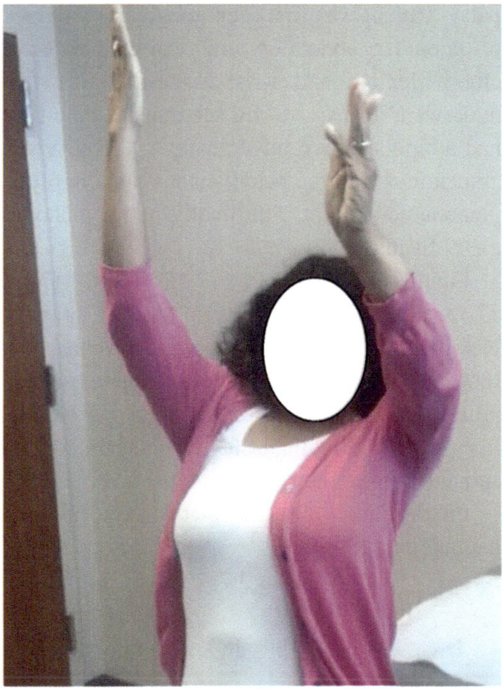

Fig. 17.7 Forward flexion

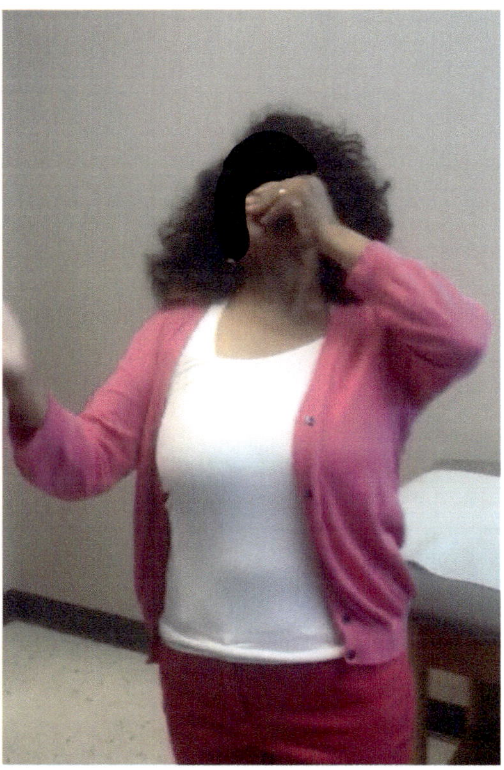

Fig. 17.8 Hand to mouth

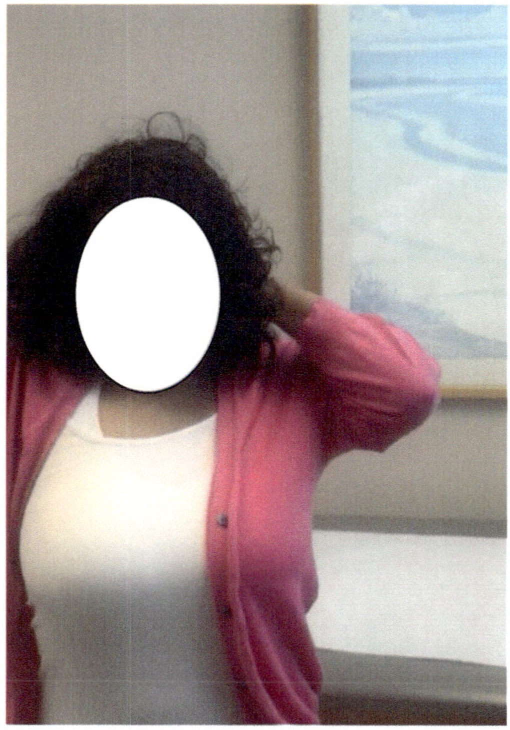

Fig. 17.9 Hand to neck

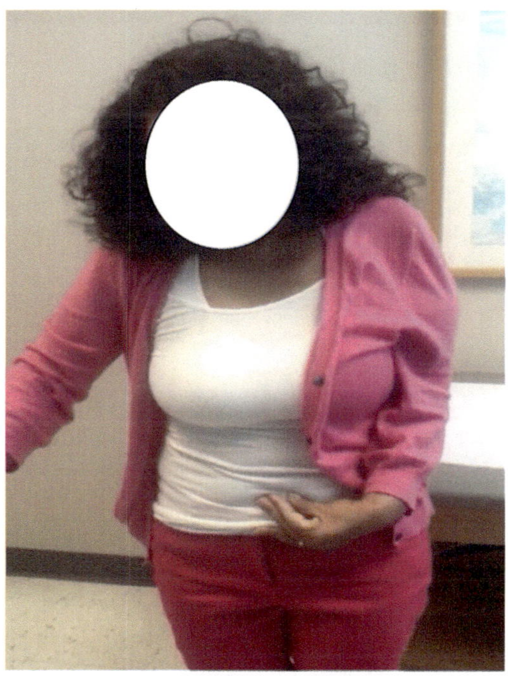

Fig. 17.10 Hand to belly

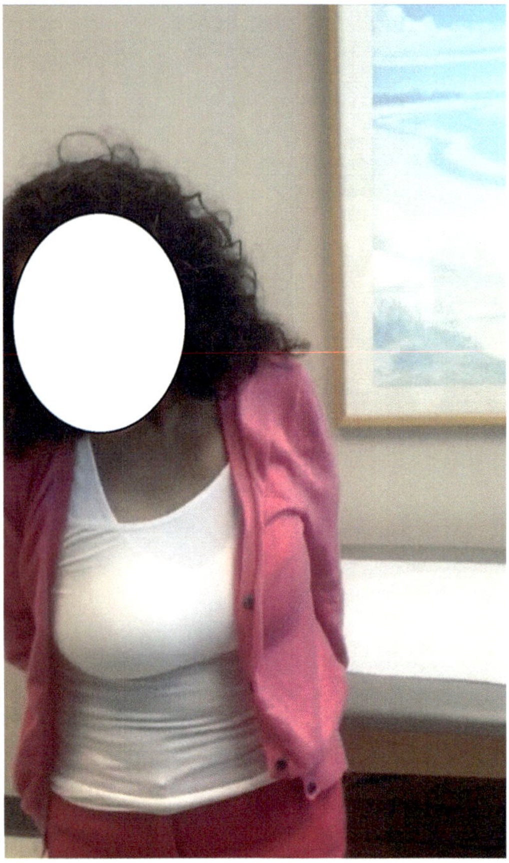

Fig. 17.11 Hand to back

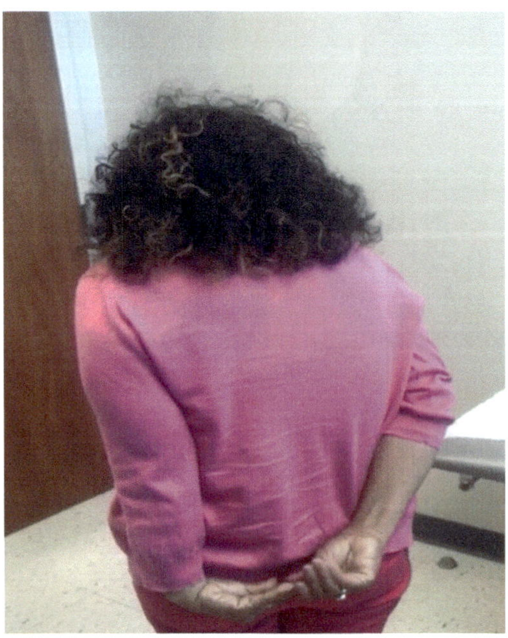

Fig. 17.12 Hand to back

palsy. Patient was first seen at age 54, with lack of shoulder abduction and external rotation, elbow flexion, and wrist extension. She first underwent an ECU to ECRB transfer. She then had a bipolar latissimus transfer to the biceps in association with the percutaneous pinning of the glenohumeral joint. She finally had a glenohumeral fusion.

Figures 17.13, 17.14, 17.15, 17.16, 17.17, 17.18, and 17.19: Results in a total brachial plexus palsy. Primary exploration revealed five root avulsions. Patient received intercostal to musculocutaneous transfer and then secondarily, free gracilis to the finger flexors, innervated with spinal accessory nerve.

Please find in attachment two movies about the outcome.

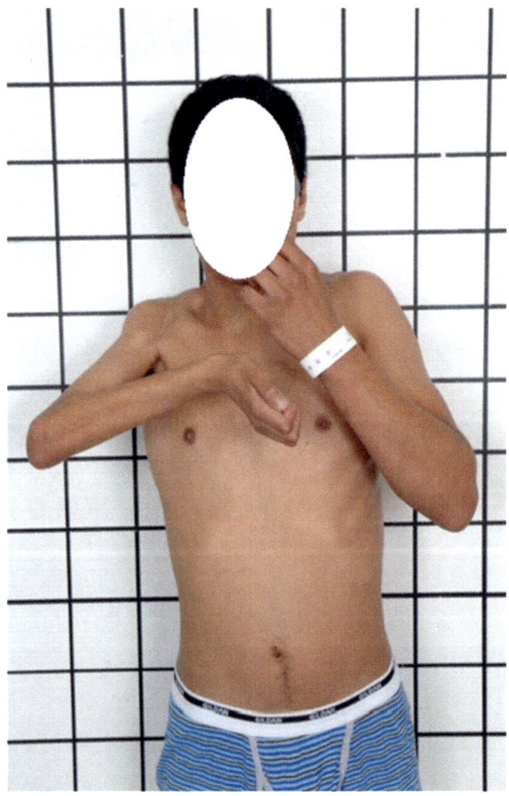

Fig. 17.13 Abduction

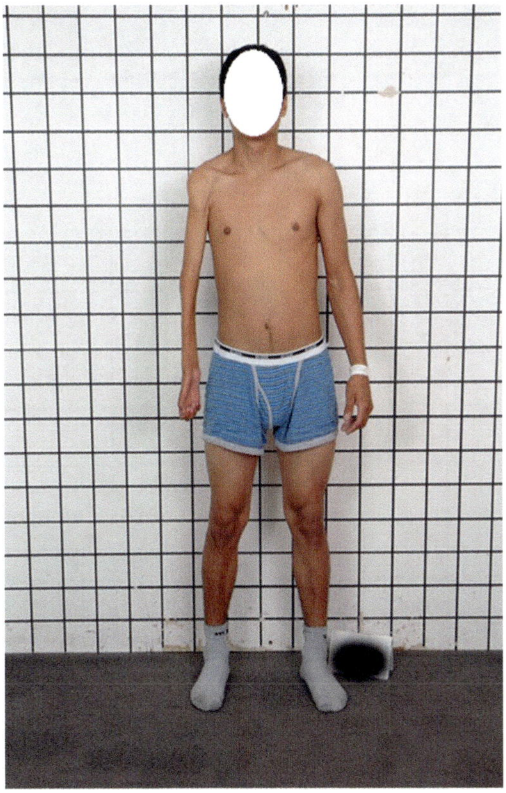

Fig. 17.14 Adduction

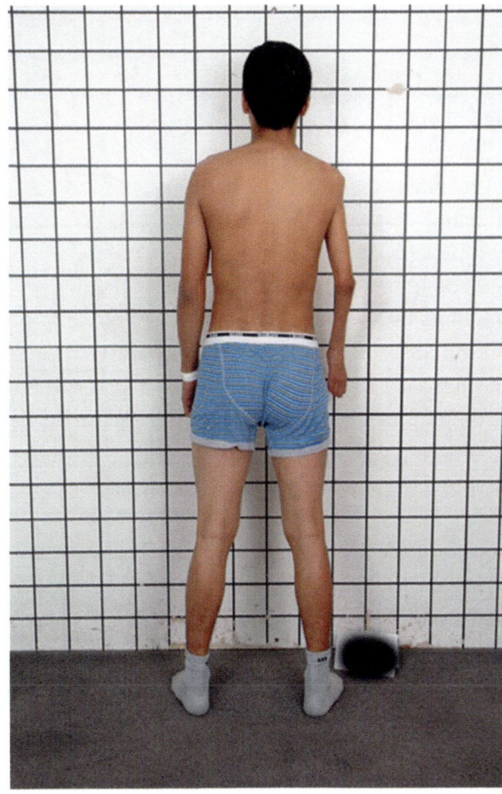

Fig. 17.15 Adduction

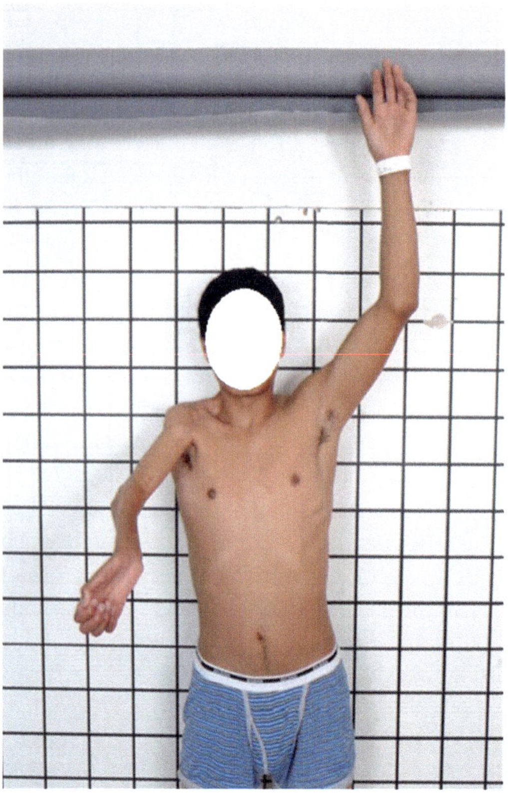

Fig. 17.16 Forward Flexion

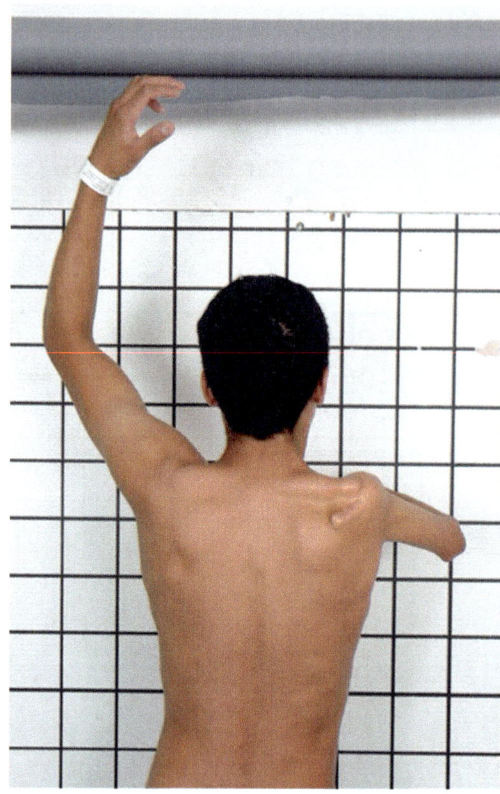

Fig. 17.17 Forward flexion

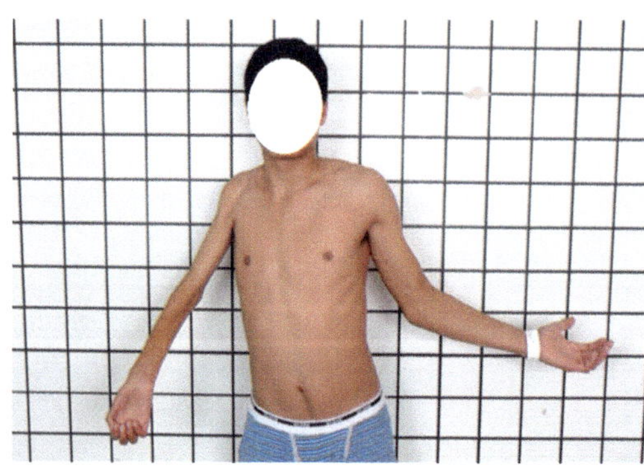

Fig. 17.18 External rotation

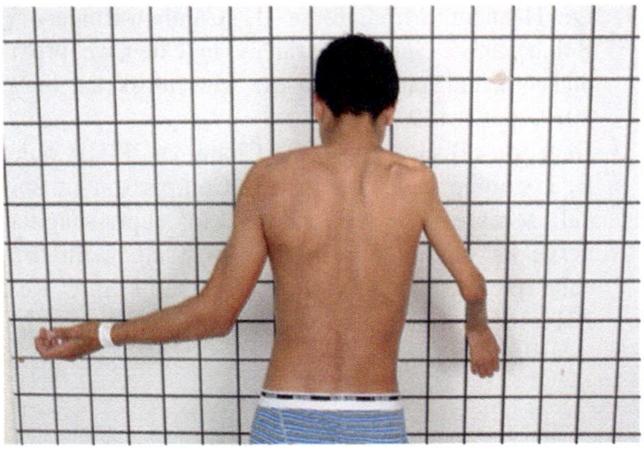

Fig. 17.19 External rotation

Bibliography

1. Clare DJ, Wirth MA, Groh GI, Rockwood CA Jr. Shoulder arthodesis. J Bone Joint Surg Am. 2001;83(4):593–600.
2. Saleh N, El-Said M. A simple method of shoulder arthodesis. J Bone Joint Surg (Br). 1998;80-B:620–3.
3. Lerch S, Berndt T, Lipka W, Rühmann O. Screw arthrodesis of the shoulder. Oper Orthop Traumatol. 2011;23(3):215–26.
4. Rouholamin E, Wootton JR, Jamieson AM. Arthrodesis of the shoulder following brachial plexus injury. Injury. 1991;22(4):271–4.
5. Emmelot CH, Nielsen HKL, Eisma WH. Shoulder fusion for paralysed upper limb. Clin Orthop Relat Res. 1997;340:95–101.
6. Atlan F, Durand S, Fox M, Levy P, Belkheyar Z, Oberlin C. Functional outcome of glenohumeral fusion in brachial plexus palsy: a report of 54 cases. J Hand Surg Am. 2012;37(4):683–8.
7. Belkheyar Z, Belkacem Djeffel A, Cambon-Binder A. Glenohumeral fusion in adults with sequelae of obstetrical brachial plexus injury: a report of eight cases. J Hand Surg Eur Vol. 2019;44(3):248–55.
8. Van Der Lingen MAJ, De Joode SGCJ, Schotanus MGM, Grimm B, Van Nie FA, Speth LAWM, Samijo SK. Satisfied patients after shoulder arthrodesis for brachial plexus lesions even after 20 years of follow-up. Eur J Orthopaed Surg Tranmatol. 2018;28:1089–94.
9. Rtaimate M, Henry E, Lariviere J, Farez E, Laffargue P. Arthrodese d'epaule pour sequelles se paralysies du plexus brachial. Revue de Chirurgie Orthopedique. 2002;88:35–40.
10. Ruhmann O, Gosse F, Wirth CJ, Schmolke S. Reconstructive operations for the paralysed shoulder in brachial plexus palsy: concept of treatment. Injury Int J Care Injured. 1999;30:609–18.
11. Sousa R, Pereira A, Massada M, Trigueros M, Lemos R, Silva C. Shoulder arthrodesis in adult brachial plexus injury: what is the optimal position? J Hand Surg Eur Vol. 2011;36E(7):541–7.
12. Richards RR, Sherman RM, Hudson AR, Waddell JP. Shoulder arthrodesis using a pelvic-reconstruction plate. A report of 11 cases. J Bone Joint Surg Am. 1988;70(3):416–21.
13. Wong ELW, Kwan MK, Loh WYC, Ahmad S. Shoulder arthrodesis in brachial plexus injuries. A review of 6 cases. Med J Malaysia. 2005;60(Supplement C):72–7.
14. Esenyel CZ, Ozturk K, Imren Y, Ayanoglu S. Shoulder arthodesis with plate fixation. Acta Orthop Traumatol Turc. 2011;45(6):412–20.
15. Lenoir H, Williams T, Griffart A, Lazerges C, Chammas M, Coulet B, Le Nen D. Arthroscopic arthrodesis of the shoulder in brachial plexus palsy. J Shoulder Elb Surg. 2017;26(5):e115–21.
16. Thangarajah T, Lambert SM. Glenohumeral arthodesis for late reconstruction of flail shoulder in patients with traumatic supraclavicular brachial plexus palsy. Shoulder Elbow. 2017;9(4):266–71.
17. Irlenbush U, Rott O, Irlenbush L. Indications, technique and long-term results after shoulder arthrodesis performed with plate fixation. Z Orthop Unfall. 2018;156777:53–61.
18. Pruitt DL, Husley RE, Fink B, Manske PR. Shoulder arthrodesis in pediatric patients. J Pediatr Orthop. 1992;12:640–5.
19. González-Díaz R, Rodríguez-Merchán EC, Gilbert MS. The role of shoulder fusion in the era of arthroplasty. Int Orthop. 1997;21(3):204–9.
20. Chammas M, Goubier JN, Coulet B, Reckendorf GM, Picot MC, Allieu Y. Glenohumeral arthodesis in upper and total brachial plexus palsy. J Bone Joint Surg Br. 2004;86(5):692–5.
21. Dávid A, Makowski S, Muhr G. Post-traumatic shoulder arthodesis. Indications, technique, results. Unfallchirurg. 1995;98(11):566–9.
22. Van Der Helm FCT, Pronk GM. Loading of shoulder girdle muscles in consequence of a glenohumeral arthrodesis. Clin Biomech. 1994;9:139–48.
23. Cofield RH, Briggs BT. Glenohumeral arthrodesis. Operative and long-term functional results. J Bone Joint Surg Am. 1979;61:668–774.
24. Neer CS. Glenohumeral arthrodesis. Philadelphia: WB Saunders; 1990. p. 438–42.
25. Hawkins RJ, Neer CS. A functional analysis of shoulder fusions. Clin Orthop. 1987;223:65–76.
26. Mah JY, Hall JE. Arthrodesis of the shoulder in children. J Bone Joint Surg Am. 1990;72:582–6.
27. Alnot JY, Daunois O, Oberlin C, Bleton R. Total paralysis of the brachial plexus caused by supraclavicular lesions. Rev Chir Orthop Reparatrice Appar Mot. 1992;78:495–504.
28. Sedel L. The results of repair of brachial plexus injuries. J Bone Joint Surg (Br). 1982;64-B:54–66.
29. Bertelli JA, Ghizoni MF. Reconstruction of C5 and C6 brachial plexus avulsion injury by multiple nerve transfers: spinal accessory to suprascapular, ulnar fascicle to biceps branch, and triceps long or lat-

eral head branch to axillary nerve. J Hand Surg Am. 2004;29:131–9.
30. Baltzer HL, Wagner ER, Kircher MF, Spinner RJ, Bishop AT, Shin AY. Evaluation of infraspinatus reinnervation and function following spinal accessory nerve to suprascapular nerve transfer in adult traumatic brachial plexus injuries. Microsurgery. 2017;37(5):365–70.
31. Leffert RD. Brachial plexus injuries: New York, Churchill Livigstone; 1985. p. 190–3.
32. Le Hanneur M, Lafosse T, Cambon-Binder A, Belkheyar Z. Surgical strategy in extensive proximal brachial plexus palsies. Musculoskelet Surg. 2019;103(2):139–48.
33. Degeorge B, Lazerges C, Chammas PE, Coulet B, Lacombe F, Chammas M. Comparison of spinal accessory nerve transfer to supra-scapular nerve vs. shoulder arthodesis in adults with brachial plexus injury. Orthop Traumatol Surg Res. 2019;105(8):1555–61.

18 Reconstructive Options for the Thumb Axis in a Brachial Plexus Injury

Rowan M. Chandler, Tod A. Clark, and Jennifer L. Giuffre

Introduction

The thumb is the first digit on the human hand and is similar to the other digits in that it is comprised of phalangeal bones whose hinge joints flex toward the palm. The thumb differs from the other digits in that it is the only digit that performs opposition. The ability of the thumb to oppose with the other four digits is due in part to the thumb's lateral position on the hand and its particularly mobile carpometacarpal (CMC) joint. This, coupled with the actions of the thenar muscles, allows for powerful precise movement in multiple directions. The role of the thumb in hand function has evolved along with the ever-increasing use and prevalence of handheld devices in the general population. The thumb, which used to function primarily as a static post against which objects were pinched, now operates independently and with greater dexterity in carrying out motions such as typing and texting [1]. Opposition and precise control of thumb interphalangeal (IP) joint flexion are particularly important for independent thumb actions [2].

Opposition has been formally defined many times by primatologists, human anatomists, and hand surgeons [3–5]. A distinction is made between opposition and apposition. Opposition is the movement by which the pulp of the thumb is placed in contact with the distal ends of one or all of the remaining digits. To achieve opposition, the thumb must abduct palmarly, flex, and pronate; this requires the use of the abductor pollicis brevis (APB), opponens pollicis (OP), and flexor pollicis brevis (FPB) muscles. Apposition refers to an extension-adduction movement (as opposed to the flexion-abduction movement of opposition) whereby the ulnar side of the distal phalanx of the thumb is brought into contact with the palm or the radial side of the index finger. Moving a digit back to its neutral position is called reposition, and a circular movement of the thumb at the carpometacarpal joint is referred to as circumduction [5].

The bones of the thumb are the first metacarpal, the proximal phalanx, and the distal phalanx. The joints of the thumb are the interphalangeal (IP) joint and the metacarpophalangeal (MCP) joint. The metacarpal of the thumb articulates with the trapezium at the wrist, thus forming the carpometacarpal (CMC) joint.

The muscles acting on the thumb can be divided into two groups: extrinsic and intrinsic.

R. M. Chandler
Section of Plastic Surgery, Department of Surgery, Winnipeg, MB, Canada

T. A. Clark
Plastic Surgery, University of Manitoba, Department of Orthopedic Surgery, Winnipeg, MB, Canada

J. L. Giuffre (✉)
Plastic Surgery, University of Manitoba, Section of Plastic Surgery, Department of Surgery, Winnipeg, MB, Canada
e-mail: jgiuffre@panamclinic.com

A. Y. Shin, N. Pulos (eds.), *Operative Brachial Plexus Surgery*,
https://doi.org/10.1007/978-3-030-69517-0_18

Those muscles with muscle bellies outside the hand are referred to as extrinsic muscles, whereas intrinsic muscles are located within the hand. The extrinsic muscles are innervated by the median and radial nerves. The flexor pollicis longus (FPL) muscle is an extrinsic muscle to the thumb which is innervated by the median nerve. The radial nerve innervates the extrinsic abductor pollicis longus (APL), extensor pollicis longus (EPL), and extensor pollicis brevis (EPB) muscles. The intrinsic muscles of the thumb are innervated by the median and ulnar nerves. The median nerve innervates the thenar muscles including the abductor pollicis brevis (APB), opponens pollicis (OP), and the superficial head of the flexor pollicis brevis (FPB), while the ulnar nerve innervates the deep head of the FPB, adductor pollicis (AP), and the first dorsal interosseous muscles.

Reconstruction of the thumb's complex movements poses a challenge to surgeons. Given the distal anatomic location of the intrinsic and extrinsic muscles of the thumb coupled with the few donor nerves available once the shoulder and elbow function have been addressed, nerve transfers alone in a patient with a brachial plexus injury are not adequate to restore thumb function. Tendon transfers are an option; however, they are limited by the level of the plexopathy. Tendon transfers reconstitute a lost function rather than restore each specific muscle lost. There have been several techniques described to appropriately reposition the digit to maximize function. First CMC joint arthrodesis and IP joint arthrodesis have been described in the treatment of the brachial plexus patient in order to improve prehension by recreating a stable post against which patients can place objects [6]. These arthrodeses are used in combination with tendon and nerve transfers to maximize thumb function.

This chapter will explore the evolution of the approach to the treatment of thumb function in the brachial plexus patient and describe surgical techniques that have been shown to have successful outcomes. This chapter will not discuss the prerequisite conditions to perform a tendon or a nerve transfer as these will be discussed in other chapters.

History

William Thorburn reported the first primary repair of a brachial plexus injury in 1900 [7]. The patient was a 16-year-old male who sustained an injury in a mill accident. Four years following the repair, the patient had good elbow and wrist function; however, he had regained minimal shoulder function and no hand function. Though much of the pioneering work on tendon transfers and the development of local flaps for upper extremity reconstruction came from the treatment of soldiers on the battlefields of the First and Second World Wars, conservative management of brachial plexus injuries was the mainstay of treatment throughout the twentieth century [8, 9]. This prevailing mindset of conservative treatment began to alter in the 1980s with publications demonstrating the work done by Millesi and Narakas [7, 10–12]. They outlined encouraging results using new microsurgical techniques in the repair of brachial plexus injuries with nerve repairs and nerve transfers. During this time, however, tendon transfers were the mainstay of treatment to restore thumb function, specifically thumb opposition. The first tendon transfer for thumb opposition was published by Steindler in 1918 [13, 14]. Today, the most commonly used opposition transfers rely on the flexor digitorum superficialis (FDS) of ring or long finger, extensor indicis proprius (EIP), palmaris longus (PL), and abductor digiti minimi (ADM) [15]. Other tendons used include extensor digiti minimi (EDM), extensor carpi ulnaris (ECU), extensor carpi radialis longus (ECRL), EPL, FPL, and pronator teres (PT) [16–19].

In the 1990s nerve transfers became popular in the treatment of nerve injuries that could not be repaired primarily or in patients with a proximal injury, significant local trauma, and scar tissue. Operating outside of the zone of injury and transferring a functional but less important redundant nerve to a distal but more important denervated nerve [20] to restore critical function gave promising results. The principles of tendon transfers influenced clinical decision-making for nerve transfers. Encouraged by the results of nerve transfers in shoulder and elbow restoration, surgeons became interested in designing motor and sensory nerve transfers for hand and thumb function.

Surgical Technique

This section will outline an approach to restoring thumb function and cover options including nerve transfer, tendon transfer, and arthrodesis. The determination of whether the thumb is reconstructed with nerve transfers and/or tendon transfers and/or arthrodesis depends on several factors: the mechanism and location of the injury, concomitant injuries (soft tissue, bone, or vasculature), donor options, and elapsed time from injury.

Complete Plexus Injury

An array of nerve transfers have been described to restore thumb and hand function in the patient with a complete brachial plexus injury. These transfers have had varying levels of success.

Contralateral C7 Use

Gu in 1986 introduced the use of the contralateral C7 (CC7), containing 25,000 myelinated motor and sensory fibers, in the reconstruction of patients with complete brachial plexus lesions [21]. In theory, because of the high cross-innervation by the contralateral C6 and C8 roots, the uninjured contralateral C7 (partial or whole) can be transferred with an ipsilateral vascularized ulnar nerve graft of the injured limb into the median nerve with the goal of restoring thumb function and grasp without leaving a permanent neurologic deficit in the donor limb.

In brief, the contralateral C7 root of the unaffected limb is identified through the traditional supraclavicular approach to the brachial plexus. The posterior superior half of the nerve root is identified and dissected distally. On the ipsilateral injured arm, the ulnar nerve is dissected in its entirety from the wrist to the axilla, while keeping its vascular pedicle intact. A subcutaneous tunnel is made across the chest to the predissected partial C7 root. The distal end of the ulnar nerve is passed across the chest, and a neurorrhaphy is performed to the contralateral C7. The proximal ulnar nerve end is divided, and a neurorrhaphy is performed to the ipsilateral median nerve at the level of the axilla.

In 1998 Gu et al. reported the results of eight CC7 nerve transfers to the median nerve with more than 2 years follow-up. Five of the eight patients achieved at least M3 recovery of the wrist, fingers, and thumb flexors [22]. Despite encouraging results, CC7 transfers have not gained universal popularity. Sammer et al. evaluated 28 patients following hemi-CC7 transfers to the median nerve using an ipsilateral pedicled vascularized ulnar nerve graft. They concluded that the outcomes of hemi-CC7 transfer for restoration of shoulder motor function or median nerve function following posttraumatic brachial plexus injury did not justify the risk of donor-site morbidity, which included possible permanent motor and sensory losses [23].

Free Innervated Gracilis Muscle Use

Unfortunately, despite favorable results for early nerve grafting and transfer techniques for shoulder and elbow function in brachial plexus injuries, results of nerve grafting or nerve transfers for thumb and hand function have been less favorable. Intrinsic muscle function of the thumb and digital movement cannot readily be restored by nerve transfers; therefore, a combination of arthrodeses and either a single or double free functioning gracilis muscle transfer or tenodesis has been proposed to augment the hand and thumb function, restore grasp and release, and position the hand adequately in space.

Doi et al. improved prehension in patients being treated for brachial plexus injuries by obtaining thumb stability with arthrodesis and performing a concomitant double free functional muscle tissue transfer for finger function [24]. The goals of the double gracilis transfer are to provide shoulder stability flexion and extension of the elbow, hand sensibility, and rudimentary hand grasp and release. In the first muscle transfer, the gracilis muscle is neurotized by the spinal accessory nerve and anastomosed to the thoracoacromial trunk to produce elbow flexion and finger or wrist extension. Proximally the gracilis is attached to the clavicle and routed distally under the brachioradialis to the radial wrist and finger extensors. In the second transfer, the gracilis is neurotized to two motor intercostal nerves and anastomosed to the thoracodorsal artery to create finger and thumb flexion. Another two motor intercostal nerves are coapted to a triceps branch to provide an agonist to the gracilis to prevent elbow flexion and allow for the gracilis to produce grasp. The sensory intercostal nerves are neurotized to the median nerve for hand sensation. Proximally the gracilis is attached to the second rib, routed subcutaneously along the medial aspect of the arm and attached distally to the flexor digitorum profundus (FDP) and FPL tendons. If successfully performed, the patient is able to activate thumb flexion at the IP joint and achieve a more functional hand [25–27].

Modifications to the gracilis free muscle transfer originally described by Doi et al. employ a single gracilis muscle to restore elbow flexion, finger flexion, and thumb flexion [6, 28, 29] (Fig. 18.1). The gracilis is secured proximally to the clavicle with several suture anchors. The muscle is tunneled into the forearm, beneath the PT to create a pulley effect, and is provisionally placed in its final position. The vascular anastomosis is preferentially performed end-to-end to the thoracoacromial trunk. The neurorrhaphy is completed with two motor intercostal nerves or alternatively the spinal accessory. Distally, the FDP and FPL tendons are identified and sutured together in a position that creates key pinch and grasp with traction. The gracilis tendon is then woven into the prepared FDP and FPL tendons using a Pulvertaft weave. The muscle flap is tensioned to allow the fingers and thumb to extend with elbow flexion and allow the fingers and thumb to close with elbow extension. In addition, the sensory intercostal nerves are neurotized to the lateral cord contribution of the median nerve to provide protective sensation to the hand, and two motor intercostal nerves are transferred into a nerve branch of the triceps for agonist for grasp.

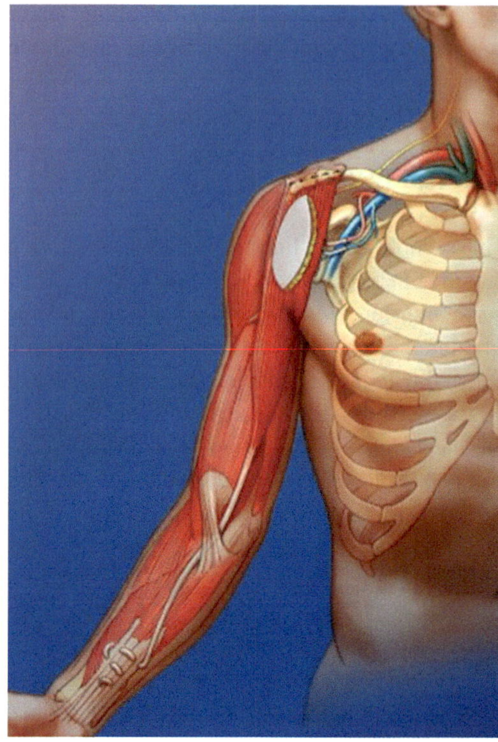

Fig. 18.1 A single free gracilis muscle transfer, secured proximally to the clavicle and distally to the flexor digitorum profundus and flexor pollicis longus tendons, restores elbow flexion and finger flexion. Options for muscle innervation include the spinal accessory nerve (as seen in the diagram) or two intercostal motor nerves

The innervated free muscle transfer offers a rudimentary straight-line pull to the finger and thumb flexors that originates in the proximal forearm. In brachial plexus injuries, several obstacles prevent this straight line of pull from being converted to an effective digital grasp and lateral pinch. The first obstacle is the lack of wrist stability. The majority of the pull from the transfer is directed to useless wrist motion instead of finger motion. The second obstacle is thumb malposition and instability. Although functional muscle transfers and tenodesis activate the FPL tendon, there are no thumb extrinsic or intrinsic muscles to help position the thumb for pinch. The imbalance of forces results in an ineffective thumb, which is supinated, hyperextended at the CMC joint, and hyperflexed at the IP joint. Therefore, despite initial surgical efforts, patients present with persistent flaccid/contracted wrists, flaccid thumbs in a supinated and extended position, poor pinch, and poor grasp.

Wrist, first CMC, and thumb IP joint arthrodeses are used as secondary adjunctive procedures to improve hand function, hand control, and appearance by increasing stability. These arthrodeses provided maximal biomechanical advantage of the tenodesis or transferred gracilis muscle by obtaining improved finger/thumb flexion through stable joints. The wrist, first CMC joint, and IP joint arthrodeses create mechanical efficiency as contraction of the transferred gracilis muscle pulls the fingers and thumb into pinch [6].

Surgical techniques for arthrodesis are no different in the thumb of the brachial plexus patient. CMC joint arthrodesis is performed using staples (3M Shapiro Staples, St. Paul, MN). Bone graft (distal radius cancellous bone harvested at Lister's tubercle) is packed between the joint surfaces. A 1.6 mm K-wire is place retrograde in the medullary canal of the thumb metacarpal and exiting the dorsal MCP joint. The thumb is placed in 35–45° of palmar abduction and 20–30° of radial abduction and pronation of the thumb so that the thumb pulp rests on the radial aspect of the index finger middle phalanx. The K-wire is advanced across the CMC joint, and Shapiro staples are placed across the CMC joint (typically two staples). A radiograph is used to confirm the position of fusion (Fig. 18.2).

IP joint arthrodesis is performed using a tension band wire technique. A burr is used to

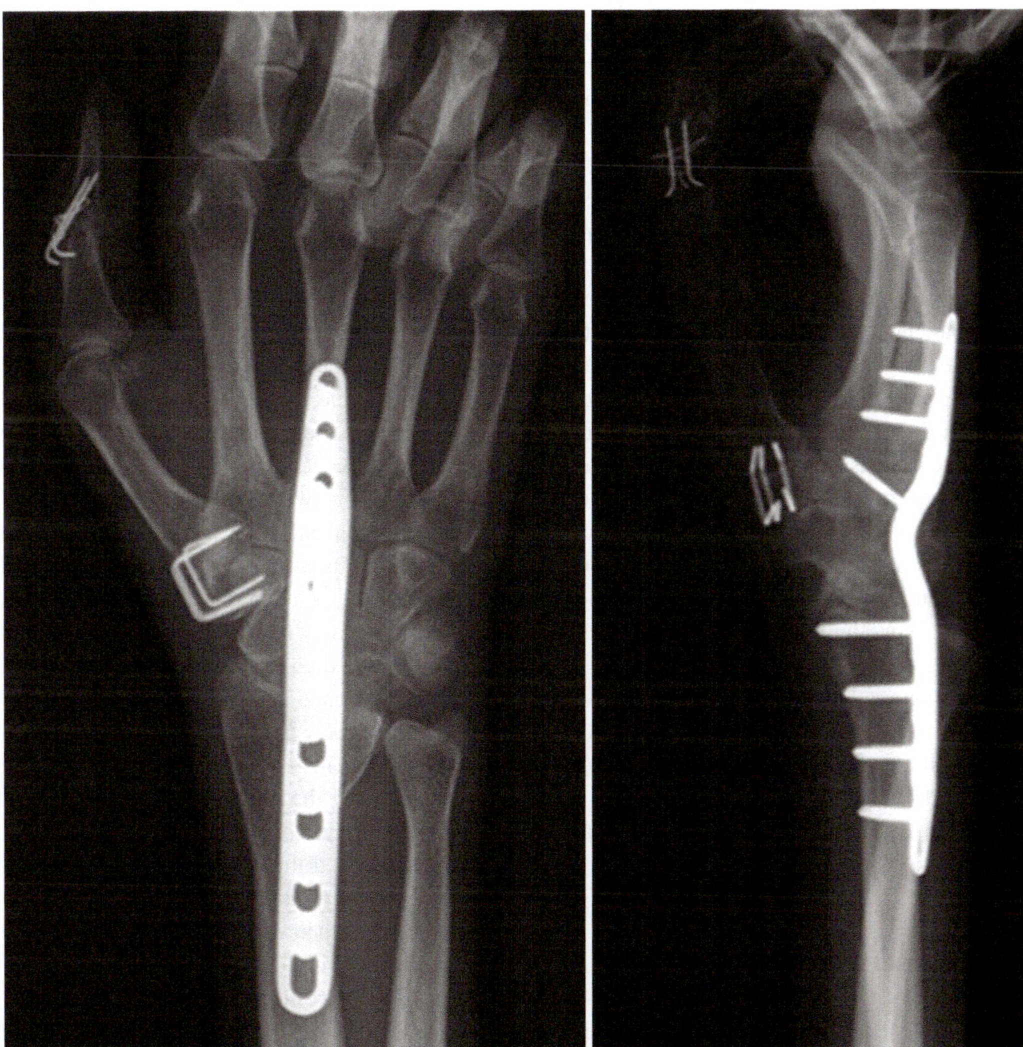

Fig. 18.2 Radiographic evidence of wrist, first CMC joint, and IP joint union by 6 weeks

remove the subchondral bone from the distal phalanx base and the head of the proximal phalanx keeping the joint surfaces congruent. The IP joint is flexed 15–35 degrees, and a tension band wire construct using 28 gauge surgical steel and 0.9 mm K-wires is used for fixation (Fig. 18.2).

Following wrist, first CMC joint, and IP joint arthrodeses, patients are immobilized in a thumb spica cast for 6–8 weeks or until radiographic union is achieved. Patients are encouraged to maintain finger range of motion after surgery. Physiotherapy and occupational therapy of the wrist and thumb begin following union.

There are very few studies that describe using first CMC joint arthrodesis and IP joint arthrodesis as part of the upper extremity reconstruction in patients with brachial plexus injuries. Giuffre el al. assessed 24 patients with brachial plexus injuries and demonstrated a statistically significant improvement in DASH scores (from 51 pre-operation to 28 post-operation), pain scores (from 5.3 pre-operation to 3.2 post-operation), as well as patient-perceived improvements in appearance, function, ease of daily cares, hygiene, pain, and satisfaction post-arthrodeses [6]. The majority of patients (84%) in the study were satisfied with the surgery. Additionally, patients in this study reported a statistically significant decrease in pain following arthrodesis. Pain pre-arthrodesis may have been associated with repetitive injuries to the paralyzed extremity due to lack of control of the flaccid thumb. The main purpose of these procedures in this population is to improve prehension and therefore elevate hand function. A stable wrist and thumb following arthrodesis alleviates the flaccid wrist and the thumb in the plane of the fingers that hinders activities of daily living.

Complications of arthrodesis are uncommon but include nonunion, infection, hardware complications, nerve complications, adjacent arthritis, impaction, impingement, and pain.

Partial Plexus Injury

In the case of a partial plexus injury, there are more transfer options available for restoration of thumb function.

The nerve that contributes to the majority of thumb sensation, flexion, and opposition is the median nerve. A low median neuropathy primarily affects true thumb opposition (palmar abduction and pronation) and sensation. A high median neuropathy results in loss of thumb opposition and thumb IP joint flexion (FPL) in addition to motor deficits of the index and long fingers FDP and FDS tendons, forearm pronation (PT and pronator quadratus (PQ)), and sensory deficits in the median innervated digits.

Nerve Transfers

Nerve transfers for low median neuropathies have been proposed [30–32] in which the terminal branch of the anterior interosseous nerve (AIN) is transferred to the median recurrent motor nerve branch; however, it requires an interpositional nerve graft and cannot be used in high median nerve injuries.

In order to perform this transfer, the nonfunctioning motor thenar nerve is identified within the carpal tunnel and dissected from the remainder of the median nerve as proximal as possible and transected. At the proximal edge of the pronator quadratus muscle, the AIN is located and traced distally into the muscle until the nerve trifurcates. An interposition nerve graft is often necessary to bridge the gap between the distal end of the AIN and the proximal end of the recurrent motor nerve branch. The medial antebrachial cutaneous (MABC) nerve or lateral antebrachial cutaneous (LABC) nerve may be used as the graft [30–32].

In a high median nerve injury, the AIN is not an available donor nerve; therefore, alternative nerve transfers for thumb opposition have been described. Bertelli et al. proposed transferring the motor branch of the ADM into the thenar recurrent motor nerve branch [33]. After surgery, patients improved thumb pronation, thenar eminence bulk, and APB. Patients recovered approximately 75% of their normal-side grasp and pinch strength with no donor deficits [33].

In addition to restoration of thumb opposition, high median neuropathies require the restoration of the AIN innervated muscles. If the injury to the median nerve is distal to the brachial plexus in the upper arm, thumb IP joint flexion (FPL) can be reestablishing by restoring the AIN through either a primary neurorrhaphy, a nerve graft if the defect is ≤6 cm, or a nerve transfer. ECRB nerve branch to AIN [34–38] and brachialis nerve branch to AIN [39] transfers have been described to restore the AIN and therefore FPL. Brachioradialis nerve to AIN with an interpositional nerve graft is another option [38].

Sensory Nerve Transfers

Sensation can be restored with either repair of the peripheral sensory nerve or nerve transfers [39]. End-to-end and end-to-side neurorrhaphies have been proposed to restore sensation in the distal radial, median, and ulnar nerve distributions. Priorities of sensation are to the ulnar side of the thumb, the radial side of the index finger, and the ulnar border of the hand. Donor nerves include the sensory intercostal nerves (to be transferred into the lateral cord contribution of the median nerve in brachial plexus injuries), LABC, distal sensory radial nerve branches [40], distal median nerve to the third webspace, and distal ulnar nerve to the fourth webspace [30]. The recovery of sensation is aimed at preventing cutaneous ulcers and restoring protective sensation [40].

Alternatives to Nerve Transfers

Tendon Transfer

If the patient's injury is such that nerve transfers are not an option, the surgeon may rely on tendon transfers to restore thumb position and function. In an isolated low median neuropathy, thumb opposition has traditionally been restored with tendon transfers using various radial or ulnar innervated muscles such as the EIP, EPL, ECU, ECRL, EDM, ADM, or high median innervated muscles (if available) such as PL or the FDS of the long or ring fingers [16].

The tetraplegia literature has provided a wealth of information on hand mechanics. The literature states that effective lateral pinch requires all three joints of the thumb to be controlled in a position of functional balance by a combination of active muscle function and capsuloligamentous stability [41]. Over time as the natural ligament and tenodesis restraints are attenuated, a zigzag collapse deformity results [42]. The CMC joint assumes an extended and supinated position, and the metacarpophalangeal joint develops a hyperflexed posture. Similar to tetraplegia patients, in brachial plexus patients, the muscles that influence thumb position and effective pinch (flexor pollicis longus, extensor pollicis longus, extensor pollicis brevis, abductor pollicis longus, three thenar muscles, adductor pollicis, and first dorsal interosseous) cannot be adequately replaced to provide thumb abduction/adduction, flexion/extension, and supination/pronation.

The most rudimentary thumb motion uses a tenodesis effect between FPL and EPL during wrist flexion and extension. If the patient has active wrist control, the FPL can produce a weak pinch when the wrist is extended. Tenodesis of the EPL can be used for release of pinch, when the wrist is flexed.

Moberg proposed a limited key pinch through tenodesis of the FPL to the volar distal radius at the proximal edge of PQ with arthrodesis of the IP joint [43]. Hentz et al. reported that Moberg's technique resulted in excessive flexion of the MCP joint and significant patient dissatisfaction [42]; therefore, Hentz further modified the Moberg procedure by tenodesing both EPB and EPL to the first metacarpal using a bone anchor [42]. House further modified the technique by prepositioning the CMC joint by arthrodesis in a lateral pinch position and IP joint arthrodesis to prevent hyperflexion [41]. Active control of the thumb was provided by tenodesis or tendon transfer to FPL. House and Shannon demonstrated strong grasp and effective lateral pinch following the modified Moberg technique with an average pinch strength of 3.3 kg and grip strength of 7.4 kg [44]. All patients were satisfied with the functional results of surgery [44].

Zancolli described a "lasso" procedure as another option to enhance thumb pinch strength and recommended a two-stage reconstruction [45, 46]. The first stage consists of extensor tenodesis of the thumb, intrinsic tenodesis using the "lasso" procedure in which a slip of FPL is reattached to itself after passing through the proximal pulley, and thumb IP joint fusion. The second stage includes ECRL to FDP tendon transfer, BR to FPL tendon transfer, a volar thumb MCP capsulodesis if the thumb MCP joint is hyperextended, and a volar tenodesis of the EPB tendon if the thumb is in excessive extension.

Discussion

Restoring thumb function in the brachial plexus patient is a challenging proposition. The valuable role the thumb plays in effective hand function places priority on at minimum achieving a stable digit against which the patient can place objects and transfer them.

In brachial plexus patients there is not a single procedure that can adequately restore all of the muscles that influence thumb position and effective pinch (FPL, EPL, EPB, APL, 3 thenar muscles, AD, and first dorsal interosseous). Combinations of tendon transfers, tenodesis, and arthrodesis procedures can be used at the CMC, MCP, and IP joints to provide effective positioning and control of the thumb to produce pinch.

Tendon transfers restore a lost function rather than restore each individual lost muscle. Tenodesis attempts to stabilize joints by anchoring the tendons that move the joint. Unlike tendon transfers or tenodeses, nerve transfers are not limited to the one tendon/one function and the "straight line of pull" principles. The major advantages of a nerve transfer are their ability to restore motor and sensory function and their ability to restore multiple muscles with a single nerve transfer. The origin and insertion of the muscles are not disrupted in a nerve transfer, so unlike in a tendon transfer or tenodesis, the original function is maintained. Arthrodesis is typically discussed in arthritis management to increase stability and decrease pain. Arthrodesis is a reliable and durable treatment with consistently good results and improved overall patient satisfaction. Arthrodesis is useful in the brachial plexus thumb to make this multiarticular digit more stable and easier to control.

A comprehensive approach, taking into consideration the patient's original injury, age, functional status, and their ability to participate in post-operative therapy, is all taken into consideration when formulating an operative plan. Restoring thumb function and giving the patient a stable digit with which to perform the functions of opposition, pinch, and release vastly improves the brachial plexus patient's quality of life and productivity. The various tools in the surgeon's arsenal in order to reach this goal have been outlined above.

References

1. Yao J, Park MJ, Davis D, Chang J. Ideal position for thumb interphalangeal arthrodesis in the era of smartphones and text communication. Orthopedics. 2012; https://doi.org/10.3928/01477447-20121023-07.
2. Arauz P, Sisto SA, Kao I. Experimental study of the optimal angle for arthrodesis of fingers based on kinematic analysis with tip-pinch manipulation. J Biomech. 2016;49(16):4009–15. https://doi.org/10.1016/j.jbiomech.2016.10.047.
3. Geissler WB, Slade JF. Green's operative hand surgery. 2011. https://doi.org/10.1016/B978-1-4160-5279-1.00018-6.
4. Curtis RM. Opposition of the thumb. Orthop Clin North Am. 1974;5(2):305–21.
5. Bunnell S. Opposition of the thumb. J Bone Jt Surg. 1938;20:269–84.
6. Giuffre JL, Bishop AT, Spinner RJ, Kircher MF, Shin AY. Wrist, first carpometacarpal joint, and thumb interphalangeal joint arthrodesis in patients with brachial plexus injuries. J Hand Surg Am. 2012; https://doi.org/10.1016/j.jhsa.2012.09.017.
7. Narakas AO, Hentz VR. Neurotization in brachial plexus injuries: indication and results. Clin Orthop Relat Res. 1988;237:43–56. https://doi.org/10.1097/00003086-198812000-00008.
8. Littler JW. The neurovascular pedicle method of digital transposition for reconstruction of the thumb. Plast Reconstr Surg. 1953; https://doi.org/10.1097/00006534-195311000-00001.
9. Hovius SER. Musculo-tendinous transfers of the hand and forearm. Clin Neurol Neurosurg. 1993; https://doi.org/10.1016/0303-8467(93)90043-G.
10. Millesi H. Brachial plexus injuries. Management and results. Clin Plast Surg. 1984;11(1):115–20.
11. Millesi H. Brachial plexus injuries. Nerve grafting. Clin Orthop Relat Res. 1988; https://doi.org/10.1097/00003086-198812000-00007.

12. Millesi H. Surgical management of brachial plexus injuries. J Hand Surg Am. 1977; https://doi.org/10.1016/S0363-5023(77)80046-4.
13. Steindler A. A muscle plasty for the relief of flail elbow in infantile paralysis. Interstate Med J. 1918;25:235–41.
14. Steindler A. Orthopaedic reconstruction work on hand and forearm. New York Med J. 1918;108:1117–9.
15. Giuffre JL, Bishop AT, Spinner RJ, Shin AY. The best of tendon and nerve transfers in the upper extremity. Plast Reconstr Surg. 2015; https://doi.org/10.1097/PRS.0000000000001071.
16. Ratner JA, Peljovich A, Kozin SH. Update on tendon transfers for peripheral nerve injuries. J Hand Surg Am. 2010; https://doi.org/10.1016/j.jhsa.2010.05.023.
17. Brandsma W, Sammut D. Update on tendon transfers for peripheral nerve injuries. J Hand Surg Am. 2011; https://doi.org/10.1016/j.jhsa.2011.01.029.
18. Kozin SH. Tendon transfers for radial and median nerve palsies. J Hand Ther. 2005; https://doi.org/10.1197/j.jht.2005.02.003.
19. Loewenstein SN, Adkinson JM. Tendon transfers for peripheral nerve palsies. Clin Plast Surg. 2019; https://doi.org/10.1016/j.cps.2019.02.004.
20. Chuang DCC. Neurotization procedures for brachial plexus injuries. Hand Clin. 1995;
21. Chen L, Gu YD. An experimental study of contralateral C7 root transfer with vascularized nerve grafting to treat brachial plexus root avulsion. J Hand Surg Am. 1994; https://doi.org/10.1016/0266-7681(94)90051-5.
22. Gu YD, Chen DS, Zhang GM, et al. Long-term functional results of contralateral C7 transfer. J Reconstr Microsurg. 1998; https://doi.org/10.1055/s-2007-1006902.
23. Sammer DM, Kircher MF, Bishop AT, Spinner RJ, Shin AY. Hemi-contralateral C7 transfer in traumatic brachial plexus injuries: outcomes and complications. J Bone Joint Surg Am. 2012;94(2):131–7.
24. Doi K, Sakai K, Kuwata N, Ihara K, Kawai S. Double free-muscle transfer to restore prehension following complete brachial plexus avulsion. J Hand Surg Am. 1995; https://doi.org/10.1016/S0363-5023(05)80097-8.
25. Doi K, Kuwata N, Muramatsu K, Hottori Y, Kawai S. Double muscle transfer for upper extremity reconstruction following complete avulsion of the brachial plexus. Hand Clin. 1999;
26. Doi K, Muramatsu K, Hattori Y, et al. Restoration of prehension with the double free muscle technique following complete avulsion of the brachial plexus Indications and long-term results. J Bone Jt Surg Ser A. 2000; https://doi.org/10.2106/00004623-200005000-00006.
27. Elzinga K, Zuo KJ, Olson JL, Morhart M, Babicki S, Chan KM. Double free gracilis muscle transfer after complete brachial plexus injury: first Canadian experience. Can J Plast Surg. 2014; https://doi.org/10.1177/229255031402200105.
28. Bishop AT. Functioning free-muscle transfer for brachial plexus injury. Hand Clin. 2005; https://doi.org/10.1016/j.hcl.2004.10.005.
29. Shin AY, Spinner RJ, Steinmann SP, Bishop AT. Adult traumatic brachial plexus injuries. J Am Acad Orthop Surg. 2005; https://doi.org/10.5435/00124635-200510000-00003.
30. Brown JM, Mackinnon SE. Nerve transfers in the forearm and hand. Hand Clin. 2008; https://doi.org/10.1016/j.hcl.2008.08.002.
31. Wang Y, Zhu S. Transfer of a branch of the anterior interosseous nerve to the motor branch of the median nerve and ulnar nerve. Chin Med J 1997;110(3):216–9.
32. Vernadakis AJ, Humphreys DB, Mackinnon SE. Distal anterior interosseous nerve in the recurrent motor branch graft for reconstruction of a median nerve neuroma-in-continuity. J Reconstr Microsurg. 2004; https://doi.org/10.1055/s-2004-818043.
33. Bertelli JA, Soldado F, Rodrígues-Baeza A, Ghizoni MF. Transfer of the motor branch of the abductor digiti quinti for thenar muscle reinnervation in high median nerve injuries. J Hand Surg Am. 2018; https://doi.org/10.1016/j.jhsa.2017.08.009.
34. Bertelli JA. Transfer of the radial nerve branch to the extensor carpi radialis brevis to the anterior interosseous nerve to reconstruct thumb and finger flexion. J Hand Surg Am. 2015; https://doi.org/10.1016/j.jhsa.2014.10.060.
35. Hsiao EC, Fox IK, Tung TH, Mackinnon SE. Motor nerve transfers to restore extrinsic median nerve function: case report. Hand. 2009; https://doi.org/10.1007/s11552-008-9128-9.
36. Murphy RKJ, Ray WZ, Mackinnon SE. Repair of a median nerve transection injury using multiple nerve transfers, with long-term functional recovery. J Neurosurg. 2012; https://doi.org/10.3171/2012.8.JNS111356.
37. Ray WZ, Yarbrough CK, Yee A, Mackinnon SE. Clinical outcomes following brachialis to anterior interosseous nerve transfers: report of 4 cases. J Neurosurg. 2012; https://doi.org/10.3171/2012.6.JNS111332.
38. García-López A, Sebastian P, Martinez F, Perea D. Transfer of the nerve to the brachioradialis muscle to the anterior interosseous nerve for treatment for lower brachial plexus lesions: case report. J Hand Surg Am. 2011; https://doi.org/10.1016/j.jhsa.2010.11.030.
39. Brunelli GA. Sensory nerves transfers. J Hand Surg Am. 2004; https://doi.org/10.1016/j.jhsb.2004.06.005.
40. Wong AH, Pianta TJ, Mastella DJ. Nerve transfers. Hand Clin. 2012; https://doi.org/10.1016/j.hcl.2012.08.007.
41. House JH. Reconstruction of the thumb in tetraplegia following spinal cord injury. Clin Orthop Relat Res. 1985; https://doi.org/10.1097/00003086-198505000-00011.
42. Hentz VR, Brown M, Keoshian LA. Upper limb reconstruction in quadriplegia: functional assessment and proposed treatment modifications. J

Hand Surg Am. 1983; https://doi.org/10.1016/S0363-5023(83)80001-X.
43. Moberg E. Surgical treatment for absent single hand grip and elbow extension in quadriplegia: principles and preliminary experience. J Bone Jt Surg Ser A. 1975; https://doi.org/10.2106/00004623-197557020-00012.
44. House JH, Shannon MA. Restoration of strong grasp and lateral pinch in tetraplegia: a comparison of two methods of thumb control in each patient. J Hand Surg Am. 1985; https://doi.org/10.1016/S0363-5023(85)80243-4.
45. Zancolli E. Structural and dynamic bases of hand surgery. Philadelphia: JB Lippincott; 1979.
46. Zancolli E. Surgery for the quadriplegic hand with active, strong wrist extension preserved. A study of 97 cases. Clin Orthop Relat Res. 1975; https://doi.org/10.1097/00003086-197510000-00013.

Wrist Arthrodesis in the Adult Brachial Plexus Patient

19

Tod A. Clark and Jennifer L. Giuffre

Introduction

Wrist arthrodesis is commonly indicated in advanced symptomatic arthritis secondary to degenerative, posttraumatic, post-infectious, or post-inflammatory conditions [1–4]. Arthrodesis is typically discussed in arthritis management to increase stability and decrease pain [5–10]. Other conditions leading to arthrodesis include burn contractures, fixed deformities, and painful instability or deformity associated with ligament or tendon injury [11]. Wrist arthrodesis has been performed to improve function, hygiene, and cosmesis in patients with contracted or flaccid wrists secondary to cerebral palsy, traumatic brain injury, or brachial plexus injuries [11, 12]. Terzis et al. [13] performed wrist arthrodesis as a secondary procedure for hand reanimation in 61 patients with posttraumatic brachial plexopathies and concluded that wrist arthrodesis offered stable, painless carpus with improved overall upper limb function [13]. Addosooki et al. [12] described their technique of wrist arthrodesis as a complementary procedure to a double free muscle transfer to restore hand prehension in patients with total brachial plexopathies [12] and concluded that wrist fusion in patients receiving double free muscle transfers resulted in improved finger range of motion and overall hand function [1]. Giuffre et al. found that a wrist, first carpometacarpal (CMC) joint, and thumb interphalangeal (IP) joint arthrodesis could be used in conjunction with other reconstructive measures to improve function and grasp in patients with complete brachial plexus injuries [14].

Useful hand function requires grasp and release and adequate positioning in space [15–17]. Methods to successfully restore elbow and shoulder function in brachial plexus injuries with early nerve grafting and nerve transfers are well documented. Results of nerve grafting and nerve transfers for the restoration of intrinsic muscle function, wrist or digital movement, pinch, and grasp have been less favorable; therefore, free functioning muscle transfers or tenodeses are currently the accepted means to restore grasp and pinch [15, 16, 18]. These transfers offer a rudimentary straight-line pull to the finger and thumb flexors that originates in the proximal forearm. In brachial plexus injuries, the lack of wrist stability prevents this straight line of pull from being converted to an effective digital grasp and lateral pinch. Instead, the majority of the pull from the transfer is lost to useless wrist motion rather than directed to useful finger motion. Unfortunately, despite initial surgical efforts, patients present

T. A. Clark
Plastic Surgery, University of Manitoba, Department of Orthopedic Surgery, Winnipeg, MB, Canada

J. L. Giuffre (✉)
Plastic Surgery, University of Manitoba, Section of Plastic Surgery, Department of Surgery, Winnipeg, MB, Canada
e-mail: jgiuffre@panamclinic.com

A. Y. Shin, N. Pulos (eds.), *Operative Brachial Plexus Surgery*,
https://doi.org/10.1007/978-3-030-69517-0_19

with persistent flaccid/contracted wrists, flaccid thumbs in a supinated and extended position, poor pinch, and poor grasp. Wrist arthrodesis is a means to provide the necessary stability to the wrist which allows all of the power and excursion of the muscle transfer to be directed to useful finger motion, grasp, and pinch.

Indications for Wrist Arthrodesis in Brachial Plexus Patients

At the time of arthrodeses, patients must be stable from their previous nerve and tendon reconstructions. Despite initial attempts at reconstruction, patients presenting with no intrinsic muscle function, a flaccid wrist or a wrist flexion contracture, poor digital grasp, a thumb in an extended and supination position with poor lateral pinch and pain would benefit from a wrist arthrodesis.

Surgical Technique

All procedures are done in an operating room under general or regional anesthesia with proximal tourniquet control. A dorsal incision is made in line with the third ray from the middle of the third metacarpal to 4–5 cm proximal to the radiocarpal joint. The extensor retinaculum is incised through the third dorsal extensor compartment. Retinacular flaps are raised radially and ulnarly to expose the second, third, fourth, and fifth dorsal extensor compartments. The retinacular flaps are used to retract the tendons radially and ulnarly. A ligament sparing dorsal wrist capsulotomy is performed to allow for adequate soft tissue to cover the plate and act as a barrier to the extensor tendons upon closure. The wrist can be fused by preparing all the carpal surfaces left intact, or a proximal row carpectomy can be performed. If a proximal row carpectomy is performed, cancellous bone from the scaphoid, lunate, and triquetrum is used for bone graft. The articular cartilage and subchondral bone of the proximal capitate and hamate, the distal articular surface of the radius, and the third CMC joints are removed with a rongeur and burr. Cancellous bone graft harvested from the proximal row carpal bones is placed within the radiocarpal, and third CMC joints. Alternatively, iliac crest bone graft or distal radius bone graft can be used. To allow for apposition of a precontoured plate on the radius, Lister's tubercle and a small portion of the dorsal distal radius is removed with an osteotome. All arthrodeses are performed using the dorsal locking wrist fusion plate (Synthes, Paoli, PA) or equivalent precontoured plate (Fig. 19.1). The proximal row carpectomy is performed to correct any fixed wrist flexion contracture and to allow the wrist to be arthrodesed in 20–25 degrees of wrist extension. Following plate placement, the dorsal capsule is repaired over the plate. The extensor tendons are replaced into their anatomic position, and the extensor retinaculum is repaired leaving extensor pollicis longus dorsal to the repair. Subsequently a first CMC joint and IP joint fusion are performed (discussed in another chapter). Following wrist, first CMC joint, and IP joint arthrodeses, patients are immobilized in a thumb spica cast for 6–8 weeks or until radiographic union is achieved. Patients are encouraged to maintain finger range of motion after surgery. Physiotherapy and occupational therapy of the wrist and thumb begin following union.

Advantages of Wrist Arthrodesis in Brachial Plexus Patients

Wrist, first CMC, and thumb IP joint arthrodeses are used as secondary adjunctive procedures to improve hand function, hand control, and appearance in patients with a brachial plexus injury by increasing stability. These arthrodeses provided the maximal biomechanical advantage of the tenodeses or transferred gracilis muscle by obtaining improved finger and thumb flexion through stable joints. Addosooki et al. [1] performed an isolated wrist arthrodesis following a double free muscle transfer and found the mean total active motion of the fingers was 39° ± 21° before arthrodesis and 49° ± 25° afterward, a statistically significant difference ($P = 0.001$). Wrist arthrodesis provides improved grasp by creating

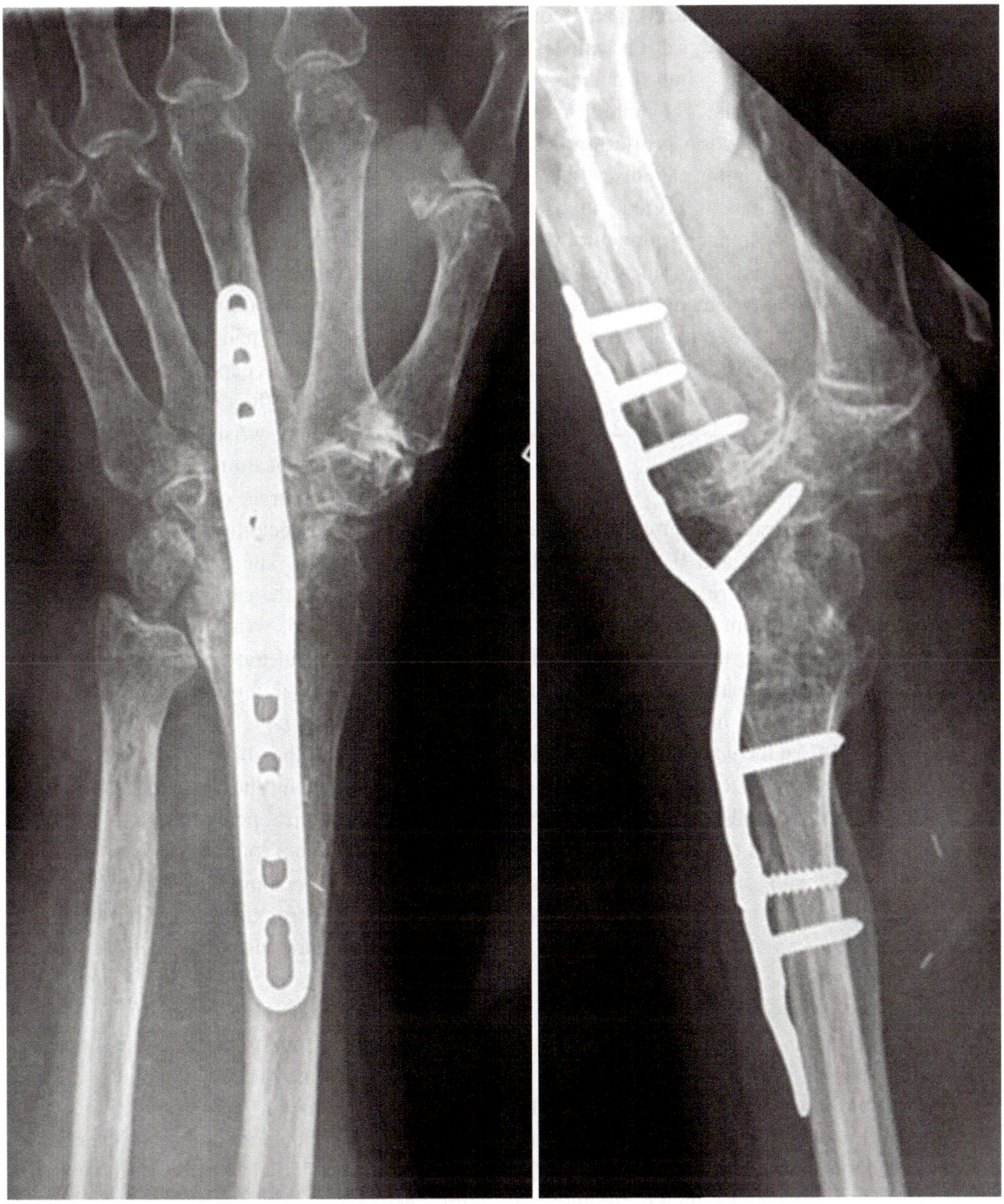

Fig. 19.1 Radiographic evidence of wrist, first CMC joint, and IP joint union by 6 weeks

mechanical efficiency as contraction of the transferred gracilis muscle pulls the fingers across a stable wrist joint. Terzis and Barmpitsioti [13] found that of 35 patients treated with wrist arthrodesis and free muscle transfer for finger flexion/extension, 31 patients had enhanced overall upper limb function with wrist arthrodesis, and 34 patients were satisfied with their achieved wrist stability [13]. The post-arthrodesis Disabilities of the Arm, Shoulder, and Hand (DASH) score was 59 ± 13 indicating moderate ability in daily activities [13]. A pre-arthrodesis DASH score was not documented. Giuffre et al. assessed 24 patients with brachial plexus injuries and demonstrated a statistically significant improvement in DASH scores (from 51 pre-operation to 28 post-operation), pain scores (from 5.3 pre-operation to 3.2 post-operation), as well as patient-perceived improvements in appearance, function, ease of daily cares, hygiene, pain, and satisfaction post-arthrodeses [14]. Several authors treating patients with brachial plexus injuries have reported improved upper extremity appearance following wrist arthrodesis [12, 13, 19, 20]. Van Heest and Strothman reported improvements in appearance and hygiene in 94–100% of patients with spastic wrist deformities [11].

Potential Complications

Most patients demonstrate radiographic evidence of wrist, first CMC joint, and IP joint union by 6 weeks (range 5–10). There is the potential for higher nonunion rates from disuse osteopenia in this population; however, this has not been the case in our brachial plexus patients. Complications of arthrodesis include nonunion (reported between 5 and 30%)at the wrist or the third CMC joint, infection, hardware complications, extensor tendon adhesions and tenosynovitis, nerve complications, adjacent arthritis, impaction, impingement, and pain [5, 21]. Wrist arthrodesis has a reported overall complication rate of 51–68% [21, 22].

Conclusion

To provide stability while the arthrodesis heals, several fixation options such as intramedullary pin or rod techniques and AO plate fixation techniques exist. Millender and Nalebuff popularized the use of a Steinmann pin as an intramedullary fixation technique for wrist arthrodesis in patients with severe bone loss secondary to rheumatoid arthritis [23]. Although the Steinmann pin is not possible in a small intramedullary canal, the Steinmann pin is drilled into the second or third intermetacarpal webspace and countersunk proximal to the metacarpal heads. Intramedullary techniques have the advantages of decreased operative time, simplicity, short recovery period, reduced cost compared to implants, and the flexibility to position the wrist in the desired position [24]. Presently pre-contoured low-contact dynamic compression titanium plates have been developed specifically for wrist arthrodesis. The plate edges are tapered to avoid prominence and the screw heads are recessed. The plates have a carpal bend to provide 10 degrees of wrist extension. Several studies indicate that power grip is maximally accomplished in slight wrist extension (10–15 degrees) and ulnar deviation [24–26]. The authors of this paper prefer plate fixation for arthrodesis as it offers reliable and reproducible fixation in slight wrist extension with minimal hardware complications post-arthrodesis.

The plate contour is designed to fit with a proximal row carpectomy and removal of the dorsal distal radius. The benefit of the proximal row carpectomy is the ease of plate application, the simplification of wrist fusion as there are a decreased number of joints to be fused, the prevention of ulnocarpal impingement, the ability to harvest cancellous bone graft from the excised carpal bones, and the ability to correct for wrist contractures allowing the wrist to be positioned in the best mechanical position to maximize grip strength. The authors' preference is to perform a proximal row carpectomy with wrist arthrodesis. Alternatively, the proximal carpal row can be incorporated into the fusion.

Incorporation of the third CMC joint within the wrist arthrodesis is controversial. Third CMC joint arthrodesis supposedly prevents micromotion across the joint, thereby potentially alleviating concerns of metal fatigue and failure of the plate over a mobile articulation. Nevertheless, painful third CMC joint nonunion after spanning arthrodesis has been reported [27], with one study reporting nonunion of the third CMC joint in up to 43% of patients [28]. Some have suggested a total wrist arthrodesis using a spanning plate, which does not fuse the CMC joint, arguing that simply bridging the joint using the compression plate is sufficient. Once the wrist is fused, the plate is removed to allow for physiologic motion of the joint [28]. Others advise not to include the third CMC joint within the wrist arthrodesis unless the CMC joint shows pre-existing pathology [28]. The authors' preferred technique is to include the third CMC joint within the fusion mass. With this patient population, we have not had any cases of nonunion.

Given the low morbidity of wrist arthrodesis and the potential for improved upper extremity grasp and pinch, at our center, all patients with complete brachial plexopathies undergo wrist arthrodesis as part of their upper extremity reconstruction. Once patients are stable from the nerve transfers and free functioning muscle transfers, a wrist arthrodesis is performed.

References

1. Addosooki A, Doi K, Hattori Y, Wahegaonkar A. Role of wrist arthrodesis in patients receiving double free muscle transfers for reconstruction following complete brachial plexus paralysis. J Hand Surg. 2012;37A:277–81.
2. Hastings H II. Wrist arthrodesis. In: Green PD, Hotchkins NR, Pederson CW, editors. Green's operative hand surgery, vol. 1. 4th ed. New York: Churchill Livingstone; 1998. p. 131–46.
3. Hayden RJ, Jebson PJ. Wrist arthrodesis. Hand Clin. 2005;21:631–40.
4. Rizzo M. Thumb arthrodesis. Tech Hand Up Extrem Surg. 2006;10:43–6.
5. Rizzo M, Moran SL, Shin AY. Long-term outcomes of trapeziometacarpal arthrodesis in the management of trapeziometacarpal arthritis. J Hand Surg. 2009;34A:20–6.
6. Stark HH, Moore JF, Ashworth CR, Byes JH. Fusion of the first metacarpotrapezial joint for degenerative arthritis. J Bone Joint Surg. 1977;59A:22–6.
7. Carroll RE, Hill NA. Arthrodesis of the carpometacarpal joint of the thumb. J Bone Joint Surg. 1973;55B:292–4.
8. Leach RE, Bolton PE. Arthritis of the carpometacarpal joint of the thumb. J Bone Joint Surg. 1968;50A:1171–7.
9. Ishida O, Ikuta Y. Trapeziometacarpal joint arthrodesis for the treatment of arthrosis. Scand J Plast Reconstr Surg Hand Surg. 2000;34:245–8.
10. Schroder J, Kerkhoffs GM, Voerman HJ, Marti RK. Surgical treatment of basal joint disease of the thumb: comparison between resection-interposition arthroplasty and trapeziometacarpal arthrodesis. Arch Orthop Trauma Surg. 2002;122:35–8.
11. Van Heest AE, Strothman D. Wrist arthrodesis in cerebral palsy. J Hand Surg. 2009;34A:1216–24.
12. Addosooki A, Doi K, Hattori Y, Wahegaonkar A. Wrist arthrodesis after double free-muscle transfer in traumatic total brachial plexus palsy. Tech Hand Up Extrem Surg. 2007;11:29–36.
13. Terzis J, Barmpitsioti A. Wrist fusion in posttraumatic brachial plexus palsy. Plast Reconstr Surg. 2009;124:2027–39.
14. Giuffre JL, Bishop AT, Spinner RJ, Kircher MF, Shin AY. Wrist, first carpometacarpal joint, and thumb interphalangeal joint arthrodesis in patients with brachial plexus injuries. J Hand Surg Am. 2012;37(12):2557–63.
15. Giuffre JL, Kakar S, Bishop AT, Spinner R. Shin AY current concepts of the treatment of adult brachial plexus injuries. J Hand Surg. 2010;35A:678–88.
16. Bishop AT. Functioning free-muscle transfer for brachial plexus injury. Hand Clin. 2005;21:91–102.
17. Shin AY, Spinner RJ, Steinmann SP, Bishop AT. Adult traumatic brachial plexus injuries. J Am Acad Orthop Surg. 2005;13:382–96.
18. Doi K, Muramatsu K, Hattori Y, Otsuka K, Tan SH, Nanda V, et al. Restoration of prehension with the double free muscle technique following compete avulsion of the brachial plexus. Indications and long-term results. J Bone Joint Surg. 2000;82A:652–66.
19. Mackenzie GI. Arthrodesis of the wrist in reconstructive surgery. J Bone Joint Surg. 1960;42:60–4.
20. Ruhmann O, Schmolke S, Bohnsack M, Carls J, Flamme C, Wirth CJ. Reconstructive operations for the upper limb after brachial plexus palsy. Am J Orthop. 2004;33:351–62.
21. Hastings H 2nd, Weiss AP, Quenzer D, Wiedeman GP, Hanington KR, Strickland JW. Arthrodesis of the wrist for post-traumatic disorders. J Bone Joint Surg. 1996;78A:897–902.
22. Zachary SV, Stern PJ. Complications following AO/ASIF wrist arthrodesis. J Hand Surg. 1995;20A:339–44.
23. Millender LH, Nalebuff EA. Arthrodesis of the rheumatoid wrist. An evaluation of sixty patients and a description of a different surgical technique. J Bone Joint Surg. 1973;55(5):1026–34.
24. Hastings H II. Arthrodesis (partial and complete). In: Green PD, Hotchkins NR, Pederson CW, Wolfe SW, editors. Green's operative hand surgery, vol. 1. 5th ed. Pennsylvania: Churchill Livingstone; 1998: Chp. 38,. p. 489.
25. Pryce JC. The wrist position between netural and ulnar deviation that facilitates the maximum power grip strength. J Biomech. 1980;13(6):505–11.
26. Rayhack JM, Wood MB. In: Cooney WP, Linscheid RL, Dobyns JH, editors. The wrist: diagnosis and operative treatment, vol. 2. Missouri: Mosby; 1998: Chp. 38.
27. Rancy SK, Ek ET, Paul S, Hotchkiss RN, Wolfe SW. Nonspanning total wrist arthrodesis with a low-profile locking plate. J Wrist Surg. 2018;7(2):127–32.
28. Nagy L, Buchler U. AO-wrist arthrodesis: with and without arthrodesis of the third carpometacarpal joint. J Hand Surg. 2002;27(6):940–7.

Part IV

Surgical Approaches

20 Supraclavicular Exposure of the Brachial Plexus

Ross C. Puffer and Robert J. Spinner

Operating Room Set-Up/Positioning

There are many aspects of a supraclavicular brachial plexus exploration and reconstruction that must be considered initially during the operating room set-up and patient positioning to ensure that there is appropriate access to all potential surgical corridors and graft harvest sites during the procedure as needed. Equipment should include a surgeon's headlight and loupes for initial exposure, both monopolar (Bovie®, Bovie Medical Corporation, Clearwater, FL) and bipolar electrocautery, an operative microscope for microsurgical repairs, intraoperative neuromonitoring/EMG to allow for motor evoked potentials (MEP), and nerve to nerve or muscle recordings. The patient will need to be secured to the operating room table using safety straps, and a normothermia system (such as the underbody 3M ™ Bair Hugger, St. Paul, MN) should be utilized as the large area of exposed skin could lead to difficulties maintaining appropriate patient temperature.

Anesthetic considerations include general anesthesia without the use of nondepolarizing muscle relaxants and/or nitrous oxide during electrodiagnostic testing portions of the procedure. Access for the anesthesiologist can be difficult, as in many cases only one extremity will be available to the anesthesia team during the case, and he/she should plan for an arterial line as well as large bore IV access in the single exposed arm. A urinary catheter should be utilized during the case. The endotracheal tube should be secured above the ears with tape and should be directed to the opposite side of the planned brachial plexus exposure.

The patient should be in the supine position on the OR table with the head turned to the opposite side of the planned neck incision with the head resting on a donut. A bump can be placed between the shoulder blades, and the neck, in some extension to facilitate the clavicle as the highest point of the exposed field. The extended neck turned to the opposite side allows for expanded access to the supraclavicular region and helps to highlight the sternocleidomastoid muscle (SCM) for incision planning. The back of the OR table is elevated, and the legs are dropped slightly, so the patient is in a semi-beach chair position. If access to the posterior shoulder is required, a bump can be placed under the torso to facilitate a semilateral position allowing access to both the supraclavicular and posterior arm/shoulder regions. The arm on the side of the planned surgery is placed in a stocking, and a non-perforating towel clamp is used to clip the stocking to the OR drapes, thus holding the arm in a slightly flexed position but allowing for active movement during

R. C. Puffer · R. J. Spinner (✉)
Mayo Clinic, Department of Neurologic Surgery, Rochester, MN, USA
e-mail: spinner.robert@mayo.edu

A. Y. Shin, N. Pulos (eds.), *Operative Brachial Plexus Surgery*,
https://doi.org/10.1007/978-3-030-69517-0_20

the case. A portable surgical instrument stand (e.g., Mayo Stand, USA Medical and Surgical Supplies, St. Louis, MO) is utilized during the case to support the arm in an abducted, externally rotated position to allow for arm/forearm exposure during reconstruction and grafting. The contralateral arm is tucked. Access of both lower limbs should be planned for harvest of sural nerve (s) and/or free functioning (gracilis) muscle.

The neck (to the ear) and the entire arm are prepped, as is the ipsilateral chest wall to midline and posterior shoulder to the mid-axillary line on the operative side. A sterile U-drape is used to drape around the operative field, and the edges of the U-drape are covered in 3M™ Ioban strips. Both legs are circumferentially prepped above the knee in the case of planned sural nerve harvest, and up to the groin when a free functioning muscle is required.

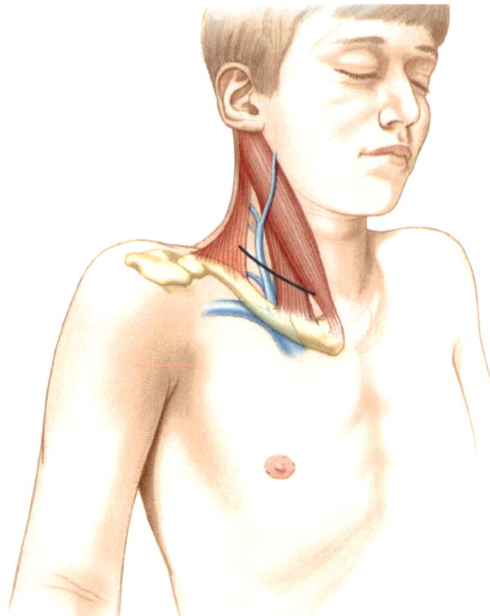

Fig. 20.1 Planned incision to the supraclavicular brachial plexus

Exposure

A transverse incision is planned in one of Langer's lines approximately 2–3 fingerbreadths above the clavicle. The incision should span from the trapezius to the SCM, usually centered on the external jugular vein which can often be seen (Fig. 20.1). Alternatively, a zig-zag incision can be planned, running parallel to the lateral border of SCM from the region just below the tip of the mastoid down to the clavicle, then running along the clavicle laterally toward the trapezius. Either the transverse or the zig-zag incisions allows for easy addition or extension of an extra incision in the deltopectoral groove to allow for incorporation of an infraclavicular brachial plexus exposure.

After incision, the platysma is divided in line with the incision. Generous subplatysmal flaps are developed both superiorly and inferiorly to improve the excursion of the exposure. The external jugular vein is encountered and can be protected in a vessel loop and retracted (Fig. 20.2). Typically, for access to the upper brachial plexus elements as in posttraumatic cases, we prefer mobilizing the external jugular vein, medially; for access to the lower brachial plexus elements

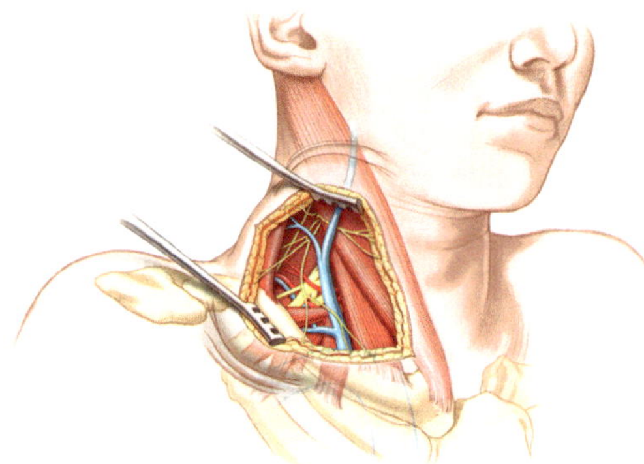

Fig. 20.2 Superficial dissection to the level of the omohyoid

as in thoracic outlet surgery, we prefer mobilizing it laterally.

In many cases, supraclavicular nerves arising from the cervical plexus are exposed and protected when possible. These nerves can be traced back to their origins at C3-C4 if necessary. Next, the cleidal attachment of the SCM should be disconnected from the clavicle. The omohyoid muscle is identified. Dissection of the omohyoid (medially toward the internal jugular vein and laterally, the suprascapular notch) enhances visualization of the relevant anatomy. It can then

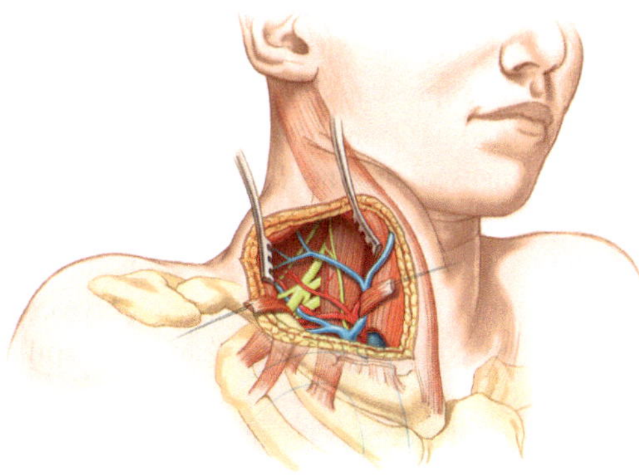

Fig. 20.3 Dissection deep to the omohyoid

either be retracted or divided with tag stitches on either end. These stitches can be pulled laterally and medially to aid in exposure (Fig. 20.3). The fat pad is then seen. Often times the plexus components can be palpated just below the fat pad. The fat pad is then cauterized (bipolar) and mobilized laterally. Dissection is then done in a perpendicular trajectory connecting the mid-point of the lateral edge of the SCM to the clavicle. Depending on the exposure needed, the clavicle can be partially exposed (or completely skeletonized, mobilized, and retracted) and subclavius divided; for brachial plexus trauma, we have not needed to osteotomize the clavicle.

The dorsal scapular and suprascapular vessels may be encountered, and they can be ligated and divided. The phrenic nerve can be visualized running along the surface of the scalene anterior muscle. It should be dissected free and protected in a vessel loop (Fig. 20.4). Confirmation of the phrenic nerve can be achieved using direct stimulation, which should cause contraction of the ipsilateral hemidiaphragm. When identified and dissected free, the phrenic nerve can be traced toward its origin at C5 and further cephalad.

After identification of C5, it can be traced distally to the upper trunk and suprascapular nerve and anterior and posterior divisions of the upper trunk. When the upper trunk is dissected free and placed in a vessel loop, C6 can be exposed by furthering the dissection proximally from the upper trunk inferior to C5.

Typically, more proximal exposure is needed. A portion of the anterior scalene muscle can be resected to allow the spinal nerves of the brachial plexus to be dissected to the foramen of the cervical spine (Fig. 20.5). The transverse processes can be carefully removed with a rongeur, but consideration must be given to the vertebral artery, which runs in close proximity to the nerves at the level of the foramen. Resecting a portion of scalene anterior is usually needed for exposure of C7. The transverse cervical artery will need to be ligated and divided. The C7 nerve and middle trunk lie medial and inferior to the upper trunk.

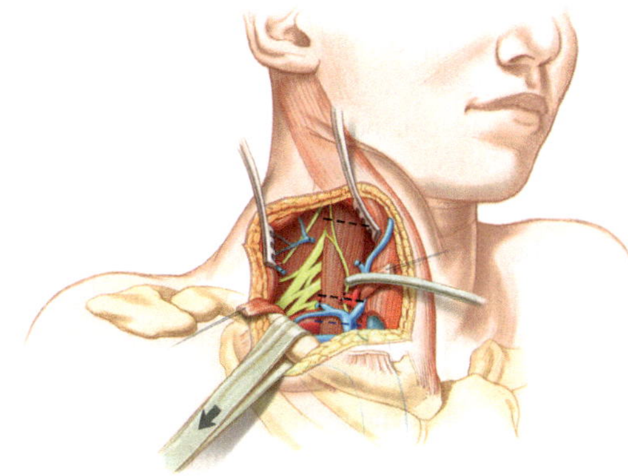

Fig. 20.4 Identification of the phrenic nerve and the brachial plexus. Dashed lines illustrate the potential resection of the scalene anterior during the exposure of the brachial plexus

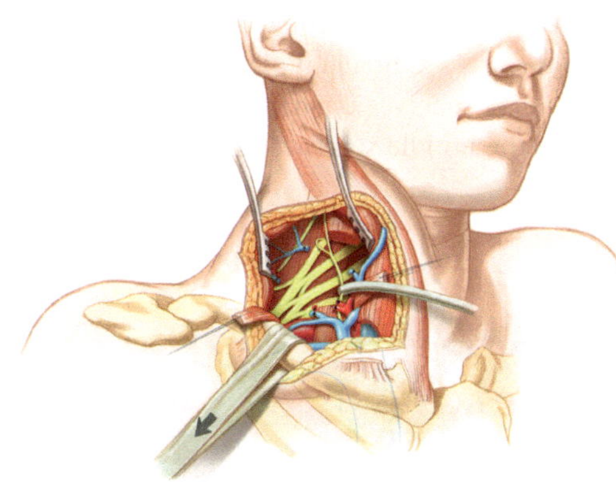

Fig. 20.5 Resection of the scalene anterior allows proximal exposure of the brachial plexus elements

Because of poor results of grafting lower trunk elements, brachial plexus exploration of C8 and T1 is not performed. If C8 and T1 are exposed, the subclavian artery will need to be identified and mobilized. The subclavian artery is posterior to the scalene anterior muscle (the subclavian vein lies anterior). The relative position of the subclavian artery to C8 and T1 is somewhat variable, but it is typically anterior and inferior. The C8 and T1 nerves and lower trunk lie deep to the C7 nerve and can be identified and isolated in vessel loops. Care must be taken to avoid injuring the pleura, which can often be visualized just below the T1 nerve [1].

In brachial plexus trauma, there may be significant scarring within the upper trunk, or even a complete rupture, making this portion of the dissection more difficult. It is best to identify normal anatomy where present and then expose proximally and distally from that point to dissect through scar tissue and identify either a neuroma in continuity or complete rupture (Fig. 20.6).

When the injury is significant and scarring is severe, C6 may not be easy to identify. The long thoracic nerve may be utilized indirectly to help lay out a scarred brachial plexus. The long thoracic nerve receives contributions from C5-C7, pierces the middle scalene, and then runs along the chest wall to innervate the serratus anterior muscle. Identifying the long thoracic nerve deep to the suprascapular nerve (lateral to the scalene medius), and tracing it proximally through the scalene medius, may provide an alternative approach to identifying the proximal C6 nerve. Contraction of the serratus anterior with stimulation of the long thoracic nerve confirms a postganglionic injury at that spinal nerve level.

In cases of neurogenic thoracic outlet syndrome, a slightly lower transverse incision is utilized. Scalene anterior is resected and then scalene medius is divided. Dissection of the entire supraclavicular brachial plexus is done with concentration on proximal dissection of the lower trunk and C8 and T1 nerves to the level of the foramina. Subclavian artery is mobilized medially toward the vertebral artery takeoff. Bony protuberances (i.e., elongated transverse process or cervical rib) are then removed.

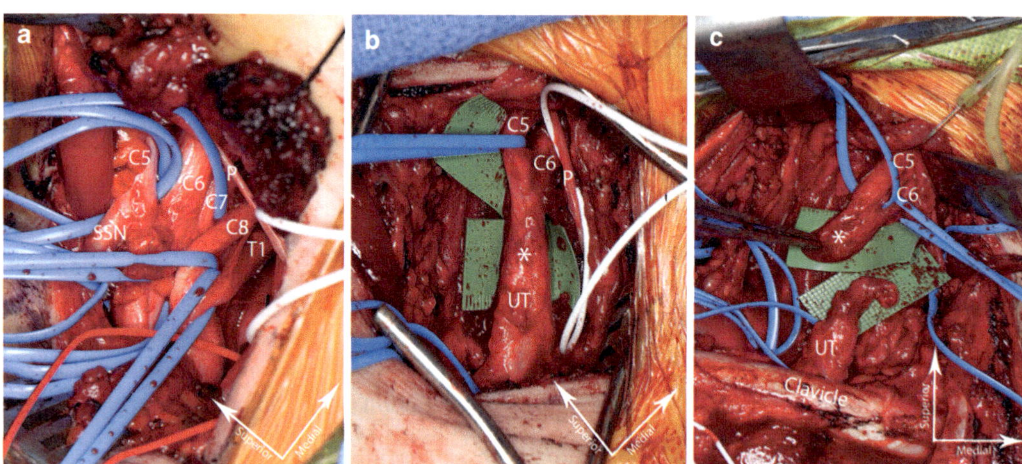

Fig. 20.6 Operative pictures: (**a**) Right brachial plexus exposure for a patient undergoing surgery for thoracic outlet syndrome. After anterior scalenectomy, there is good exposure of all spinal nerves (C5-T1) of the brachial plexus; phrenic (P) and suprascapular nerves (SSN). (**b**) Right brachial plexus exposure with a neuroma in continuity (asterisk) of the upper trunk (UT). The suprascapular nerve is seen (just above the retractor blade) at its takeoff just at the inferior margin of the neuroma. The suprascapular nerve can then be used as a distal target for grafting or transfer. (**c**) Right brachial plexus exposure with rupture (asterisk) of the upper trunk (UT). The suprascapular nerve is in a vessel loop just above the clavicle. The rupture has caused the upper trunk to retract distally underneath the clavicle. Phrenic nerve is not seen in this photograph

Spinal Accessory Nerve

The spinal accessory nerve is created by a combination of cranial and spinal nerves. It descends in the posterior triangle of the neck in an oblique fashion. It can be identified more cranially approximately 1.5 cm above the great auricular nerve as it wraps around the SCM. From this point, the spinal accessory nerve traverses obliquely toward the trapezius muscle where it runs along the medial border before diving deep along the muscle to provide its innervation. We prefer to identify the spinal accessory nerve several centimeters above the clavicle on the medial border of the trapezius muscle during supraclavicular brachial plexus exploration. Intraoperative stimulation can be useful to identify the nerve. When identified, it can be dissected both proximally and distally along its course to obtain adequate length for either direct nerve transfer or as a donor with interpositional grafting. If using as a neurotizer, major proximal branches to the trapezius should be preserved in order to avoid complete denervation of the trapezius muscle.

Reference

1. Kim DH, Hudson AR, Kline DG. Atlas of peripheral nerve surgery. Philadelphia: Elsevier; Chapter 2: the brachial plexus. 2013.

Infraclavicular Exposure of the Brachial Plexus

21

Shelley S. Noland and Pelagia Kouloumberis

Indications for Use

The infraclavicular brachial plexus comprises the cords that result from the anterior and posterior divisions as well as the terminal branches. Indications for infraclavicular brachial plexus exposure are not as common as the supraclavicular approach, as traumatic injuries in this area are infrequent. Surgical exposure of the infraclavicular brachial plexus may be used for resection of tumors, repair of traumatic lacerations, and nerve grafting.

Operating Room Set-Up and Positioning

Operating room set-up/positioning/anesthetic considerations and equipment are as described in the previous chapter. The patient should be in the supine position on the OR table with the head turned to the opposite side of the planned arm incision. The head should be resting comfortably on a head support such as a gel donut. The arm for the planned surgery is placed on a hand table attached to the OR table. The contralateral arm is tucked. Access of both lower limbs should be planned for possible harvest of sural nerve(s) and/or free-functioning (gracilis) muscle. Prepping and draping are as described in the previous chapter. The entire neck and upper quadrant of the chest should be prepped and draped in the event that a supraclavicular dissection is needed [1–4].

Exposure

The skin incision is marked along the deltopectoral groove, from the junction of the middle and lateral thirds of the clavicle to the anterior axillary fold (Fig. 21.1). Abduction of the arm can facilitate identification of the deltopectoral groove. The surgeon may opt to use a local anesthetic/epinephrine infiltration to facilitate hemo-

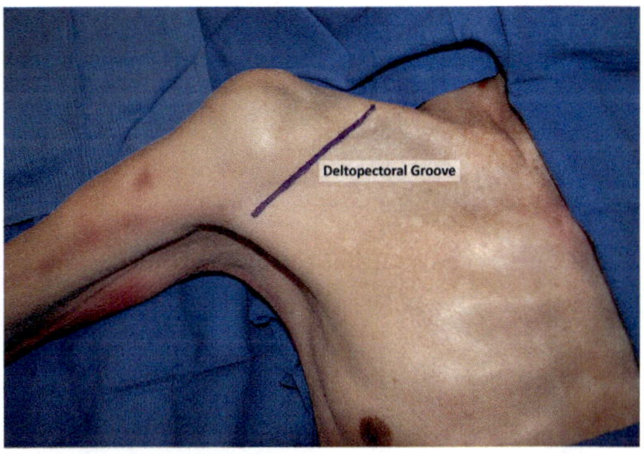

Fig. 21.1 Deltopectoral groove

S. S. Noland (✉) · P. Kouloumberis
Plastic & Orthopedic Surgery, Peripheral Nerve/Brachial Plexus Clinic, Mayo Clinic College of Medicine, Mayo Clinic Arizona, Phoenix, AZ, USA
e-mail: Noland.Shelley@mayo.edu; Kouloumberis.Pelagia@mayo.edu

A. Y. Shin, N. Pulos (eds.), *Operative Brachial Plexus Surgery*,
https://doi.org/10.1007/978-3-030-69517-0_21

stasis (1% lidocaine with 1:200,000 epinephrine is common).

The skin is incised; the first structure identified is the cephalic vein, which resides in the deltopectoral groove (Fig. 21.2). This is an important landmark to confirm that the dissection is proceeding in the proper location. The cephalic vein should be mobilized and preserved (i.e., for possible future free functioning muscle venous outflow) but can be safely ligated and transected if necessary. The interval between the deltoid and pectoralis muscle is identified and bluntly retracted to identify the clavipectoral fascia, the coracoid, and the pectoralis minor tendon (Fig. 21.3). This tendon can be identified as it inserts onto the coracoid process. The superior and inferior portions of the pectoralis minor tendon are identified, and the tendon is divided and tagged such that it can be repaired at the end of the surgery. If additional exposure is necessary, the deltoid and pectoralis major muscles can be elevated off the clavicle (typically done in conjunction with a supraclavicular approach). Medial retraction of the divided pectoralis minor muscle will allow for identification of the cords of the brachial plexus. The lateral cord (formed from the anterior divisions of the upper and middle trunks, C5-C7) is typically the most anterior cord and should be the first cord to be identified (Fig. 21.4). A vessel loop is placed around the lateral cord and it is dissected distally. The surgeon may encounter the small lateral pectoral nerve which branches off the lateral cord in this region. Further distally, the lateral cord divides into the musculocutaneous nerve (Fig. 21.5) and the lateral cord contribution to the median nerve. The lateral cord contribution to the median nerve is the sensory component and may have fibers to flexor carpi radialis and pronator teres. These two structures (the muscu-

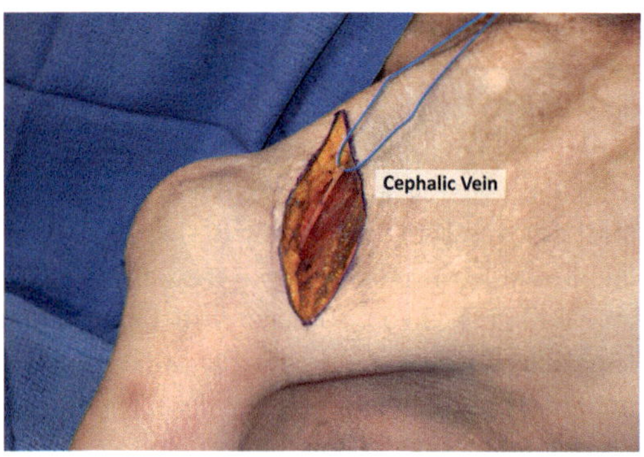

Fig. 21.2 Cephalic vein in deltopectoral groove

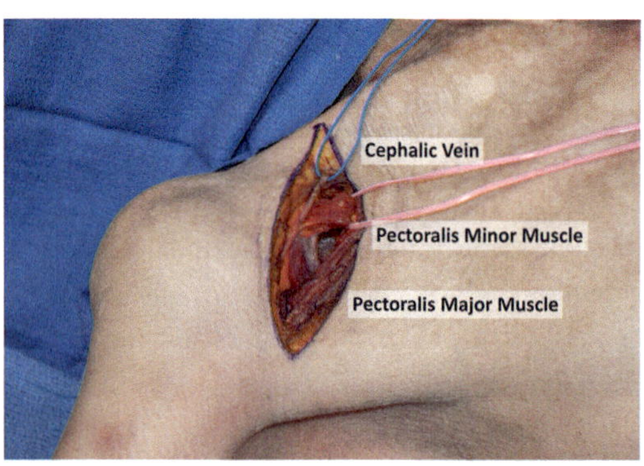

Fig. 21.3 Pectoralis minor tendon

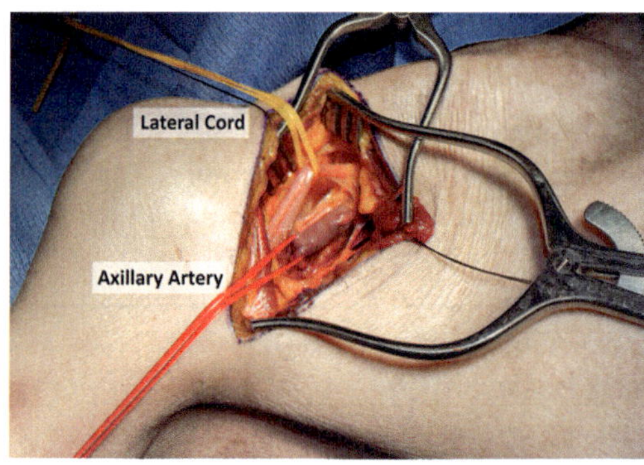

Fig. 21.4 Lateral cord of the brachial plexus (yellow vessel loop) and axillary artery (red vessel loop)

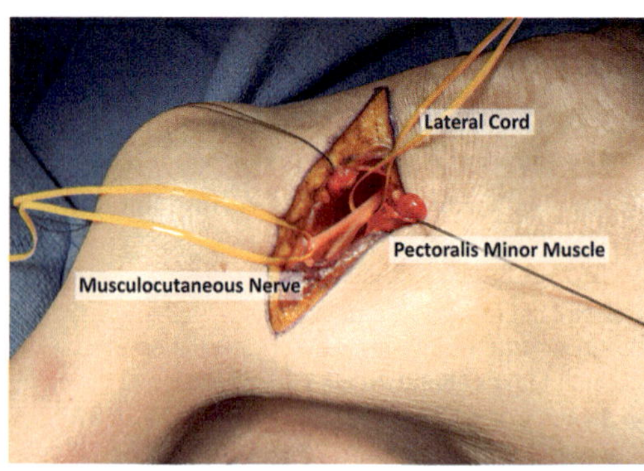

Fig. 21.5 Lateral cord (proximal) with musculocutaneous nerve (distal)

locutaneous nerve and the lateral cord contribution to the median nerve) comprise the lateral ½ of the "M" classically described infraclavicular plexus. If the patient is not paralyzed, and there is no nerve injury, handheld stimulation of the identified nerves can confirm their function. The musculocutaneous nerve is very important clinically, as it provides biceps and brachialis function and is critical for elbow flexion. This nerve is a common recipient for nerve transfers to restore elbow flexion [1–4].

The lateral cord (named relative to its position in relation to the axillary artery) is then retracted laterally, and the axillary artery can be identified and looped medial to the lateral cord (Fig. 21.4). Care is taken to avoid compression, stretching, or violation of the axillary artery, and it is handled delicately throughout the surgery. During dissection, it may be necessary to ligate branches of the axillary artery [1–4].

Once the axillary artery has been identified and is looped, the surgeon can carefully and gently retract it (along with the lateral and medial cords) medially to identify the posterior cord which is also looped (Fig. 21.6). The posterior cord (formed from the posterior divisions of upper, middle, and lower trunks, C5-T1) is then traced distally, in a similar fashion to the lateral cord, to identify the radial nerve, axillary nerve, thoracodorsal nerve, and subscapular nerve (Fig. 21.7). The most clinically relevant components of the posterior cord are the radial and axillary nerves as these are commonly used in nerve transfer surgery. The axillary nerve is typically the most difficult to identify as it loops posteriorly deep in the axilla. The easiest way for the surgeon to identify this nerve is to trace the branches of the posterior cord along the axillary artery. With gentle traction of the axillary artery, a large posterior humeral circumflex branch can be identified. This branch loops posteriorly through the quadrangular space, and *immediately superior* to it lies the axillary artery. The axillary artery can be gently identified using a single looped finger above this artery. The surgeon may consider using a Doppler to help identify the posterior circumflex humeral artery if needed. Once identified, the axillary nerve is looped, and gentle retraction will reveal its four branches. The four branches include the sensory branch (the smallest and most inferior branch), the teres minor branch, and the anterior and posterior axillary nerve branches. The axillary nerve proper is a common recipient for nerve transfers designed to reinnervate the deltoid muscle [1–4].

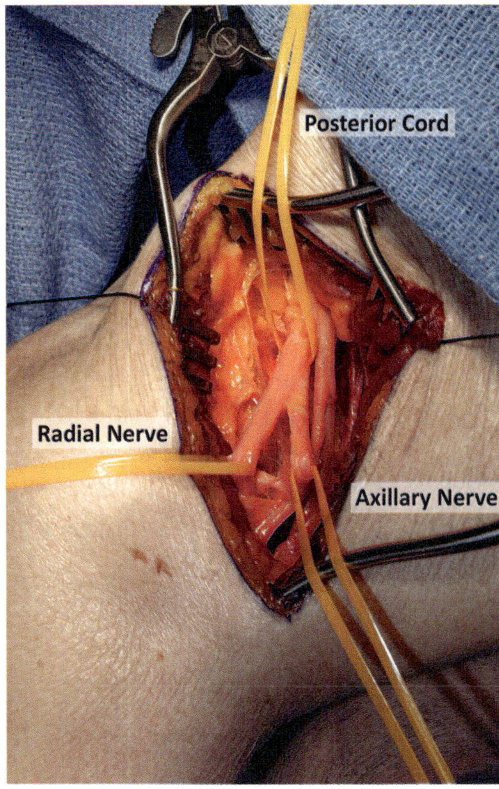

Fig. 21.7 Posterior cord with axillary and radial nerve branches (axillary artery removed)

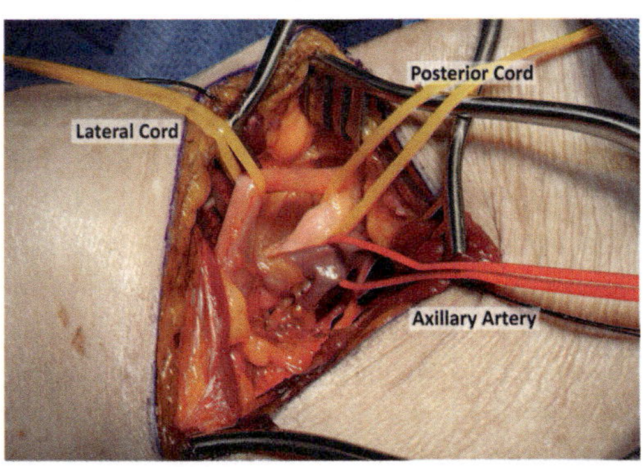

Fig. 21.6 Posterior cord of the brachial plexus (between lateral cord and axillary artery)

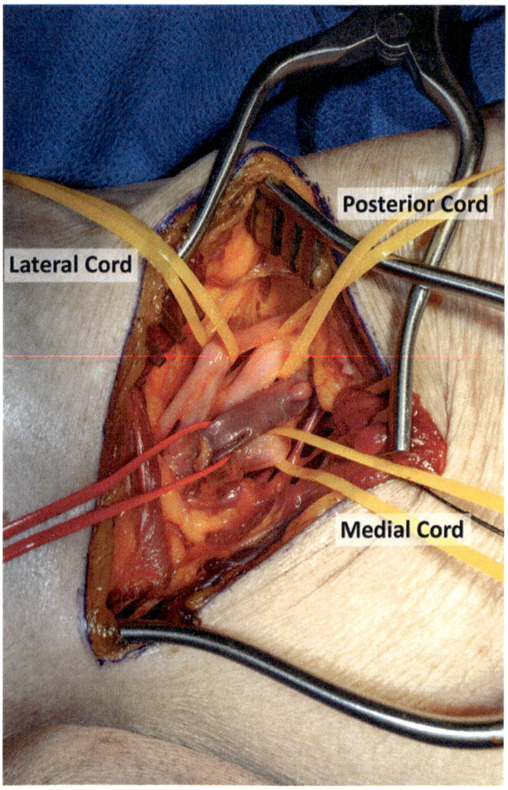

Fig. 21.8 Lateral, posterior, and medial cords of the brachial plexus

Medial to the axillary artery, the medial cord is identified and looped (Fig. 21.8). The medial cord (formed from the anterior division of the lower trunk, C8-T1) will give off the medial pectoral nerve and the medial brachial and antebrachial cutaneous nerves before terminating in the ulnar nerve and medial cord contribution to the median nerve. The medial pectoral nerve is clinically relevant as it can be used as a donor nerve for nerve transfer. There are several branches of this nerve that can be identified entering the undersurface of the pectoralis minor muscle. These must be handled delicately as they are very small branches. If not paralyzed, nerve stimulator can facilitate identification. The medial brachial and antebrachial cutaneous nerves can be used as nerve grafts if they are not functioning as sensory nerves. The medial antebrachial cutaneous nerve can be identified running along the basilic vein in the upper arm. The medial cord contribution to the median nerve is the motor

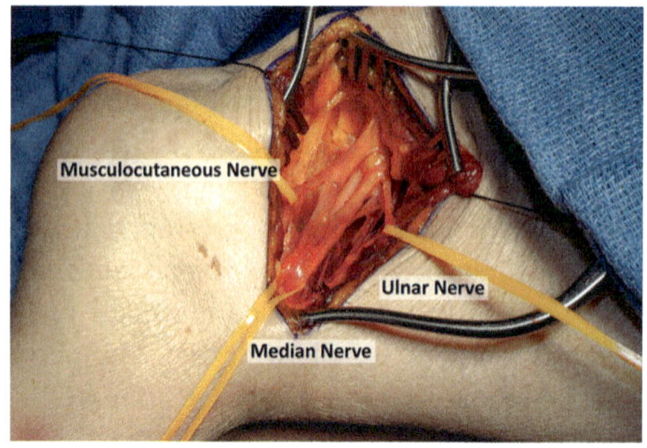

Fig. 21.9 Lateral and medial cord contributions to the median nerve (with M-shape overlay)

component. The medial cord contribution to the median nerve and the ulnar nerve comprise the medial ½ of the medial component of the "M" formation. The median nerve (with contributions from both the lateral and medial cords) forms the center of the "M" (Fig. 21.9). This "M" configuration is very helpful for the surgeon to identify the major components of the brachial plexus and give confidence that the dissection is progressing as planned [1–4].

If additional exposure is needed superiorly, the clavicle can be looped with an umbilical tape and gently retracted superiorly to identify the divisions of the brachial plexus, or extension of the incision parallel to the clavicle can be undertaken as described in the supraclavicular exploration chapter. After dissection and surgery is completed, the surgeon may opt to repair the pectoralis minor tendon before closing the skin.

The surgeon will undoubtedly discover anatomic variations and this can confuse dissection. In the infraclavicular region, there are some commonly encountered variations. The thoracodorsal nerve, for example, can branch off of the axillary nerve rather than the posterior cord. The ulnar nerve can receive contribution from the lateral cord in some patients. The median nerve may receive more than one contribution from the lateral cord or may receive a contribution from the posterior cord or the musculocutaneous nerve. On occasion, the lateral cord may receive contribution from C7. Of course, the surgeon may encounter additional variations and needs to be consider this possibility if the dissection is not straightforward. With experience, patterns emerge, and the surgeon can confidently identify structures, even in the setting of variations.

Complication Avoidance

Complication avoidance in brachial plexus surgery begins with a thorough understanding of the anatomy and normal variants that may be encountered. Developing a normal anatomic plane during repeat procedures is crucial in avoiding injury to the underlying nerves and vasculature. Use of intraoperative stimulation may also mitigate injury to important structures. We prefer to use a handheld stimulator which allows direct stimulation of structures and may decrease the cost and user error associated with other forms of conventional monitoring.

As with most procedures, meticulous dissection and hemostasis may help avoid vascular injury or the formation of a post-operative surgical site hematoma.

References

1. Maniker AH. Operative exposures in peripheral nerve surgery. New York: Thieme Medical Publishers, Inc; 2005. p. 15–21.
2. Midha R, Zager EL. Surgery of peripheral nerves. New York: Thieme Medical Publishers, Inc; 2008. p. 15.
3. Nader R, Berta SC, Gragnaniello C, Sabbath AJ, Levy ML. Neurosurgery tricks of the trade: spine and peripheral nerves. New York: Thieme Medical Publishers, Inc; 2014. p. 423–5.
4. Socolovsky M, Rasulic L, Midha R, Garozzo D. Manual of peripheral nerve surgery. Stuttgart: Georg Thieme Verlag KG; 2018. p. 3.

Posterior Approach for Spinal Accessory to Suprascapular Nerve Transfer

22

Nikhil K. Murthy and Robert J. Spinner

Rationale

The reconstruction of shoulder function is difficult because of the complexity of joint movement carried out by many different muscle groups. Typically, reconstructive efforts target only the deltoid, supraspinatus, and infraspinatus muscles that are critical in stabilization of the joint as well as abduction and external rotation [14]. The two spinati muscles are innervated by the suprascapular nerve with dysfunction of this nerve often being associated with upper brachial plexus injuries. A common nerve transfer is the spinal accessory nerve to the suprascapular nerve; this is performed when proximal reconstruction options are unavailable (such as in avulsion injuries) or when a nerve transfer is selected preferentially over nerve grafting. The spinal accessory nerve transfer to the suprascapular nerve can be accomplished from either anterior or posterior approaches. The anterior approach, first described by Lurje in 1948, is generally used at the time of brachial plexus exploration in cases of multiple nerve or pan-plexus disruption where an anterior approach would have already been used [5]. The posterior approach was first documented in the literature by Bahm et al. in 2005 to address obstetric brachial plexus lesions in children who had recovery of other functions, but lacked clinical improvement of shoulder abduction and external rotation [1]. An advantage of the posterior approach would be decreasing the distance of the nerve transfer to the target muscle(s), but at the disadvantage of having fewer available axons in the terminal branch (1328 proximally versus 817 axons terminally) [16]. The posterior approach has been recommended in cases of predicted double crush injury of the nerve such as with the possibility of compression at the suprascapular notch, as well as the concomitant need for axillary nerve reconstruction in a posterior approach. Some are favoring use of the distal nerve transfer to target the infraspinatus specifically, as it is hypothesized that the supraspinatus muscle preferentially takes the majority of axons during spinal accessory nerve to suprascapular nerve transfer [12, 17].

Technique

The patient is placed prone with the upper back and ipsilateral arm prepped and draped. The spinous processes of the thoracic spine, medial border of the scapula, and acromion are identified both visually and by palpation, and subsequently

N. K. Murthy
Department of Neurological Surgery, Northwestern Memorial Hospital, Chicago, IL, USA
e-mail: nkmurthy@kellogg.northwestern.edu

R. J. Spinner (✉)
Mayo Clinic, Department of Neurologic Surgery, Rochester, MN, USA
e-mail: spinner.robert@mayo.edu

A. Y. Shin, N. Pulos (eds.), *Operative Brachial Plexus Surgery*,
https://doi.org/10.1007/978-3-030-69517-0_22

marked. A point along the incision at 40% from the midline to the acromion along the superior border of the scapula is also marked to indicate the expected region of the distal spinal accessory nerve branches [3]. A midpoint between the acromion and the superior angle of the scapula are also marked to indicate the expected region of the suprascapular notch (Fig. 22.1).

A transverse incision is made along the superior border of the scapula between the acromion and the thoracic spinous processes. Alternatively, two incisions can be used – a medial incision to first find the spinal accessory nerve and a second to find the suprascapular nerve (Fig. 22.2). Dissection is carried out through the subcutaneous layers, fat, and superficial fascia. The trapezius muscle is then encountered and split along its fibers to encounter the sub-trapezius deep fascia. This deep fascia is then dissected to identify another layer of fat within which the distal spinal accessory nerve and branches are found. A nerve stimulator initially set at two milliamps is used within the area of the deep fascia and fat to identify trapezius muscle contraction and therefore identify the areas of distal spinal accessory nerve branches.

Attention is then given to finding the suprascapular notch, which is expected to be midpoint between the medial border of the scapula and the acromion, along the superior border of the scapula (the coracoid anteriorly is a good landmark for the notch). The medial aspect of the notch is identified through further blunt soft tissue dissection with a Kittner, as to avoid the more laterally and superficially located suprascapular vessels. The suprascapular nerve is expected to be deep to the superior transverse scapular ligament (which effectively makes the notch into a foramen). This suprascapular ligament is cut on its medial aspect, and further soft tissue dissection is done to identify the suprascapular nerve (Fig. 22.3).

The donor distal spinal accessory nerve branch is identified and confirmed with the use of a nerve stimulator. Sufficient length of the donor nerve is dissected distally to reach the recipient suprascapular nerve without tension. Direct end to end neurorrhaphy with standard microsurgical technique is performed.

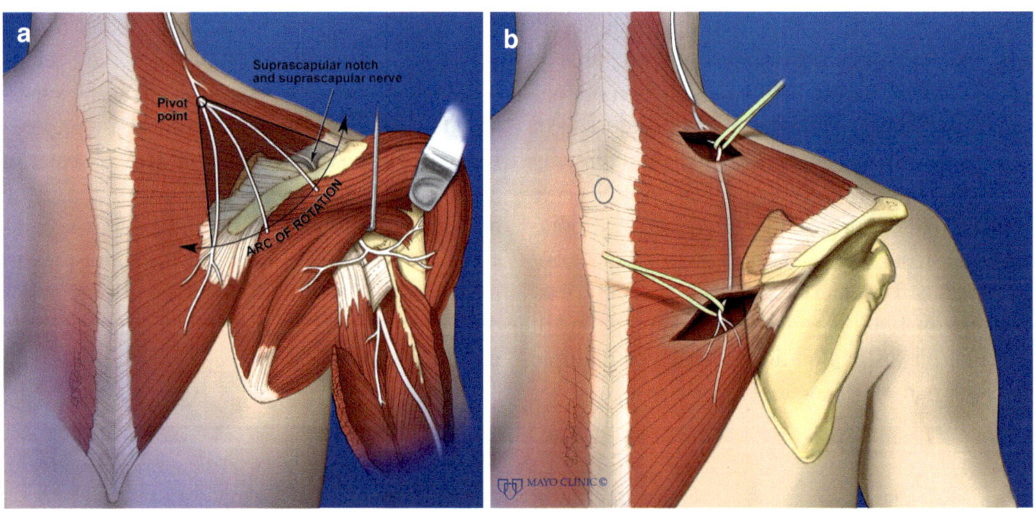

Fig. 22.1 (**a**) Illustration of arc of rotation of distal spinal accessory nerve when estimating sufficient length for transfer to suprascapular nerve. (**b**) Incisions for extended spinal accessory nerve harvest with identification of distal and more proximal portions of the nerve

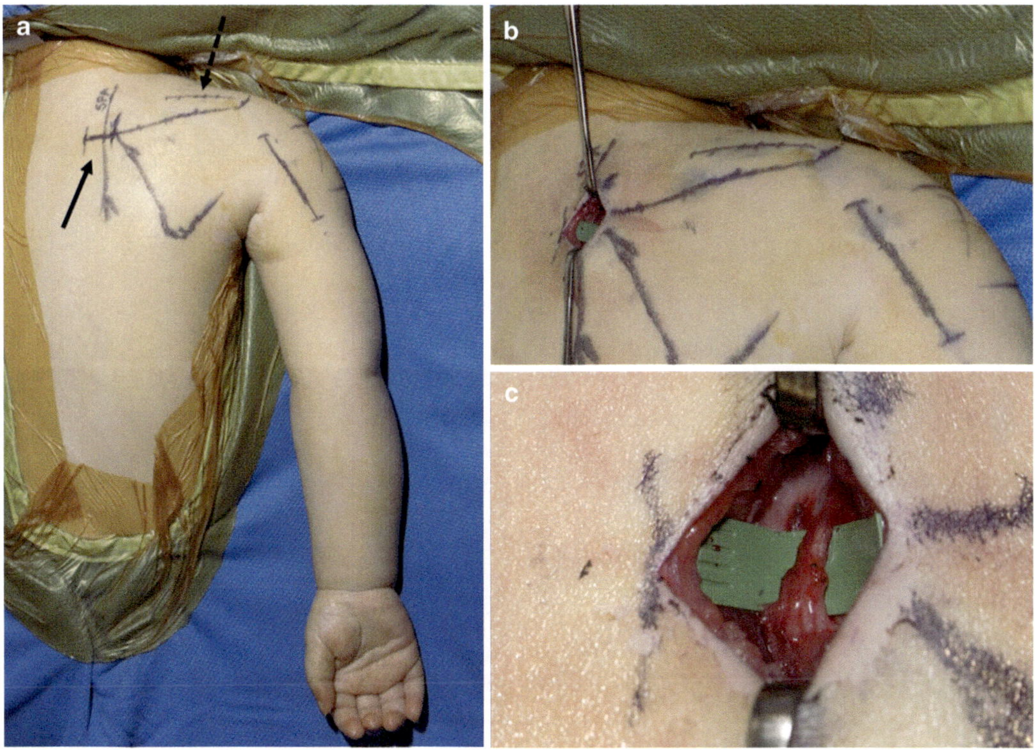

Fig. 22.2 (**a**) Positioning and marking for posterior approach for distal spinal accessory nerve to suprascapular nerve transfer. Two smaller incisions used in this pediatric patient. Solid arrow indicating region in which spinal accessory nerve will be found. Dashed arrow indication incision for identification of suprascapular nerve. (**b**) Initial incision made to dissect and identify distal spinal accessory nerve. (**c**) Distal spinal accessory nerve after circumferential dissection

Outcomes

Overall, the spinal accessory to suprascapular nerve transfer is beneficial in improving shoulder motion in both adults and pediatric patients using anterior or posterior approaches; however, the outcomes may be overestimated and suboptimal [6, 7]. Bertelli et al. reported that up to 95% of patients achieved at least 30 degrees of shoulder abduction in patients with an average age of 26 years old [2]. Malessy et al. reported electromyographic reinnervation of the supraspinatus in 85% of patients and infraspinatus reinnervation in 70% of patients. For strength testing, MRC of grade 3 or 4 for supraspinatus and infraspinatus occurred in 24% and 14% of patients, respectively [6]. From an anterior approach, 76% of patients were able to have direct coaptation of the spinal accessory to suprascapular nerve. Of these patients with direct coaptation, only 25% were able to achieve 60 to 90 degrees of total functional abduction (suprascapular nerve innervated function plus thoracoscapular rotation) [6]. In pediatric cases, anterior and posterior approaches both show some improvements in functional outcomes, although no difference in outcome between approaches was reported [11]. Patients without sufficient shoulder external rotation, who have otherwise recovered spontaneously, are recommended to undergo spinal accessory nerve to suprascapular nerve transfer even in a delayed fashion [15]. However, with an anterior approach in these patients, there is risk of losing previous gains in supraspinatus shoulder abduction,

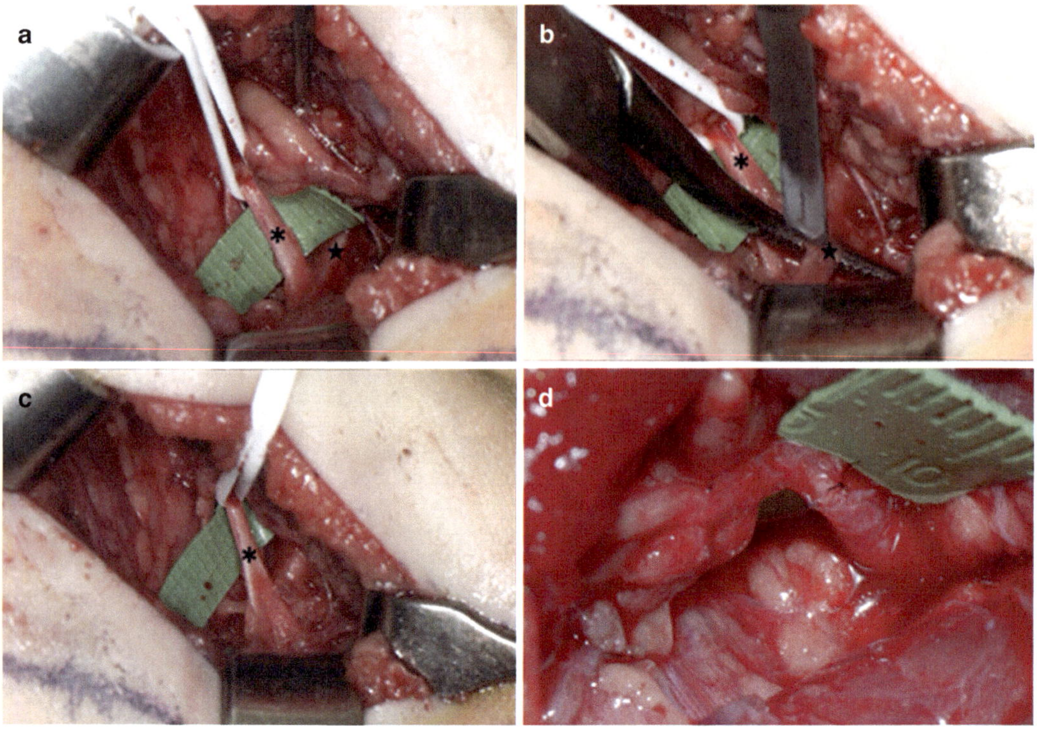

Fig. 22.3 (**a**) Exposure of suprascapular nerve at transverse scapular ligament. (**b**) Release of transverse scapular ligament. (**c**) Appearance of suprascapular nerve after release of ligament. (**d**) Completed transfer of distal spinal accessory nerve to suprascapular nerve. Suprascapular nerve indicated by asterisk. Transverse scapular ligament indicated by star

whereas a posterior approach can offer the potential of saving this function if done distally enough on the suprascapular nerve [12].

The literature is overall mixed as to differences in outcomes between anterior and posterior approaches, although all studies show that the posterior approach is at least equivalent or possibly superior to the anterior approach for specific functional outcomes relating to shoulder function. Electromyographic outcomes were shown to be similar in infraspinatus recovery between approaches [10]. Guan et al. found that a posterior approach was associated with earlier improvement in shoulder abduction and greater degrees of shoulder abduction than the anterior approach, while preserving upper trapezius function [4]. Souza et al. found no difference in the improvement of shoulder abduction, but better results in external arm rotation using a posterior approach compared to the anterior approach [13]. While unclear if either approach is better, the benefits of the posterior approach may be related to the nerves being coapted closer to target muscles, as well as addressing the possibility of double injury at the level of the suprascapular notch as reported in the literature [8, 9].

In summary, both approaches can improve shoulder function. Each has advantages and disadvantages, but outcomes thus far are similar. The anterior approach has been used in cases of multi-nerve reconstruction as part of a supraclavicular brachial plexus exploration. A distal injury to the suprascapular nerve at the notch may be missed. If needed, even a posterior approach for the triceps branch transfer to the anterior division of the axillary nerve can still be done by adducting the arm. The posterior approach can be done if nerve transfers to shoulder targets are being performed without brachial plexus exploration or at a separate posterior stage – e.g., for spinal accessory to suprascapular nerve transfer by itself or in combination with triceps branch to axillary nerve transfer. Performing the spinal accessory nerve transfer posteriorly in a prone position is more anatomic than doing this procedure in a lateral decubitus position.

References

1. Bahm J, Noaman H, Becker M. The dorsal approach to the suprascapular nerve in neuromuscular reanimation for obstetric brachial plexus lesions. Plast Reconstr Surg. 2005;115:240–4.
2. Bertelli JA, Ghizoni MF. Results of spinal accessory to suprascapular nerve transfer in 110 patients with complete palsy of the brachial plexus. J Neurosurg Spine. 2016;24:990–5. https://doi.org/10.3171/2015.8.SPINE15434.
3. Colbert SH, Mackinnon S. Posterior approach for double nerve transfer for restoration of shoulder function in upper brachial plexus palsy. Hand (N Y). 2006;1:71–7. https://doi.org/10.1007/s11552-006-9004-4.
4. Guan SB, Hou CL, Chen DS, Gu YD. Restoration of shoulder abduction by transfer of the spinal accessory nerve to suprascapular nerve through dorsal approach: a clinical study. Chin Med J. 2006;119:707–12.
5. Lurje A. Concerning surgical treatment of traumatic injury to the upper division of the brachial plexus (Erb's type). Ann Surg. 1948;127:317–26.
6. Malessy MJ, de Ruiter GC, de Boer KS, Thomeer RT. Evaluation of suprascapular nerve neurotization after nerve graft or transfer in the treatment of brachial plexus traction lesions. J Neurosurg. 2004;101:377–89. https://doi.org/10.3171/jns.2004.101.3.0377.
7. Merrell GA, Barrie KA, Katz DL, Wolfe SW. Results of nerve transfer techniques for restoration of shoulder and elbow function in the context of a meta-analysis of the English literature. J Hand Surg Am. 2001;26:303–14. https://doi.org/10.1053/jhsu.2001.21518.
8. Mikami Y, Nagano A, Ochiai N, Yamamoto S. Results of nerve grafting for injuries of the axillary and suprascapular nerves. J Bone Joint Surg Br. 1997;79:527–31. https://doi.org/10.1302/0301-620x.79b4.7481.
9. Nagano A. Treatment of brachial plexus injury. J Orthop Sci. 1998;3:71–80. https://doi.org/10.1007/s007760050024.
10. Rui J, Zhao X, Zhu Y, Gu Y, Lao J. Posterior approach for accessory-suprascapular nerve transfer: an electrophysiological outcomes study. J Hand Surg Eur Vol. 2013;38:242–7. https://doi.org/10.1177/1753193412447495.
11. Segal D, Cornwall R, Little KJ. Outcomes of spinal accessory-to-suprascapular nerve transfers for brachial plexus birth injury. J Hand Surg Am. 2019;44:578–87. https://doi.org/10.1016/j.jhsa.2019.02.004.
12. Sommarhem AJ, Grahn PM, Nietosvaara YA. Selective neurotization of the infraspinatus muscle in brachial plexus birth injury patients using the accessory nerve. Plast Reconstr Surg. 2015;136:1235–8. https://doi.org/10.1097/PRS.0000000000001761.
13. Souza FH, Bernardino SN, Filho HC, Gobbato PL, Martins RS, Martins HA, Silva-Neto RP. Comparison between the anterior and posterior approach for transfer of the spinal accessory nerve to the suprascapular nerve in late traumatic brachial plexus injuries. Acta Neurochir. 2014;156:2345–9. https://doi.org/10.1007/s00701-014-2222-6.
14. Terzis JK, Kostas I. Suprascapular nerve reconstruction in 118 cases of adult posttraumatic brachial plexus. Plast Reconstr Surg. 2006;117:613–29. https://doi.org/10.1097/01.prs.0000203410.35395.fa.
15. van Ouwerkerk WJ, Uitdehaag BM, Strijers RL, Frans N, Holl K, Fellner FA, Vandertop WP. Accessory nerve to suprascapular nerve transfer to restore shoulder exorotation in otherwise spontaneously recovered obstetric brachial plexus lesions. Neurosurgery. 2006;59:858–67.; discussion 867-859. https://doi.org/10.1227/01.NEU.0000232988.46219.E4.
16. Vathana T, Larsen M, de Ruiter GC, Bishop AT, Spinner RJ, Shin AY. An anatomic study of the spinal accessory nerve: extended harvest permits direct nerve transfer to distal plexus targets. Clin Anat. 2007;20:899–904. https://doi.org/10.1002/ca.20545.
17. Wyles CC, Maldonado AA, Wagner ER, Houdek MT, Lachman N, Spinner RJ. Proposed surgical technique to facilitate targeted reinnervation of the infraspinatus: a cadaveric feasibility study. Clin Anat. 2019;32:131–6. https://doi.org/10.1002/ca.23310.

Surgical Approach: Axillary Posterior

23

Somsak Leechavengvongs
and Navapong Anantavorasakul

Surgical Approach for Axillary Nerve (Posterior)

Lurje [1] was the first in the English literature who describe the technique of using the triceps fascicles of the radial nerve transfer to the axillary nerve without nerve grafting in a patient with Erb's palsy. Nath and Mackinnon subsequently reported using Lurje's technique in five patients with satisfactory results [2]. In 2003, we reported nerve transfer to the anterior branch of the axillary nerve using the nerve to the long head of triceps [3, 4].

Relevant Anatomy

The axillary nerve is the terminal branch of the posterior cord of the brachial plexus. It usually carries the nerve fibers from C5 and C6. The axillary nerve travels through the quadrangular space along with the posterior circumflex humeral artery and vein. At this level, it typically divides into two main branches: the anterior branches (which may have up to three separate branches) and one posterior branch. The posterior branch is located more superficially than the anterior branch and divides into the superior lateral cutaneous nerve of arm and a branch to the posterior part of deltoid muscle. The posterior branch also provides branches that supply the teres minor.

The anterior branch of the axillary nerve ascends around the surgical neck of the humerus before supplying the anterior and middle parts of the deltoid muscle. Our cadaveric study demonstrated that in most cases (91.5%) the anterior branch of the axillary nerve also supplies the posterior part of the deltoid [5]. Therefore, nerve transfer to the anterior branch of the axillary nerve will restore not only the anterior and middle parts but also the posterior part of the deltoid in most cases. Crouch et al. demonstrated that even if the posterior part of the deltoid muscle was not reinnervated, other muscles crossing the shoulder such as the middle part of the deltoid and the latissimus dorsi could compensate in shoulder extension which is provided by the posterior part of the deltoid. They concluded that the reconstruction of the anterior branch of the axillary nerve only is an appropriate technique for restoring shoulder abduction after isolated axillary nerve injury [6].

We deliberately avoid doing nerve transfer to the posterior branch of the axillary nerve so that no axons are wasted on the superior lateral cutaneous nerve or the teres minor. The teres minor is not only an external rotator of the shoulder but also a strong shoulder adductor which is antagonist to the desired functional restoration. We believe that shoulder external rotation in patients

S. Leechavengvongs (✉) · N. Anantavorasakul
Upper Extremity and Reconstructive Microsurgery Unit, Institute of Orthopaedics, Lerdsin Hospital, Bangkok, Thailand

A. Y. Shin, N. Pulos (eds.), *Operative Brachial Plexus Surgery*,
https://doi.org/10.1007/978-3-030-69517-0_23

treated with combined nerve transfer is restored partly from the transfer to suprascapular nerve which reanimates the infraspinatus and partly from the reinnervation of the posterior part of the deltoid muscle.

At the triangle interval in the posterior arm (defined by the teres major, the lateral head, and the long head of triceps), the radial nerve gives branches to the triceps muscle. The first branch is the nerve to the long head of triceps which is given off about 1 cm proximal to the inferior edge of the teres major. The second branch is more variable and may go to the upper medial head (38%), the medial head (10.1%), the upper lateral head (44.3%), or the lateral head of triceps (7.6%) [7]. Subsequently, the nerve to the lateral head of the triceps and the nerve to the medial head of the triceps have been promoted as the donor nerve [8–11]. We prefer the nerve to the long head of the triceps because of its constant branching point, proximity to the recipient, and the similar diameter offering the best size match to the recipient nerve [7].

In addition, if the nerve to the long head of the triceps was sacrificed, the functional loss would be minimal as it plays the least important role in elbow extension and could easily be compensated for by the remaining two heads of the triceps.

Preoperative Planning

Triceps muscle power has to be at least M4. Good passive range of motion of the shoulder is essential.

Preparation and Patient Positioning

The patient is placed in the supine position with the sandbag beneath the scapula of the affected upper extremity. The affected arm is placed across the chest thus exposing the posterior aspect of the shoulder.

Surgical Approach and Procedure

A curved incision is made along the posterior border of the deltoid (Fig. 23.1). As the deltoid is atrophic, the posterior border can be elevated easily without having to detach its origin from the scapular spine. The interval between the long and the lateral heads of the triceps is then developed to expose the quadrilateral space and the triangular interval. The teres major is the key structure, which divides the quadrilateral space from the triangular interval. Next, the radial nerve at the triangular interval is isolated, and the first branch of the nerve, which usually comes off at about 1 cm proximal to the inferior edge of teres major, is identified as the nerve to the long head of the triceps (Fig. 23.2). The axillary nerve is accompanied by the posterior circumflex humeral artery and vein within the quadrilateral space. After

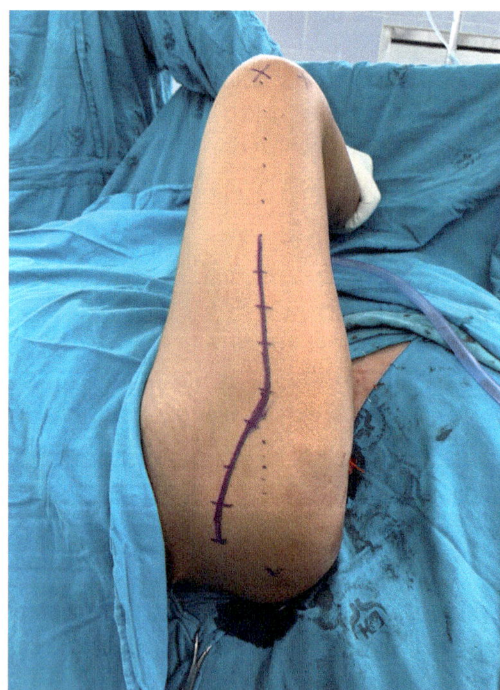

Fig. 23.1 Surgical incision along the border of the posterior deltoid proximally and mid posterior of the left arm distally

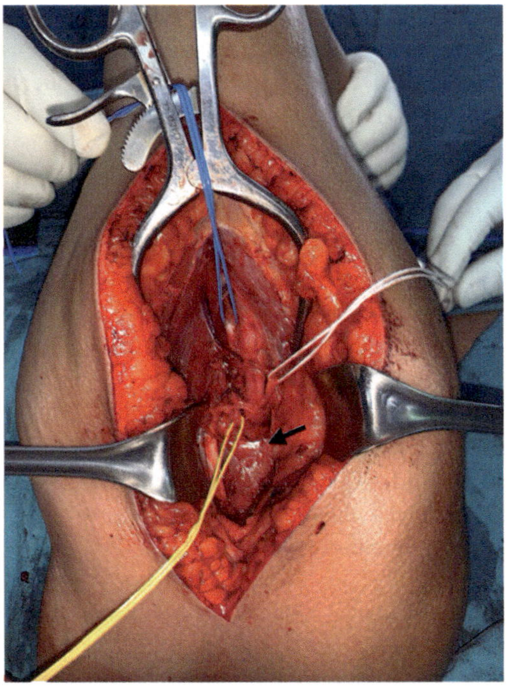

Fig. 23.2 Intraoperative view of radial nerve at triangular interval below the inferior edge of the teres major muscle (black arrow). Nerve to long head of triceps (yellow loop), to lateral head of triceps (white loop) and to medial head of triceps (blue loop)

emerging from the space, the axillary nerve gives a branch to the teres minor and then divides into one to three anterior branch(es) and one posterior branch (Fig. 23.3). The anterior branches, which are the major motor branches to the deltoid muscle, are dissected free as proximally as possible. Electrical stimulation of the identified nerves is used to confirm paralysis of the deltoid and strong contraction of the triceps. The nerve to the long head of the triceps (donor) is cut as distally as possible just before it enters the muscle and flipped 180° to coapt to the anterior branch of the axillary nerve (recipient) which is transected as proximally as possible. In our experience, this always provides sufficient length for a tension-free and direct neurorrhaphy with 9-0 nylon sutures with the aid of the operating microscope (Figs. 23.4 and 23.5). The site of nerve transfer was reinforced with fibrin glue (Tisseel, Baxter Inc.). A technical tip to increase mobility of the donor nerve, though rarely required, is to incise the inferior edge of teres major for approximately 1 cm.

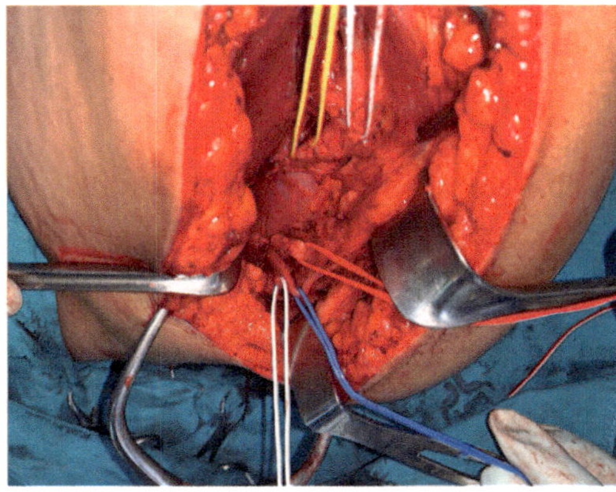

Fig. 23.3 Intraoperative view of the anterior branch (red loop) and the posterior branch of the axillary nerve. The posterior branch is more superficial and smaller than the anterior branch and divided into branch to posterior deltoid muscle (lower white loop) and superolateral cutaneous nerve of the arm (blue loop)

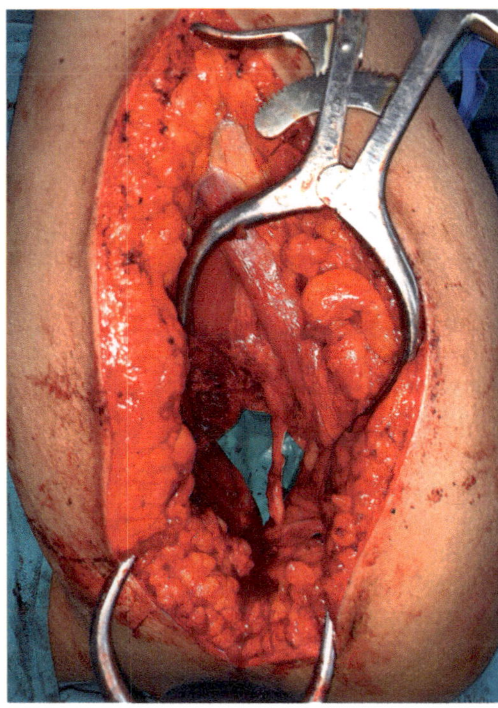

Fig. 23.4 Intraoperative view of the transfer to the anterior branch of the axillary nerve from the nerve to the long head of triceps

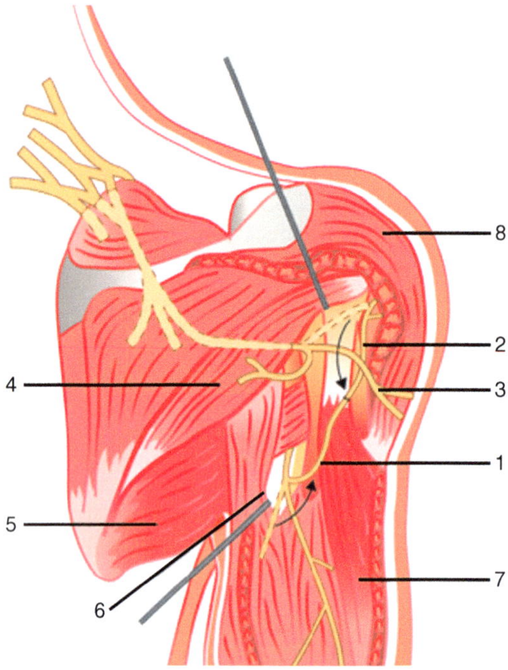

Fig. 23.5 The right shoulder from the posterior aspect. Nerve transfer to the anterior branch of the axillary nerve using the nerve to the long head of the triceps. (1) The nerve to the long head of the triceps, (2) the anterior branch of the axillary nerve, (3) the posterior branch of the axillary nerve, (4) teres minor muscle, (5) teres major muscle, (6) the long head of the triceps, (7) the lateral head of the triceps, and (8) deltoid muscle (cut)

Postoperative Care and Rehabilitation

The patient's arm is placed in a sling for 3 weeks. Gentle passive mobilization is then performed to prevent joint stiffness starting with pendulum exercise and then progressing to passive full range of shoulder motion in all directions. No specific motor re-education is necessary.

Clinical Results

In our first series of seven patients, who had dual nerve transfers of SAN to SSN and the branch to long head of the triceps of radial nerve to the anterior branch of axillary nerve, all patients achieved M4 deltoid function with mean abduction of 124° [4]. Bertelli and Ghizoni reported their results of dual nerve transfers in 10 patients with C5 and C5-C6 injuries [10]. Three patients achieved M4 and seven patients achieved M3 shoulder abduction. The mean abduction was 92° and the mean external rotation was 93° (from full internal rotation). In 2006, we reported another series of 15 patients with C5 and C6 injuries. Thirteen patients achieved M4 deltoid function and two patients regained M3. The mean shoulder abduction was 115° and the mean external rotation was 97° [12].

A recent review of 21 patients with an isolated axillary nerve injury treated with a nerve to the long head of triceps transfer resulted in 16 patients who obtained M3 or greater recovery of deltoid muscle strength [13].

References

1. Lurje A. Concerning surgical treatment of traumatic injury of the upper division of the brachial plexus (Erb's-type). Ann Surg. 1948;127(2):317–26.
2. Nath RK, Mackinnon SE. Nerve transfers in the upper extremity. Hand Clin. 2000;16(1):131–9, ix.
3. Witoonchart K, Leechavengvongs S, Uerpairojkit C, Thuvasethakul P, Wongnopsuwan V. Nerve transfer to deltoid muscle using the nerve to the long head of the triceps, part I: an anatomic feasibility study. J Hand Surg Am. 2003;28(4):628–32.
4. Leechavengvongs S, Witoonchart K, Uerpairojkit C, Thuvasethakul P. Nerve transfer to deltoid muscle using the nerve to the long head of the triceps, part II: a report of 7 cases. J Hand Surg Am. 2003;28(4):633–8.
5. Leechavengvongs S, Teerawutthichaikit T, Witoonchart K, Uerpairojkit C, Malungpaishrope K, Suppauksorn S, et al. Surgical anatomy of the axillary nerve branches to the deltoid muscle. Clin Anat. 2015;28(1):118–22.
6. Crouch DL, Plate JF, Li Z, Saul KR. Biomechanical contributions of posterior deltoid and teres minor in the context of axillary nerve injury: a computational study. J Hand Surg Am. 2013;38(2):241–9.
7. Uerpairojkit C, Ketwongwiriya S, Leechavengvongs S, Malungpaishrope K, Witoonchart K, Mekrungcharas N, et al. Surgical anatomy of the radial nerve branches to triceps muscle. Clin Anat. 2013;26(3):386–91.
8. Bertelli JA, Ghizoni MF. Nerve transfer from triceps medial head and anconeus to deltoid for axillary nerve palsy. J Hand Surg Am. 2014;39(5):940–7.
9. Colbert SH, Mackinnon S. Posterior approach for double nerve transfer for restoration of shoulder

function in upper brachial plexus palsy. Hand (N Y). 2006;1(2):71–7.

10. Bertelli JA, Ghizoni MF. Reconstruction of C5 and C6 brachial plexus avulsion injury by multiple nerve transfers: spinal accessory to suprascapular, ulnar fascicles to biceps branch, and triceps long or lateral head branch to axillary nerve. J Hand Surg Am. 2004;29(1):131–9.
11. Kostas-Agnantis I, Korompilias A, Vekris M, Lykissas M, Gkiatas I, Mitsionis G, et al. Shoulder abduction and external rotation restoration with nerve transfer. Injury. 2013;44(3):299–304.
12. Leechavengvongs S, Witoonchart K, Uerpairojkit C, Thuvasethakul P, Malungpaishrope K. Combined nerve transfers for C5 and C6 brachial plexus avulsion injury. J Hand Surg Am. 2006;31(2):183–9.
13. Lee JY, Kircher MF, Spinner RJ, Bishop AT, Shin AY. Factors affecting outcome of triceps motor branch transfer for isolated axillary nerve injury. J Hand Surg Am. 2012;37(11):2350–6.

Anterior Approach for Axillary Nerve Reconstruction

24

Jorge Francisco Clifton Correa,
Alejandro Muset Lara, Anil Ghanshyam Bhatia,
Tarek Abdalla El-Gammal, Rafael Reynoso Campo,
and Leonardo Lopez Almejo

Principles

Blunt trauma to the shoulder, dislocation of the glenohumeral joint, and shoulder surgeries have been suggested as a frequent etiology for an isolated axillary nerve injury [1–5]. They can occur in 6% of all brachial plexus injuries [1, 6]. Shoulder function is compromised following axillary nerve injury. The most common complaints are limitations in active shoulder range of motion, weakness, and deltoid atrophy (Fig. 24.1). Tenderness and a positive Tinel's sign can be helpful if noted but are not always present at the site of injury which is typically at the infraclavicular region or the quadrilateral space. The nerve injury can be minor and may recover spontaneously [7], or it can be severe requiring nerve reconstruction. Nerve grafting is still considered the gold standard with good results [8].

Posterior cord injuries are not common [9] and present with the axillary nerve and the radial nerve dysfunction. A few reports of this injury type have been published. The posterior cord injuries are usually associated with high energy trauma and with another associated cord or nerve injuries (i.e., musculocutaneous nerve).

In upper brachial plexus injury with C5 and C6 injury, there are paralysis of shoulder abduction and external rotation, elbow flexion, and forearm supination. In this situation many authors

J. F. Clifton Correa (✉)
Brachial Plexus International School, Barcelona, Spain

Department of Hand, Micro and Nerve Surgery, Universidad Autonoma De Guadalajara, Universidad Autonoma de Coahuila Sede Torreon, Real San Jose: UAG, Guadalajara Jalisco, Hospital Universitario Dr. Joaquin Del Valle Sanchez, Torreon Coahuila, Zapopan, Jalisco, Mexico

A. M. Lara
Brachial Plexus and Birth Palsy Surgery, Muset Institute and Brachial Plexus International School, Barcelona, Spain

A. G. Bhatia
Brachial Plexus International School, Barcelona, Spain

Department of Brachial Plexus Surgery, Deenanath Mangeshkar Hospital, Pune, Maharashtra, India

T. A. El-Gammal
Brachial Plexus International School, Barcelona, Spain

Department of Brachial Plexus and Microsurgery, Assiut University Hospitals, Assiut, Egypt

R. R. Campo
Brachial Plexus International School, Barcelona, Spain

Department of Plastic Surgery and Microsurgery, Hospital General de México, Ciudad de México, Mexico

L. L. Almejo
Brachial Plexus International School, Barcelona, Spain

Department of Brachial Plexus and Microsurgery, Universidad Autonoma de Coahuila, Hospital Universitario, Torreon, Coahuila, Mexico

A. Y. Shin, N. Pulos (eds.), *Operative Brachial Plexus Surgery*,
https://doi.org/10.1007/978-3-030-69517-0_24

have reported good results with the use of nerve transfers after an irreparable upper brachial plexus injury (i.e., avulsions); however nerve grafting of viable nerve roots remain a good option for restoration of axillary nerve function [10–12].

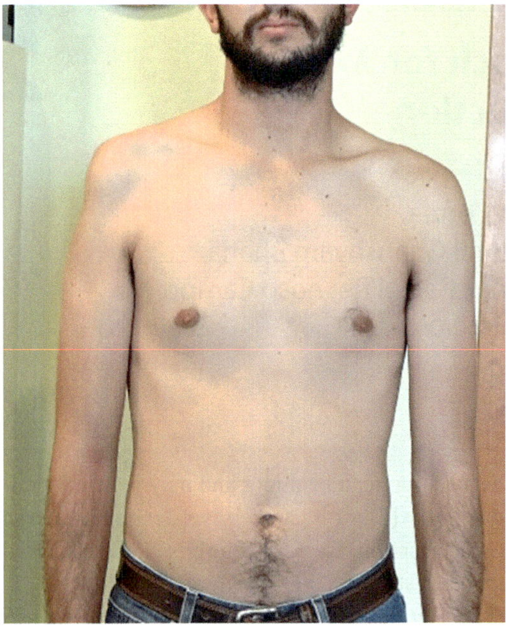

Fig. 24.1 Deltoid atrophy demonstrated in a patient with an isolated axillary nerve injury

History

In 1911 Adolf Stoffel described the anterior axillary approach to perform a triceps nerve fascicles transfer into the axillary nerve (Fig. 24.2) [13]. This procedure was later used by Lurje in 1948 to reconstruct a patient with Erb's palsy with good reported results [14]. The anterior deltopectoral approach has been used for exploration and reconstruction of the posterior cords and axillary nerves with nerve grafts and nerve transfers [15]. Borrero published a technique using a small anterior infraclavicular incision to expose the proxi-

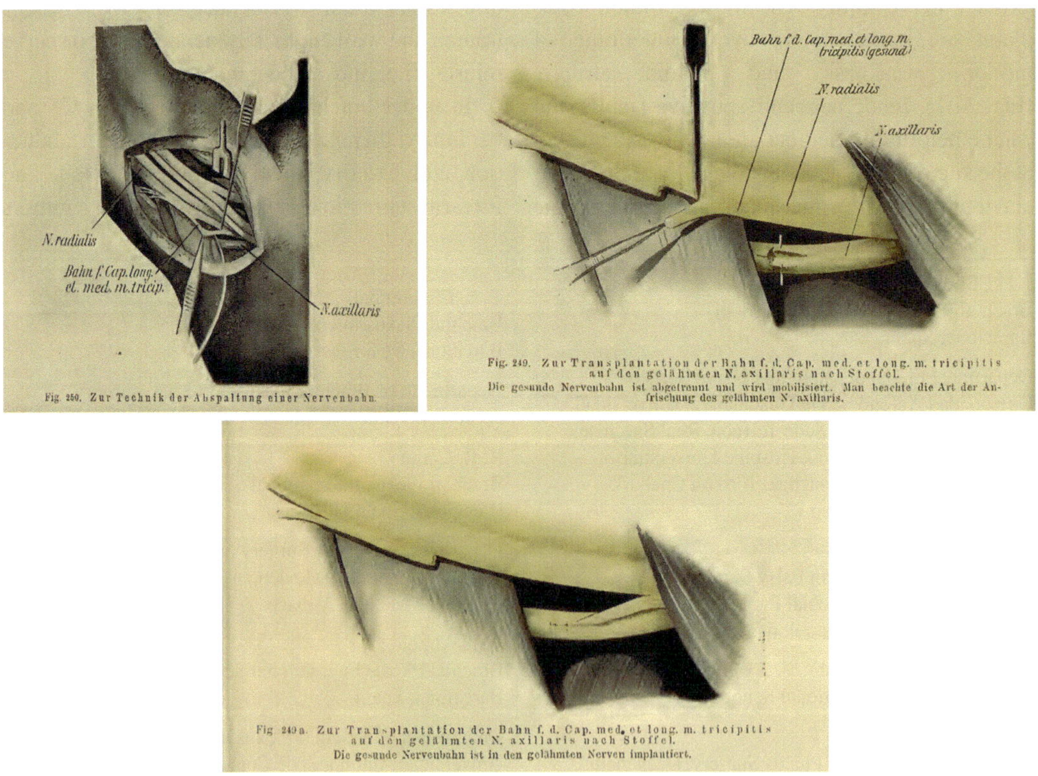

Fig. 24.2 Original description of the transfer of triceps branch to axillary nerve in 1911 by Adolf Stoffel. Top left: Nerve fibers of the triceps branches are identified and dissected. Top right: The axillary nerve is identified, and the triceps branches are mobilized and divided distally. Bottom: The triceps branches are implanted into the axillary nerve

mal segment of the axillary nerve [16] as an alternative to the deltopectoral incision.

Leechavengvongs published in 2003 a posterior approach where the triceps long head branch was transferred to the anterior division of the axillary nerve [17–19]. This technique has become quite popular in the past several years. In 2004 Bertelli published a posterior approach and recommended to include the branch of the teres minor muscle to improve the shoulder external rotation [20], and in 2006, Mackinnon described a posterior approach and similar to Bertelli recommended including the branch of the teres minor muscle [21]. In 2007 Bertelli reported an anterior axillary approach that gives a direct visualization of the axillary nerve and major vessels [22]. In this approach, the triceps to axillary nerve transfer could be performed, and there was direct access to other potential donor nerves such as the thoracodorsal nerve, the medial pectorals nerve, and the intercostal nerves [22, 23].

Clinical Evaluation

The history is important in planning the treatment of patients who may have an axillary nerve injury. The initial physical exam should include not only active and passive range of motion, abduction, internal and external rotation, strength, swelling, and but also a complete neurologic examination of the extremity. Even with a history of shoulder anterior dislocation, trauma, or shoulder surgery, a young athletic patient may be able to compensate for complete deltoid paralysis and can often perform activities of daily living with limited disability (Fig. 24.3). There are specific physical exam tests to evaluate the posterior deltoid (Fig. 24.4) [24]. The abduction-in-internal-rotation test is also useful to isolate the deltoid [25]. In posterior cord injuries, the axillary nerve and the radial nerve are typically affected; however other lateral or medial cord nerves can be affected as well. If pain precedes the loss of motor function, the diagnosis may be a brachial neuritis (i.e., Parsonage-Turner syndrome). Upper trunk brachial plexus injury will result in

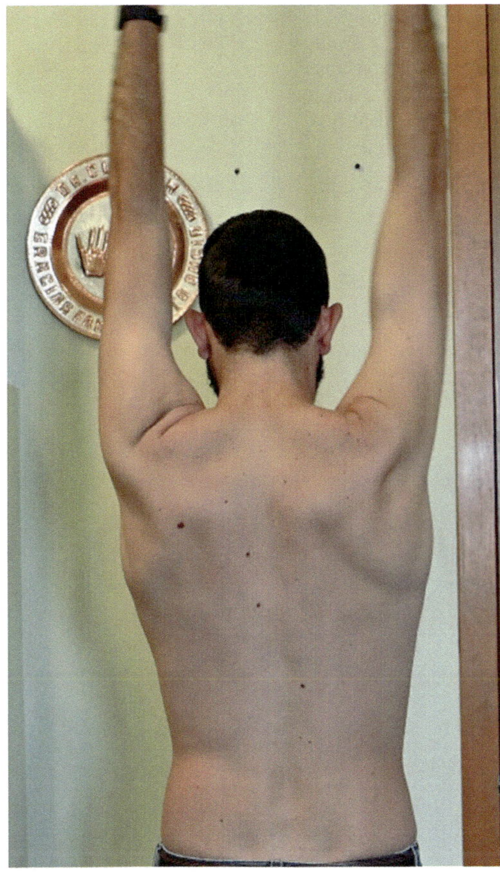

Fig. 24.3 Patients with isolated axillary nerve injury can have full range of motion secondary to strong rotator cuff function. A careful exam needs to be performed to evaluated the deltoid. This patient demonstrates full abduction with an axillary nerve injury

paralysis of shoulder abduction and external rotation, elbow flexion, and forearm supination [26, 27]. Osseous injuries should be ruled out with radiographs. An EMG 3 weeks after injury and repeated at 10 or 12 weeks is recommended if no clinical improvement occur.

If there is no reinnervation by 12 weeks, exploration with reconstruction should be considered [5].

Surgical Anatomy

The axillary nerve is a branch from the posterior cord of the brachial plexus (Fig. 24.5), with contributions from C5 and C6 roots (Fig. 24.6). It

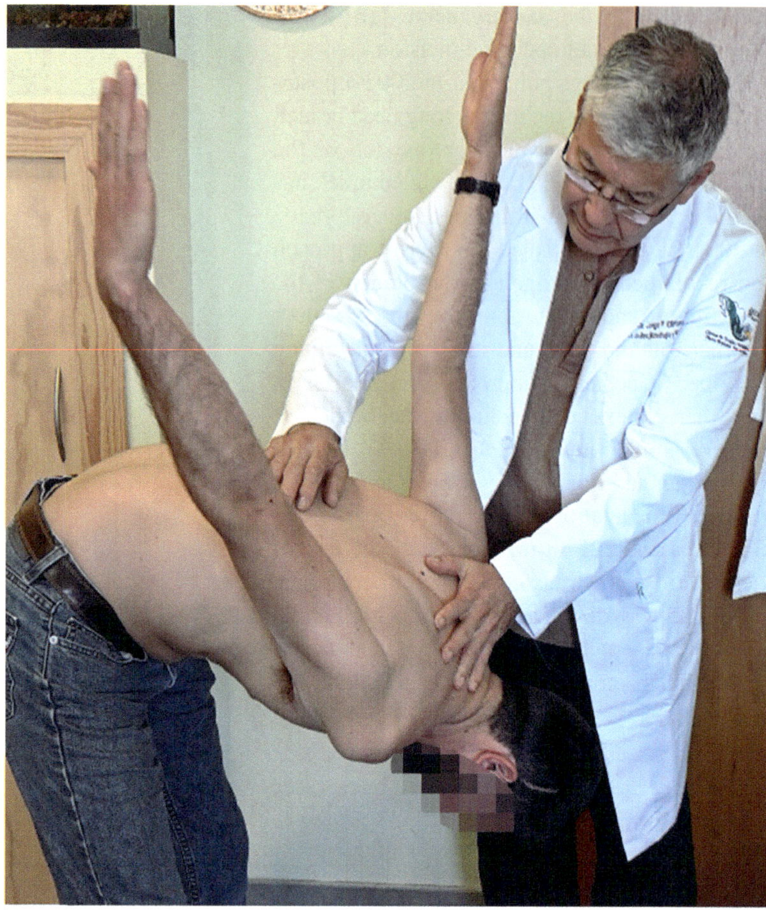

Fig. 24.4 Deltoid extension lag or swallow tail test is demonstrated. The lag of full extension is helpful to identify posterior deltoid weakness

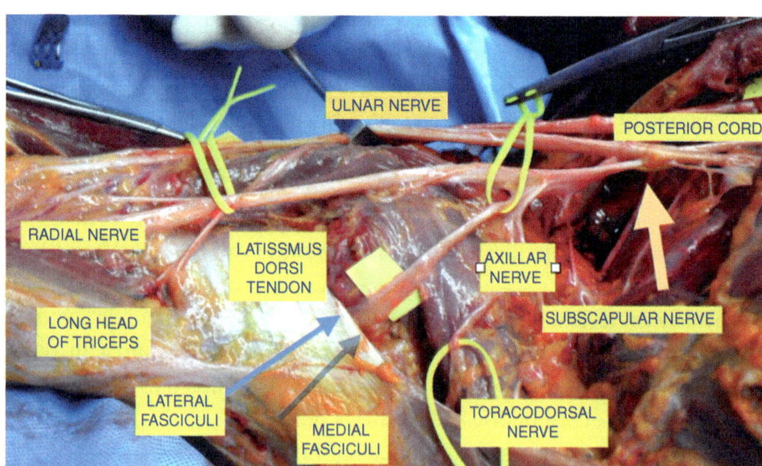

Fig. 24.5 Posterior cord branches with their respective labels in a fresh cadaver specimen

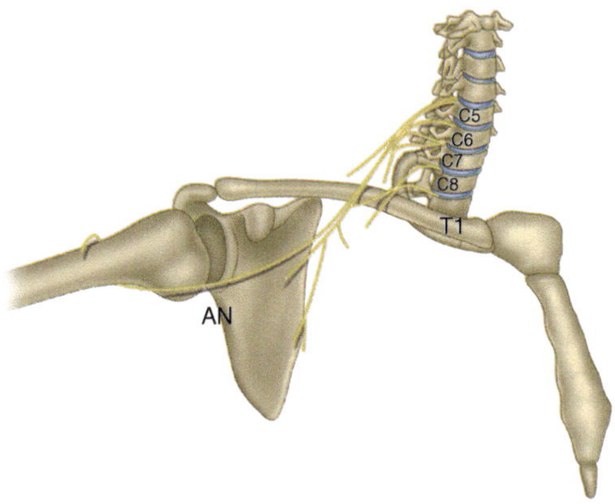

Fig. 24.6 C5 and C6 root contribution to axillary nerve

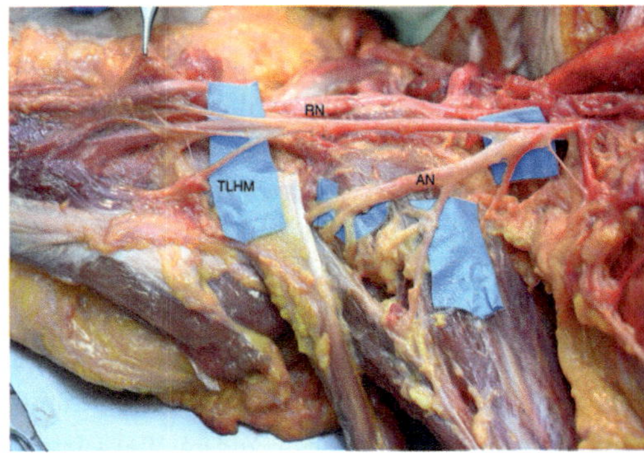

Fig. 24.8 The radial nerve demonstrated in a cadaver specimen. (RN radial nerve, AN axillary nerve, TLHM triceps long head muscle)

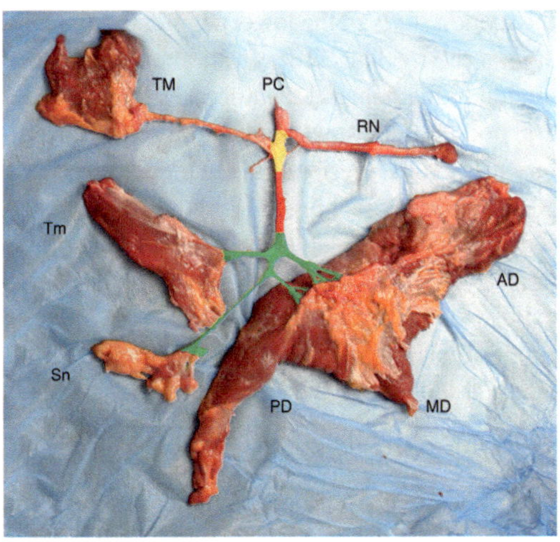

Fig. 24.7 Axillary nerve provides innervation to the deltoid, teres major and minor, as well as sensory innervation to the skin. PC posterior cord, RN radial nerve, TM teres major muscle, Tm teres minor muscle, Sn sensory branch, PD posterior deltoid, MD middle deltoid, AD anterior deltoid

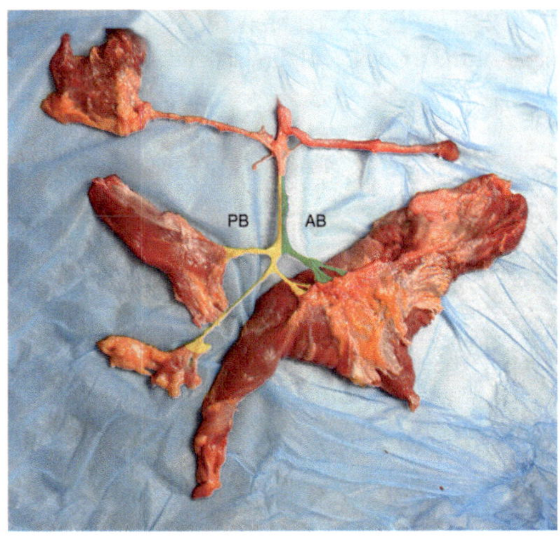

Fig. 24.9 The axillary nerve portion to the deltoid includes the anterior branch and posterior branch (AB anterior branch (green), PB posterior branch (yellow))

arises medial and inferior to the coracoid process [28–30] and contains approximately 6700 nerve fibers [31]. There are three segments of the posterior cord (Fig. 24.7) [32]. The first is from the posterior cord to the subscapularis muscle, and at this level there is only one nerve trunk and usually without nerve branches, but occasionally the inferior subscapular nerve comes from this segment (Fig. 24.8); the second segment is anterior to the subscapular muscle, and at this level the nerve fasciculi begin to form two groups, the lateral and the medial fasciculi groups that are separated only by a loose perineurium [33]. Finally, the third segment is at the inferior border of the subscapular muscle and is the axillary nerve. At this level the axillary nerve has an anterior branch and posterior branch, which are a continuation of the lateral and medial fasciculi groups, respectively, at the quadrangular space. The motor branch is deep, and the branch to the teres minor and the sensory branch are superficial. The anterior branch contains all the fibers that innervate the anterior and middle deltoid muscle, and in 91.5% of cases it will also innervate the posterior deltoid (Fig. 24.9) [34, 35]. The posterior branch divides into the superior lateral brachial cutaneous nerve, the posterior deltoid, and the teres minor motor branch. The axillary nerve has an intimate relation with the inferior aspect of the glenoid and shoulder joint capsule. A surgical blind zone of the axillary nerve has been described, a 1.6 cm segment of the nerve anterior to the quadrilateral space in direct proximity to the glenohumeral joint [36,37]. The teres minor motor branch consistently reached the teres minor muscle by its anterior and medial surface (Fig. 24.10) [22].

The radial nerve gives branch to innervate all three heads of the triceps brachii, the first and lower branch is the nerve to the long head of triceps (Fig. 24.11), the second branch goes to the medial head of the triceps, and the last and more superior goes to the lateral head of the triceps. Each of the triceps motor branch might be considered a donor for transfer to the axillary nerve; because of their proximal origin in the axilla, the triceps long head and the upper branch to the medial head are ideal nerves to be transferred to the axillary nerve by an anterior axillary approach [23].

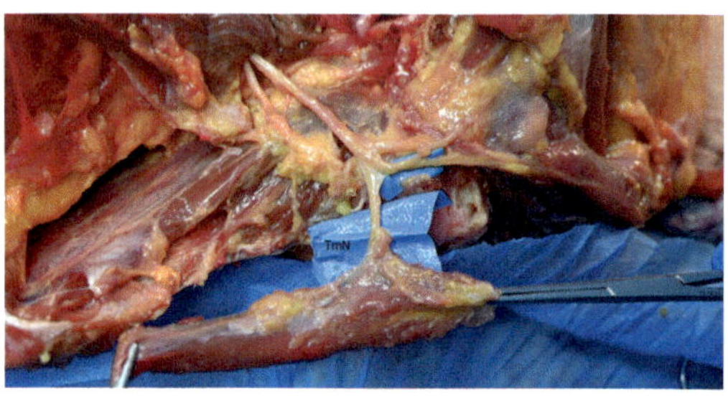

Fig. 24.10 The nerve to the teres minor is shown as a branch of the posterior branch of the axillary nerve (TmN teres minor nerve)

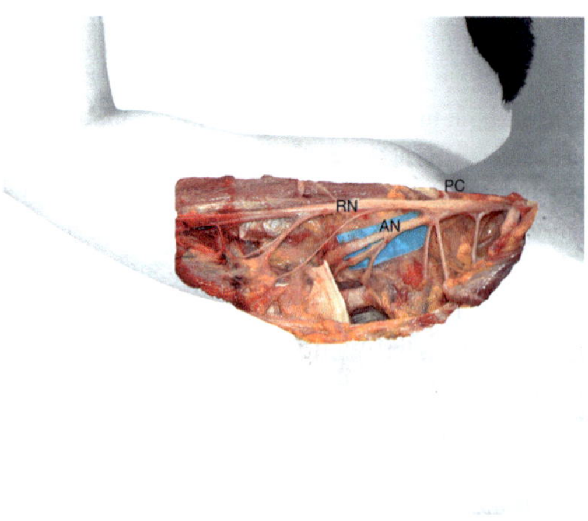

Fig. 24.11 Cadaver dissection illustration of the elements of the posterior cord. (PC posterior cord, RN radial nerve, AN axillary nerve)

Surgery

With the patient in supine position under general anesthesia, with the arm abducted and externally rotated, an "L" shape (Fig. 24.12) is used that follows the axillary crease from the pectoral major inferior border to the latissimus tendon. Dissection starts in the lower segment of the incision at the medial border of the latissimus dorsi tendon to the humeral tendon insertion at the lateral border of the subscapularis muscle. The axillary nerve runs inferior of the humeral head along with the posterior humeral circumflex artery. A retractor is placed at the medial border of the latissimus dorsi and teres major muscles to expose the axillary nerve branches at the entrance of the quadrangular space. The branch of the anterior deltoid and the teres minor motor branch are dissected as far proximal as possible. The nerve is divided and turned distally. The radial nerve and the triceps long head motor branch can be found inferior to the latissimus dorsi tendon. The triceps long head branch divides in two branches to reach the triceps muscle (Fig. 24.13).

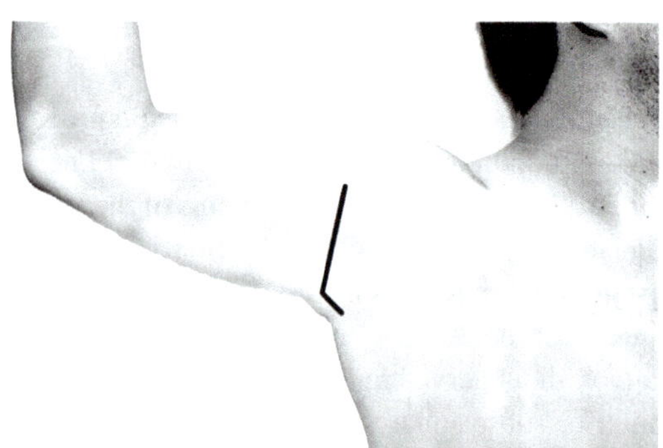

Fig. 24.12 Anterior approach to axillary nerve – skin incision

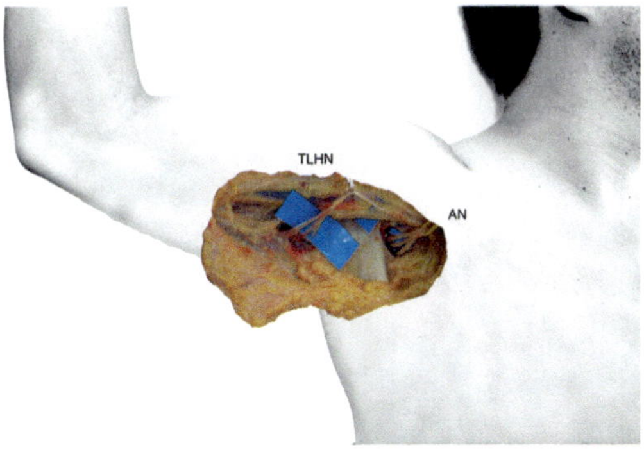

Fig. 24.13 The posterior cord and axillary nerve are identified in preparation for nerve transfer (AN axillary nerve, TLHNB triceps long head nerve branch)

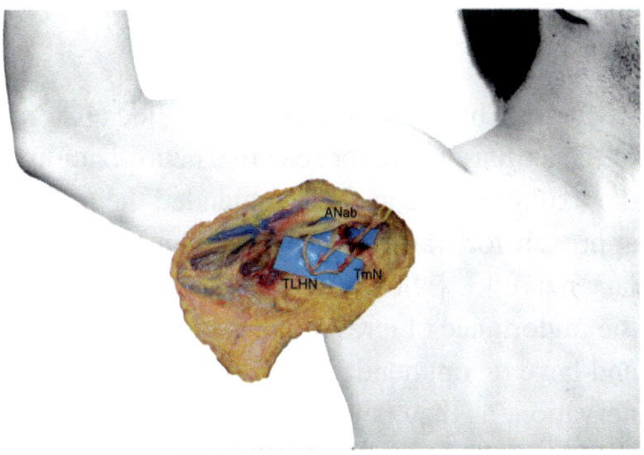

Fig. 24.14 The triceps long head branch is transferred to the anterior axillary nerve branch as well as to the nerve to the teres minor. (ANab axillary nerve anterior branch, SB sensory branch, TmN teres minor nerve, TLHN triceps long head nerve)

At this level it is stimulated to verify triceps strength, then divided distally, and coapted to the anterior axillary nerve branch and teres minor branch tension free under magnification using 9-0 nylon (Fig. 24.14). Intraoperative full passive shoulder range of motion is confirmed to verify a tension free repair.

Postoperative

Following upper extremity nerve reconstruction, a shoulder sling is applied for 2 weeks followed by full passive range of motion in a rehabilitation program.

Motor re-education following nerve transfer is similar to the strategies used after tendon transfers, and generally synergistic muscle actions are easier to recruit and re-learn.

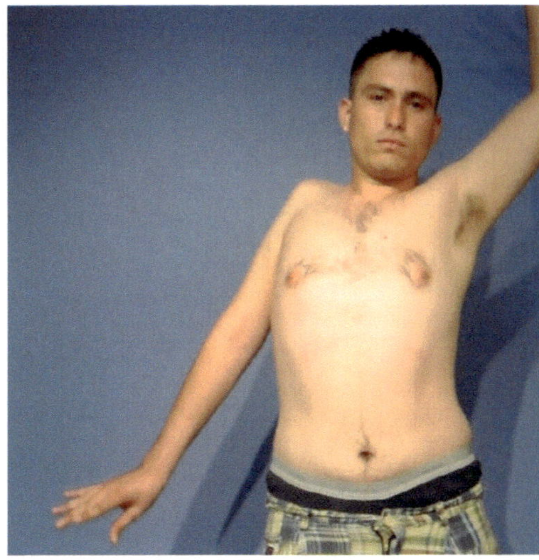

Fig. 24.15 Preoperative upper brachial plexus injury with axillary nerve injury

Reinnervated muscles will be weaker and fatigue more quickly compared with uninjured muscles. Frequent short exercise sessions are optimal to have then best possible outcome. A patient with an upper brachial plexus injury preoperative (Fig. 24.15) and 18 months postoperative after two nerve transfers for shoulder function (Figs. 24.16 and 24.17), and two for elbow flexion, is an example of an excellent outcome.

Discussion

Although the first report of axillary nerve transfer was reported in 1911 [38], the last two decades have witnessed new approach and a better understanding of shoulder nerve anatomy [26, 32, 33, 36–39], biomechanics [40], and surgery [11, 12, 17–20]. Isolated axillary nerve injury can compromise shoulder function, and fortunately most of these injuries will recovered spontaneously (85%). The most common indication for surgery is to improve shoulder abduction and forward flexion. In isolated axillary nerve injuries, the nerve might be injured at the level of the pectoral minor muscle or lower pectoral major inferior border or at the quadrilateral space (Fig. 24.18).

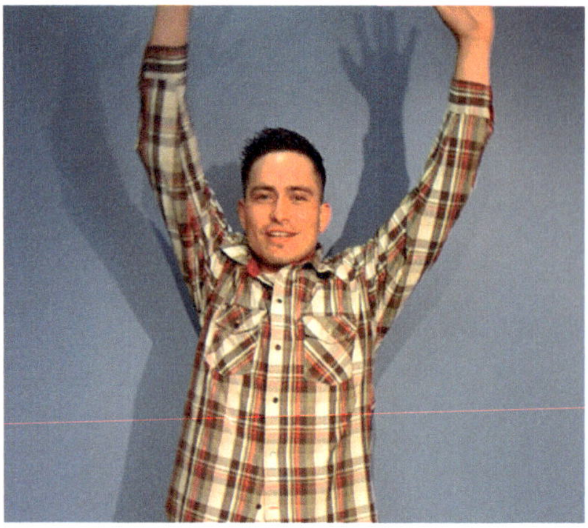

Fig. 24.16 Postoperative full abduction after anterior triceps branch transfer to the anterior axillary branch and teres minor

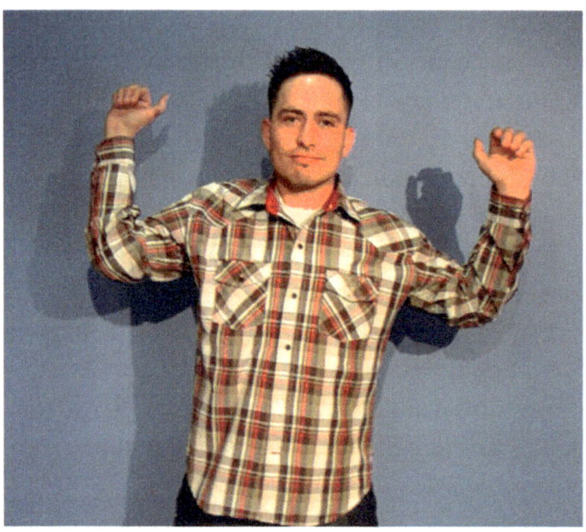

Fig. 24.17 Postoperative full shoulder external rotation in abduction through a spinal accessory to suprascapular nerve transfer

If a healthy distal stump should be found at the level of the injury, a nerve graft should be considered if prior to 6–8 months from injury [2, 3, 8, 11, 12]. While shoulder nerve transfers have become an accepted and popular method for treatment [17, 19, 20], there has been controversy regarding the ideal donor and recipient branches (i.e., inclusion of teres minor branch).

Different approaches have been described to repair the axillary nerve: anterior axillary, deltopectoral, posterior, anterior infraclavicular, and combined anterior/posterior approaches.

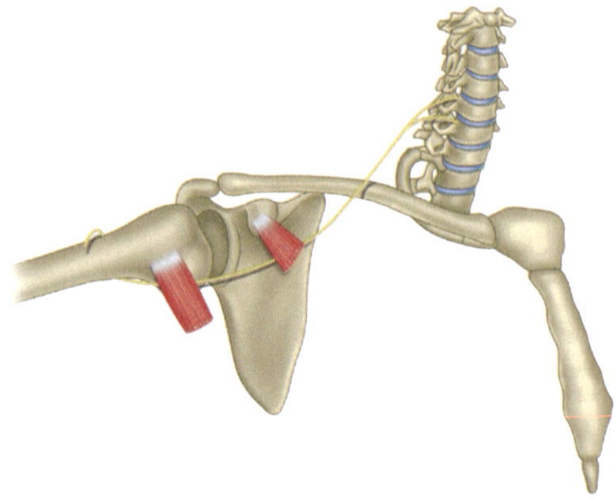

Fig. 24.18 Drawing of course of axillary nerve: AN axillary nerve, Pm pectoral minor muscle, LDt latissimus dorsi tendon, QS quadrangular space

Recently, Zhao et al. studied the applied anatomy of the axillary nerve for selective neurotization of the axillary nerve and recommended the axillary approach for transfer triceps branch to the axillary nerve [33]. Some surgeons have diminished the importance of teres minor in external rotation and have recommended against teres minor reinnervation, as they believe the teres minor to be a shoulder adductor [17–19]. The posterior deltoid and teres minor have biphasic function and function as either an abductor or adductor depending on the humeral position [38]. The teres minor is an adductor in early-mid abduction and an abductor beyond 45 degrees of abduction [39–41]) with a mean maximum abduction moment arm at abduction angle greater than 60 degrees. The teres minor is one of the four rotator cuff muscles and has the lowest profile. It contributes to 20% of normal external rotation strength [41], and its function may become more important with large tears of the infraspinatus or when the infraspinatus is weak. A compensatory hypertrophy of the teres minor occurs to augment or assist with external rotation strength [42].

An argument against the teres minor reinnervation is that there are not enough axons in the triceps long head to reinnervate both the anterior deltoid branch and teres minor motor branch. The optimal donor to recipient nerve axon count radio for restoring function is controversial. Animal studies of partial nerve sectioning suggest that as few as 20% of remaining motor units can provide suitable contractility and less than 50% of the axons will result in a poor functional result [43]. The main axillary nerve has 7887 axons, the anterior branch has 4052 axons, the posterior branch has 1242 axons, and the teres minor branch has 1242 axons. Donor nerves: the long head of triceps has 2302 axons, medial head of triceps has 2198 axons, and lateral head of triceps has 1462 axons [44].

Thus the anterior axillary branch and teres minor muscle branch have a combined 5300 axons. The long head of triceps branch has 2300 axons or 43% of axons. If a portion of the medial head of triceps can be used, there may be enough axons to have greater than 50% [45].

Timing of surgery is also important. Early repair generally results in improved clinical outcome from timely reinnervation of motor endplates compared to late reconstruction. Younger patients have greater regeneration capacity and better outcome compared with the elderly.

Restoration of shoulder stability, abduction, and external rotation are as important as elbow flexion. In a posterior cord nerve injury and upper trunk brachial plexus injury, there is the added challenge of needing longer nerve grafts, which may lead to poorer functional recovery secondary to the distance from the reconstruction site and the motor endplate. Nerve transfers have gained popularity for reducing the reinnervation time as well as injury zone. Despite this, we prefer to perform a brachial plexus exploration and nerve graft reconstruction when feasible. When not feasible, double nerve transfers for shoulder reinnervation (spinal accessory nerve to suprascapular nerve, and the triceps long head and/or the upper medial head motor branch to the anterior axillary branch and the branch to the teres minor muscle) are performed for shoulder reconstruction.

A wide variety of donor nerves have been used to reinnervate the axillary nerve (spinal accessory nerve, phrenic nerve, thoracodorsal nerve, medial pectoral nerve, triceps branch, IC nerves, median nerve, ulnar nerve, and also the contralateral C7), and these transfers can be performed through an anterior axillary approach [46, 47].

Conclusion

After an isolated axillary nerve injury, shoulder function can be severely compromised, with deltoid and teres minor muscle palsy. Several considerations should be taken when planning to do an axillary nerve reconstruction, nerve grafting is considered the standard of care with good results, and an attractive alternative can be a nerve transfer. Our preference is to reinnervate the axillary nerve by means of the long head of the triceps or the medial head of triceps to the anterior axillary and teres minor motor branch, using the anterior axillary approach.

References

1. Petrucci FS, Morelli A, Raimondi PL. Axillairy nerve injuries—21 cases treated by nerve graft and neurolysis. J Hand Surg Am. 1982;7(3):271–8.
2. Bonnard C, Anastakis DJ, Van Melle G, Narakas AO. Isolated and combined lesions of the axillary nerve. J Bone Jt Surg Ser B. 1999;81(2):212–7.
3. Steinmann SP, Moran EA. Axillary nerve injury: diagnosis and treatment. J Am Acad Orthop Surg. 2001;9:328–35.
4. Kline DG, Kim DH. Axillary nerve repair in 99 patients with 101 stretch injuries. J Neurosurg. 2003;99:630–6.
5. Coene LNJEM, Narakas AO. Operative management of lesions of the axillary nerve, isolated or combined with other nerve lesions. Clin Neurol Neurosurg. 1992;94(SUPPL):64–6.
6. Lee JY, Kircher MF, Spinner RJ, Bishop AT, Shin AY. Factors affecting outcome of triceps motor branch transfer for isolated axillary nerve injury. J Hand Surg Am. 2012;37(11):2350–6.
7. Okazaki M, Shawi A, Gschwind CR, Warwick DJ, Tonkin MA. Outocome of axillary nerve injuries treated with nerve grafts. J Hand Surg. 2011;36:535–40.
8. Wolfe SW, Johnsen PH, Lee SK, Freinberg JH. Long-nerve grafts and nerve transfers demonstrate comparable outcomes for axillary nerve injuries. J Hand Surg Am. 2014;4:245–56.
9. Oberlin C, Chino J, Belkheyar Z. Surgical treatment of brachial plexus posterior cord lesion: a combination of nerve and tendon transfers, about nine patients. Chir Main. 2013;32(3):141–6.
10. Koshy JC, Agrawal NA, Seruya M. Nerve transfer versus interpositional nerve graft reconstruction for posttraumatic, isolated axillary nerve injuries: a systematic review. Plast Reconstr Surg. 2017;140(5):953–60.

11. Garg R, Merrell GA, Hillstrom HJ, Wolfe SW. Comparison of nerve transfers and nerve grafting for traumatic upper plexus palsy: a systematic review and analysis. J Bone Joint Surg Am. 2011;93:819–29.
12. Baltzer HL, Kircher MF, Spinner RJ, Bishop AT, Shin AY. A comparison of outcomes of triceps motor branch-to-axillary nerve transfer or sural nerve interpositional grafting for isolated axillary nerve injury. Plast Reconstr Surg. 2016;138(2):256e–64e.
13. Vulpius O, Stoffel A. Orthopädische operationslehre, vol. 1. Stuttgart: Verlag Von Ferdinand Enke; 1913. p. 241–91.
14. Lurge A. Concerning surgical treatment of traumatic injury of the upper division of the brachial. Ann Surg. 1948;127(2):317–26.
15. Baltzer HL, Spinner RJ, Bishop AT, Shin AY. Axillary nerve reconstruction: anterior-posterior expopsure with sural nerve cable graft pull-trough technique. Tech Hand Surg. 2015;19:168–75.
16. Borrero J. Surgical technique, infraclavicular approach, obstetrical brachialm plexus paralysis: Progressive Communications; 2002. p. 58–9.
17. Witoonchart K, Leechavengvongs S, Uerpairojkit C. Nerve transfer to deltoid muscle using the nerve to the long head of the triceps, part I: an anatomic feasibility study. J Hand Surg Am. 2003;28A(4):628–32.
18. Leechavengvongs S, Witoonchart K, Uerpairojkit C. Nerve transfer to deltoid muscle using the nerve to the long head of the triceps, part II: a report of 7 cases. J Hand Surg Am. 2003;28A(4):633–8.
19. Maldonado AA, Bishop AT, Spinner RJ, Shin AY. Five operations that give the best results after brachial plexus injury. Plast Reconstr Surg. 2017;140(3):545–56.
20. Bertelli JA, Ghizoni MF. Reconstruction of C5 and C6 brachial plexus avulsion injury by multiple nerve transfers: spinal accessory to suprascapular, ulnar fascicles to biceps branch, and triceps long or lateral head branch to axillary nerve. J Hand Surg Am. 2004;29(1):131–9.
21. Colbert SH, Mackinnon S. Posterior approach for double nerve transfer for restoration of shoulder function in upper brachial plexus palsy. Hand. 2006;1:71–7.
22. Bertelli JA, Paulo RK, Santos MA. Axillary nerve repair by triceps motor branch transfer through an axillary access: anatomical basis and clinical results. J Neurosurg. 2007;107:370–7.
23. Bertelli JA, Santos MA, Kechele PR, Ghizoni M, Duarte H. Triceps motor nerve branches as a donor or receiver in nerve transfers. Oper Neurosurg. 2007;61(November):333–9.
24. Hertel RH, Lambert SM, Ballmer FT. The deltoid extension lag sign for diagnosis and grading of axillary nerve palsy. J Shoulder Elb Surg. 1998;7:97–9.
25. Bertelli JA, Ghizoni MF. Nerve transfer from triceps medial head and anconeus to deltoid for axillary nerve palsy. J Hand Surg Am. 2014;39(5):940–7.
26. Kostas-agnantis I, Korompilias A, Vekris M, Lykissas M, Gkiatas I, Mitsionis G, et al. Shoulder abduction and external rotation restoration with nerve transfer. Int J Care Inj. 2013;44(3):299–304.
27. Bertelli JA, Ghizoni MF. Results and current approach for brachial plexus reconstruction. J Brachial Plex Peripher Nerve Inj. 2011;6(2):1–8.
28. Aszmann OC, Dellon AL. The intraneural topography of the axillary nerve: an anatomic and histologic study as it relates to microsurgery. J Reconstr Microsurg. 1996;12(6):359–63.
29. Apaydin N, Tubbbs RS, Loukas M, Dupare F. Review of the surgical anatomy of the axillary nerve and the anatomic basis of its iatrogenic and traumatic injury. Surg Radiol Anat. 2010;32:193–201.
30. Bonnel F. Microscopic anatomy of the adult human brachial plexus: an anatomical and histological basis for microsurgery. Microsurgery. 1984;5(3):107–17.
31. Bonnel F, Rabischong P. Anatomie et systématisation du plexus brachial de l'adulte. Anat Clin. 1980;2(3):289–98.
32. Uz A, Apaydin N, Bozkurt M, Elhan A. The anatomic branch pattern of the axillary nerve. J Shoulder Ellbow Surg. 2007;16:240–4.
33. Zhao X, Phil M, Hung LK, Zhang GM, Phil M, Lao J. Applied anatomy of the axillary nerve for selective neurotization of the deltoid muscle. Clin Orthop Relat Res. 2001;390:244–51.
34. Leechavengvongs S, Teerawutthichaikit T, Witoonchart K, Uerpairojkit C, Malungpaishrope K, Suppauksorn S, et al. Surgical anatomy of the axillary nerve branches to the deltoid muscle. Clin Anat. 2014;00(September 2013):118–22.
35. Rastogi P, Stewart DA, Lawson RD, Tremblay DM, Smith BJ, Tonkin MA. Cadaveric dissection of the axillary nerve: an investigation of extra- muscular and intra-muscular branching patterns. J Hand Surg. 2018;23:533–8.
36. Maldonado AA, Howe BM, Lawton R, Bishop AT, Shin AY, Spinner RJ. Anatomical study of the axillary nerve: description of a surgical blind zone. Plast Reconstr Surg. 2016;138(2):419–26.
37. Maldonado AA, Spinner RJ, Bishop AT, Shin AY, Elhassan BT. Effectiveness of the extended surgical approach to visualize the axillary nerve in the blind zone in an arthroscopic axillary nerve injury model. J Plast Reconstr Aesthetic Surg. 2016;69(12):1697–703.
38. Hik F, Ackland DC. The moment arms of the muscles spanning the glenohumeral joint: a systematic review. J Anat. 2019;234(1):1–15.
39. Ackland DC, Pak P, Richardson M, Pandy MG. Moment arms of the muscles crossing the anatomical shoulder. J Anat. 2008;213:383–90.
40. Crouch DL, Plate JF, Li Z, Saul KR. Biomechanical contributions of posterior deltoid and Teres minor in the context of axillary nerve injury: a computational study. J Hand Surg Am. 2013;38(2):241–9.
41. Gerber C, Blumenthal S, Curt A, Werner I. Effect of selective experimental supraescapular nerve block on abduction and external rotation strength of the shoulder. J Shoulder Elbow Surg. 2007;16:815.820.

42. Kikukawa K, Ide J, Terakawa Y, Takada K, Morita M, Hashimoto K, Mizuta H. Hypertrophic teres minor restores shoulder strength and range of external rotation in posterosuperior rotator cuff tears. J Shoulder Elb Surg. 2016;25:1882–8.
43. Cederna PS, Youssef MKH, Asato H, Urbanchek MG, Kuzon WM. Skeletal muscle reinnervation by reduced axonal numbers results in whole muscle force deficits. Plast Reconstr Surg. 2000;105(6):2003–9.
44. Khair MM, Schreiber JJ, Rosenblatt L, Byun DJ, Lee SK, Wolfe SW. Axon counts yield multiple options for triceps fascicular nerve to axillary nerve transfer. J Hand Surg Am. 2016;41(11):e405–10.
45. Bertelli JA, Ghizoni MF. Nerve root grafting and distal nerve transfers for C5-C6 brachial plexus injuries. J Hand Surg Am. 2010;35:769–75.
46. Tung TH, Weber RV, Mackinnon SE. Nerve transfers for the upper and lower extremities. Oper Tech Orthop. 2004;14(3):213–22.
47. Power DM, Parthiban S, Nassimizadeh M. The evolution of nerve transfer restoration of shoulder function. J Musculoskelet Surg Res. 2019;3:47–52.

Upper Brachium Approach: The "Ulnar-Biceps Median-Brachialis" Double Nerve Transfer

25

Zoubir Belkheyar, Adeline Cambon-Binder, and Christophe Oberlin

Principles

The goal is to reinnervate the two most powerful elbow flexors using regional donor nerves [1, 2]. To shorten the function recovery, the distance between elbow flexors motor endplates and regional donor motor branches has to be as short as possible. Oberlin first described the technique of nerve transfer from one fascicule of the ulnar nerve to the biceps motor branch in 1994 [1], then added a transfer of one fascicule of the median nerve to the motor branch of the brachialis muscle [3], with better results in term of elbow flexion strength [4, 5].

Briefly, branches of division of the musculocutaneous nerve are neurotized by selected fasciculi of respectively the median and the ulnar nerves at the level of the arm (Fig. 25.1). Donor branches should be redundant motor branches for wrist flexion or forearm pronation, avoiding branches for intrinsic muscles of the hand and finger flexors. Finally, the two nerve sutures have to be tensionless.

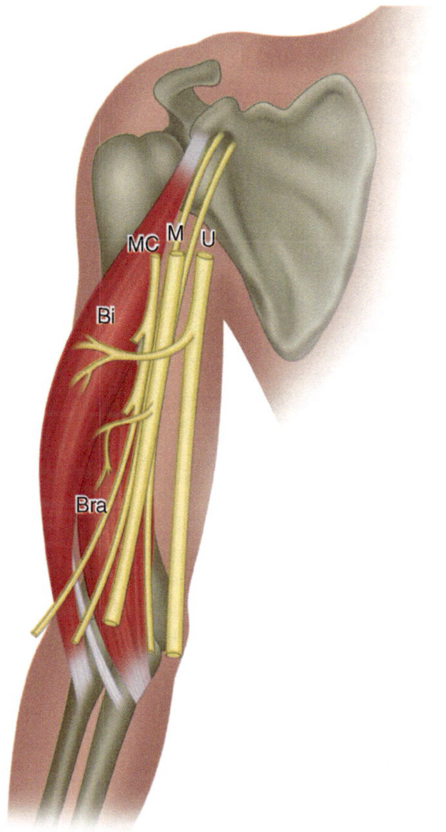

Fig. 25.1 Principle of the "Ulnar-Biceps Median-Brachialis" double transfer. Bi, biceps brachii; Bra, brachialis; MC, musculocutaneous nerve; M, median nerve; U, ulnar nerve

Z. Belkheyar · C. Oberlin
Clinique du Mont Louis, Paris, France

A. Cambon-Binder (✉)
Sorbonne University, Orthopaedic and Traumatology Surgery Department, Saint-Antoine Hospital, Paris, France

A. Y. Shin, N. Pulos (eds.), *Operative Brachial Plexus Surgery*,
https://doi.org/10.1007/978-3-030-69517-0_25

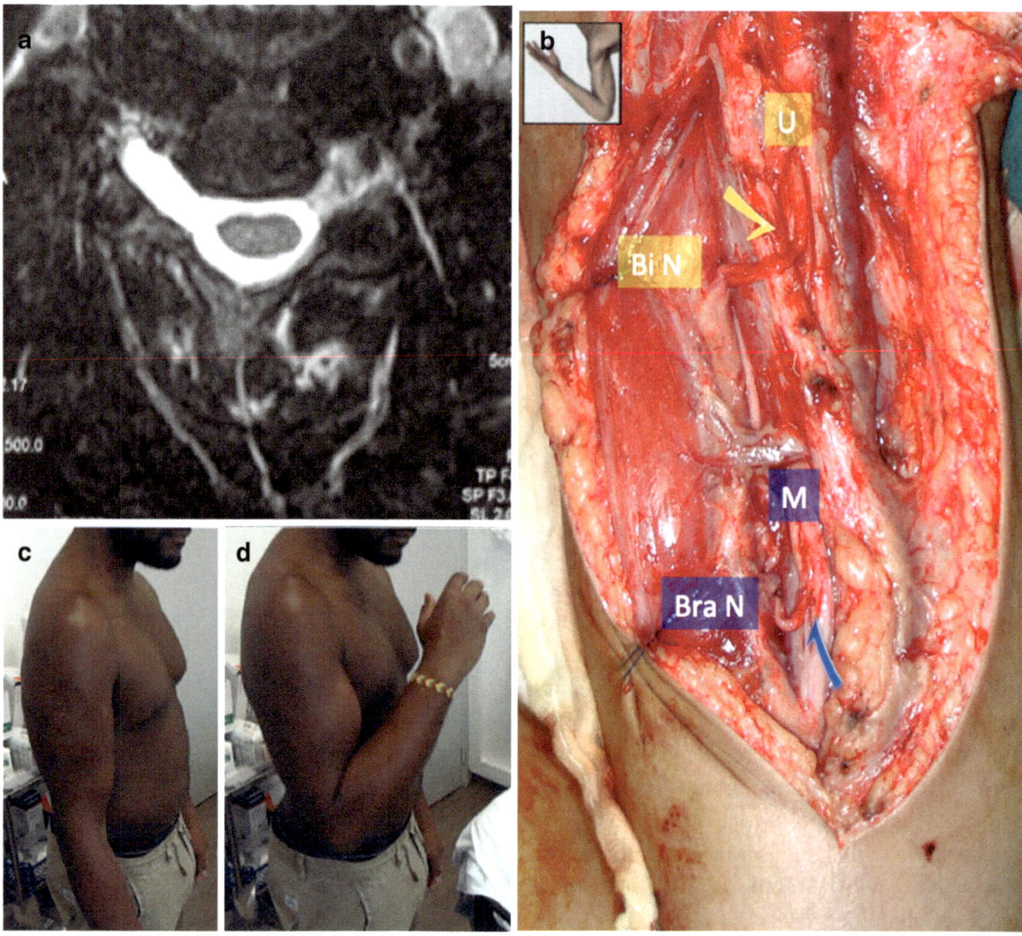

Fig. 25.2 Traumatic avulsion of C5 and C6 brachial plexus roots in a 32-year-old man: medullar resonance magnetic imaging showing pseudomeningoceles (**a**); peri-operative view of the Ulnar-Biceps (yellow arrow) Median-Brachialis (blue arrow) double nerve transfer (**b**); outcome 18 months postoperatively with elbow flexion strength score of M4 (**c**, **d**). UN ulnar nerve, MN median nerve, Bi N biceps brachii nerve branch, Bra N Brachialis nerve branch

Provided all these precautions are observed, the outcomes of this double nerve transfer are satisfactory [4] (Fig. 25.2).

Operative Technique

The patient is supine under general anesthesia with an arm table. The entire affected limb is included in the operative field.

Incision is on the anteromedial aspect of the proximal half of the arm. It descends 8–10 cm from the lower edge of the pectoralis major tendon along the bicipital sulcus. The skin, subcutaneous fat, and fascia of the biceps muscle are open to retract the biceps muscle and expose the musculocutaneous nerve (MCN). The MCN lies between the bellies of the biceps muscle and brachialis muscle and is dissected from proximal to distal in order to identify its main terminal branches (Fig. 25.3). In most of patients those branches involve one (or two) for the biceps muscle, one for the brachialis muscle, and the lateral cutaneous antebrachial nerve [6]. In case of several motor branches for the same muscle, dissection is continued proximally to a common trunk. Motor branches for the biceps exit from the MCN between 37% and 52% of the arm length, defined

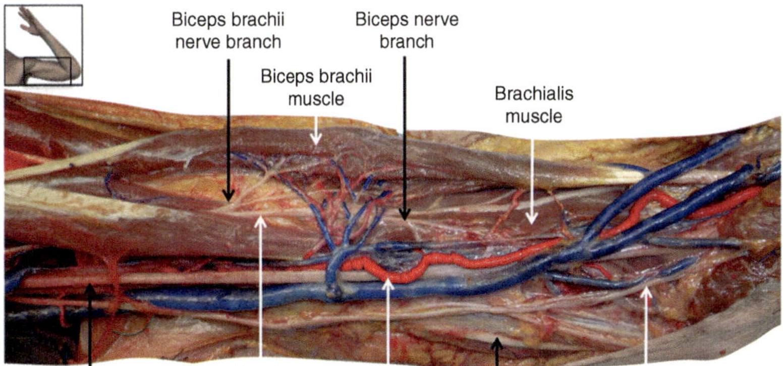

Fig. 25.3 Anatomy of the brachium. Personal dissection of the left brachial area (ACB) in a fresh cadaver, after intravascular latex injection by L. Bourcheix

by distance between the coracoid process and the tip of the lateral epicondyle [6]. For the brachialis muscle, branches arose from 52% to 62% of the arm length.

The two identified main motor branches are then stimulated to confirm paralysis, with the nerve stimulator used by anesthesiologist colleagues to perform motor loco-regional anesthesia. Branches are separated proximally from the musculocutaneous nerve by approximately 2 cm before being sectioned. This dissection is conducted under microscope with microsurgical instruments.

The medial intermuscular septum of the arm is then opened to identify the ulnar nerve at the level of the biceps motor branch. The epineurium of the ulnar nerve is incised, and intraneural dissection is performed to isolate a motor fascicle of similar diameter to the biceps motor branch. Neurostimulator helps to select a motor branch supplying the flexor carpi ulnaris, which is frequently located on the anterolateral side of the ulnar nerve. Branches for intrinsic muscles of the hand should be avoided. Sufficient residual ulnar nerve function is verified via stimulation of the remaining fascicules. The chosen fascicle is then dissected distally for 2 cm, divided and turned laterally.

Internal neurolysis of the median nerve is performed as well at the level of the motor branch of the musculocutaneous nerve for the brachialis muscle in order to isolate a motor fascicle of similar diameter, dedicated to the pronator teres muscle and/or to the palmaris longus muscle.

In rare cases, a communication between the MCN and the median nerve occurs. The principles of the technique are preserved: nerve stimulation should help to identify donor fascicules and recipient motor branches.

Once the ulnar and medial fascicles had been proximally dissected approximately 2 cm and distally cut, direct ulnar-biceps and medial-brachial (so-called "UB-MB") transfers were performed. Nerve sutures are performed without tension using simple epiperineural stitches of single-strand nonabsorbable 9.0 suture (Ethilon, Ethicon, Somerville, NJ, USA) and coadapted with biological fibrin-based glue (Tisseel ™, Baxter, Deerfield, IL, USA).

Postoperatively, the shoulder is splinted in abduction with the elbow in flexion at 90° for 6 weeks, when rehabilitation begins.

References

1. Oberlin C, Béal D, Leechavengvongs S, Salon A, Dauge MC, Sarcy JJ. Nerve transfer to biceps muscle using a part of ulnar nerve for C5 C6 avulsion of the brachial plexus. Anatomical study and report of 4 cases. J Hand Surg [Am]. 1994;19(2):232–7.
2. Oberlin C, Ameur NE, Teboul F, Beaulieu JY, Vacher C. Restoration of elbow flexion in brachial plexus injury by transfer of ulnar nerve fascicles to the nerve to the biceps muscle. Tech Hand Up Extrem Surg. 2002;6:86–90.
3. Goubier JN, Teboul F. Technique of the double nerve transfer to recover elbow flexion in C5, C6, or C5 to C7 brachial plexus palsy. Tech Hand Up Extrem Surg. 2007 Mar;11(1):15–7.

4. Donnelly MR, Rezzadeh KT, Vieira D, Daar D, Hacquebord J. Is one nerve transfer enough? A systematic review and pooled analysis comparing ulnar fascicular nerve transfer and double ulnar and median fascicular nerve transfer for restoration of elbow flexion after traumatic brachial plexus injury. Microsurgery. 2020;40(3):361–9.
5. Sneiders D, Bulstra LF, Hundepool CA, Treling WJ, Hovius SER, Shin AY. Outcomes of single versus double fascicular nerve transfers for restoration of elbow flexion in patients with brachial plexus injuries: a systematic review and meta-analysis. Plast Reconstr Surg. 2019;144(1):155–66.
6. Cambon-Binder A, Leclercq C. Anatomical study of the musculocutaneous nerve branching pattern: application for selective neurectomy in the treatment of elbow flexors spasticity. Surg Radiol Anat. 2015;37(4):341–8.

Intercostal Nerve Harvest in Brachial Plexus Injuries

26

Anil Ghanshyam Bhatia, Alejandro Muset Lara, Jorge Francisco Clifton Correa, Tarek Abdalla El-Gammal, and Pablo Zancolli

Surgical treatment for closed traction injuries of the brachial plexus has been established over the past several decades. A large majority of these lesions affect the supraclavicular elements of the brachial plexus (roots, trunks, and divisions). Root avulsions are frequently seen. The techniques of nerve reconstruction have changed over the past few decades. The pioneering efforts of Millesi, Narakas, and their associates brought confidence in restoration of function in the paralyzed upper limbs following nerve grafting from ruptured root stumps. With root avulsions, alternatives to nerve grafting are necessary, and nerve transfers were developed and designed. Intercostal nerves are typically spared (apart from associated rib fractures) and are, hence, available for transfer to suitable target nerves in the paralyzed arm. Since the initial report by Seddon [1], who cited three cases operated upon by Yeoman using intercostals bridged by ulnar nerve grafts to the musculocutaneous nerve, this transfer has been popularized worldwide. Currently, in root avulsion scenarios where there is no available intraplexual nerve transfer to restore biceps function, direct nerve transfer of several intercostal motor nerves to the musculocutaneous nerve is a potential option to restore elbow flexion [2].

A. G. Bhatia (✉)
The International School of Brachial Plexus Surgery, Pune, Maharashtra, India

Department of Brachial Plexus Surgery, Deenanath Mangeshkar Hospital, Pune, Maharashtra, India

A. M. Lara
Brachial Plexus and Birth Palsy Surgery, Muset Institute and Brachial Plexus International School, Barcelona, Spain

J. F. C. Correa
The International School of Brachial Plexus Surgery, Guadalajara, Mexico

Department of Hand, Micro and Nerve Surgery, Universidad Autonoma De Guadalajara, Universidad Autonoma de Coahuila Sede Torreon, Real San Jose: UAG, Guadalajara Jalisco, Hospital Universitario Dr. Joaquin Del Valle Sanchez, Torreon Coahuila, Zapopan, Jalisco, Mexico

T. A. El-Gammal
Hand and Reconstructive Microsurgery Unit, Assiut University Hospitals and School of Medicine, Assiut, Egypt

P. Zancolli
Fundacion Favaloro, Buenos Aires, Argentina

Technique of Harvest

Incision Harvest of third to the sixth intercostal nerves is possible through an incision from the lower border of the pectoralis major along the sixth rib. However, isolation of the target nerve (musculocutaneous or radial branches to the triceps) requires extension laterally. Early reports have described exposure of the musculocutaneous nerve via a separate incision over the anterior aspect of the arm [3].

A. Y. Shin, N. Pulos (eds.), *Operative Brachial Plexus Surgery*,
https://doi.org/10.1007/978-3-030-69517-0_26

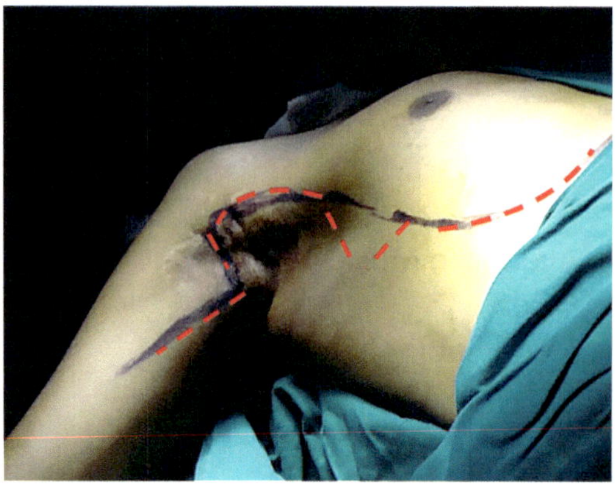

Fig. 26.1 The chest incision is performed from the lower border of the pectoralis major along the sixth rib laterally. A "V" shape anteriorly based at the lower border of the pectoralis major muscle helps to avoid skin edges maceration at the axilla as the arm is immobilized during the postoperative period (red line shows the V shape modification from previous incision)

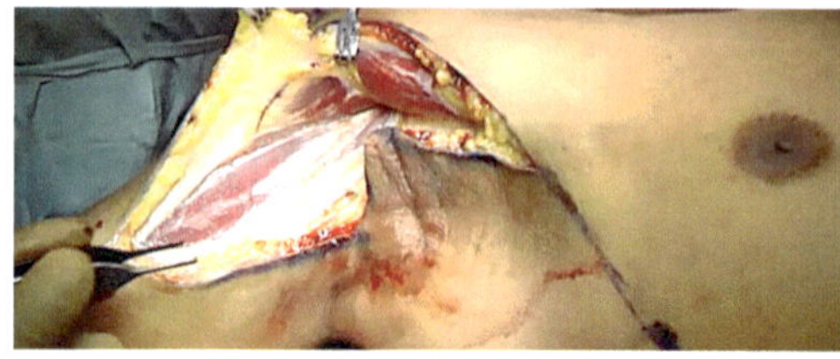

Fig. 26.2 First the recipient nerve is identified before harvesting the intercostal nerves. The musculocutaneous nerve is easily identified between the heads of the biceps at the proximal arm

Continuing the chest incision laterally would impose a stagger at the level of the axillary crease. This can be in the form of a "V" based anteriorly (Fig. 26.1). The skin edges along this portion of the incision tend to get macerated as the arm is immobilized in adduction for 3–4 weeks after this transfer. Hence, the actual preference is to locate the "V" further medially at the lower border of the pectoralis major muscle. Making separate incisions with a subcutaneous tunnel at the axillary crease leads to loss of length of the lower intercostals, and the repair has to be performed in less abduction to enable visualization of the ends of the intercostal nerves in the arm wound.

Target Nerves The musculocutaneous nerve is easily identified between the heads of the biceps (Fig. 26.2). Occasionally, the origin of the musculocutaneous nerve may vary. It may arise from the lateral aspect of the median nerve behind or just distal to the insertion of the pectoralis major muscle. In very few cases, the musculocutaneous nerve gives branches to the biceps, brachialis, and the lateral cutaneous nerve of the forearm and continues distally as the lateral root of the median nerve.

Exposure of the Ribs We have not found it necessary to detach the pectoralis major at the humeral insertion. Medially, one might need to divide a portion of the pectoralis major to expose the costochondral junctions of the fifth and sixth ribs. The insertions of the pectoralis minor (second to fourth ribs) and the serratus anterior are visualized. Cutaneous branches from the upper intercostal nerves can be noted winding around the margin of the pectoralis major laterally to reach the skin over the deltopectoral region. These are consistently accompanied by an artery and two veins that might need to be clipped and divided. The intercostobrachial nerve can be seen as it crosses the axilla to reach the skin on the medial aspect of the arm. This must be protected as it is, often, the sole source of sensation in the paralyzed arm.

The exposure of the nerves starts by tracing the margin of the insertion of the slip of the serratus anterior at the sixth rib. This helps to expose the costo-chondral junction and the insertion of the rectus abdominis muscle (Fig. 26.3). The serratus anterior is detached from the rib, and the plane between the muscle and the rib is developed. As we proceed laterally, the junction with the adjacent slip of the serratus anterior is seen, and the muscle can be split laterally between the fibers of these converging slips to expose the rib up to the anterior axillary line (Fig. 26.4). The long thoracic vessels and nerve can be seen on the surface of the muscle at the mid-axillary line, and the nerve branches to the serratus anterior are protected. The rib can be exposed up to the posterior axillary line passing deep to the serratus anterior. The periosteum is incised between the superior and inferior margins of the rib and, then, stripped off the bone around the lower margin to detach the intercostal muscles from the rib. Care is taken to

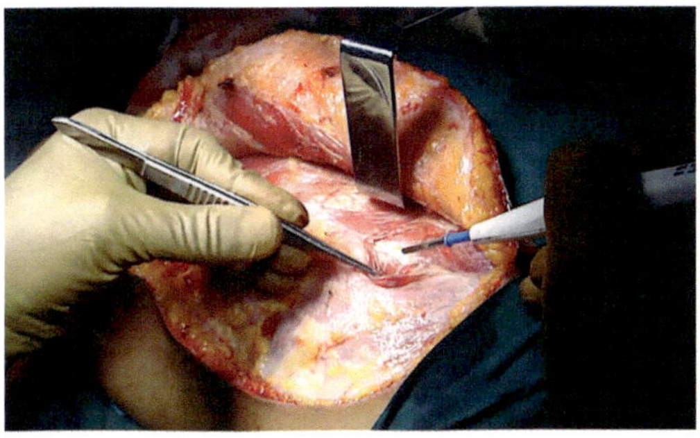

Fig. 26.3 Exposure of the nerves starts by tracing the margin of the insertion of the slip of the serratus anterior at the sixth rib (muscle retracted with the pick-ups). This helps to expose the costo-chondral junction and the insertion of the rectus abdominis muscle

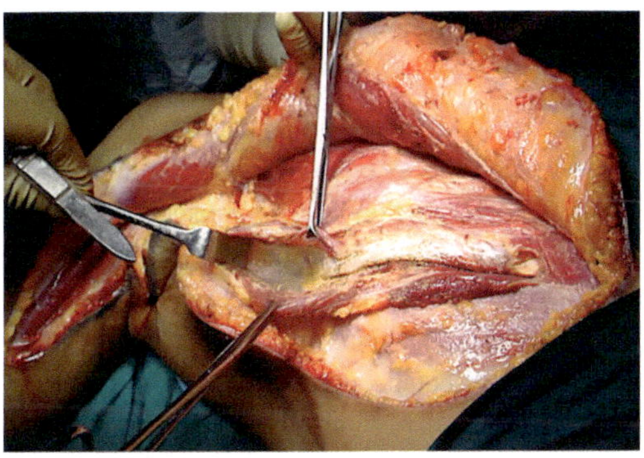

Fig. 26.4 As we proceed laterally, the junction with the adjacent slip of the serratus anterior is seen, and the muscle can be split laterally between the fibers of these converging slips to expose the rib up to the anterior axillary line

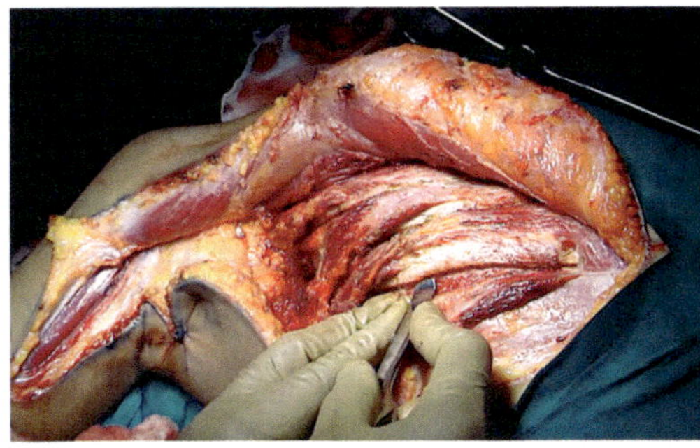

Fig. 26.5 The use of a curved periosteum elevator with a rounded margin helps to stay flush with the rib while separating the periosteum off the inner aspect avoiding accidental injury to the parietal pleura

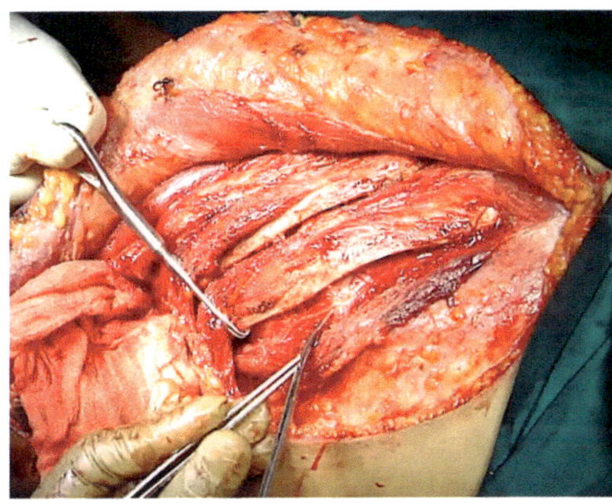

Fig. 26.6 The terminal anterior motor component can be viewed through the transparency as it runs along the margins of the intercostal muscles

stay flush with the rib while separating the periosteum off the inner aspect. Use of a curved periosteum elevator with a rounded margin helps in avoiding accidental injury to the parietal pleura (Fig. 26.5). This separation of the periosteum starts anteriorly and proceeds laterally and posteriorly. The margin of the periosteum then carries the combined insertions of the external and middle intercostal muscles. This step is repeated for each rib. At the fourth and third ribs, it is necessary to separate the serratus from the pectoralis minor and the latter muscle can be partly detached. The sixth rib is then retracted superiorly using a blunt-tipped curved retractor (like a cat's paw) while the edge of the periosteum is grasped and pulled inferiorly. The intercostal vessels and nerve can, then, be visualized at the margin of the intercostal muscles in the anterior axillary line. A large lateral cutaneous branch is regularly found separating from the intercostal nerve at this level. It is seen penetrating the intercostal muscles on its way to the dermis infero-medially. The trunk of the intercostal nerve can, thus, be identified. The terminal anterior motor component can be viewed through the transparency as it runs along the margins of the intercostal muscles (Fig. 26.6). Eversion of the flap of the periosteum facilitates this. The nerve can be easily traced along this course with careful division of the tiny branches to the muscles. The pleura is not at risk in this step. The nerve is separated from the muscles and from the underlying pleura. We try to achieve adequate length to reach the musculocutaneous nerve in the axilla. This necessitates shifting the pivot point almost up to the posterior axillary line. It is difficult to separate the cutaneous and motor branches over such a distance, and, hence, the branch noted at the anterior axillary line has, most often, to be sacrificed [4]. Passage to the axilla around the margin of the serratus anterior would lead to loss of length. Hence, the muscle is split at a level posterior to the long thoracic nerve, and the nerves are passed laterally through the gap created. Usually, we can approximate the intercostal nerves to the trunk of the musculocutaneous nerve in the axilla with the arm in 60 degrees abduction. However, reaching the terminal motor branches for the biceps and brachialis involves dissection of the intercostals medial to the costochondral junctions with, evidently, reduction in the axon content. Alternatively, we need to plan the repair in less abduction.

Repair

The diminishing content of motor fibers along the course of each intercostal nerve prompted techniques that involved division of the nerve at the level of the mid-axillary line and bridging them to suitable target nerves with nerve grafts [5].

Tsuyama and Hara first proposed dissection of the nerves up to the costochondral junctions for direct transfers to the musculocutaneous nerve [6]. David Chuang [7] described his experience in a large series of cases whom intercostals were transferred directly to the musculocutaneous nerve.

In general, each intercostal is approximated to the target nerve with 2–3 epineural sutures using 9/0 or 10/0 nylon (Fig. 26.7). In the absence of tension at the repair site, application of tissue glue provides strength to the repair, and handling of the nerve ends for suturing is reduced.

The cross-sectional area of the intercostal nerves is much less than that of the trunk of the musculocutaneous nerve. Approximation of the predominantly motor intercostal nerves to the mixed musculocutaneous nerve would, inevitably, lead to loss of axons passing along the component heading for the lateral cutaneous nerve of the forearm. An attempt has been made to overcome this hurdle by coaptation of the intercostals to the lateral portion of the musculocutaneous nerve, which would lead to the terminal motor branches to the biceps and brachialis [8].

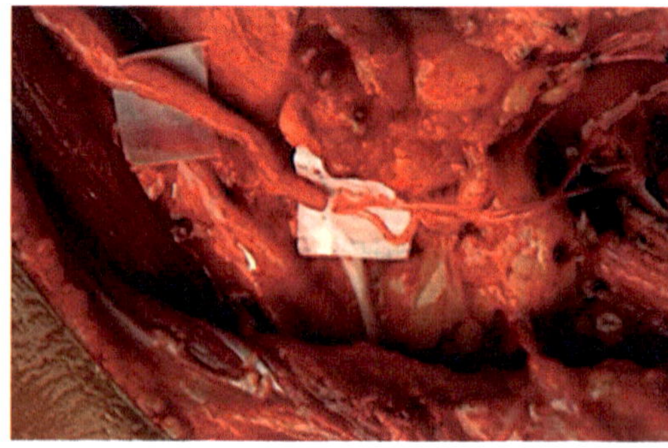

Fig. 26.7 The intercostal nerves are approximated to the trunk of the musculocutaneous nerve in the axilla with the arm in 60 degrees abduction. Neurorraphy of each intercostal nerve is performed with 2–3 epineural sutures using 9/0 or 10/0 nylon. Coaptation of the intercostals to the lateral portion of the musculocutaneous nerve would lead to the terminal motor branches to the biceps and brachialis

Brandt and Mackinnon [21] had proposed turning the lateral cutaneous branch back to be buried into the muscle. They published it for avoiding loss of axons along the sensory pathways and to augment the innervation of the biceps following transfer of the medial pectoral nerve to the musculocutaneous nerve. In the discussion, they have mentioned use of the technique in cases of intercostal nerve transfers to the musculocutaneous nerve as well. They have also mentioned exclusion of the branch to the coracobrachialis as that does not contribute to flexion of the elbow. It's our standard practice to transfer intercostal nerves to the trunk of the musculocutaneous nerve distal to the branch to the coraco-brachialis.

Postoperative Care

The arm is supported against the chest in an arm pouch sling for a month. Some surgeons prefer use of encircling bandages or even a spica cast. However, that would interfere with care of the axilla and, in my opinion, isn't necessary. Mobilization of the shoulder is limited to 30 degrees in any direction for a further period of a month to avoid excessive traction on the delicate repair of the intercostal nerves.

Galvanic stimulation of the biceps may be instructed to slow down the atrophy of the denervated muscle. The patient is instructed to flex the elbow passively 15–20 times per day to avoid stiffness while awaiting reinnervation. Malessy [9] has described the stages in re-appearance of function in the biceps following transfer of intercostal nerves. Initially, there is tenderness on pinching the muscle. Later, one can observe contraction of the distal portion of the muscle on deep inspiration. This can be made more evident by supporting the elbow at 90 degrees flexion and asking the patient to lift his head and look at the affected arm while lying supine. This exercise has been shown to be most effective in activation of the biceps via the intercostal nerve transfer [9, 10].

These early signs of reinnervation of the biceps are seen at 6–8 months after the repair. This contraction of the muscle should be demonstrated to the patient and his attendant so that the same maneuver can be repeated at home as well. Usually, the patient is instructed to practice contraction of the biceps in this way 100 times on waking up in the morning and, again, 100 times before going to bed (in groups of 3 repetitions each time). Progressive strengthening of the biceps is monitored and increased by adding resistance by tying weights at the wrist (50 g on wards). By this method, one can observe ability to flex the elbow against gravity by 6 months after the first appearance of contraction of the biceps. Surface EMG has been described as part of a biofeedback for re-education and strengthening. This was initially proposed for free functioning muscle transfers and can also be applied for intercostal nerve transfers to the musculocutaneous.

Utility of Intercostal Transfers in Reconstruction of Brachial Plexus Injuries

The availability of intercostal nerves as donors in the presence of root avulsions was known for a long time. Initial descriptions of their use are depicted in the designs published in the archives of Narakas and in the monograph of the GEM (1990) and show one or two intercostals being transferred to the musculocutaneous, pectoral, long thoracic, axillary, radial, and, even, median and ulnar nerves. Repeated studies of morphometry have revealed the limited content of motor fascicles in each intercostal nerve. Experience has shown that nerve transfers provide useful function when they are dedicated for one or, at most, two synergistic actions.

Elbow Flexion

Intercostal nerve transfers are most commonly utilized for the restoration of elbow flexion. The trunk of the musculocutaneous nerve contains 6000 myelinated fibers Bonnel et al. [11]. Freilinger et al. [12] reported on the number of motor and sensory fibers in each intercostal nerve. The number of motor fibers was approximately 45% at the level of the intervertebral foramen, and it dropped to 30% from the mid-axillary line forward for the upper intercostal nerves (up to the fourth) and as low as 15% for the lower intercostals (represented by the seventh). The drop in cross-sectional area of each intercostal nerve along its course was studied by Asfazadourian et al. [22]. They found that three intercostals (third to fifth) could effectively cover only a third of the cross-section of the musculocutaneous nerve and hypothesized that use of an additional intercostal would be more suitable. However, they also pointed to the greater difficulty faced in trying to achieve direct approximation of the next (sixth) intercostal nerve in the axilla. The correct number of intercostal nerves necessary for successful restoration of elbow flexion against gravity is not certain. The initial publications from Japan [17] referred to the use of two intercostals and even mentioned that they did not find a significant difference in the success rate with the use of three nerves. Most publications, however, refer to the use of three intercostals for the musculocutaneous nerve. The Mayo Clinic [20] has described the use of two intercostals for the nerve to the biceps and simultaneous transfer to two intercostals to innervate a gracilis for restoration of finger flexion (that also contributes to elbow flexion as it passes anterior to the elbow).

Elbow Extension

Doi [23] has stressed on the importance of reinnervating the triceps in his strategy of using two functioning free muscle transfers in the reconstruction of total palsies. Hence, the second stage includes use of two intercostals for the gracilis for finger flexion along with two intercostals for the long head of the triceps. Goubier and Teboul [13] have also reported their satisfaction with the use of three intercostals for the long head of the triceps (8/10 cases). On the other hand, Zheng et al. reported insufficient elbow extension against gravity in all 7 patients who had undergone the transfer of 2 to 3 intercostal nerves to the triceps branch of the radial nerve. In their series, the phrenic nerve had been used for restoration of elbow flexion [14].

In my own experience, innervation of the triceps using intercostal nerves could be documented. However, the patients with partial palsies, inevitably, regained some function in the triceps spontaneously. Close observation at long term revealed that the portion of the triceps innervated by the intercostals was not utilized when the patients reached out for objects. The absence of visual feedback of the effect of straining could be responsible for this as the patient cannot see the triceps contract.

Pectoral Nerve

Narakas had referred to the transfer of the third intercostal nerve to one of the pectoral nerves. We have preferred to use this technique in addition to the transfer of three intercostal nerves to the musculocutaneous nerve [15]. Useful contraction of the pectoralis major has been noted in 90% of patients, and this is synergistic with elbow flexion. The patients appear to have better stability of the shoulder joints, and the muscle also provides better control in patients in whom the shoulder was fused subsequently.

Long Thoracic Nerve

Doi [24] described the transfer of intercostals to the long thoracic nerve to augment the shoulder function in cases of avulsions of the C5-6-7 roots. In my own experience of 26 patients, the combined transfer of spinal accessory to suprascapular with two intercostals (fifth and sixth) to the long thoracic nerve has consistently restored external rotation in such patients with extensive partial palsies.

Axillary Nerve

It is known that the results for abduction can be improved by providing for reinnervation of the deltoid in addition to reconstruction of suprascapular function. A transfer from the triceps branches of the radial nerve is not feasible in extensive partial palsies. Leechavengvongs et al. proposed the simultaneous use of two intercostals for the triceps and two for the deltoid in such patients [16]. However, he has, now, abandoned that technique. In my own experience, contraction of the deltoid is seen with deep inspiration, but the range of abduction does not improve as the patient seems unable to harness the muscle during that action.

Outcomes (Intercostals to MC for Elbow Flexion Function)

Studies show variable results of elbow flexion after intercostal nerve transfer to the musculocutaneous nerve. An MRC-3 grade or more result ranges from 59.5% to 79.3% according to the literature with nerve transfer [18, 19].

In my study of 232 from 279 patients with total and near-total brachial plexus injuries, three intercostal nerves (ICN) were transferred to the main trunk of the musculocutaneous (MCN) for restoration of the biceps. These included 200 patients of total palsies (flail upper limbs) and 32 partial palsies. 31 of the partial palsies had sustained injuries to the roots with week residual hand function that precluded use of intraplexual nerve transfers (ulnar/

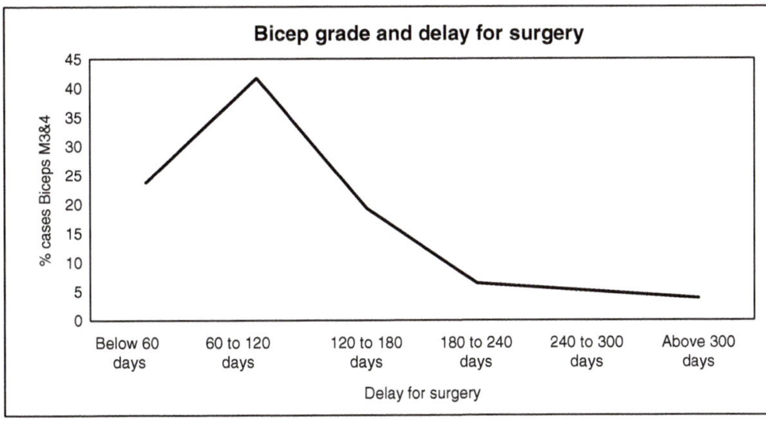

Fig. 26.8 Percentage of cases with biceps grade M3 and 4 and time delay for surgery ($n = 232$)

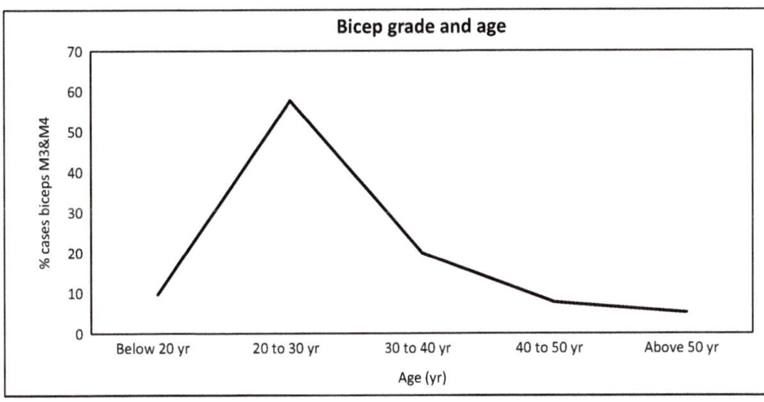

Fig. 26.9 Percentage of cases with biceps grade M3 and 4 and age ($n = 232$)

median). Patients who underwent surgery within 180 days had a successful outcome (MRC grade 3 and above) more often who were underwent surgery at a longer delay (72.1% vs 49.0%) (Fig. 26.8). This difference between patients operated upon beyond 6 months was found to be statistically significant ($p = 0.002$) (Table 26.1).

Age is another important factor to consider during nerve reconstructions. Significant association ($p < 0.005$) was observed between age and follow-up biceps grades in patients with total or near total brachial plexus injuries that underwent three intercostal nerves transfer (ICN) to musculocutaneous. Patients younger than 30 years old had better outcomes (MRC grade 3 and above) than older patients (Fig. 26.9). The percentage of a successful outcome (MRC grade 3 and greater) in patients younger than 30 years was significantly better (80.2%) in patients with less than 30 years than in older patients (50.5%) (Table 26.2).

Table 26.1 Association between follow-up biceps grade and delay for surgery ($n = 232$)

	Biceps grades at follow-up		
Delay in surgery in days	0–2 ($n = 76$)	3 and 4 ($n = 156$)	Chi-square value (p)
<180 ($n = 183$)	51 (27.9%)	132 (72.1%)	9.405 ($P = 0.002$)
>180 ($n = 49$)	25 (51.0%)	24 (49.0%)	

Table 26.2 Association between follow-up biceps grade and age at surgery in patients who underwent intercostal nerve transfer ($n = 232$)

	Biceps grades at follow-up		
Age at surgery	0–2 ($n = 76$)	3 & 4 ($n = 156$)	Chi-square value (p)
≤30 years ($n = 131$)	26 (26.1%)	105 (80.2%)	22.77 ($p < 0.005$)
>30 years ($n = 101$)	50 (49.5%)	51 (50.5%)	

References

1. Yeoman PM, Seddon HJ. Brachial plexus injuries: treatment of the flail arm. J Bone Joint Surg. 1961; 43B:3. https://doi.org/10.1302/0301-620X.43B3.493.
2. Waikakul S, Wongtragul S, Vanadurongwan V. Restoration of elbow flexion in brachial plexus avulsion injury: comparing spinal accessory nerve transfer with intercostal nerve transfer. J Hand Surg. 1999;24A:571–7. https://doi.org/10.1053/jhsu.1999.0571.
3. Nagano A, Yamamoto S, Mikami Y. Intercostal nerve transfer to restore upper extremity functions after brachial plexus injury. Ann Acad Med Singap. 1995;1995(24):42–5.
4. Malungpaishrope K, Leechavengvongs S, Witoonchart K, Uerpairojkit C, Boonyalapa A, Janesaksrisakul DJ. Simultaneous intercostal nerve transfers to deltoid and triceps muscle through the posterior approach. Hand Surg Am. 2012;37(4): 677–82. https://doi.org/10.1016/j.jhsa.2011.
5. Dolenc VV. Reconstruction of individual peripheral nerves with intercostal nerves in avulsions of all five roots of the brachial plexus. Clin Plast Surg. 1984;11:144.
6. Tsuyama N, Hara T. Intercostal nerve transfer in the treatment of brachial plexus injury of root avulsion type. Exerpta Medica. 1972;29(01):35.
7. Chuang DC, Yeh MC, Wei FC. Intercostal nerve transfer of the musculocutaneous nerve in avulsed brachial plexus injuries. Evaluation of 66 patients. J Hand Surg. 1992;17(5):822–8.
8. Ochial N, Mikami Y, Yamamoto S, Nakagawa T, Nagano A. A new technique for mismatched nerve suture in direct intercostals nerve transfers. J Hand Surg Br. 1993;18(3):318–9.
9. Malessy MJ, Thomeer RT. Evaluation of intercostal to musculocutaneous nerve transfer in reconstructive brachial plexus surgery. J Neurosurg. 1998;88:266–71.
10. Chalidapong P, Sananpanich K, Klaphaione J. Electromyographic comparision of various exercises to improve elbow flexion following intercostal nerve transfer. J Bone Joint Surg Br. 2006;88(5):620–2.
11. Bonnel FR. P. Anatomie et systématisation du plexus brachial de l'adulte. Anatomia Clin. 1980;2:289–98.
12. Freilinger G, Holle J, Sulzgruber SC. Distribution of motor and sensory fibers in the intercostal nerves. Plast Reconstr Surg. 1978;62:240–4.
13. Goubier JN, Teboul F. Technique of the intercostals nerves to the nerve of the long head of the triceps to recover elbow extension in brachial plexus palsy. Tech Hand Up Extrem Surg. 2007;11:139–41.
14. Zheng MX, Xu WD, Qiu YQ, Xu JG, Gu YD. Phrenic nerve transfer for elbow flexion and intercostals nerve transfer for elbow extension. J Hand Surg. 2010;35A:1304–9.
15. Narakas AO. The surgical treatment of traumatic brachial plexus lesions. Int Surg. 1980;65:521–7.
16. Malungpaishrope K, Leechavengvongs S, Witoonchart K, Uerpairojkit C, Boonyalapa A, Janesaksrisakul D. Simultaneous intercostal nerve transfers to deltoid and triceps muscle through the posterior approach. J Hand Surg. 2012;37A:677–82.
17. Nagano A, Naoichi T, Naoyuki O, Tetsuya H, Masataru T. Direct nerve crossing with the intercostal nerve to treat avulsion injuries of the brachial plexus. J Hand Surg. 1989;14(6):980–5.
18. Socolovsky M, Paez MD. A literature review of intercostal-to-musculocutaneous-nerve transfers in brachial plexus injuries patients: does body mass index influences results in Eastern versus Western countries? Surg Neurol Int. 2013;4:152. Published online 27 Nov 2013.
19. Bulstra LF, Shin AY. Nerve transfers to restore elbow function. Hand Clin. 2016;32(2):165–74.
20. Maldonado AA, Kircher MF, Spinner RJ, Bishop AT, Shin AY. Free functioning gracilis muscle transfer with and without simultaneous intercostal nerve transfer to musculocutaneous nerve for restoration of elbow flexion after traumatic adult brachial panplexus injury. J Hand Surg. 2017;42(4):293–7.
21. Brandt KE, Mackinnon SE. A technique for maximizing biceps recovery in brachial plexus reconstruction. J Hand Surg. 1993;18(4):726–33.
22. Asfazadourian H, Tramond B, Dauge MC, Oberlin C. Morphometric study of the upper intercostal nerves-practical application for neurotisations in traumatic brachial plexus palsies. Ann Chir Main (Ann Hand Surg). 1999;18(4):243–53.
23. Double free-muscle transfer to restore prehension following complete brachial plexus avulsion. J Hand Surg 1995;20(3):408–14.
24. Yamada T, Doi K, Hattori Y, Hoshino S, Sakamoto S, Arakawa Y. Long thoracic nerve neurotisation for restoration of shoulder function in C5-7 brachial plexus pre-ganglionic injuries-case report. J Hand Surg. 2010;35A:1427–31.

Sural Nerve Harvest

27

Christine Oh, Nicholas Pulos,
and Alexander Y. Shin

Introduction

For grafting of mixed and motor nerve segments, autologous sural nerve remains the gold standard. The sural nerve can reliably provide 30 cm of usable nerve graft from one lower extremity with minimal donor site morbidity. Advances in minimally invasive harvest techniques in sural nerve graft harvest continue to improve donor site morbidity.

Anatomy

The sural nerve originates from nerve roots S1 and S2 and provides sensation to the distal posterolateral leg. It is formed by the confluence of the medial sural cutaneous nerve from the posterior tibial nerve and the lateral sural cutaneous nerve from the common peroneal nerve. The site of sural nerve origin is approximately 8 cm below the bifurcation of the sciatic nerve. The medial sural nerve continues on to exit from the subfascial plane deep to the gastrocnemius fascial raphe in the midline and will meet the lateral sural which is subcutaneous at approximately 20 cm proximal from the lateral malleolus. Anatomic variations are possible in approximately 20 percent of cases, with absent branching or more proximal branching possible [12]. The sural nerve will course within the subcutaneous plane in the posterolateral leg. Its distal continuation via the lateral calcaneal and lateral dorsal cutaneous branches provides sensation to the posterolateral aspect of the foot. Its contribution to the plantar foot sensation is insignificant and thus is acceptable for nerve graft harvest. For nerve harvest, the sural nerve can be identified between the lateral malleolus and Achilles tendon at the midpoint between the two structures 2 cm superior to the lateral malleolus in the subcutaneous plane. The lesser saphenous vein runs adjacent to the sural nerve and is typically located just posterior to the nerve. It can be useful as a marker for the nerve.

Total length of the sural nerve harvest may be longer than 30 cm. Sural nerve fibers are isolated from the other tibial and sciatic nerve fibers beyond its anatomical origin with a thin layer of epineurium [13]. Reidl et al. described an additional 14 cm of length, which may be harvested when an epineurolysis is performed proximally within the tibial nerve to separate the sural nerve fascicles. There is a potential risk associated with dissection adjacent to the important motoneurons

C. Oh · N. Pulos
Department of Orthopedic Surgery, Mayo Clinic, Rochester, MN, USA
e-mail: oh.christine@mayo.edu

A. Y. Shin (✉)
Department of Orthopedic Surgery, Mayo Clinic, Rochester, MN, USA
e-mail: shin.alexander@mayo.edu

A. Y. Shin, N. Pulos (eds.), *Operative Brachial Plexus Surgery*,
https://doi.org/10.1007/978-3-030-69517-0_27

of the tibial and sciatic nerve, but with meticulous, tension free dissection, the perineurium and nerve fibers remain uninjured [9, 13].

Blood Supply

The ideal nerve graft is a conduit that promotes rapid axon regeneration, and thus blood supply of the graft is a critical consideration for success [15]. Adequate vascularity is associated with the retention of Schwann cells and funicular architecture to facilitate the ingrowth and maturation of axons. In 1939 Sterling Bunnell first used thin autogenous grafts transferred to a healthy vascular bed for successful grafting [1]. Subsequently, in 1972 cable nerve grafting was refined by Millesi et al. allowing accurate interfascicular placement of grafts [11]. Nerve grafts are revascularized in a centripetal fashion and require a healthy recipient bed, evolving to the use of cable nerve grafting. Hence, the conventional nerve grafts of today rely on free cable grafts of thin long peripheral sensory nerves instead of a single large nerve graft to prevent central necrosis. The blood supply to a traditional nerve graft is provided with the longitudinal vessels which course axially on the surface of the nerve, supplying the epineurium, perineurium, and endoneurium with an anastomotic vascular network [16]. With the advent of microsurgery, Taylor et al. first described the free vascularized nerve graft utilizing the contralateral superficial radial nerve to reconstruct the median nerve in the setting of a patient with Volkmann's ischemic contracture [16]. This was then expanded upon by Gilbert and Doi who described the vascularized sural nerve graft in 1984 [4, 6]. Vascularized nerve grafts are reported to allow faster nerve regeneration, averaging 2.4 mm per day compared to a standard 1 mm per day [15].

In a study comparing vascularized versus conventional nerve graft within a well-vascularized wound bed, no difference in speed of recovery or final outcome was noted for axillary nerve defects. However, for long nerve gaps between 7 and 14 cm in patients with ulnar or radial nerve lesions, earlier and improved functional recovery with vascularized nerve grafts than conventional grafts has been reported [5]. Doi et al. conclude that consideration for vascularized nerve graft should be given in the case of a nerve gap larger than 6 cm associated with a skin defect or compromised wound bed [5]. Doi described a technique for harvesting a vascularized sural nerve. The procedure is challenging and time consuming with a steep learning curve. Most reports are in the setting of large nerve gaps where the recipient bed is heavily scarred and also requires the transfer of a thick nerve; thus the applications of a vascularized sural nerve graft are quite limited [15]. If a patient necessitates vascularized nerve graft, it is likely best served with a different donor nerve, such as vascularized ulnar nerve [4].

Operative Techniques

Patient positioning varies depending on the surgical situation. Prone positioning is the most conducive for sural nerve harvest, but often does not facilitate the primary operation. The patient may be lateral decubitus or supine. If supine, an assistant can either maintain positioning of the lower extremity. Downsides to this can include congestion of the operating room space secondary to the additional assistant and if a trainee, whether medical student or resident, is holding the extremity, precludes visualization of the procedure and compromises intraoperative education. Our preference is to use a lower extremity limb positioner (SPIDER2 Limb Positioner, Smith and Nephew, Andover, MA) during nerve harvest. The limb positioner may be used with an ankle distractor accessory to elevate the leg and provide exposure to the posterior lower leg without the need to reposition the patient.

The traditional open technique of sural nerve harvest uses a single longitudinal incision along the lower leg in line with the course of the nerve beginning distally within the groove between the Achilles tendon and the lateral malleolus. The lesser saphenous vein is identified, preserved, and retracted. Once the nerve is identified, it is mobilized tagged with a vessel loop, which provides identification, gentle handling, and mild traction. The dissection is carried out proximally to the level of the popliteal fossa. This open approach provides visualization of the entire sural nerve anatomy, especially of the lateral branch which can be harvested if additional length is needed. The main advantages of this approach are that the direct visualization allows for meticulous hemostasis, careful handling of the nerve, and proper treatment of any diverging nerve branches. However, a stocking seam incision may be excessively morbid for some patients, and minimally invasive techniques have been described [3]. Starting distally, several (typically 3–4) 2–3 cm "stair-step" or counter incisions can be made along the length of the nerve until the popliteal fossa is reached with the nerve transected distally and then proximally. This technique can limit incision burden, yet the scars can still be unsightly.

An alternative would be to use a nerve or tendon stripper. With these devices, a limited distal incision is made, and the stripper is passed through the end of the nerve and then gently passed proximally in a rotary maneuver until the tip of the instrument can be palpated near the popliteal fossa [8]. This technique allows for two total incisions (distal and proximal). Potential complications of using a stripper include injury to the nerve during dissection as well inadvertent transection of the sural nerve graft. The communicating branch of the peroneal nerve is transected in a potentially traumatic, avulsing manner with this technique since it is not directly visualized. The entire dissection is completed without any direct visualization, and just by proprioception and when resistance is met, typically at the site of nerve branching, inadvertent force could potentially transect the nerve. It is critical to understand the expected anatomic course of the nerve and position the instrument in the direction toward the primary nerve and not any lateral branch points.

To circumvent such a complication, endoscopic sural nerve harvest is a technique to allow direct visualization of the dissection. A limited (1–2 cm) distal incision is made and the sural nerve identified; a vessel loop may be placed around the nerve for gentle traction. There are variations in harvest technique—the number of incisions and preferred dissecting instruments (tenotomy, endoscopic scissor, nerve or tendon stripper, or Foley catheter balloon) [2, 7, 10, 14]. A cone tip endoscopic dissector typically used for vessel harvest in vascular surgery such as the VasoView (Guidant Co., Natick, MA) is used with a 0 degree, 5 mm endoscope (Storz Instruments, San Dimas, CA). The VasoView conical dissectors seem to be the optimal instrument for endoscopic sural nerve harvest compared to the Foley catheter or standard endoscopic view port. The cone dissector is inserted from the distal incision and CO2 is used for light insufflation. Dissection is directly visualized and carried out throughout the length of the sural nerve using only the cone dissector. This is a rapid and facile dissection with minimal bleeding. No additional endoscopic instruments are necessary. The nerve can be free circumferentially from the surrounding subcutaneous tissue to allow full mobilization and carried up to the popliteal fossa where the medial and lateral sural nerve join. A counter incision is then made at the level approximately 2 cm below the popliteal fossa in a transverse fashion to allow for harvesting of the sural nerve proximally under direct visualization using the endoscope. The lateral sural nerve branch may be separated at this time and either harvest in conjunction or left in place. A transverse incision at this level takes advantage of the skin tension lines in this area and will optimize scar healing. The sural nerve is then extracted through the distal wound. The endoscopic technique allows for shorter incisions, less visible scarring, decreased post-operative pain, and shorter recovery [2, 3]. In pediatric patients especially, a standard telescope can even be utilized to facilitate endoscopic dissection if a cone tip dissector is not available given the shorter length of the pediatric limb.

Complications

The sural nerves can provide an abundant source of graft material with minimal branching and functional deficit associated with harvest. It is easily accessible and has large fascicles to facilitate successful grafting. Complications associated with nerve graft harvest include injury to the nerve during dissection, primarily with traction and handling, which may compromise the quality of the nerve graft. This emphasizes the importance of gentle handling of the nerve throughout the harvest and using as atraumatic a technique as possible. When harvesting additional length beyond the popliteal fossa, there is the potential for injury to the sciatic or tibial nerves. When additional length is necessary after bilateral harvest, proximal dissection should be done under direct visualization as with open harvest. There is the risk of symptomatic neuroma at the remaining stump of the sural nerve. However, by harvesting the nerve proximal to its course within the gastrocnemius fascia, the remaining nerve stump may be buried within the muscle belly and is rarely symptomatic.

References

1. Bunnell S, Boyes JH. Nerve grafts. Am J Surg. 1939;44(1):64–75. ISSN 0002-9610, https://doi.org/10.1016/S0002-9610(39)90934-7. (https://www.sciencedirect.com/science/article/pii/S0002961039909347).
2. Butler DP, Johal KS, Wicks CE, Grobbelaar AO. Objective sensory and functional outcomes at the donor site following endoscopic-assisted sural nerve harvest. J Plast Reconstr Aesthet Surg. 2017;70:659–65.
3. Capek L, Clarke HM, Zuker RM. Endoscopic sural nerve harvest in the pediatric patient. Plast Reconstr Surg. 1996;98:884–8.
4. Doi K, Kuwata N, Kawakami F, Tamaru K, Kawai S. The free vascularized sural nerve graft. Microsurgery. 1984;5:175–84.
5. Doi K, Tamaru K, Sakai K, Kuwata N, Kurafuji Y, Kawai S. A comparison of vascularized and conventional sural nerve grafts. J Hand Surg Am. 1992;17:670–6.
6. Gilbert A. Vascularized sural nerve graft. Clin Plast Surg. 1984;11:73–7.
7. Hadlock TA, Cheney ML. Single-incision endoscopic sural nerve harvest for cross face nerve grafting. J Reconstr Microsurg. 2008;24:519–23.
8. Hill HL, Vasconez LO, Jurkiewicz MJ. Method for obtaining a sural nerve graft. Plast Reconstr Surg. 1978;61:177–9.
9. Jaroszynski G, Johnston GH. Harvesting of the sural nerve with a tendon stripper. Microsurgery. 1996;17:217–20.
10. Koh KS, Park S. Endoscopic harvest of sural nerve graft with balloon dissection. Plast Reconstr Surg. 1998;101:810–2.
11. Millesi H, Meissl G, Berger A. The interfascicular nerve-grafting of the median and ulnar nerves. J Bone Joint Surg Am. 1972;54:727–50.
12. Ortiguela ME, Wood MB, Cahill DR. Anatomy of the sural nerve complex. J Hand Surg Am. 1987;12:1119–23.
13. Riedl O, Koemuercue F, Marker M, Hoch D, Haas M, Deutinger M. Sural nerve harvesting beyond the popliteal region allows a significant gain of donor nerve graft length. Plast Reconstr Surg. 2008;122:798–805.
14. Spinks TJ, Adelson PD. Pediatric sural nerve harvest: a fully endoscopic technique. Neurosurgery. 2009;64:360–3; discussion 363–4.
15. Taylor GI. Free vascularized nerve transfer in the upper extremity. Hand Clin. 1999;15:673–95, ix–x.
16. Taylor GI, Ham FJ. The free vascularized nerve graft. A further experimental and clinical application of microvascular techniques. Plast Reconstr Surg. 1976;57:413–26.

Contralateral C7 Nerve Transfer in the Treatment of Adult Brachial Plexus Injuries and Spastic Hemiplegia

28

Yun-Dong Shen and Wen-Dong Xu

Introduction

Contralateral C7 nerve root transfer surgery is one of the most important surgical methods in treating brachial plexus avulsion injury, which was first reported by Dr. Gu in 1986. In this surgery, the C7 nerve on the healthy side was transferred to the injured side to establish a connection between the ipsilateral motor cortex and the affected limb and restore limb function. With long-term follow-up and experimental studies, it was found that contralateral C7 nerve root transfer could trigger a series of brain plasticity and indicated that one hemisphere has potential in controlling bilateral upper limb after nerve transfer. Based on these discoveries, the contralateral C7 nerve root transfer has been extended to treat hemiplegic paralysis and gets much achievement.

Y.-D. Shen · W.-D. Xu (✉)
Department of Hand Surgery, Huashan Hospital, Shanghai Medical College, Fudan University, Shanghai, China
e-mail: wendongxu@fudan.edu.cn

Part I: Adult Brachial Plexus Injuries: Restoration of Hand Function in the Pan Plexus Injury— CC7

Brief History of Contralateral C7 Nerve Root Transfer

In the case of brachial plexus avulsion injury (BPAI), nerve transfer is the optimal method for restoration of critical motor or sensory function in the injured limb. In a nerve transfer procedure, total or partial of an intact but less important nerve is coapted to the distal of an injured peripheral nerve to reconstruct a more important motor or sensory function. However, for patients with complete root avulsion of the brachial plexus, intraplexus donor nerves are not available to be used for restoring the function of the injured upper extremity; thus all the donor nerves are from extraplexus origins. Extraplexus donor nerves that are most commonly used for transfer include the accessory nerve, phrenic nerve, intercostal nerves, contralateral C7 (CC7) nerve, and motor branches of the cervical plexus. The contralateral C7 nerve is a relatively new, controversial but valuable donor.

The seventh cervical nerve root transfer from the contralateral healthy side was first performed in 1986 for treatment of total BPAI [1]. Since then, this procedure has been increasingly adopted and has been one of the major treatments

A. Y. Shin, N. Pulos (eds.), *Operative Brachial Plexus Surgery*,
https://doi.org/10.1007/978-3-030-69517-0_28

for BPAI. Although there have been controversies on cutting off a normal nerve root without any neurologic sequelae to the donor limb, this technique has been gaining wider and wider acceptance as increasing experiences have been acquired to verify its efficiency and safety.

Surgical Anatomy of C7 Nerve

The C7 nerve has its unique anatomic features that make it an efficient and safe donor nerve for transfer:

1. The C7 nerve contains 27,213 ± 5417 myelinated nerve fibers which are more than the total number of all extraplexus donor nerves available for transfer [2]. It is a mixed nerve root that consists of both motor and sensory fibers, and the histochemical studies of C7 in cadavers have revealed that the posterior division of C7 mainly contains motor fibers while the anterior division mainly contains sensory fibers. In the anterior division particularly, the sensory fibers are mostly located in the anterior and medial part.
2. The C7 nerve root independently forms the middle trunk of brachial plexus, while the C5-C6 nerve roots form the upper trunk and the C8-T1 nerve roots form the lower trunk, respectively. Further studies suggested that the C7 nerve root mostly joins the lateral cord (44–44.2%) and posterior cord (44.6–44.8%) of brachial plexus. The motor fibers mainly innervate the medial head of triceps, extensor carpi radialis brevis, and extensor digitorum communis. The sensory fibers mostly distribute to the lateral arm and forearm and the digits centered on the index finger.
3. There is cross-innervation from the upper or lower trunk of brachial plexus in C7-innervated muscles; thus no single muscle is dominated by C7 alone. Muscles controlled by C7 can be compensated for by other nerve roots; for example, latissimus dorsi is also innervated by C6 and C8, triceps by C5, 6, and 8 and T1, and flexor carpi ulnaris and extensor digitorum communis by C8 and T1 [3]. Accordingly, the function of C7 nerve could be compensated either by the upper trunk or the lower trunk while it is injured or cut off. Microdissection and histochemical studies of the C7 nerve root indicated that motor fibers of the C7 nerve root are dispersive and only half of the fibers from the thoracodorsal nerve originate from the C7 root. These findings confirmed that the innervation of motor fibers in the C7 root is dependent and compensable, which provides a scientific evidence for the safety of contralateral C7 nerve root transfer. Therefore, cutting off the entire or partial C7 nerve root isolatedly does not result in significant functional loss of any individual muscle [4, 5].

Indications for Contralateral C7 Transfer

1. Patients who had traction injury of unilateral upper extremity with complete palsy and total root avulsions. They should have no associated injury with the contralateral upper extremity or around the shoulder.
2. Contralateral C7 nerve root transfer could be indicated as one of the series of multiple nerve transfer for treatment of total or severe BPAI, together with other nerve transfers such as accessory nerve, phrenic nerve, and intercostal nerves transfer. Besides that, contralateral C7 nerve could also be a donor nerve of free muscle transplantation, such as free gracilis muscle transplantation by innervated median nerve.

Preparation of Contralateral C7 Nerve Root

The patient is placed in supine position with the head toward the affected side after execution of general anesthesia. A ~7 cm transverse incision is made 2 cm parallel to and above the contralateral clavicle. The transverse cervical vessels and omohyoid muscle are ligated or retracted to one side. All five roots are explored, and the anatomic configuration of brachial plexus is identified by gross observation. The C7 nerve root is determined by detecting action potentials elicited from the latissimus dorsi muscle and the triceps as well as observing shoulder adduction, elbow, and wrist extension by using intraoperative microstimulation with direct current stimulator [3]. Thereafter, the contralateral C7 is dissected as distally as possible and then severed for transfer.

Preparation of Nerve Grafts

1. Ulnar nerve graft with vessel anastomosis

In order to ensure sufficient blood supply of long grafted nerve, some authors suggested vessel anastomosing with ulnar nerve graft. In this procedure, the ulnar artery and ulnar vein were harvested accompany with the ulnar nerve, and then the ulnar artery and vein were anastomosed with the transverse cervical artery and vein, respectively. The proximal end of the ulnar nerve is coapted to the target nerve such as the median nerve in the upper arm of the affected side.

2. Pedicled ulnar nerve graft

In a more recent time, with the development of anatomy, it is suggested that the superior ulnar collateral artery with cross section diameter of more than 0.5 mm is capable of providing sufficient blood supply for the ulnar nerve with a width/length ratio of 1/45, and the pedicled ulnar nerve could be harvested for grafting without anastomosing the ulnar artery or vein. Based on this, an equally satisfactory outcome could be achieved without anastomosing vessels in pedicled ulnar nerve grafted contralateral C7 nerve transfer. Therefore, for a simplified procedure, the superior ulnar collateral artery that is located above the elbow and provides blood supply for the upper segment of ulnar nerve was also harvested with the ulnar nerve.

A two-stage surgery is suggested to connect the contralateral C7 nerve root to the injured brachial plexus via pedicled ulnar nerve graft to maintain a good blood supply for the grafting ulnar nerve.

In the first stage, the ulnar nerve and its dorsal cutaneous branch on the affected side are severed at the wrist level and dissected proximally to the level of superior ulnar collateral artery (Fig. 28.1a). The distal end of the ulnar nerve is then drawn to the supraclavicular region on the contralateral side through a cross-chest subcutaneous tunnel. The distal end of the ulnar nerve is coapted to the C7 nerve root (Fig. 28.1b) in the first stage of this surgery while the proximal end of the pedicled ulnar nerve is coapted to the recipient nerve, such as the median nerve, radial nerve, and musculocutaneous nerve of the injured side at the second stage.

The second stage could be performed when nerve regeneration has reached the axilla of the affected side as decided by clinical and physiological studies as follows: i) tapping along the route of ulnar nerve until the Tinel's sign could be elicited at ipsilateral axilla; ii) sensory evoked potential (SEP) could be elicited from scalp while stimulating along the route of subcutaneous ulnar nerve, which demonstrates successful nerve regeneration; iii) based on previous experiences and the nerve growth rate of 1 mm per day, the average time for nerve regeneration to the axilla was 4–20 months (mean 10.5 months) in adults [1, 6].

According to previous studies, no significant difference was found in terms of motor recovery in the forearm and hand using a vascularized ulnar nerve graft with vessel anastomosing, compared with a pedicled ulnar nerve graft which involved only the superior ulnar collateral vessels [5]. Therefore, the pedicled ulnar nerve grafted contralateral C7 transfer is suggested over the one with vessel anastomosing.

3. Sural nerve graft

With respect to avulsion of both the upper and the middle trunk of brachial plexus with partial injury of the lower trunk, the ulnar nerve on the affected side is not suitable to be harvested for grafting because it has the possibility of continuous functional recovery. In these circumstances, free or vascularized sural nerve grafts are harvested for bridging the donor and recipient nerves.

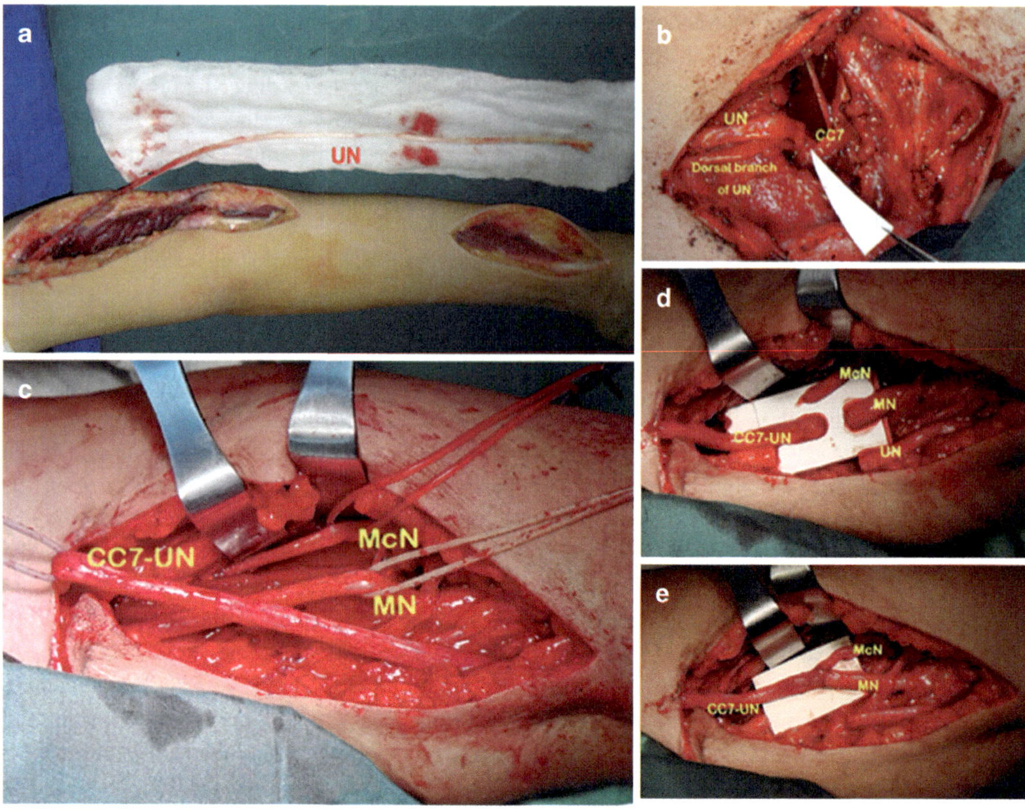

Fig. 28.1 (**a**) Preparation of pedicled ulnar nerve graft. The ulnar nerve and its dorsal cutaneous branch on the affected side are severed at the wrist level and dissected proximally. The superior ulnar collateral artery of upper arm segment is also harvested together with the ulnar nerve. The distal end of the ulnar nerve is then drawn to the supraclavicular region on the unaffected side through a cross-chest subcutaneous tunnel. UN ulnar nerve. (**b**) The distal end of the ulnar nerve is drawn to the supraclavicular region on the contralateral side through a cross-chest subcutaneous tunnel. The distal end of the ulnar nerve is coapted to the C7 nerve root in the first stage of this surgery. CC7 contralateral C7 nerve, UN ulnar nerve. (**c**) Exploration of affected upper arm at the second stage of CC7 nerve transfer. The reversed UN is dissected and then transected for transfer. MN median nerve, McN musculocutaneous nerve, UN ulnar nerve, CC7 contralateral C7 nerve. (**d**) The proximal UN was ready for coaptation with the distal McN and MN. MN median nerve, McN musculocutaneous nerve, UN ulnar nerve, CC7 contralateral C7 nerve. (**e**) The coaptation of proximal UN with McN and MN simultaneously at the second stage of CC7 nerve transfer (through pedicled ulnar nerve graft). MN median nerve, McN musculocutaneous nerve, UN ulnar nerve, CC7 contralateral C7 nerve

(i) Free sural nerve graft

Free sural nerve that matches the defect length between contralateral C7 nerve and the recipient nerve is dissected and harvested from either leg. Two to four strands of the harvested sural nerve are arranged passing though subcutaneous tunnel in the upper chest region depending on the cross-sectional area of the contralateral C7 nerve root.

(ii) Vascularized sural nerve graft

The grafted sural nerve is harvested together with the small saphenous vein. The proximal end of the small saphenous vein is anastomosed with the transverse cervical artery and the distal end to the thoracoacromial artery while the nerve grafting is performed.

4. Direct neurorrhaphy to the lower trunk

In 2010, Feng et al. introduced a new route for contralateral C7 nerve root transfer to the injured lower trunk or the C8-T1 nerve roots of brachial plexus via a subcutaneous tunnel across the anterior surface of the chest and neck. Direct neurorrhaphy was performed in two patients and nerve grafts of 4.5 cm in length were used in the other two patients [7].

In contrast with traditional route, the regenerating distance in this procedure was greatly shortened, and ulnar nerve harvesting with extensive scar was avoided. Therefore, it might be a possible alternative to regain better wrist flexion, finger flexion, and hand sensation for total BPAI patients. Nevertheless, a long-term follow-up with more cases involved is still needed to validate this new surgical procedure over the traditional approaches.

Selection of Recipient Nerves

1. Single recipient nerve

In order to ensure a satisfactory recovery, the entire contralateral C7 root is frequently used, and usually a single target is reconstructed. In most of the patients, the contralateral C7 root is directed to musculocutaneous nerve, radial nerve, or median nerve of the affected limb [1]. The median nerve is the mostly recommended single recipient nerve because both the C7 nerve and the median nerve consist of mixed nerve fibers including sensory and motor fibers. With this combination of nerve, both motor and sensory functional recoveries of a single recipient nerve are reconstructed [4, 5, 8]. In others, they preferred to repair the suprascapular nerve or the posterior cord first as a part of double free muscle transfer procedure for a further reconstruction of prehension function with innervated free muscles [9].

2. Multiple recipient nerves

The contralateral C7 root could be transferred to neurotize median nerve and triceps branches of radial nerve or both the musculocutaneous nerve and the median nerve of the affected side (Fig. 28.1c–e).

In a recent report of selective contralateral C7 transfer by Terzis, the anterior division of contralateral C7 was used to neurotize flexors and median nerve while the posterior division was transferred to extensor targets. Usually, neurotized free muscles were transferred in a staged reconstruction to enhance the upper extremity function. Free muscles for elbow flexion or finger flexion were neurotized from the anterior division, and free muscles for elbow or finger extension were from the posterior division [10].

Postoperative Monitoring

After surgery, the head, neck, and the affected upper extremity are immobilized with a brace for 3–4 weeks with arm against the chest, elbow flexed, and neck in neutral position.

Nerve regeneration is tested by advancing Tinel's sign along the nerve route and the sensory evoked potential (SEP) elicited from the scalp while stimulating the subcutaneous nerve graft. And needle electromyography (EMG) examination confirms successful reinnervation of the nerve by compound muscle action potential (CMAP) in the target muscles.

Rehabilitation protocol is performed instantly after removal of the splint. It contains four aspects: (1) passive range of motion of the affected upper extremity; (2) slow-pulse electrical stimulation on the nerve regenerating route; (3) simultaneous motions of abducting, internally rotating, and extending the shoulder and the elbow of the contralateral upper extremity while contracting of the reinnervated muscles; (4) conscious reeducation of voluntary motions of affected upper extremity without initiation of contralateral limb should be performed to promote an interhemispheric cerebral reorganization.

Potential Complications

1. Sensory abnormality

In the literature, most researchers reported that a majority of the patients experienced temporary paresthesia in the median nerve area of the donor limb. In Songcharoen et al.'s report, nearly all patients (97%) had sensory deficits transiently, which resolved completely within 7 months [4]. Paresthesia, mostly numbness, frequently affects the distal index finger followed by thumb and middle finger. In a few cases, paresthetic area also includes the ring finger, volar palm, and radial area of the contralateral forearm. But the sensory abnormalities spontaneously recovered postoperatively although the recovery duration varied in different studies. Liu et al. reported a period of 1.5–2 years is needed for disappearance of sensory abnormalities [11], but in Sungpet and his associates' report, it took only 3 months for all but 1 patient to resolve this paresthesia [12]. In Chuang's series of 21 patients with more than 2 years' follow-up, 48% of the patients had no significant sensory changes, and most patients (81%) were free of motor weakness in the contralateral limb. In his observation, sensory and motor function abnormalities mostly recovered within 3 months postoperatively [13].

2. Temporary motor deficit

Motor deficits of extensor weakness in the elbow, wrist, or fingers in the contralateral limb are also the main complication after operation but less common than sensory deficit. Temporary mild weakness of the strength of the extensor muscles occurs shortly after operation, but muscle strength may return to normal in the long run [14]. Chuang reported a motor deficit in 19% of patients after entire contralateral C7 transection [13]. Other reports of contralateral C7 root transfer also confirm the absence of any long-term functional deficits [5]. In another study of hemi-contralateral C7 nerve transfer, there were only 3% of the patients reported transient motor deficit [4]. Nearly all the motor deficits recovered to normal within 6–12 months. Usually, complete functional recovery was noted within 6 months after surgery.

3. Anatomic variation associated upper extremity paralysis

Theoretically, the anatomic variation of prefixed or postfixed brachial plexus with involvement of C4 or T2 contribution may result in considerable complications of limb paralysis after contralateral C7 transfer. Although this anatomic variation is rare, adequate exposure of all five roots and intraoperative EMG tests were effective and necessary preventions to avoid function deficits in the donor limb.

Results and Outcomes from the Literature

In the contralateral C7 transfer to the median nerve with pedicled ulnar nerve grafting, 62.5% of 8 patients with 2-year follow-up regained M3 for wrist flexion and finger flexion [15]. In a relatively recent report of long-term follow-up, functional recovery reached M3 or greater in 50% for the finger flexors and S3 or greater in 12 patients after median nerve neurotization.

In Hierner et al.'s report, 25% of 4 patients with 1.5-year follow-up regained M3 of target muscle strength [16]. Waikakul et al. and Songcharoen et al., respectively, reported that 21% of 96 patients and 28.6% of 21 patients gained M3 for both wrist flexion and finger flexion after contralateral C7 to median nerve transfer [4, 5].

Better recoveries in our series may be contributed to the fact that the entire contralateral C7 was used in most of our patients while in a majority of other studies only partial or half of the contralateral C7 nerve was used.

With respect to other recipient nerves, in a 2-year follow-up of pedicled ulnar nerve grafted contralateral C7 transfer, the ulnar nerve was coapted to the musculocutaneous nerve in six cases, with recovery of biceps up to M3 in four and S3 in five cases; the ulnar nerve was coapted to the median nerve in eight cases, with recovery of the wrist and finger flexors to M3 in five and S3 in six cases; the ulnar nerve was coapted to the radial nerve in four cases, with recovery of the triceps to M4 in two and S3 in three cases; and the ulnar nerve was coapted to the thoracodorsal nerve in two cases, with recovery of the latissimus dorsi to M4 in one case. Overall, the total muscle recovery rate (≥M3) of the series was 60%, and the sensory recovery rate (≥S3) was 78% [14]. In a relatively recent study of a population of 32 patients with an adequate follow-up (more 2 years), the entire C7 root was transferred in most of their patients (17 cases), followed by the posterior division (12 cases) and the anterior division (three cases). The neurotizations were directed to musculocutaneous, radial, and median nerves. Functional recovery reached M3 or greater in 80% of patients for the biceps, in 66% for the wrist and finger extensors, and in 50% for the finger flexors, and S3 or greater in 12 patients (85.7%) after median nerve neurotization. In Hattori et al.'s series, all five patients with the posterior cord repair achieved more than M2 recovery of triceps function, which contributed to stability of the elbow joint in reconstruction of prehension by a double free muscle transfer procedure [9]. Four patients with nerve repair of the suprascapular and musculocutaneous nerve achieved M3 or M2 recovery.

There are several factors that may affect results of contralateral C7 transfer. It is suggested that operation delay of more than 1 year after injury may lead to poor functional results of contralateral C7 transfer [14]. Waikakul et al. revealed that a timely repair of contralateral C7 transfer in patients within 18 years could finally acquire effective recovery in 50–60% of them [5]. In Chen et al.'s report, 3 of 8 of infant patients who underwent contralateral C7 nerve transfer to median nerve failed to regain satisfactory motor recoveries. The reasons may be attributed to surgical delay of more than 1 year. But good muscle strength for the elbow could still be gained even when the surgery was delayed for 14 months after injury [6]. These indicated that the timing of this procedure for the shoulder and elbow may not be as critical as in adults. In Terzis et al.'s study, she revealed that patients who were younger than 18 years or underwent this surgery within 9 months after injury are more likely to regain better recovery results [10].

Brain Plasticity After Contralateral C7 Transfer

Clinically, after contralateral C7 transfer to the injured median nerve for treatment of BPAI, only about half of the patients regained sensation of the median nerve innervated area in the affected hands and can flex their wrists and fingers. But the synchronous motion and sensation in both hands almost always occurred after surgery because C7 comes from the contralateral side [15]. Finally, some patients can control their affected limb independently after long-time reeducation. However, before independent limb control appeared, the movement of the affected limb could only be initiated by movement of the healthy limb.

In a recent study of adult rats, the motor representation map constructed by intracortical microstimulation revealed a dynamic process of the transhemispheric functional reorganization in the motor cortex after transferring the C7 nerve root from the contralateral healthy side to the injured limb for treatment of BPAI. Initially the ipsilateral motor cortex activated the injured forepaw for 5 months after the operation. Then, bilateral cerebral hemispheres of the cortex activated the movement of the injured side of forepaw at the seventh month postoperatively, and finally the contralateral cortex exclusively controlled the injured forepaw after 10 months [17, 18]. It suggested that original contralateral functional area in the cerebral cortex was reactivated, so some patients could regain independent movement finally. In contrast with the motor reorganization, the sensory reorganization remains within the ipsilateral cortex which may be the possible explanation of existence of synchronous sensitivity in patients after contralateral C7 transfer to the median nerve [19]. In the PET imaging study of adults after contralateral C7 transfer, the transhemispheric reorganization in the cortex and finally the median nerve innervated area in the affected limb was also reactivated [20].

Therefore, contralateral C7 transfer is a complex procedure referable to cerebral plasticity, and the final results could be attributed to involvement of both peripheral regeneration and brain reorganization.

Part II: Contralateral C7 Nerve Transfer in the Treatment of Spastic Hemiplegia

The Mechanism of Contralateral C7 Nerve Transfer in Treating of Spastic Hemiplegia

Central neurological injury (e.g., brain trauma, stroke, and cerebral palsy) is an important cause of long-term functional disability, especially spastic hemiplegia [21–23]. Some studies have demonstrated that contralesional hemispheric compensation may be an important recovery mechanism of motor function recovery [24, 25]. However, the ipsilateral fibers only account for 10 ~ 20% or even less of all corticospinal projections, which limits this compensatory capacity.

In the contralateral C7 nerve transfer, 20% of the nerve fibers that innervate the intact upper extremity were severed and transferred to the paralyzed limb. Thus, the quantity of the connection between the contralesional hemisphere and the paralyzed limb could be significantly enhanced and it amplifies signal exchanges, both afferent and efferent motor control over the paretic limb improves.

Clinical Trials of Contralateral C7 Nerve Transfer in Treating of Spastic Hemiplegia

We originally applied the contralateral C7 nerve transfer in the treatment of spastic extremity paralysis due to injury to a cerebral hemisphere from stroke, traumatic brain injury, or cerebral palsy, and finished the world's first clinical case in 2008 and got encouraging result [26]. Then we further applied this surgery in a series of hemiplegic patients and succeeded in spastic releasing and motor function restoration [27]. In the latest single-center clinical trial [28], it was showed that contralateral C7 nerve transfer is associated with a greater improvement in function and reduction of spasticity than physical rehabilitation alone. After the surgery and subsequent rehabilitation, the Fugl-Meyer score in paralyzed limb significantly improved (17.7 ± 5.6 points in the surgery group vs. 2.6 ± 2.0 points in the control group), and a majority of patients were able to use the paralyzed hand to perform three or more of the tasks of dressing, tying shoes, wringing out a towel, and operating a mobile phone.

Indications for Contralateral C7 Transfer

1. Spastic hemiplegia following different causes of central neurologic injury, such as stroke, traumatic brain injury, and cerebral palsy, principally presenting as difficulty in hand opening.
2. Central neurologic injury only involving the hemisphere contralateral to the paralyzed hand.

Exclusion

1. Presence of severe systemic diseases such as diabetes mellitus or cardiopulmonary diseases, contraindicating surgery.
2. Patient at high risk of recurrent stroke.

Surgical Technique

Detailed description and operative figures were presented in the recent article [29].

The patient is placed in a supine position with the head turned away from the operative side and a pillow under the shoulders for sufficient exposure of the brachial plexus. A transverse incision approximately 15 cm in length is made parallel to the clavicle and 2 cm superior.

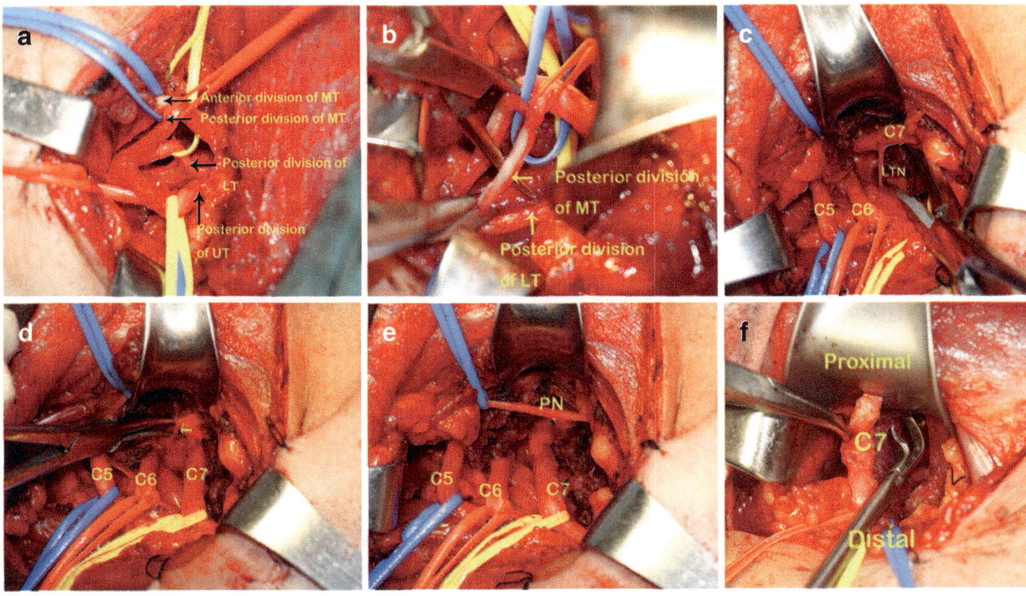

Fig. 28.2 (**a**) Picture showing the anterior division of C7 nerve jointing to lateral cord, and the posterior division jointing to posterior cord. UT upper trunk, MT middle trunk, LT lower trunk. (**b**) After anterior division is transected, the posterior division of C7 nerve, as well as the posterior division of lower trunk, could be seen. The posterior division of lower trunk is functionally important and should be carefully protected during operation. MT middle trunk, LT lower trunk. (**c**) Picture showing motor nerve branch of C7 root jointing to the long thoracic nerve. When performing contralateral C7 nerve transfer, this branch needs to be transected. LTN long thoracic nerve. (**d**) Picture showing tiny nerve branch (arrow) entering to the paraspinal muscle. This branch is emitted after C7 root runs out the foramen intervertebrale, which also, should be transected in operation. (**e**) Phrenic nerve runs above the C7 root. In operation, much more care should be taken. PN Phrenic nerve. (**f**) The paralyzed-sided C7 root is transected nearby the foramen intervertebrale. Picture shows a custom-made surgical scissor with orthogonal, grooved tip

1. Preparation of Bilateral C7 Nerve

The patient was placed in a supine position with the head turned away from the operative side and a pillow under the shoulders for sufficient exposure of the brachial plexus. A transverse incision approximately 15 cm in length is made parallel to the clavicle and 2 cm superior.

First, a layered exploration is performed. The external jugular vein is ligated and the omohyoid muscle is retracted to one side. The transverse cervical vessels are ligated. The C5-T1 nerve roots and the anterior scalenus muscle could be seen. Be careful with the phrenic nerve on the surface of anterior scalenus muscle and protect it. After partial transection of the anterior scalene muscle, the C5-T1 nerve roots are visualized.

Second, track the C7 nerve on the nonparalyzed side distal to the back of clavicle. The anterior and posterior divisions are transected at its distal end. In this process, some tiny nerve branches that come from the upper and lower trunks should be protected. The merging point between posterior divisions of middle and lower trunk is variable. Besides, the posterior division of lower trunk is relatively thin but functionally important. Therefore, much more care should be taken to prevent damage (Fig. 28.2a, b).

Third, track the C7 nerve proximal to the foramen intervertebrale. Some details are mentioned as follows. C7 nerve root is exposed after cutting partial anterior scalenus muscle. When tracking C7 root proximally, tiny branches that joint to the long thoracic nerve or enter to the paraspinal muscle could be seen. Those small branches should be sacrificed when performing contralateral C7 nerve transfer (Fig. 28.2c–e).

Fourth, the C7 nerve in paralyzed body side is exposed by similar processes. However, in this side, the motor branch of C7 root, jointing to the long thoracic nerve, should be preserved (Fig. 28.2f).

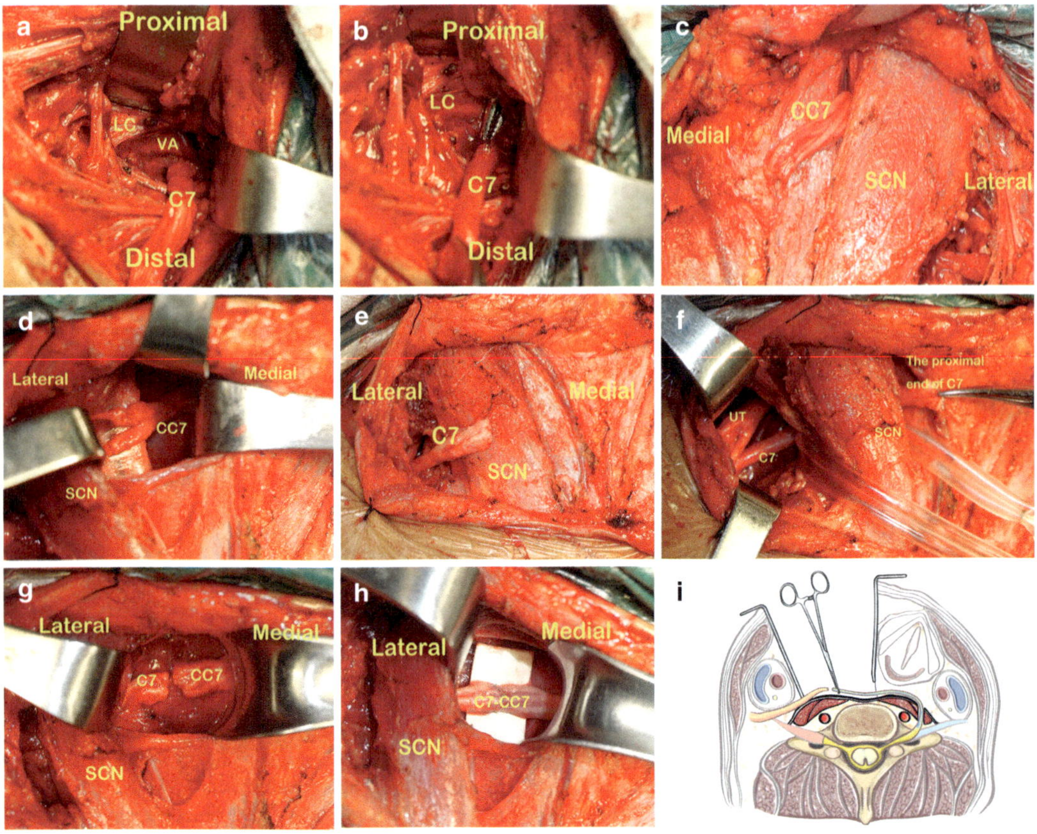

Fig. 28.3 (**a**) Picture showing the C7 nerve and the vertebral artery. VA vertebral artery, LC long colli muscle. (**b**) Picture showing the tip of the forceps reaching the C7 root. LC long colli muscle. (**c**) After penetrating the paraspinal muscle, the contralateral C7 nerve is guided to the space between the sternocleidomastoid and the esophagus and trachea in the healthy side. CC7 contralateral C7 nerve, SCN sternocleidomastoid muscle. (**d**) The contralateral C7 nerve is guided to the paralyzed side through the space between esophagus and cervical vertebra. CC7 contralateral C7 nerve, SCN sternocleidomastoid muscle. (**e**) The paralyzed-sided C7 nerve is transected. SCN sternocleidomastoid muscle. (**f**) The paralyzed-sided C7 nerve is guided deep through the carotid sheath to the medial space of ipsilateral sternocleidomastoid and meets with the nonparalyzed-sided C7 nerve. UT upper trunk, SCN sternocleidomastoid muscle. (**g**) Pictures showing bilateral C7 nerve before anastomosis. CC7 contralateral C7 nerve. (**h**) Pictures showing bilateral C7 nerve after anastomosis. CC7 contralateral C7 nerve. (**i**) Illustrations showing anastomosis between bilateral C7 nerves in front of cervical vertebra

2. Approach Build

In the contralateral side, the vertebral artery and its accompanying vein run upward in front of the C7 root (Fig. 28.3a). Carefully expose it and cut the tendon behind it, which is part of the tendon of longus colli ending to the transverse process of seventh cervical vertebra.

Separate the space between the sternocleidomastoid and the esophagus and trachea, and pull the carotid sheath outward. Through this space, the cervical vertebra and paraspinal muscle can be seen. At the superior margin of C7 vertebra, we use a vascular forceps to penetrate the paraspinal muscle downward and outward. Then, the tip of the forceps can reach the site of C7 root (Fig. 28.3b).

Use the forceps to expand the route longitudinally and cut the tendon around for prevention of potential nerve entrapment.

The contralateral C7 nerve was transferred to the space behind the esophagus and trachea via the longus colli-traverse approach (Fig. 28.3c), and further directed to the space behind the carotid sheath in injury side (Fig. 28.3d).

In the paralyzed side, the C7 passes through the deep side of the carotid artery and is leaded to the medial side of the sternocleidomastoid muscle (Fig. 28.3e, f).

Finally, the nonparalyzed-sided C7 nerve is anastomosed to the paralyzed-sided C7 nerve directly and tension freely (Fig. 28.3g, h and i).

Postoperative Monitoring

It is the same as contralateral C7 nerve transfer in treating BPAI, the neck and the should be immobilized with a brace for 3 weeks with arm against the chest, elbow flexed, and neck in neutral position. And rehabilitation protocol is performed instantly after removal of the splint.

Recovery Process Following Surgery

There were two recovery stages after the surgery. The initial phase of recovery after surgery was characterized by the release of spasticity, which usually started as early as the first postoperative day and continued to 12 months (Fig. 28.4). This release of spasticity may have been a result of sectioning of the proximal C7 nerve, which contains nerve fibers from gamma motor neurons that innervate muscle spindles and maintain muscle tone. The scores on the Modified Ashworth Scale, a measure of spasticity, correspondingly started to decrease in the paralyzed elbows and wrists immediately after surgery. The second phase of recovery was characterized by improvements in muscle power and motor function, which were most evident beginning at approximately month 10, possibly reflecting the time course of nerve fiber regeneration through the gap between the distal end of the transplanted nerve and most distally, on the side of the paralyzed hand.

The progress of nerve fiber regeneration could be estimated by physical examination of Tinel's sign, tapping C7 nerve targeting muscles and nerves (pectoralis major muscle, latissimus dorsi muscle, radial nerve groove, or supinator tunnel of radial nerve in the forearm). The patient would report a slight tingling sensation in the tips of the unaffected thumb, index, and middle fingers while tapping these sites. Along with nerve regeneration, from the proximal to the distal, a positive Tinel's sign was induced by testing the pectoralis major muscle (about post-operative month 4), latissimus dorsi muscle (about post-operative month 4), the radial nerve groove in the upper arm (about post-operative month 6), and the supinator tunnel of radial nerve in the forearm (about post-operative month 8) of the paralyzed side. These findings indicated that nerve fiber regeneration had reached the forearm at post-operative month 8 and the muscle power and motor function started to improve. The electromyography (EMG) and transcranial magnetic stimulation (TMS) evoked responses also verified the completion of nerve fiber regeneration. Therefore, at post-operative month 10, all patients showed significantly increased Fugl-Meyer scores. But the extent of recovery differed among patients.

Complications

The most common complications following contralateral C7 nerve transfer surgery in the treatment of spastic hemiplegia were slight weakness in elbow/wrist extension and numbness in thumb, index, and middle fingers. Some patients also reported temporary pain and foreign body sensation while swallowing.

In our phase II clinical trial, treatment-related adverse events included limb or shoulder pain in 13/18 surgery patients (72.2%) and in 8/18 control patients (44.4%); foreign body sensation while swallowing in 12/18 surgery patients (66.7%); fatigue in 15/18 (83.3%) and numbness in 16/18 (88.9%) surgery patients; decreased power of elbow extension in 15/18 (83.3%) and wrist extension in 16/18 (88.9%), and attenuated sensory function in 16/18 (88.9%) surgery patients. In the surgery group, weakness disappeared in 13 of the 15 patients, and numbness disappeared in 15 of the 16 patients within 3 months. Sensorimotor changes were absent in all patients at month 6. There were no significant differences in sensorimotor functions between baseline and post-operative month 12 in the non-paralyzed limb except for a decrease in sensory function in the index finger. Based on our clinical

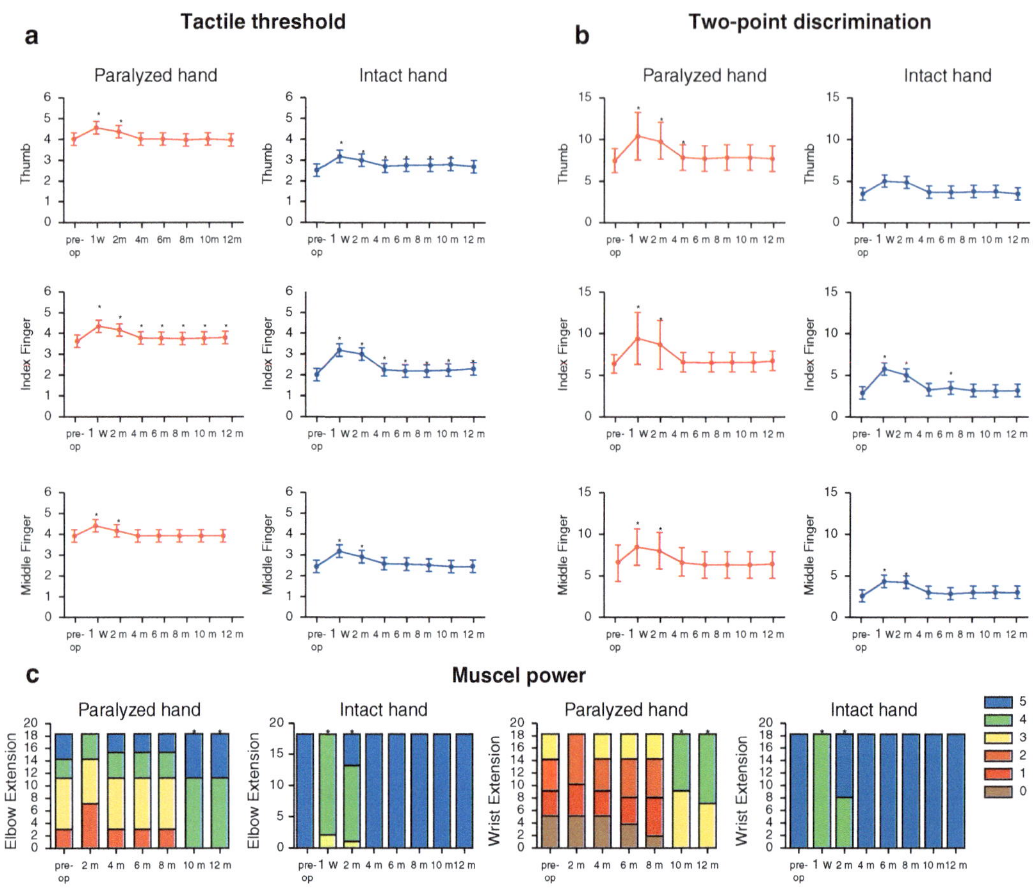

Fig. 28.4 Sensorimotor functions of bilateral hands of 12 months follow-up in the contralateral C7 nerve transfer surgery group [28]. (**a**, **b**) The tactile threshold and two-point discrimination (2-PD) results in the surgery group (mean ± SD). *significant difference in the intergroup comparison of the incremental value (comparing with baseline value) at each follow-up visit; Φ significant difference in the intergroup comparison of the incremental value (comparing with 2-month post-op value) at each follow-up time ($P < 0.05$). (**c**) The frequency chart of patient number in each muscle power level in elbow and wrist extension. *significant difference in the intergroup comparison of category changes (comparing with baseline value); Φ significant difference in the intergroup comparison of category changes (comparing with 2-month post-op value) ($P < 0.05$)

experiences in more than 400 cases, it is a safe surgical procedure.

Progresses

The major mechanism for motor recovery following contralateral nerve transfer was enhancing the contralesional hemisphere's control over the hemiplegic extremity. Therefore, we further applied this concept to the hemiplegic lower extremity. In our experimental study, contralateral L6 transfer was applied in the treatment for hemiplegic hindlimbs after unilateral hemisphere injury in adult rats. Behavioral evidence from beam and ladder rung walking tests and CatWalk gait analysis was employed to verify its feasibility. It indicated that contralateral L6 nerve transfer could be a promising and safe surgical approach for improving motor recovery of the hemiplegic hindlimb following unilateral central neurologic injury in adult rats [30].

Clinically, we used contralateral hemi-L5 nerve transfer for the treatment of incomplete spinal cord injury patients with unilateral lower limb dysfunction in two male patients. Muscle strength transiently decreased in the donor-side before recovery within 12 months postoperatively. Muscle strength significantly improved 2 years postoperatively. The Fugl-Meyer score increased from 7 to 14 and 15, respectively. And the patients regained independent walking ability with crutches. The study suggested that contralateral hemi-L5 nerve transfer was safe and could benefit incomplete spinal cord injury patients with unilateral lower limb dysfunction [31].

References

1. Gu YD, Zhang GM, Chen DS, et al. Seventh cervical nerve root transfer from contralateral healthy side for treatment of brachial plexus root avulsion. J Hand Surg (Br). 1992;17:518–21.
2. Chuang DC. Neurotization procedures for brachial plexus injuries. Hand Clin. 1995;11:633–45.
3. Gu YD. Functional motor innervation of brachial plexus roots. An intraoperative electrophysiological study. J Hand Surg (Br). 1997;22:258–60.
4. Songcharoen P, Wongtrakul S, Mahaisavariya B, et al. Hemi-contralateral C7 transfer to median nerve in the treatment of root avulsion brachial plexus injury. J Hand Surg (Am). 2001;26:1058–64.
5. Waikakul S, Orapin S, Vanadurongwan V. Clinical results of contralateral C7 root neurotization to the median nerve in brachial plexus injuries with total root avulsions. J Hand Surg (Br). 1999;24:556–60.
6. Chen L, Gu YD, Hu SN, et al. Contralateral C7 transfer for the treatment of brachial plexus root avulsions in children- a report of 12 cases. J Hand Surgery (Am). 2007;32:96–103.
7. Feng J, Wang T, Gu Y, et al. Contralateral C7 transfer to lower trunk via a subcutaneous tunnel across the anterior surface of chest and neck for total root avulsion of the brachial plexus: a preliminary report. Neurosurgery. 2010;66:252–63.
8. Grundy DJ, Silver JR. Combined brachial plexus and spinal cord trauma. Injury. 1983;15:57–61.
9. Hattori Y, Doi K, Toh S, et al. Short-term results of contralateral C7 transfer for brachial plexus reconstruction. J Jpn Soc Surg Hand. 2001;18:213–7.
10. Terzis JK, Kokkalis ZT. Selective contralateral C7 transfer in posttraumatic brachial plexus injuries: a report of 56 cases. Plast Reconstr Surg. 2009;123:927–38.
11. Liu J, Pho HW, Kour AK, et al. Neurologic deficit and recovery in the donor limb following cross-C7 transfer in brachial-plexus injury. J Reconstr Microsurg. 1997;13:237–42.
12. Sungpet A, Suphachatwon C, Kawinwonggowit V. Sensory abnormalities after the seventh cervical nerve root transfer. Microsurgery. 1999;19:287–8.
13. Chuang DC, Cheng SL, Wei FC, et al. Clinical evaluation of C7 spinal nerve transection: 21 patients with at least 2 years' follow-up. Br J Plast Surg. 1998;51:285–90.
14. Gu YD, Chen DS, Zhang GM, et al. Long-term functional results of contralateral C7 transfer. J Reconstr Microsurg. 1998;14:57–9.
15. Gu Y, Xu J, Chen L, Wang H, et al. Long-term outcome of contralateral C7 transfer: a report of 32 cases. Chin Med J (Engl). 2002;115:866–8.
16. Hierner R, Berger AK. Did the partial contralateral C7-transfer fulfill our expectations results after 5 year experience. Acta Neurochir Suppl. 2007;100:33–5.
17. Jiang S, Li ZY, Hua XY, et al. Reorganization in motor cortex after brachial plexus avulsion injury and repair with the contralateral C7 root transfer in rats. Microsurgery. 2010;20:314–20.
18. Lou L, Shou T, Li Z, et al. Transhemispheric functional reorganization of the motor cortex induced by the peripheral contralateral nerve transfer to the injured arm. Neuroscience. 2006;138:1225–32.
19. Wang M, Li ZY, Xu WD, et al. Sensory restoration in cortical level after a contralateral C7 nerve transfer to an injured arm in rats. Neurosurgery. 2010;67:136–43.
20. Zuo CT, Hua XY, Guan YH, et al. Long-range plasticity between intact hemispheres after contralateral cervical nerve transfer in humans. J Neurosurg. 2010;113:133–40.
21. Sauser K, Burke JF, Reeves MJ, Barsan WG, Levine DA. A systematic review and critical appraisal of quality measures for the emergency care of acute ischemic stroke. Ann Emerg Med. 2014;64(3):235–244. e5.
22. Lo AC, Guarino PD, Richards LG, et al. Robot-assisted therapy for long-term upperlimb impairment after stroke. N Engl J Med. 2010;362:1772–83.
23. Olawale O, Gbiri C, Isaac S. Burden of care among informal caregivers of stroke survivors is influenced by intrinsic and extrinsic factors: a multi-centre analytical survey. Physiotherapy. 2015;101(Suppl 1):e1135–6. abstract.
24. Turton A, Wroe S, Trepte N, Fraser C, Lemon RN. Contralateral and ipsilateral EMG responses to transcranial magnetic stimulation during recovery of arm and hand function after stroke. Electroencephalogr Clin Neurophysiol. 1996;101(4):316–28.
25. Netz J, Lammers T, Hömberg V. Reorganization of motor output in the non-affected hemisphere after stroke. Brain. 1997;120(Pt 9):1579–86.
26. Xu WD, Hua XY, Zheng MX, Xu JG, Gu YD. Contralateral C7 nerve root transfer in treatment of cerebral palsy in a child: Case report. Microsurgery. 2011;31(5):404–8.
27. Hua XY, Qiu YQ, Li T, Zheng MX, Shen YD, Jiang S, Xu JG, Gu YD, Xu WD. Contralateral peripheral neurotization for hemiplegic upper extremity after central neurologic injury. Neurosurgery. 2015;76(2):187–95.

28. Zheng MX, Hua XY, Feng JT, et al. Trial of Contralateral Seventh Cervical Nerve Transfer for Spastic Arm Paralysis. N Engl J Med. 2018;378(1):22–34.
29. Xu WD. Surgical technique of Xu's CC7 procedure "Contralateral C7 to C7 cross nerve transfer through a trans longus colli, prespinal route for treating spastic arm". Oper Neurosurg (Hagerstown, MD). 2020; https://doi.org/10.1093/ons/opaa325.
30. Zheng MX, Hua XY, Jiang S, Qiu YQ, Shen YD, Xu WD. Contralateral peripheral neurotization for a hemiplegic hindlimb after central neurological injury. J Neurosurg. 2018;128(1):304–11.
31. Yu BF, Qiu YQ, Du MX, et al. Contralateral hemi-fifth-lumbar nerve transfer for unilateral lower limb dysfunction due to incomplete traumatic spinal cord injury: A report of two cases. Microsurgery. 2020;40(2):234–40.

The Harvest of a Free Innervated Functional Gracilis Muscle and Its Use in Brachial Plexus Injuries

29

Jennifer L. Giuffre and Alexander Y. Shin

Introduction

Reconstructive surgery has been revolutionized by the discovery of muscle and myocutaneous flaps. One of the first flaps to be recognized and utilized was the gracilis muscle. The entire muscle could be elevated reliably on its dominant vascular pedicle and transposed locally around the perineal and pelvic region. Pickerell et al. used the gracilis muscle to correct anal incontinence and later urinary incontinence [1, 2]. Historically, the gracilis flap was used to cover a variety of defects including the sole of the foot [3], reconstruct the penis [4], and repair perineal fistulas and sinuses [5, 6]. McCraw et al. reported the first large "island" myocutaneous flap experience in which they employed the gracilis muscle for vaginal reconstruction [7].

The discrete and independent myocutaneous vascular territory of the gracilis muscle and the overlying skin was initially delineated by injecting a thin latex suspension into the major muscular arteries of 12 live mongrel dogs [8]. Subsequently, similar latex injections were performed in human specimens [8]. In 1976, Harii et al. employed the direct transfer of a free gracilis musculocutaneous flap by microvascular anastomosis for the reconstruction of three different defects: a facial defect, an unstable scar over the tibia, and a scalp defect [9].

The use of the gracilis muscle evolved from being used for coverage to being used for function. Manktelow and McKee in 1978 described the use of a free, innervated functioning gracilis muscle to replace finger flexor musculature destroyed by Volkmann's ischemic contracture in 1975 [10]. Harii et al. similarly described use of a free functional gracilis muscle to replace muscles of facial expression in long-standing Bell's palsy [11]. Ikuta et al. in 1979 described the first application of using a free functioning gracilis muscle flap to restore elbow flexion in a boy with a 10-year-old brachial plexus injury [12]. Since then, the use of the free innervated myocutaneous gracilis flaps in brachial plexus reconstruction has become an invaluable tool to restore elbow flexion, prehension, and rudimentary grasp. In a complete brachial plexus injury, Doi et al. reported the restoration of finger flexion and extension as well as elbow flexion and extension with a double free gracilis muscle transfer in conjunction with multiple nerve transfers [13].

J. L. Giuffre (✉)
Plastic Surgery, University of Manitoba, Section of Plastic Surgery, Department of Surgery, Winnipeg, MB, Canada
e-mail: jgiuffre@panamclinic.com

A. Y. Shin
Department of Orthopedic Surgery, Mayo Clinic, Rochester, MN, USA
e-mail: shin.alexander@mayo.edu

A. Y. Shin, N. Pulos (eds.), *Operative Brachial Plexus Surgery*,
https://doi.org/10.1007/978-3-030-69517-0_29

Gracilis Muscle Anatomy

The gracilis muscle is situated in the medial thigh and is the most superficial of the adductor muscle group (Fig. 29.1). It originates from the lower half of the symphysis pubis and the medial portion of the inferior pubic ramus by a thin aponeurosis. This muscle is flat proximally and courses distally and longitudinally ending in a round tendon which passes posterior to the medial condyle of the femur and inserts into the medial surface of the proximal portion of the tibia at the pes anserine. The gracilis acts as an adductor of the thigh and also flexes and medially rotates the leg. It is the smallest of the three adductors, which also includes the adductor magnus and adductor longus muscles.

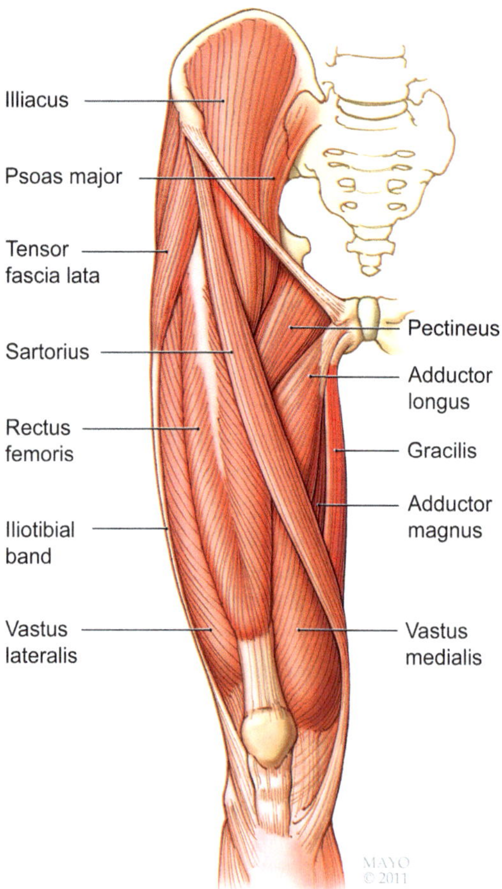

Fig. 29.1 The gracilis muscle is situated in the medial thigh and is the most superficial of the adductor muscle group. (Reproduced with permission of the Mayo Foundation, Copyright 2011)

Gracilis Muscle Vascular Anatomy

The gracilis muscle is a type 2 muscle (one dominant pedicle and minor pedicle(s)) per the Mathes and Nahai classification of the vascular anatomy of muscles [14]. The larger dominant vascular pedicle is capable of sustaining the circulation to the muscle after the elevation of the flap and division of the distal and minor pedicles (Fig. 29.2).

Located proximally, the dominant vascular pedicle is the medial femoral circumflex artery and venae comitantes, which originate from the profunda femoris artery and vein. Typically this vascular pedicle to the gracilis is approximately 7–12 cm from the groin crease but can be quite variable. There are many vascular variations in the origin of the nutrient vessels to the gracilis muscle. They may branch directly from either the profunda

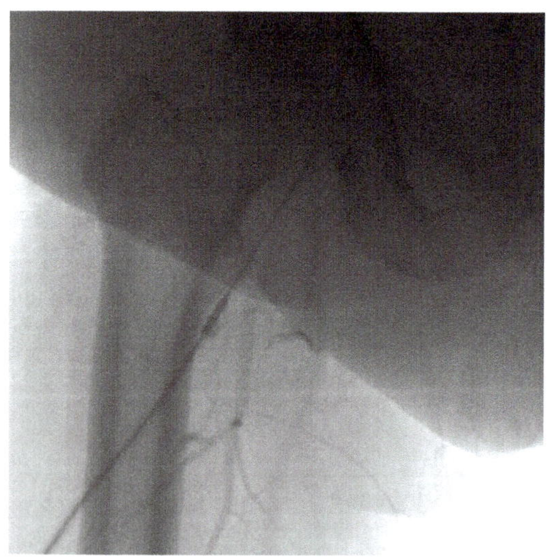

Fig. 29.2 The medial circumflex artery is the dominant vascular pedicle to the gracilis that courses beneath the adductor longus muscle and superficial to the adductor magnus muscle, entering the medial, deep aspect of the gracilis muscle, approximately 10 cm inferior to the pubic tubercle. The angiogram depicts the dominant artery arising directly from the profunda femoris artery. (Pictures courtesy of Drs. T.E. Hayakawa and E.W. Buchel from the University of Manitoba, Canada)

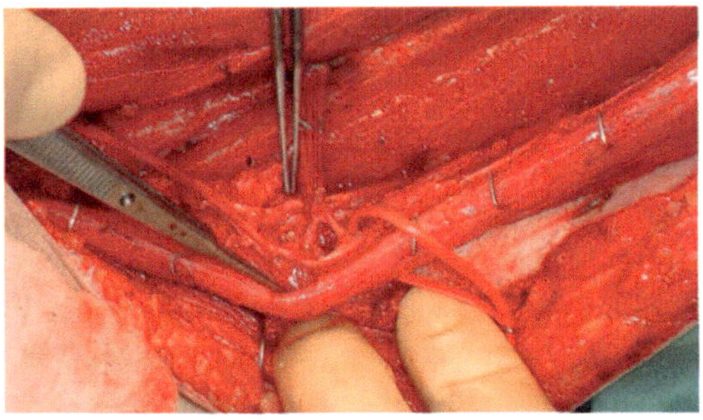

Fig. 29.3 The pedicle terminates as two or three branches entering the medial, deep aspect of the gracilis muscle, approximately 10 cm inferior to the pubic tubercle. (Pictures courtesy of Drs. T.E. Hayakawa and E.W. Buchel from the University of Manitoba, Canada)

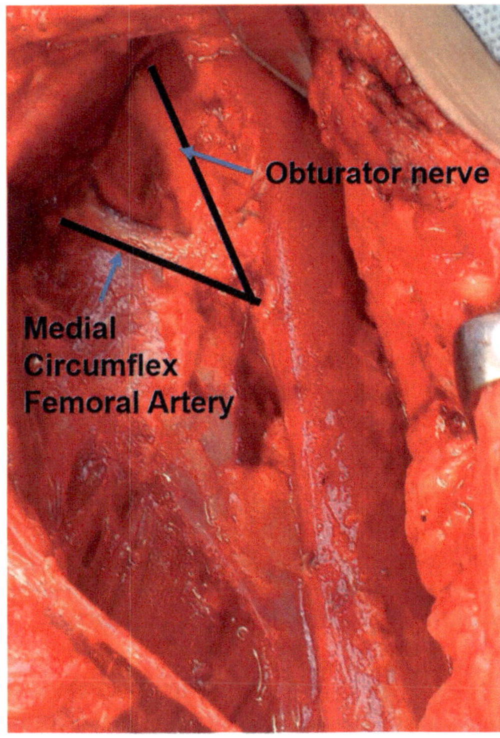

Fig. 29.4 The nerve enters the muscle approximately 2–3 cm superior to the point of entrance of the major vascular pedicle and nearly constantly at a 45 degree angle to the muscle

femoris vessels or the medial circumflex femoral vessels [9]. Without exception, the pedicle courses beneath the adductor longus muscle and superficial to the adductor magnus muscle, providing branches to each of these muscles. The pedicle terminates as two or three branches entering the medial, deep aspect of the gracilis muscle, approximately 10 cm inferior to the pubic tubercle (Fig. 29.3). The length of the pedicle is 6–8 cm from the profunda femoris vessels and has a vessel diameter of approximately 1.6–1.8 mm.

The veins of the gracilis muscle are located with the arterial pedicle as paired venae comitantes. The entire muscle and proximal half of the cutaneous territory are adequately drained by the paired venae comitantes associated with the medial femoral circumflex artery. The venae eventually drain into the deep veins associated with profunda femoris artery. The proximal veins of the dominant pedicle have an external lumen diameter of 1.5–2.5 mm and a pedicle length of 6–8 cm.

The minor vascular pedicle(s) include one or two branches of the superficial femoral artery and venae comitantes. These pedicles are approximately 2 cm in length and 0.5 mm in diameter. They are located within the distal half of the muscle.

Gracilis Muscle Neural Anatomy

The motor nerve of the gracilis muscle is the anterior branch of the obturator nerve (L2, L3, L4). The nerve enters the muscle approximately 2–3 cm superior to the point of entrance of the major vascular pedicle and nearly constantly at a 45 degree angle to the muscle (Fig. 29.4). The motor nerve may be dissected proximally between the adductor longus and adductor magnus muscles to increase donor nerve length. This motor nerve gives branches to the adductor muscles as well. To further increase the length of the nerve harvested with the gracilis muscle, in cases where a long nerve pedicle is required, the nerve branches to the adductor muscles can be carefully dissected from the gracilis motor branch in an interfascicular fashion.

The motor nerve runs with the sensory nerve along the medial surface of the adductor longus muscle. There are small sensory branches from the obturator nerve that enter the medial thigh skin, although no specific sensory branch can be located consistently. The skin territory of the gracilis is innervated by branches of the anterior femoral cutaneous nerve of the thigh (L2 and L3).

Gracilis Muscle Flap and Myocutaneous Flap

Gracilis Muscle Flap Dimensions

The gracilis muscle measures approximately 5–6 cm in width and 24–30 cm in length and has an additional 10–12 cm of tendon (Fig. 29.5). If the gracilis muscle is harvested with a cutaneous portion, the musculocutaneous flap reliably measures 6–8 cm in width and 24 cm in length. The muscle is thin and flat proximally (measuring 2–5 cm in thickness, depending on the size of the individual), becomes round in the midportion, and tapers to the size of the gracilis tendon distally.

Gracilis Muscle Flap Skin Territory

The medial thigh skin is not entirely vascularized by musculocutaneous perforating vessels from the gracilis. The clinically reliable island of skin based on the gracilis measures 8 × 24 cm and is usually designed over the proximal two-thirds of the muscle [8, 15]. Survival of the proximal cutaneous territory requires adequate localization of the skin territory over the muscle and careful preservation of the musculocutaneous perforating vessels. Perforating musculocutaneous arteries are small, are less than 0.5 mm in diameter, and are distributed mostly over the proximal portion of the muscle [15]. The skin over the distal third of the muscle is not reliable with division of the minor pedicles(s). Local transposition or free transfer of the gracilis with the proximal two-thirds skin island is a reliable flap.

McCraw and Dibbell described the relationship of cutaneous blood supply to subadjacent muscle vascular territories by injecting a thin latex suspension into human specimens [8]. They demonstrated hundreds of minute vessels passing to the skin through the deep fascia. At the level of the deep fascia (not the investing muscular fascia), there is a dense lateral arborization of vessels on either side of the fascia. These minute vessels form a plexus on the superficial surface of the deep fascia. From this location, the vessels pass perpendicularly outward to the skin. To help improve the survival of the skin flap, it is best to include the fascia within the flap [8].

Innervated Free Functional Gracilis Flap

The strength of a muscle is directly proportional to the physiological cross-sectional area of the muscle fibers. It has been suggested that following transplantation, the muscle will atrophy to 25–50% of the pre-transfer size [9, 16].

It can be estimated that, with maximum contraction, a muscle can shorten between 40% and 57% of its fully stretched length [17, 18]; therefore, the degree of shortening of the gracilis, with a 30 cm long muscle belly, would be at least

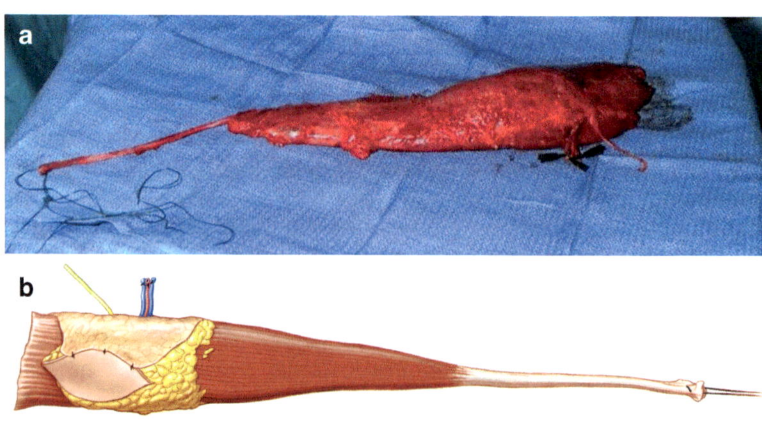

Fig. 29.5 (**a**) The gracilis muscle measures approximately 5–6 cm in width, 24–30 cm in length and has an additional 10–12cm of tendon. (**b**) The vascular pedicle and the nerve are illustrated entering the deep surface of the muscle. Printed with permission of the Mayo Foundation for Medical Education and Research. All rights reserved, copyright 2010

12 cm of its normal state (30 cm × 40%) [10]. This allows for a rough calculation of a muscle's contractile range by measuring the muscle fiber length. In a strap muscle, such as the gracilis, the muscle fibers are arranged parallel to the line of pull of the muscle and the bundles of muscle fibers run the full length of the muscle.

Manktelow explained that a muscle develops its greatest contractile force at its physiological stretched resting length and has less amount of contractile force as the muscle shortens [10]. As such he recommended that if the gracilis is to be used as a functional muscle for finger flexion, it is desirable to insert the muscle into the forearm so that it is stretched maximally when the fingers and wrist are extended. This will give the desired contractile force when the wrist and fingers are in a neutral position. He also noted that if the full range of contraction is employed, the last portion of the range of contraction usually cannot be carried out against significant resistance; therefore, the last few centimeters of contraction should not be expected to be useful in finger flexion where the requirement is for good strength at full finger flexion. A muscle should then be selected that normally has an amplitude of motion greater than the desired range of motion in its transplanted site [10].

The Technique of Gracilis Muscle Flap Harvest

The gracilis flap may be designed with or without a cutaneous portion for local or distant coverage of defects or as a functional muscle. The gracilis musculocutaneous flap requires careful planning since the muscle is narrow and the overlying skin is not adherent to the muscle.

Although there are many different methods of harvest, a majority if not all harvest methods begin proximally. The indication of the gracilis flap will determine the technique of harvest. If a small innervated gracilis is needed for facial reanimation, a proximal incision is used. If the complete length of the gracilis muscle and tendon with or without a skin paddle is required for restoration of elbow flexion or prehension in patients with brachial plexus injuries, it has been the experience of the authors to commence with a distal dissection either at the distal insertion of the gracilis at the pes anserine or at the distal medial thigh at the myotendinous junction. This method of harvest allows reliable identification of the overlying skin paddle, particularly in patients who have redundant or obese medial thighs. The following section will describe the distal-incision-first technique.

In the standing position, the gracilis muscle can be topographically identified by drawing a line between the proximal pubic tubercle and the distal gracilis muscle tendinous insertion at the pes anserine. Before the patient is placed in lithotomy or any other position involving flexion of the knee and hip, the topographic guideline should be drawn onto the patient as the landmarks may migrate and become inaccurate with posture changes. If a cutaneous portion of the flap is to be included, it is outlined slightly posterior to the line drawn from the pubic tubercle to the pes anserine of the knee. The anterior border of the skin paddle should lie on this topographic line and may be extended posterior 6–9 cm to allow for primary closure. The skin paddle should be centered over the gracilis muscle and contain a cutaneous perforator that is detected with an audible handheld Doppler signal. The skin paddle design is confirmed once the distal gracilis tendon has been identified as described later in the chapter. The location of the dominant vascular pedicle into the medial muscle belly, approximately 10 cm from the pubic tubercle, must be considered in the design of the skin island on the muscle belly. In the operating room, the patient is positioned supine with the legs externally rotated and abducted.

Distal Dissection First (Full-Length Myocutaneous Innervated Flap) Technique

If a full-length gracilis is needed, the gracilis tendon at the pes anserine can be identified via a 3 cm longitudinal incision over the pes anserine and a 4 cm longitudinal incision in the distal medial thigh (Fig. 29.6). At the pes anserine, the gracilis tendon can be easily palpated as the most superior tendinous insertion. The inferior tendon

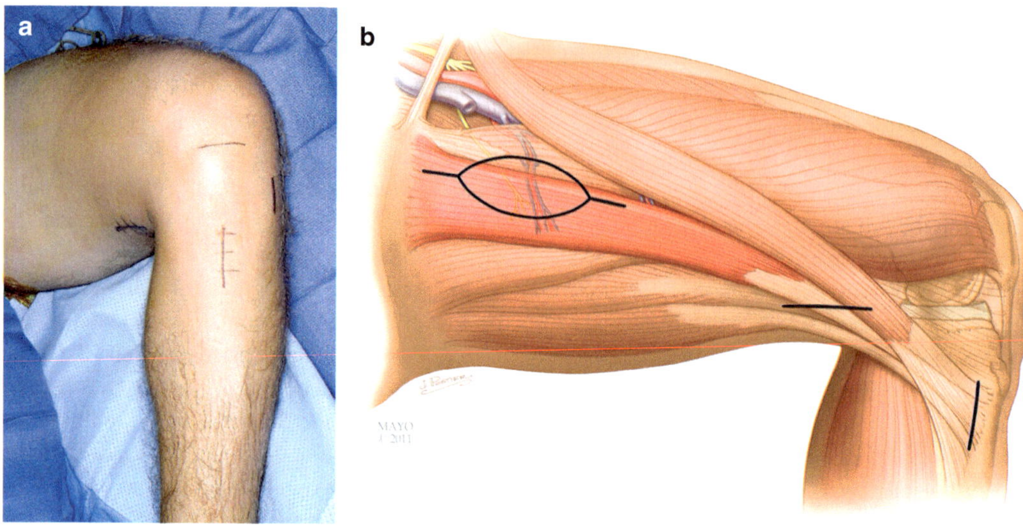

Fig. 29.6 When a full length gracilis is needed, the harvest begins distally where the gracilis tendon at the pes anserine can be identified via. (**a**) 3 cm longitudinal incision over the pes anserine and a 4 cm longitudinal incision in the distal medial thigh and (**b**) A proximal thigh incision/skin paddle. Printed with permission of the Mayo Foundation for Medical Education and Research. All rights reserved, copyright 2010

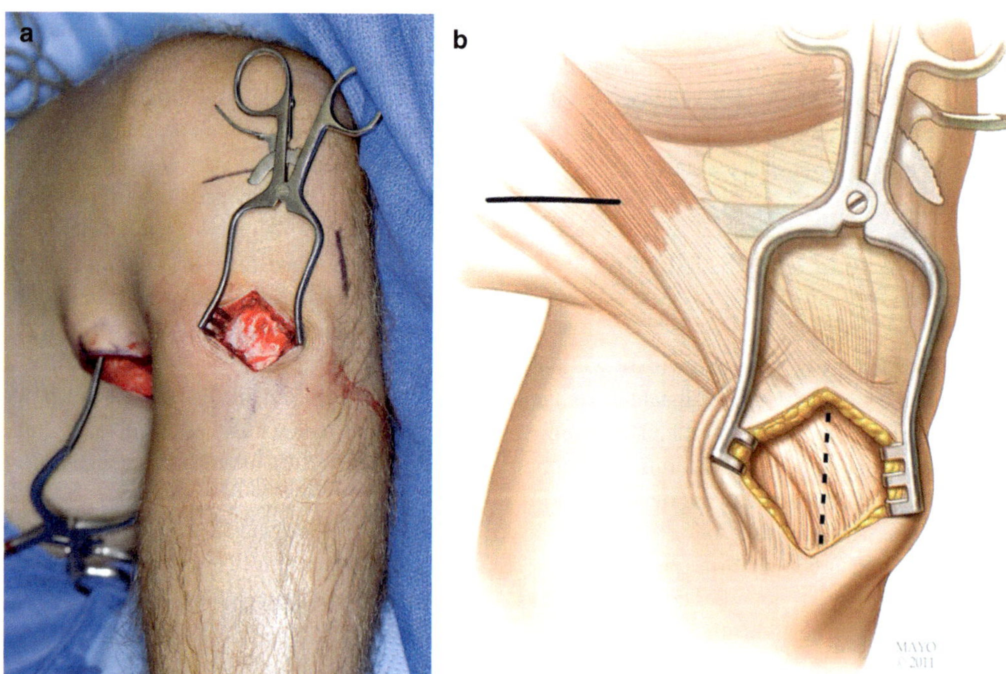

Fig. 29.7 The gracilis and semitendinosis tendons are covered by sartorius fascia which is demonstrated in. (**a**) An intraoperative photo as well as. (**b**) A line drawing. Printed with permission of the Mayo Foundation for Medical Education and Research. All rights reserved, copyright 2010

at the pes anserine is the semitendinosus tendon. The gracilis and semitendinosus tendons are covered by sartorius fascia (Fig. 29.7). A longitudinal incision is made over the tendons and the sartorius fascia is incised. Dissection is carried between the tendons until the medial collateral ligament of the

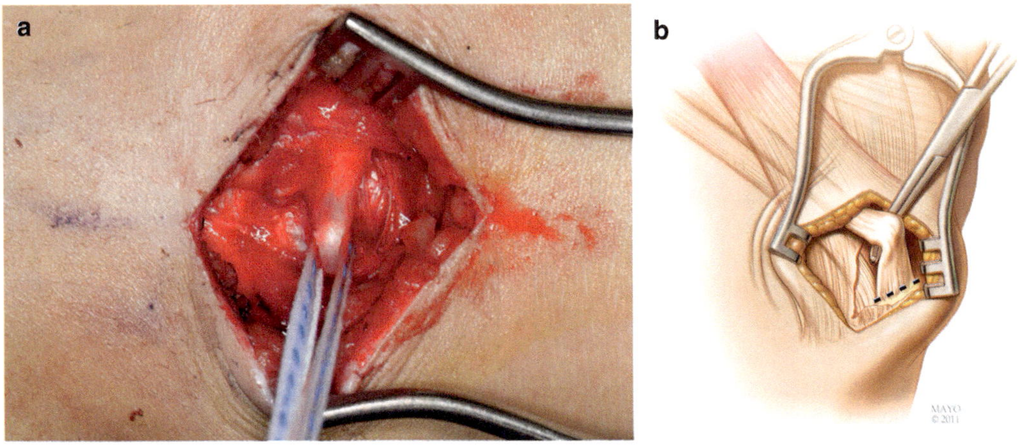

Fig. 29.8 (**a**) Once the overlying sartorius fascia is divided, umbilical tape is placed around the superior, gracilis tendon, and the multiple soft tissue attachments to the gracilis tendon are divided. (**b**) At the pes anserine, the gracilis tendon is the most superior tendinous insertion while the inferior tendon is the semitendinosis tendon. Printed with permission of the Mayo Foundation for Medical Education and Research. All rights reserved, copyright 2010

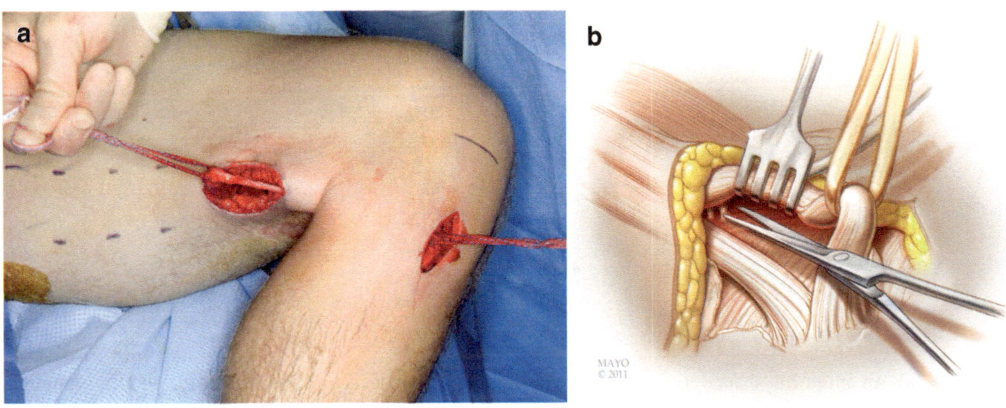

Fig. 29.9 All soft tissues attachments to the gracilis are divided between the two incisions at the pes anserine and the distal medial thigh as seen in. (**a**) An intraoperative photo as well as. (**b**) A line drawing. Printed with permission of the Mayo Foundation for Medical Education and Research. All rights reserved, copyright 2010

knee is visualized. Umbilical tape is placed around the superior, gracilis tendon, and the multiple soft tissue attachments to the gracilis tendon are divided (Fig. 29.8). A 4 cm incision is made over the distal medial thigh, where the myotendinous portion of the gracilis is identified. The gracilis is pulled to confirm the gracilis tendon previously identified inserting into the proximal tibia. All soft tissue attachments to the gracilis are divided between these two incisions (Fig. 29.9).

Once the gracilis muscle/tendon has been identified distally, traction can be applied to the muscle/tendon proximally, causing the entire muscle to “bowstring,” thus outlining the specific area of cutaneous territory overlying the muscle that may be incorporated into the musculocutaneous flap if required (Fig. 29.10). When the skin island is placed directly over the muscle, the skin dimensions include the proximal two-thirds of the medial thigh skin with a maximum width of 8 cm. The location of the dominant vascular pedicle into the medial muscle belly, approximately 10 cm from the pubic tubercle, must be considered in the design of the skin island on the muscle belly. A handheld, sterile Doppler device can be used to identify and mark skin perforators overlying the proximal gracilis muscle (Fig. 29.11). An elliptical-shaped incision is drawn slightly anterior to

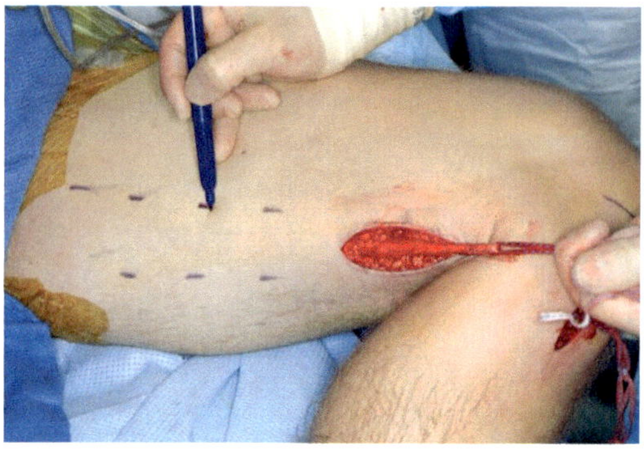

Fig. 29.10 Once the gracilis muscle/tendon has been identified, traction can be applied to the muscle/tendon proximally, causing the entire muscle to "bowstring," thus outlining the specific area of cutaneous territory overlying the muscle that may be incorporated into the musculocutaneous flap if required

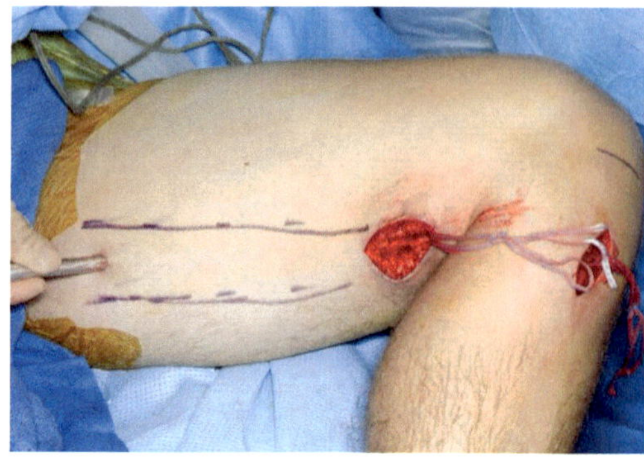

Fig. 29.11 A handheld, sterile Doppler device can be used to identify and mark skin perforators overlying the proximal gracilis muscle

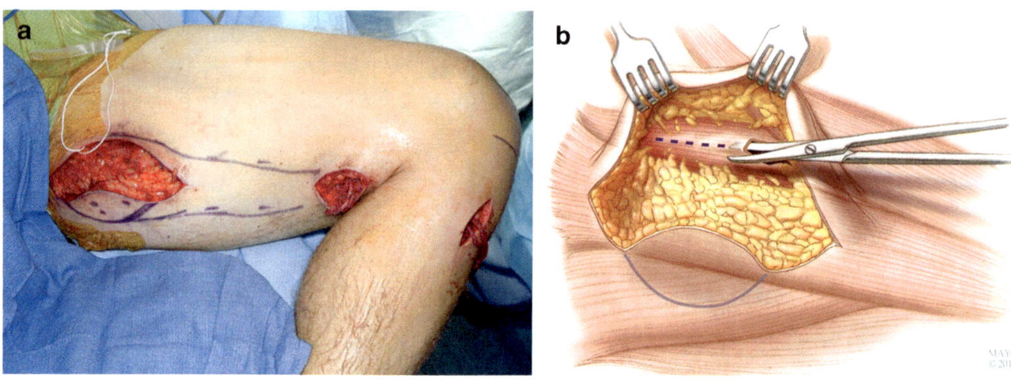

Fig. 29.12 (**a**) An elliptical shaped incision is drawn slightly anterior to the anterior border of the gracilis muscle, centered about the identified skin perforators. The proximal thigh incision is made along the anterior border of the skin paddle and dissection is carried towards the adductor longus. (**b**) The fascia of the adductor longus is incised longitudinally. Printed with permission of the Mayo Foundation for Medical Education and Research.

the anterior border of the gracilis muscle, centered about the identified skin perforators.

The proximal thigh incision is made along the anterior border of the skin paddle, and dissection is carried towards the adductor longus (Fig. 29.12). The fascia of the adductor longus is incised longitudinally, and the fascial edge is sewn to the skin paddle edge to avoid shear and traction on musculocutaneous perforating vessels (Fig. 29.13). In the interval between the adductor longus and gracilis muscles, the fascia of the adductor longus is gently retracted to expose the obturator nerve and the dominant proximal artery and venae comitantes. The adductor longus muscle is retracted medially and superiorly, while the vascular perforators to the adductor longus are carefully dissected and ligated. Caution to aggressive dissection should be made as the medial femoral circumflex vessels are tented up against the adductor longus and can be iatrogenically injured. Once the perforators to the adductor longus are ligated, the vessels are dissected to the profunda femoral artery and vein. The artery and vein are isolated proximally, and vessel loops are placed around each vessel. For an innervated flap to be used, the obturator nerve is identified entering the deep surface of the gracilis obliquely to the vascular pedicle and stimulated with a disposable nerve stimulator to verify contraction. A vessel loop is placed around the nerve, and the dissection pro-

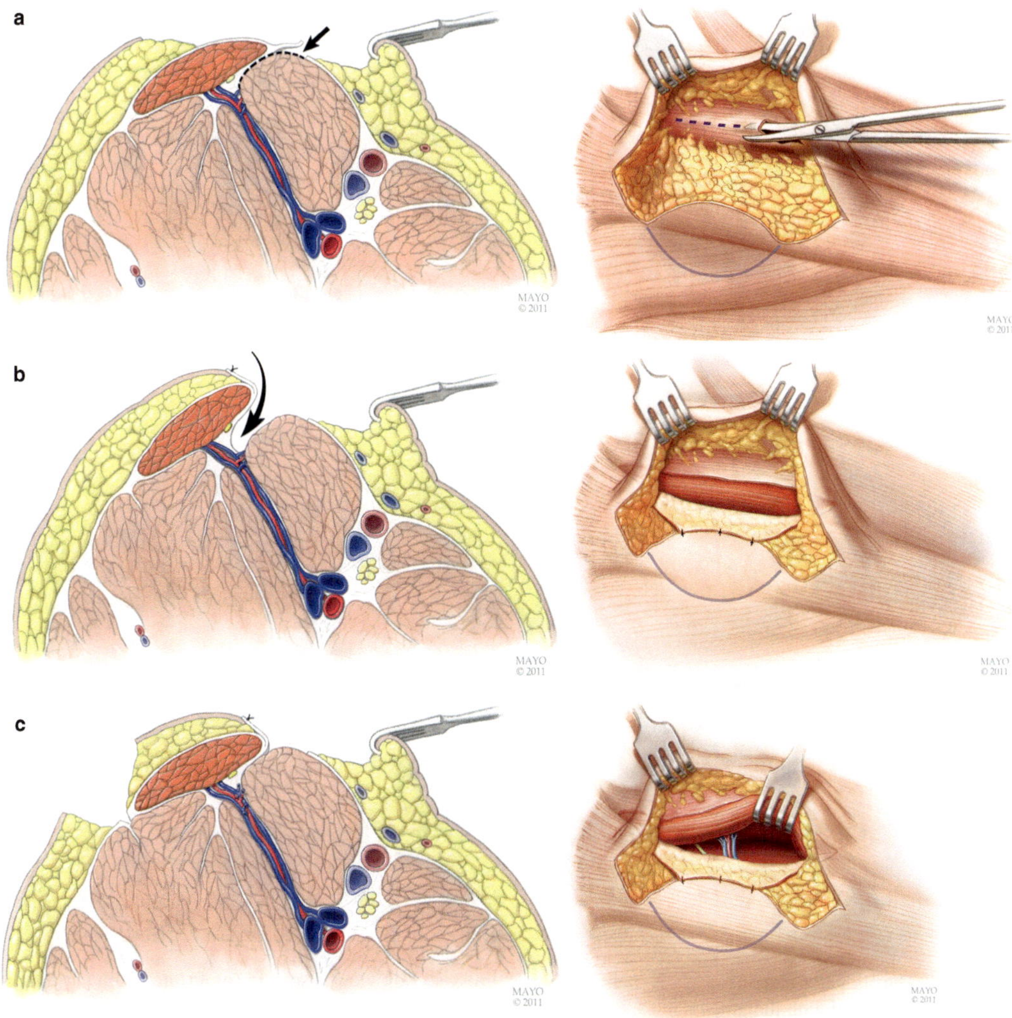

Fig. 29.13 (**a**) The fascia of the adductor longus is incised longitudinally and (**b**) The fascial edge is sewn to the skin paddle edge to avoid shear and traction on musculocutaneous perforating vessels. (**c**) In the interval between the adductor longus and gracilis muscles, the fascia of the adductor longus is gently retracted to expose the obturator nerve and the dominant proximal artery and venae commitantes. A cross-section view is seen on the left of the figure. Printed with permission of the Mayo Foundation for Medical Education and Research. All rights reserved, copyright 2010

gresses as far proximal as possible. To gain nerve length, the nerve branches to the adductor muscles are carefully dissected in an interfascicular fashion from the gracilis motor branch. Typically, a nerve pedicle of 8–12 cm can be obtained.

The posterior skin paddle incision is made, and dissection is carried to the level of the adductor magnus muscle. The adductor magnus fascia is incised longitudinally and reflected with the gracilis muscle (Fig. 29.14). Care should be made not to expose the gracilis or perforate the gracilis fascia. Ultimately a fascial sleeve around the proximal gracilis (the adductor longus, adductor magnus, and semitendinosus fascia) and its skin paddle remain.

Between the two thigh incisions, blunt finger dissection is performed in a subfascial plane. The secondary pedicle can often be felt or seen and is ligated. The distal tendon of the gracilis is then detached from the pes anserine and passed first into the distal thigh incision and then passed to the proximal thigh incision. The gracilis muscle is gently delivered out of the proximal incision (Fig. 29.15). The fascia of the adductor

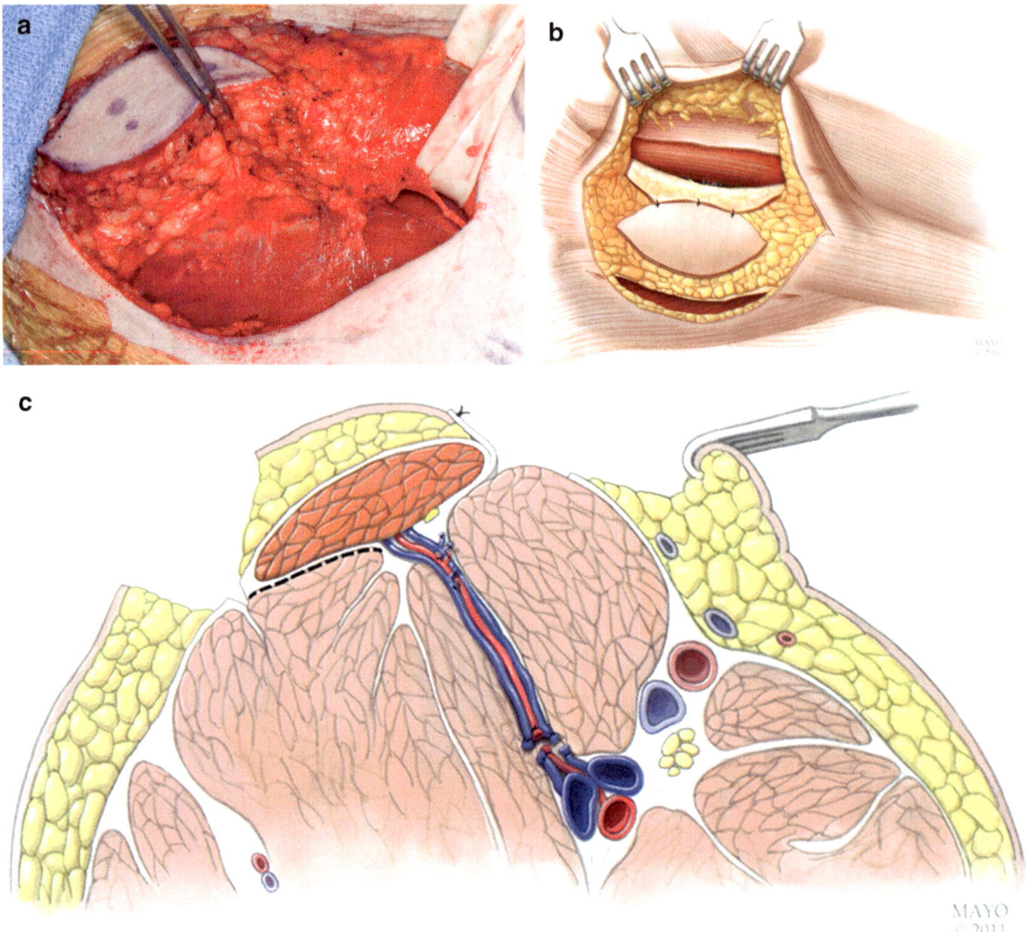

Fig. 29.14 The adductor magnus fascia is incised longitudinally and reflected with the gracilis muscle as seen in an intraoperative photo (**a**) and a line drawing (**b**). A cross-section view is seen in (**c**). Printed with permission of the Mayo Foundation for Medical Education and Research. All rights reserved, copyright 2010

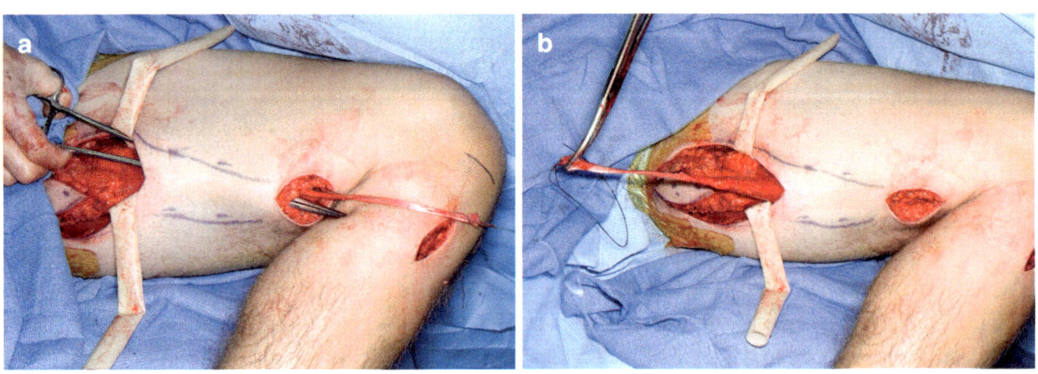

Fig. 29.15 (**a**) The distal tendon of the gracilis is then detached from the pes anserine and passed first into the distal thigh incision, and then passed to the proximal thigh incision. (**b**) The gracilis muscle is gently delivered out of the proximal incision. Printed with permission of the Mayo Foundation for Medical Education and Research. All rights reserved, copyright 2010

magnus is transversely divided at the distal edge of the gracilis. At this point, the only attachments of the gracilis are to the tendinous origin at the pubic tubercle and the vascular pedicle (Fig. 29.16).

The gracilis muscle is replaced back into its native bed, and the proximal attachment is addressed. The proximal attachment is tendinous laterally and more muscular medially. The tendon is dissected off the adductor longus tendon, and using an angled electrocautery tip, the gracilis tendon is detached from the pubic rami (Fig. 29.17). The flap harvest is now complete and is perfusing from its pedicle. A papaverine-soaked sponge is placed over the vessels until the recipient site has been prepared. Once the recipient site is ready for the transfer, the pedicle of the gracilis is ligated.

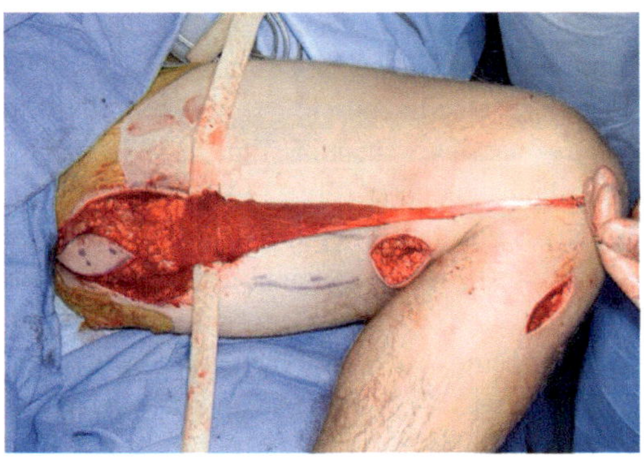

Fig. 29.16 The only attachments of the gracilis are to the tendinous origin at the pubic tubercle and the vascular pedicle

The three donor site incisions are closed primarily over suction drains. The donor deficit is minimal, and the three small donor scars are acceptable in the medial thigh.

Insetting of the Free Innervated Gracilis Flap

The application of the free innervated gracilis flap will determine how it is inset, what vessels are used, and what nerve will innervate the flap. Secure and strong proximal attachments of the gracilis at the recipient site are first performed followed by vascular anastomosis. Reestablishment of vascular flow within 60 minutes of ischemia time is ideal. Following vascular anastomosis, coaptation of the donor motor nerve to the obturator branch of the gracilis is performed under an operating microscope. Finally, tensioning of the gracilis is performed. Placement of sutures every 5 cm into the muscle to obtain ideal resting length of the muscle has been recommended by Manktelow and McKee [10]. In brachial plexus reconstructions, however, the authors found that tensioning the gracilis flap such that the elbow is maintained in 30 degrees of flexion at rest is a reliable way of tensioning the muscle.

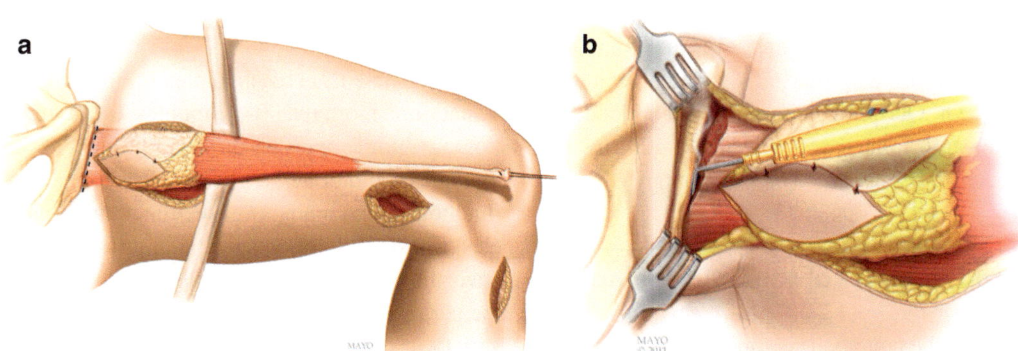

Fig. 29.17 (a) The proximal attachment is tendinous laterally and more muscular medially. (b) The tendon is dissected off the adductor longus tendon and adductor magnus muscles, and using an angled electrocautery tip (bent by the surgeon), the gracilis tendon is detached from the pubic rami. Printed with permission of the Mayo Foundation for Medical Education and Research. All rights reserved, copyright 2010

Advantages of the Gracilis Flap

The gracilis muscle harvested as a flap is reliable, and the anatomy is consistent with few anatomic variants. The muscle is pliable, with minimal bulk and can be tailored to fill the dimensions of a small defect. A cutaneous skin paddle may be incorporated into the flap to supplement the reconstruction or monitor the flap. Alternatively, the gracilis muscle can be harvested without a cutaneous component and covered by a skin graft. During harvest of the gracilis muscle flap, a simultaneous recipient site may be prepared. The gracilis muscle flap may be innervated for functional use in facial reanimation or upper extremity movement restoration. The muscle may even be split as is required in facial muscle replacement. The donor site is closed with an acceptable medial thigh scar and without a donor site functional deficit.

Prerequisites for using a free, functional, innervated flap in the upper extremity include a recipient site with a suitably located artery and vein to be used for anastomosis to the muscle's vessels; a donor muscle supplied by a single major neurovascular pedicle (i.e., gracilis or equivalent muscle); an available donor motor nerve to innervate the transferred muscle; a donor muscle with adequate excursion, strength, and contractility; and an expendable donor muscle. Additional factors affecting the speed and extent of muscle recovery following transfer appear to be related to the ischemia time, the distance from the neurorrhaphy to the muscle flap motor end plates, and the technical adequacy of the neurorrhaphy. The maximum ischemia time of a muscle at room temperature is unknown. Our preference is to restore blood flow within 60 minutes; however, 90–120 minutes appears to be safe based on the literature.

Disadvantages of the Gracilis Flap

Without the cutaneous component of the gracilis flap, the muscle is covered with a skin graft. The skin graft can be unsightly and cause tethering of the muscle thereby inhibiting muscle excursion and glide. The muscle power and bulk may be excessive in facial reconstruction but not adequate enough in upper extremity reconstruction. An occasional complaint of patients has been hyperesthesia, particularly in the distal thigh, presumably caused by iatrogenic injury to the cutaneous branch of the obturator nerve, which courses near the vascular pedicle. Patients may also complain of the scarring to the medial aspect of the thigh.

Indications for the Gracilis Flap

A functional gracilis flap has been described for facial reanimation, elbow flexion, and finger and wrist flexion and extension in brachial plexus injury patients. Recently, TUG (transverse upper gracilis) flaps have been described for breast reconstruction following a skin-sparing mastectomy. The gracilis muscle has also been used to restore quadriceps function (Fig. 29.18) and anterior tibialis function (Fig. 29.19). Other reconstructive indications for this flap include coverage of any small defects, vaginal and penile reconstruction, coverage of pressure sores in the groin and perineum, rectal sphincter reconstruction, reconstruction of urethrocutaneous and vesicocutaneous fistulas as well as vesicovaginal and rectovaginal fistulas, and correction of intractable vaginal prolapse (Table 29.1).

Elbow Flexion in Brachial Plexus Patients

When the time from brachial plexus injury to presentation is more than 9–12 months, a free functioning muscle transfer in conjunction with an extraplexal motor nerve transfer to restore elbow function is recommended. Free functioning muscles transferred for a specific purpose should have the strength and excursion comparable to the paralyzed muscles they are replacing [31]. A variety of free functioning muscles can be transferred, including the latissimus dorsi (thoracodorsal nerve), the rectus femoris (femoral nerve), and the gracilis (anterior division of the obturator nerve). The gracilis has become a com-

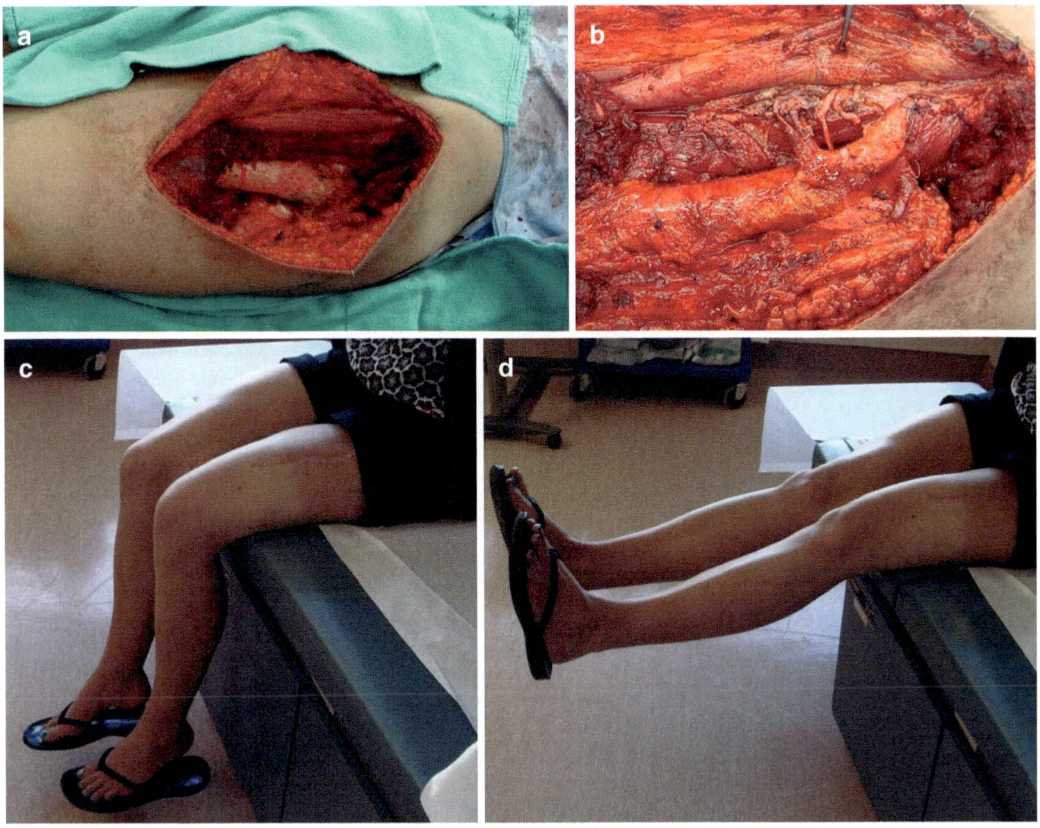

Fig. 29.18 Reconstruction of a quadriceps muscle using a free functioning innervated gracilis muscle from the contralateral leg. The debrided quadriceps muscle is seen in (**a**) the free functioning innervated gracilis attached proximally into the origin of the rectus femoris muscle and distally into the remnant of the quadriceps tendon in the bottom left picture (**b**). Postoperative pictures taken at 18 months (**c** and **d**). (Pictures courtesy of Drs. T.E. Hayakawa and E.W. Buchel from the University of Manitoba, Canada)

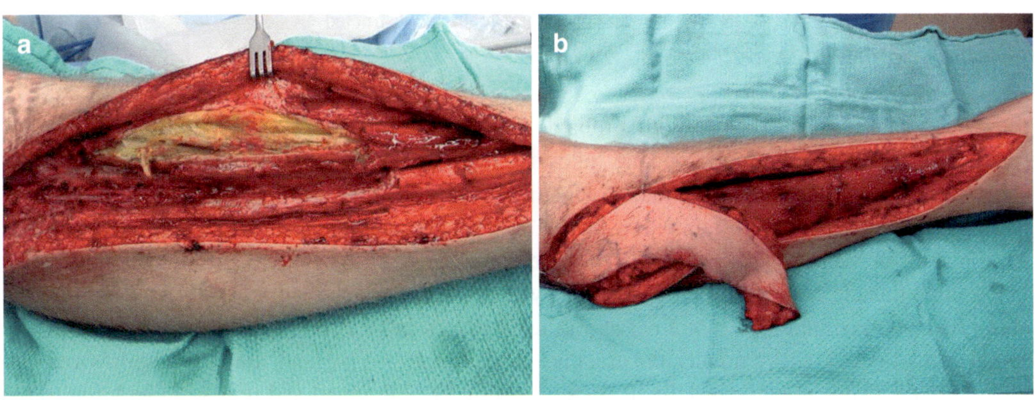

Fig. 29.19 (**a**) Complete necrosis of the anterior tibialis muscle following anterior compartment syndrome. (**b**) Reconstruction of anterior tibialis muscle using an innervated free functioning gracilis muscle. (Pictures courtesy of Drs. T.E. Hayakawa and E.W. Buchel from the University of Manitoba, Canada)

Table 29.1 Indications for gracilis flap

	References	Advantages	Disadvantages
Genitourinary reconstruction Vaginal reconstruction Penile reconstruction Anal sphincter reconstruction	McCraw et al. [7] Cronje and Van Zyl [19] Soper et al. [20] Nahai [21] Mathes and Nahai [15] Orticochea [3, 4] Hester et al. [22] Song et al. [23]	Brings vascularity and bulk to fill the soft tissue deficit Pliable Epithelial surface in musculocutaneous flaps for lining Hastens recovery after radical ablative surgery for tumor resection, especially in cases with adjunctive radiotherapy	Location and bulk of the vascular pedicle may hinder flap mobility Upper thigh bulge of tissue secondary to rotated gracilis flap Atrophy Aesthetics Possible prolapse
Small wound defect coverage Perineal and pelvis Extremity Facial defects (orbital exenteration, maxillectomy) Contour defects (hemifacial atrophy)	Mathes and Nahai [15] Conway and Griffith [24] Foster et al. [25]	Promotes healing by introducing vascular supply Has greater bulk for obliterating dead space	Muscle is more susceptible to ischemic necrosis than the skin or subcutaneous tissue
Facial reanimation	Frey [26] Harii et al. [9, 11] Harii and Asato [27] Zuker [28]	Muscle fibers are parallel and show a long amplitude of contraction Thin muscle with minimal bulk A portion of the muscle can be used	Muscle power and bulk may be excessive for facial reanimation
Upper extremity movement restoration	Ikuta et al. [12] Manktelow and McKee [10] Doi et al. [29] Shin et al. [30] Bishop [31]	Long tendon length Able to achieve M4 muscle strength Adequate excursion and contractility	Not all patients achieve M4 muscle strength
Breast reconstruction	Yousif et al. [32] Furnas [33] Wechselberger and Schoeller [34]	Can be an option in thin women without adequate abdominal, buttock, or back subcutaneous tissue used in other flaps Discrete donor site scarring Allows aesthetic shaping, contouring, and projection of the reconstructed breast	For reconstruction of small- to medium-sized breasts Possible complications of wound dehiscence and lymphedema Upper thigh contour defect

monly transferred muscle because of its reliable, proximally based neurovascular pedicle (allows earlier reinnervation) and its long tendon length (which has the potential to restore elbow flexion, wrist extension, or finger flexion) [30]. The free functioning muscle transfers may be powered by either two to three intercostal motor nerves or the spinal accessory nerve. Proximally, the gracilis is secured to the clavicle, while distally the gracilis tendon is woven into the biceps tendon (Fig. 29.20). 79% of the gracilis free functioning muscle transfers for elbow flexion alone achieved at least M4 strength [31].

Hand Function Restoration in Brachial Plexus Patients

Despite favorable results for early nerve grafting and transfer techniques for the shoulder and elbow function, reported results of grafting or nerve transfers for hand function have been less favorable [31]. Hand function requires restoration of both grasp and release in addition to the adequate positioning of the hand in space. Intrinsic muscle function and wrist or digital movement cannot readily be restored by nerve transfers; therefore, either a single or double

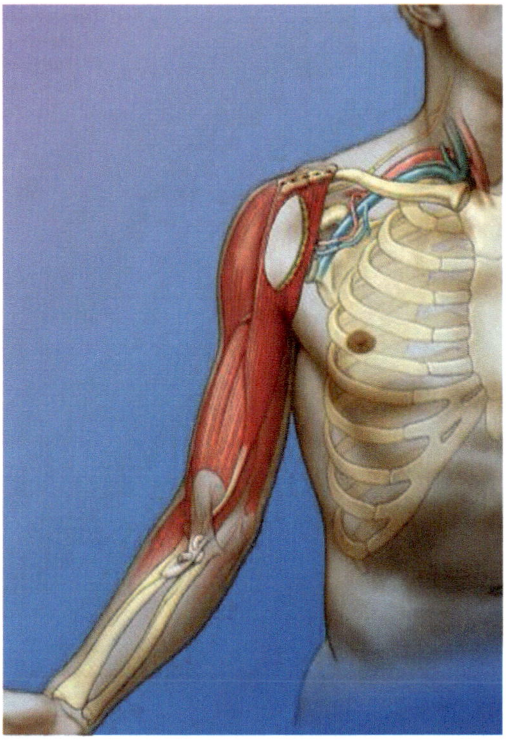

Fig. 29.20 Proximally the gracilis is secured to the clavicle, while distally the gracilis tendon is woven into the biceps tendon. (Printed with permission of the Mayo Foundation for Medical Education and Research. All rights reserved)

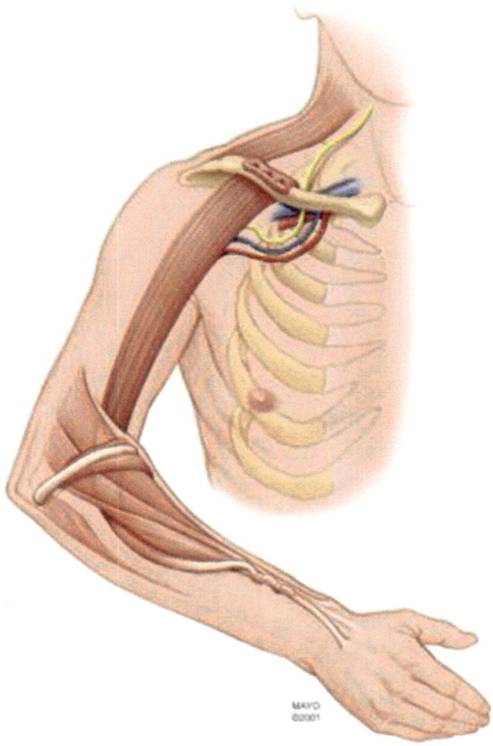

Fig. 29.21 In Doi et al.'s [35] first muscle transfer, the gracilis is attached to the clavicle proximally and routed distally under the brachioradialis to the radial wrist and finger extensors. (Printed with permission of the Mayo Foundation for Medical Education and Research. All rights reserved)

gracilis free functioning muscle transfer has been proposed.

Doi et al. described a double gracilis transfer to provide shoulder stability and function combined with flexion and extension of the elbow, hand sensibility, and rudimentary hand grasp and release [35]. In the first muscle transfer, the gracilis muscle is neurotized by the spinal accessory nerve and anastomosed to the thoracoacromial trunk to produce elbow flexion and finger or wrist extension. Proximally, the gracilis is attached to the clavicle and routed distally under the brachioradialis to the radial wrist and finger extensors (Fig. 29.21). In the second transfer, the gracilis is neurotized to motor intercostal nerves and anastomosed to the thoracodorsal artery to create finger flexion (Fig. 29.22). The sensory intercostal nerves are neurotized to the lateral cord contribution to the median nerve for hand sensation. Proximally, the gracilis is attached to the second rib, routed subcutaneously along the medial aspect of the arm, and attached to the finger flexor tendons.

The author (AYS) and his colleague (Dr. A.T. Bishop) have made modifications to the gracilis free muscle transfer originally described by Doi et al. A single gracilis muscle transfer is performed to restore elbow flexion and finger flexion. The gracilis is secured proximally to the clavicle with several suture anchors. The muscle is tunneled into the forearm, beneath the pronator teres to create a pulley effect, and is provisionally placed in its final position. The vascular anastomosis is preferentially performed end to end to the thoracoacromial trunk. The neurorrhaphy is completed with two motor intercostal nerves or, alternatively, the spinal accessory. Triceps reanimation is necessary and is typically accomplished

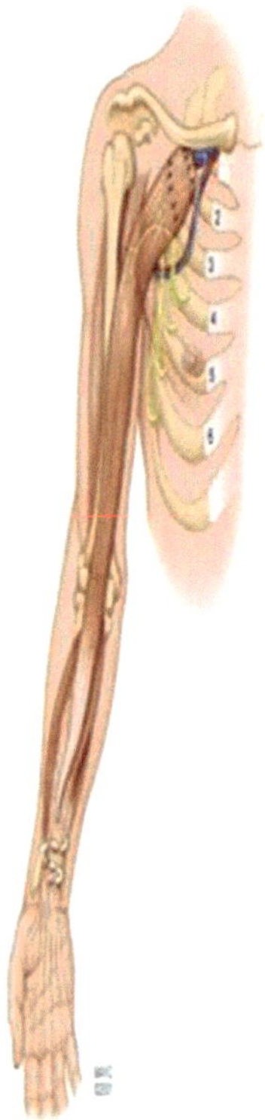

Fig. 29.22 In Doi et al.'s [35] second transfer, the gracilis is neurotized to motor intercostal nerves and anastomosed to the thoracodorsal artery to create finger flexion. (Printed with permission of the Mayo Foundation for Medical Education and Research. All rights reserved)

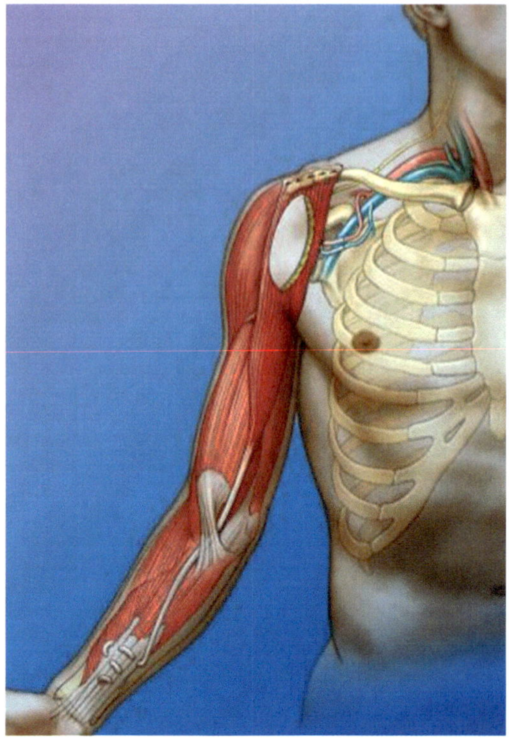

Fig. 29.23 The graft is tensioned to allow the fingers to extend with elbow flexion and allow the fingers and thumb to close with elbow extension. (Printed with permission of the Mayo Foundation for Medical Education and Research. All rights reserved)

by a spinal accessory to triceps transfer with an interposition sural nerve graft. Triceps allows agonist function to allow grasp to occur. Distally, the flexor digitorum profundus and flexor pollicis longus tendons are identified and sutured together in a position that creates key pinch and grasp with traction. The gracilis tendon is then woven into the prepared flexor digitorum profundus and flexor pollicis longus tendons using a Pulvertaft weave. The graft is tensioned to allow the fingers to extend with elbow flexion and allow the fingers and thumb to close with elbow extension (Fig. 29.23). At a second stage, wrist, first carpometacarpal, and thumb interphalangeal joint arthrodeses are used as adjunctive procedures to improve hand function, hand control, and appearance by increasing stability [36].

Conclusion

Regardless of the technique in harvesting the flap, the gracilis muscle flap is a reliable, versatile, expendable muscle which can be used for static coverage of wounds and as a dynamic muscle transfer. Recent advances in the harvest of the gracilis flap have concentrated on reducing the length of the scars to the medial thigh for aesthetic improvement.

Various minimally invasive techniques have been proposed, all of which aim to reduce scar formation. An endoscopic free gracilis muscle harvest has been described. Lin et al. (2000) compared the conventional gracilis harvest to that of an endoscopic harvest [37]. They found the endoscopic technique to be safe, relatively simple, and cost-effective with shorter scar length (6.5 cm compared with 15 cm in the conventional technique) and reduced donor site morbidity. They state, however, that the endoscopic technique requires training and an extensive learning period. Due to the drawbacks of endoscopic techniques including the steep learning curve as well as the need for special equipment, Bannasch (2009) described a semi-open approach to the gracilis muscle flap, without endoscopic assistance [38]. This approach involves a short inconspicuous transverse incision in the groin area with a counter incision distally. The mean incision length was 8.8 cm. The authors of this paper prefer to harvest the gracilis muscle with three small incisions: a 2–3 cm longitudinal incision at the pes anserine, a 2–3 cm transverse incision in the medial-posterior aspect of the distal thigh, and an incision approximately 7 cm in length to remove the muscle and skin paddle in the medial thigh.

References

1. Pickerell K, Broadbent TR, Masters FW, Metzger JT. Construction of a rectal sphincter and restoration of anal continence by transplanting the gracilis muscle. Ann Surg. 1952;135:853.
2. Pickerell K, Georgiade N, Crawford H, Maguire C, Boone A. Gracilis muscle transplant for correction of urinary incontinence in male children. Ann Surg. 1956;143:239.
3. Orticochea M. The musculocutaneous flap method: an immediate and heroic substitute for the method of delay. Brit J Plast Surg. 1972;25:106.
4. Orticochea M. A method of total reconstruction of the penis. Brit J Plast Surg. 1972;25:347.
5. Pers M, Medgyesi S. Pedicle muscle flaps and their application in the surgery of repair. Br J Plast Surg. 1973;26:313.
6. Bartholdson L, Hulten L. Repair of persistent perineal sinuses by means of a pedicle flap of musculus gracilis. Scand J Plast Reconstr Surg. 1975;9:74.
7. McCraw JB, Massey FM, Shanklin KD, Horton CE. Vaginal reconstruction with gracilis myocutaneous flaps. Plast Reconstr Surg. 1976;58:176–83.
8. McCraw JB, Dibbell DG. Experimental definition of independent myocutaneous vascular territories. Plast Reconst Surg. 1977;60(2):212–20.
9. Harii K, Ohmori K, Sekigughi J. The free musculocutaneous flap. Plast Reconstr Surg. 1976;57(3):294–303.
10. Manktelow R, McKee N. Free muscle transplantation to provide active finger flexion. J Hand Surg. 1978;3(5):416–26.
11. Harii K, Ohmori K, Torii S. Free gracilis muscle transplantation with microneurovascular anatomoses for the treatment of facial paralysis. Plast Reconstr Surg. 1976;57:133.
12. Ikuta Y, Yoshioka K, Tsuge K. Free muscle graft as applied to brachial plexus injury-case report and experimental study. Ann Acad Med Singap. 1979;8(4):454–8.
13. Doi K, Sakai K, Kuwata N, Ihara K, Kawai S. Double free-muscle transfer to restore prehension following complete brachial plexus avulsion. J Hand Surg Am. 1995;20(3):408–14.
14. Mathes SJ, Nahai F. Classification of the vascular anatomy of muscles: experimental and clinical correlation. Plast Reconstr Surg. 1981;67(2):177.
15. Mathes SJ, Nahai F. Clinical applications for muscle and musculocutaneous flaps. St Louis: The C.V. Mosby Company; 1982.
16. Terzis JK, Dykes RW, Williams HB. Recovery of function in free muscle transplants using microneurovascular anatomoses. J Hand Surg. 1978;3:37–59.
17. Haines R. The laws of muscle and tendon growth. J Anat. 1932;66:578.
18. Pfuhl W. Anatomy for surgeons: back and limbs, vol. 23. New York: Harper & Row, Publishers; 1969.
19. Cronje HS, Van Zyl JS. Resurfacing the vulva and vagina. Int J Gynecol Obstet. 1988;27:113.
20. Soper JT, Larson D, Hunter VJ, et al. Short gracilis myocutaneous flaps for vulvovaginal reconstruction after radical pelvic surgery. Obstetr Gynecol. 1989;74(5):823.
21. Nahai F. Muscle and musculocutaneous flaps in gynecologic surgery. Clin Obstet Gynecol. 1981;24:1277.
22. Hester TR, Hill HL, Jurkiewicz MJ. One stage reconstruction of the penis. Br J Plast Surg. 1978;31:279.
23. Song R, Song Y, Yu Y. Anal reconstruction by a modified Pickerell procedure. Clin Plast Surg. 1982;9:109.
24. Conway H, Griffith BH. Plastic surgery for closure of decubitus ulcers in patients with paraplegia: based on experience of 1000 cases. Am J Surg. 1956;91:946.
25. Foster RD, Anthony JP, Lathes SJ, et al. Flap selection as a determinant of success in pressure sore coverage. Arch Surg. 1997;132(8):868.
26. Frey M. Smile reconstruction using the gracilis muscle. Oper Tech Plast Reconstr Surg. 1999;6(3):180–9.
27. Harii K, Asato H. Grabb's encyclopedia of flaps volume I: head and neck section I: head and neck reconstruction. Chp 149. Microneurovascular free gracilis muscle transfer for facial reanimation. 2008.
28. Zuker R. Grabb's encyclopedia of flaps volume I : head and neck section I: head and neck reconstruction. Chp 150. Microneurovascular free transfer of a partial gracilis muscle to the face. 2008.
29. Doi K, Muramatsu K, Hattori Y, et al. Restoration of prehension with the double free muscle technique

following complete avulsion of the brachial plexus. Indications and long-term results. J Bone Joint Surg Am. 2000;82:652–6.
30. Shin AY, Spinner RJ, Steinmann SP, Bishop AT. Adult traumatic brachial plexus injuries. J Am Acad Orthop Surg. 2005;13:382–96.
31. Bishop AT. Functioning free-muscle transfer for brachial plexus injury. Hand Clin. 2005;21(1):91–102.
32. Yousif NJ, Matloub HS, Kolachalam R, Grunert BK. Sanger. The transverse gracilis musculocutaneous flap. Ann Plast Surg. 1992;29(6):482–90.
33. Furnas HJ. Re: the transverse gracilis musculocutaneous flap. Ann Plast Surg. 1993;30(5):480.
34. Wechselberger G, Schoeller T. The transverse myocutaneous gracilis flap: a valuable tissue source in autologous breast reconstruction. Plast Reconstr Surg. 2004;114(1):69–73.
35. Doi K, Muramatsu K, Hattori Y, et al. Restoration of prehension with the double free muscle technique following compete avulsion of the brachial plexus. Indications and long-term results. J Bone Joint Surg. 2000;82A:652–66.
36. Giuffre JL, Bishop AT, Spinner RJ, Kircher MF, Shin AY. Wrist, first carpometacarpal joint, and thumb interphalangeal joint arthrodesis in patients with brachial plexus injuries. J Hand Surg Am. 2012;37(12):2557–63.
37. Lin CH, Wei FC, Lin YT. Conventional versus endoscopic free gracilis muscle harvest. Plast Reconstr Surg. 2000;105:89–93.
38. Bannasch MA. The semi-open approach to the gracilis muscle flap: aesthetic refinements in gracilis muscle harvest. J Reconstr Microsurg. 2009;25(1):63–7.

Part V

Management of Specific Injury Patterns

Management of C5–6 Injuries

30

Chairoj Uerpairojkit and Piyabuth Kittithamvongs

Traumatic C5 and C6 brachial plexus injuries result in denervation of the biceps, brachialis, deltoid, and the rotator cuff muscle. The patients in this group incur loss of elbow flexion, forearm supination, shoulder abduction, and external rotation. Some of them also have winged scapula [1]. The sensation over the dorsoradial area of the hand may be lost in some patients, and/or they can experience neuropathic pain in that area [2]. In case of intact and healthy nerve root stump, one of the treatment options is nerve grafting. The intact C5 and/or C6 root can be grafted to the trunk, cord, or peripheral nerve by means of an autogenous graft. Intraoperative determination of the root stump's viability for grafting can be subjective, and an incorrect decision can potentially subject the patient to a long and unsuccessful recovery period [3]. Recently, a systematic review by Merrel et al. demonstrated that for patients with complete upper trunk palsy, without clinical or electromyographic evidence of recovery at 3–6 months after the injury, the functional outcomes for restoration of elbow flexion and shoulder function are better by using the nerve transfers procedure compared to autogenous nerve grafts [4]. On the other hand, Bertelli et al. recommended combined use of nerve transfers and root grafting which may enhance outcomes in the reconstruction of C5–C6 injuries of the brachial plexus [5].

In our opinion, if the proximal root stumps are not available for grafting (i.e., avulsed) or are questionably viable, our treatment recommendation is for nerve transfers.

Our strategy of nerve transfers in this injury is as follows:

- Spinal accessory nerve (SAN) transfer to suprascapular nerve (SSN) for shoulder abduction
- The nerve to long head triceps transfer to the anterior branch of the axillary nerve for deltoid reconstruction (shoulder abduction)
- Double fascicular nerve transfer for elbow flexion (ulnar and median nerve fascicle to biceps motor and brachialis motor branch)
- Thoracodorsal nerve transfer to the long thoracic nerve in case of winged scapula
- End-to-side nerve transfer from superficial radial nerve to median nerve in case of pain and numbness in the dorsoradial aspect of the hand.

Spinal Accessory Nerve Transfer to Suprascapular Nerve

The SAN is a pure motor nerve, which innervates the sternocleidomastoid and trapezius muscles. When used as a donor nerve, it is important to

C. Uerpairojkit (✉) · P. Kittithamvongs
Upper Extremity and Reconstructive Microsurgery Unit, Institute of Orthopaedics, Lerdsin Hospital, Bangkok, Thailand

A. Y. Shin, N. Pulos (eds.), *Operative Brachial Plexus Surgery*,
https://doi.org/10.1007/978-3-030-69517-0_30

isolate the distal branch while preserving the proximal branches to the upper and middle trapezius to preserve some trapezius function. Interposition nerve graft should be avoided because it will require two neurorrhaphy sites for a single transfer, thereby compromising the potential outcome.

Surgical Technique

The patient is placed in a supine position with a sandbag beneath the ipsilateral scapula. The head is turned to the contralateral side, and the upper part of the body is elevated slightly to reduce venous congestion (relaxed beach chair position).

Our preferred exposure of the supraclavicular plexus is through a V-shaped incision (Fig. 30.1). We use the lateral portion of the transverse limb, which lies 1 cm above and parallel to the clavicle, for exploration of the SAN. The medial-most aspect of the lateral upper trapezius is detached from the distal clavicle for 1–2 cm. Dissection is then performed on the anterior surface of the trapezius muscle several centimeters above the clavicle. The landmark for detecting the nerve is the transverse cervical vessels that accompany the nerve. An electrical stimulator can be used around the vessels to identify the distal part of the SAN. One of the key points in obtaining the SAN donor is not to be confused with the nerve branches from the cervical plexus, a pure sensory nerve which will not elicit any muscle response when stimulated. A small branch of the SAN to the upper trapezius should be preserved (Fig. 30.2). The terminal branch of the nerve should be dissected as far distally as possible.

The SSN is normally found arising from the upper trunk 2–3 cm above the clavicle (Fig. 30.3). However, the nerve can be difficult to find following traction injury to the plexus. A technical tip is asking the assistant to pull the patient's affected arm downward while the surgeon palpates a tented structure on the most lateral aspect of the brachial plexus with his or her finger. This

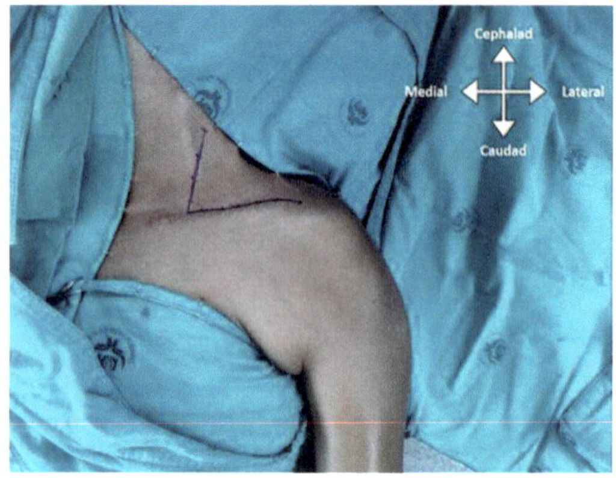

Fig. 30.1 The authors preferred incision for exposure of the supraclavicular brachial plexus is depicted

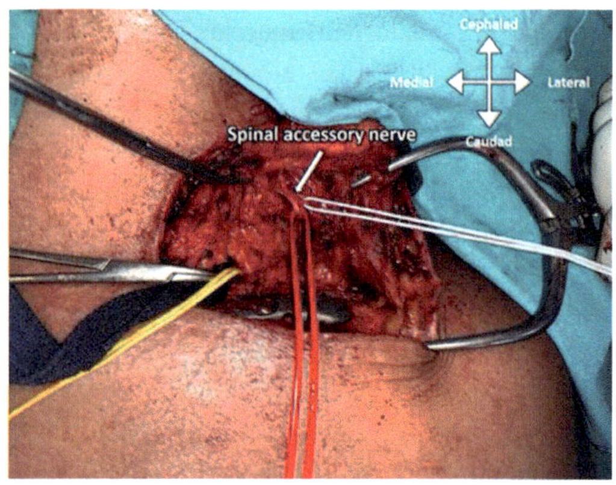

Fig. 30.2 The spinal accessory nerve (SAN) is identified and a branch to the upper trapezius (white loop) is identified and preserved. The terminal branch (red loop) is traced distally as possible to reach the suprascapular nerve

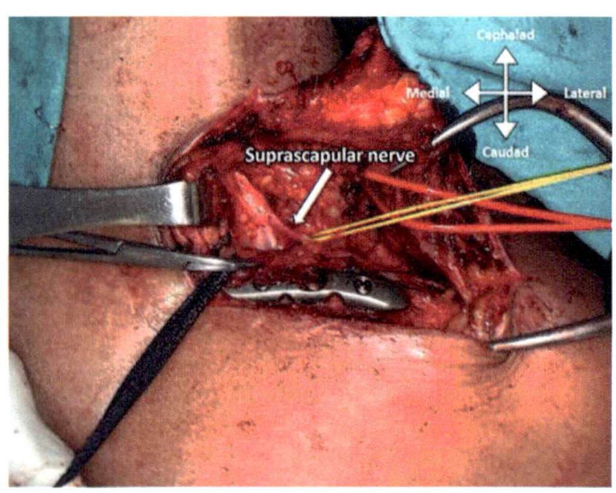

Fig. 30.3 The suprascapular nerve (SSN) is identified arising from the upper trunk

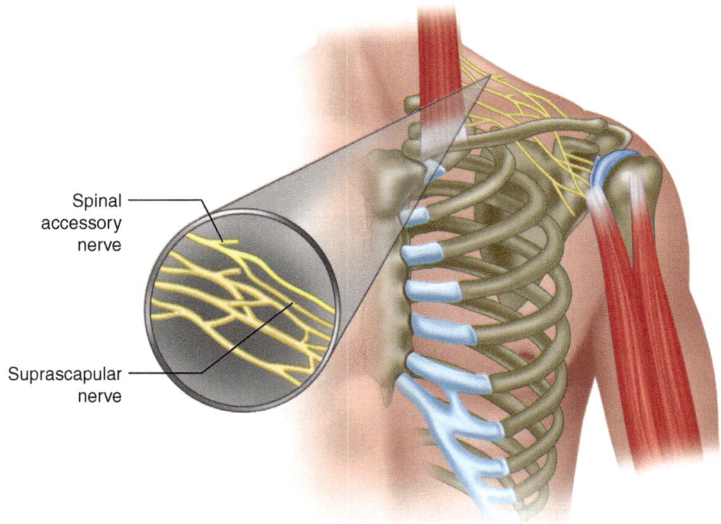

Fig. 30.4 Transfer of the spinal accessory nerve to the suprascapular nerve by anterior approach

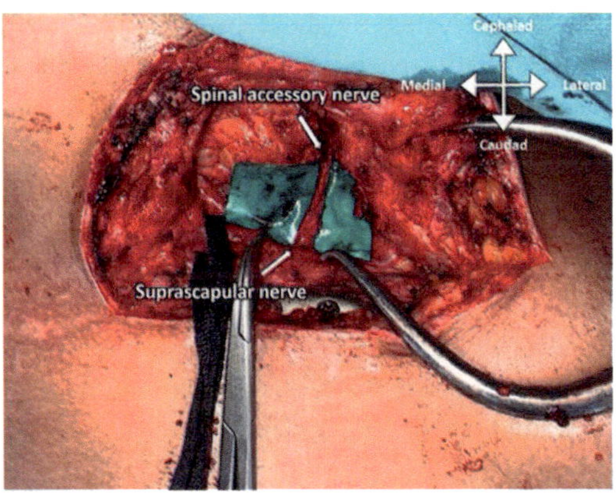

Fig. 30.5 Intraoperative view of a transfer to the suprascapular nerve (SSN) from the spinal accessory nerve (SAN)

is then followed with further blunt finger dissection down to the scapular notch where the integrity of the nerve is confirmed. The SSN is then traced from distal to proximal and disconnected from the upper trunk before coaptation with the donor SAN (Figs. 30.4 and 30.5). Interposition nerve graft should be avoided due to the additional neurorrhaphy sites, which may compromise the potential outcome. It is also important to mobilize enough nerve length to avoid suturing the nerves under tension.

The Nerve to Long Head Triceps Transfer to the Anterior Branch of the Axillary Nerve

The technique was described in the Chap. 11.

Double Fascicular Nerve Transfer (Double Oberlin Nerve Transfer)

In 1994, Oberlin et al. described the partial transfer of the ulnar nerve to the biceps motor branch [6]. This nerve transfer has stood the test of time and remains one of the most successful nerve transfers [7, 8]. Subsequently, double nerve transfer in which appropriate motor fascicles were harvested from the median and ulnar nerves transfer to motor branches to biceps and brachialis muscles was also proposed [9, 10].

Theoretically, the double nerve transfers decrease the chance of a poor result if one of the nerve transfers fails and may improve the strength of the elbow flexion in a heavy arm. Therefore, it is our preference to perform a double nerve transfer for restoration of elbow flexion whenever sufficient donors exist.

Surgical Technique

An incision is made on the anteromedial aspect of the arm starting just distal to the anterior axillary fold and continuing 15 cm distally. The branch of the musculocutaneous nerve supplying the biceps muscle is identified. It is usually located approximately four fingerbreadths below the anterior axillary fold. The branch to brachialis, usually located at midlevel of the line between the anterior axillary fold and the medial epicondyle, is then dissected distally as it enters the brachialis muscle.

The ulnar nerve and the median nerve are approached at the same level as the origin to the motor branch to the biceps and brachialis, respectively. We used a microelectric nerve stimulator to select the motor fascicle(s) predominately going to the wrist flexors. For the ulnar nerve, the typical donor fascicle is the fascicle innervating the FCU muscle and is usually located on the medial side of the ulnar nerve. The typical donor fascicle from the median nerve is the fascicle innervating the FCR muscle and is also usually located on the medial side of the median nerve. The chosen fascicles from the ulnar nerve and the median nerve are dissected distally for 2 cm and then divided, turned laterally, and sutured to the nerve of the biceps and brachialis under a microscope (Fig. 30.6).

The combined nerve transfer has shown over 80% recovery of ≥ M4 elbow flexion strength with minimal donor morbidity [4, 9–12]. However, Carlson et al. found that there was no significant improvement in elbow strength using the double compared to the single nerve transfer and recommended sparing the median nerve for others use [13]. Another prospectively study by Martins et al. also found no significant difference in elbow strength between the single and double transfer [14].

Thoracodorsal Nerve Transfer to Long Thoracic Nerve in Case of Winged Scapula

Palsy of the serratus anterior muscle causes pain, weakness, limitation of shoulder movements, and winging of the scapula [15] (Fig. 30.7). The muscle is innervated by the long thoracic nerve, which usually receives nerve fibers from C5 to C7 roots. However, some patients with C5 and C6 brachial plexus injury in whom there is no C7 contribution to the serratus anterior muscle or in those who have sustained partial injury to C7 root can present with deficit of the muscle. In these situations, the thoracodorsal nerve, which is a pure motor nerve and receives nerve fibers from C7 to C8 roots, is still preserved and may be used as a donor nerve for transfer.

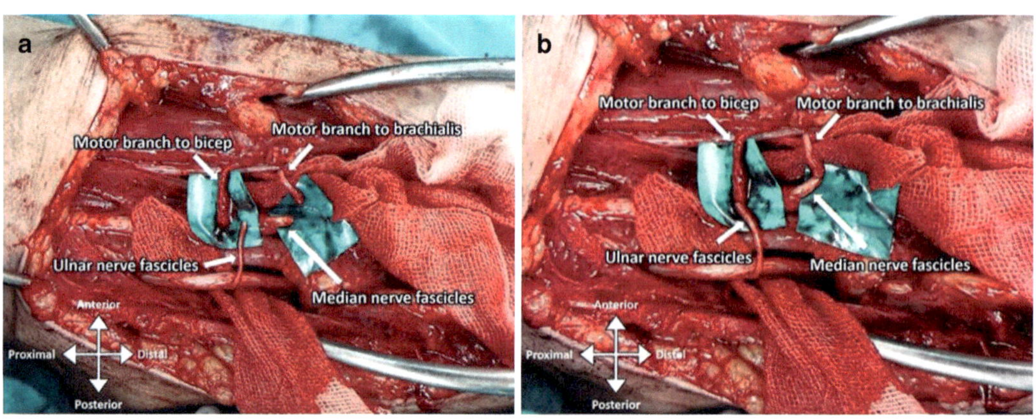

Fig. 30.6 Intraoperative view of double Oberlin nerve transfer. (**a**) Before neurorrhaphy. (**b**) After neurorrhaphy

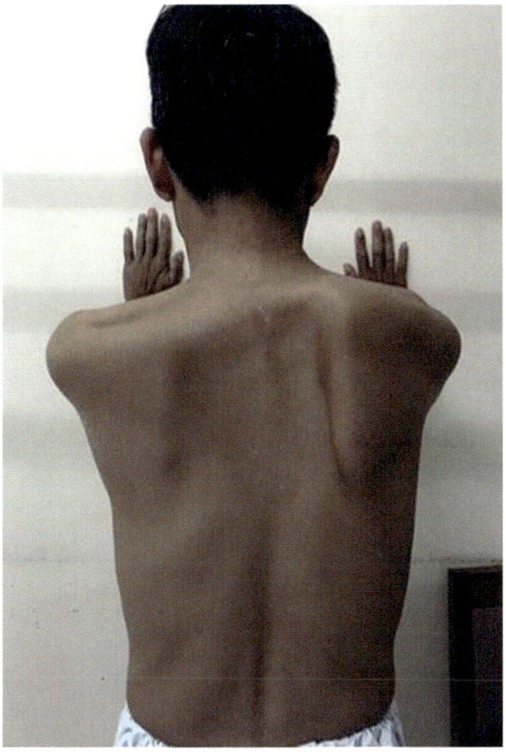

Fig. 30.7 Prominent, medial-winged right scapula evident as the patient attempts to push forward against resistance

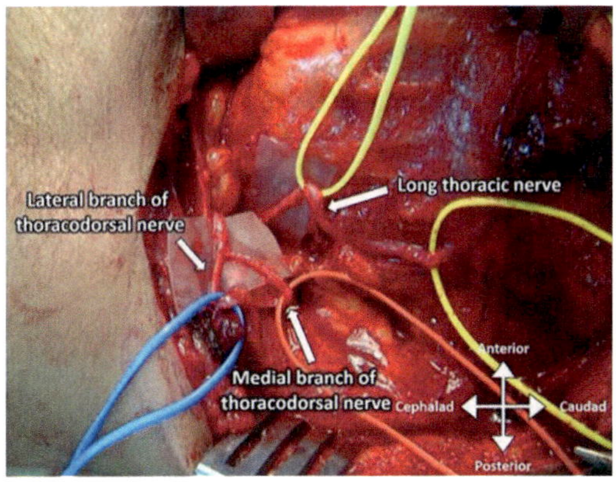

Fig. 30.8 Intraoperative view of the lateral branch and the medial branch of the thoracodorsal nerve

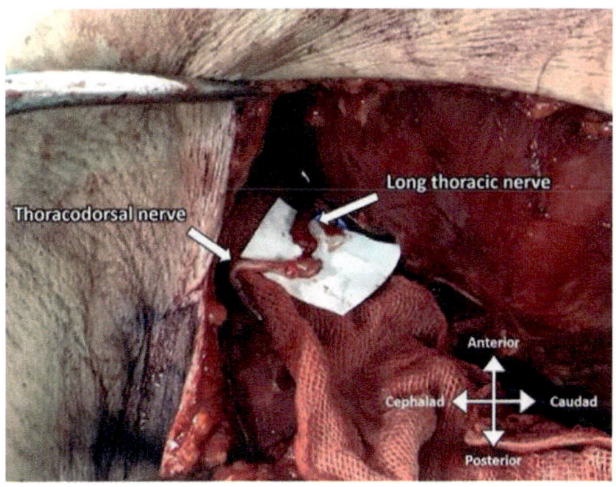

Fig. 30.9 Intraoperative view of the transfer to the long thoracic nerve from the lateral branch nerve of the thoracodorsal nerve

Surgical Technique

A 12-cm longitudinal incision is made along the posterior axillary fold, which represents the anterior margin of latissimus dorsi. The plane between the latissimus dorsi and pectoralis major was created bluntly by using fingers of the surgeon. The latissimus dorsi is then retracted posteriorly to expose the thoracodorsal and long thoracic nerves. Dissection around the anterior border of latissimus dorsi will reveal the thoracodorsal nerve and vessels. There are two main branches of the thoracodorsal nerve, the medial and the lateral (Fig. 30.8). The lateral branch runs parallel to the lateral border of the muscle, and the medial branch course runs parallel the upper muscle border and separates from the lateral branch at the neurovascular hilum at an angle of 45 degree. We use the nerve stimulator to select the branch that reveals the stronger contraction. The selected branch, usually the lateral, is then cut as distal as possible. The long thoracic nerve appears as a fine silvery white structure situated slightly anterior to the mid-axillary line on the lateral chest wall. In some instances, the fatty tissue around this area may obscure the nerve and make dissection difficult. In this situation, blunt dissection using fingers is useful. The overlying fascia is released, taking care not to damage the accompanying fine vessels which may easily bleed. Once the paralysis of serratus anterior is confirmed, the nerve is transected as proximal as possible to maximize the amount of muscle that can be reinnervated and to facilitate a tension-free neurorrhaphy with the thoracodorsal nerve (Figs. 30.9 and 30.10).

Novak and Mackinnon transferred the medial branch of the thoracodorsal nerve to the long

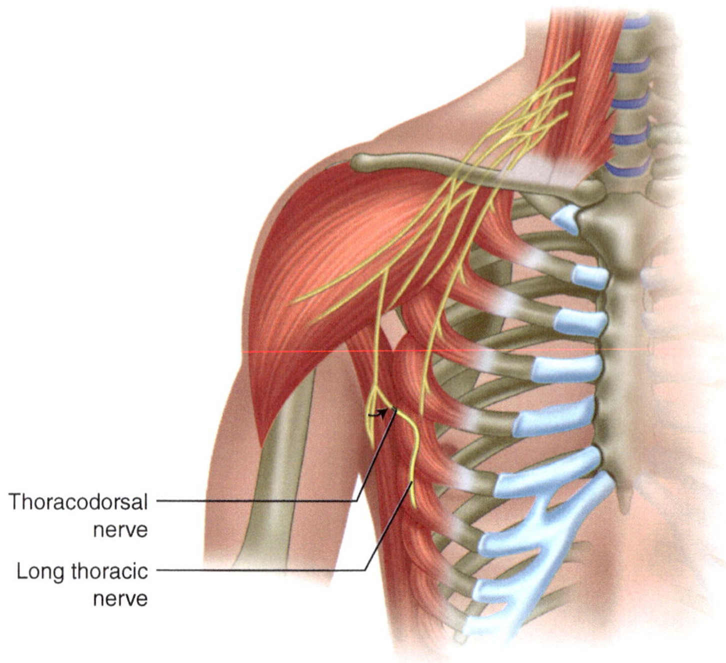

Fig. 30.10 The right shoulder showing nerve transfer to the long thoracic nerve from the lateral branch of the thoracodorsal nerve

thoracic nerve in a patient with idiopathic serratus anterior muscle weakness. At 7-year follow-up, there was full range of motion of the shoulder without winging of the scapula [16]. Tomaino reported a case of long thoracic nerve injury following axillary lymph node dissection. He transferred the medial pectoral nerve to the long thoracic nerve via a 11-cm sural nerve graft. At 18 months, the scapular winging improved [17]. In our series, five patients with C5–C6 brachial plexus injury with winged scapula due to paralysis of the serratus anterior confirmed clinically and electromyographically underwent the thoracodorsal nerve transfer to the long thoracic nerve. At a mean follow-up of 28 months, two patients had no winging, while three had mild winging. The mean arc of shoulder abduction was 134 degree. The mean arc of external rotation from full internal rotation was 124 degree. No patient complained of any functional deficit from harvesting a branch of the thoracodorsal nerve. The overall results were excellent in two patients, good in two patients, and fair in one patient [1]. The outcomes appeared to be better than in our previous patients with similar injuries but who had not undergone the additional thoracodorsal nerve transfer [18].

End-to-Side Nerve Transfer from Superficial Radial Nerve to Median Nerve

In our experience, the pain on the dorsal radial aspect of the hand which correlated with the superficial radial nerve distribution occurs in about one-third of patients with C5 and C6 root avulsion. Some of them have severe pain which is one of the most important obstacles in rehabilitation. In 2011, we described the end-to-side superficial radial nerve to median nerve transfer to restore sensation and relieve pain in C5 and C6 nerve root avulsion [2]. All eight patients in our series perceived at least one number lower of Semmes-Weinstein filament at the dorsoradial aspect of the affected hand. Before surgery, the mean VAS of pain was 6.1. After surgery, all patients reported relief pain within 2 weeks, with a mean VAS of

3.7. At the last follow-up, five patients reported no pain and the mean VAS was 0.5 [2].

Surgical Technique

A 6-cm longitudinal incision is made 4 cm proximal to the radial styloid on the dorsoradial site of the wrist. The superficial radial nerve is identified and trace as proximal as possible. Another 6-cm longitudinal incision is made 1 cm proximal to the wrist crease along the median nerve location. The fascicle of the median nerve over the ulnovolar side approximately 4 cm proximal to the wrist crease which corresponded to the fascicles of the third web space sensation is identified and used as the donor nerve. The distal part of the superficial radial nerve is then transferred subcutaneously and coapted end to side into the ulnovolar of the median nerve by an epineurial window technique. This technique provided enough length for a nerve suture under microscope without tension (Figs. 30.11 and 30.12)

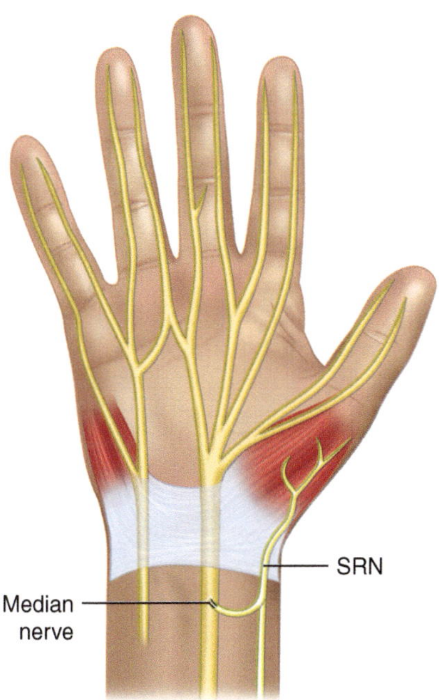

Fig. 30.11 Diagram of end-to-side nerve transfer of the superficial radial nerve into the ulnovolar part of the median nerve

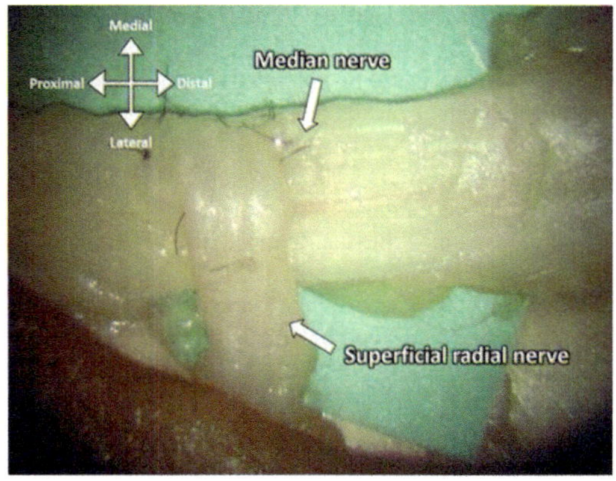

Fig. 30.12 Intraoperative picture showing epineurial window end-to-side nerve transfer of the superficial radial nerve into the ulnovolar part of the median nerve of the right upper extremity. The median nerve was of the right upper extremity

References

1. Uerpairojkit C, Leechavengvongs S, Witoonchart K, Malungpaishorpe K, Raksakulkiat R. Nerve transfer to serratus anterior muscle using the thoracodorsal nerve for winged scapula in C5 and C6 brachial plexus root avulsions. J Hand Surg Am. 2009;34(1):74–8.
2. Leechavengvongs S, Ngamlamiat K, Malungpaishrope K, Uerpairotkit C, Witoonchart K, Kulkittiya S. End-to-side radial sensory to median nerve transfer to restore sensation and relieve pain in C5 and C6 nerve root avulsion. J Hand Surg Am. 2011;36(2):209–15.
3. Garg R, Merrell GA, Hillstrom HJ, Wolfe SW. Comparison of nerve transfers and nerve grafting for traumatic upper plexus palsy: a systematic review and analysis. J Bone Joint Surg Am. 2011;93(9):819–29.
4. Merrell GA, Barrie KA, Katz DL, Wolfe SW. Results of nerve transfer techniques for restoration of shoulder and elbow function in the context of a meta-analysis of the English literature. J Hand Surg Am. 2001;26(2):303–14.
5. Bertelli JA, Ghizoni MF. Nerve root grafting and distal nerve transfers for C5-C6 brachial plexus injuries. J Hand Surg Am. 2010;35(5):769–75.
6. Oberlin C, Beal D, Leechavengvongs S, Salon A, Dauge MC, Sarcy JJ. Nerve transfer to biceps muscle using a part of ulnar nerve for C5-C6 avulsion of the brachial plexus: anatomical study and report of four cases. J Hand Surg Am. 1994;19(2):232–7.
7. Leechavengvongs S, Witoonchart K, Uerpairojkit C, Thuvasethakul P, Ketmalasiri W. Nerve transfer to biceps muscle using a part of the ulnar nerve in brachial plexus injury (upper arm type): a report of 32 cases. J Hand Surg Am. 1998;23(4):711–6.

8. Teboul F, Kakkar R, Ameur N, Beaulieu JY, Oberlin C. Transfer of fascicles from the ulnar nerve to the nerve to the biceps in the treatment of upper brachial plexus palsy. J Bone Joint Surg Am. 2004;86(7):1485–90.
9. Liverneaux PA, Diaz LC, Beaulieu JY, Durand S, Oberlin C. Preliminary results of double nerve transfer to restore elbow flexion in upper type brachial plexus palsies. Plast Reconstr Surg. 2006;117(3):915–9.
10. Tung TH, Novak CB, Mackinnon SE. Nerve transfers to the biceps and brachialis branches to improve elbow flexion strength after brachial plexus injuries. J Neurosurg. 2003;98(2):313–8.
11. Mackinnon SE, Novak CB, Myckatyn TM, Tung TH. Results of reinnervation of the biceps and brachialis muscles with a double fascicular transfer for elbow flexion. J Hand Surg Am. 2005;30(5):978–85.
12. Ray WZ, Pet MA, Yee A, Mackinnon SE. Double fascicular nerve transfer to the biceps and brachialis muscles after brachial plexus injury: clinical outcomes in a series of 29 cases. J Neurosurg. 2011;114(6):1520–8.
13. Carlsen BT, Kircher MF, Spinner RJ, Bishop AT, Shin AY. Comparison of single versus double nerve transfers for elbow flexion after brachial plexus injury. Plast Reconstr Surg. 2011;127(1):269–76.
14. Martins RS, Siqueira MG, Heise CO, Foroni L, Teixeira MJ. A prospective study comparing single and double fascicular transfer to restore elbow flexion after brachial plexus injury. Neurosurgery. 2013;72(5):709–14; discussion 14–5; quiz 15.
15. Warner JJ, Navarro RA. Serratus anterior dysfunction. Recognition and treatment. Clin Orthop Relat Res. 1998;349:139–48.
16. Novak CB, Mackinnon SE. Surgical treatment of a long thoracic nerve palsy. Ann Thorac Surg. 2002;73(5):1643–5.
17. Tomaino MM. Neurophysiologic and clinical outcome following medial pectoral to long thoracic nerve transfer for scapular winging: a case report. Microsurgery. 2002;22(6):254–7.
18. Leechavengvongs S, Witoonchart K, Uerpairojkit C, Thuvasethakul P, Malungpaishrope K. Combined nerve transfers for C5 and C6 brachial plexus avulsion injury. J Hand Surg Am. 2006;31(2):183–9.

Management of C5–7 Injuries

31

Kanchai Malungpaishrope
and Detchporn Putthiwara

The C5–C7 root injury of the brachial plexus is the combination of upper and middle trunk injury. The incidence is approximately 20–35% [1]. These patients have deficits in shoulder abduction, shoulder external rotation, elbow flexion, and forearm supination as a component of the C5–C6 root injury and also variable deficiencies of the elbow, wrist, and finger extension because of the C7 root or middle trunk injuries (Figs. 31.1, 31.2, and 31.3). The priorities for reconstruction are restoration of elbow flexion, shoulder abduction, and shoulder external rotation. In addition, the elbow extension and wrist and finger extension should be addressed. Generally, the injury of the brachial plexus is classified as pre-ganglionic lesion or post-ganglionic lesion. In the patients with post-ganglionic lesions, when proximal root(s) is(are) available, we advocate cable grafting with autologous nerve grafts. In the case of a pre-ganglionic lesion, nerve transfer is our preference.

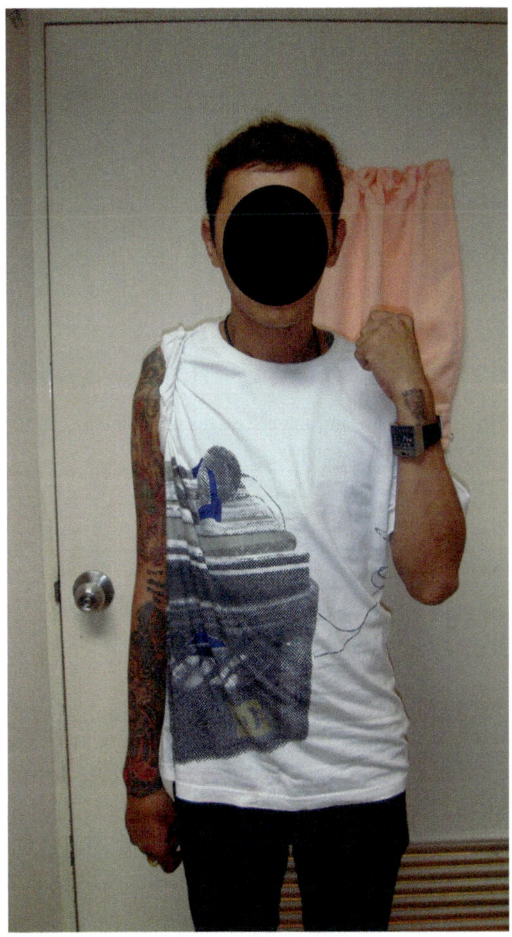

Fig. 31.1 Shoulder abduction and elbow flexion deficiency in the patient with C5–C7 injury

K. Malungpaishrope (✉) · D. Putthiwara
Upper Extremity and Reconstructive Microsurgery Unit, Institute of Orthopaedics, Lerdsin Hospital, Bangkok, Thailand

A. Y. Shin, N. Pulos (eds.), *Operative Brachial Plexus Surgery*,
https://doi.org/10.1007/978-3-030-69517-0_31

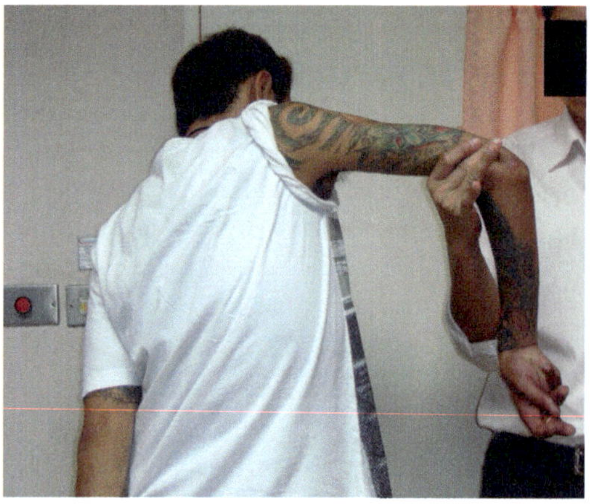

Fig. 31.2 Elbow extension deficiency in the patient with C5–C7 injury

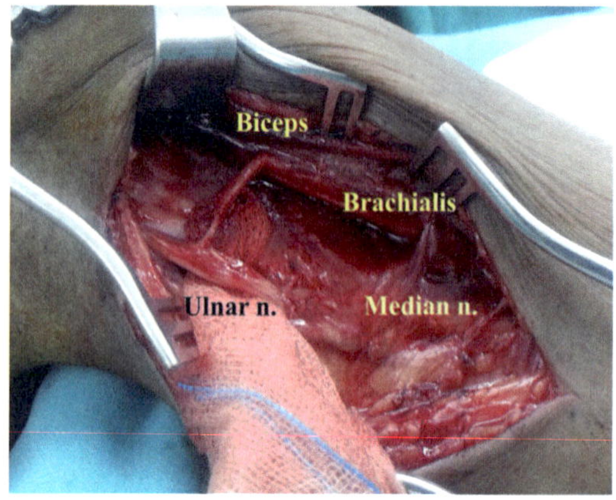

Fig. 31.4 A fascicle of the ulnar nerve transfer to the biceps branch and a fascicle of the median nerve transfer to the brachialis branch

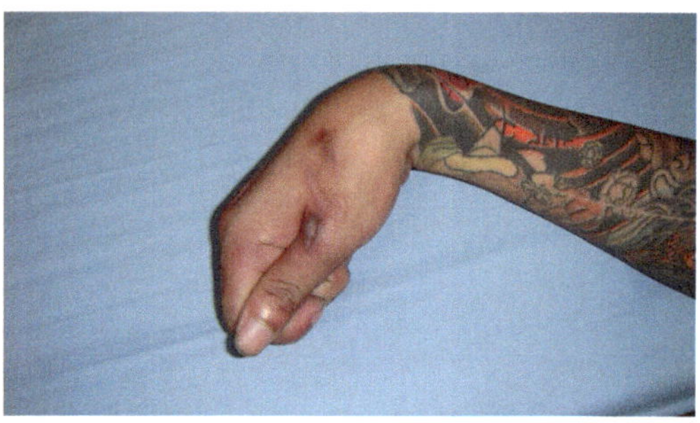

Fig. 31.3 Wrist and fingers extension deficiency in the patient with C5–C7 injury

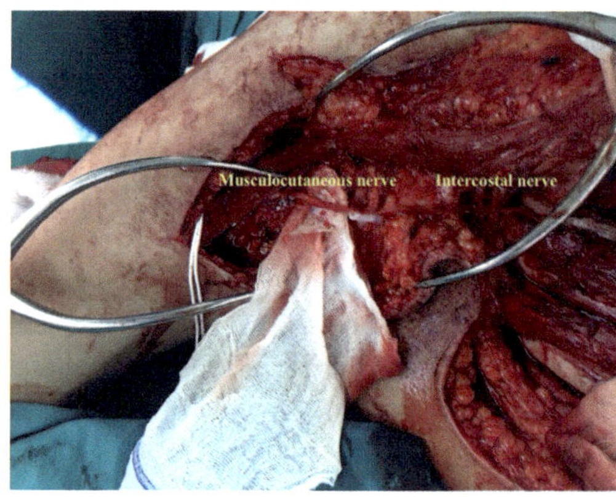

Fig. 31.5 Intercostal nerves transfer to the musculocutaneous nerve

Strategies for Reconstruction of the Elbow Flexion in C5–C7 Root Injury

We classify the patients with C5–C7 injuries into two groups: those with and without C8–T1 root injury. Careful preoperative evaluation of the median nerve and ulnar nerve is mandatory. In patients with normal C8–T1 root function, we prefer the double fascicular transfer which is a fascicle of the ulnar nerve transfer to biceps muscle and a fascicle of median nerve transfer to brachialis muscle [2] (Fig. 31.4). Studies reported MRC grade 3 or higher elbow flexion recovery in 97% to 100% with this technique [2–5]. In cases of C8–T1 root involvement, the reconstruction of the elbow flexion using the injured fascicle of the ulnar nerve to biceps branch provides a poor result. The extra-plexus donor nerve such as intercostal nerve, phrenic nerve, spinal accessory nerve, medial pectoral nerve, thoracodorsal nerve, and hypoglossal nerve is an available donor nerve to transfer for the elbow flexion [6]. Intercostal nerves are one of the most common nerves used to restore elbow flexion [7–13] (Fig. 31.5). Recently, studies reported variable results of elbow flexion from 33% to 89% of elbow flexion MRC grade 3 strength or better [14–18]. Phrenic nerve is also one of the donor nerves in nerve transfer for elbow reconstruction [19–21]. Overall effective rate of the transfer of the phrenic nerve was 70–85% (MRC $\geq$ 3) [6].

We do not use spinal accessory nerve transfer to the biceps muscle. We prefer using spinal accessory nerve to reconstruct the shoulder abduction.

Double Oberlin Nerve Transfer

The technique is described in the Chap. 30.

Intercostal Nerve Transfer to the Musculocutaneous Nerve

An incision is curved along the 6th rib through the lateral border of the pectoralis major to the medial aspect of the upper arm. The pectoralis major and pectoralis minor are elevated to identify the 3rd, 4th, and 5th ribs. Rib periosteum elevator is used to incise along the inferior border of each rib. The intercostal nerve is dissected meticulously. To ensure that the length of the nerve is adequate, we dissect the intercostal nerves from the costochondral junction to the anterior axillary line. At the anterior axillary line, the sensory branch of each intercostal nerve is divided to enhance mobility. At the medial of the upper arm, the musculocutaneous nerve is exposed underneath the biceps muscle. Proximal dissection of the musculocutaneous nerve should be performed to enhance the length of the transferred intercostal nerves without tension. The coaptation is usually performed directly under the microscope without nerve graft with 45 degrees of shoulder abduction and external rotation.

Phrenic Nerve Transfer to the Biceps Motor Branch

Phrenic nerve can be identified through the supraclavicular approach. The incision is made along the posterior border of the sternocleidomastoid muscle to the supraclavicular area. The platysma is incised. The external jugular vein is retracted medially. The cervical fat pad is retracted. The omohyoid muscle and transverse cervical vessels are identified and retracted. The upper trunk is identified and dissected medially. Phrenic nerve is found on the anterior surface of the anterior scalene muscle. Dissection of the biceps motor branch is performed as previously described. Use of the phrenic nerve requires a sural interposition nerve graft. The graft length is usually 30–35 cm long. The nerve graft is passed subcutaneously. The coaptation is performed under a microscope.

Strategies for the Reconstruction of the Shoulder Function in C5–C7 Root Injury

Loss of shoulder abduction and external rotation are commonly seen in C5–C7 root injuries as a result of paralysis of the rotator cuff and deltoid muscles. Simultaneous nerve transfers to both suprascapular and axillary nerve have been recommended [22–26]. To reconstruct the axillary nerve, the radial nerve branch of the triceps is one of the most commonly used transfers [24, 25]. In C5–C7 root injury, the radial nerve branch of the triceps cannot be used because of the injury to its main component from the C7 root. Many studies reported variable outcomes of the transfer of the spinal accessory nerve to the suprascapular nerve alone with the average degrees of shoulder abduction varying from 45 to 122 degrees [27–31]. In 2012, we reported a nine-case series after combined nerve transfer of the spinal accessory nerve to the suprascapular nerve and two intercostal nerves to the anterior axillary nerve via the posterior approach with average 69 degrees of shoulder abduction and 42 degrees of external rotation [32, 33] (Fig. 31.6).

Recently, the importance of reconstruction of the shoulder external rotation is increasingly recognized [34]. The results of spinal accessory nerve transfer to suprascapular nerve in the patients with C5–C7 root injury are not as effective as in C5–C6 root injury but better than in patients with panplexus injury. Baltzer reported 37% useful recovery of shoulder external rotation after transfer of the spinal accessory nerve to the suprascapular nerve in the patients with C5–C7 root injury compared with 76% in C5–C6 root injury and 26% in pan-

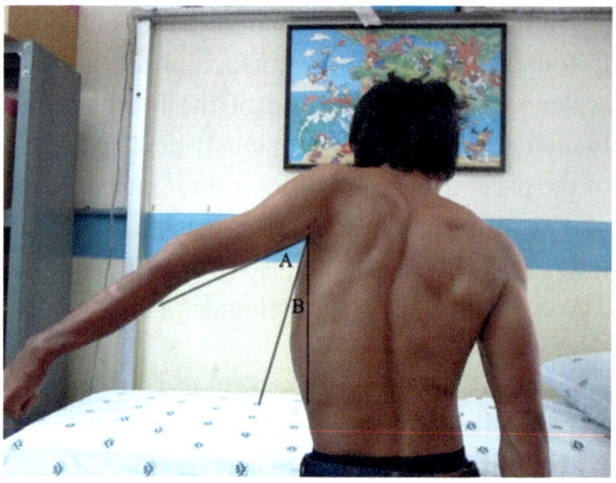

Fig. 31.6 Shoulder abduction after combined nerve transfer of spinal accessory nerve to suprascapular nerve and intercostal nerves to axillary nerve

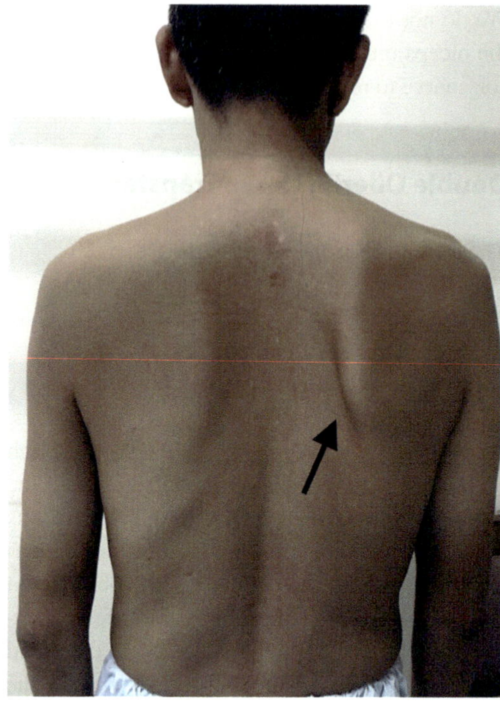

Fig. 31.7 Arrow indicates winged scapula in the patient with C5–C7 root injury

plexus injury [35]. They advocated sparing the spinal accessory nerve for later tendon transfer of lower trapezius for the patients with extensive brachial plexus injury. At our institution, we also found the shoulder external rotation after transfer of the spinal accessory nerve to the suprascapular nerve in the patients with C5–C7 root injury is poorer compared with the patients with C5–C6 root injury. However, we still prefer the spinal accessory nerve transfer to the suprascapular nerve in the patients with C5–C7 root injury because this is an effective transfer for reconstruction of the shoulder abduction.

Beside the glenohumeral motion, winged scapula is commonly seen in the patient with C5–C7 root injury (Fig. 31.7). Serratus anterior is an essential scapular stabilizer. Injury of the long thoracic nerve results in winged scapula which limits the shoulder movement. As the stability of the scapula is fundamental for optimal shoulder function, Suzuki recommended reanimation of the paralyzed serratus anterior muscle [27]. The transfer of the medial branch of the thoracodorsal nerve to the long thoracic nerve was reported to transfer for treatment of the paralysis of the serratus anterior [36–38]. However, in C5–C7 root injury, the thoracodorsal nerve cannot be used due to its components of C7 and C8 root. Yamada reported a successful case of intercostal nerve transfer to long thoracic nerve in a patient with C5–C7 root injury [39].

Recently, in cases of C5–C7 root injury who have no winged scapula, we reconstruct the shoulder stabilization with spinal accessory nerve transfer to the suprascapular nerve alone. We spare three intercostal nerves for reconstruction of the elbow extension. In the patients with C5–C7 root injury who have winged scapula, we prefer combined spinal accessory nerve transfer to the suprascapular nerve with 6th–7th intercostal nerve transfer to the long thoracic nerve (Fig. 31.8). In some patients who have partially recovered the triceps to M3, we transfer the spinal accessory nerve to the suprascapular nerve combined with the 3rd and 4th intercostal nerve to the anterior axillary nerve via the axillary approach.

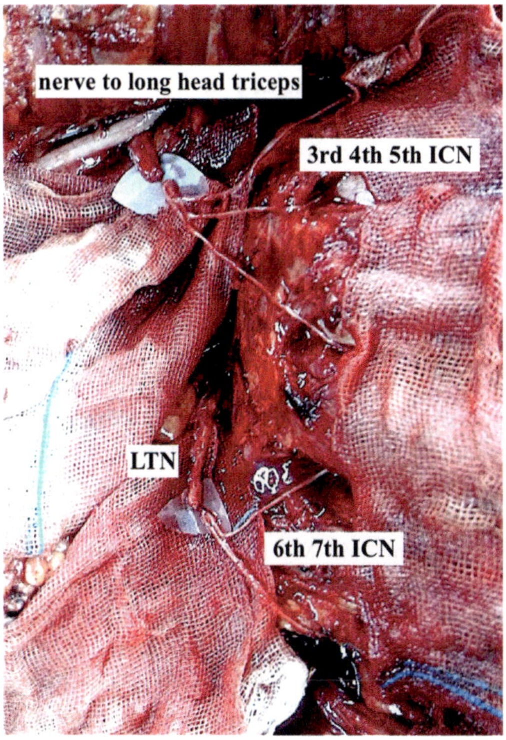

Fig. 31.8 Combined three intercostal nerves to the nerve of long head triceps and two intercostal nerves to the long thoracic nerve

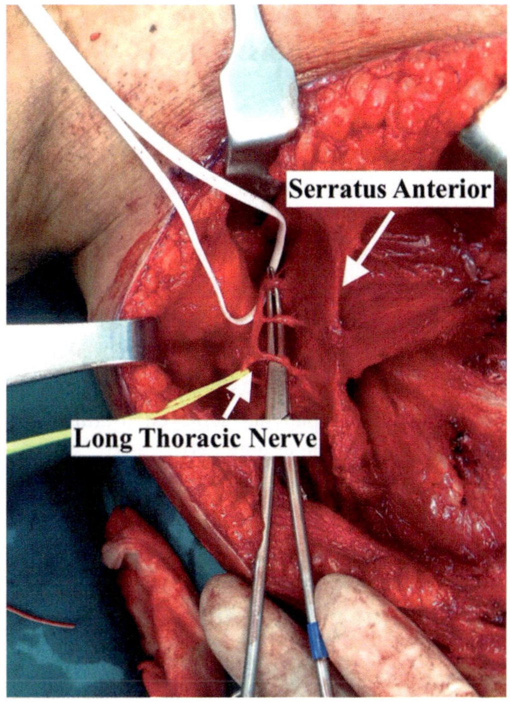

Fig. 31.9 Long thoracic nerve located on the serratus anterior muscle

Surgical Technique: Spinal Accessory Nerve Transfer to Suprascapular Nerve

The technique is described in the Chap. 30.

Surgical Technique: The 6th and 7th Intercostal Nerve Transfer to Long Thoracic Nerve

From the same approach, the latissimus dorsi muscle is identified and retracted posteriorly. The serratus anterior muscle is usually located on the chest wall. The long thoracic nerve is identified. It is usually found on the serratus anterior muscle (Fig. 31.9). The electrical nerve stimulation is performed to confirm no contraction of the serratus anterior muscle. The long thoracic nerve is dissected and divided as proximally as possible. The 6th and the 7th intercostal nerves are transected at the level of midclavicular line. The coaptation of the intercostal nerves to the long thoracic nerve is performed under an operating microscope.

Surgical Technique: The 3rd and 4th Intercostal Nerve Transfer to the Anterior Axillary Nerve

The technique to approach the intercostal nerve is the same as described previously. At the anterior axillary line, the sensory branch of each intercostal nerve was cut to enhance mobility. At the axillary region, we identified the common axillary nerve which was located proximally to superior border of the teres major muscle. The anterior axillary nerve is identified and separated from the common axillary nerve and cut as proximally as possible. The 3rd and 4th intercostal nerves are transected at the costochondral junction. Nerve coaptation is performed under an operating microscope.

Strategies for Reconstruction of the Elbow Extension in C5–C7 Root Injury

Recently reconstruction of the elbow has gained attention. To achieve useful restoration of the upper extremity's ability to reach out in space, the power of the elbow extension is required. Moreover, future reconstruction of the hand function requires a stable elbow flexion and extension. In 2011, Goubier et al. reported the case series of the intercostal nerve transfer to the nerve of the long head of the triceps [40]. Nine of 11 patients achieved useful elbow extension against the gravity (MRC $\geq$ 3).

Surgical Technique: The 3rd, 4th, and 5th Intercostal Nerve Transfer to the Nerve of Long Head Triceps

The 3rd to 5th intercostal nerves from the costochondral junction to the anterior axillary line are harvested. Through the same incision, the radial nerve branch of the long head the triceps is located beneath the brachial artery distally to the inferior border of the teres major muscle in the axillary region. The 3rd, 4th, and the 5th intercostal nerves are transected at the costochondral junction. The radial nerve branch of the long head of the triceps and the long thoracic nerve were cut as proximally as possible and coated directly under an operating microscope (Fig. 31.10).

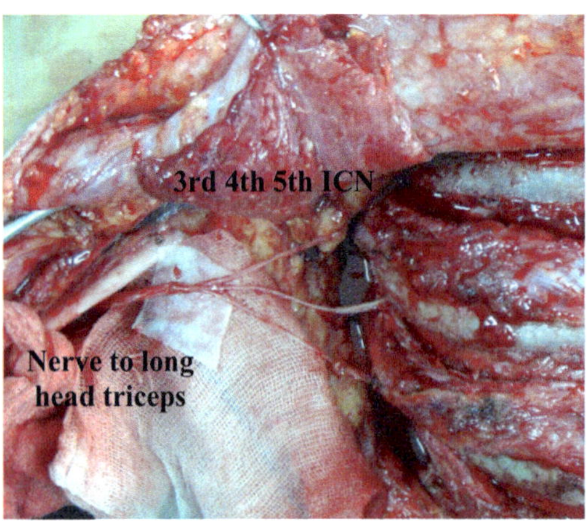

Fig. 31.10 Three intercostal nerve to nerve to long head triceps

Strategies for Reconstruction of the Wrist and Finger Extension in C5–C7 Root Injury

Reconstruction of the wrist and finger extension with nerve transfer in the patients with C5–C7 root injury is challenging. In 2007, Ray et al. reported a case series of successful reconstruction of the wrist and finger extension using fascicles of the median nerve (innervating flexor digitorum superficialis and flexor carpi radialis to the nerve to extensor carpi radialis brevis (ECRB) and the posterior interosseous branches of the radial nerve) [41]. In 2009, Ukrit et al. conducted an anatomical feasibility study and reported two cases of C5–C7 injury who had M4 recovery and 30 and 70 degrees of wrist extension after transferring of the proximal FDS motor branch to the ECRB motor branch [42]. Bertelli transferred the pronator quadratus motor branch to the ECRB motor branch in 28 patients with C5–C8 injury. Twenty-five of 28 patients recovered active wrist extension, scoring M4 [43]. Since our preference is to use the fascicle of the median nerve for reconstruction of the elbow flexion, it is our preference to perform late reconstruction of the wrist and fingers extension using tendon transfers or arthrodesis.

In summary, our strategy of reconstruction in the C5–C7 root avulsion is divided into two groups as follows:

Group 1: C5–C7 Root Avulsion with Normal C8–T1 Root

- Double Oberlin nerve transfer for elbow flexion
- Spinal accessory nerve transfer to suprascapular nerve for shoulder abduction and external rotation
- 6th and 7th intercostal nerves nerve to long thoracic nerve
- 3rd ,4th and 5th intercostal nerves to the nerve of long head triceps for elbow extension
- Late reconstruction of wrist and finger extension with tendon transfer

Group 2: C5–C7 Root Avulsion with C8–T1 Root Involvement

- Extraplexal (three intercostal nerves or phrenic nerve) transfer for elbow flexion
- Spinal accessory nerve transfer (SAN) to suprascapular nerve (SSN) for shoulder abduction
- Late reconstruction of wrist and finger extension with tendon transfer or arthrodesis

References

1. Kim DH, Murovic JA, Tiel RL, Kline DG. Mechanisms of injury in operative brachial plexus lesions. Neurosurg Focus. 2004;16(5):E2.
2. Liverneaux PA, Diaz LC, Beaulieu JY, Durand S, Oberlin C. Preliminary results of double nerve transfer to restore elbow flexion in upper type brachial plexus palsies. Plast Reconstr Surg. 2006;117(3):915–9.
3. Mackinnon SE, Novak CB, Myckatyn TM, Tung TH. Results of reinnervation of the biceps and brachialis muscles with a double fascicular transfer for elbow flexion. J Hand Surg Am. 2005;30(5):978–85.
4. Ray WZ, Pet MA, Yee A, Mackinnon SE. Double fascicular nerve transfer to the biceps and brachialis muscles after brachial plexus injury: clinical outcomes in a series of 29 cases. J Neurosurg. 2011;114(6):1520–8.
5. Tung TH, Novak CB, Mackinnon SE. Nerve transfers to the biceps and brachialis branches to improve elbow flexion strength after brachial plexus injuries. J Neurosurg. 2003;98(2):313–8.
6. Bulstra LF, Shin AY. Nerve transfers to restore elbow function. Hand Clin. 2016;32(2):165–74.
7. Minami M, Ishii S. Satisfactory elbow flexion in complete (preganglionic) brachial plexus injuries: produced by suture of third and fourth intercostal nerves to musculocutaneous nerve. J Hand Surg Am. 1987;12(6):1114–8.
8. Friedman AH, Nunley JA 2nd, Goldner RD, Oakes WJ, Goldner JL, Urbaniak JR. Nerve transposition for the restoration of elbow flexion following brachial plexus avulsion injuries. J Neurosurg. 1990;72(1):59–64.
9. Chuang DC, Yeh MC, Wei FC. Intercostal nerve transfer of the musculocutaneous nerve in avulsed brachial plexus injuries: evaluation of 66 patients. J Hand Surg Am. 1992;17(5):822–8.
10. Nagano A, Ochiai N, Okinaga S. Restoration of elbow flexion in root lesions of brachial plexus injuries. J Hand Surg Am. 1992;17(5):815–21.
11. Malessy MJ, Thomeer RT. Evaluation of intercostal to musculocutaneous nerve transfer in reconstructive brachial plexus surgery. J Neurosurg. 1998;88(2):266–71.
12. Songcharoen P, Wongtrakul S, Spinner RJ. Brachial plexus injuries in the adult. Nerve transfers: the Siriraj Hospital experience. Hand Clin. 2005;21(1):83–9.
13. Xiao C, Lao J, Wang T, Zhao X, Liu J, Gu Y. Intercostal nerve transfer to neurotize the musculocutaneous nerve after traumatic brachial plexus avulsion: a comparison of two, three, and four nerve transfers. J Reconstr Microsurg. 2014;30(5):297–304.
14. Samardzic M, Rasulic L, Grujicic D, Milicic B. Results of nerve transfers to the musculocutaneous and axillary nerves. Neurosurgery. 2000;46(1):93–101; discussion –3.
15. Bhatia A, Shyam AK, Doshi P, Shah V. Nerve reconstruction: a cohort study of 93 cases of global brachial plexus palsy. Indian J Orthop. 2011;45(2):153–60.
16. Moiyadi AV, Devi BI, Nair KP. Brachial plexus injuries: outcome following neurotization with intercostal nerve. J Neurosurg. 2007;107(2):308–13.
17. Terzis JK, Barbitsioti A. Primary restoration of elbow flexion in adult post-traumatic plexopathy patients. J Plast Reconstr Aesthet Surg. 2012;65(1):72–84.
18. El-Gammal TA, Fathi NA. Outcomes of surgical treatment of brachial plexus injuries using nerve grafting and nerve transfers. J Reconstr Microsurg. 2002;18(1):7–15.
19. Monreal R. Restoration of elbow flexion by transfer of the phrenic nerve to musculocutaneous nerve after brachial plexus injuries. Hand (N Y). 2007;2(4):206–11.
20. Siqueira MG, Martins RS. Phrenic nerve transfer in the restoration of elbow flexion in brachial plexus avulsion injuries: how effective and safe is it? Neurosurgery. 2009;65(4 Suppl):A125–31.
21. Gu YD, Wu MM, Zhen YL, Zhao JA, Zhang GM, Chen DS, et al. Phrenic nerve transfer for brachial plexus motor neurotization. Microsurgery. 1989;10(4):287–9.
22. Merrell GA, Barrie KA, Katz DL, Wolfe SW. Results of nerve transfer techniques for restoration of shoulder and elbow function in the context of a meta-analysis of the English literature. J Hand Surg Am. 2001;26(2):303–14.
23. Chuang DC, Lee GW, Hashem F, Wei FC. Restoration of shoulder abduction by nerve transfer in avulsed brachial plexus injury: evaluation of 99 patients with various nerve transfers. Plast Reconstr Surg. 1995;96(1):122–8.
24. Leechavengvongs S, Witoonchart K, Uerpairojkit C, Thuvasethakul P, Malungpaishrope K. Combined nerve transfers for C5 and C6 brachial plexus avulsion injury. J Hand Surg Am. 2006;31(2):183–9.
25. Bertelli JA, Ghizoni MF. Reconstruction of C5 and C6 brachial plexus avulsion injury by multiple nerve transfers: spinal accessory to suprascapular, ulnar fascicles to biceps branch, and triceps long or lateral head branch to axillary nerve. J Hand Surg Am. 2004;29(1):131–9.
26. Malungpaishrope K, Leechavengvongs S, Uerpairojkit C, Witoonchart K, Jitprapaikulsarn S, Chongthammakun S. Nerve transfer to deltoid muscle using the intercostal nerves through the posterior

approach: an anatomic study and two case reports. J Hand Surg Am. 2007;32(2):218–24.
27. Suzuki K, Doi K, Hattori Y, Pagsaligan JM. Long-term results of spinal accessory nerve transfer to the suprascapular nerve in upper-type paralysis of brachial plexus injury. J Reconstr Microsurg. 2007;23(6):295–9.
28. Bertelli JA, Ghizoni MF. Transfer of the accessory nerve to the suprascapular nerve in brachial plexus reconstruction. J Hand Surg Am. 2007;32(7):989–98.
29. Cardenas-Mejia A, O'Boyle CP, Chen KT, Chuang DC. Evaluation of single-, double-, and triple-nerve transfers for shoulder abduction in 90 patients with supraclavicular brachial plexus injury. Plast Reconstr Surg. 2008;122(5):1470–8.
30. Malessy MJ, de Ruiter GC, de Boer KS, Thomeer RT. Evaluation of suprascapular nerve neurotization after nerve graft or transfer in the treatment of brachial plexus traction lesions. J Neurosurg. 2004;101(3):377–89.
31. Songcharoen P. Brachial plexus injury in Thailand: a report of 520 cases. Microsurgery. 1995;16(1):35–9.
32. Malungpaishrope K, Leechavengvongs S, Witoonchart K, Uerpairojkit C, Boonyalapa A, Janesaksrisakul D. Simultaneous intercostal nerve transfers to deltoid and triceps muscle through the posterior approach. J Hand Surg Am. 2012;37(4):677–82.
33. Elhassan B, Bishop AT, Hartzler RU, Shin AY, Spinner RJ. Tendon transfer options about the shoulder in patients with brachial plexus injury. J Bone Joint Surg Am. 2012;94(15):1391–8.
34. Langer JS, Sueoka SS, Wang AA. The importance of shoulder external rotation in activities of daily living: improving outcomes in traumatic brachial plexus palsy. J Hand Surg Am. 2012;37(7):1430–6.
35. Baltzer HL, Wagner ER, Kircher MF, Spinner RJ, Bishop AT, Shin AY. Evaluation of infraspinatus reinnervation and function following spinal accessory nerve to suprascapular nerve transfer in adult traumatic brachial plexus injuries. Microsurgery. 2017;37(5):365–70.
36. Novak CB, Mackinnon SE. Surgical treatment of a long thoracic nerve palsy. Ann Thorac Surg. 2002;73(5):1643–5.
37. Tomaino MM. Neurophysiologic and clinical outcome following medial pectoral to long thoracic nerve transfer for scapular winging: a case report. Microsurgery. 2002;22(6):254–7.
38. Uerpairojkit C, Leechavengvongs S, Witoonchart K, Malungpaishorpe K, Raksakulkiat R. Nerve transfer to serratus anterior muscle using the thoracodorsal nerve for winged scapula in C5 and C6 brachial plexus root avulsions. J Hand Surg Am. 2009;34(1):74–8.
39. Yamada T, Doi K, Hattori Y, Hoshino S, Sakamoto S, Arakawa Y. Long thoracic nerve neurotization for restoration of shoulder function in C5-7 brachial plexus preganglionic injuries: case report. J Hand Surg Am. 2010;35(9):1427–31.
40. Goubier JN, Teboul F, Khalifa H. Reanimation of elbow extension with intercostal nerves transfers in total brachial plexus palsies. Microsurgery. 2011;31(1):7–11.
41. Ray WZ, Mackinnon SE. Clinical outcomes following median to radial nerve transfers. J Hand Surg Am. 2011;36(2):201–8.
42. Ukrit A, Leechavengvongs S, Malungpaishrope K, Uerpairojkit C, Chongthammakun S, Witoonchart K. Nerve transfer for wrist extension using nerve to flexor digitorum superficialis in cervical 5, 6, and 7 root avulsions: anatomic study and report of two cases. J Hand Surg Am. 2009;34(9):1659–66.
43. Bertelli JA, Ghizoni MF, Tacca CP. Results of wrist extension reconstruction in C5-8 brachial plexus palsy by transferring the pronator quadratus motor branch to the extensor carpi radialis brevis muscle. J Neurosurg. 2016;124(5):1442–9.

32 Strategies for Pan-Brachial Plexus Reconstruction: The Mayo Clinic Brachial Plexus Team Approach

Anthony J. Archual and Alexander Y. Shin

The field of brachial plexus surgery requires the cooperation of surgeons with other physicians and providers from multiple subspecialties. Synergy of these providers results in a team that is more than the sum of its parts. The collaboration of neurosurgeons, orthopedic hand surgeons, plastic surgeons, microvascular surgeons, and general surgeons with the singular focus of improving the patient has led to reconstructive outcomes that have surpassed what each could accomplish alone. The addition of non-surgical physicians further improves the team by addressing patient's non-surgical needs (rehabilitation, pain management, etc.). A team approach to treating brachial plexus injuries improves communication, surgical efficiency, and decision-making and brings the best innovations of each specialty to the patient in a single setting. The Brachial Plexus Clinic model we have assembled is a team of primary surgeons who evaluate acute and chronic injuries and perform the necessary nerve or reconstructive procedures together. Our current primary team includes two orthopedic surgeons with subspecialty training in hand and microvascular surgery and a neurosurgeon with subspecialty training in peripheral nerve surgery. These surgeons are responsible for evaluation, education, reconstructive decision-making, and determining if additional consultations are necessary. A group of ancillary surgeons and physicians associated with the team is available to address paralytic shoulder issues, pediatric orthopedic problems, pain management, and rehabilitation and occupational therapy needs. A dedicated brachial plexus team coordinator is highly recommended to organize and facilitate consultation schedules, testing, follow-up care, outcome data recording, video/photography documentations, and operative schedules.

Preoperative Evaluation

Much of the preoperative evaluation including history and patient exam, neurodiagnostic evaluation, and imaging has been detailed in previous chapters. After such information is obtained and reviewed, the patient's expectations and goals are evaluated. An educational discussion on the natural history of nerve injuries and the risks and benefits of all available options is undertaken. A series of standardized illustrations is used during this discussion and provided to the patient for further review after they depart the clinic (Fig. 32.1). This conversation not only provides the patient with information but also builds

A. J. Archual
Indiana University, Indianapolis, IN, USA

A. Y. Shin (✉)
Department of Orthopedic Surgery, Mayo Clinic, Rochester, MN, USA
e-mail: shin.alexander@mayo.edu

A. Y. Shin, N. Pulos (eds.), *Operative Brachial Plexus Surgery*,
https://doi.org/10.1007/978-3-030-69517-0_32

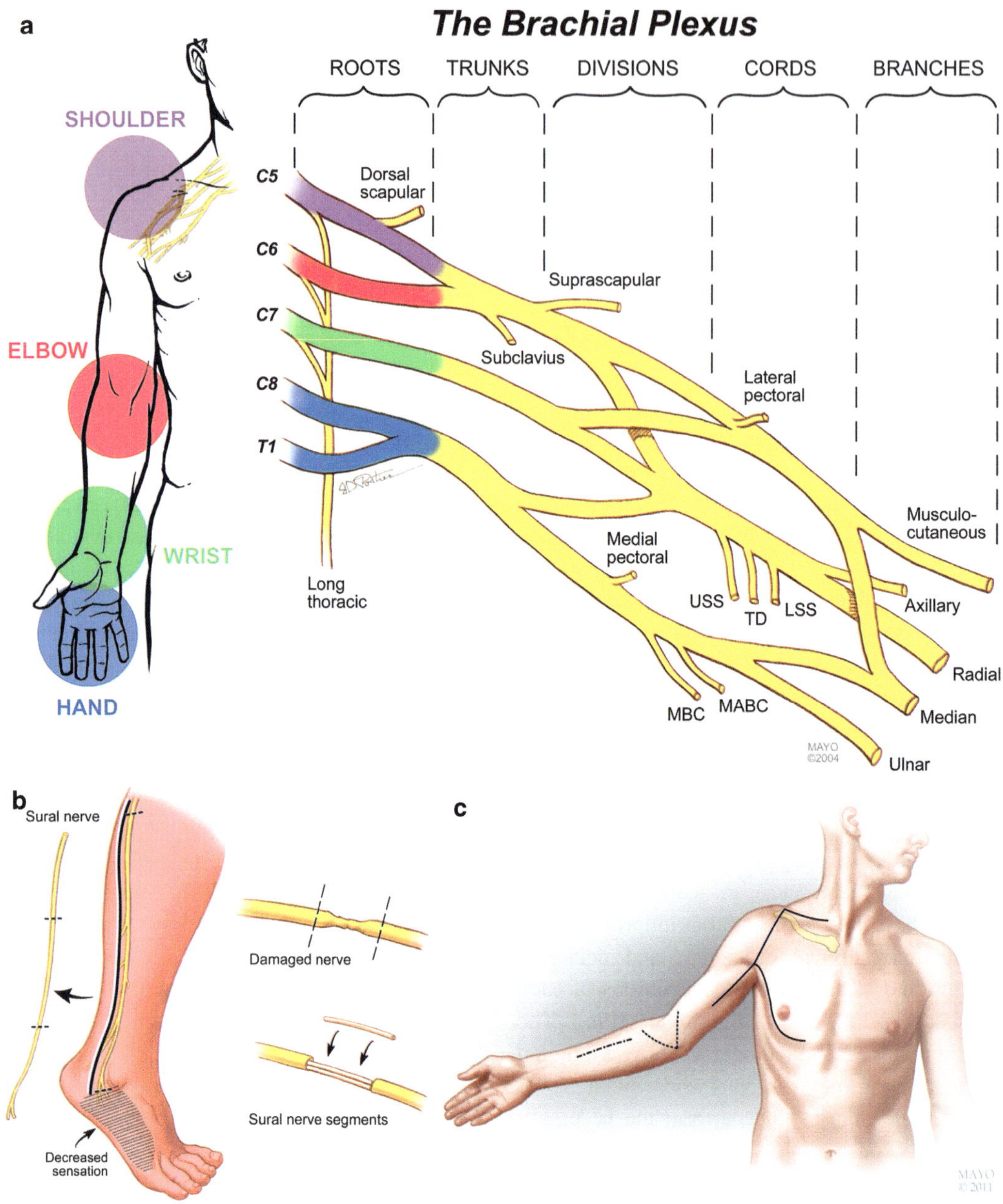

Fig. 32.1 (**a**) Educational illustration of the brachial plexus and types of brachial plexus injuries that are used to explain the injury to patients. (With permission of the Mayo Foundation, Copyright 2004). (**b**) Illustration of sural nerve graft harvest, area of numbness, and how the sural graft is used. (With permission of the Mayo Foundation, Copyright 2004). (**c**) Illustration of potential incisions for reconstruction. (With permission of the Mayo Foundation, Copyright 2011)

rapport with the patient and their loved ones. It is important to understand that the volume of information the patient and his/her family receives can be overwhelming and much of what is conveyed may be forgotten or misinterpreted. Having three reconstructive surgeons with three different styles of communication allows patients to have the information repeated and explained in different ways thereby facilitating a better understanding of their complex problem.

The patient's expectations of the outcomes of surgical reconstruction must be addressed both with respect to function and pain. In the pan-plexus patient, a frank discussion of the expected outcomes of surgery must be undertaken to gain the patients trust and prevent future dissatisfaction. Our discussions emphasize the goal of creating the best possible helper arm/hand possible and that a return to normal upper extremity function is rarely feasible. The outcomes discussed in previous chapters for specific nerve transfers/grafting or free functioning muscle procedures are reviewed. The role of hybrid type operations, combining nerve grafting/transfers with microvascular free tissue transfers (FFMT), is explained. The etiology of pain, especially neuropathic pain, is detailed, and referral to our pain specialist is recommended if indicated.

The priorities of reconstruction are reviewed with the patient as they are detailed in previous chapters. These priorities include elbow flexion, shoulder stability with external rotation, rudimentary grasp, and protective sensation. While there are multiple options for obtaining each individual function, combining them all in a single reconstruction can be daunting. It is explained that there is no right or wrong answer for a patient's reconstructive goals and that reconstruction is highly individualized. Some patients express limited or stepwise goals, beginning with restoration of elbow flexion and shoulder stability with the potential for further procedures in the future. Others request "everything possible" be done to restore as much function as possible at the index procedure. It is the responsibility of the surgeon to discuss the rationale for and outcomes of such choices and to empower the patient to make an educated decision. This includes explaining the implications of procedures on future use of myoelectric devices should the patient eventually express the desire for amputation. In these circumstances, establishing some functional control of upper arm muscles may improve the outcomes of myoelectric prosthetics. In patients who request primary amputation, it is important to delve into the patient's rationale for desiring amputation. If it is with the intention of relieving neuropathic pain, the patient needs to be educated on the etiology of the neuropathic pain, explaining that it is likely a result of avulsions of nerve roots from the spinal cord and thus amputation at any level would be unlikely to relieve this pain.

Available Options in the Pan-Plexus Patient

During the evaluation period, all data must be considered including clinical exam findings, electrodiagnostic studies, and imaging (CT myelogram, MRA or angiography, ultrasound (US)), and/or consultations (neurology, vascular surgery, etc.), to determine the availability of resources for reconstruction. The reconstructive plan should take into account all available nerve and muscle donors and techniques including nerve grafting, nerve transfers, free functioning muscles, tendon transfers, and joint arthrodeses.

Ipsilateral Intraplexal Nerves With the goal using of all viable intraplexal nerve donors, exploration of the supraclavicular brachial plexus is performed to determine if any viable intraplexal ipsilateral donor roots are present. Though some authors report that C5 nerve root is always viable [1], we have not had the same experience over the past 20 years. Thus if any viable roots are identified and viability confirmed with intraoperative SSEP/MEP, they are used as donor nerves with nerve grafts to targets as is detailed below. The phrenic nerve has been described as a donor for nerve transfers [2, 3]. If the C5 nerve root is avulsed, this could theoretically make phrenic nerve transfer less reliable as the phrenic nerve receives contributions from C3, C4, and C5. The phrenic nerve has not been routinely utilized in our practice as a great majority of our patients are pan-avulsion. Additionally, the generally high BMI of the patients in our region and our frequent use of intercostal nerves (ICN) may put respiratory function at risk if a normal phrenic nerve is used as a donor.

Ipsilateral Extraplexal Nerves The spinal accessory nerve is a common source of donor nerve axons in brachial plexus reconstruction, especially in the pan-plexus-injured patient, as it provides voluntary motor control with minimal donor site morbidity [4]. An uninjured spinal accessory nerve is available for use as a donor in 94% of cases [5] and can be easily identified in the supraclavicular approach. Intercostal nerves also serve as a valuable ipsilateral extraplexal source of axons under volitional control as well as sensory donors, but harvesting them can be challenging and carries morbidity. While rib fractures are a common concomitant injury occurring with brachial plexus injuries, Kovachavich et al. found that the intercostal nerves are still suitable for grafting in 92% of patients [6]. The sensory portions of these nerves can be used to reestablish protective sensation in the median distribution by transfer to the lateral cord contribution of the median nerve.

Contralateral Intraplexal Donors The C7 nerve root or hemi-root can be extended with a free graft or transferred via the retropharyngeal route to reinnervate contralateral targets [7]. Our experience with the use of contralateral C7 has not been as encouraging as the published reports. We reviewed the outcomes of hemi-contralateral C7 for hand function and reported dismal outcomes [8]. When used for shoulder re-animation, the outcomes were good. However, patients never regained independent function and required the contralateral extremity to activate to initiate shoulder function on the injured side making use more of an academic success and clinical failure. Almost all patients found this lack of independence precluded the usefulness of the transfer [8]. As such, using contralateral C7 as a donor in our practice for adult pan-plexus reconstruction has been largely abandoned by our group.

Free Functioning Muscle Transfer The transfer of a free functioning muscle is a powerful technique for reconstruction after a brachial plexus injury, with the gracilis muscle being the workhorse of our practice. These flaps have been described to power elbow flexion, wrist/finger flexion, and wrist/finger extension. Some authors advocate for the use of two flaps in two to three separate operations, to reestablish a grasp and elbow function [9, 10]. A single-stage procedure to obtain rudimentary grasp is more attractive to our patients and medical insurance system. As such, we have pursued a single-stage procedure utilizing a single gracilis to restore elbow flexion and rudimentary grasp (Fig. 32.2).

Tendon Transfers If nerve transfers, nerve grafting, and free muscle transfers are not an option, as is the case in the reconstruction of shoulder external rotation in some pan-plexus injury patients, tendon transfers can be considered. In these cases, the spinal accessory nerve is spared in the nerve reconstruction plan and the lower trapezius tendon is transferred to the infraspinatus tendon for external rotation [11]. Transfer of the contralateral trapezius tendon in a turnover fashion can be performed if the ipsilateral trapezius muscle is not suitable for use [12].

Arthrodesis Arthrodesis procedures of the shoulder, wrist, or small joints are generally done as secondary procedures. These may be part of the initial plan but performed in a staged fashion or added to the plan later as part of the fine-tuning that occurs after primary reconstruction. Shoulder fusion is reserved for instances where no other reconstructive options are available or previous attempts at reestablishing stability have failed (see "Shoulder Fusion" chapter). Wrist fusion can optimize free functioning muscle transfer for grasp and is generally well tolerated by patients [13]. Similarly, arthrodesis of the small joints of the hand can optimize the function of other reconstruction. For example, we commonly fuse the interphalangeal joint of the thumb to bolster rudimentary pinch [13].

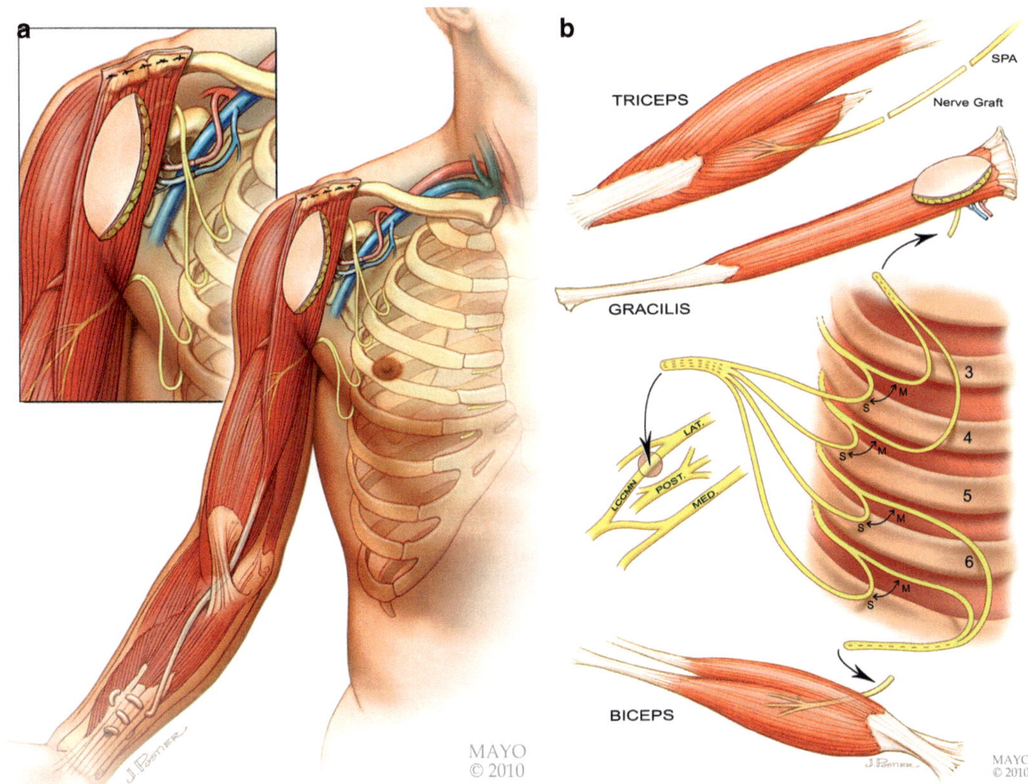

Fig. 32.2 A single stage free functioning gracilis muscle can be used to obtain rudimentary grasp, elbow flexion, and elbow extension. (**a**) Illustration of inset of the gracilis muscle to lateral clavicle and extended to the finger and thumb flexors (with permission of the Mayo Foundation, Copyright 2010). (**b**) The triceps is typically innervated by the spinal accessory nerve (SPA), the gracilis with two intercostal nerves, and the biceps with two intercostal nerves, and sensation is restored with transfer of sensory intercostal nerves to the lateral cord contribution to the median nerve. (With permission of the Mayo Foundation, Copyright 2010)

Common Presentations and Our Strategies

A variety of strategies are available depending on the goals of the patient and the experience and preferences of the surgeon/surgical team. Listed below are general strategies for our patients. It is imperative to understand that a donor unit or structure can typically only be used for one purpose (e.g., a lower trapezius tendon transfer cannot be performed if the spinal accessory nerve has been previously utilized as a nerve donor). Additionally, each patient is unique and their available nerve resources, general medical condition, concomitant injuries, and goals. These factors should be carefully considered when choosing a reconstructive strategy (Tables 32.1 and 32.2).

Pan-plexus: C5 Available

No Vascular Injury The C5 root is grafted to suprascapular and posterior division of the upper trunk (axillary nerve) to restore shoulder function. A free functioning muscle transfer

Table 32.1 Our algorithm for Pan Brachial Plexus reconstruction when viable roots are available

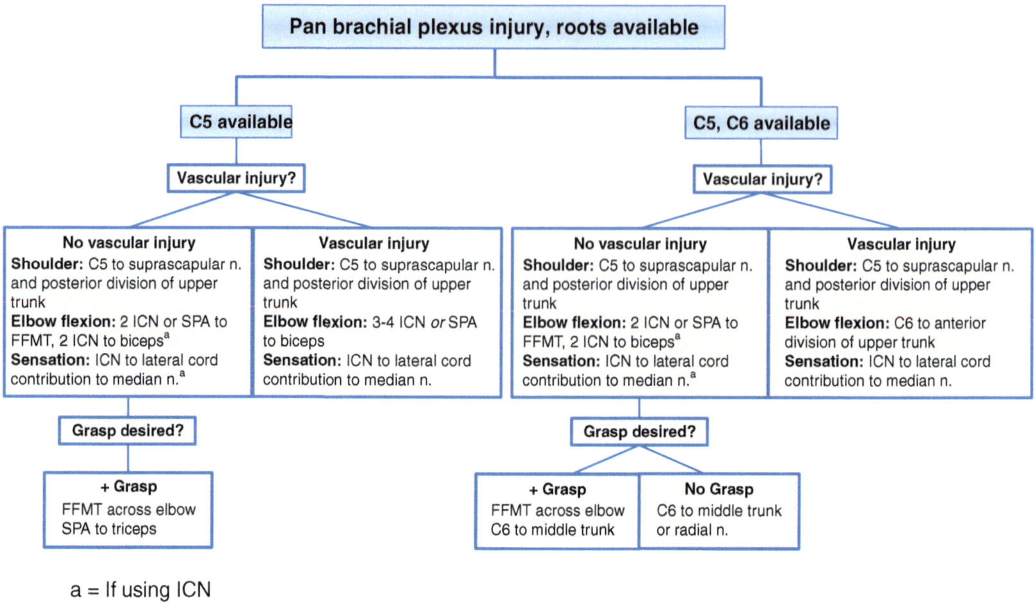

Table 32.2 Our algorithm for Pan Brachial Plexus reconstruction with there are no available roots

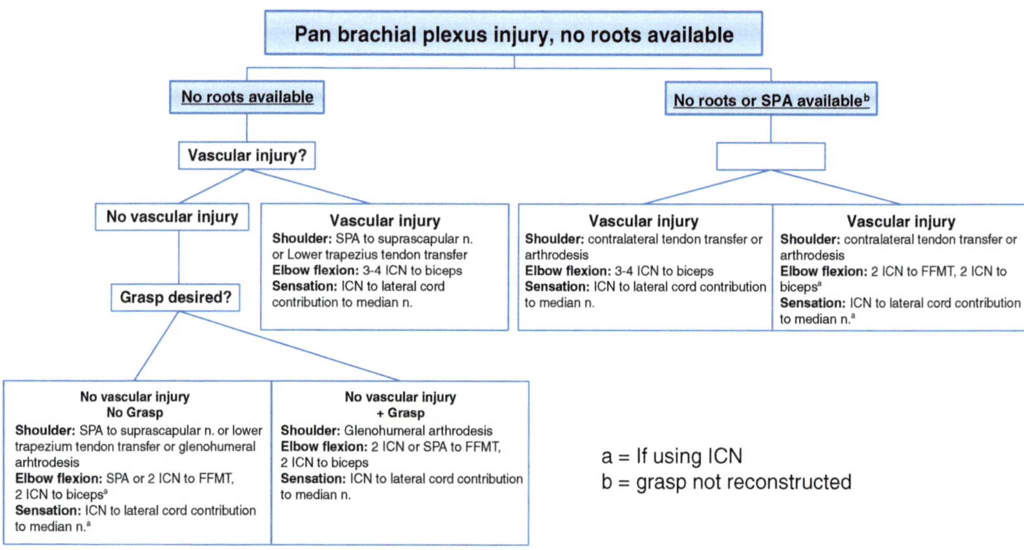

innervated by two intercostal nerves is performed for elbow flexion which is augmented with two intercostal nerves transferred to the biceps motor branch. The free functioning muscle may be inset across the elbow to simultaneously power rudimentary grasp if desired. If the FFMT is utilized for grasp, the spinal accessory nerve is grafted to the triceps to act as an agonist [14] . Otherwise, the SPA may be used to power the FFMT or saved for potential lower trapezius tendon transfer at a later time. Intercostal sensory nerves can be transferred to the lateral cord contribution of the median nerve for protective sensation.

With Vascular Injury If a vascular injury is present, FFMT is not performed. The C5 root is grafted to suprascapular and/or axillary nerve to restore shoulder function. Three to four intercostal nerves are transferred to the biceps motor branch, or the spinal accessory nerve can be grafted to the biceps motor branch with a sural nerve intervening graft. Consideration can be given triceps reinnervation. Sensory reconstruction with sensory intercostals can be performed if intercostals are used.

Pan-plexus: C5 and C6 Available

This is a very rare situation and the limiting factor is the availability of donor autograft nerve. Bilateral sural nerves are used in addition to the ipsilateral superficial branch of the radial nerve. Many permutations of grafting exist, and a few options are described below.

No Vascular Injury The C5 root is grafted to suprascapular and posterior division of the upper trunk (axillary nerve) to restore shoulder function. As above, an FFMT is performed for elbow flexion and innervated by intercostal nerves or SPA. If the FFMT is used to provide grasp, the second viable root is grafted to reinnervate the triceps muscle via grafting to the middle trunk or directly to triceps branches. If the FFMT is performed for elbow flexion only, the second root is grafted to the middle trunk or radial nerve. Alternatively, in all nerve reconstruction with C5 to the shoulder and C6 to the anterior division of the upper trunk (elbow flexion), use of ICN for triceps can be considered, saving SPA for future use with a FFMT in case the reconstruction failed to restore elbow flexion.

With Vascular Injury If a vascular injury is present, an FFMT is not performed. The C5 root is grafted to the suprascapular and posterior division of the upper trunk (axillary nerve) to restore shoulder function, and the C6 root is grafted to the anterior division of the upper trunk for elbow flexion. The ICN and SPA can be used as previously described. In this situation, there is no future FFMT.

Pan-plexus: No Roots

No Vascular Injury If no viable roots are available for grafting, shoulder function is addressed in one of several ways. In cases where the spinal accessory nerve is normal, it is transferred to the suprascapular nerve. Shoulder external rotation may be reestablished by a delayed lower trapezium tendon transfer. In such cases, the SPA is not used in the nerve reconstruction. Finally, a glenohumeral arthrodesis can be performed in the future, allowing use of valuable nerve resources for other functions. If rudimentary grasp is desired, the shoulder is left alone for future arthrodesis, ICN are used to power FFMT for grasp and elbow flexion, and SPA is transferred to a triceps branch. Sensory ICN provide protective sensation as previously described.

With Vascular Injury If a vascular injury is present and therefore no FFMT can be performed, the SPA is grafted to the suprascapular nerve, and intercostal nerves are transferred to the biceps motor branch. Alternatively, the shoulder may be reconstructed with a tendon transfer and ICN transferred to reinnervate the biceps. If the shoulder is to be fused, SPA is available to be used as a nerve donor.

Pan-plexus: No Roots, No SPA

No Vascular Injury An FFMT is performed for elbow flexion and is innervated by intercostal nerves. In this situation, we generally do not reconstruct grasp as there is a lack of options to reinnervate elbow extension. The shoulder is addressed with either a contralateral tendon transfer or fusion.

With Vascular Injury If a vascular injury is present and thus no FFMT can be performed, elbow flexion is reestablished by transferring intercostal nerves to the biceps motor branch, and the shoulder is addressed with a fusion or contralateral tendon transfer.

Author's Preferences

The overall surgical plan is developed with both salvage options and secondary adjustment procedures in mind. Some authors advocate saving a donor nerve and/or vessel for a potential salvage reconstruction with a FFMT should the initial reconstruction fail to give satisfactory results. Prior to proceeding, the implications of saving a donor nerve/vessel for future salvage must be thoroughly discussed with the patient as it may limit the resources available during the initial reconstruction. Secondary procedures are always discussed with patients. The need for future "tune-up" procedures (such as arthrodesis, tendon transfers, or tenodesis) to improve or augment function might be planned at the initial evaluation or need of them determined as function returns.

We begin the operative treatment of any pan-brachial plexus injury with exploration of the plexus. Even if preoperative imaging suggests root avulsions, exploration and evoked potential testing may reveal viable roots suitable for grafting. Occasionally, the somatosensory evoked potential (SSEP) will be absent and motor evoked potential (MEP) may be present. In this case, an intraoperative decision needs to be made regarding whether the root should be used. In these instances with no other viable roots, using the MEP positive but SSEP negative root for shoulder stability is considered. Grafting of this root to the suprascapular nerve and posterior division of the upper trunk (to restore axillary nerve function) with a sural nerve graft is preferred.

Routine primary application of FFMT for improving elbow flexion with the potential for adding finger flexion or wrist extension has been supported by multiple authors [10, 15–17]. Addition of a free functioning gracilis muscle when possible has improved outcomes of elbow flexion in our experience. In patients desiring rudimentary grasp, the use of either a double free functioning muscle or single free functioning muscle is considered. Our preference is use of a single FFMT for grasp as detailed in a previous chapter. When the gracilis crosses the anterior elbow and is used for distal function (finger flexion or wrist/finger extension), it is imperative to reinnervate the triceps to provide antagonist function to obtain the distal function [14].

Our coordinated brachial plexus team allows for up to three separate surgical teams to operate simultaneously. Typically, one team explores the supraclavicular plexus and performs intraoperative nerve testing, a second team performs the infraclavicular plexus exploration (including exploration of donor vessels) and intercostal nerve harvest, and a third team harvests a free functioning gracilis or sural nerves as needed. Each of the team's three core surgeons is capable of this portion of the operation and is interchangeable for all nerve exploration and reconstructive procedures. Two members of the team are microsurgeons and perform the transfer of the FFMT when indicated. All decisions are made as a team. The team approach has allowed us to perform more complex surgical procedures in a shorter period of time, which significantly benefits the patients. Shorter operative time results in less anesthesia, less blood loss, and less cost. When intraoperative complexities or anatomic anomalies are seen, the team works together to navigate the problem, working toward the best outcome for the patient.

Conclusion

Patients with pan-brachial plexus injuries represent one of the most challenging populations for the reconstructive surgeon to treat. A team approach to diagnosis and treatment and good surgeon-patient communication concerning goals and expectations are essential to improving patient outcomes. While many challenges remain in the management of these patients, advances in nerve transfers, microsurgery, and growing understanding of the "nerve economics" practiced in planning reconstruction have improved outcomes for these patients over the last several decades.

References

1. Bertelli JA, Ghizoni MF. Results and current approach for brachial plexus reconstruction. J Brachial Plex Peripher Nerve Inj. 2011; https://doi.org/10.1186/1749-7221-6-2.
2. Cardoso MDM, Gepp RDA, Mamare E, Guedes-Correa JF. Results of phrenic nerve transfer to the musculocutaneous nerve using video-assisted thoracoscopy in patients with traumatic brachial plexus injury: series of 28 cases. Oper Neurosurg. 2019; https://doi.org/10.1093/ons/opy350.
3. Siqueira MG, Martins RS. Phrenic nerve transfer in the restoration of elbow flexion in brachial plexus avulsion injuries: how effective and safe is it? Neurosurgery. 2009; https://doi.org/10.1227/01.NEU.0000338865.19411.7F.
4. Hems T. Nerve transfers for traumatic brachial plexus injury: advantages and problems. J Hand Microsurg. 2016; https://doi.org/10.1007/s12593-011-0031-1.
5. Bertelli JA, Ghizoni MF. Combined injury of the accessory nerve and brachial plexus. Neurosurgery. 2011; https://doi.org/10.1227/NEU.0b013e318201d7d9.
6. Kovachevich R, Kircher MF, Wood CM, Spinner RJ, Bishop AT, Shin AY. Complications of intercostal nerve transfer for brachial plexus reconstruction. J Hand Surg Am. 2010; https://doi.org/10.1016/j.jhsa.2010.09.013.
7. Vu AT, Sparkman DM, van Belle CJ, Yakuboff KP, Schwentker AR. Retropharyngeal contralateral C7 nerve transfer to the lower trunk for brachial plexus birth injury: technique and results. J Hand Surg Am 2018. doi:https://doi.org/10.1016/j.jhsa.2017.12.001.
8. Sammer DM, Kircher MF, Bishop AT, Spinner RJ, Shin AY. Hemi-contralateral C7 transfer to the median nerve: outcomes and complications. J Hand Surg Am. 2009; https://doi.org/10.1016/s0363-5023(09)60109-x.
9. Doi K, Muramatsu K, Hattori Y, et al. Restoration of prehension with the double free muscle technique following complete avulsion of the brachial plexus. Indications and long-term results. J Bone Jt Surg – Ser A. 2000; https://doi.org/10.2106/00004623-200005000-00006.
10. Doi K, Hattori Y, Sakamoto S, Dodakundi C, Satbhai NG, Montales T. Current procedure of double free muscle transfer for traumatic total brachial plexus palsy. JBJS Essent Surg Tech. 2013; https://doi.org/10.2106/jbjs.st.m.00010.
11. Elhassan B, Bishop AT, Hartzler RU, Shin AY, Spinner RJ. Tendon transfer options about the shoulder in patients with brachial plexus injury. J Bone Jt Surg – Ser A. 2012; https://doi.org/10.2106/JBJS.J.01913.
12. Elhassan BT, Wagner ER, Spinner RJ, Bishop AT, Shin AY. Contralateral trapezius transfer to restore shoulder external rotation following adult brachial plexus injury. J Hand Surg Am. 2016; https://doi.org/10.1016/j.jhsa.2015.12.026.
13. Giuffre JL, Bishop AT, Spinner RJ, Kircher MF, Shin AY. Wrist, first carpometacarpal joint, and thumb interphalangeal joint arthrodesis in patients with brachial plexus injuries. J Hand Surg Am. 2012; https://doi.org/10.1016/j.jhsa.2012.09.017.
14. Doi K, Shigetomi M, Kaneko K, et al. Significance of elbow extension in reconstruction of prehension with reinnervated free-muscle transfer following complete brachial plexus avulsion. Plast Reconstr Surg. 1997; https://doi.org/10.1097/00006534-199708000-00013.
15. Doi K. New reconstructive procedure for brachial plexus injury. Clin Plast Surg. 1997;
16. Giuffre JL, Bishop AT, Shin AY. Harvest of an entire gracilis muscle and tendon for use in functional muscle transfer: a novel technique. J Reconstr Microsurg. 2012; https://doi.org/10.1055/s-0032-1313767.
17. Maldonado AA, Kircher MF, Spinner RJ, Bishop AT, Shin AY. Free functioning Gracilis muscle transfer with and without simultaneous intercostal nerve transfer to musculocutaneous nerve for restoration of elbow flexion after traumatic adult brachial pan-plexus injury. J Hand Surg Am. 2017; https://doi.org/10.1016/j.jhsa.2017.01.014.

Lower-Type Injuries of the Brachial Plexus (C6–T1, C7–T1, and C8–T1 Root Involvement)

33

Jayme Augusto Bertelli, Neehar Patel, and Francisco Soldado

Lower-type injuries are the rarest of lesions of the brachial plexus. In our own series, it corresponded to 3% of all cases. Others reported rates between 4% and 8% of all cases of brachial plexus traumatic injuries [1–3]. Differently from complete or upper type lesions, the most common mechanism of injury is a car accident, possibly related to forceful anterior shoulder compression by the seat belt. Forced arm suspended after falling into a hole and obese patients who fall and hit the ground with the shoulder completely abducted are other potential causes of lower-type injuries [4] (Fig. 33.1).

The major deficits in lower-type injuries of the brachial plexus are related to hand function. In all patients, shoulder motion and elbow flexion are normal as well as wrist flexion and extension and forearm prono-supination. A few cases of lower-type root injury are initially a complete paralysis in which the upper roots recovered spontaneously.

We have recognized three patterns of paralysis based on root involvement:

- C8–T1 root injury (30% of the cases): Finger flexion is the major deficit here. Despite some preserved motion, finger flexion is very weak and needs reconstruction.
- C7–T1 root injury (60% of the cases): Finger flexion-extension and intrinsic muscle of the hand are all paralyzed (Fig. 33.2).
- C6–T1 root injury (10% of the cases): C6 root might be partially involved, and along with finger flexion-extension and intrinsic muscle paralysis, elbow extension is lost and needs reconstruction.

Sensory abnormalities are related to the ulnar side of the arm, forearm, and hand (Fig. 33.3). Contrary to upper-type lesions with preserved hand radial side sensation due to overlapping of upper and lower roots dermatomes, in lower-type injuries of the brachial plexus, there is a complete anesthesia on ulnar side of the hand because upper roots do not overlap in the ulnar nerve territory [5]. Despite the common avulsion of the lower roots, hand pain is not a predominant complaint as compared to complete root lesions [5]. Patients who complain about pain are those in

J. A. Bertelli (✉)
Center of Biological and Health Sciences, Department of Neurosurgery, University of the South of Santa Catarina (Unisul), Tubarão, SC, Brazil

Department of Orthopedic Surgery, Governador Celso Ramos Hospital, Florianópolis, SC, Brazil

N. Patel
Bombay Hospital Institute of Medical Sciences, New Marine Lines, Mumbai, Maharashtra, India

F. Soldado
Pediatric Hand Surgery and Microsurgery Unit, Barcelona University Children's Hospital HM Nens, HM Hospitales, Barcelona, Spain

Pediatric Hand Surgeryand Microsurgery Unit, Vall d'Hebron Barcelona Hospital Campus, Barcelona, Spain

A. Y. Shin, N. Pulos (eds.), *Operative Brachial Plexus Surgery*,
https://doi.org/10.1007/978-3-030-69517-0_33

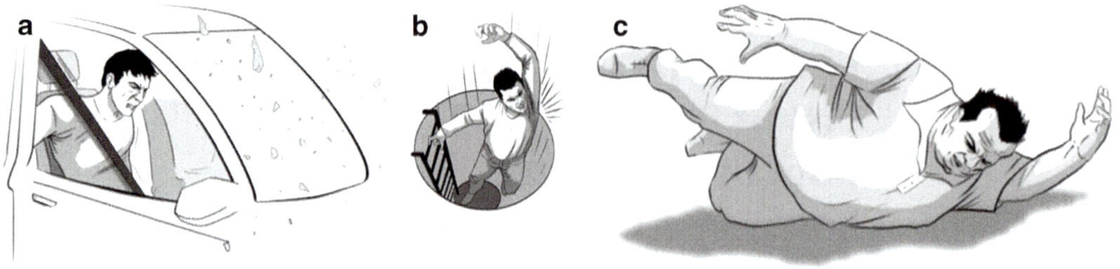

Fig. 33.1 Mechanisms of lower type brachial plexus root injury. In (**a**), the most common mechanism of injury. Car accident and seatbelt injury. In (**b**), a fall with the armout-strecthed. In (**c**), 0bese patients with a fall from their own heigth with the arm outstreched

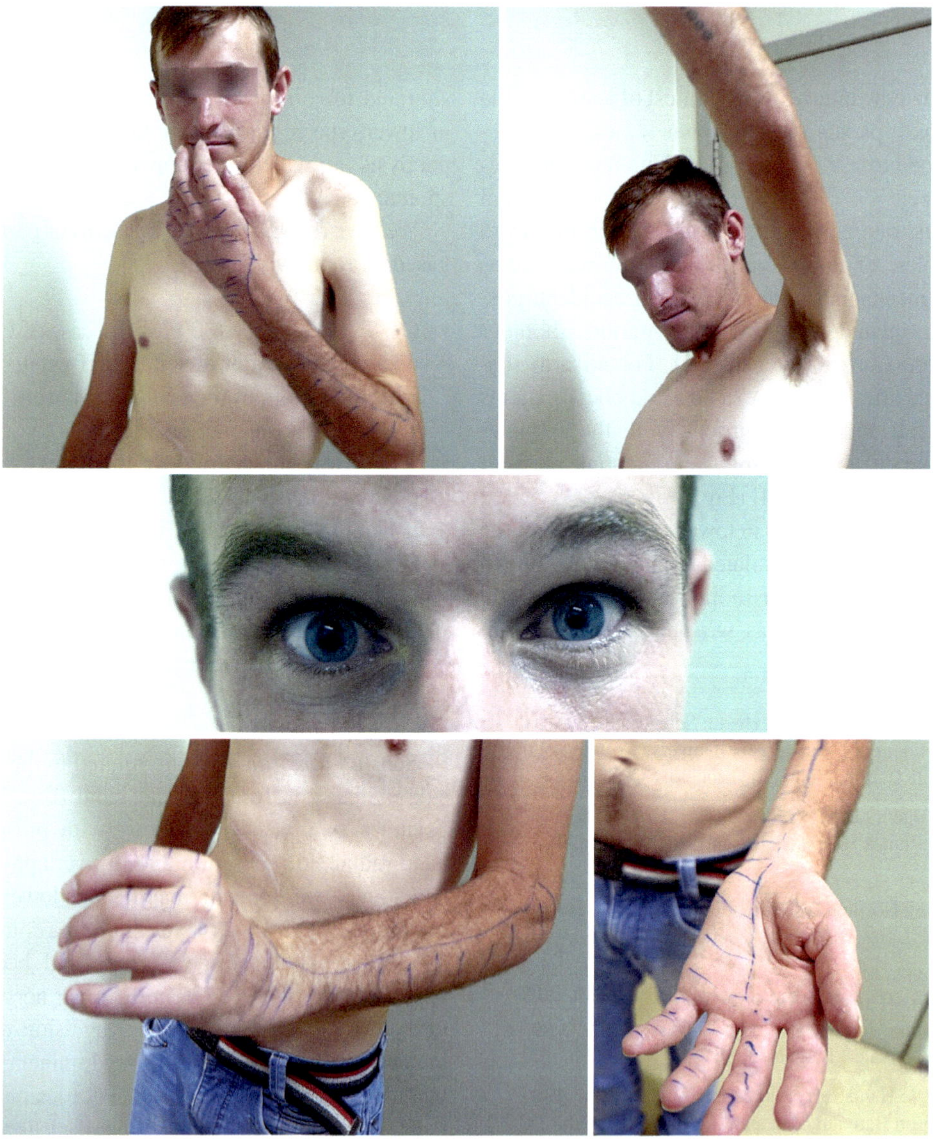

Fig. 33.2 Typical findings in a patient with C7–T1 root injury. Preserved shoulder, elbow, and wrist motion while finger motion is paralyzed. This injury is associated with avulsion injury, which is reflected by the Horner sign. Note miosis on the left eye

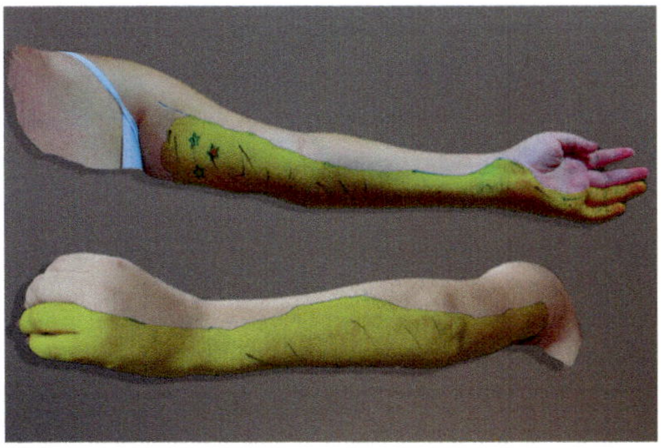

Fig. 33.3 Typical zone of anesthesia (yellow overlay) in a C7–T1 root avulsion

whom initially the paralysis was complete, but the upper roots recovered fortuitously.

Diagnosis

Diagnosis of lower-type brachial plexus injury is evident on clinical examination. Because the lower roots are often avulsed, Horner's sign is a prominent finding. Horner's sign can predict lower root avulsion in 94% of the cases [6]. MRI or CT myelogram is recommended to demonstrate lower roots avulsion and to propose immediate treatment since spontaneous recovery would be unexpected [7–9]. In the absence of a Horner's sign and normal imaging studies, hand paralysis might be related to an infraclavicular lesion of the brachial plexus. At our department, for all types of brachial plexus paralysis, we do not rely on electrophysiological studies for our surgical planning.

Treatment

Motor reconstruction

Acute and subacute cases

This encompasses patients seen within 1 year of their accident. There is no rationale in exploring the lower roots because surgery would be very demanding and risky; the roots are generally avulsed, and even in the cases of rupture, grafting will be unsuccessful secondary to the long distance that the axons need to regenerate to reach forearm muscles. In this group of patients, we advocate early nerve transfer according to the function needed to be restored. The current guidelines we use are those also employed in the treatment of tetraplegia with intact C6 level because of the similarity of the clinical deficits [10, 11].

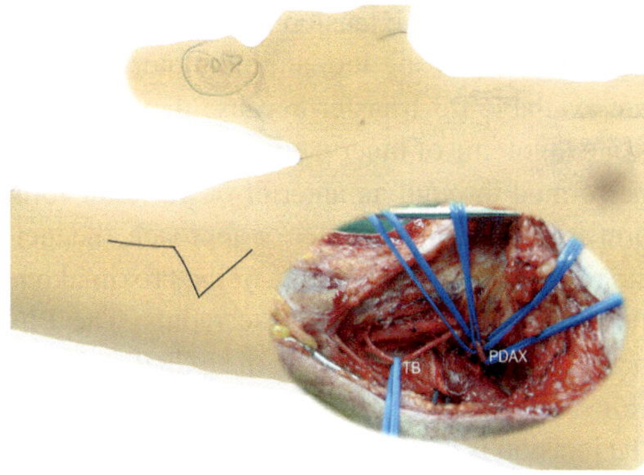

Fig. 33.4 Schematic representation of the axillary approach for transferring the posterior division of the axillary nerve (PDAX) to triceps motor branches (TB)

Elbow Extension

If elbow extension needs reconstruction, we propose transferring the posterior division of the axillary nerve to the triceps motor branches [12]. The axillary approach (Fig. 33.4) is our preference [13], although this nerve transfer has been reported through the posterior arm approach as well [14]. M4 elbow extension is normally obtained. Alternatively, the branch to the brachialis can be used to reinnervate the triceps long and medial heads [15, 16].

Thumb and Finger Extension

For the reconstruction of finger extension, we rely on the transfer of the supinator motor branches to the posterior interosseous nerve

(PIN) [5]. If wrist extension is strong, the supinator muscle is strong too, and its motor branches are available for transfer because they share the same myotome of innervation [5]. Surgery can be performed through an anterior or posterior forearm approach. In the posterior approach, the incision is in the posterior aspect of the proximal one third of the forearm, over the radius. The PIN nerve is approached between the ECRB and EDC (Figs. 33.5 and 33.6). In the anterior approach, the incision is on the antecubital fossa and is preferred when a nerve transfer is concomitantly planned for finger flexion reconstruction (Fig. 33.6). Two motor branches innervate the supinator muscle flanking the PIN proximally to the arcade of Frohse. The lateral one is bigger and innervates the superficial head, whereas the medial branch is smaller and innervates the deep head. On some occasions, a single branch is identified in general on the lateral side of the PIN, which divides to innervate the superficial and deep heads of the supinator muscle (Figs. 33.7 and 33.8). The average number of myelinated fibers in the supinator branches is 550 whereas that in the PIN is 750 [17]. Despite fewer fibers in the donor than in the recipient nerve, the results of this nerve transfer are being reported to be predictable and good [7, 10, 18, 19]. This probably relates not only to the fact that strength is not needed for thumb and finger extension but also because wrist flexion, by the tenodesis effect, can boost range of motion. Patients just need to position the fingers and thumb for grasping. An interesting point on this technique is that it also addresses the issue of stability of the CMC joint, thus avoiding the need to do a CMC joint arthrodesis. In addition, reinnervation of the extensor carpi ulnaris entails rebalancing of wrist radial deviation. In our experience, motion control is quickly learned, but there is no independent control of thumb and finger extension.

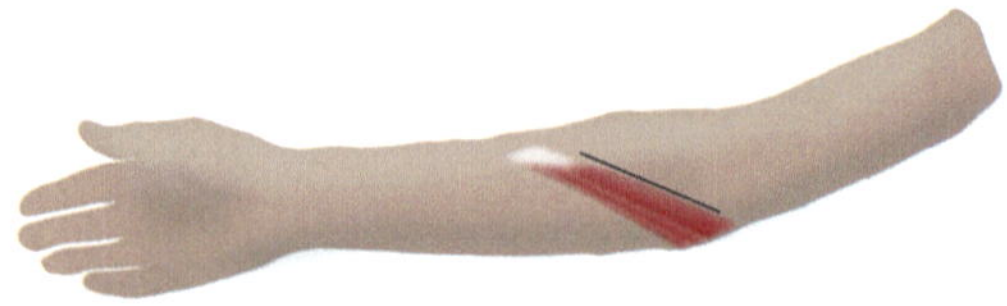

Fig. 33.5 Design of the surgical incision for transferring the branches of the supinator muscle to the posterior interosseous nerve via a posterior forearm approach

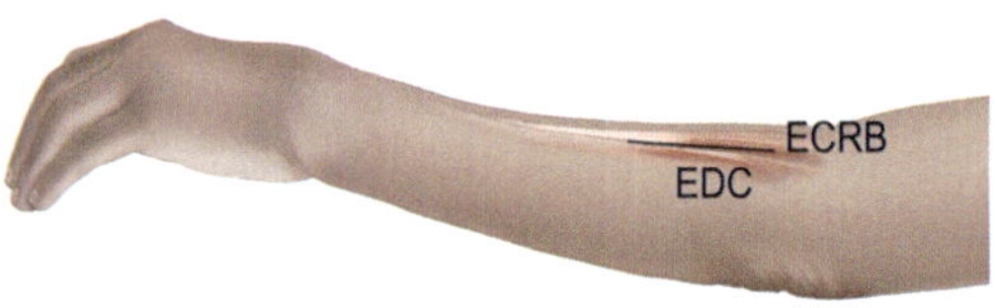

Fig. 33.6 Cadaveric dissection of the posterior aspect of the right forearm depicting the posterior interosseous nerve (PIN) and its branches to the supinator muscle (NS), to the extensor carpi ulnaris (ECU) and extensor digiti quinti (EDQ), and its terminal division into a deep (DBPIN) and a superficial branch (SPIN). The DBPIN innervates thumb muscles, whereas the SPIN innervates the extensor digitorum communis. The superficial head of the supinator muscle has been divided to expose the PIN. Surgery consists of dividing the branches to the supinator at the muscle entrance and dividing the PIN just distal to the emergence of the branches to the supinator in order to get an extra nerve length on the donor and recipient nerves to avoid tension. Then the nerves to supinator are sutured to the PIN

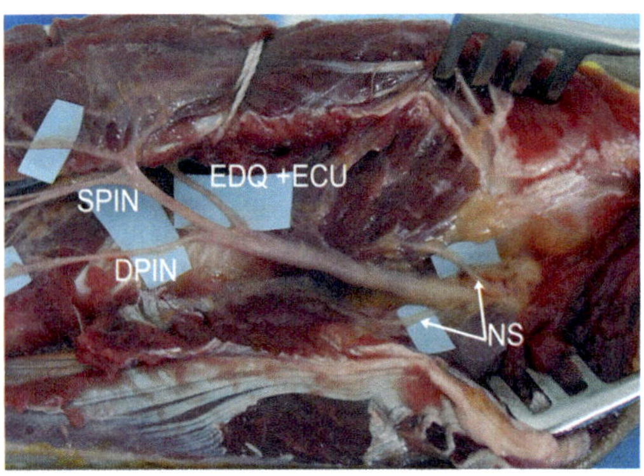

Fig. 33.7 Design of the surgical incision for transferring the branches to the supinator muscle to the posterior interosseous nerve via an anterior forearm approach. Through the same incision, other nerve transfers are performed to reconstruct thumb and finger flexion. The incision design borders the proximal margin of the pronator teres

Finger Flexion

Finger flexion is attained by the reconstruction of the anterior interosseous nerve (AIN). AIN reinnervation also addresses flexion of the ulnar fingers because of nerve interconnections within the flexor digitorum profundus (FDP) and/or because of a drag effect on FDP tendons [20]. Either the motor branch of the extensor carpi radialis brevis

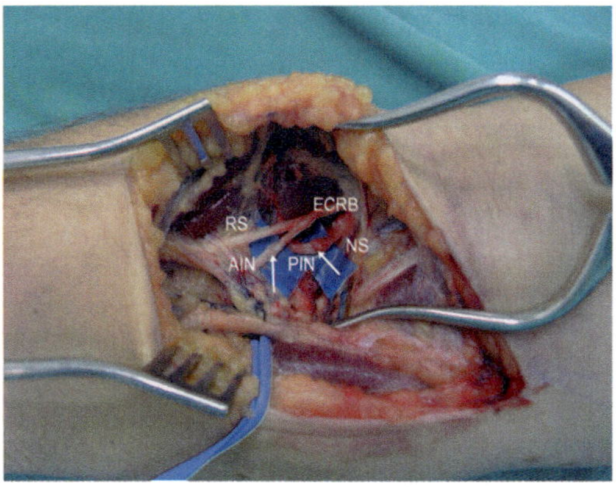

Fig. 33.8 Intraoperative view of the transfer of nerves to supinator (NS) to the posterior interosseous nerve (PIN) and the extensor carpi radialis brevis motor branch (ECRB) to the anterior interosseous nerve (AIN). (RS) radial superficial nerve. Arrows indicate the site of nerve coaptation

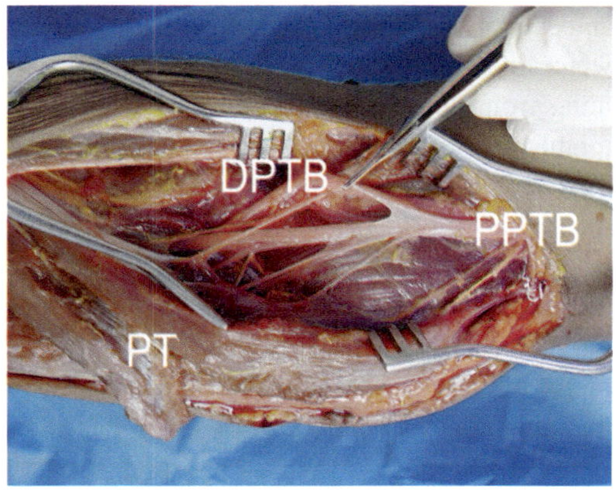

Fig. 33.10 Cadaveric dissection of the right antecubital fossa depicting the motor branches of the pronator teres (PT). The forceps holds the distal pronator teres motor branch (DPTB). Proximal pronator teres motor branch (PPTB)

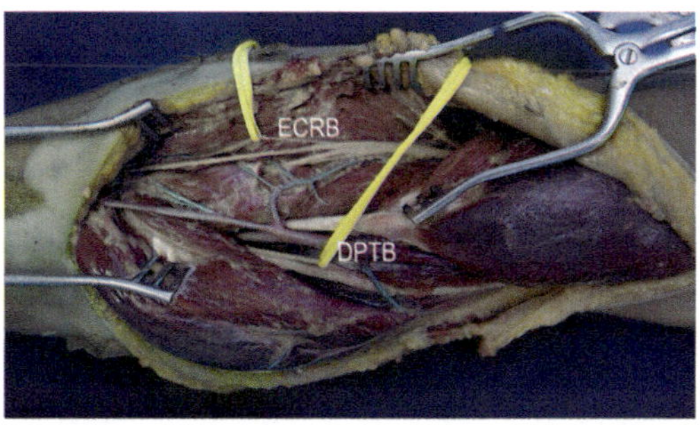

Fig. 33.9 Cadaveric dissection of the right antecubital fossa depicting the extensor carpi radialis brevis motor branch (ECRB) and the distal branch of the pronator teres (DPTB)

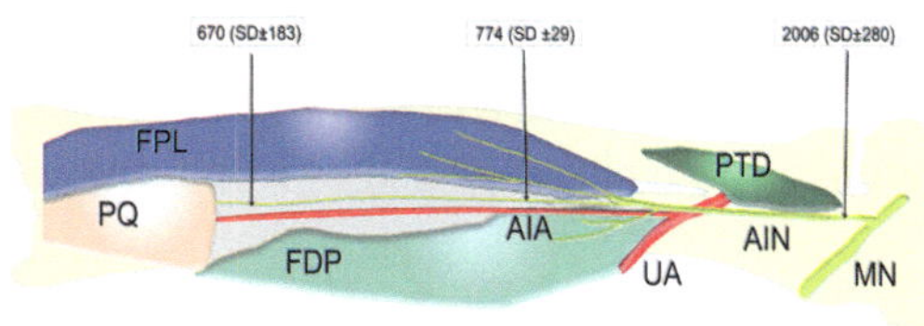

Fig. 33.11 Schematic representation of the anterior interosseous nerve (AIN) and number of myelinated fibers at different levels. (FPL) Flexor pollicis longus, (PQ) pronator quadratus, (FDP) flexor digitorum profundus, (AIA) anterior interosseous artery, (UA) ulnar artery, (PTD) pronator teres deep branch, and (MN) median nerve

(ECRB) or one branch of the pronator teres (PT) can be coapted to the AIN (Fig. 33.9). The PT has two motor branches: (a) a proximal one (PPTB), which arises from the anterior aspect of the median nerve at the level of the medial epicondyle and innervates the superficial head of the PT, and (b) a distal one (DPTB which is longer), which originates on the anterior aspect of the median nerve, travels on the top of the median nerve (along its course), and innervates predominantly the deep head of the PT. (Fig. 33.10). The AIN has in average 2000 fibers but approximately only 1300 fibers but approximately only 1300 fibers are devoted to finger and thumb flexion (Fig. 33.11). The remainder of the fibers is destined to innervate the pronator quadratus [21]. The ECRB motor branch has in average 457 nerve fibers, whereas the proximal and the distal PT motor branch have an average of 646 and 563 nerve fibers, respectively [22]. Because the number of motor fibers in recipient and donor nerves does not match, endurance and strength recovery tend to be suboptimal. In general, grasping strength recovery is around 5 kg, whereas pinch strength is 2 kg. However, functional reconstruction is largely predictable and easy to reeducate [8, 19]. Transfer of one of the PT motor branches was able to restore finger flexion in three among four patients [23, 24]. Using either the ECRB or the distal PT, which has our preference because it is longer than the proximal PT motor branch, surgery is performed with an anterior incision on the antecubital fossa. Special care should be taken when dividing the AIN. A motor branch stemming from the AIN proximal to the PT muscle might innervate the flexor carpi radialis (FCR). This motor branch must be preserved either by internal neurolysis of by sectioning the AIN distal to it. In lower-type injuries of the brachial plexus, the FCR is the only wrist flexor functioning. Our preference now is to connect the ECRB motor branch with the AIN and the DPTB with the main branch of the FDS. By using this strategy, we can not only increase grasping strength but also ensure reinnervation of the FDS that could be used to treat clawing, if needed (Figs. 33.12 and 33.13).

To establish independent control of radial and ulnar fingers, we have transferred the motor branch of the brachialis to the ulnar nerve. This technique was not reliable because of difficulties in motion control and long interval of at least 3 years to start motion relying on the nerve to brachialis. In those cases, resisted elbow flexion was a facilitator

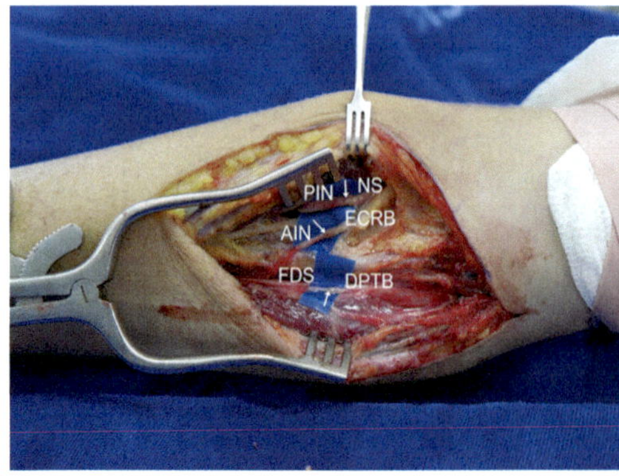

Fig. 33.12 Intraoperative view of the right antecubital fossa depicting our current approach to reconstruct thumb and finger motion in a lower-type injury of the brachial plexus. The incision used follows the guideline on Fig. 33.7. Nerves to supinator (NS) are transferred to the posterior interosseous nerve (PIN) for thumb and finger extension reconstruction. For thumb and finger flexion reconstruction, the extensor carpi radialis brevis motor branch (ECRB) is transferred to the anterior interosseous nerve (AIN), while the distal pronator teres motor branch (DPTB) is transferred to a branch of the flexor digitorum superficialis (FDS). Pronation is preserved because the proximal branch of the pronator teres is retained

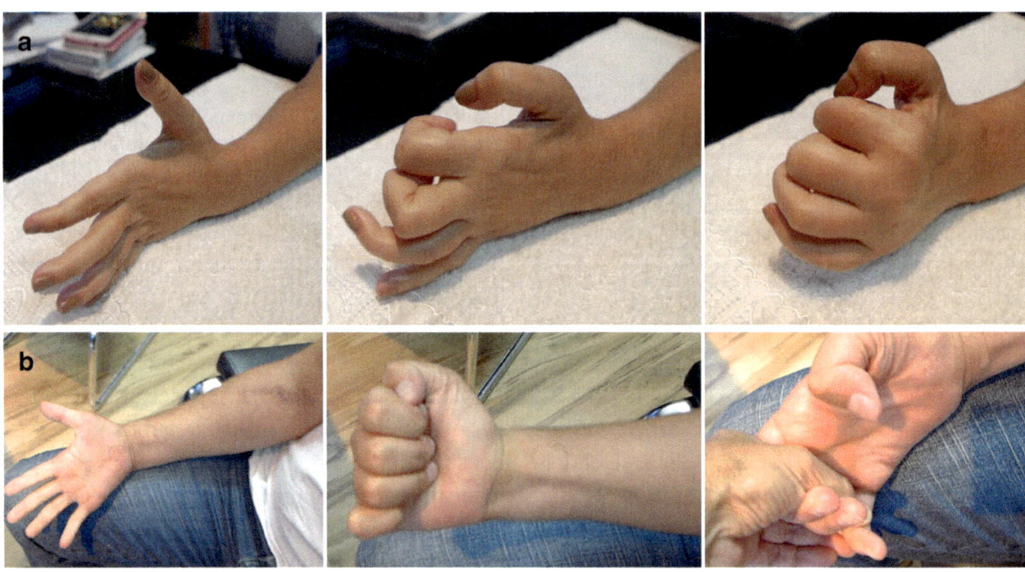

Fig. 33.13 Postoperative view of the hand of two different patients 36 months after surgery. In Case **a**, we transferred the extensor carpi radialis motor branch to the anterior interosseous nerve and the nerve to supinator to the posterior interosseous nerve. In Case **b**, in addition to the nerve transfers performed in Case **a**, we transferred the distal pronator motor branch to a FDS branch. Full finger flexion-extension was obtained in both patients. However, in Case **a**, there was a predominant flexion of the thumb and radial fingers, while this was less evident in Case **b**. In both patients, when resisting finger flexion, the flexor pollicis longus contracted as well. This can be observed in the image on the right side at the bottom. Note that despite no intrinsic muscle reconstruction, proximal interphalangeal joint extension was almost complete

movement for finger motion [12]. Alternative donor nerves for transfer to the AIN are the nerve to brachialis [25] and nerve to brachioradialis [26]. We do not advocate those nerve transfers because our results were not encouraging when we employed either one or the other [11].

Intrinsic Muscle Reconstruction

Not all patients need intrinsic muscle reconstruction related to the inability to fully extend the PIP joint, but when needed, surgery is a great challenge. We have unsuccessfully tried the transfer of the ECRB tendon prolonged with tendon grafts to the lateral band of the extensor tendons as reported elsewhere and have abandoned this technique [27, 28]. We have removed a ellipse on the distal palmar crease and sutured the A1 pulley to the proximal dermis. Although this maneuver prevented MP hyperextension, it did not keep the MP flexed, consequently not improving PIP extension dramatically. We have tried to centralize the lateral bands of the extensor tendon by releasing the sagittal bands from the volar plate at the PIP joint and suturing them over the extensor tendons without much benefit. The only cases in which we observed improvement was when the FDS was functional and one slip was transferred dorsally to the central band of the extensor tendon at the PIP joint. We observed improvement of PIP extension but with some limitation of PIP flexion. Difficulties in correcting PIP extension lag are related to (a) suboptimal strength of the EDC after reinnervation, (b) central band elongation, and (c) in most cases the lack of the FDS to use as a donor for tendon transfer. This is the reason why we now advocate reinnervation of the FDS by a nerve transfer using the distal PT motor branch as donor.

Chronic Cases

Elbow Extension

In long-standing lesions, more than 2 years, elbow extension should be reconstructed by muscle transfer similar to those used for the treatment of tetraplegia. However, if biceps to triceps tendon transfer is chosen and if the nerve to the supinator is to be used for reconstruction of thumb and finger extension, supination will be lost. Posterior deltoid is an alternative, but results are less encouraging [29]. More recently, the use of the lower trapezius was described as a method for elbow extension reconstruction [30–32].

Thumb and Finger Extension

In lower-type injuries, the only preserved wrist flexor is the FCR, and it should be preserved. In our hands, when we transferred the ECRL or the brachioradialis to the extensor tendons, results were not impressive. Finger flexors are paralyzed, and very few alternatives remain available. Tenodesis of the EDC to the dorsal side of the radius or to the FDS through the interosseous membrane can improve hand span; however, the wrist should be at least in 30 of flexion [33]. Because of this drawback, some surgeons propose no reconstruction for thumb and finger extension if the only option is tenodeses [34]. In this situation of complete lack of donor tendons for transfer, we suggest a free gracilis muscle transfer reinnervated by the nerve to supinator [35]. We advocate attaching the gracilis muscle a little bit tight to take advantage of the tenodesis effect of wrist flexion.

Finger and Thumb Flexion

In patients with injuries between 1 and 2 years, if young, we still consider nerve transfers for finger flexion and extension reconstruction. However, in this situation, the donor nerve imperatively is one branch of the PT, because the radial wrist extensors should be preserved for use for tendon transfer for finger flexion reconstruction in case of nerve transfer failure.

In long-standing paralysis, either ECRB or ECRL tendon is useful for finger flexion reconstruction. It seems that strength provided by these tendon transfers are higher than with nerve transfer [33]. We observed, however, that tendon

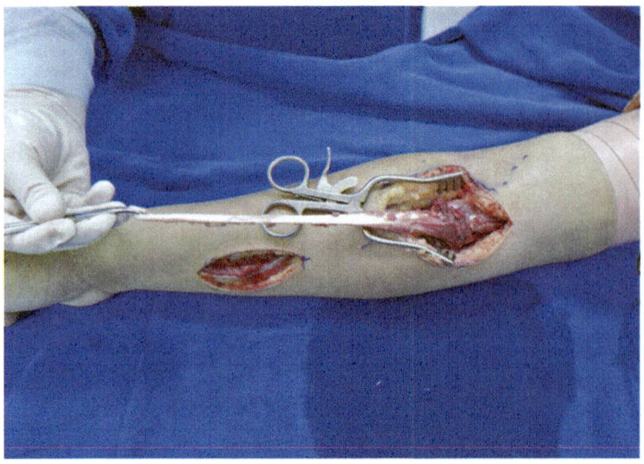

Fig. 33.14 Intraoperative view of transferring the brachialis muscle prolonged with a tendon graft, which will reach the distal forearm by tunneling between the flexor digitorum superficialis and flexor digitorum profundus (FDP) to be sutured to the FDP and flexor pollicis longus. Because graft and tendons can be attached with strong sutures, there is no need for postoperative casting. Motion can be started promptly

transfer augmented the deficit of PIP extension. Another alternative is the transfer of the brachialis muscle prolonged with a tendon graft to the FDP and FPL (Figs. 33.13 and 33.14). Recovery of ROM for finger flexion may not be complete, but it is useful and strong. Finger flexion strength, however, depends on elbow position [36–38].

Ancillary Procedures

In some patients with tendon transfer procedures for finger flexion reconstruction, stabilization of the thumb IP joint in extension is important on two grounds: (a) to prevent nail to nail pinch with the index finger and (b) to prevent the flexed thumb from missing the index finger platform. To achieve this, we transfer one half of the FPL to the EPL at the proximal phalanx of the thumb as proposed elsewhere [39]. In some patients with C8–T1 root injury, extensor tendons are not paralyzed, and if the ECU is working, it can be transposed for thumb opposition. Concomitantly, the ECRB can be prolonged with a tendon graft passed between the first and second metacarpals and attached to the medial side of the thumb MP to mimic the adductor pollicis function. The intention of this transfer is not only to increase pinch strength but also to increase thumb adduction ROM, which allows thumb motion towards the ulnar fingers.

Sensory Reconstruction

Pain and Touch

Sensory reconstruction should address the ulnar side of the hand. Two recipient nerves should be considered: (a) dorsal branch of the ulnar nerve and (b) the proper palmar ulnar digital nerve (PPUDN) of the little finger. In the case of reinnervation of the DBUN, the donor nerve is the palmar cutaneous branch of the median nerve. Protective sensibility is restored on the dorsoulnar side of the hand but not on the ulnar side of the little finger. When the recipient nerve is the PPUDN of the little finger, the donor nerves are the cutaneous branches that innervate the skin just distal to the thenar eminence. To consider these nerves as donors, preoperatively we must check to ensure that sensations in this zone are preserved. Expected results are much less than normal. Usually patients recover light touch and pain perception. Two-point discrimination is not restored. We reinforce, however, that the goal of surgery is to reconstruct protective sensibility [40]. When patients request, also sensibility on the ulnar side of the forearm can be reconstructed by transferring the lateral antebrachial cutaneous nerve to the ulnar nerve or to the medial antebrachial cutaneous nerve [41].

A very interesting point about nerve transfer in lower-type injuries of the brachial plexus is that sensibility can be restored even in long-standing paralysis, years after accident. The reason for this is that lower-type paralysis is associated with root avulsion, i.e., pre-ganglionic lesion. Because in the sensory system the sensory neurons are located in the DRG, there is no degeneration in the peripheral nerve (Fig. 33.15). Consequently, somatosensory potentials can be recorded in the ulnar nerve in a paretic and anesthetized limb [42]. In a single case, even after 14 years of trauma, we have successfully restored sensibility on the ulnar side of the forearm and wrist by transferring the lateral antebrachial cutaneous nerve to the ulnar nerve.

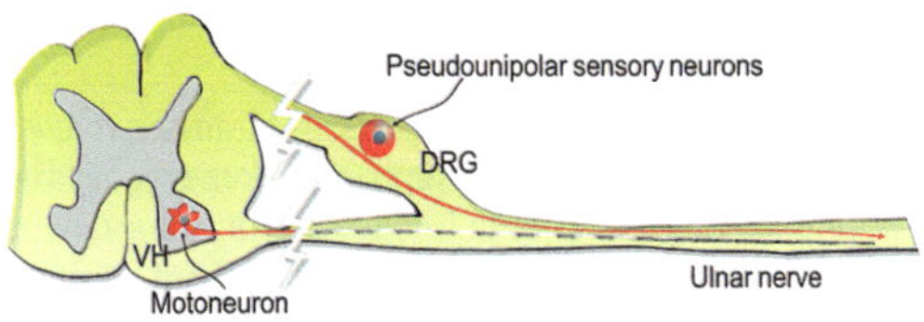

Fig. 33.15 Schematic representation of a transverse section of the spinal cord depicting an avulsion injury. Note that sensory axons do not degenerate in contrast to motoneurons. The location of sensory neurons, distal to the site of lesion, at the dorsal root ganglion (DRG), maintain viable axons in the peripheral nerves

References

1. Millesi H. Brachial plexus injuries. Management and results. Clin Plast Surg. 1984;11(1):115–20.
2. Kim DH, Cho YJ, Tiel RL, Kline DG. Outcomes of surgery in 1019 brachial plexus lesions treated at Louisiana State University Health Sciences Center. J Neurosurg. 2003;98(5):1005–16.
3. Dubuisson AS, Kline DG. Brachial plexus injury: a survey of 100 consecutive cases from a single service. Neurosurgery. 2002;51(3):673–82; discussion 682–673
4. Soldado F, Ghizoni MF, Bertelli J. Injury mechanisms in supraclavicular stretch injuries of the brachial plexus. Hand Surg Rehabil. 2016;35(1):51–4.
5. Bertelli JA. Upper and lower trapezius muscle transfer to restore shoulder abduction and external rotation in longstanding upper type palsies of the brachial plexus in adults. Microsurgery. 2011;31(4):263–7.
6. Bertelli JA. Brachialis muscle transfer to the forearm muscles in obstetric brachial plexus palsy. J Hand Surg Br. 2006;31(3):261–5.
7. Walker AT, Chaloupka JC, de Lotbiniere AC, Wolfe SW, Goldman R, Kier EL. Detection of nerve rootlet avulsion on CT myelography in patients with birth palsy and brachial plexus injury after trauma. AJR Am J Roentgenol. 1996;167(5):1283–7.
8. Yamazaki H, Doi K, Hattori Y, Sakamoto S. Computerized tomography myelography with coronal and oblique coronal view for diagnosis of nerve root avulsion in brachial plexus injury. J Brachial Plex Peripher Nerve Inj. 2007;2:16.
9. Echalier C, Teboul F, Dubois E, Chevrier B, Soumagne T, Goubier JN. The value of preoperative examination and MRI for the diagnosis of graftable roots in total brachial plexus palsy. Hand Surg Rehabil. 2019;38(4):246–50.
10. Bertelli JA, Ghizoni MF. Nerve transfers for elbow and finger extension reconstruction in midcervical spinal cord injuries. J Neurosurg. 2015;122(1):121–7.
11. Bertelli JA, Ghizoni MF. Nerve transfers for restoration of finger flexion in patients with tetraplegia. J Neurosurg Spine. 2017;26(1):55–61.
12. Soldado F, Ghizoni MF, Bertelli J. Reconstruction of a C7-T1 brachial plexus lower root injury by transferring multiple nerves and a free gracilis muscle: Case report. Microsurgery. 2020;40(6):696–9.
13. Bertelli JA, Tacca CP, Winkelmann Duarte EC, Ghizoni MF, Duarte H. Transfer of axillary nerve branches to reconstruct elbow extension in tetraplegics: a laboratory investigation of surgical feasibility. Microsurgery. 2011;31(5):376–81.
14. Klika BJ, Spinner RJ, Bishop AT, Kircher MF, Shin AY. Posterior branch of the axillary nerve transfer to the lateral triceps branch for restoration of elbow extension: case report. J Hand Surg Am. 2013;38(6):1145–9.
15. Bertelli JA, Soldado F, Ghizoni MF, Rodriguez-Baeza A. Transfer of the musculocutaneous nerve branch to the brachialis muscle to the triceps for elbow extension: anatomical study and report of five cases. J Hand Surg Eur Vol. 2017;42(7):710–4.
16. Bertelli JA, Ghizoni MF. Transfer of nerve branch to the brachialis to reconstruct elbow extension in incomplete tetraplegia: case report. J Hand Surg Am. 2012;37(10):1990–3.
17. Bertelli JA, Kechele PR, Santos MA, Besen BA, Duarte H. Anatomical feasibility of transferring supinator motor branches to the posterior interosseous nerve in C7-T1 brachial plexus palsies. Laboratory investigation. J Neurosurg. 2009;111(2):326–31.
18. Bertelli JA, Ghizoni MF. Transfer of supinator motor branches to the posterior interosseous nerve in C7-T1 brachial plexus palsy. J Neurosurg. 2010;113(1):129–32.
19. van Zyl N, Hill B, Cooper C, Hahn J, Galea MP. Expanding traditional tendon-based techniques with nerve transfers for the restoration of upper limb function in tetraplegia: a prospective case series. Lancet. 2019;394(10198):565–75.
20. Bertelli JA, Ghizoni MF, Tacca CP. The median nerve consistently drives flexion of the distal phalanx of the ring and little fingers: interest in finger flexion reconstruction by nerve transfers. Microsurgery. 2015;35(3):207–10.
21. Bertelli JA, Tacca CP, Winkelmann Duarte EC, Ghizoni MF, Duarte H. Transfer of the pronator quadratus motor branch for wrist extension reconstruction in brachial plexus palsy. Plast Reconstr Surg. 2012;130(6):1269–78.
22. Bertelli JA, Nehete S, Winkelmann Duarte EC, Patel N, Ghizoni MF. Distal pronator teres motor branch transfer for wrist extension restoration in radial nerve paralysis. J Neurosurg. 2020, 17:1–7.
23. Yang J, Jia X, Yu C, Gu Y. Pronator teres branch transfer to the anterior interosseous nerve for treating C8T1 brachial plexus avulsion: an anatomic study and case report. Neurosurgery. 2014;75(4):375–9. discussion 379
24. Li Z, Reynolds M, Satteson E, Nazir O, Petit J, Smith BP. Double distal intraneural fascicular nerve transfers for lower brachial plexus injuries. J Hand Surg Am. 2016;41(4):e15–9.

25. Ray WZ, Yarbrough CK, Yee A, Mackinnon SE. Clinical outcomes following brachialis to anterior interosseous nerve transfers. J Neurosurg. 2012;117(3):604–9.
26. Garcia-Lopez A, Sebastian P, Martinez F, Perea D. Transfer of the nerve to the brachioradialis muscle to the anterior interosseous nerve for treatment for lower brachial plexus lesions: case report. J Hand Surg Am. 2011;36(3):394–7.
27. Revol M, Servant JM. Paralysis of the intrinsic muscles of the hand. Chir Main. 2008;27(1):1–11.
28. Sapienza A, Green S. Correction of the claw hand. Hand Clin. 2012;28(1):53–66.
29. Kozin SH, D'Addesi L, Chafetz RS, Ashworth S, Mulcahey MJ. Biceps-to-triceps transfer for elbow extension in persons with tetraplegia. J Hand Surg Am. 2010;35(6):968–75.
30. Bertelli JA. Lower trapezius muscle transfer for reconstruction of elbow extension in brachial plexus injuries. J Hand Surg Eur Vol. 2009;34(4):459–64.
31. Alrabai HM, Gesheff MG, Hammouda AI, Conway JD. Trapezius muscle transfer for restoration of elbow extension in a traumatic brachial plexus injury. J Hand Surg Am. 2018;43(9):872.e871–6.
32. Nehete S, Bertelli JA. Lower trapezius muscle transfer for elbow extension reconstruction after failed nerve transfer for tetraplegia. J Hand Surg Am. 2020;45(6):558.e1–558.e4.
33. Goubier JN, Teboul F. Management of hand palsies in isolated C7 to T1 or C8, T1 root avulsions. Tech Hand Up Extrem Surg. 2008;12(3):156–60.
34. Lamb D. The paralyzed hand. London: Churchill Livingstone; 1987.
35. Soldado F, Bertelli J. Free gracilis transfer reinnervated by the nerve to the supinator for the reconstruction of finger and thumb extension in longstanding C7-T1 brachial plexus root avulsion. J Hand Surg Am. 2013;38(5):941–6.
36. Bertelli JA, Ghizoni MF. Brachialis muscle transfer to reconstruct finger flexion or wrist extension in brachial plexus palsy. J Hand Surg Am. 2006;31(2):190–6.
37. DeGeorge BR Jr, Becker HA, Faryna JH, Spinner RJ, Bishop AT, Shin AY. Outcomes of muscle brachialis transfer to restore finger flexion in brachial plexus palsy. Plast Reconstr Surg. 2017;140(2):307e–17e.
38. Shen YD, Zheng MX, Hua XY, Qiu YQ, Hu KJ, Xu WD. Brachialis muscle transfer for reconstructing digital flexion after brachial plexus injury or forearm injury. J Hand Surg Eur Vol. 2018;43(3):259–68.
39. Mohammed KD, Rothwell AG, Sinclair SW, Willems SM, Bean AR. Upper limb surgery in tetraplegia. J Hand Surg (Br). 1992;74:873–9.
40. Bertelli JA. Distal sensory nerve transfers in lower-type injuries of the brachial plexus. J Hand Surg Am. 2012;37(6):1194–9.
41. Bertelli JA, Ghizoni MF. Nerve transfer for sensory reconstruction of C8-T1 dermatomes in tetraplegia. Microsurgery. 2016;36(8):637–41.
42. Deletis V, Morota N, Abbott IR. Electrodiagnosis in the management of brachial plexus surgery. Hand Clin. 1995;11(4):555–61.

Part VI

Restoration of Hand Function in Pan Plexus Injury

34 Restoration of Hand Function in Pan Plexus Injury – Double Free Functioning Muscle Transfer

Kazuteru Doi, Yasunori Hattori, Sotetsu Sakamoto, Kota Hayashi, Abdullah Alawadhi, and Abdullah Albazzaz

Rationale

Prehensile function is the most advisable reconstruction for patients with pan-brachial plexus injury (BPI). Several surgical approaches have been developed for this strategy [1–4]. Conventional surgical reconstructions such as combined nerve transfer (NT) and contralateral C7 transfer (CC7) excluding double free muscle transfer (DFMT) procedures [5–8] did not attain desired hand function. Simple NTs to median or ulnar nerve displayed far too much gap between nerve suture site and neuromuscular units of the targeted forearm muscle as well as numerous branches of distal nerve, which can result in misdirection of regenerating nerve fibers. Even though NT and CC7 provided random innervations to the forearm muscles, it did not recover reliable prehension [9–11]. DFMT was advantageous as the nerve suture site was within proximity to the neuromuscular unit and the distal nerve had only one motor branch, which promoted early and certain innervations to the transferred muscle [12].

The DFMT did not restore key pinch like Moberg-type simple hand grip reconstruction, which is used as the standard technique for patients with spinal cord injury. However, the weak pinch function by synergistic action was ineffective for patients with brachial plexus injury [12, 13], because BPI patients have normal contralateral upper limb and can perform most activities of daily living. This is very different for patients with spinal cord injury. Patients with complete brachial plexus palsy need reconstruction of few important two-handed activities, such as lifting a heavy box with both hands or holding a bottle while opening its cap. These require a powerful grip independent of the contralateral limb as well as the use of both hands. Direct activation of finger flexion and extension is imperative for a powerful grip.

Based on these rationales, we introduced the double free muscle transfer (DFMT) procedure in 1995 [5] and added several modifications [14, 15].

Outline of Current Double Free Muscle Transfer

Stage 1 consisted of surgical exploration of the brachial plexus and intraoperative diagnosis using electrophysiological testing and nerve repair for reconstruction of the shoulder function

K. Doi (✉) · Y. Hattori · S. Sakamoto · K. Hayashi
A. Alawadhi · A. Albazzaz
Department of Orthopedic Surgery, Ogori Daiichi General Hospital, Yamaguchi City, Yamaguchi Prefecture, Japan
e-mail: doimicro@saikyo.or.jp

A. Y. Shin, N. Pulos (eds.), *Operative Brachial Plexus Surgery*,
https://doi.org/10.1007/978-3-030-69517-0_34

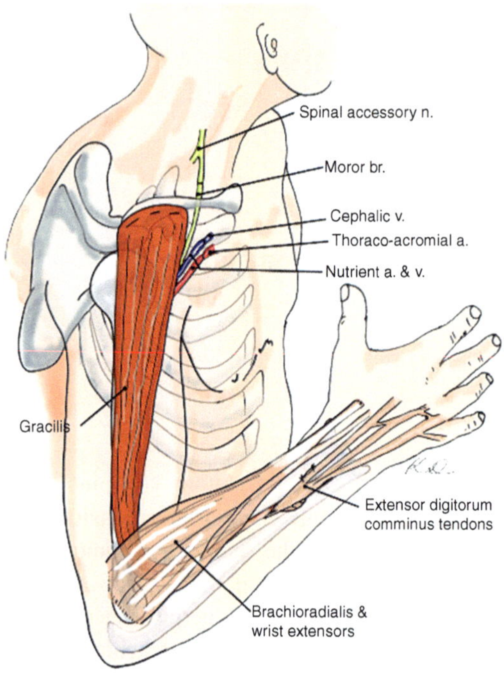

Fig. 34.1 Stage 2 of the procedure, in which the first gracilis muscle graft is used to restore elbow flexion and finger extension. (Reuse according to STM guideline from the author's article [12])

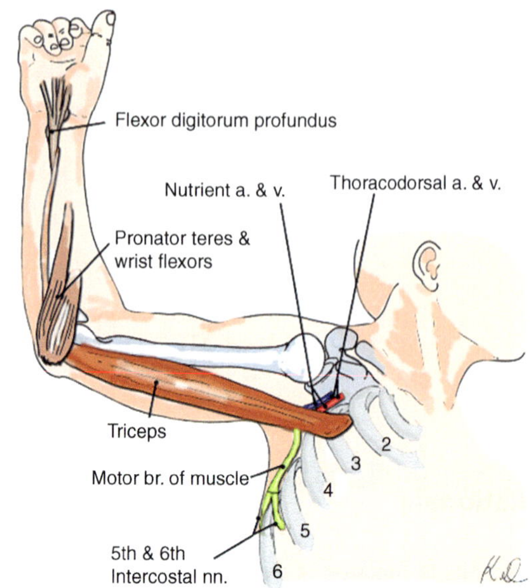

Fig. 34.2 Stage 4 of the procedure, in which the second gracilis muscle graft is used to restore elbow flexion and finger flexion. (Reuse according to STM guideline from the author's article [12])

when the patients presented less than 6 months from injury.

Stage 2 was to perform the first FFMT to restore elbow flexion and finger extension (Fig. 34.1).

Stage 3 comprised of the second FFMT to restore finger flexion (Fig. 34.2), nerve transfers of the third and fourth intercostal nerves to the motor branch of the triceps to restore elbow extension (Fig. 34.3), and transfer of the sensory rami of intercostal nerve to the median nerve to restore hand sensibility.

Stage 4 consisted of supplemental procedures of wrist fusion (Fig. 34.4) and Zancolli's capsulodesis (Fig. 34.5).

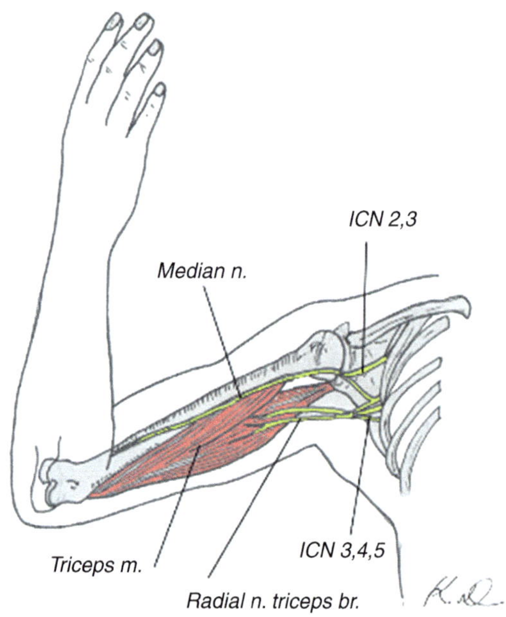

Fig. 34.3 Stage III of the procedure: sensory restoration of the hand with nerve transfer of the intercostobrachial nerve and sensory rami of the second and third intercostal nerves to the median nerve and reconstruction of elbow extension with nerve transfer of the third and fourth intercostal nerves to the long-head branches of the triceps brachii muscle of the radial nerve

Indication

Not all patients with a pan-BPI are candidates for DFMT. Currently the indications for DFMT are as follows:

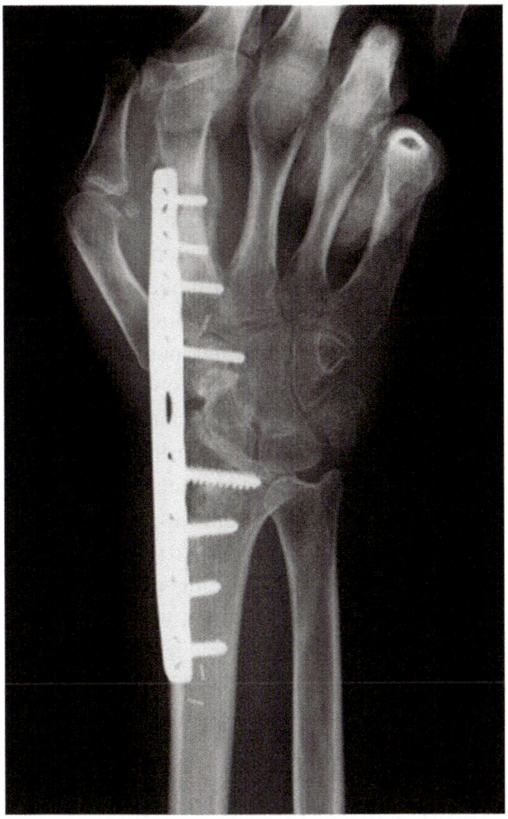

Fig. 34.4 Wrist fusion with a dynamic compression plate and screws

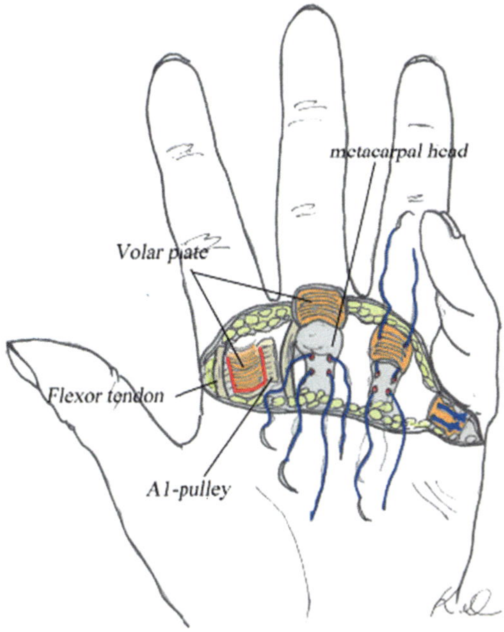

Fig. 34.5 Capsulodesis of the metacarpophalangeal joint for static correction of claw finger deformity, by proximal advancement of the distally based flap of the volar plate. The volar plate is anchored to the metacarpal neck

Indications

- Pan-paralysis of the brachial plexus, and *selected cases of lower-type BPI with no available muscles for tendon transfer in the forearm*
- Acute cases that are less than 6 months after injury
- Failed or chronic cases exceeding 7 months after injury with available donor motor nerves from the spinal and intercostal nerves
- Patients younger than 50 years but more preferably patients younger than 40 years old
- Financial support and patient's motivation to continue postoperative rehabilitation longer than 1 year
- *BMI less than 25*

Contraindications

- Patients older than 60 years
- Accompanying serious systemic injury such as head and spinal cord injury
- Injury of subclavicular artery without available recipient artery
- *BMI greater than 30*

Surgical Procedure

Stage 1: Shoulder Reconstruction

The priority for donor nerve for shoulder reconstruction was C5 nerve root, of which availability was judged by preoperative magnetic resonance imaging (MRI) and intraoperative electrical stimulation. After surgical exploration, SSN will be connected with sural nerve graft. When the C5 root was found to be unusable (i.e., avulsion), the priority shifted to SSN reinnervation in DFMT using CC7 before 2006 and phrenic nerve (PN) transfer after 2007.

All patients underwent exploration of the C5 to T1 nerve roots through the transverse cervical and supraclavicular incisions, and the availability of C5 nerve root was decided after direct electric nerve stimulation. When the serratus anterior muscle contracted, it was decided to use the C5 nerve root to connect to the distal SSN nerve stump with sural nerve graft. And when C5 was found to be beyond repair, posterior divisions of CC7 from the contralateral neck were transected and transferred through a subcutaneous tunnel in the upper chest region, and the distal end of CC7 was connected to SSN utilizing vascularized ulnar nerve graft. The PN was harvested distally from beneath the sternal attachment of the sternocleidomastoid muscle with direct coaptation to SSN.

Excluding CC7 transfer, nerve grafting of C5 to SSN or NT of PN to SSN was performed simultaneously with stage 2 operation.

Stage 2: 1st FFMT for Elbow Flexion and Finger Extension (Fig. 34.1)

After exploration of the spinal accessory nerve through the lateral transverse supraclavicular incision with detachment of the trapezius muscle from the clavicle and acromion, division of the distal branch of the spinal accessory nerve and transfer to the supraclavicular fossa, the thoracoacromial artery, and the cephalic vein were explored through additional deltopectoral skin incision. A subcutaneous tunnel between the deltopectoral skin incision and the anterior cubital skin incision was made to pass the muscle graft in the anterior upper arm, and a pulley was created underneath the brachioradialis and long wrist extensor muscles. The extensor digitorum communis (EDC) tendons were dissected through the additional dorsal forearm skin incision.

Harvesting the Gracilis Muscle

The donor gracilis muscle from the proximal origin to the distal attachment in the contralateral thigh was harvested as the ultimate location of the neurovascular bundle matched the site of the donor vessels for the 1st FMT and in the ipsilateral thigh for the 2nd FMT. The length of gracilis muscle under the maximal traction should be measured before detaching the pubic origin to adjust correct tension of muscle at suturing (see chapter on "Gracilis Harvest").

Transfer the 1st Muscle Graft (Fig. 34.1)

The transferred muscle to the acromion and lateral clavicle was sutured, ensuring it lay superficially over the anterior portion of the deltoid muscle and pass the distal tendon of the muscle graft into the subcutaneous tunnel in the upper arm and the pulley described above.

The nutrient vessels of the muscle to the thoracoacromial artery and cephalic vein were anastomosed individually, and the motor nerve of the gracilis was passed underneath the clavicle and sutured to the SAN in the supraclavicular region. After neurovascular anastomoses, the distal tendon of the gracilis was sutured to the EDC tendon using two weaves of interlacing suture maintaining the finger in full extension, with the wrist in neutral position and the elbow in −30°of flexion allowing the elbow in 90° flexion with the fingers fully flexed and the wrist in neutral extension.

Stage3: Nerve Transfer for Elbow Extension and Sensory Restoration (Fig. 34.3)

Stage 4: 2nd FFMT for Elbow Flexion and Finger Flexion (Fig. 34.2)

Steps 3 and 4 were done at the same operation.

Through the skin, an incision extending from the longitudinal medial upper arm, the midaxillary line, and the transverse incision over the sixth rib until the costochondral junction was made to expose the second to sixth ribs. The 3rd to 6th intercostal nerves in the lateral chest region and the tricep branches of the radial and median nerve were dissected. Bypassing the nonabsorbable sutures through four holes made in the second and third ribs to fix the origin of the second muscle graft. The subcutaneous tunnel and the pulley underneath the pronator teres and long wrist flexor muscles were constructed using the same process as mentioned within stage 2 in the medial upper arm. The flexor digitorum profundus (FDP) tendon was dissected through a volar forearm skin incision. The nerve transfer of the intercostal brachial and sensory rami of the third intercostal nerve to median nerves was done for sensory restoration of the hand, and the third and fourth intercostal nerves should be transferred to the motor branch of the triceps muscles to activate the elbow extension. These were completed before the second muscle was detached from the donor site (Fig. 34.3).

Transfer of the 2nd Muscle Graft

The harvested donor gracilis muscle was transferred from its proximal origin to the distal attachment in the ipsilateral thigh to the recipient site. After suturing the proximal end of the muscle graft to the second and third ribs and passing the muscle under pulley of the pronator teres and long wrist flexors, anastomosis was done to the nutrient vessels of the thoracodorsal artery and vein. Following this, suture the fifth and sixth intercostal nerves to the motor nerve of the second muscle transplant. Finally, the distal portion of the muscle graft was coapted to the FDP tendon (Fig. 34.2) after determining muscle tension with the principles described above.

Postoperative Monitoring of the Muscle Vascularity

The use of skin flap as a monitoring tool cannot sensitively reflect the vascularity of a FFMT and may result in delayed detection of vascular compromise. We routinely use the compound muscle action potentials (CMAPs) as a supplemental method in the monitoring of free gracilis transfers [16, 17]. The clinical critical values of CMAP amplitude changes for vascular compromise are more than 40% sudden decrease and continued decrease. This technique has proved clinical significance in current vascular compromised cases.

Postoperative Management

After each muscle transfer, the upper limb should be immobilized with the shoulder in 30° of abduction and flexion and 60 °of internal rotation, the elbow in 100° of flexion, the wrist maintained at neutral position, and the fingers in forced flexion or extension. This should be done using an arm brace and cast for 4 weeks, and, subsequently, a sling can be used to prevent subluxation of the glenohumeral joint until recovery of the shoulder girdle muscles.

Rehabilitation

Early passive mobilization is started to prevent adhesion of the muscle-tendon unit 1 week after free muscle transfer and continued to active movement of fingers [18] (Fig. 34.6).

Documentation of reinnervation of the transferred muscle usually performed between 3 and 8 months postoperatively by electromyographic feedback techniques using small portable myotrainers with surface electrodes is initiated to train the transferred muscles to move the elbow and fingers (Fig. 34.7) as patients usually have difficulty contracting each muscle effectively. After recovery of active elbow and finger movements, electromyographic feedback to train independent finger flexion and extension is commenced, and simultaneous flexion of the elbow should be negated by the antagonist action of the triceps brachii. This depends on reinnervation from the third and fourth intercostal nerves. The patients are taught a home program to activate the individual transferred gracilis and triceps muscles.

Usually, patients stay in the hospital for 2 months after the second free muscle transfer and then attend a nearby rehabilitation center two to three times a week and visit our clinic every 1–3 months for another 1 1/2–2 years.

Ultimately, most patients with satisfactory recovery of active finger motion develop an intrinsic-minus finger deformity but are able to use their hand for hook grip. Patients undergo a progressive resistance excessing consisting of strengthening finger flexion, elbow flexion, and shoulder adduction with pulleys and weights, in order to increase the strength of the hook grip and arm-trunk prehension. The patients are then started on skilled activities, such as lifting, holding, carrying, and pinching.

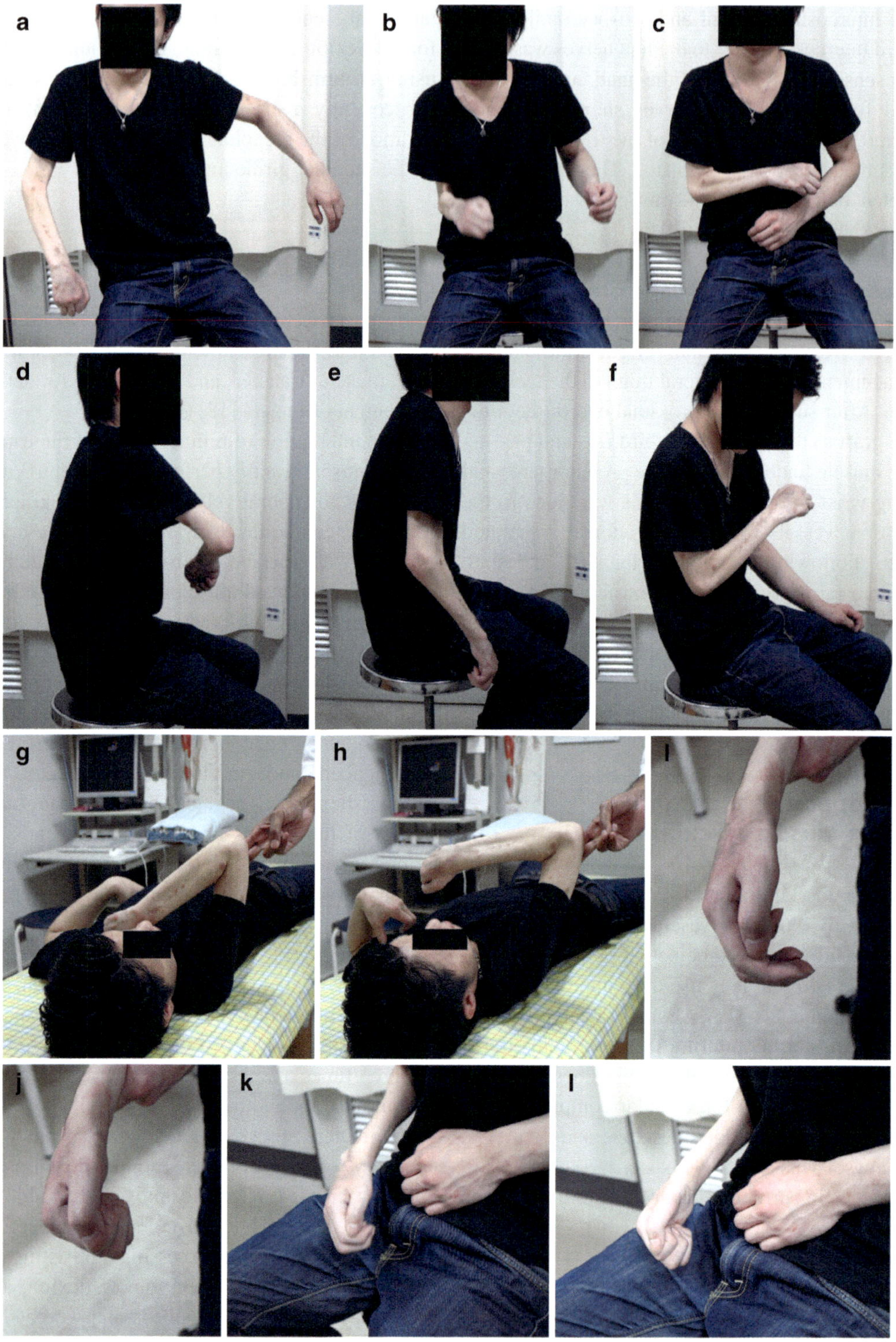

Fig. 34.6 Illustrated case with right pan BPI. (**a**) shoulder abduction, (**b**, **c**) shoulder external and internal rotation, (**d**) shoulder flexion, (**e**, **f**) elbow extension and flexion, (**g**, **h**) elbow flexion and extension in supine position showing M2 power of elbow extension, (**i**, **j**) finger flexion and extension with stability of elbow to prevent simultaneous elbow flexion by double transferred muscles, (**k**, **l**) finger flexion and extension without any support of contra lateral normal hand

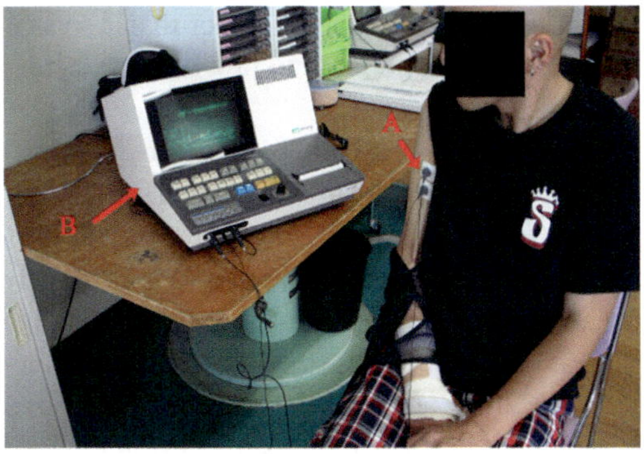

Fig. 34.7 Electromyographic feedback techniques using small portable myotrainers (*B*) with surface electrodes (*A*)

Secondary Reconstruction

Wrist Fusion

When the wrist remains unstable following wrist splinting, the wrist joint is fused in the neutral position or mild dorsiflexion using dynamic compression plate (Fig. 34.4) [14, 19].

Correction of Intrinsic-Minus Deformity

Claw finger deformity is frequently observed after satisfactory recovery of finger flexion and extension. This should be prevented by applying a plastic static volar splint, but most patients require secondary procedures, including wrist fusion with Zancolli's MCP joint capsulodesis (Fig. 34.5) [14] or transient interphalangeal joints fixation with K-wires which depends on the patient's selection under a preoperative trial with a simulation splint[4].

Current Outcomes Summarized

Out of the 114 patients with more than 24 months postoperative follow-up, excluding 3 postoperative vascular compromises, 3 children, and 3 foreign patients, there were only 4 females and the remainders were males. Median age of the patients was 24 years old (range: 15–55 years). Except for five patients who presented to us very late (>100 months from injury), the median time to first intervention was 3 months (range: 1–56 months). Median follow-up after the second FFMT was 30 months (range: 24–164 months).

Median range of shoulder motions were 30° (range: 0–100°) in abduction and − 20° (range: −80–45°) in external rotation individually. Median range of elbow flexion was 120° (range: 80–155°).

Power of elbow flexion according to BRMC grading was noted as M4 in 62, M3 in 48, and M2 in 4. Power of elbow extension in 53 patients who underwent INC-triceps branch transfer was M3 in 12, M2 in 21, M1 in 15, and M0 in 5.

TAM of finger joints was recorded as excellent (>60°) in 114 patients, good (30–55°) in 51 patients, fair (5–25°) in 24 patients, and poor (0°) in 5 patients. Quantitative isokinetic measurements of elbow flexion done in 77 patients revealed that the reconstructed limb regained a concentric elbow flexion of 5 Newton meters (12% of contralateral normal limb) and eccentric elbow flexion of 7 Newton meters (15% of contralateral normal limb).

Illustrated Case

A 16-year-old male with right pan BPI underwent DFMT procedure including nerve transfer of the phrenic nerve to suprascapular nerve at stage 1 with standard DFMT, wrist fusion, and Zancolli's techniques and obtained excellent functional recovery (Fig. 34.6).

Discussion

We have reported several times the long-term results of DFMT to provide prehension for patients with traumatic total brachial plexus injury [5–8, 12, 14, 15]. Presently, the number of cases with DFMT exceeds 130 cases. Owing to the increase in number of cases, the conclusion has been changed a little. In the other hand, few articles, of other authors, have published the DFMT outcomes [20–23].

Besides our long-term results of DFMT, the Mayo Clinic Brachial Plexus Team have reported on the long-term results of DFMT in 30 patients [22]. The functional outcome of prehension according to the authors' findings was excellent in 6 patients (which implies restoration of more than 90 degrees of elbow flexion, dynamic stability of the elbow while moving the fingers, and more than 60 degrees of total active motion of the fingers), good (similar to excellent, except for total active motion of 30–60 degrees) in 11 patients, fair (total active motion of less than 30 degrees) in 3 patients, and poor in 10 patients. Satisfactory results (excellent and good) were achieved in 17 out of 30 patients (57%). Half the patients recovered sensitivity of the palm and adequate positional sense. However, protective sensation in the ulnar side of the hand and fingers showed no recovery in the other half of patients. Minor injury and burns can easily occur in these parts of the hand.

Despite reported success of double FFMT for prehension, it remains a daunting undertaking for both the surgeon and patient. Two to three major surgeries followed by significant dedicated rehabilitation may prove to be both financially and emotionally challenging for patients. They changed their procedure to single muscle transfer which is described in the next chapter of this textbook.

We are aware that other surgeons did not achieve as successful outcomes as we reported utilizing the DFMT technique [20–23]. The major reason for inferior outcomes following DFMT is the postoperative rehabilitation, which comprised of two sessions – early passive mobilization of transferred muscle-tendon junction to prevent adhesion [18] and long-term rehabilitation. The former session required daily attendance at the rehabilitation center until the transferred muscle starts moving which is at around 5 or 6 months post-operation, and the latter session continued for 1 or 1.5 post-operation [12, 14, 15]. It is understandable that such long-term rehabilitation cannot be implemented in other countries, excluding Japan, unless it is for special insurance like worker's care. The patient's financial support and motivation to undertake postoperative rehabilitation longer than 1 year is the foremost requirement to provide satisfactory outcomes.

The current outcome also discloses that one-third of patients with DFMT attained satisfactory finger function (total active finger motion). Additionally, according to our current data, daily use of the reconstructed hand is directly related to the range of elbow flexion, TAM, and sensory recovery of the hand. The detailed QoL outcomes and patients' satisfaction results will not appear in this chapter, as it will soon be published separately in journal articles. The TAM is also dependent on the patient's age and body mass index (BMI). Our current indication of DFMT is based on a limit of patients younger than 39 years with a BMI of less than 23.

In conclusion, although we can't deny that long hours of DFMT surgery are strenuous for both the surgeon and the patient, the functional possibility of prehension by DFMT resulted in hook grip which not only need finger flexion but also minimal opening of fingers. Based on our experiences from single muscle transfer, the patients end up never using the reconstructed hand because of the closed finger grip.

References

1. Carlstedt T. Central nerve plexus injury. London: Imperial College Press; 2007. p. 139–66.
2. Chuang DCC, Ma HS, Borud LJ, Chen HC. Surgical strategy for improving forearm and hand function in late obstetric brachial plexus palsy. Plast Reconstr Surg. 2002;109:1934–46.
3. Liang C, Yu-Dong G, Hu S-N, Xu J-G, Xu L, Yang F. Contralateral C7 transfer for the treatment of brachial plexus root avulsion in children – a report of 12 cases. J Hand Surg. 2007;32A:96–103.
4. Songcharoen P, Wongtrakul S, Mahaisavariya B, Spinner RJ. Hemi-contralateral C7 transfer to median nerve in the treatment of root avulsion brachial plexus injury. J Hand Surg. 2001;26A:1058–64.
5. Doi K, Sakai K, Kuwata N, Ihara K, Kawai S. Double free-muscle transfer to restore prehension following complete brachial plexus avulsion. J Hand Surg Am. 1995;20(3):408–14.
6. Doi K, Muramatsu K, Hattori Y, Otsuka K, Tan SH, Nanda V, Watanabe M. Restoration of prehension with the double free muscle technique following complete avulsion of the brachial plexus. Indications

and long-term results. J Bone Joint Surg Am. 2000;82(5):652–66.
7. Dodakundi C, Doi K, Hattori Y, Sakamoto S, Fujihara Y, Takagi T, Fukuda M. Outcome of surgical reconstruction after traumatic total brachial plexus palsy. J Bone Joint Surg Am. 2013;95(16):1505–12.
8. Satbhai NG, Doi K, Hattori Y, Sakamoto S. Functional outcome and quality of life after traumatic total brachial plexus injury treated by nerve transfer or single/double free muscle transfers: a comparative study. Bone Joint J. 2016;98-B(2):209–17.
9. Arnal M, Cambon A, Marcheix PS, Belkhayar Z. Restoration of elbow and hand function in total brachial plexus palsy with intercostal nerves and C5 root neurotization. Results in 21 patients. Hand Surg Rehabil. 2016;35(4):283–7.
10. Li WJ, He LY, Chen SL, Lyu YW, Wang SF, Yong Y, Tian W, Tian GL, Gu YD. Contralateral C7 nerve root transfer for function recovery in adults: a meta-analysis. Chin Med J. 2017;130(24):2960–8.
11. Wang GB, Yu AP, Ng CY, Lei GW, Wang XM, Qiu YQ, Feng JT, Li T, Chen QZ, He QR, Ding F, Cui SS, Gu YD, Xu JG, Jiang S, Xu WD. Contralateral C7 to C7 nerve root transfer in reconstruction for treatment of total brachial plexus palsy: anatomical basis and preliminary clinical results. J Neurosurg Spine. 2018;29(5):491–9.
12. Doi K. Management of total paralysis of the brachial plexus by the double free-muscle transfer technique. J Hand Surg Eur Vol. 2008;33(3):240–51.
13. Takka S, Doi K, Hattori Y, Kitajima I, Ikeda K, Guafen C. Selection of grip function in double free gracilis transfer procedures after complete paralysis of the brachial plexus. Ann Plast Surg. 2005;54(6):610–4.
14. Doi K, Hattori Y, Sakamoto S, Dodakundi C, Satbhai NG, Montales T. Current procedure of double free muscle transfer for traumatic total brachial plexus palsy. JBJS Essent Surg Tech. 2013;3(3):e16.
15. Hentz VR, Doi K. Traumatic brachial plexus palsy. In: Green DP, editor. Operative hand surgery. 5th ed. New York: Churchill Livingstone; 2005. p. 1353–4.
16. Khater AM, Doi K, Hattori Y, Sakamoto S, Yonemura H, Kumar K. The use of compound muscle action potentials (CMAP) for postoperative monitoring of free functioning gracilis muscle transfer: a preliminary report. J Plast Reconstr Aesthet Surg. 2015;68(7):e137–46.
17. Dodakundi C, Doi K, Hattori Y, Sakamoto S, Yonemura H, Fujihara Y. Postoperative monitoring in free muscle transfers for reconstruction in brachial plexus injuries. Tech Hand Up Extrem Surg. 2012;16(1):48–51.
18. Doi K, Hattori Y, Yamazaki H, Wahegaonkar AL, Addosooki A, Watanabe M. Importance of early passive mobilization following double free gracilis muscle transfer. Plast Reconstr Surg. 2008;121(6):2037–45.
19. Addosooki A, Doi K, Hattori Y, Wahegaonkar A. Wrist arthrodesis after double free-muscle transfer in traumatic total brachial plexus palsy. Tech Hand Up Extrem Surg. 2007;11(1):29–36.
20. Barrie KA, Steinmann SP, Shin AY, Spinner RJ. Bishop AT Gracilis free muscle transfer for restoration of function after complete brachial plexus avulsion. Neurosurg Focus. 2004;16(5):E8.
21. Elzinga K, Zuo KJ, Olson JL, Morhart M, Babicki S, Chan KM. Double free gracilis muscle transfer after complete brachial plexus injury: first Canadian experience. Plast Surg (Oakv). 2014;22(1):26–9.
22. Spinner RJ, Shin AY, Hebert-Blouin MN, Elhassan BT, Bishop AT. Traumatic brachial plexus injury. In: Wolfe SW, Hotchikiss RN, Pederson WC, Kozin SH, editors. Green's operative hand surgery. 6th ed. Philadelphia: Elsevier Churchil Livingstone; 2011. p. 1270–5.
23. Tu Y, Ueng S. Double free functioning muscle transfer FFMT) for the reconstruction of brachial plexus injury. 2nd Congress of the World Society for Reconstructive Microsurgery. Germany: Reconstr Microsurg; 2003:297–301.

35 Restoration of Active Grasp Function in Total Brachial Plexus Avulsion Injury

Shu-feng Wang, Yun-hao Xue, Peng-cheng Li, Wen-jun Li, and Feng Li

Total brachial plexus avulsion injury, which is the most severe type of brachial plexus injury, refers to the avulsion of all five spinal roots of the brachial plexus from the spinal cord, resulting in complete paralysis of the affected upper limb. Due to the lack of proximal residual nerve roots, reconnection of the spinal roots to the spinal cord does not lead to regeneration of nerve fibers from the spinal cord (Fig. 35.1). Extra plexus nerve transfers have been clinically confirmed to be an effective treatment and have achieved good efficacy in restoring shoulder and elbow function [1, 2]. Currently, the donor nerves available for transfer in clinical practice mainly include the accessory nerve, intercostal nerve, phrenic nerve, and contralateral cervical 7 (CC7) nerve . However, except for the CC7, all of these donor nerves are small and, consequently, neurotization can recover only partial function of the affected limb. No breakthrough has been discovered to restore hand function distal to the elbow joint, and restoration of hand function in patients with total brachial plexus avulsion injuries remains an aspiration of hand surgeons. To restore the active pick-up function of the paralyzed upper limb in patients with total brachial plexus avulsion injuries, the upper limb should at least have the following basic functions: active shoulder abduction, active elbow flexion and extension, and a stable wrist joint and active finger flexion and extension [3]. Restoring as many functions as possible using the limited donor nerve resources is the goal of related clinical research.

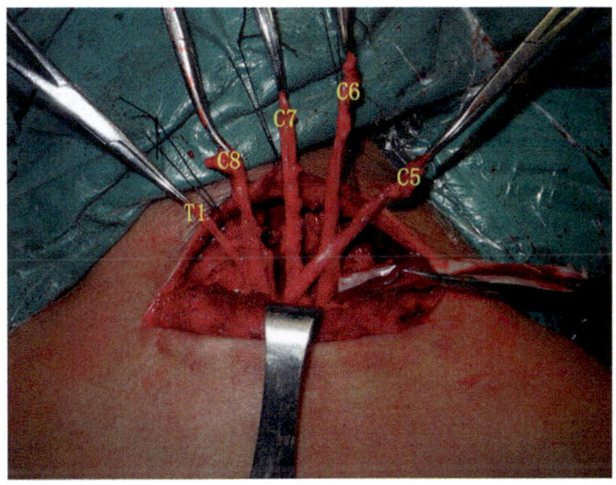

Fig. 35.1 Supraclavicular surgical exploration demonstrates five nerve root (C5-T1) avulsion injury from the spinal cord

In 1989, Yudong Gu designed the method of CC7 nerve transfer and confirmed that severing the CC7 did not significantly affect contralateral upper extremity function, which has been verified by scholars worldwide [4–7]. However, the traditional method of reconstructing finger

Supplementary Information The online version of this chapter (https://doi.org/10.1007/978-3-030-69517-0_35) contains supplementary material, which is available to authorized users.

S.-f. Wang (✉) · Y.-h. Xue · P.-c. Li · W.-j. Li · F. Li
The Department of Hand Surgery, Beijing Jishuitan Hospital, Beijing, China

A. Y. Shin, N. Pulos (eds.), *Operative Brachial Plexus Surgery*,
https://doi.org/10.1007/978-3-030-69517-0_35

flexion function by CC7 nerve transfer involves dividing the ulnar nerve at the level of the wrist. The proximal ulnar nerve is retrogradely dissected to the middle level of the upper arm and then is reversed to the contralateral neck through a subcutaneous tunnel in the neck and chest and used to anastomose to the CC7 in phase I of the surgery. When the regenerated nerve fibers from the CC7 grow and reach the middle level of the upper arm, phase II of the surgery is performed. The ulnar nerve is severed at the reversed site and coapted to the median nerve to restore the function of finger flexion. This entire procedure is equivalent to bridging a long segment of the ulnar nerve (about 35 cm), and the regenerated nerve fibers must pass through two anastomoses and then pass a distance of approximately 20 cm to reach the forearm muscle . The duration of nerve regeneration from the CC7 to the forearm muscle is long. In most cases, the fingers can only move slightly, and the final recovered finger flexion strength is not satisfactory [8, 9].

Based on the experience of previous researchers, we designed a new method in May 2004 in which the CC7 is transferred to the lower trunk directly via the shortest prespinal route to restore finger flexion, and the CC7 is synchronously bridged with the medial antebrachial cutaneous nerve continued (MABCN) from the lower trunk to regenerate to the musculocutaneous nerve and restore elbow flexion [10]. In 2013, a study of 73 patients with more than 4 years of follow-up showed that more than 64% of the patients had finger flexor muscle strength reaching level 3+ or higher, and 60% of the patients had elbow flexor muscle strength reaching level 3+ or higher [11]. The therapeutic efficacy of this new method is significantly improved compared to that of the conventional method. This technology was named the "Wang technique" at the 8th International Brachial Plexus Conference in India in November 2015, and some researchers in India have reproduced the same result [12].

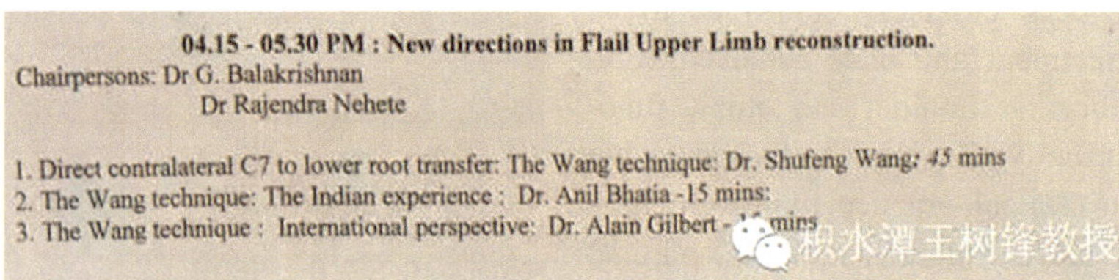
04.15 - 05.30 PM : New directions in Flail Upper Limb reconstruction.
Chairpersons: Dr G. Balakrishnan
Dr Rajendra Nehete

1. Direct contralateral C7 to lower root transfer: The Wang technique: Dr. Shufeng Wang: 45 mins
2. The Wang technique: The Indian experience : Dr. Anil Bhatia -15 mins:
3. The Wang technique : International perspective: Dr. Alain Gilbert - [illegible] mins

Following these achievements in the recovery of finger flexion, restoring finger extension has become another obstacle to overcome. In addition to the CC7, the remaining donor nerves, such as the spinal accessory nerve and the phrenic nerve, are small, have limited nerve fibers, and cannot ensure the recovery of finger extension if used to regenerate the radial nerve. Theoretically, if a functional bundle that mainly innervates finger extension can be found in the brachial plexus, then the limited regenerated nerve fibers can be concentrated in the finger extensor muscles through direct coaptation, which can thus solve the mismatch problem between the donor nerve and the recipient nerve. However, such a functional nerve bundle remains to be identified. Clinical studies have shown that patients with completely injured upper and middle trunks (C5-7 injuries) and a normal lower trunk have normal finger flexion and extension, and their elbow extensor muscle strength is about grade 4. This finding suggests that finger flexor muscle and interosseus muscle are derived from innervation of the anterior division of the lower trunk (through the medial cord to the medial head of the median nerve and ulnar nerve) and that elbow and finger extension is derived from the innervation of the posterior division (through the posterior cord to the radial nerve). Through many clinical observations and electrophysiological studies, we have confirmed that the posterior division of the lower trunk (PDIT) is the main functional nerve tract that innervates the finger extensor muscles (and is more important than the posterior division of C7)

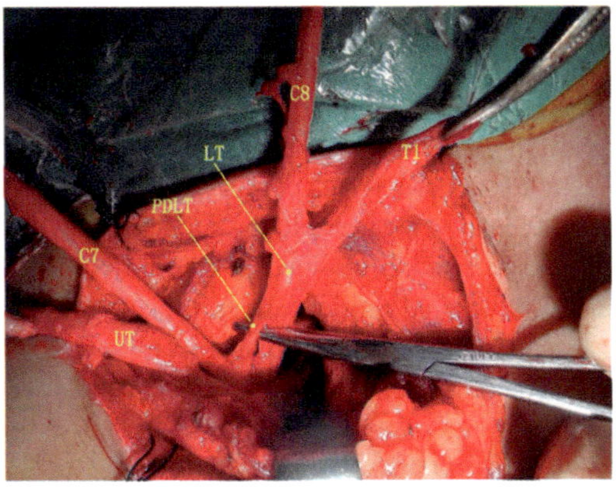

Fig. 35.2 Intraoperative photograph showing the posterior division of the lower trunk (PDLT) of the brachial plexus exposed through the supraclavicular incision. LT lower trunk, UT upper trunk

and innervates the long head of the triceps [13] (Fig. 35.2). Based on this finding, we designed a surgical procedure that directly coapts the phrenic nerve with the posterior division of the lower trunk to restore elbow and finger extension, which was first applied clinically in June 2005. In 2015, we reported 27 patients with total brachial plexus injuries who underwent this surgery and were followed up for more than 4 years [14]. Our results showed that 81.5% and 48% of the patients regained M3 or greater muscle power for elbow and finger extension, respectively.

Since November 2006, we have used modified multiple nerve transfer methods to restore active pick-up function in patients with total brachial plexus avulsion injuries. In one surgical procedure, three groups of nerve transfers are used to restore five functions, including accessory nerve transfers to neurotize the suprascapular nerve and restore shoulder abduction and external rotation, CC7 nerve transfers via the prespinal route for direct coaptation with the lower trunk to restore finger flexion and wrist flexion, medial antebrachial cutaneous nerve transfers to neurotize the musculocutaneous nerve to restore the function of elbow flexion, and phrenic nerve transfers to neurotize the posterior division of the lower trunk to restore elbow and finger extension [15]. Conventional multiple nerve transfers usually require three to four surgeries, whereas the newly designed method can be completed in one procedure, which reduces medical costs, shortens the duration of muscle denervation, and facilitates the recovery of function of the affected limb.

If muscle strength can be recovered for all restored functions described above following nerve transfers ($\geq$3 years for adults after surgery and $\geq$ 2 years for children), then hand function reconstruction including wrist arthrodesis, opponensplasty or carpometacarpal (CMC) fusion, and volar metacarpophalangeal (MP) joint capsulodesis can restore the active pick-up function of the affected upper limb in some patients.

Modified Multiple Nerve Transfers

Supraclavicular Exploration

A transverse supraclavicular incision parallel to the clavicle is made. A skin flap including the platysma is raised as much as possible superiorly and inferiorly. The posterior margin of the sternocleidomastoid muscle is exposed, and the external jugular vein is ligated. The supraclavicular sensory nerve branch is exposed and retracted for protection. The cervical fascia is incised and the omohyoid muscle is exposed and retracted for protection. The transverse cervical vessels are severed and ligated. Medially, the phrenic nerve is located on the anterior surface of the anterior scalene muscle. In most cases, a dense scar mass is present at the interscalene space and extend to the behind of clavicle. The supraclavicular brachial plexus is usually covered by the scar tissue and difficult to expose. Under this circumstance, we prefer to identify the distal of suprascapular nerve firstly, which is located behind and deep to the origin of omohyoid muscle. Then, the suprascapular nerve is dissected retrogradely to its origin from the posterior division of the upper trunk, which is used as a mark to identify the anterior division of the upper trunk and the upper trunk. Using the upper trunk as a marker, the middle and lower trunks are then exposed sequentially. Avulsion injury can be determined by observing the ganglion of the nerve root by tracing it to the corresponding intervertebral foramen proximally along the nerve trunk. After exposing the avulsed lower trunk, the PDLT can be exposed by dissecting distally and then the PDLT is dissected retrogradely to the proximal and severed at the origin. The distal end of the PDLT is labeled for subsequent use. If the lower trunk is avulsed distally behind the clavicle, or the PDLT originates distally, the PDLT should be explored inferior to the clavicle [14].

The phrenic nerve is isolated toward the mediastinum through the thoracic outlet. The dissected level of the phrenic nerve should be as long as possible so that it can be directly coapted to the posterior division of the lower trunk. Since the phrenic nerve travels close to the large blood vessels in the mediastinum, especially the right phrenic nerve, which is located in the mediastinum on the side wall of the superior vena cava, harvesting of the phrenic nerve in the mediastinum should be performed under direct visualization. In order to clearly expose the upper segment of the phrenic nerve at the mediastinum, the clavicle should be lifted forward with a goiter retractor, and the thoracic outlet should be separated bluntly. When the upper segment of the phrenic nerve at the mediastinum is exposed, the phrenic nerve is pulled proximally using a nerve hook and dissected as distally as possible using a pair of long-handled tissue scissors. Generally, incision of the phrenic nerve at a depth of 2 cm in the mediastinum is safe.

Notes of supraclavicular surgical exploration: if no ganglion is observed on the ruptured nerve root, and which is significantly shorter than its natural length, in this situation it usually indicated that the related nerve root probably ruptured other than avulsed. We should review the preoperative magnetic resonance imaging (MRI) of the brachial plexus again to see whether there is a residual nerve root present, and carefully surgical exploration should be traced to the corresponding intervertebral foramen. Additionally, for a small number of patients who suffered with total brachial plexus preganglionic injures, no obvious abnormalities are detected when exploring the brachial plexus above the clavicle. Almost no dense scar tissue around the nerve roots can be detected, and the appearance of the nerve roots outside the intervertebral foramen obviously is not abnormal, and no avulsed ganglion around the exit of intervertebral foramen can be visualized. This situation is probably caused by a shift of the spinal cord, which causes breakage of rootlets of the affected nerve in the spinal canal when the cervical spine is subjected to severe trauma, and the ruptured rootlets are still inside the spinal canal [16]. Some unique manifestations of this type of brachial plexus injury are evident on MRI in these patients, the pseudodural cysts in the cervical spinal canal extend from C5 to T1 on the affected side, and the filling defects can be found in the pseudodural cysts. Edema is present in the brachial plexus outside the vertebral foramen, but continuity of the brachial plexus is noted (Fig. 35.3a, b). An X-ray examination often shows that the cervical transverse and spinous processes of the cervical vertebrae are fractured. The specificity of the injuries should be fully considered before surgery for this type of patient. Although a pseudodural cyst is present within the spinal canal, especially at C8 and T1, the anterior and posterior rootlets of the corresponding nerves may still be partially continuous. These patients should be observed for at least 3 months after injury, and surgical exploration should be performed if no functional recovery is noted.

Infraclavicular Brachial Plexus Exploration – Mobilization of Lower Trunk and Posterior Division of the Lower Trunk Through the Infraclavicular Approach

Infraclavicular brachial plexus is exposed through the deltopectoral groove approach. After skin incision, the deltopectoral interval was maneuvered to expose the cephalic vein. The infraclavicular plexus was explored by detaching the tendinous insertion of the pectoralis major and minor muscle. The musculocutaneous nerve, the lateral head of the median nerve, the ulnar nerve, the medial head of the median nerve, and the medial antebrachial cutaneous nerve were exposed. Dissecting proximally along the medial cord to the lower trunk behind the clav-

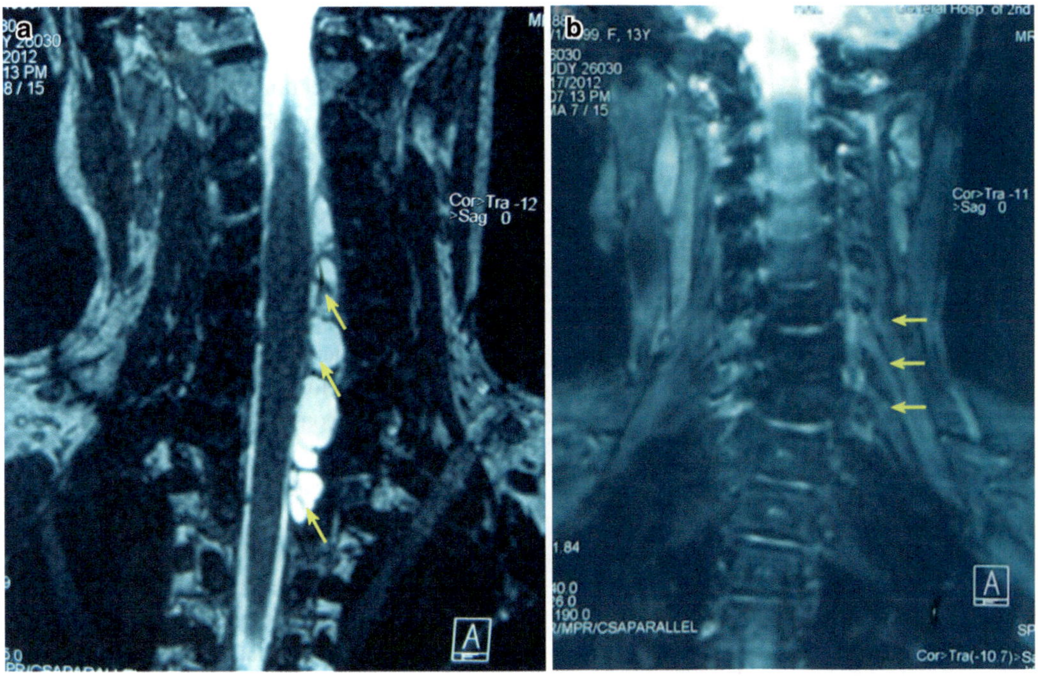

Fig. 35.3 (**a**) MRI demonstrates that the pseudodural cysts extend from C5 to T1 on the affected side, and the filling defects (arrow head) can be found in pseudodural cysts. (**b**) Nerve roots of the injured brachial plexus (arrow head) outside the intervertebral foramen are in continuity (same case with the **a**)

icle and getting through the supraclavicular and the infraclavicular incision, the lower trunk was delivered from the supraclavicular into the infraclavicular incision. Then, the PDLT originating from the lower trunk can be clearly exposed and severed at the origin. The proximal end of PDLT can be separated and removed from the full LT using micro-intrafascicular dissection surgical technique, but they could not be taken out from the C8 and T1 nerve roots because the nerve fascicles interweave. The authors chose to exclude the PDLT from the lower trunk in order to direct all the axons toward the medial root of the median nerve and the ulnar nerve for restoration of the wrist and finger flexion. The lower trunk, medial cord, medial head of the median nerve, main trunk of the median nerve, ulnar nerve, and MABC nerve were dissected distally until reaching the middle level of the upper arm (Fig. 35.4). The medial pectoral nerve and medial brachial cutaneous nerve were severed at their origins, and the MABC nerve was cut at the middle level of the upper arm for subsequent use [11]. The lower trunk or the medial cord is used as a receptor nerve to restore finger flexion. One main factor that affects the postoperative outcome is whether the lower trunk is injured. In addition to observation under the operating microscope during surgery, the preoperative electrophysiological examination is also very helpful for determining the quality of the lower trunk. If preoperative electrophysiological examination indicated that the somatosensory evoked potential (SEP) of the ulnar nerve is absent and SNAP is present, then preganglionic avulsion injury of the lower truck can be considered [17], and coaptation with the CC7 nerve can be performed at any level.

The musculocutaneous nerve is severed close to the origin. The affected shoulder joint is set at 0° of adduction and 0–10° of anterior flexion. The lower trunk is pulled proximally. If the proximal end of the lower trunk reaches the cervical midline, then the lower trunk can be coapted with the CC7 nerve without tension [18]. If tension after direct anastomosis of the nerves is expected, the lower trunk can be relatively extended by short-

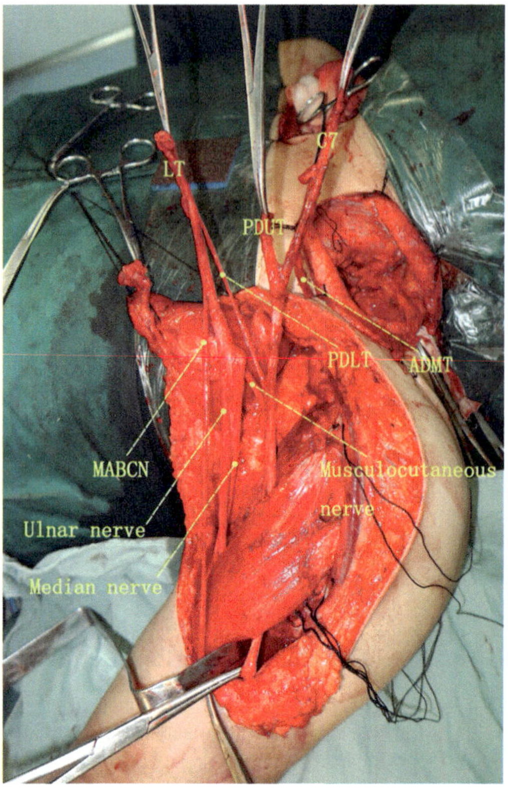

Fig. 35.4 Intraoperative photography showing the full freed lower trunk, posterior cord, and its branches. LT lower trunk, MABCN medial antebrachial cutaneous nerve, PDLT posterior division of lower trunk, PDUT posterior division of upper trunk, ADMT anterior division of upper trunk

ening the humerus. The periosteum is removed at the lateral edge of the biceps and the distal end of the deltoid muscle, and a shortening osteotomy of humerus is performed with a wire saw. A locking compression plate is fixed on the medial side of the humerus, and the tendinous part of the biceps is tightened and sutured. The length of the osteotomy is generally not greater than 4 cm for adults and 3 cm for children (Figs. 35.5a, b, 35.6, and 35.7). Otherwise, a nerve graft is essential.

The phrenic nerve was measured to determine whether it can be directly coapted with the PDLT. If direct coaptation cannot be completed, then the PDLT should be isolated distally until reaching the posterior cord, and the remaining two posterior divisions that arose from the C7 and upper trunk, respectively, are severed simultaneously. Isolation of the posterior cord distally to the proximal segment of radial nerve can be continued. After cutting the axillary nerve, thoracodorsal nerve, upper subscapular nerve, and lower subscapular nerve, the PDLT can be moved proximal to complete direct coaptation with the phrenic nerve.

Notes of infraclavicular surgical exploration: Exploration of the supraclavicular and infraclavicular brachial plexus and dissection of the lower trunk generally do not require osteotomy of the clavicle. However, inexperienced surgeon can perform osteotomy of the clavicle such that the lower trunk is easier to expose and mobilize, which can reduce the risk of subclavian artery injury.

The presence of the radial artery pulse in the affected limb must be assessed before surgery for patients with total brachial plexus injury. If the radial artery pulse is weak or absent, then angiography of the subclavian artery and axillary artery should be performed. For patients with a blocked subclavian artery or axillary artery, ligation of the artery branches should be minimized when exploring and isolating the brachial plexus above and below the clavicle to prevent ischemia of the affected limb. The subclavian artery or axillary artery can also be restored by vascular grafting. Normally, the autologous great saphenous vein is selected for transplantation rather than using an artificial blood vessel because anticoagulation treatment is required after artificial blood vessel transplantation, and a hematoma can easily form after surgery. For patients with subclavian artery or axillary artery blockage, if vascular restoration is not performed during surgery, then clavicle osteotomy should be avoided as much as possible to reduce damage to the collateral circulation.

The Harvest of the CC7 Nerve Root

A similar supraclavicular transverse incision is made on the contralateral side. The contralateral brachial plexus above the clavicle is exposed by layers through a transverse incision. The contralateral C7 nerve root was identified, and its anterior and posterior divisions were dissected as far

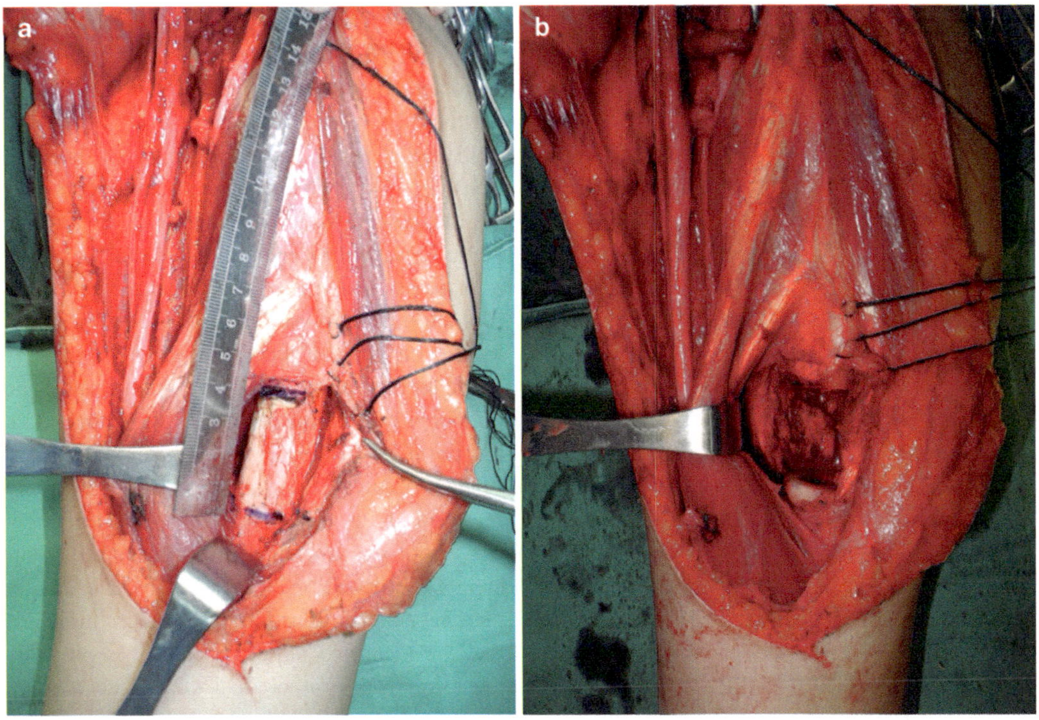

Fig. 35.5 (**a**, **b**) Intraoperative photography showing humeral shortening osteotomy just distal to the insertion of the deltoid muscle

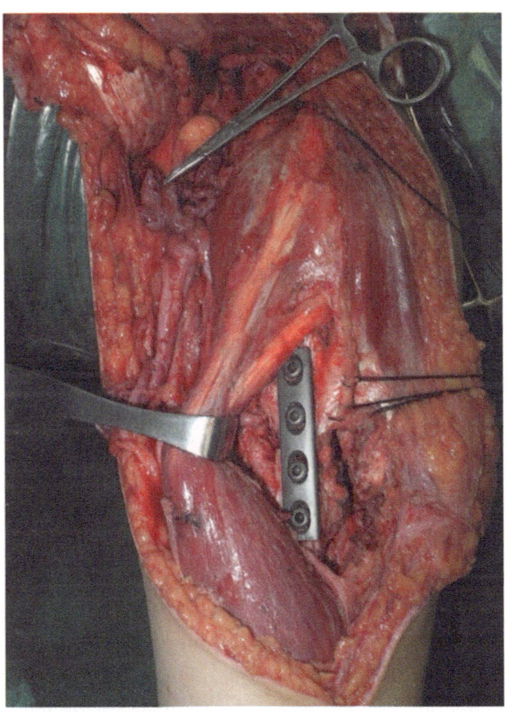

Fig. 35.6 Apply locking compression plate (LCP) to the medial aspect of the humerus for stable fixation

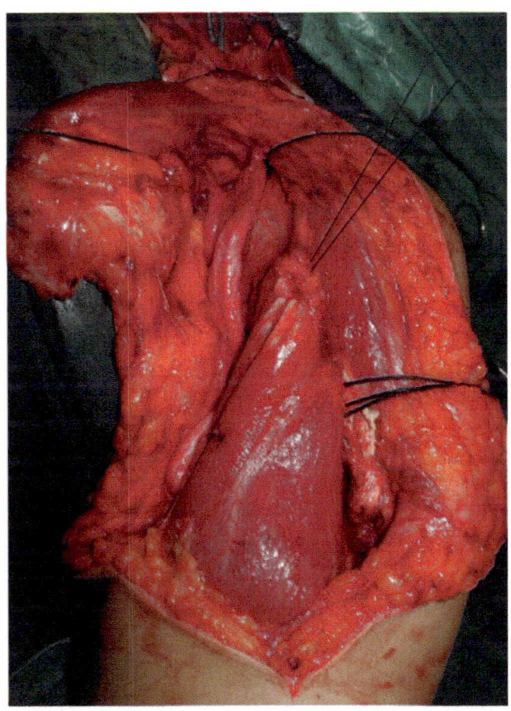

Fig. 35.7 Retighten the suture of the tendon of the biceps

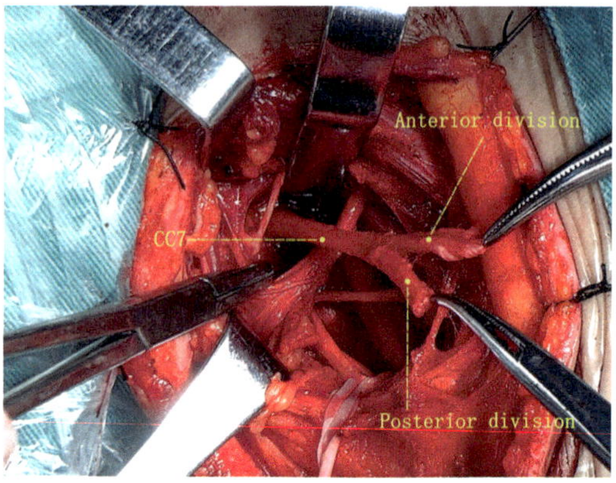

Fig. 35.8 Intraoperative photography showing the CC7 transectioned at the distal end of anterior and posterior divisions and dissected up to the intervertebral foramen

distally as possible; it was divided at the junction between divisions and cords. Then the contralateral C7 nerve root was dissected proximally to the neuroforamina (Fig. 35.8).

Notes of Harvest of the CC7 Nerve Root:

Avoiding Mis-identification of the CC7 Nerve Root

Generally, identifying CC7 is relatively simple during the surgical operation. However, due to the existence of anatomical variation of brachial plexus, it is necessary to carefully identify whether the target nerve root was just as exactly as the CC7. After the brachial plexus in the health side was exposed, the suprascapular nerve, which originates at the origin of the posterior division of the upper trunk, should be identified first. Accordingly, the anterior division of the upper trunk and the C5 and C6 nerve roots can be identified, and subsequently the C7 nerve root can be exposed on the deep side. After preliminary identification, the anterior and posterior divisions originating from the C7 nerve root can be observed and fused with the anterior and posterior divisions of the upper trunk, respectively. Special attention is required if the target C7 nerve root is inconsistent with the normal anatomical structure described above, in case the target C7 nerve root may be mistakenly identified. In this situation, the lower trunk and C8 and T1 nerve roots should be exposed to confirm whether the target nerve root is the C7 nerve root. Additionally, if the diameter of the target nerve root is too small, then it should be considered whether variation exists in the target nerve. The authors once encountered a case in which two independent nerve roots exiting the one intervertebral foramen formed the C6 nerve root, the upper part join the C5, and the inferior part was mistakenly regarded as the C7 root. However, the correct C7 nerve root was still located on the deep side, which could have easily led to an incorrect cutting [19]. Additionally, the C7 nerve root is not inferior to the upper trunk but posterior to the upper trunk in some cases. In this circumstance, the lower trunk is easily regarded as the C7 nerve root. When the target nerve root was dissected distally, and the diameter of the posterior division is obvious smaller than the anterior division, this variance indicated that the identified target nerve root is probably the lower trunk rather than the C7 nerve root. Therefore, the deep side should be explored further to determine whether other nerve roots are present. Absence of the nerve roots indicates that the lower trunk was mistakenly identified as the C7. For the beginner, when the target C7 nerve root is found, you can give mechanical or electrical stimulation to see if there will be elbow or wrist extension action elicited.

Prevention of Iatrogenic Injury of the Posterior Division of Lower Trunk

After identifying the CC7 nerve root, its anterior and posterior divisions were dissected distally and then proximally until reaching the intervertebral foramen. Rarely, the posterior division of lower trunk joins the C7 nerve root at a very high level (prior to the C7 bifurcation of the anterior and posterior divisions). In this situation, if the C7 was sectioned at the distal end, it is equivalent to cutting off PDLT together, which can cause finger extension deficient of the healthy hand. Therefore, only after confirming that no PDLT joins the C7 in proximal level, the C7 nerve root was severed at its utmost distal end. In addition, since the posterior division of the C7 nerve root is deeply located, severing the posterior division of the C7 nerve root should prevent accidental injury of the PDLT [19, 12].

Prevention of Iatrogenic Injury of the Long Thoracic Nerve

The composition of long thoracic nerve comes from the branches of C 7 and C 5, 6 nerve roots. The branch arising from C 7 is small and long, and this branch needs to be cut off. In a few cases, this branch arising from C7 is very short, and the main trunk of the long thoracic nerve is closely attached to the posterior surface of C7 nerve root. It is easy to mistakenly sever the main trunk of the long thoracic nerve if it is incorrectly identified as the C7 branch of the long thoracic nerve (Fig. 35.9). As a result, a contralateral winged scapula may occur postoperatively.

Contraindication of Contralateral C7 Harvest

Physical examination of the sensory and motor function of the healthy upper limb should be carried out carefully pre-operation. Patients with the following conditions should not undergo CC7 nerve transfer: (a) patients with partial injury of the contralateral brachial plexus or those with elbow and finger extensor muscle strength lower than grade M4; (b) patients with cervical spinal cord injury and MRI test showing a high signal at the cervical spinal cord and those with a positive pathological reflex of the affected upper limb or the muscle strength of the contralateral limb decreased.

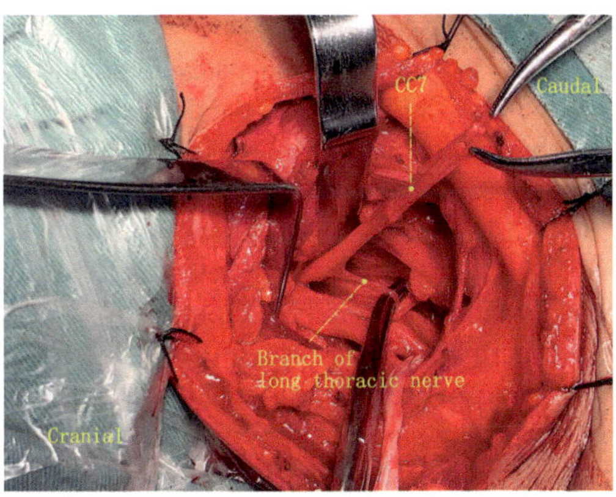

Fig. 35.9 Intraoperative photography showing the branch of the long thoracic nerve, which arises from the CC7

Preparation of Shortest Presipnal Route

Direct coaptation of the CC7 nerve root with the lower trunk or the medial cord without tension was based on the following prerequisites: **A**. The CC7 nerve is harvested to the maximum length. **B**. The shortest route is required for CC7 nerve transfer to the affected side. **C**. The lower trunk or the medial cord is used instead of the median nerve as the receipt nerve. The shortest prespinal routes consist of the CC7 to the paravertebral body and the retro-esophagus route. Surgical techniques to make this shortest route are gradual improving. After continuous optimization, the final shortest prespinal route has been established, and the surgical techniques are as follows.

1. The preparation of CC7 nerve root to the paravertebral body route: The interval space (angular space) between the medial margin of the anterior scalene muscle (Fig. 35.10) and the lateral margin of musculus longus colli was bluntly separated from the anterior to the deep until to the CC7 at the exit of intervetebral foramen. The CC7 nerve root emerging from the intervertebral foramen can be observed by pulling the anterior scalene muscle outward (Fig. 35.11).

Mobilize the contralateral C7 nerve root to the anterior aspect of the scalenus anterior through this expanded angular space (Fig. 35.12). After completing this step, the fibrous band attached at the exit of intervertebral foramen should be carefully examined to determine whether it is pressed against the CC7; if this is the case, then the fibrous band should be divided such that the pathway is sufficiently wide.

The vertebral artery and its accompanying vein are exposed in the angle space simultaneously (Fig. 35.13). The lateral part of the lon-

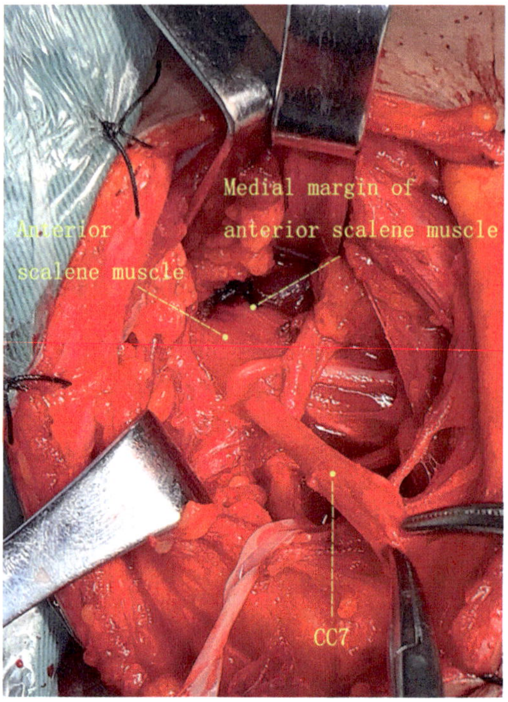

Fig. 35.10 Intraoperative photography showing the medial margin of anterior scanlene muscle. The angle space between the deep of the medial margin of anterior scanlene muscle and lateral margin of longus colli muscle

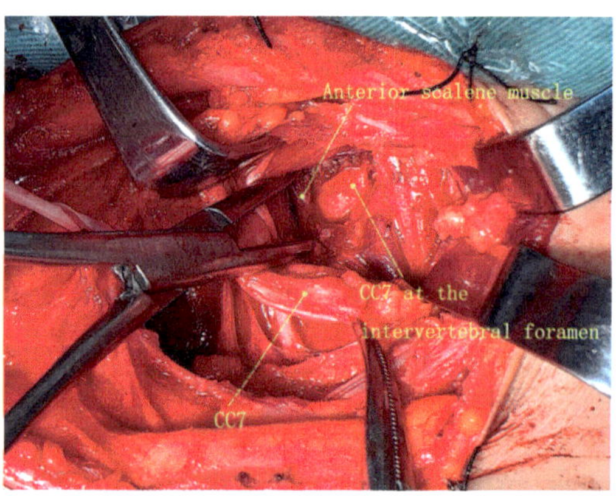

Fig. 35.11 Exposing the CC7 at the exit of intervertebral foramen through the angle space

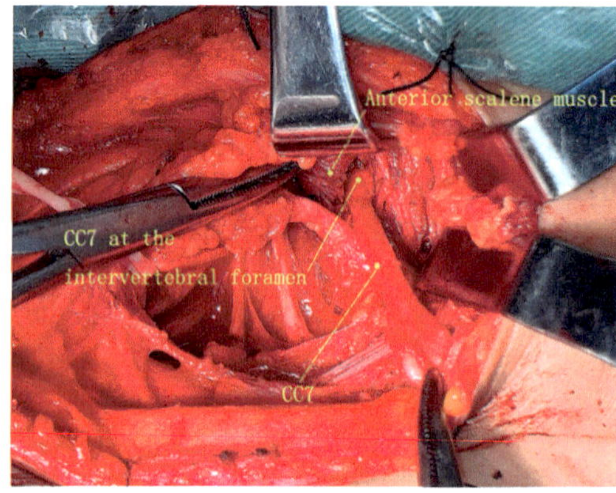

Fig. 35.12 Intraoperative photography showing the mobilization of the CC7 nerve root to the anterior aspect of the scalenus anterior through this expanded angular space

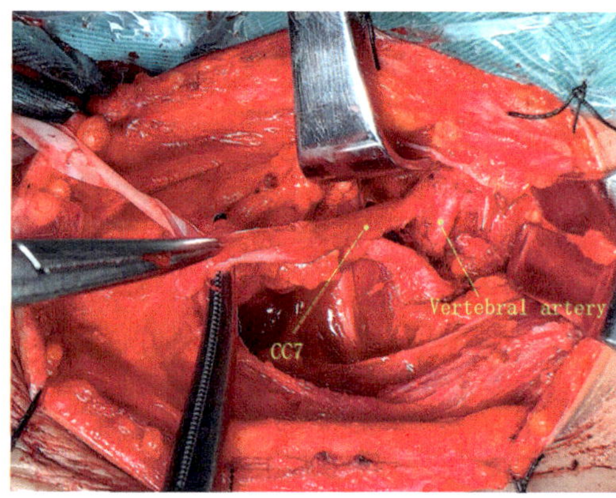

Fig. 35.13 The vertebral artery and the exit at the intervertebral foramen of CC7

gus colli is severed to form a deep groove and to fully visualize the vertebral artery and vein. The posterior space of the vertebral artery and vein is separated by using right angle forceps, and the vertebral artery and vein were fully freed. Then the CC7 is guided to the paravertebral body space by passing it through the deep side of the vertebral artery and the groove formed by dividing the lateral parts of longus colli (Figs. 35.14 and 35.15).

The above steps are completed under direct visualization. The vertebral artery and vein may bleed during isolation, which is usually caused by rupture of the venous branch. Bleeding can be stopped by bipolar coagulation after applying pressure with the tip of the finger. If the length of the CC7 is ≥7 cm, then the vertebral artery and vein may not be exposed, and the CC7 can pass through the front of the vertebral artery and vein.

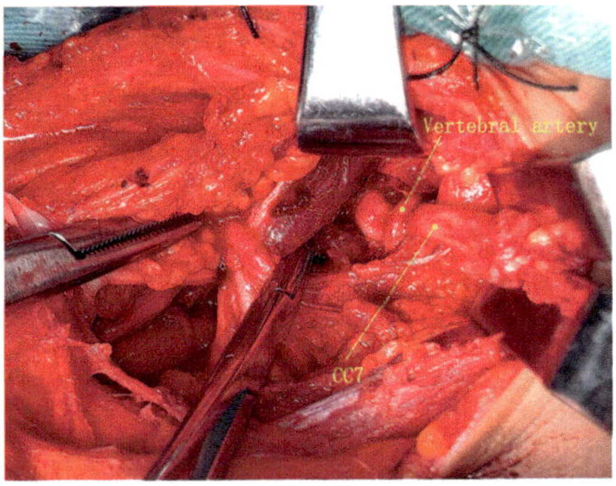

Fig. 35.14 Intraoperative photography showing the CC7 nerve root pass behind the vertebral artery

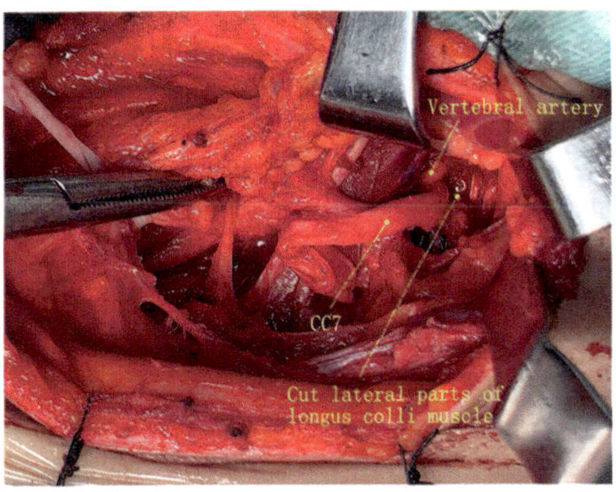

Fig. 35.15 Intraoperative photography showing the groove formed by divided the lateral parts of longus colli muscle, and the CC7 passed behind the vertebral artery

2. Preparation of the retro-esophagus route: In the supraclavicular incision of the affected side, dissection was performed along the anterior surface of the anterior scalene muscle from the lateral to the medial until reaching the space between the esophagus and the anterior vertebral body of the affected side. The pathway is temporarily filled with gauze. In some cases, the anterior aspect of anterior scalene muscle adheres to the posterior wall of internal jugular vein because of dense scar, and the boundary between the posterior aspect of internal jugular vein and the anterior aspect of anterior scalene muscle is difficult to identify. So it can break the internal jugular vein and cause serious bleeding when creating retro-esophagus route. The key point to prevent the above-mentioned adverse complication is to identify the anterior surface of the anterior scalene muscle accurately, and the dissection was performed closely along its anterior surface. On the contralateral, uninjured side, continue to dissect the anterior surface of the longus colli muscle bluntly until to the retro-esophagus space. The retro-esophagus route of the healthy side and affected side was connected by using long forceps under direct inspection from both side. Pass a plastic tube with a diameter of approximately 5 mm through the prefabricated prespinal tunnel from the injured side to the healthy side. Insert the contralateral C7 nerve root into the plastic tube and suture it in place (Fig. 35.16). Then, pass the contralateral C7 nerve root to the injured side using the plastic tube as a guide. Generally, the CC7 nerve can reach the midline or more lateral of the scalenus anterior muscle on the injured side (Figs. 35.17, 35.18, and 35.19).

In rare cases, the length of the CC7 nerve root is shorter than 6 cm or the patient's neck is very short and thick; therefore, the ultimate reach of the CC7 could only be at the medial border of the affected scalenus anterior muscle. Consequently, the process of completion of CC7 nerve direct anastomosis with lower trunk is very difficult due to the deep position of CC7 nerve in the above-

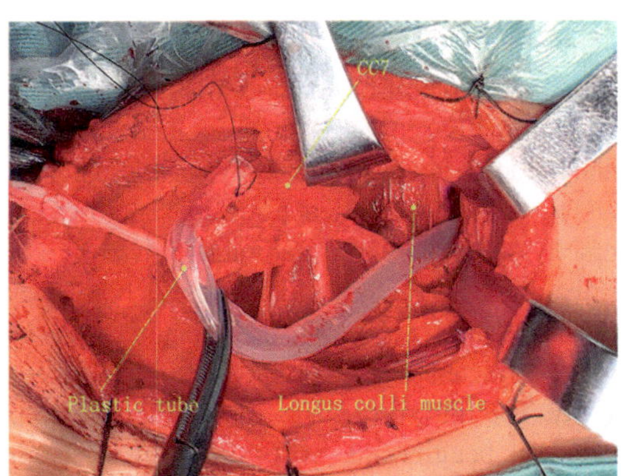

Fig. 35.16 The CC7 wrapped in the plastic tube and sutured in place

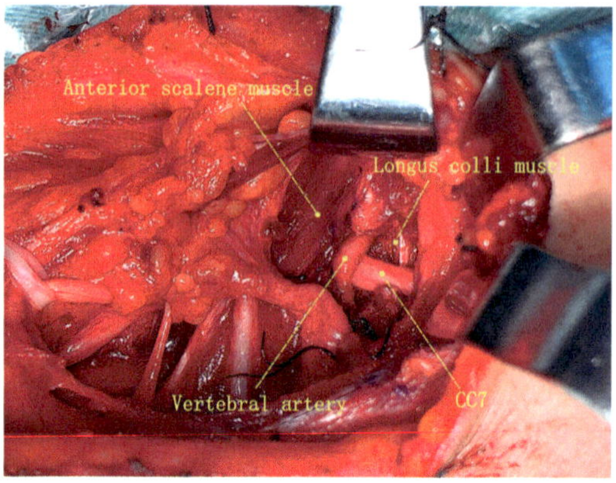

Fig. 35.17 On the healthy side, the CC7 passed the behind of vertebral artery and through the groove formed by divided the lateral parts of longus colli muscle

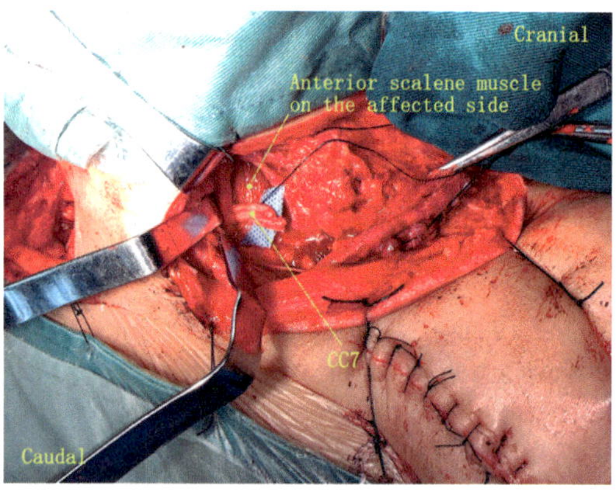

Fig. 35.18 The CC7 transferred to the injured side via the shortest prespinal route

mentioned circumstance, and the solution is to extend the supraclavicular incision to the medial until it reaches the medial margin of the sternocleidomastoid muscle on the affected side and longitudinally separated along its medial border and retracted lateral. The omohyoid was exposed, and then the deep cervical fascia that encloses the omohyoid medial to the carotid sheath was carefully divided. The anterior vertebral body was exposed while the carotid sheath and esophagus were retracted laterally and medially, respectively. The retro-esophagus route of the affected side and healthy side was connected by blunt dissection under direct inspection. The CC7 nerve root was transferred to the interval space between the carotid sheath and esophagus on

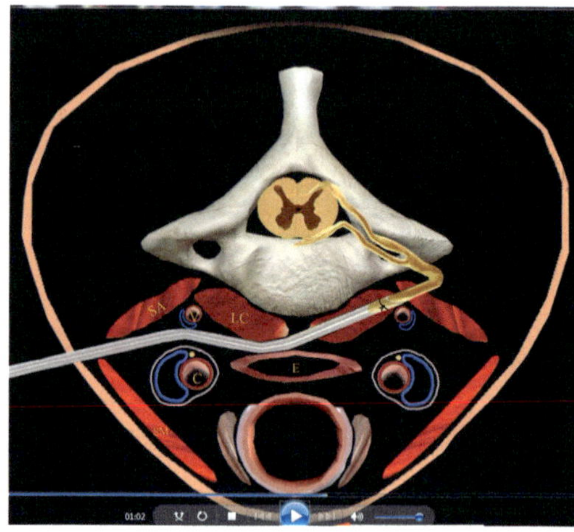

Fig. 35.19 Schematic illustration of the contralateral C7 nerve transfer via the shortest prespinal route. LC longus colli muscle, SA scalenus anterior muscle, E esophagus, C carotid sheath, V vertebral artery, SM sternocleidomastoid

the injured side by using a plastic tube as in the above-mentioned method, and the lower trunk of the affected side is pulled into this space through the back of the sternocleidomastoid [20]. Direct coaptation of CC7 with the lower trunk can be completed at this space.

Sequence of Nerve Anastomosis and Postoperative Management

After the CC7 nerve has been transferred to the injured side through the shortest prespinal route, in the infraclavicular incision, one band of sural nerve graft together with the medial antebrachial cutaneous nerve which is divided at the appropriate level of the injured upper arm is first coapted with the musculocutaneous nerve. Then the other end of the grafted sural nerve together with the PDLT and the freed lower trunk is pulled to the supraclavicular incision from behind the clavicle, and the infraclavicular incision is closed first. Then the affected upper limb is wrapped with sterile dressing and positioned with the shoulder in 0° of adduction and 0–10°of anterior flexion, the elbow in 90°of flexion, and the forearm placed on the abdomen. This position is maintained until the operation is finished and a prefabricated brace is applied. The sequence of nerve repair in the supraclavicular incision was as follows: the terminal branch of the accessory nerve was directly coapted with the suprascapular nerve. Then the phrenic nerve was directly coapted with the PDLT. Finally, the freed lower trunk is preferably divided just distal to where the PDLT arises, and direct coaptation of the CC7 nerve with the injured lower trunk is performed with use of 8–0 nylon. The other end of the grafted sural nerve is coapted with the lateral pectoral nerve, which originates from the anterior division of the CC7 such that the musculocutaneous nerve is connected to more nerve fibers (Fig. 35.20).

After surgery, a prefabricated brace was used to hold the patient's head in the neutral position and the entire upper extremity is immobilized with the shoulder in 0 °of adduction and 0–10° of anterior flexion, the elbow in 90° of flexion, and the forearm placed on the abdomen for 6 weeks (Fig. 35.21). Passive hand and wrist exercises were performed during that period.

After removing the brace, the affected limb is suspended with a sling with the elbow in 90° of flexion for 1 week. Passive activities of the shoulder, elbow, wrist, and finger are then initiated, together with electrical stimulation therapy. Patients are asked to perform active shoulder adduction training of the contralateral side 2000 times each day, as well as deep breathing training. Patients are also asked to follow-up every 2–3 months. Since the recovery of finger extension is slower than finger flexion, patients should wear finger extension brace immediately after recovering from finger flexion function. Otherwise, finger flexion contracture will occur due to the lack of finger extension antagonism, which will eventually lead to relaxation of the central slip and slipping of the lateral slip, thereby complicating the reconstruction of hand function in the later stage.

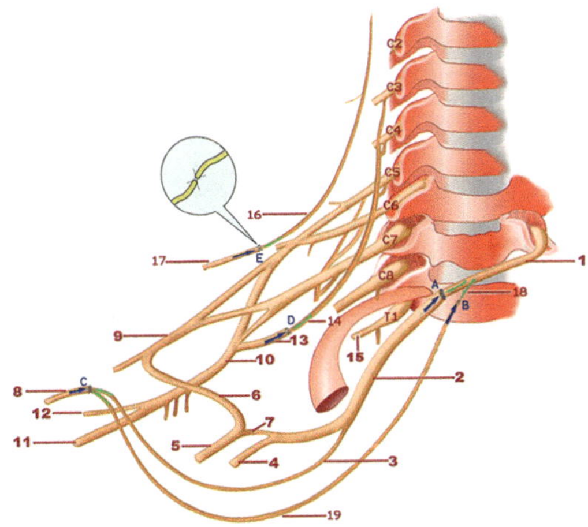

Fig. 35.20 Schematic illustration of the modified multiple nerve transfers, which were performed in all of the patients in this group. 1: contralateral C7 nerve root (CC7), 2: lower trunk, 3: medial antebrachial cutaneous nerve, 4: ulnar nerve, 5: median nerve, 6: lateral cord of median nerve, 7: medial cord of median nerve, 8: musculocutaneous nerve, 9: lateral cord, 10: posterior cord, 11: radial nerve, 12: axillary nerve, 13: posterior division of lower trunk (PDLT), 14: phrenic nerve, 15: T1 nerve root, 16: spinal accessory nerve, 17: suprascapular nerve, 18: lateral pectoral nerve originating from anterior division of CC7, 19: grafting sural nerve. A: coaptation between CC7 and lower trunk, B: coaptation between lateral pectoral nerve and sural nerve, C: coaptation between sural nerve and medial antebrachial cutaneous nerve and musculocutaneous nerve, D: coaptation between phrenic nerve and PDLT, E: coaptation between spinal accessory nerve and suprascapular nerve. Note: A and C show that the CC7 was transferred to the lower trunk with direct coaptation to restore lower trunk function (A) and the CC7 was also transferred to the musculocutaneous nerve with interpositional bridging by medial antebrachial cutaneous nerve arising from the lower trunk to restore elbow flexion (C). To enhance the strength of elbow flexion, we also transfer the lateral pectoral nerve onto the musculocutaneous nerve using sural nerve as a graft (B and C). (Copyright of Fig. 35.20 need the permission of Ref. [15])

Secondary Hand Function Reconstruction

Patients with total brachial plexus avulsion injuries first underwent modified multiple nerve transfers in one stage. These included transfer of the accessory nerve onto the suprascapular nerve to recover shoulder abduction, contralateral C7 nerve onto the lower trunk or medial cord via the shortest prespinal route with direct coaptation to restore finger flexion and onto the musculocutaneous nerve with interpositional bridging by medial antebrachial cutaneous nerve arising from lower trunk together with the sural graft to restore elbow flexion, and the phrenic nerve onto the posterior division of lower trunk to

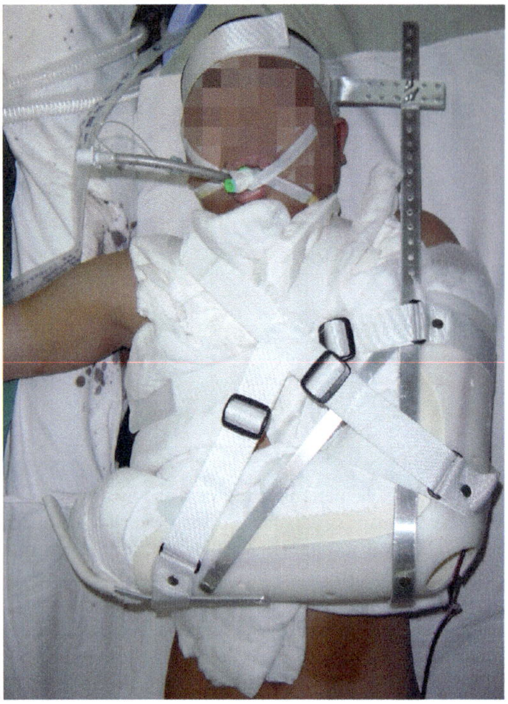

Fig. 35.21 A prefabricated brace to hold the head in the neutral position and immobilize the injured limb

recover elbow and finger extension. However, the patients still could not complete the active pick-up function using the affected limb even if the above mentioned five functions are effectively reconstructed. Only after the additional secondary hand procedures could the patients complete active pick-up objects in daily life. So, secondary hand function reconstruction procedures are critical for restoring active pick-up function of the affected hand.

Prerequisites for Secondary Hand Function Reconstruction Procedures

At least 3 years in adults or 2 years in children after the modified multiple nerve transfers, the secondary hand reconstruction surgeries were only indicated in cases when the nerve transfers had resulted in effective recovery, including a degree of shoulder abduction of 30°or better; elbow, wrist, and finger flexion strength grade of M4 or better; and elbow and finger extension strength grade of M3 or better and normal passive activity of the MP and interphalangeal joints. Muscle strength is assessed according to the muscle grading system of the British Medical Research Council (BMRC) [21].

Secondary Hand Function Reconstruction Procedures

The patients with total brachial plexus nerve avulsion injury who underwent modified multiple nerve transfers can achieve satisfactory results of the finger and wrist flexion and finger extension; however, the patients still cannot use their hand to complete the active grasping function due to the difficult reorganization and remodeling of the cerebral cortex after the primary procedure of multiple nerve transfers. We observed that the restored function of wrist and finger flexion contract simultaneously, since both function were restored by CC7 direct repair the lower trunk that is, the patient unable to complete the independent finger flexion or wrist flexion, even after long-term rehabilitation training. In the above-mentioned situation, wrist motions are difficult to play a synergistic role to the finger flexion or extension. Therefore, without the stability of the wrist, it is impossible to complete the active pick-up function of the hand. Wrist arthrodesis is one of the prerequisites for patients to complete active grasp after multiple nerve transfers in total brachial plexus avulsion injuries. In addition to the wrist arthrodesis, the secondary hand reconstruction procedures include claw-finger correction and thumb opposition.

Wrist Arthrodesis

If the patient is younger than 14 years old, wrist fusion is not suitable as the epiphyses of distal radius and carpus were not closed. We usually select the procedure of wrist tenodesis, or use the wrist brace until the children is older than 14 years and then select the wrist fusion.

Wrist Fusion

The traditional procedure of wrist fusion is through the dorsal middle approach of the wrist (between the third and fourth extensor tendon sheaths) [22] .The deficiency of this approach was that it exposed the common extensor tendons widely and easily caused the complication of tendon adhesion after the operation. Consequently, the patients would lose their function of finger extension. In order to overcome the above-mentioned complication, a modified approach of wrist fusion was designed through the ulnar dorsal of the wrist. This approach is through the wrist joint at the ulnar side of the extensor carpi ulnaris. Approximately 1.5–2 cm of the distal ulnar head was resected and the triquetrum was removed. The articular cartilage of the distal radius, scaphoid, lunate, capitate, hamate trapezium, and trapezoid was removed. The resected ulnar head was modified and implanted between the proximal end of the hamate and the distal end of the radius. The distal end of the pre-bent plate was located on the ulnar side or dorsal side of the fifth metacarpal, and the proximal end was on the ulnar side of the radius (Fig. 35.22). The angle of wrist fusion must be determined comprehensively according to the specific conditions of preoperative finger flexor and extensor strength. If finger flexor strength is strong and extensor strength is weak, the wrist joint can be integrated at 0° or a slightly flexed position.

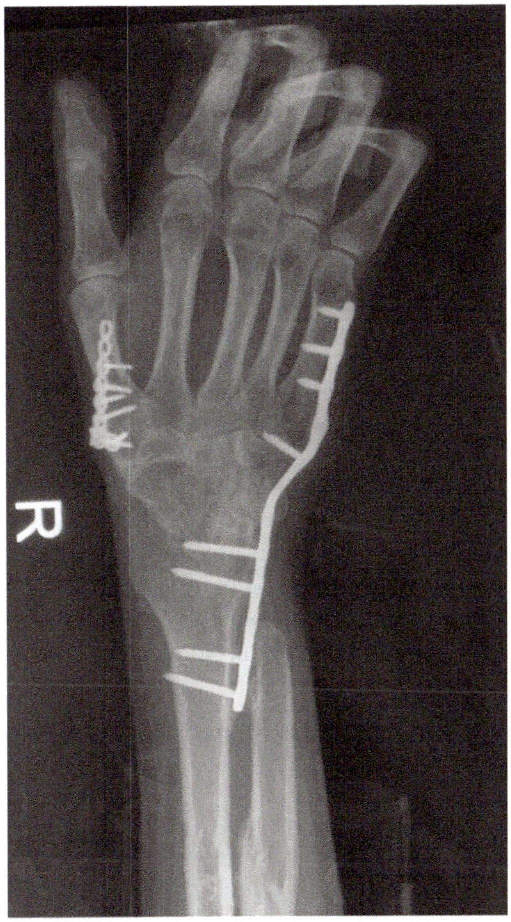

Fig. 35.22 The wrist fusion through the ulnar dorsal side approach of the wrist

Wrist Tenodesis in Children

For the wrist tenodesis, a dorsoradial incision on the distal forearm is made. An osseous tunnel was created through the distal radius, and the flexor carpi radialis was cut at the more proximal level. The distal end of flexor carpi radialis was passed through the prefabricated bone tunnel from the anterior to the posterior and sutured to the distal part of extensor carpi radialis longus using pulvertaft technique, and then the distal part of extensor carpi radialis longus was covered with periosteum. The child was immobilized with a plaster of Paris cast with finger inclusion for 6 weeks and protected with a palmar splint without finger inclusion for another 8 weeks.

Correction of Claw Finger

Palmar capsulodesis of the metacarpophalangeal joints (MPJ) was performed on the index, middle, ring, and small fingers but not the thumb, because our patients did not have an obvious deformity there. For patients with serious PIP joint flexion deformity of the fingers, isolated palmar capsulodesis of MPJ could not successfully correct the claw-finger deformity completely, and PIP joint central tendon shortening suture was performed simultaneously. If the finger flexor and extensor strengths are balanced, then the claw finger deformity is mild and does not need to be corrected.

Reconstruction of Thumb Opposition

The flexor carpi ulnaris (FCU) strength usually recovers well; therefore, we prefer to select FCU transfer for thumb opponensplasty. As the first carpometacarpal (CMC) joint is not stable because of imbalanced forces (i.e., thenar muscles, abductor pollicis longus, and extensor brevis pollicis are paralyzed), after this transfer, a palmar flexion deformity of the thumb maybe occurred. Therefore, the abductor pollicis longus tendon was fastened and inserted into the brachioradialis tendon simultaneously to stabilize the first CMC joint. Additionally, the first CMC joint fusion can be performed for patients with poor outcomes after dynamic thumb opposition reconstruction.

Results of This Surgical Procedures

According to our follow-up data, 48 patients with total brachial plexus avulsion injuries underwent modified multiple nerve transfers between 2006 and 2009 [14]. Forty patients were followed up for more than 3 years and had complete data: an average age of 25 years (4–44 years) and an average interval between injury and surgery of 3 months (1–11 months) . The mean follow-up was 53 months (range 37–76 m.s). The average shoulder abduction was 51° (range 0–90°). Meaningful recovery of elbow extension (M3 or better) was achieved in 29 cases (72.5%) and motor strength of finger extension was attained (M3 or better) in 15 cases (37.5%). In 25 cases (62.5%), strength for finger flexion (M4 or better) was achieved, and meaningful recovery of wrist flexion and elbow flexion (M4 or better) was achieved in 28 cases (70%) and 24 cases (60%), respectively.

Twelve patients (30%) achieved elbow, wrist, and finger flexion strength of M4 or better, elbow and finger extension strength of M3 or better, and 50–90°shoulder abduction. These patients underwent secondary hand reconstruction. Overall, active pick-up function was recovered in 10 patients (25%) in this series (Fig. 35.23a–e and Video 35.1; Fig. 35.24a–d and Videos 35.2 and 35.3).

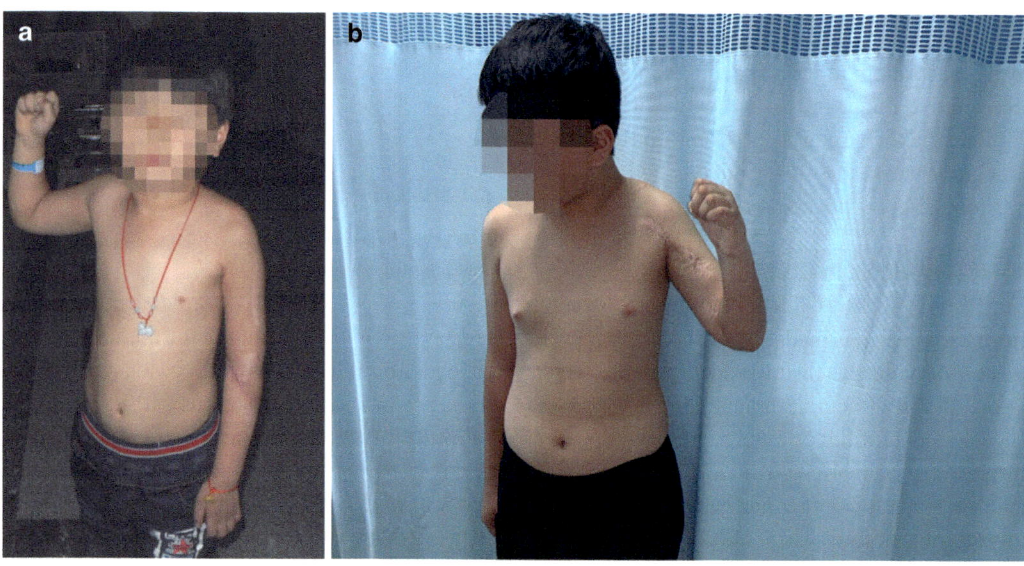

Fig. 35.23 (**a**) A 7-year-old patient sustained a left total brachial plexus injury following a traffic accident on August 20, 2012. The patient underwent surgical exploration and nerve repair on December 3, 2012. Complete C5 to T1 avulsion injuries were confirmed. The reconstructive procedure included transfer of accessory nerve onto the suprascapular nerve, direct coaptation of phrenic nerve with the posterior division of lower trunk, transfer of the CC7 onto the lower trunk via the shortest prespinal route with direct coaptation and also onto the anterior division of upper trunk (for recovering the elbow flexion) with interpositional bridging by the medial antebrachial cutaneous nerve arising from lower trunk, and one band sural graft connected to the lateral pectoral nerve that arose from the anterior division of CC7. About 7 years after the first surgical procedure, the patient underwent the secondary hand function reconstruction, which included wrist fusion and the flexor carpi ulnaris transfer for thumb opposition reconstruction. (**b**) Preoperative CTM examination indicated the C5-T1 nerve roots avulsion injuries. (**c**) Eighty-eight months after the first operation, follow-up demonstrated satisfactory recovery of elbow flexion and finger flexion. (**d**) Eighty-eight months after the first operation, follow-up demonstrated satisfactory recovery of shoulder abduction, elbow extension, and finger extension. (**e**) Limited wrist fusion, the epiphysis of the distal radius was not injured and was not closed

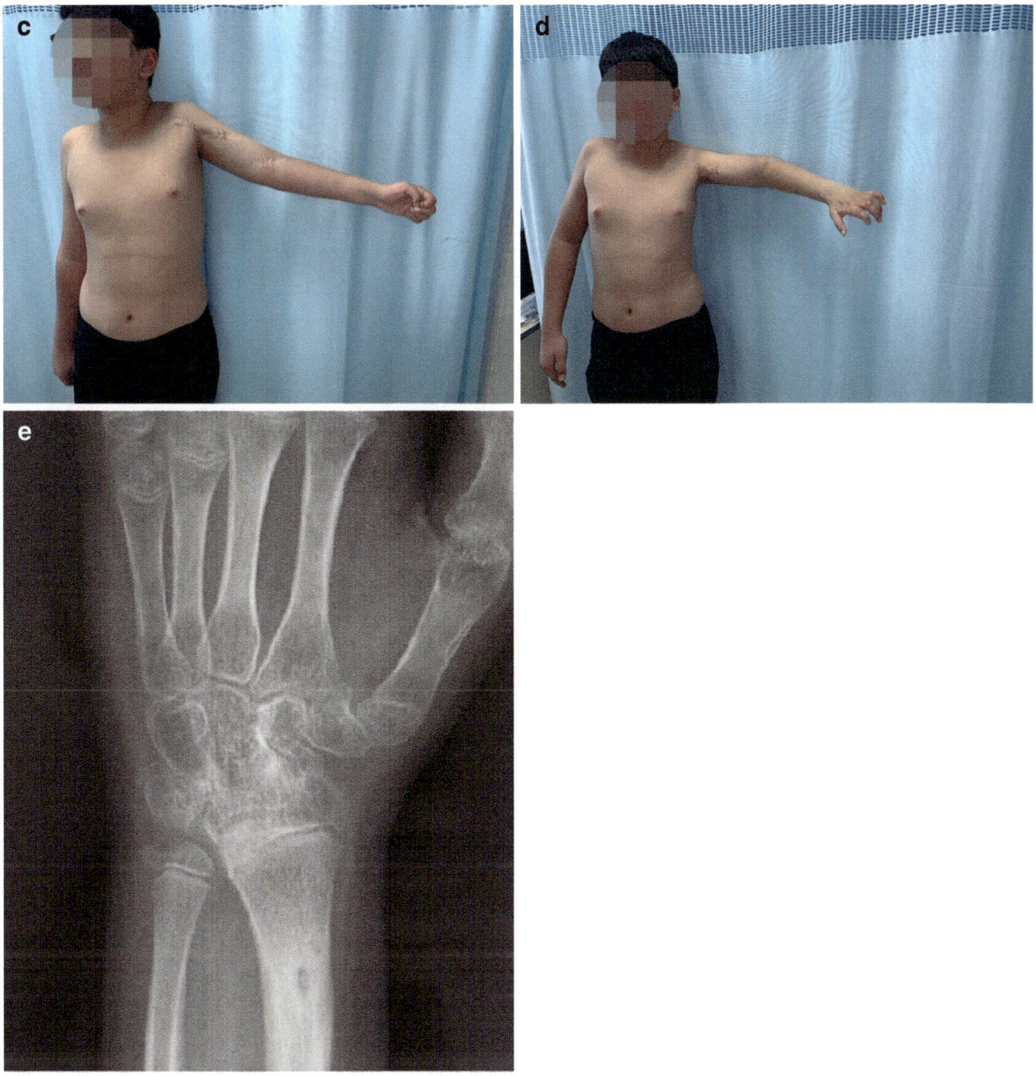

Fig. 35.23 (continued)

Overall Evaluation and Problems of this Surgical Procedure

The newly designed multiple nerve transfer procedure has contributed to substantial progress in hand function reconstruction. Currently, some patients have recovered active pick-up function in completely paralyzed upper limbs, indicating that they can use the restored hand to complete active grasping function. The efficacy of this reconstruction procedure was satisfactory in younger people especially in adolescents and children, and the procedure has substantially helped patients in their daily and professional lives. However, in general, the rate of active pick-up function recovery remains low. One of the main factors contributing to this low rate is that finger extension after nerve transfers is not adequately restored. The focus of future research will be to improve the efficacy of surgery to restore finger extension, which is extremely difficult to restore than finger flexion.

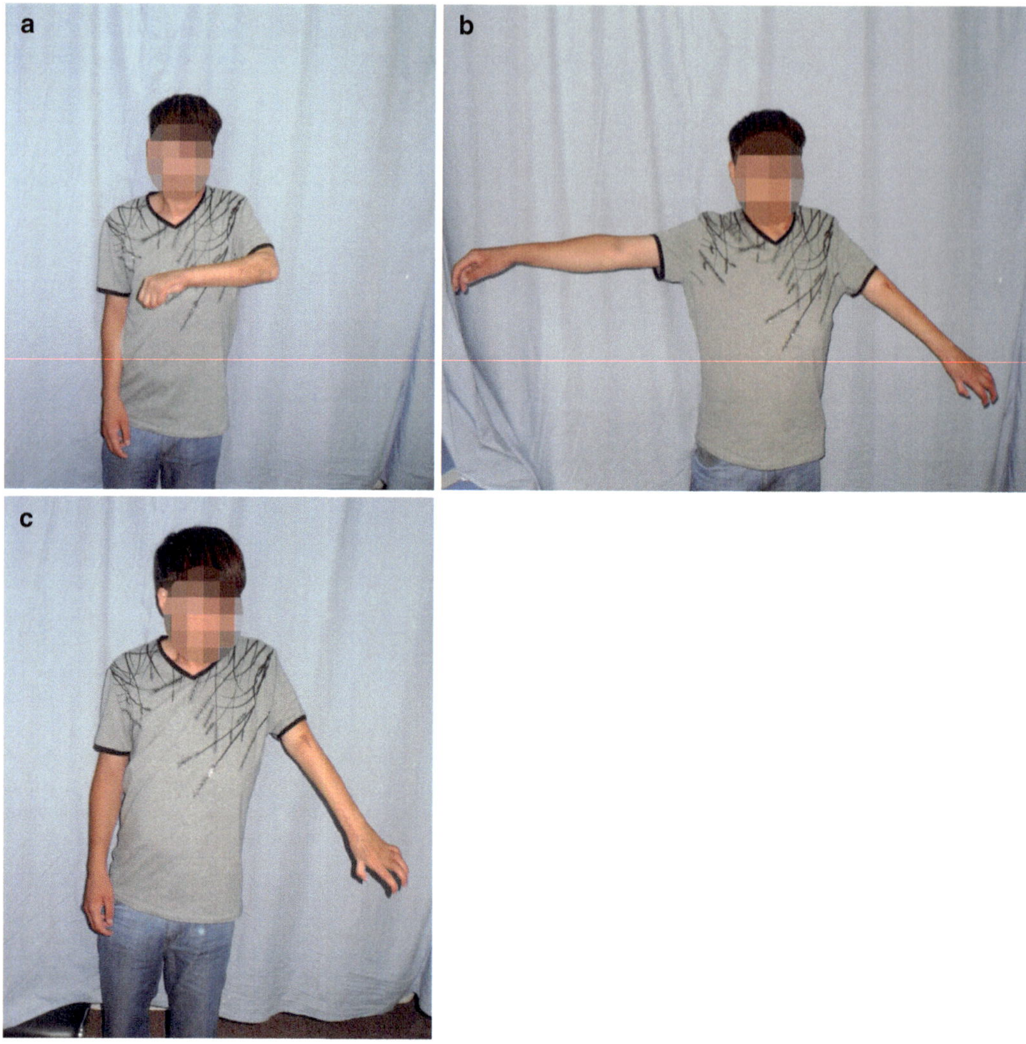

Fig. 35.24 (**a**) A 25-year-old patient suffered a left total brachial plexus avulsion injury after a motorcycle accident on December 23, 2008. The patient underwent surgical exploration and nerve reconstruction 3 months after the injury. Completely total brachial plexus avulsion injury was confirmed. Nerve transfers were performed. The distal accessory nerve was used to neurotize the suprascapular nerve . Phrenic nerve transfer to the posterior division of lower trunk with direct coaptation. CC7 nerve root was transferred via the shortest prespinal route to be directly coapted with the lower trunk. The musculocutaneous nerve was also neurotized by the CC7 through the medial antebrachial cutaneous nerve bridging. The humerus was shorten 4 cm and refixed by locking compress plate. On September 18, 2012, the patient underwent the secondary hand function reconstruction, which included wrist fusion and the thumb opposition reconstruction by flexor carpi ulnaris transfer for thumb opposition reconstruction, and the first CMC joint tenodesis. (**b**) Follow-up demonstrated satisfactory functional recovery of shoulder abduction about 50° 4 years after the first operation. (**c**) Follow-up demonstrated satisfactory functional recovery of finger extension at 4-year follow-up after first operation

The efficacy of nerve transfers is closely related to patient age and the time interval from injury to surgery. This modified multiple nerve transfer procedure is not suitable for patients older than 50 years. Direct restoration of the lower trunk by CC7 nerve transfer and restoration of the PDLT by phrenic nerve transfer are not recommended for patients with the delay from injury to surgical operation over 8 months, patients with forearm ischemic muscle contracture, and patients with damaged forearm muscles.

Since the motor donor nerves for this modified multiple nerve transfers are from the extra of brachial plexus, especially after CC7 nerve transfer, they require retraction of the contralateral upper limb with force to be induced. So, the functional reorganization of the cerebral cortex after this modified multiple nerve transfer was very difficult. Additionally, effective recovery of the intrinsic muscle was very difficult to achieve, and the forearm has no rotation function; thus, the active grasping function of the affected hand is not flexible.

We propose the concept of the active pick-up function, which is defined as actively touching a target object without the help of the contralateral hand, grabbing it, moving it to another place, and putting it down. Depending on the size and weight of the objects tested, the active pick-up function can be more or less difficult. Therefore, assessment criteria need to be further defined and validated in further studies [15].

References

1. Chuang DC. Neurotization procedures for brachial plexus injuries. Hand Clin. 1995;11:633–45.
2. Narakas AO, Hentz VR. Neurotization in brachial plexus injuries. Indication and results. Clin Orthop Relat Res. 1988;(237):43–56.
3. Doi K. Management of total paralysis of the brachial plexus by the double free-muscle transfer technique. J Hand Surg Eur. 2008;33:240–51.
4. Gu YD, Zhang GM, Chen DS, Yan JG, Cheng XM, Chen L. Seventh cervical nerve root transfer from the contralateral healthy side for treatment of brachial plexus root avulsion. J Hand Surg Br. 1992;17:518–21.
5. Gu Y, Xu J, Chen L, Wang H, Hu S. Long term outcome of contralateral C7 transfer: a report of 32 cases. Chin Med J. 2002;115(6):866–8.
6. Terzis JK, Kokkalis ZT. Selective contralateral C7 transfer in posttraumatic brachial plexus injuries: a report of 56 cases. Plast Reconstr Surg. 2009;123(3):927–38.
7. Gu YD. Contralateral C7 root transfer over the last 20 years in China. Chin Med J. 2007;120(13):1123–6.
8. Waikakul S, Orapin S, Vanadurongwan V. Clinical results of contralateral C7 root neurotization to the median nerve in brachial plexus injuries with total root avulsions. J Hand Surg Br. 1999;24(5):556–60.
9. Sammer DM, Kircher MF, Bishop AT, Spinner RJ, Shin AY. Hemi-contralateral C7 transfer in traumatic brachial plexus injuries: outcomes and complications. J Bone Joint Surg Am. 2012;94(2):131–7.
10. Wang SF, Hu Q, Pan YW. Feasibility of direct anastomosis of contralateral C7 transferred through prespinal route with lower trunk in patient with brachial plexus root avulsion. Chinese J Pract Hand Surg. 2005;119:67–9.
11. Wang SF, Li PC, Xue YH, Yiu HW, Li YC, Wang HH. Contralateral C7 nerve transfer with direct coaptation to restore lower trunk function after traumatic brachial plexus avulsion. J Bone Joint Surg Am. 2013;95:821–7.
12. Bhatia A, Doshi P, Koul A, Shah V, Brown JM, Salama M. Contralateral C-7 transfer: is direct repair really superior to grafting? Neurosurg Focus. 2017;43(1):E3. 1-9
13. Li WJ, Wang SF, Li PC, et al. Electrophysiological study of the dominant motor innervation to the extensor digitorum communis muscle and long head of triceps brachii at posterior divisions of brachial plexus. Microsurgery. 2011;31(7):535–8.
14. Wang SF, Li PC, Xue YH, Zou JY, Li WJ, Li YC. Direct coaptation of the phrenic nerve with the posterior division of the lower trunk to restore finger and elbow extension function in patients with total brachial plexus injuries. Neurosurgery. 2016;78:208–15.
15. Li F, Wang SF, Li PC, Xue YH, Zou JY, Li WJ. Restoration of active pick-up function in patients with total brachial plexus avulsion injuries. J Hand Surg (E). 2018;43(2):269–74.
16. Moran SL, Steinmann SP, Shin AY. Adult brachial plexus injuries: mechanism, patterns of injury, and physical diagnosis. Hand Clin. 2005;21:13–24.
17. Harper CM. Preoperative and intraoperative electrophysiologic assessment of brachial plexus injuries. Hand Clin. 2005;21:39–46.
18. Sunderland IR, Brenner MJ, Singham J, Rickman SR, Hunter DA, Mackinnon SE. Effect of tension on nerve regeneration in rat sciatic nerve transection model. Ann Plast Surg. 2004;53(4):382–7.
19. Li WJ, Wang SF, Zho JY, Rahman MF, Li YC, Li PC, Xue YH. Complications of contralateral C-7 transfer through the modified prespinal route for repairing brachial plexus root avulsion injury: a retrospective study of 425 patients. J Neurosurg. 2014;12:1–8.
20. Wang SF, Yiu HW, Li PC, Li YC, Wang HH, Pan YW. Contralateral C7 nerve root transfer to neurotize the upper trunk via a modified prespinal route in repair of brachial plexus avulsion injury. Microsurgery. 2012;32:183–8.
21. James MA. Use of the Medical Research Council muscle strength grading system in the upper extremity. J Hand Surg Am. 2007;32:154–6.
22. Terzis JK, Barmpitsioti A. Wrist fusion in posttraumatic brachial plexus palsy. Plast Reconstr Surg. 2009;124:2027–39.

Intercostal Nerve Transfer for Sensory Reconstruction of the Hand Following Complete Avulsion of the Brachial Plexus

36

Yasunori Hattori

Introduction

Functional reconstruction of the hand following complete avulsion of the brachial plexus has been the main focus in the treatment of brachial plexus injury (BPI).

For this purpose, several procedures, including nerve transfer to the median nerve using contralateral seventh cervical nerve root (CC7) transfer and combined functioning free muscle transfer (FFMT), have been reported [1–5]. Although the recovery of motor function has been the main focus in brachial plexus reconstruction, restoration of basic sensory function of the hand is imperative when hand function is restored after irreparable BPI.

For sensory reconstruction of the hand, the median nerve should be the recipient nerve because of its wider sensory cutaneous distribution. There are several previous reports that focus on the results of sensory recovery after brachial plexus reconstruction [2, 4, 6–10] (Table 36.1). The intercostal nerve, supraclavicular nerve, and CC7 have been the primary donors for sensory fibers. Although we used the supraclavicular nerve for sensory reconstruction in earlier series of double free muscle transfer, the priority of the donor sensory nerve has been changed to the intercostal nerve in our current strategy of double free muscle transfer. The intercostal nerve transfer has demonstrated superior results with regard to sensory recovery and has easier access in the axillary dissection [5]. The whole nerve trunk or only the sensory ramus of the intercostal nerve can be used for sensory reconstruction.

Surgical Technique

Motor reconstructions such as nerve transfer or FFMT were performed, and sensory reconstruction is performed during the same surgery. A curved longitudinal incision was made from medial upper arm to anterior chest along the anterior axillary line. Fatty tissue in the axillar region was dissected and carefully mobilized. Sensory rami of intercostal nerves are identified within this adipose tissue. Sensory rami of the second and third intercostal nerves are frequently used. Sensory rami are transected distally and reflected towards the infraclavicular space to reach the median nerve. Sensory rami of the intercostal nerves and median nerve were sutured in the infraclavicular region using three or four 10-0 nylon stitches under an operative microscope (Fig. 36.1).

Y. Hattori (✉)
Department of Orthopedic Surgery, Ogori Daiichi General Hospital, Yamaguchi City, Yamaguchi Prefecture, Japan
e-mail: yhattori@saikyo.or.jp

A. Y. Shin, N. Pulos (eds.), *Operative Brachial Plexus Surgery*,
https://doi.org/10.1007/978-3-030-69517-0_36

Table 36.1 Results of sensory recovery in previous studies

Author(s), year	Number of patients/donor(s)	Results
Ihara et al., 1996	13/ICNs in 3 and SCN in 10	S2 in 3 patients using ICNs and S2 in 2 patients using SCN
Gu et al., 1998	8/CC7	S3 in 6 patients
Songchaoren et al., 2001	21/CC7	S3 in 10 patients, S2 in 7 patients
Terzis et al., 2008	29/CC7	S3 in 12 patients, S2 in 10 patients
Hattori et al., 2009	17/ICNs	S2+ in 2 patients, S2 in 9 patients, S1 in 6 patients
Gao et al., 2013	22/CC7	S3 in 10 patients
Foroni et al., 2017	11/ICNs	S3 in 2 patients, S2+ in 2 patients, S2 in 6 patients, S1 in 1 patient

CC7 contralateral C7, *ICNs* intercostal nerves, *SCN* supraclavicular nerve

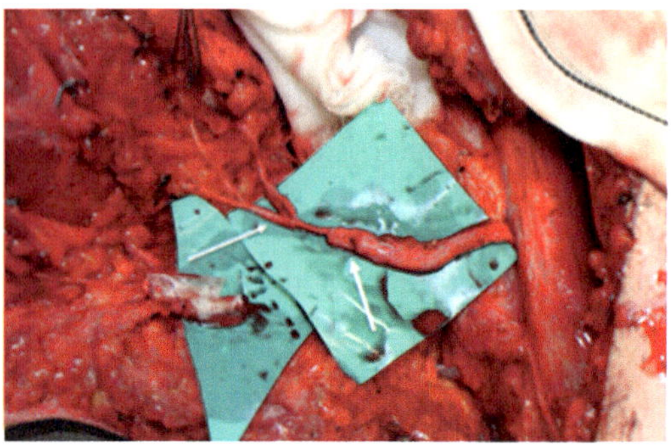

Fig. 36.1 Intraoperative view of intercostal nerve transfer to the median nerve. The large arrow indicates the median nerve and the small arrows indicate the intercostal nerves

Discussion

Nerve transfer to the median nerve has been performed for more than 30 years in an attempt to reconstruct sensibility to the hand in patients with complete BPI [11, 12]. In 1977, Millesi reported the recovery of protective sensation in 15 of 18 patients who underwent sensory reconstruction by nerve graft or intercostal nerve crossing after complete BPI with multiple roots avulsion [11]. In 1988, Kawai et al. reported S2 recovery in 5 of 13 cases in which intercostal nerve crossing was performed for both sensory and motor reconstruction [13]. In 1996, Ihara et al. reported the results of 13 cases in which the sensory rami of the intercostal nerves (3 cases) or the supraclavicular nerve (10 cases) had been used for sensory reconstruction [6]. The intercostal nerve provided S2 recovery in all cases, whereas the supraclavicular nerve provided S2 recovery in only two of ten patients. Ihara et al. reported that a possible explanation for the inferior results of the supraclavicular nerve is that the site of nerve crossing is 10 cm more proximal and that there are fewer sensory fibers present [6].

Hattori et al. reported the long-term results with 17 patients who underwent sensory reconstruction of the hand with intercostal nerve transfer to the median or ulnar nerve [8]. All patients underwent double free muscle transfer to restore the prehensile function of the hand. All patients perceived at least the 6.65 filament at the territory of the median or ulnar nerve. Best result on Semmes-Weinstein monofilament test was perception of the 4.31 filament in two patients. None of the patients had two-point discrimination. Vibration with 30-cycles/second stimuli was perceived in 12 patients, whereas vibration with 256-cycles/second stimuli was perceived in only 6 patients. Eight patients had perception of warmth, and 13 patients had perception of cold. Seven patients felt sensation in the cutaneous distribution of the repaired nerve of the hand in situ. Recently, Foroni et al. reported the satisfactory results of this procedure in 11 patients with BPI [10]. According to Highet's scale, sensation was recovered to S3 in two patients, to S2+ in two patients, to S2 in six patients, and S0 in one patient.

The results of these studies indicated the achievement of the uppermost limit of sensory recovery under the current methodology using the intercostal nerve as a donor for sensory reconstruction. The overall conclusion was that sensory reconstruction with intercostal nerve transfer could provide limited sensibility of the hand which is useful for activities of daily living in severely handicapped patients with BPI.

References

1. Gu Y-D, Zhnag G-M, Chen D-S, Yan J-G, Cheng X-M, Chen L. Seventh cervical nerve root transfer from the contralateral healthy side for treatment of brachial plexus root avulsions. J Hand Surg (Br). 1992;17:518–21.
2. Gu Y-D, Chen D-S, Zhang G-M, et al. Long-term functional results of contralateral C7 transfer. J Reconstr Microsurg. 1998;14:57–9.
3. Chuang DC-C, Wei F-C, Noordhoff MS. Cross-chest C7 nerve grafting followed by free muscle transplantations for the treatment of total avulsed brachial plexus injuries: a preliminary report. Plast Reconstr Surg. 1993;92:717–25.
4. Songcharoen P, Wongtrakul S, Mahaisavariya B, Spinner RJ. Hemi-contralateral C7 transfer to median nerve in the treatment of root avulsion brachial plexus injury. J Hand Surg [Am]. 2001;26:1058–64.
5. Doi K, Sakai K, Kuwata N, Ihara K, Kawai S. Double free muscle transfer to restore prehension following complete brachial plexus avulsion. J Hand Surg [Am]. 1995;10:408–14.
6. Ihara K, Doi K, Sakai K, Kuwata N, Kawai S. Restoration of sensibility in the hand after complete brachial plexus injury. J Hand Surg [Am]. 1996;21:381–6.
7. Terzis JK, Kokkalis ZT, Kostopoulos E. Contralateral C7 transfer in adult plexopathies. Hand Clin. 2008;24(4):389–400.
8. Hattori Y, Doi K, Sakamoto S, Yukata K. Sensory recovery of the hand with intercostal nerve transfer following complete avulsion of the brachial plexus. Plast Reconstr Surg. 2009;123(1):276–83.
9. Gao K, Lao J, Zhao X, Gu Y. Outcome of contralateral C7 transfer to two recipient nerves in 22 patients with the total brachial plexus avulsion injury. Microsurgery. 2013;33(8):605–11.
10. Foroni L, Siqueira MG, Martins RS, Heise CO, Neto SH, Imamura AY. Good sensory recovery of the hand in brachial plexus surgery using intercostobrachial nerve as the donor. Arq Neuropsiquiatr. 2017;75(11):796–800.
11. Millesi H. Surgical management of brachial plexus injuries. J Hand Surg [Am]. 1977;2:367–78.
12. Narakas AO, Hentz VR. Neurotization of brachial plexus injuries. Clin Orthop. 1988;237:43–56.
13. Kawai H, Kawabata H, Masada K, et al. Nerve repairs for traumatic brachial plexus palsy with root avulsion. Clin Orthop. 1988;237:75–86.

Management of Neuropathic Pain

37

Keith A. Bengtson

Abbreviations

BPA	Brachial plexus avulsion
BPI	Brachial plexus injury
DN4	Douleur Neuropathique en 4 Questions
DREZ	Dorsal root entry zone
NeuPSIG	Neuropathic Pain Special Interest Group
rTMS	Repetitive transcranial magnetic stimulation
SNRIs	Selective norepinephrine reuptake inhibitors
TCAs	Tricyclic antidepressants
VAS	Visual analog scale

Introduction

Patients with brachial plexus injuries (BPIs) often have severe neurologic deficits and functional difficulties. Despite their physical challenges, the main concern of many patients is their severe life-altering pain. The pain makes it impossible for them to sleep more than 30 minutes at a time. It can stop conversations mid-sentence. Patients become socially isolated and depressed to the point of suicide. Pain becomes the center of their lives. As surgeons, therapists, and physicians, we have been trained to focus on improving the function of the injured limb. However, the patient may be so intensely focused on their pain that they ignore the efforts of their health providers to improve the function of their injured extremity.

A BPI can produce pain from many different sources. The trauma which leads to a BPI produces disruption of nerve tissue as well as surrounding structures. Pain from the trauma to the neural structures is labeled as "neuropathic." Pain from the surrounding non-neural structures are termed "mechanical" or "nocioceptive." The neuropathic pain is divided further into central and peripheral components and will be discussed later.

The reported prevalence of pain varies widely but is generally thought to be present in 54–92% of patients with traumatic brachial plexus injuries at 3 months after their injury [1–4]. Unfortunately, the treatment of pain in BPIs is more art than science. Very few studies have been published on the subject secondary to the low volume of patients at any single institution. Moreover, the treatment is challenging with many patients recalcitrant to medications, modalities, and surgeries.

K. A. Bengtson (✉)
Physical Medicine and Rehabilitation, Mayo Clinic, Rochester, MN, USA
e-mail: bengtson.keith@mayo.edu

A. Y. Shin, N. Pulos (eds.), *Operative Brachial Plexus Surgery*,
https://doi.org/10.1007/978-3-030-69517-0_37

Avulsion Injuries

A recurring issue in the study of BPI is the differences between nerve root avulsions (preganglionic injuries) and more post-ganglionic injuries. The treatment, natural course, and outcomes of nerve root avulsions are quite different from that of post-ganglionic injuries. Unfortunately, many studies fail to describe how the diagnosis of a nerve root avulsion is established. From a surgical perspective, the treatment of brachial plexus injuries depends heavily on the location of the injury and whether or not a nerve root has been avulsed. In a similar fashion, the source of pain in brachial plexus injuries depends on injury location and the presence or absence of an avulsion. Unfortunately, the literature is not necessarily specific regarding the presence or absence of a nerve root avulsion and how this may have been verified. In fact, the term "brachial plexus avulsion" (BPA), whether referring to "injury" or "pain," is often used loosely to refer not only to true nerve root avulsion but also the more distal lesions. In a critical review of the literature, it is often difficult to determine how the term "brachial plexus avulsion" is being used. In contrast, in an earlier paper, Wynn Parry clearly defines the criteria for the diagnosis of nerve root avulsion:

> The criteria for diagnosis of an avulsion is one or more of the following: (1) actually visualizing the avulsed root at open operation in which the posterior root ganglion can clearly be seen in the wound; (2) the presence of radiological evidence of root avulsion, either a diverticulum or a pouch of medial lateral to the nerve root, a cystic arachnoid accumulation of dye limited to the spinal canal and extending for several segments or an elongation or Excedrin ray shin of the nerve root sleeve; (3) the presence of electrical conduction in the peripheral nerve supplying the anesthetic areas; (4) the presence of an N9, either normal or attenuated, on the spinogram [1].

Demographics

The reported prevalence of pain in traumatic brachial plexus injuries varies widely. Classically, Wynn Perry's large cohort of 275 patients with greater than 3 years follow-up from 1980 presents the most comprehensive picture of pain and brachial plexus injuries [2]. Of the 108 patient's with one or more nerve root avulsions, 98 (91%) had pain. Moreover, after 11 years, 17% of patients still reported pain. Interestingly, 12 patients experienced increasing pain over time. In 1996, a long-term follow-up on 122 patients with avulsion injuries (including some patients from the original cohort) found 112 patients (92%) with pain initially after their injury, 48 (39%) with pain after 3 years, and only 22 (18%) with pain after 7 years [3]. Recent demographic studies from different world regions have a variable experiences with BPI pain. Studies from Brazil [4] and China [5] have more carefully characterized the pain experienced by patients with BPIs into neuropathic and nocioceptive (musculoskeletal) pain by using the Douleur Neuropathique en 4 Questions (DN4) [6]. In a cross-sectional study of 65 patients with BPIs, Santana found 49 patients (75%) with pain and 38 (54%) specifically with neuropathic pain [4]. The pain was located mostly in the forearm and hand with a definite distal greater than proximal pattern. Similarly, a second study of 77 patients with BPIs utilizing the DN4 found 41 (55%) with neuropathic pain [5]. In Germany, a long-term follow-up of 70 patients after brachial plexus reconstruction surgery found 60 (80%) with ongoing pain [7]. In strong contradistinction, an Argentinian study [8] found incredible improvements in pain as measured by the Visual Analog Scale (VAS) following surgical reconstruction. Within 3 months after surgery, the VAS decreased on average from 9.1 to 2.5 out of 10 in 28 patients. None of those reports differentiated between patients with or without avulsion injuries.

Traditionally, patients with brachial plexus birth injury or obstetrical palsy were thought to be relatively free of neuropathic pain. However, three retrospective studies [9–10] have shown a substantial prevalence of pain in those with brachial plexus birth injury. An English review of 36 adults with brachial plexus birth injury found 33 (92%) with pain, although not necessarily neuropathic [9]. A study out of Finland reported 35/122 (31%) with pain after undergoing surgery. Of these patients, nine had nonunion of the clavicle which was thought to be the source of pain. Otherwise, there was no correlation with the extent of injury, type of surgery, radiographic findings, or secondary operations [11]. A Canadian survey of 283 children (ages 6–18 years) used the pain face scale and the adolescent pediatric pain tool to determine the prevalence of pain in brachial plexus birth injury patients [12]. Pain was reported in 65/283 (23%) of the subjects. However, the average level of pain was 2/10. In a less formal study of brachial plexus birth injuries out of Sweden, 70 patients were observed and only 1 patient was found to have "neuropathic pain" requiring medication [13]. However, they stated that "most" had some discomfort in their arm with exercise of their shoulder or elbow.

Mechanisms

Patients with brachial plexus injury describe a variety of pain symptoms that likely stem from the wide variety of injuries that they have suffered. Wynn Parry presents a classic description of BPI pain in his large cohort of patients. He states that most patients describe a "burning pain" primarily in their hands as if their "hands were on fire." A minority described paroxysmal pain [2].

Traditionally, the pain from BPIs has been divided into three sources. The injury to the peripheral nerve, either pre-ganglionic or post-ganglionic, should produce a peripheral neuropathic pain. If there is a nerve root avulsion, either partial or complete, there is an injury to the cervical spinal cord which should create a central neuropathic pain. The subsequent neurologic deficit could also produce a third type of pain stemming from the mechanical workings of the shoulder and arm. Additionally, the trauma from the initial injury may have also damaged the structure of the ipsilateral shoulder girdle producing a post-traumatic mechanical pain. These mechanical pains would result from abnormal stresses on the joints, ligaments, muscles, and tendons of the upper extremity. A fourth hybrid type of pain could also be considered based on the traction of the nerves secondary to the subluxation of the weakened shoulder.

Brachial plexus nerve root avulsion uniquely affects the area where the peripheral and central nervous systems intersect, and there is likely injury to both the peripheral and central nerves. Perhaps this is why the neuropathic pain from brachial plexus avulsion is somewhat unique and more refractory to treatment than injury to only one of the systems. Lamina I and II of the dorsal horn of the spinal cord (Lissauer's tract and the substantia gelatinosa, respectively) are the most superficial area of the dorsal root entry zone (DREZ) and are the most likely areas to be a damaged by brachial plexus avulsion injuries (Fig. 37.1). Lissauer's tract is composed of fibers that travel up and down the spinal cord one or more segments. Approximately 1/3 of these are afferent fibers (peripheral nerves) originating in the dorsal root ganglia. The remaining 2/3 are fibers whose cell bodies originate within the dorsal horn (central neurons). These nerve groups are inhibitory sensory fibers. Injuries to these areas lead to lack of inhibition and increase excitation of sensory fibers. It has been suggested that the paroxysmal pain is peripheral neuropathic pain and the more stable baseline pain is central neuropathic pain [14].

Treatment

The neuropathic pain which results from BPIs, particularly avulsion injuries, is multifaceted and complex. As such, the treatment of this neuropathic pain may be confusing, unsatisfying, and difficult. However, as previously stated, not all pain from brachial plexus avulsion injury is neuropathic in nature. The direct and indirect results of brachial plexus trauma often encompass the surrounding non-neural structures of the neck and shoulder regions. Pain from these non-neural structures is labeled as "mechanical" or "nociceptive." Therefore, the treatment of BP pain must address both neuropathic and nociceptive pain. Moreover, the treatment of the neuropathic pain may be further divided into the treatment of both central and peripheral neuropathic pain.

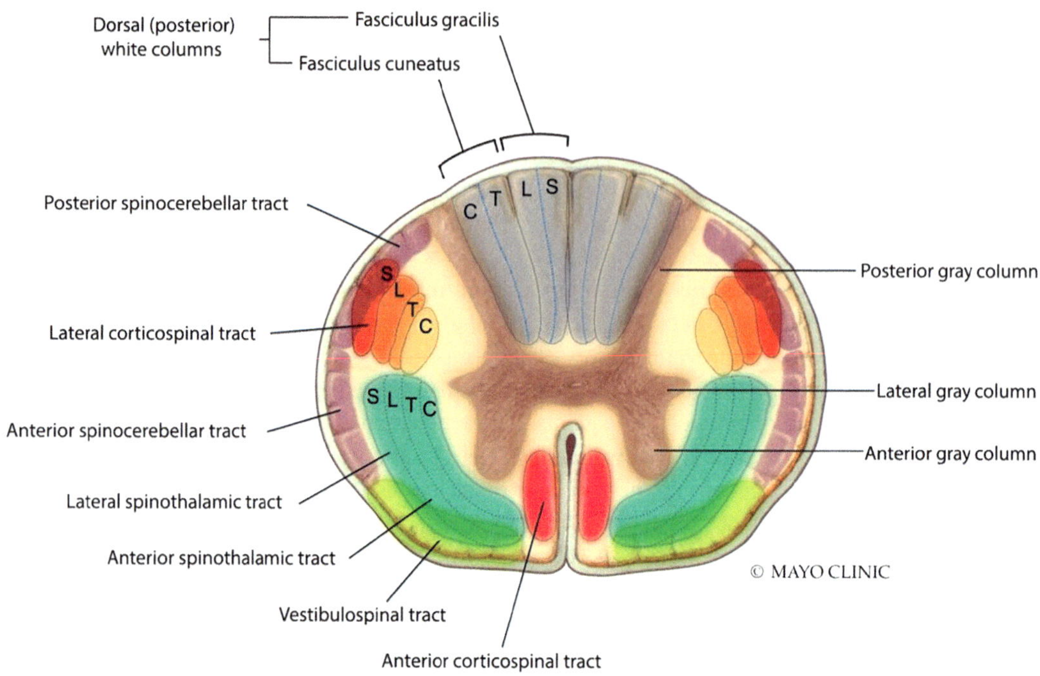

Fig. 37.1 Cross section of cervical spinal cord

Neuropathic Pain

Very few studies have been published regarding the specific medical treatment of brachial plexus pain. A small study out of England in 2004 looked at nabilone, a synthetic tetrahydrocannabinol (THC) analog [15]. This was used as an oral mucosal spray both in its pure form and a 1:1 mixture with cannabidiol (CBD). A crossover study with 50 patients was employed with only 3 subjects withdrawing from the study. Patients had some improvement in pain as measured on a visual analog scale (VAS) but less than two points on a 10-point scale. Patients did report improved quality of sleep as well. A second study from India looked at the use of preoperative gabapentin for BPI neuropathic pain [16]. This was a placebo-controlled trial with 20 patients. Gabapentin was given 2 hours before surgery for brachial plexus reconstruction. Interestingly, the treatment group displayed a decrease in intraoperative fentanyl consumption. Additionally, patients used less rescue analgesic with decreases in their VAS pain score both at rest and with movement.

Aside from these two studies, the literature is wanting and we are left to treat brachial plexus pain as an analog of both central and peripheral neuropathic pain. Fortunately, the literature is resplendent with studies and recommendations for both of these pains states. Many neuropathic pain treatment guidelines have been published by various groups interested in pain treatment, such as pain societies, pain journals, and various National Health Services. The Neuropathic Pain Special Interest Group (NeuPSIG) regularly publishes guidelines for the treatment of neuropathic pain based on a meta-analysis of the literature, the latest of which was published in 2015 [17]. More recent meta-analyses were put out by the Canadian Pain Society [18] and by the Journal of Pain Medicine [19]. Fortunately, there is almost complete consensus as to the first-line and second-line drugs in the past decade. There is more disagreement on the third- and fourth-line drugs which have much

Table 37.1 Medications for neuropathic pain

1st line medications	Gabapentinoids
	Gabapentin
	Pregabalin
	SNRIs
	Duloxetine
	Venlafaxine
	Milnacipran
	TCAs
	Amitriptyline
	Nortriptyline
2nd line medications	Capsaicin 8% patches
	Lidocaine patches
	Tramadol
3rd line medications	Other anticonvulsants
	Topiramate
	Lamotrigine
	Carbamazepine
	Strong opioids
	N-methyl-D-aspartate (NMDA) antagonists
	Ketamine

Adapted from Finnerup et al. (2015) [17].

less evidence for efficacy. The guidelines are summarized in the Table 37.1.

From a practical standpoint, a prescriber would typically start by treating patients with one of the first-line drugs [gabapentinoids, tricyclic antidepressants (TCAs), and selective norepinephrine reuptake inhibitors (SNRIs)] with an upward dose titration until the optimum efficacy/side effect ratio is achieved. Generally, medications with high side effect profiles such as TCAs are titrated more slowly than medications with less bothersome side effects. If the patient has good pain relief, but also experiences intolerable side effects, then it is logical to switch to another drug in the same category starting with a low dose and titrating upwards. However, if the patient has no pain relief despite large dosages of a certain medication, then it would be logical to switch to a medication in a different category with a different mechanism of action. One must take into account other practical aspects such as drug costs, availability, and ease of dosing. Patient characteristics such as allergies, previous medication experience, and coexisting medical problems must be considered when choosing medications.

Beyond first-line drugs, one could proceed to trials of second-line drugs. Alternatively, one could use a combination of two first-line drugs from different categories, thus avoiding overlapping mechanisms of action. The evidence for combination therapy is unclear; however, a Cochran review of combination therapies [20] indicates that combination therapy can be effective. In fact, there are multiple studies which show higher pain relief with two drugs than with a single drug. Unfortunately, given the multitude of possible drug combinations, no single combination has been shown effective in two or more studies. Although it seems likely that combination therapy can be more effective than monotherapy, one must take into consideration the problem of additive side effects and the increased toxicity of polypharmacy.

Central Pain

The vast majority of guidelines and studies address the treatment of peripheral neuropathic pain (although often not specified in the title), and the treatment of central neuropathic pain is poorly addressed. However, similar guidelines do exist for the treatment of central neuropathic pain. The Canadian Pain Society assembled an international expert panel to address guidelines for the treatment of pain in spinal cord injury [21]. There are fewer studies on central neuropathic pain, so the recommendations are much less robust than for peripheral neuropathic pain. However, the first-line medications are similar with a notable absence of SNRIs. Lamotrigine is also recommended as a second-line drug, and this often falls to a third- or fourth-line drug in peripheral neuropathic pain recommendations. Often, general neuropathic pain clinical practice guidelines recommend that the treatment of central neuropathic pain utilizing the same recommendations as those for peripheral neuropathic pain, with the exception of certain situations where strong evidence exists.

Cannabinoids are at the periphery of all clinical practice guidelines. Cannabinoids may actually be the most highly used medication for control of peripheral neuropathic pain, yet they are the least studied. This is largely because of political and legal forces that have historically banned or discouraged the study of cannabinoids in medical terms. As the legal environment changes, further studies may change the place of cannabinoids in the clinical practice guidelines.

Surgical Treatment

The most common surgical procedure used for the treatment of brachial plexus avulsion pain is the ablation of the dorsal root entry zone (DREZ). This is known as the "DREZ procedure" or the "DREZ-otomy." Three large studies have been published (two out of the same institution) on using the DREZ procedure for the treatment of BPA pain [22, 23]. An older study by Wynn Parry in 1984 [2] reviewed his experience in 24 patients treated with DREZ ablation.

In the Lyon, a single institution has reviewed two decades of experience. Their first series reviewed 55 patients treated before January 2000 with 44 patients having greater than 1 year follow-up [22]. Their second series included 29 new patients that were treated from 2000 to 2009 [23]. Impressively, their initial experience found 66% of patients had near total relief of pain indicated by complete discontinuation of pain medications. The 1 year follow-up is fairly short, and there have been reports of gradual recurrence of pain over the years following surgery. The next largest case series [24] included 14 patients with BPAs among a group of 51 pain patients treated with a DREZ procedure. They indicated a much less favorable outcome with only 10/14 patients reporting a result of "good" or "fair." The mean follow-up was 76 months which is much longer than the Lyon series. Wynn Parry in his exhaustive study of brachial plexus patients [2] also reviewed 24 patients who underwent DREZ lesioning for BPA pain. Although the details are sparse, he reported 16/24 patients with excellent relief with follow-up period unspecified.

Spinal Cord Stimulation

The second most common procedure for treating brachial plexus avulsion pain involves implantation of an electrical stimulator at the level of the spinal cord or cerebral cortex. No large series exist but rather a number of small case series. Moreover, the case series for electrical stimulation at the brain level consists of disparate diagnoses with only a few treating pain from BPIs – avulsions or otherwise.

The published experience for spinal cord stimulation is very optimistic with a number of studies showing greater than 50% success rate [25–28]. In total, only 12 patients were reported overall with impressive results. This contrasts with this author's personal experience with over 150 patients undergoing spinal cord stimulation trials and only 2 patients going on to actual implantation. Despite the minimal evidence as to its efficacy, spinal cord stimulation is likely the most common procedure used to address pain from BPIs. This is a fairly simple procedure that is well-known to pain practitioners. Therefore, it is a tool within the easy reach of a typical pain physician. In practice, an electrical lead is placed in the epidural space at the level of the cervical spinal cord which corresponds to the patient's pain, typically at or above the affected nerve roots. A needle is introduced at the midthoracic level through which the electrical lead is passed in a cephalad direction through the epidural space. Many patients with brachial plexus injuries have suffered injuries to the cervical and thoracic spine which may impede the passage of the electrical lead. Therefore, cross-sectional imaging must be obtained to rule out such an impediment.

Alternatively, one may insert a long rectangular lead called a paddle lead through a cervical laminectomy (see Fig. 37.2). Although this is a much more invasive procedure, this approach has the advantage of clear visualization of the cord as well as the ability to secure the lead in place, thus preventing movement of the lead with excessive movement of the cervical spine.

As a technology of spinal cord stimulation evolves, more options for electrical parameters

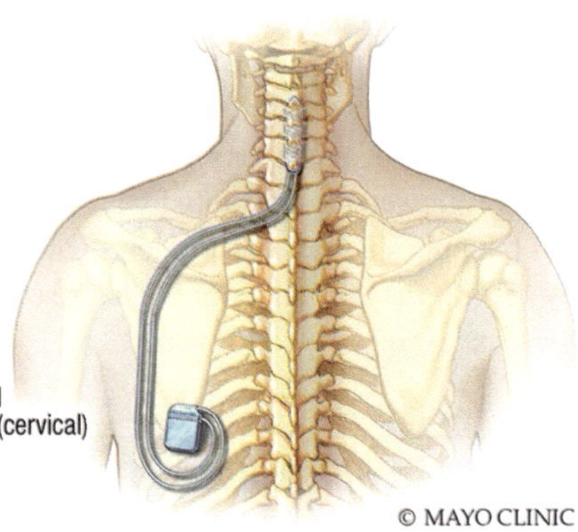

Fig. 37.2 Cervical spinal cord stimulator

are becoming available. In particular, higher-frequency stimulation may allow the stimulation to penetrate deeper into the spinal cord and stimulate different tracks and neurons than previously possible. Moreover, a larger variety of stimulation patterns are being offered with more individualized programmable options. One may expect these advancements to change our approach to treatment significantly.

Brain Stimulation

In contrast to spinal cord stimulator implantation, electrical stimulation at the level of the cerebral cortex is much more complex and limited in use. The target of stimulation is the motor cortex rather than the sensory cortex. Perhaps this seems less than intuitive. However, the concept originally came from a cat pain model where thalamic hyperactivity was recorded with pain stimulation. Subsequent stimulation of various regions within the cortex was only successful in decreasing the thalamic hyperactivity when stimulating the motor cortex. As such, the motor cortex has been the primary target of brain stimulation for pain control throughout most of its history. Bipolar stimulation is used with the cathode on the motor cortex and the anode on the sensory cortex. The motor cortex may be stimulated either transcranially with the magnetic field (repetitive transcranial magnetic stimulation or rTMS), with an electric mat placed on the surface of the motor cortex (either epidural or subdural), or with a single lead inserted into the thalamus (deep brain stimulation).

The use of repetitive transcranial magnetic stimulation (rTMS) is attractive because it is non-invasive. However, it also requires ongoing use over time in order to be effective. The efficacy has not been verified, but the modality has some positive studies for various neuropathic pain states. A meta-analysis of 7 controlled trials on 144 patients indicated pain reduction in multiple central and peripheral neuropathic pain conditions [29]. There is a definite trend towards increased pain relief for central states (spinal cord injury, trigeminal neuralgia, and stroke) over those pain states from a peripheral nerve source. Unfortunately, none of the patient's studied had BPA pain. In addition to using rTMS as a primary pain treatment, there may be a role for using rTMS as a trial modality before attempting surface electrode placement. A positive result with rTMS may indicate a more favorable result with surface stimulation.

The invasive methods of motor cortex stimulation include surface stimulation (both epidural and subdural) and deep brain thalamic stimulation. Surface stimulation is much more common than deep stimulation. Only a small number of controlled studies have been published for surface stimulation. A meta-analysis of 9 studies of 155 patients showed a tendency towards greater efficacy in central pain states over peripheral nerve pathology as was seen in rTMS. If the treatment was defined as successful when there is a 40% decrease in visual analog scale, the overall success was 75% for trigeminal neuralgia and 60% for both spinal cord injury and stroke pain. Treatment efficacy in phantom limb and BPI pain was successful for only 53% and 45%, respectively [30]. A meta-analysis of 14 uncontrolled case series with a total of 195 patients showed a similar response. If a good response was defined as greater than or equal to 40–50% pain relief, then the response rate for trigeminal neuralgia was 68% with the response of central pain secondary to brain or spinal cord injury equal to 54%. Phantom limb pain produced a 60% response and brachial plexus avulsion pain only

45% [31]. Adverse events included seizures in the immediate postoperative period in 29 patients, infection in 9 patients, skin ulceration at the implant site in 2 patients, and subdural hematoma in 2 patients (both with subdural implants). One patient also developed phantom pain. The advantage of subdural stimulation over epidural stimulation is that one can more easily reach the central sulcus which corresponds to the more caudal regions of the body. The epidural placement of the electrode most likely has less chance of CSF leakage.

Peripheral Nerve Stimulation

A third target for electrical stimulation is the peripheral nerve. This technique would only apply to injuries distal to the nerve root where the peripheral nerve could be stimulated proximal to the level of injury [32]. Kim reported two cases using peripheral nerve placement of stimulation electrodes for the post-ganglionic lesions confirmed by nerve conduction findings. They suggested that the patients with shoulder paresis would have better outcomes since lack of shoulder movement would ensure better stability of the peripheral stimulating electrode placement.

Amputation

The role of upper extremity amputation for the treatment of brachial plexus injury pain remains controversial [33–35]. As far back as 1980, Rorabeck reported on eight patients who underwent upper extremity amputations specifically for pain relief. Only three patients reported pain relief, and those were all performed within the first 12 months after injury [34]. At such an early date of intervention, it is possible that the decreased pain represented the natural course of pain resolution in these patients. Given these poor results, the role of amputation for pain relief has remained controversial. Siquiera suggested amputation in the case of a flail arm mostly for functional reasons [35]. However, he also thought that the amputation would address the nociceptive pain source. More recently, Hrubet et al. reported on seven patients who underwent amputation followed immediately by prosthetic fitting. All patients showed a decrease in pain measured by VAS as they began progressive use of the prosthesis at 10 months follow-up.

Treatment of Mechanical Pain

Musculoskeletal or nocioceptive pain is caused by mechanical forces on the shoulder girdle and upper limb. Traumatic BPIs involve high force injuries and may injure structures beyond the brachial plexus. Pain from these structural injuries may contribute to the patient's pain state. Additionally, the muscle weakness resulting from the nerve injuries may cause traction forces on the injured nerves as well as the supporting structures of the shoulder and arm. This appears to be particularly problematic in the area of the shoulder girdle muscles and structures. Weakness of the rotator cuff muscles results in subluxation of the glenohumeral joint causing traction on the traversing tendons, ligaments, and capsular structures. The result is further nocioceptive sources such as tendinopathies, muscle spasms, and arthritis. Nocioceptive pain is much less common distally. Perhaps this is because the more distal structures have much less mechanical stressors, particularly if the hand is not being used for functional activities. Although no studies exist on the treatment of such pain sources, one can proceed with standard musculoskeletal techniques. Modalities, such as heat, ice, massage, traction, chiropractic manipulation, and surface electrical stimulation, may all be used in a standard fashion. Acupuncture and dry needling may help with myofascial components of pain as well. Medications such as acetaminophen and nonsteroidal anti-inflammatories may be used. Injections in the peritendinous areas or trigger points can be effective as well.

Mechanically, it is difficult to support the weight of the arm with any type of shoulder sling. Patients may feel more comfortable with the shoulder subluxation reduced and often find themselves holding their injured arm with the unaffected side, trying to push the humeral head back into the glenoid fossa. Various forms of balanced forearm orthoses have been utilized. Theoretically, one may use a forearm trough to hold the distal upper limb horizontally. This is then suspended from a shoulder cap and harness from a point on the proximal forearm. The weight of the hand is used to push the humerus upwards and reduce glenohumeral subluxation. Unfortunately, this fine balancing act is difficult to maintain in normal daily activities. In more active individuals, it is much more practical to use a sling and swath device which is most effective with the elbow at an acute angle placing the hand at the level of the contralateral clavicle. This allows the sling to suspend most of the weight of the upper limb with direct force on the flexed elbow. If the sling is secured to the torso using a wide swath which extends superiorly to the midthoracic level, the patient may participate in active sports such as running, skiing, and skydiving to name a few. Surgeries such as shoulder fusion [36] and shoulder tendon transfers about the shoulder girdle [37] have been to help control mechanical pain associated with brachial plexus injuries as well.

Conclusion

In summary, the treatment of pain following brachial plexus injuries is challenging. Pain is often recalcitrant to standard medication regimens for both nociceptive and neuropathic pain. The patients are often overcome by both types of pain, and pain remains at the center of their lives.

The tools for treating brachial plexus pain are essentially the standard tools for the treatment of neuropathic pain in general. Medication protocols are taken directly from neuropathic pain treatment guidelines. Modalities for nociceptive pain are derived from experiences treating musculoskeletal pain of other etiologies. Finally, surgical treatment for pain is modestly successful and remains controversial.

References

1. Parry WCB. Pain in avulsion lesions of the brachial plexus. Pain. 1980;9:41–53.
2. Wynn Parry CB. Pain in avulsion of the brachial plexus. Neurosurgery. 1984;15:960–5.
3. Berman J, Anand P, Chen L, Taggart M, Birch R. Pain relief from preganglionic injury to the brachial plexus by late intercostal nerve transfer. J Bone Joint Surg. 1996;78-B:759–60.
4. Santana MV, et al. High prevalence of neuropathic pain in the hand of patients with traumatic brachial plexus injury: a cross-sectional study. Arq Neuropsiquiatr. 2016;74:895–901.
5. Zhou Y, Liu P, Rui J, Zhao X, Lao J. The associated factors and clinical features of neuropathic pain after brachial plexus injuries: a cross-sectional study. Clin J Pain. 2017;33:1030–6.
6. Bouhassira D, Attal N, Alchaar H, Boureau F, Brochet B, Bruxelle J, Cunin G, Fermanian J, Ginies P, Grun-Overdyking A, Jafari-Schluep H, Lantéri-Minet M, Laurent B, Mick G, Serrie A, Valade D, Vicaut E. Comparison of pain syndromes associated with nervous or somatic lesions and development of a new neuropathic pain diagnostic questionnaire (DN4). Pain. 2005;114:29–36.
7. Kretschmer T, et al. Patient satisfaction and disability after brachial plexus surgery. Neurosurgery. 2009;65:A189–96. https://doi.org/10.1227/01.NEU.0000335646.31980.33.
8. Bonilla G, Di Masi G, Battaglia D, Otero JM, Socolovsky M. Pain and brachial plexus lesions: evaluation and initial outcomes after reconstructive microsurgery and validation of a new pain severity scale. Acta Neurochir. 2010;153:171–6.
9. Partridge C, Edwards S. Obstetric brachial plexus palsy: increasing disability and exacerbation of symptoms with age. Physiother Res Int. 2004;9:157–63.
10. Hosomi K, Saitoh Y, Kishima H, Oshino S, Hirata M, Tani N, Shimokawa T, Yoshimine T. Electrical stimulation of primary motor cortex within the central sulcus for intractable neuropathic pain. Clin Neurophysiol. 2007;119:993–1001.
11. Kirjavainen M, et al. Long-term results of surgery for brachial plexus birth palsy. J Bone Joint Surg Am. 2007;89:18–26.

12. Holbech JV, et al. Combination treatment of neuropathic pain: Danish expert recommendations based on a Delphi process. J Pain Res. 2017;10:1467–75. https://doi.org/10.2147/JPR.S138099.
13. Strombeck C, Remahl S, Krumlinde-Sundholm L, Sejersen T. Long-term follow-up of children with obstetric brachial plexus palsy II: neurophysiological aspects. Dev Med Child Neurol. 2007;49:204–9.
14. Blumenkopf B. Neuropharmacology of the dorsal root entry zone. Neurosurgery. 1984;15:900–3.
15. Berman JS, Symonds C, Birch R. Efficacy of two cannabis based medicinal extracts for relief of central neuropathic pain from brachial plexus avulsion: results of a randomised controlled trial. Pain. 2004;112:299–306.
16. Prabhakar H, Arora R, Bithal PK, Rath GP, Dash HH. The analgesic effects of preemptive gabapentin in patients undergoing surgery for brachial plexus injury--a preliminary study. J Neurosurg Anesthesiol. 2007;19:235–8.
17. Finnerup NB, et al. Pharmacotherapy for neuropathic pain in adults: a systematic review and meta-analysis. Lancet Neurol. 2015;14:162–73. https://doi.org/10.1016/S1474-4422(14)70251-0.
18. Mathieson S, et al. Trial of pregabalin for acute and chronic sciatica. N Engl J Med. 2017;376:1111–20. https://doi.org/10.1056/NEJMoa1614292.
19. Bates D, Carsten Schultheis B, Hanes MC, Jolly SM, Chakravarthy KV, Deer TR, Levy RM, Hunter CW. A comprehensive algorithm for management of neuropathic pain. Pain Med. 2019;20:S2–S12.
20. Chaparro LE, Wiffen PJ, Moore RA, Gilron I. Combination pharmacotherapy for the treatment of neuropathic pain in adults. Cochrane Database Syst Rev. 2012;2012(7):CD008943.
21. Guy SD, Mehta S, Casalino A, Côté I, Kras-Dupuis A, Moulin DE, Parrent AG, Potter P, Short C, Teasell R, Bradbury CL, Bryce TN, Craven BC, Finnerup NB, Harvey D, Hitzig SL, Lau B, Middleton JW, O'Connell C, Orenczuk S, Siddall PJ, Townson A, Truchon C, Widerström-Noga E, Wolfe D, Loh E. The CanPain SCI Clinical Practice Guidelines for rehabilitation management of neuropathic pain after spinal cord: recommendations for treatment. Off J Int Spinal Cord Soc. 2016;54:S14–23.
22. Sindau MP, Blondet E, Emery E, Mertens P. Microsurgical lesioning in the dorsal root entry zone for pain due to brachial plexus avulsion: a prospective series of 55 patients. J Neurosurg. 2005;102:1018–28.
23. Aichaoui F, Mertens P, Sindou M. Dorsal root entry zone lesioning for pain after brachial plexus avulsion: results with special emphasis on differential effects on the paroxysmal versus the continuous components. A prospective study in a 29-patient consecutive series. Pain. 2011;152:1923–30. https://doi.org/10.1016/j.pain.2011.03.037.
24. Rath SA, Braun V, Soliman N, Antoniadis G, Richter HP. Results of DREZ coagulations for pain related to plexus lesions, spinal cord injuries, and postherpetic neuralgia. Acta Neurochir. 1996;138:364–9.
25. Bennett MI, YMA T. Cervical dorsal column stimulation relieves pain of the brachial plexus avulsion. J R Soc Med. 1994;87:5–6.
26. Brill S, Aryeh I. Neuromodulation in the management of pain from brachial plexus injury. Pain Physician. 2008;11:81–5.
27. Lai HY, Lee C-Y, Lee ST. High cervical spinal cord stimulation after failed dorsal root entry zone surgery for brachial plexus avulsion pain. Surg Neurol. 2009;72:286–9.
28. Piva B, Shaladi A, Saltari R, Gilli G. Spinal cord stimulation in the management of pain from brachial plexus avulsion. Neuromodulation. 2003;6:27–31.
29. Leung A, Donohue M, Xu R, et al. rTMS for suppressing neuropathic pain: a meta-analysis. J Pain. 2009;10:1205–16.
30. Nguyen JP, Nizard J, Keravel Y, Lefaucheur JP. Invasive brain stimulation for the treatment of neuropathic pain. Nat Rev Neurol. 2011;7:699–709.
31. Fontaine D, Hamani C, Lozano A. Efficacy and safety of motor cortex stimulation for chronic neuropathic pain: critical review of the literature. J Neurosurg. 2009;110:251–6.
32. Kim JH, Ho Shi S, Rong LY. Ultrasound-guided peripheral nerve stimulation for neuropathic pain after brachial plexus injury: two case reports. Clin Rep. 2017;31:453–7.
33. Hruby LA, Sturma A, Mayer JA, Pittermann A, Salminger S, Aszmann OC. Algorithm for bionic hand reconstruction in patients with global brachial plexopathies. J Neurosurg. 2017;127:1163–71.
34. Rorabeck CH. The management of the flail upper extremity in brachial plexus injuries. J Trauma Inj Infect Crit Care. 1980;20:491–3.
35. Siqueira MG, Martins RS, Heise CO, Foroni L. Elective amputation of the upper limb is an option in the treatment of traumatic injuries of the brachial plexus? Arq Neuropsiquiatr. 2017;75:667–70. https://doi.org/10.1590/0004-282X20170096.
36. Richards RR, Waddell JP, Hudson AR. Shoulder arthrodesis for the treatment of brachial plexus palsy. Clin Orthop Relat Res. 1985:250–8.
37. Elhassan B, Bishop AT, Hartzler RU, Shin AY, Spinner RJ. Tendon transfer options about the shoulder in patients with brachial plexus injury. J Bone Joint Surg Am. 2012;94:1391–8. https://doi.org/10.2106/JBJS.J.01913.

Prosthetics and Orthotics in Brachial Plexus Injury: Background, Historical Perspective, and Role of Amputation and Prosthetic Fitting

38

Andrew Nelson, Brandon Sampson, and Andrés A. Maldonado

Prosthetics in Brachial Plexus – Background and Historical Perspective

Traumatic brachial plexus injuries can have devastating effects on upper extremity function [1]. Historically, prosthetic and orthotic treatment options for brachial plexus injury have varied greatly, with results of treatment being poor to limited. Following World War II, the traditional approach was surgical reconstruction involving shoulder fusion, elbow bone block, and finger tenodesis [2]. With limited functional outcomes, surgical intervention shifted in the 1960s to transhumeral amputation and shoulder fusion in a slight abducted and flexed position, treated with body-powered prosthetics [3]. The shoulder fusion increases the biomechanical leverage on the scapula from the weight of the arm and prosthesis [4]. In 1961, Yeoman and Seddon [5] reported 36 patients treated for flail arm in brachial plexus. Reconstruction versus amputation and shoulder arthrodesis versus no treatment were compared. Improved functional result was described by amputation-arthrodesis than either reconstruction or no operation. The loss of glenohumeral motion due to suprascapular and axillary nerve involvement limited the effectiveness of body-powered prostheses [5]. The limited effectiveness relates to the lack of bi-scapular abduction, shoulder depression, and extension required to operate the terminal device or elbow position, as the excursion necessary to generate output greatly exceeds the physiological capacity of the user. Additionally, the maximum effort to create excursion greatly reduces the ability for proportional control to the terminal device. Yeoman and Seddon's article noted patients tended to be "one-handed" within 2 years of the injury and that primitive surgical reconstruction outcomes yielded less satisfactory results compared to amputation and shoulder fusion that occurred within 24 months of injury.

In 1977, Ransford and Hughes [6] reviewed 20 patients, 13 of whom were treated with amputation after brachial plexus injuries. Amputation did not relieve pain, and the prosthesis was not frequently used. In 1980, Rorabeck et al. [7] pub-

A. Nelson (✉) · B. Sampson
Prosthetics and Orthotics, Limb Lab,
Rochester, MN, USA
e-mail: Andrew@limblab.com;
Brandon@limblab.com

A. A. Maldonado
Peripheral Nerve and Brachial Plexus Unit,
Department of Plastic Surgery, University Hospital
Getafe, Madrid, Spain
e-mail: mail@andresmaldonado.es

A. Y. Shin, N. Pulos (eds.), *Operative Brachial Plexus Surgery*,
https://doi.org/10.1007/978-3-030-69517-0_38

lished 23 patients with complete brachial plexus lesions and 3 treatment approaches: no surgery, amputation, and amputation with shoulder arthrodesis. Return to employment and prosthetic wearing were best achieved with early amputation. In 2005, Bedi et al. [8] described their combined glenohumeral arthrodesis and above-elbow amputation technique for the flail limb following a complete post-traumatic brachial plexus injury. According to their clinical experience, the combination of these procedures resulted in an improved pain level, enhanced shoulder stability, and encouraged functional rehabilitation via prosthetic fitting and was associated with high patient satisfaction.

The enthusiasm for early elective amputation as a treatment option for severe brachial plexus lesions has been tempered with the introduction of more sophisticated nerve transfers, free functioning muscle transfers, and intraplexal nerve grafting. Narakas [9] published in 1978 a series of 508 patients with traction injuries of the brachial plexus over a period of 11 years. Only three secondary amputations were reported. Sedel [10] in 1982 had no amputations in his 139 cases. Allieu et al. [11] in 1988 published a series of 28 patients with complete brachial plexus paralysis after at least four years of follow-up. According to the authors, the preservation of the limb was always preferable to amputation, which was only requested by one patient. A series of 750 patients was published by Wilkinson et al. [12], where elective amputation was performed in 13 cases at the patient's request and as a possible element of rehabilitation. The pain of preganglionic injury was not relieved by amputation. According to Terzis et al., amputation should no longer be considered an option even in the face of global root avulsion [13].

A more recent study by Maldonado et al. [14] analyzed retrospectively all the amputations performed at the Mayo Clinic after traumatic brachial plexus injury. Out of more than 2000 brachial plexus injuries, only 9 underwent an amputation. Three conditions were observed in all nine patients: (1) all were pan-plexus injury; (2) non-recovery (mid-humeral amputation) or elbow flexion recovery only (forearm amputation) 1 year after all other surgical options were performed; and (3) at least one chronic complication (chronic infection, nonunion fractures, full-thickness burns, chronic neck pain with arm weight, etc.). Pain improvement was found in five patients. Two more details are important from this study: (1) all patients requesting amputation were exposed to the amputation scenario before surgery by a multidisciplinary team – long discussions with the surgeons, rehabilitation staff, psychologists, prosthetists, and contact with previous amputee patients, and (2) neuropathic pain and shoulder subluxation pain should be properly distinguished and discussed in detail with the patient understanding that neuropathic pain will not be addressed with an amputation.

With improved surgical techniques, flail arm reconstruction versus amputation offers two different approaches to restore function to pan-plexus-injured patients. Restoration of reliable elbow flexion and primitive prehension of the hand is now possible. Elective amputation after brachial plexus injury should be considered as an option in the above specific circumstances [14]. Regardless of surgical approach, further developed prosthetic and orthotic technology offers lighter, faster, and more intricate prehension that greatly exceeds the historical outcomes.

Prosthetic Advances and Application to Patients with Upper Motor Neuron Injury

With widespread advancement and application of externally powered prosthetic components, limited body excursion for patients with upper motor neuron injury is now less problematic. Technologic advances with componentry, materials, and myoelectric inputs paired with design concept advances have opened the possibilities for brachial plexus-injured patients to actuate the control of a prosthesis. This includes control to the terminal device with open-close, wrist supination-pronation, and elbow flexion-extension. Additionally, with a greater number of individuals surviving motor vehicle accidents, which is the leading cause of brachial plexus injury [15], more successful clinical experience and collaboration has taken place improving technology and functional outcomes.

During the initial appointment, the prosthetist should complete a thorough evaluation to understand the abilities and deficiencies of the patient. Assessing sound side and amputated side range of motion, manual muscle testing, and shoulder stability should occur, gathering necessary information to consider when designing the prosthesis. If shoulder subluxation is a concern, incorporating offloading harnessing techniques and reducing the weight of the device should be prioritized.

Evaluating the patient to determine the control strategy and design that is most appropriate based upon the level of injury and amputation is required. Myotesting will determine which muscles can generate the greatest electromyography (EMG) potential for prosthetic control, which is the most important aspect for successful operation of the myoelectric prosthesis. The electrode should be placed matching the long axis of the muscle fiber, making even contact to assure accurate transcutaneous detection. The patient should be asked to contract and relax their muscles at normal effort and maximum effort. Visual feedback should be used with the patient, showing the EMG graph for a better understanding of myoelectric control. The prosthetist and occupational therapist should work together to identify which muscles produce consistent, reliable outputs that can be assigned to functions for myoelectric control. The muscle groups selected should be assigned their natural movement, often a flexor and an extensor. Very weak muscles may still produce viable signals to operate externally powered prostheses. Based upon the level nerve involvement and myotesting results, various control strategies can be used, including:

- Dual-site differential control: Motor power is determined by the stronger of the two signals, where the stronger signal is listened to by the terminal device.
- Dual-site first-over control: Motor power is determined by the first input signal to cross the threshold. The second signal is ignored until both open and close signals drop below the threshold.
- Single-site alternating control: Motor power is controlled by alternating the muscle contraction. The signal must cross the threshold for the movement and must drop below the threshold before another signal is detected to move in the opposite direction. This control strategy is used if only one viable muscle site can be detected.
- Single-site voluntary close: The hand is fully opened at rest, and motor power will ensue for hand close when the signal crosses the threshold. The signal must remain above the threshold if the hand is desired to stay in the closed position.
- Single-site voluntary open: The hand is fully closed at rest, and motor power will ensue for hand open when the signal crosses the threshold. The signal must remain above the threshold if the hand is desired to stay in the opened position.

If myotesting does not detect adequate, reproducible signals, a linear transducer should be considered. The linear transducer requires excursion less than 10 mm, usually produced through bi-scapular abduction, replacing the functional inputs of the electrodes. The patient uses a figure-9 harness with axilla loop around the non-amputated side, which connects to the linear transducer. The linear transducer switch uses a variety of control strategies, including "alternating open-close" and "slow-close, quick-open." The "slow-close, quick-open" option uses a slow bi-scapular abduction movement to close the terminal device and a quick bi-scapular abduction movement to open. This option allows for proportional control of the terminal device, controlling the speed of the terminal device by controlling the strength of the signal. Proportional control will allow for grasping of delicate objects gently, avoiding damage and distortion of the object. The linear transducer requires significantly less excursion in comparison with traditional body-powered control, resulting in reduced energy expenditure and compensatory movements.

Once the control strategy is determined, identifying the appropriate suspension technique is required. If surface electrodes are being used, skin-fit suction suspension is preferred to create

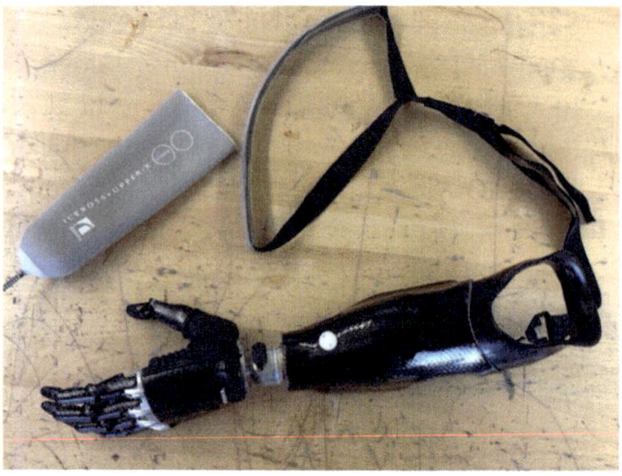

Fig. 38.1 Transradial prosthesis with flexible supracondylar cuff, figure-9 harness with linear transducer excursion. Silicone liner with pin suspension. Manual flexion-extension wrist. Externally powered terminal device

direct contact to the electrodes. Direct contact of skin to electrode is required for EMG detection and control of the myoelectric prosthesis. A residual limb "pull sock" or "parachute sock" may be required for donning the prosthesis to fully seat the residual limb in the socket.

If a linear transducer is being used due to poor EMG signals on the residual limb, a silicone pin-locking liner is donned over the residual limb. The silicone liner provides an interface of protection between residual limb and prosthesis, as those with upper motor neuron involvement may have impaired sensation. Additionally, the pin-locking mechanism creates a secure lock for adequate prosthetic suspension (Fig. 38.1).

With appropriate control strategy and suspension determined, terminal device options should be considered. Discussion with the patient regarding their goals, work requirements, hobbies, and expectations should occur. This conversation will aid the prosthetist in selecting the necessary componentry, pairing the appropriate technology with the design of the prosthesis that will best meet the goals, needs, and lifestyle of the patient. When it comes to a loss or amputation of the upper extremity, it is very important the prosthetist communicates that there is truly no replacement for the part of the hand or arm that has been lost and that can mechanically accomplish the intricate movements and intuitive control found in the human body. There is no one device or one prosthetic hand or prosthetic hook or control strategy that will completely restore function. At best, the referring physician will prescribe a prosthetic system that will be used as a tool to help restore some level of function for the patient's life. Although myoelectric terminal devices differ in appearance, including resembling the anatomic hand or presenting as a hook, each device functions off a similar principle, being a functional tool.

Advancements in technology has had the greatest impact in myoelectric terminal devices, especially in comparison with the historical predecessors. No longer providing only rudimentary prehension grip, myoelectric hands are now capable of a multitude of grip patterns, including but not limited to opposition, precision pinch, three-jaw chuck, and cylindrical. Furthermore, recent advancements have now incorporated customizable grips, where the patient can select a specific grip for a given activity by programming each digit to move at a certain speed, endpoint, and time. Outside of muscle triggers, grips can be accessed in a variety of ways including Bluetooth grip chips, gesture control, and mobile application. Bluetooth grip chips can be placed in strategic locations with pre-programmed grips associated to each chip. When in vicinity of the grip chip, the Bluetooth connection will automatically activate the programmed grip, creating ease and quick activation of a specified grip. Gesture control offers an additional means of control strategy, creating intuitive interaction between the patient and prosthesis. Gesture control enables specific grips by moving the myoelectric hand in one of four directions, which is sensed by the gyroscope and actuators imbedded in the device. Mobile application control can be activated when using a smartphone or tablet, allowing for instant access of multiple grips. These improvements have created an expanded functional capacity of use, offering more features to restore function to the amputated extremity.

There are numerous manufacturers designing and producing externally powered prosthetic hands and hooks that are readily available on the market. Each device offers a different capability of speed, grip patterns, grip force, opening width, operating voltage, waterproof or water-resistant features, and battery capacity. Working closely with the patient, physician, occupational therapist, physical therapist, and prosthetist will assure the componentry selected will best meet the functional goals of the patient.

Further Considerations

Simpson states the prerequisites for upper limb function include proximal stability, placement in space, and functional grasp [16]. Proximal stability of the shoulder should be achieved for improved prosthetic outcomes. The weight of the prosthesis needs to be considered when designing and constructing the device, selecting materials, and incorporating techniques to reducing further subluxation or instability. Material advancements include synthetic carbon fiber, fiberglass, and nyglass. These materials create strong, durable prostheses with minimal weight. Keeping the weight proximal is important, including housing the batteries, charging ports, and myoelectric controls in a strategic manner to reduce the perceived weight. Additionally, enhanced axilla harnessing can assist in reducing shoulder subluxation.

Placement in space refers to the functional envelope in which the prosthesis will operate. Patients with upper motor neuron involvement tend to have limited ability to control external rotation at the shoulder and, thus, internally rotate at the shoulder. For transhumeral patients, anterior and posterior proximal socket trimline extensions at the shoulder will improve shoulder control and pre-positioning of the prosthesis. Incorporating a socket extension panel on the anterior proximal trimline of the prosthesis will create an endpoint of contact, improving the socket alignment and pre-position in a functional space (Fig. 38.2). Adversely, a posterior proximal socket extension panel will promote external rotation at the shoulder (Fig. 38.3).

Additionally, harnessing techniques can encourage external rotation alignment, creating an external control strap added to the figure-9 harness. With most tasks being performed at or near midline, assuring the alignment is conducive

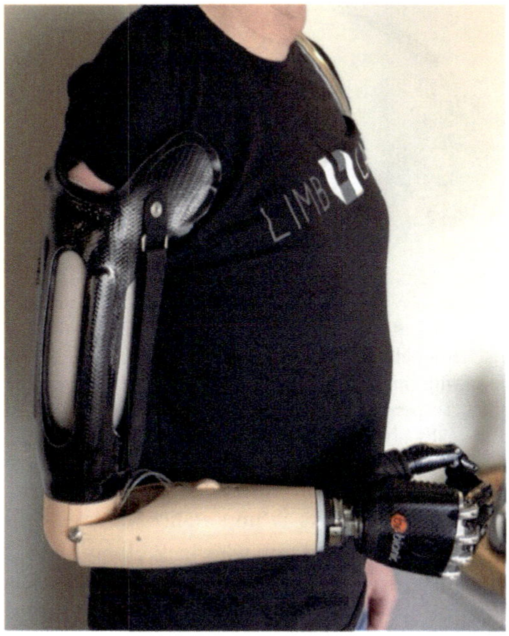

Fig. 38.2 Transhumeral prosthesis with anterior proximal extension at the shoulder, improving the positioning of the terminal device in a functional space. Externally powered terminal device

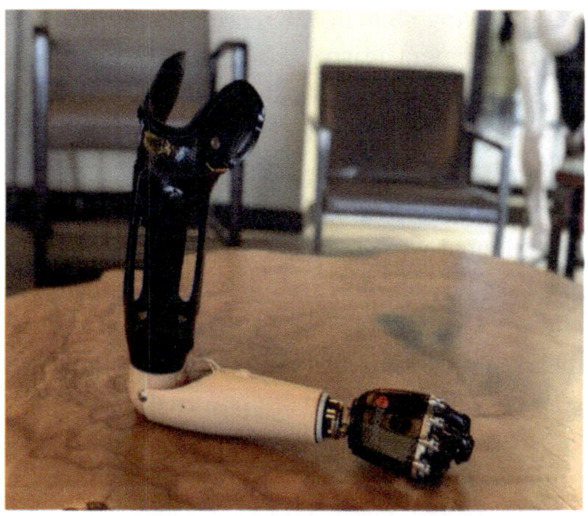

Fig. 38.3 Transhumeral prosthesis with anterior and posterior proximal extension at the shoulder, improving the positioning of the terminal device in a functional space and promoting external rotation at the shoulder. High-Fidelity socket design. Figure-9 harness with linear transducer excursion. Manual locking elbow. Manual flexion-extension wrist

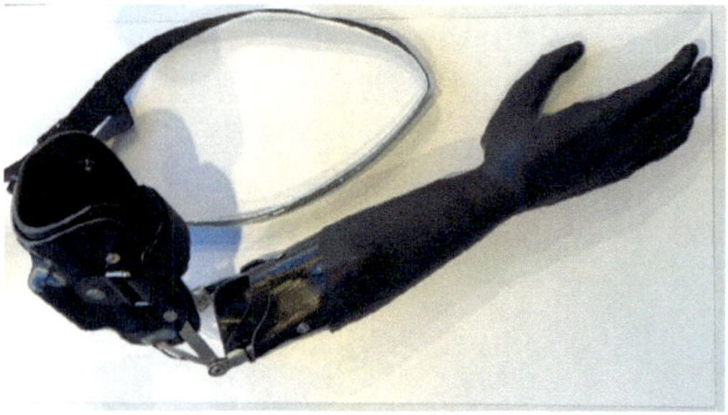

Fig. 38.4 Transradial prosthesis with humeral cuff, ratcheting elbow lock joint on medial side, figure-9 harness with linear transducer excursion. Silicone liner with pin suspension. Manual flexion-extension wrist. Externally powered terminal device

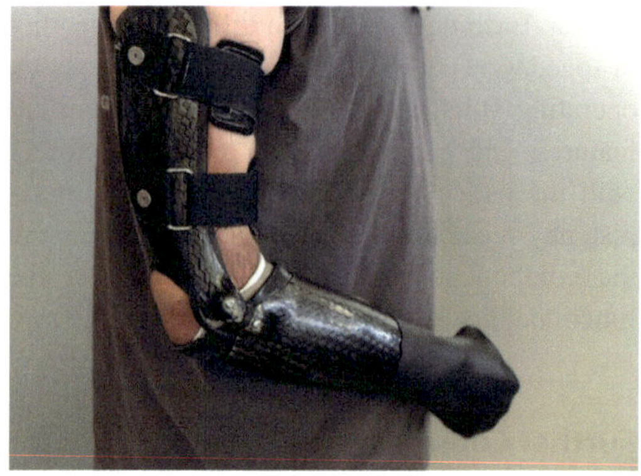

Fig. 38.5 Transradial prosthesis with humeral cuff, free motion joint on elbow, silicone liner pin suspension. Biceps and triceps electrodes housed in the humeral cuff for myoelectric control. Externally powered terminal device. Resting position at or near midline for improved function

for functional tasks is important. For transradially amputated patients who lack elbow flexion sustainability, incorporating a humeral cuff with ratcheting step-up locking elbow joints with set increments will help pre-position the prosthesis in a functional capacity (Fig. 38.4). The ratcheting lock feature can be positioned on or off, whether free motion or locking assistance is desired.

Achieving functional grasp relates closely with placement in space (Fig. 38.5). Some features that may improve the efficiency of functional grasp include wrist flexion and extension, manual wrist rotation, powered wrist rotation, manual elbow flexion, and powered elbow flexion. Manual wrist rotation, manual wrist flexion, and manual elbow flexion requires manipulation with the sound side hand (Fig. 38.3). Although these manual functions are less intuitive in comparison with the externally powered technological advancements, the benefit of reduced weight often creates a functional advantage. However, some patients may benefit from externally powered features to the wrist and elbow. For example, externally powered wrist supination and pronation can help the patient position the terminal device in the optimal position unilaterally while maintaining grasp of an object on their sound side (Fig. 38.6). Additionally, transhumeral patients may benefit from externally powered elbow flexion and extension, positioning the terminal device in an advantageous functional capacity while maintaining hold on their sound side. Each externally powered component requires an additional control source, which can be accessed using specific muscles inputs including "hold open," "double impulse," "triple impulse," or "co-contraction."

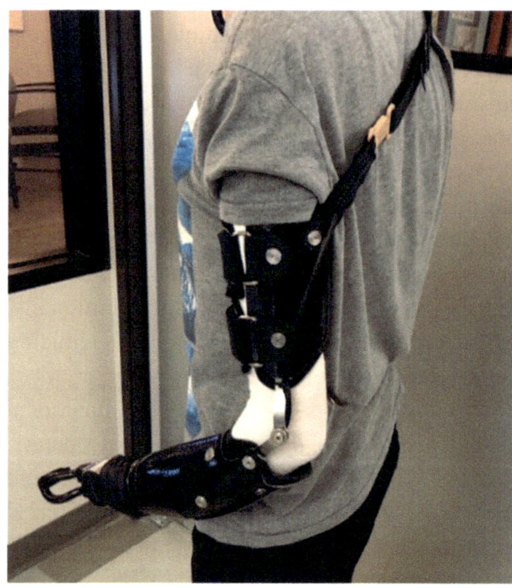

Fig. 38.6 Transradial prosthesis with humeral cuff, ratcheting elbow lock on medial side, figure-9 harness with linear transducer excursion. Silicone liner with pin suspension. Externally powered wrist pronation-supination. Externally powered terminal device

Prosthetic technological advances and increased clinical experience in managing patients with upper motor neuron injury have greatly improved the ability to perform bimanual activities, which prevents overuse injury of the sound side and limits compensatory movements, restoring functional outcomes that surpass the previous approach. Using a hybrid approach of myoelectric components with manual positioning additions will optimize function while minimizing weight, though externally powered additions can improve functional capacity if weight can be tolerated. Combining the technological advancements with a well-designed prosthesis that provides enhanced suspension and rotational control will improve the prosthetic outcome.

Orthotics in Brachial Plexus Injury

Patients with upper motor neuron involvement have historically been offered rudimentary orthotic options. A standard sling, hemisling, Wilmer carrying orthosis, and hinged tenodesis splint have been the standard for treatment. These options offer advantages of reduced cost and ease of donning and doffing. Conventional static orthoses, though applicable in some instances, are less sophisticated options that lack the coveted dynamic functional movement many patients desire. Recent application of technology used in myoelectric prosthetic design has been utilized in externally powered orthotic devices, restoring elbow flexion, elbow extension, hand open, and hand close using muscle signals produced by the patient. Incorporating technology that provides visual and physical feedback allows the patient to reproduce muscle activation and thus restore functional movements.

Myomo, a medical robotics company based in Cambridge, Massachusetts, developed an externally powered myoelectric orthosis named the MyoPro (Fig. 38.7). Originally developed at MIT and Harvard Medical School, the MyoPro is a custom-fabricated orthosis that helps restore dynamic function to those with intact arms affected by upper motor neuron injury. The MyoPro translates EMG signals detected by electrodes at the biceps, triceps, wrist flexors, and wrist extensors into movement of the extremity. These muscle signals are read via transcutaneous detection and amplified to produce physiological elbow and hand motion.

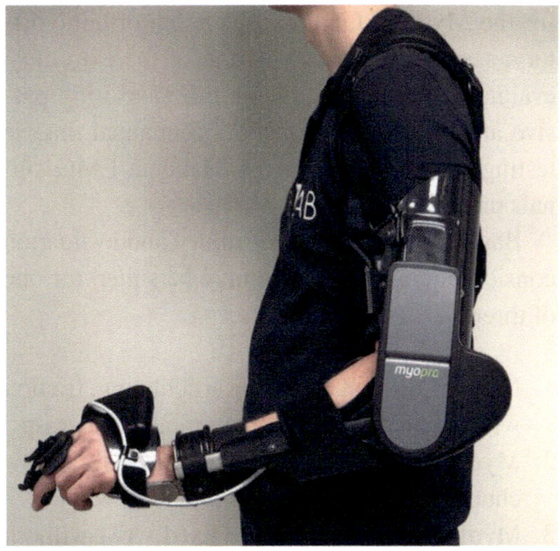

Fig. 38.7 The MyoPro Motion G custom-fabricated myoelectric orthosis. The electrodes are housed within the humeral cuff and forearm cuff, reading the muscle signals from the biceps, triceps, wrist flexors, and wrist extensors. The multi-articulating wrist allows for passive pronation, supination, wrist flexion, and wrist extension. Velcro closures are applied at the hand, forearm section, humeral section, chest strap, and axilla saddle. Donning begins distally at the hand and moves proximal, working one joint segment at a time to assure proper positioning and alignment

The MyoPro software can be programmed for each individual to refine the sensitivity and proportional control to the device, using gain, boost, threshold, and range of motion settings to create optimal function. Furthermore, programming can be adjusted as strength and reinnervation occurs. The MyoPro elbow motor offers approximately 7 Newton-meters of torque. For Motion G, the grasp motor offers approximately 1.1 Newton-meters of torque [17]. Each device uses interchangeable rechargeable batteries. The MyoPro device is currently the only commercially available externally powered upper extremity orthosis.

A thorough evaluation of the patient must be completed by the orthotist to assure candidacy for the MyoPro. Gathering detailed orthotic history, assessing resting position of the extremity, evaluating shoulder subluxation, measuring passive and active range of motion, manual muscle testing, and myotesting for adequate EMG signals must be completed.

Based upon the level of injury and evaluation considerations, the patient may be suited for one of three MyoPro options:

1. MyoPro Motion W: Multi-articulating, friction wrist-jointed model without motorized grasp
2. MyoPro Motion G: Motorized three-jaw chuck grasp with multi-articulating wrist
3. MyoPro Motion E: Static fixed wrist without motorized grasp

There are eight different modes that can be readily accessed in the Motion G, while only four different modes for Motion W and E. Each mode can be accessed via the device or in the software (Fig. 38.8). Patients require only one viable EMG location to be considered a candidate for the MyoPro, though additional myosites will allow for multiple modes to be used.

Different control strategies based on level of involvement and myotesting results include:

- Elbow:
  - Standby Mode: The device is powered on. The elbow motor will not respond to EMG signals.
  - Bicep Mode: The elbow motor will respond to the bicep EMG signal. When the bicep EMG signal is relaxed, the device is extended. When the bicep EMG signal crosses the threshold, the device will flex.
  - Triceps Mode: The elbow motor will respond to the triceps EMG signal. When the triceps EMG signal is relaxed, the device is flexed. When the triceps EMG signal crosses the threshold, the device will extend.
  - Dual Mode: The elbow motor will respond to both bicep and triceps EMG signals. When the bicep EMG signal crosses the threshold, the device will flex, as long as the bicep EMG signal is greater than the triceps EMG signal. When the triceps EMG signal crosses the threshold, the device will extend, as long as the triceps EMG signal is greater than the bicep EMG signal.
- Hand (Motion G only):
  - Standby Mode: The device is powered on. The hand motor will not respond to EMG signals.
  - Open Mode: The hand motor will respond to the wrist extensor EMG signal. When the wrist extensor EMG signal is relaxed, the device is closed. When the wrist extensor EMG signal crosses the threshold, the device will open.
  - Close Mode: The hand motor will respond to the wrist flexor EMG signal. When the wrist flexor EMG signal is relaxed, the device is opened. When the wrist flexor EMG signal crosses the threshold, the device will close.

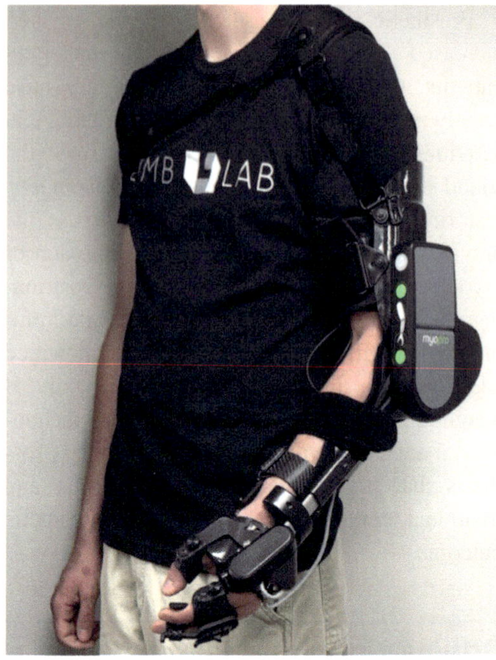

Fig. 38.8 The MyoPro Motion G, incorporating a three-jaw chuck grasp with multi-articulating wrist. The battery source is located on the lateral portion of the device. The various modes to the elbow and hand can be readily accessed by clicking the green buttons. Mode options include elbow only, hand only, or both elbow and hand. Electrodes need to make direct contact to the skin for accurate detection of the muscle signal. The gain, boost, and threshold settings can be adjusted within the software for consistent, reproducible outputs that will restore physiological elbow and hand motion

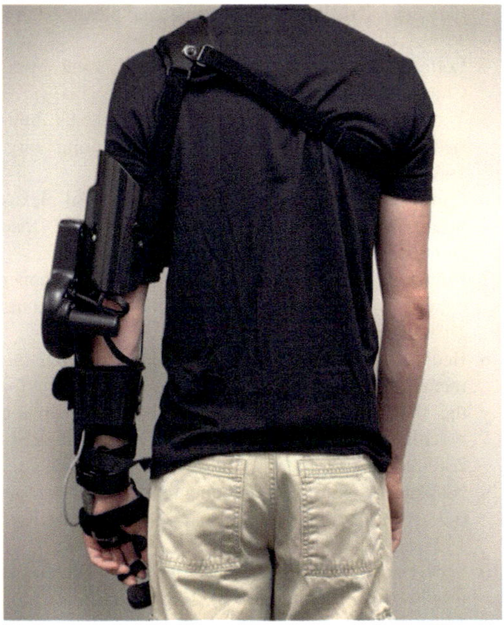

Fig. 38.9 Axilla saddle harnessing is required to reduce shoulder subluxation concerns and provide support to the weakened shoulder muscles. The axilla harness will load weight proximally, reducing the perceived weight of the 4.5 lb. device. Custom harnessing should be considered for significant shoulder instability. An external shoulder rotation strap can be applied if necessary, attaching from the D-ring posteriorly to the axilla strap at or near the inferior angle of the scapula. Secure strap once the desired tension of external rotation is achieved

- Dual Mode: The hand motor will respond to both wrist extensor and wrist flexor EMG signals. When the wrist extensor EMG signal crosses the threshold, the device will open, as long as the wrist extensor EMG signal is greater than the wrist flexor EMG signal. When the wrist flexor EMG signal crosses the threshold, the device will close, as long as the wrist flexor EMG signal is greater than the wrist extensor EMG signal.

Shoulder and elbow harnessing must be incorporated into the device to create alignment in a functional capacity. Axilla saddle supports are required due to shoulder subluxation concerns and shoulder girdle weakness (Fig. 38.9). External rotation straps are used if shoulder weakness or instability occurs, better positioning the arm in a functional space. This will limit the tendency for the arm to be internally rotated upon use. Customized harnesses should be considered for significant shoulder instability or inability to preform external rotation. Contraindications for the MyoPro include shoulder subluxation greater than two finger-widths, inadequate EMG signal at both biceps and triceps, elbow contractures, and any uncontrollable pain.

Multidisciplinary Approach

Regardless of prosthetic or orthotic treatment, a multidisciplinary approach is required for the best outcomes for the patient. Each member of the care team contributes specific knowledge in their discipline, improving the function and proficiency for the patient.

- Physician/surgeon: Documenting surgical intervention, including specification on targeted muscle reinnervation, nerve transfer, or free muscle transfer, will assist the prosthetist, orthotist, occupational therapist, and physical therapist on proper considerations for device and therapy training. Additionally, documentation supporting the prescribed device, including justification and rational of the componentry and socket design concepts, will ultimately provide the insurance company better understanding and increase the likelihood of approval. Prescribing physical therapy and occupational therapy appointments for the patient will improve proficiency and function.
- Prosthetist and orthotist: The prosthetist and orthotist design, fabricate, and fit the appropriate device based off the injury or amputation. They assure appropriate fit of the device, adjusting myoelectric settings for accurate and efficient function, including adjusting the amplification, sensitivity, and threshold. Additionally, determining optimal placement of electrodes, assessing the control strategy, and optimizing the prehension and speed of the terminal device is necessary. Lastly, assuring appropriate suspension, harnessing location, and alignment needs to be monitored.
- Physical therapist and occupational therapist: During the rehabilitation phase, pre-prosthetic

training should be performed. This includes training to use specific muscle movements within the residual limb to mimic grip patterns, which will improve the intuitiveness of the prosthetic control strategy and utilization. Additionally, strength and range of motion exercises should be covered. Following orthotic or prosthetic fitting, donning and doffing strategies need to be discussed and attempted with the patient, determining the most effective option based on the level of injury or amputation. Education and exercises focusing on activating and differentiating isometric muscle groups, along with co-contraction and proportional control training, will aid in efficient control techniques. Strategies for managing bimanual activities and reducing compensatory movements need to be emphasized. Assuring the appropriate amount of therapy sessions have been scheduled for the patient is required, increasing the effectiveness and success while minimizing frustration and rejection. With advanced physical therapy and occupational therapy, the patient will require less cognitive effort and movements will become more natural.

References

1. Rohde RS, Wolfe SW. Nerve transfers for adult traumatic brachial plexus palsy (brachial plexus nerve transfer). HSS J Springer-Verlag. 2007;3(1):77–82.
2. Hendry HAM. The treatment of residual paralysis after brachial plexus lesions. J Bone Joint Surg. 1949;31B:42.
3. Fletcher I. Traction lesions of brachial plexus. Hand. 1969;1:129–36.
4. Leffert RD. Brachial plexus injuries. New York: Churchill Livingstone; 1985.
5. Yeoman PM, Seddon HJ. Brachial plexus injuries: treatment of the flail arm. J Bone Joint Surg. 1961;43B:493–500.
6. Ransford AO, Hughes SP. Complete brachial plexus lesions: a ten-year follow-up of twenty cases. J Bone Joint Surg Br. 1977;59-B(4):417–20.
7. Rorabeck CH. The management of the flail upper extremity in brachial plexus injuries. J Trauma. 1980;20(6):491–3.
8. Bedi A, Miller B, Jebson PJL. Combined glenohumeral arthrodesis and above-elbow amputation for the flail limb following a complete posttraumatic brachial plexus injury. Tech Hand Up Extrem Surg. 2005;9(2):113–9.
9. Narakas A. Surgical treatment of traction injuries of the brachial plexus. Clin Orthop Relat Res. 1978;133:71–90.
10. Sedel L. The results of surgical repair of brachial plexus injuries. J Bone Joint Surg Br. 1982;64(1):54–66.
11. Allieu Y, Cenac P. Is surgical intervention justifiable for total paralysis secondary to multiple avulsion injuries of the brachial plexus?. Hand clinics 4.4 (1988): 609–618.
12. Wilkinson MC, Birch R, Bonney G. Brachial plexus injury: when to amputate? Injury. 1993;24(9):603–5.
13. Terzis JK, Vekris MD, Soucacos PN. Brachial plexus root avulsions. World J Surg. 2001;25(8):1049–61.
14. Maldonado AA, Kircher MF, Spinner RJ, Bishop AT, Shin AY. The role of elective amputation in patients with traumatic brachial plexus injury. J Plast Reconstr Aesthet Surg. 2016;69(3):311–7.
15. Narakas A. The treatment of brachial plexus injuries. Int Orthop. 1985;9:29–36.
16. Simpson DC. The hand/arm system. In: Murdoch G, editor. Prosthetic and orthotic practice. London: E Arnold; 1968.
17. MyoPro Orthosis & Prosthetics Clinical Resources. 2017. Retrieved from https://myomo.com/op-resources/.

The Role of Therapy: Pre- and Post-surgery Protocols

39

Kimberly Jensen and Stephanie Kannas

Introduction

One of the most anxiety-provoking topics for occupational and physical therapists is learning and understanding the complex anatomy of the brachial plexus. Knowing the proper rehabilitation techniques to treat adults with a brachial plexus lesion is essential. It must be communicated with the therapist the rehabilitation needs from the time of first evaluation through the post-surgical reconstruction period, including lifetime restrictions and expectations.

Common therapy interventions for all patients with brachial plexus injuries include:

1. Range of motion
2. Gravity-eliminated motion/strengthening
3. Slings and/or orthotics
4. Manual therapies for scar management and edema control
5. Graded motor imagery
6. Neuromuscular reeducation and activation techniques
7. Modalities
8. One-handed activities of daily living, work, and leisure

K. Jensen (✉) · S. Kannas
Physical Medicine & Rehabilitation, Mayo Clinic, Rochester, MN, USA
e-mail: Jensen.Kimberly@mayo.edu; Kannas.Stephanie@mayo.edu

Preoperative Rehabilitation

Therapy plays a critical role in a patient's care after a brachial plexus injury. Even if an injury to the brachial plexus has not been ascertained, the care team should be suspicious especially, when a patient sustains multi-trauma and requires sedation with significant injuries to the shoulder girdle, first rib, or axillary arteries [1]. The surgeon should ideally be in close communication with the therapist during the acute phase. In the acute phase of the injury, the therapist needs to consider instructing the patient and caregivers in a self-care management program that includes range of motion exercises, edema management, sling use, orthotic use, graded motor imagery, one-handed activities of daily living, pain management address psychosocial concerns [2].

Range of motion needs to be maintained after the initial injury. Emphasis should be placed on maintaining shoulder external rotation, shoulder elevation, elbow flexion, forearm supination, metacarpal phalangeal joint flexion, and first web space abduction while being mindful of other injuries which may preclude motion (Figs. 39.1, 39.2, 39.3, 39.4, 39.5, and 39.6). Motion can progress from passive to active assisted to active range of motion based on the pattern of injury. Even in a complete avulsion, it is imperative to maintain full passive finger range of motion to allow for future surgical reconstruction efforts if

A. Y. Shin, N. Pulos (eds.), *Operative Brachial Plexus Surgery*,
https://doi.org/10.1007/978-3-030-69517-0_39

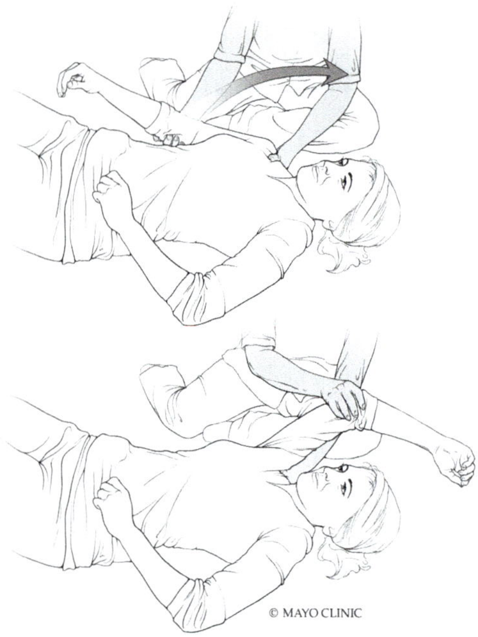

Shoulder flexion

Fig. 39.1 Passive range of motion for shoulder elevation/flexion

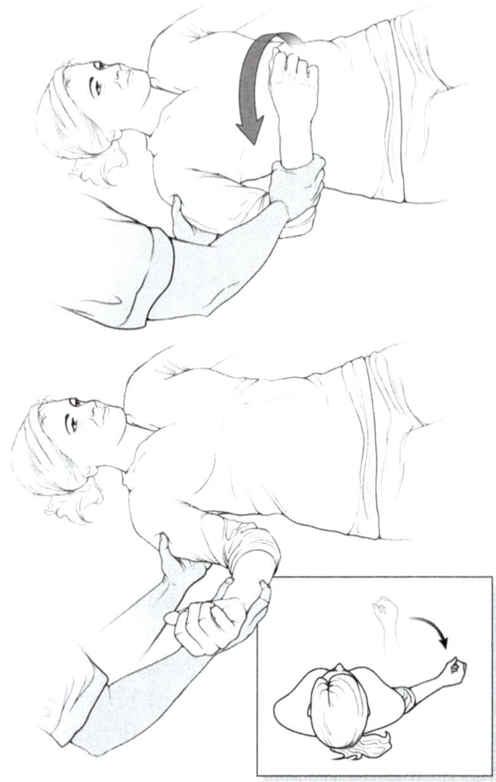

Shoulder external rotation

Fig. 39.2 Passive range of motion for shoulder external rotation

necessary [3]. A self-management program at home is optimal to achieve the best results [3].

As nerve function returns (either spontaneously or post-surgically), a gravity-eliminated strengthening program needs to be initiated. Once the patient can perform 10–15 repetitions without fatigue or substitution patterns, resistance in the form of weights (wrist cuff, dumbbell) can be added to the gravity-eliminated position. Progression of the amount of weight should continue in the gravity-eliminated position until the patient reaches approximately 8 pounds of resistance. Working up to 8 pounds of resistance in a gravity-eliminated plane will replicate the weight of the forearm once the patient can progress to the against gravity plane. The patient can then change positions to an against gravity position without weight in the affected extremity.

Strengthening of potential donor muscles for potential future nerve or tendon transfers is also very important. For example, if the surgeon is planning on using a branch of the triceps radial nerve to the axillary nerve, the preoperative therapy should focus on strengthening of the triceps.

Sling use is important for patients with panplexal or upper trunk injuries to support the paralyzed arm, mitigate inferior glenohumeral subluxation, and maintain the length-tension relationship of the involved muscles' sarcomeres to allow each muscle to generate appropriate force [4, 5]. Common slings used include universal slings, envelope slings, or hemi slings (Figs. 39.7, 39.8, 39.9, and 39.10). The sling should position the head of the humerus in normal alignment to a slightly elevated position in

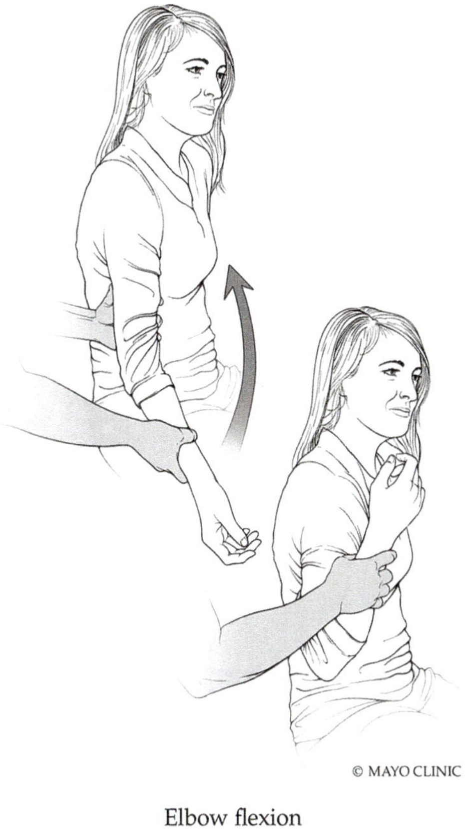

Fig. 39.3 Passive range of motion for elbow flexion

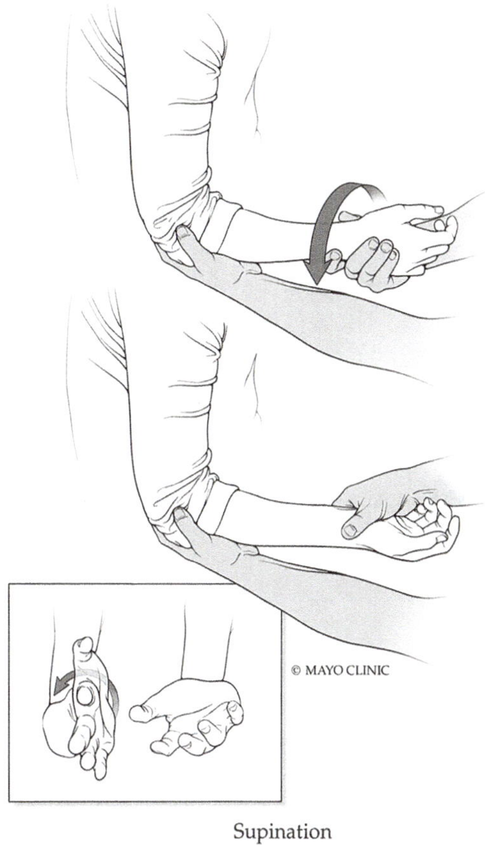

Fig. 39.4 Passive range of motion for forearm supination

the glenoid [3]. If a patient wants more security in a sling, a swath component may be included to keep the arm positioned close to the body. Another sling option is the Wilmer Carrying Orthosis and modifying the forearm component for custom wrist support. This sling has a pulley that allows for positioning the elbow in various degrees of flexion (Fig. 39.11).

Upper extremity orthoses help maintain joint alignment in a functional position and maintain the length-tension relationship of each muscle. An intrinsic plus resting orthosis should be fabricated to keep the wrist in extension, metacarpal phalangeal joints in flexion, interphalangeal joints in extension, and the thumb in palmer abduction (Fig. 39.12). This orthosis should be fabricated if the patient has lower trunk involvement or noted joint contractures in the hand. By diligently keeping full passive range of motion, the patients may not need additional procedures by such as joint manipulations under anesthesia, capsulotomies, or intrinsic tendon transfers. If the patient is beginning to lose passive range of motion, dynamic orthoses or static progressive orthoses should be considered. Common motions that become limited over time include shoulder external rotation, forearm supination, metacarpal phalangeal joint flexion, and first web space abduction. Common orthoses fabricated in our clinic include the intrinsic plus resting orthosis with thumb in palmer abduction (Fig. 39.12), web spacer or C-bar (Fig. 39.13), and dynamic

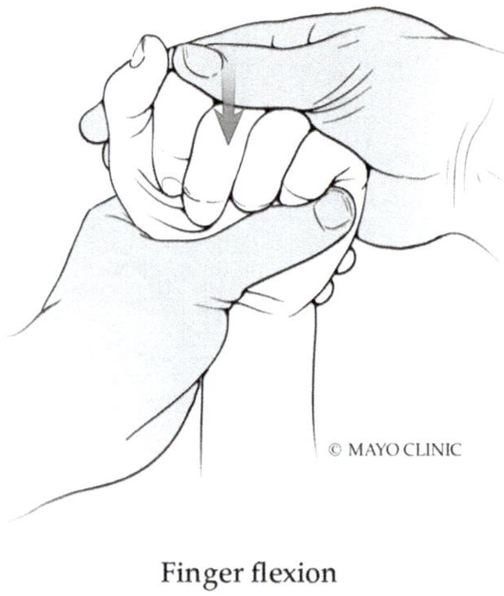

Fig. 39.5 Passive range of motion for metacarpal phalangeal joint flexion

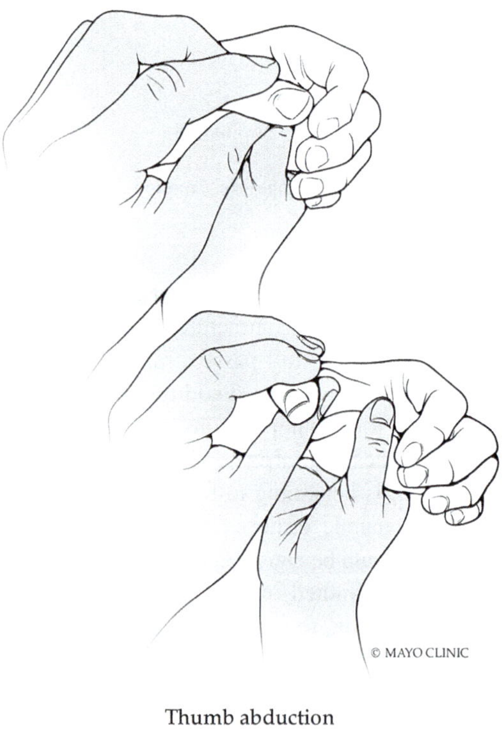

Fig. 39.6 Passive range of motion for first web space stretch

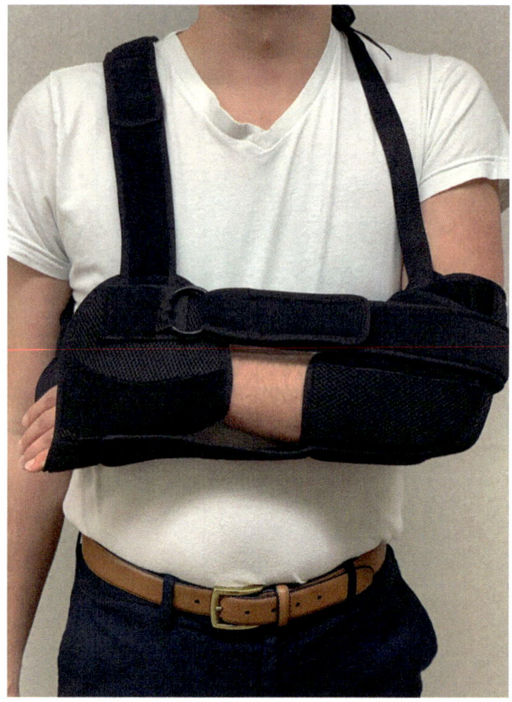

Fig. 39.7 Hely & Weber The UpLift Support Sling

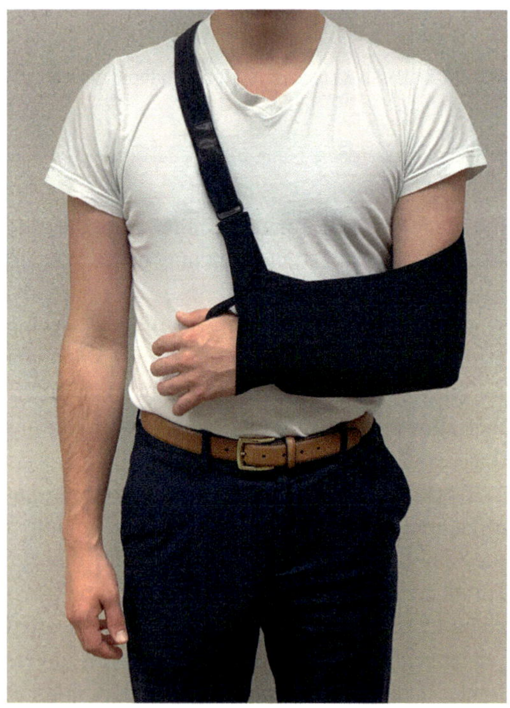

Fig. 39.8 The Ultimate Arm Sling

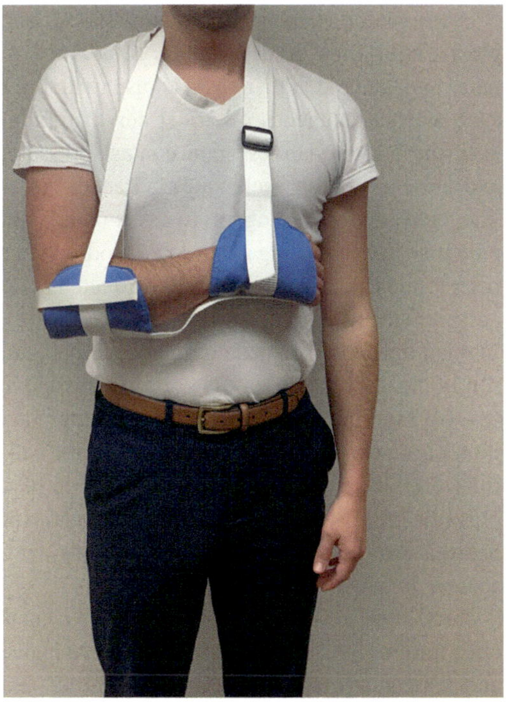

Fig. 39.9 The Universal Sling

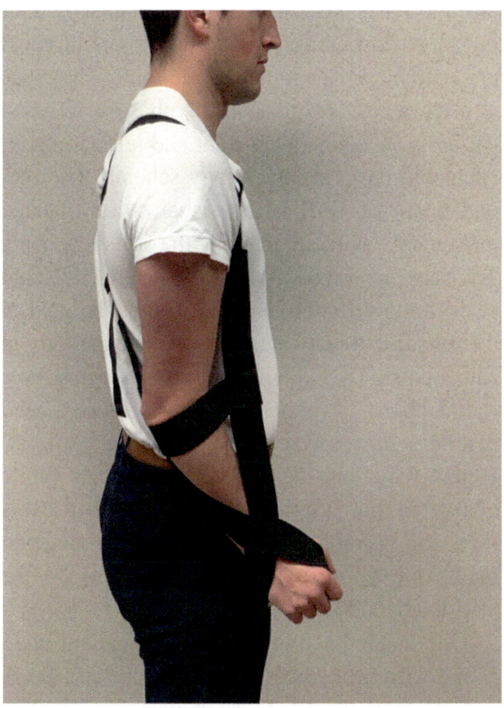

Fig. 39.10 The GivMohr Sling

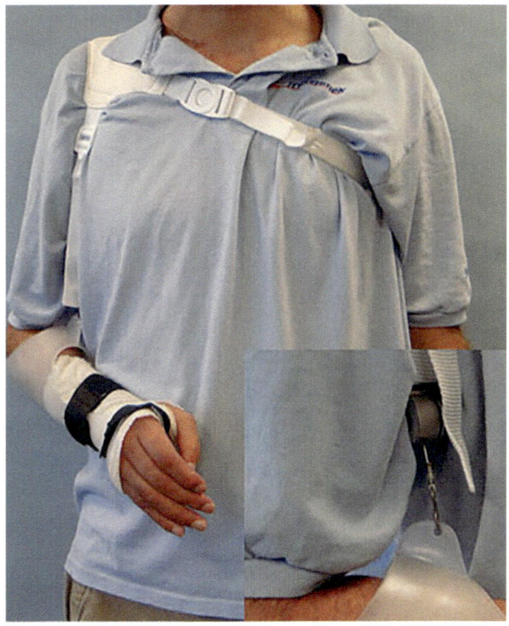

Fig. 39.11 Modified Wilmer Carrying Orthosis

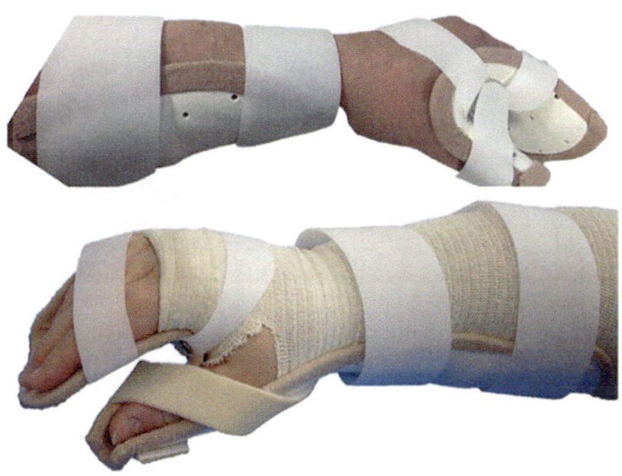

Fig. 39.12 Intrinsic plus resting hand orthoses

metacarpal phalangeal joint flexion orthosis (Fig. 39.14).

Cortical changes occur directly after an injury to the brachial plexus [6]. In a primate model, once the nerve has been injured, the somatosensory cortex for that nerve becomes silent. Corresponding areas in the somatosensory cortex will attempt to take over this silent region. If the nerve can regenerate or is repaired, the somatosensory cortex will have continued reorganization in the silent area [6]. The primary motor

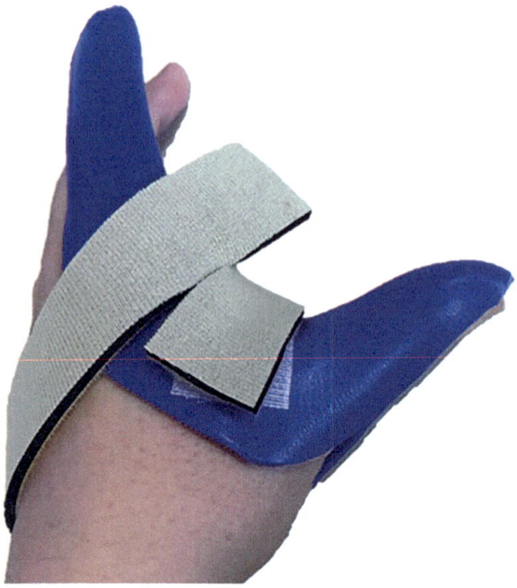

Fig. 39.13 Web spacer or C-bar orthosis

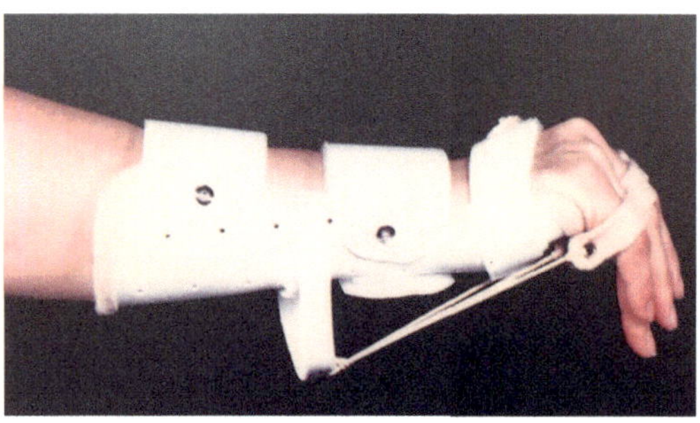

Fig. 39.14 Dynamic metacarpal phalangeal joint flexion orthosis

cortex has plasticity during motor skill acquisition. Research has shown in the adult primary motor cortex to be slowly changing and ever adapting to new motor learning [7]. If possible during the preoperative visit, neuromuscular reeducation of the potential nerve transfer should begin [4, 6]. For example, if a patient is to have a spinal accessory nerve transfer to the suprascapular nerve, activating the trapezius upper, middle, and lower should be emphasized while the patient visualizes shoulder elevation and external rotation of the arm before surgery. Adherence to the home exercise program for neuromuscular reeducation to achieve the best results is also emphasized [4, 6].

Neuropathic pain after a traumatic brachial plexus injury can be devastating. In addition to pain management, a therapist can use modalities such as transcutaneous electrical nerve stimulation, thermal modalities, total contact pressure, and desensitization techniques. Graded motor imagery (GMI) is a program to assist patients in pain management using a top-down model. It has been found that chronic pain in the affected body part influences cortical changes in the brain [8]. In phantom limb pain and complex regional pain syndrome, the somatosensory cortex is less active [8–10]. Another key concept of using graded motor imagery is the mirror neurons. Mirror neurons are active in both motor execution and observation [10]. It is thought that these mirror neurons do not fire correctly in patients with chronic pain [8].

Graded motor imagery has three phases: laterality training, visualization of hand movements, and mirror visual feedback (Figs. 39.15 and 39.16). This three-step program is used to activate the cortical motor networks and improve cortical reorganization. In the laterality phase, the patient identifies right versus left hands through flashcards. Increasing difficulty by adding more flashcards, increasing the rate of cards presented, and changing orientation of the cards is performed. The goal of this phase is to assist the brain in establishing right and left hand concepts and have an intact body schema. The second phase of GMI is the visualization of hand movements without moving the affected hand. The patient is asked to visualize the affected hand performing different hand positions. The goal of this phase is to activate the motor cortex without causing pain [8, 11]. The last phase is mirror box. In this phase, the patient places the affected hand behind a mirror box while observing the unaffected hand in the mirror reflection. While observing the mirror reflection, the patient is receiving visual feedback that not all hand movements are painful in what appears to be the affected hand [8].

One-handed activities with each patient diagnosed with a brachial plexopathy are discussed, and the patient should be educated with one-handed aids and tools. Despite advances in recon-

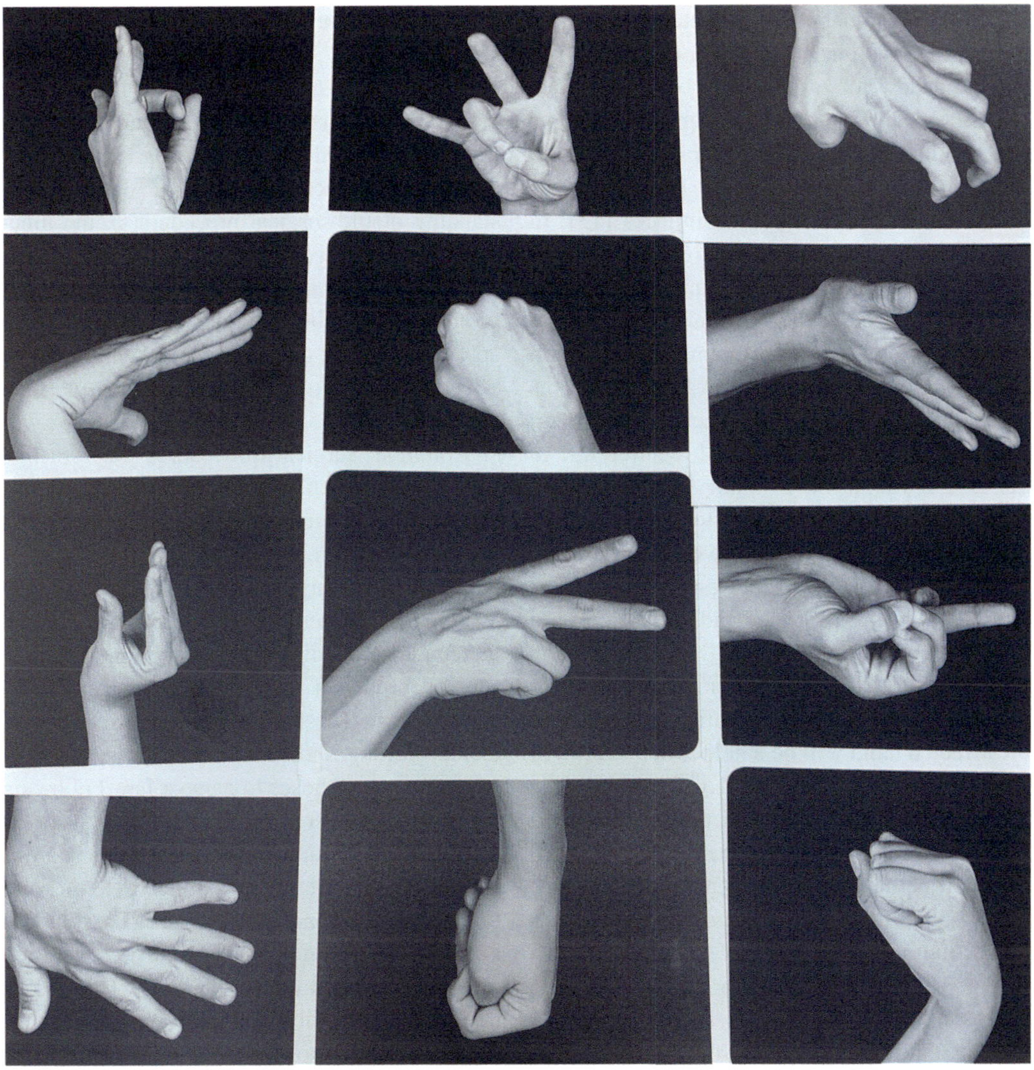

Fig. 39.15 Phase 1 of graded motor imagery: laterality cards

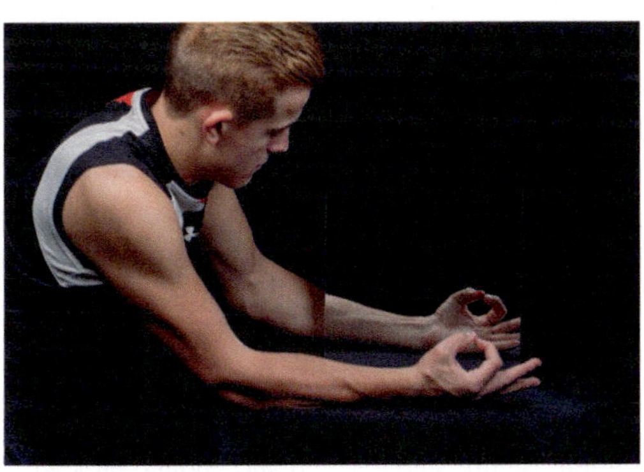

Fig. 39.16 Phase 3 of graded motor imagery: mirror box

structive procedures, the affected hand becomes a helper hand after the injury. In a study by Mancuso et al. [12], the authors encouraged rehabilitation efforts to support therapies for both the affected and unaffected extremities. It may be beneficial to have the therapies for each upper extremity separate from each other to allow the patient to fully participate in one-handed activities of daily living in one session while focusing on the affected extremity in another session [12]. Hand dominance affects the intensity of therapy for one-handed activities and compensatory techniques using adaptive equipment. Common themes in our clinic for difficult daily activities include handwriting, donning a bra for women, tying shoes, zipping a coat, and cracking an egg.

Psychosocial concerns and patient expectations impact rehabilitation outcomes for patients with brachial plexus injuries [13]. In one qualitative study assessing psychosocial factors and discussing patient expectations prior to surgery, the patients expected a decrease in pain and improvement in function for self-care, leisure, and work. These patients reported mental health effects of anxiety, depression, anger, and suicidal ideation due to the BPI. Patients have major life changes in education or employment due to the devastating injury. Finances after injury were also a major stress factor [14]. It is important to use a holistic approach as appearance and body image are important to our patients [13]. During therapy sessions, for pan-plexal, lower trunk injuries or complex injuries, it is imperative to stress that the affected hand will be a helper hand and will not return to the prior level of function. This helps set up realistic expectations for each patient. The therapist often becomes the advocate for patients who are having difficulties coping with injury and recommends visits with rehabilitation psychologists.

Preoperative rehabilitation needs a holistic approach to treat each patient. Rehabilitation needs a multidisciplinary approach to address all concerns. These concerns range from regaining range of motion and strengthening, fabricating orthoses, and fitting of slings to maintaining the length-tension relationship of muscles, beginning neuromuscular reeducation techniques for future reconstructive surgery options, assisting with pain management strategies, increasing function with daily occupations, and advocating for each patient with psychosocial concerns. It is crucial to maintain close contact with the referring surgeon to consistently keep the message the same that the affected extremity will be a helper hand and not return to normal. It is the goal of rehabilitation providers want to help increase the patient's function through the unaffected and affected extremity.

Postoperative Rehabilitation

Proper physical and occupational therapy after brachial plexus reconstructive surgery is of great importance to aid the patient in achieving their best possible functional outcome. A keen understanding of the surgical procedure(s), the timeline for healing, the future neuromuscular reeducation techniques, and the specific surgeon protocols should be communicated with the therapy team. When the surgeon and therapist are effective as a team, the optimal therapy plan can be formulated.

Common surgical procedures for brachial plexus reconstruction include nerve grafts, nerve transfers, free functioning muscle transfers (FFMT), tendon transfers, and joint fusions.

Ideally the surgical team will immediately involve the services of physical and occupational therapy postoperatively. It is important to follow surgical protocols for early immobilization and allowed range of motion. Immobilization may include casting, shoulder immobilizers, slings, or custom-made orthoses to name a few. Following immediate post-surgical immobilization, it is important that patients with upper trunk injuries continue with a hemi-sling to decrease the subluxation of the glenohumeral joint. This sling can be discontinued once appropriate reinnervation to the supraspinatus has occurred. The patient may need education in passive and/or active range of motion to the unaffected joints to be completed multiple times a day. Udina and colleagues [15] found that performing active and passive exercises of the involved limb slightly improved the amount of nerve reinnervation by increasing trophic factor release in rats. Therefore, it may be important for our patients to begin range of motion exercises of the involved joint(s) as soon as safely possible after surgery. The patient may need appropriate edema control measures immediately postoperative. The patient should be instructed in proper education in scar management techniques. In the case of a nerve transfer surgery, it is extremely important that the patient is educated early in and understands what donor muscle(s) needs to be "fired" to send the proper signal to the receiving muscle [4]. Once it is safe to do so, the patient needs to practice frequent activation techniques with the donor muscle to promote neural activation and growth [4]. The patient would also benefit from a supportive discussion regarding the short- and long-term rehabilitation expectations postoperatively. The patient needs to understand that recovery is a long, slow process and strength gains vary among individuals and may take several years for good results [4].

After EMG confirmation of reinnervation, we begin patient neuromuscular reeducation in a progressive gravity-eliminated (GE) exercise program for all brachial plexus reconstruction surgeries. The progression is as follows: (1) exercises in GE positions on low friction surfaces, (2) GE with added friction or light resistance once the patient achieves a functional arc of motion, (3) against gravity exercises without resistance after the patient builds strength in GE, and lastly (4) against gravity strengthening and eventual dissociation of the donor muscle with recipient muscle co-contraction. It is important to keep in mind as reinnervation to the targeted muscles begins, the patient will be very weak and fatigue quickly due to decreased number of muscle units available and the recovering muscle physiology. Sessions should be of short duration (5–10 minutes possibly) and completed several times a day [16]. Trick motions or substitution patterns and undesired muscle co-contractions during all phases of the rehabilitation process should be watched for and corrected. Once the patient has good strength in the reinnervated muscle(s) and can use the arm functionally, they often still will note significant fatigue with repetitive tasks and with activities needing sustained contraction [17].

Through the neuromuscular reeducation program, a patient will establish new cortical mapping to gain functional use of the affected extremity [18]. A GMI program can be started with a patient before any surgical procedure to stimulate the premotor cortex and should continue after surgery. If the patient has not participated in a GMI program prior to surgery, he/she should be instructed in the process by a physical or occupational therapist shortly after surgery.

Therapy Programs for Specific Neurotizations

Spinal Accessory Nerve (SAN) to Suprascapular Nerve (SSN)

The spinal accessory nerve (SAN) to suprascapular nerve (SSN) transfer is used to help restore shoulder function. The distal portion of the SAN, which provides motor innervation to the middle and lower trapezius, is transferred to the SSN (Fig. 39.17). Immediately following surgery, the patient will be in an immobilized for 3 weeks to allow nerve coaptation to heal and should work on maintaining passive range of motion of all other available joints except the shoulder. It is important that the patient return to wearing a hemi-sling to support the glenohumeral joint while awaiting reinnervation to the supraspinatus muscle. Early neuromuscular rehabilitation begins with activation of the upper and middle trapezius muscles (shoulder rolls and shoulder blade squeezes). Detailed neuromuscular reeducation will begin with noted EMG reinnervation, typically around

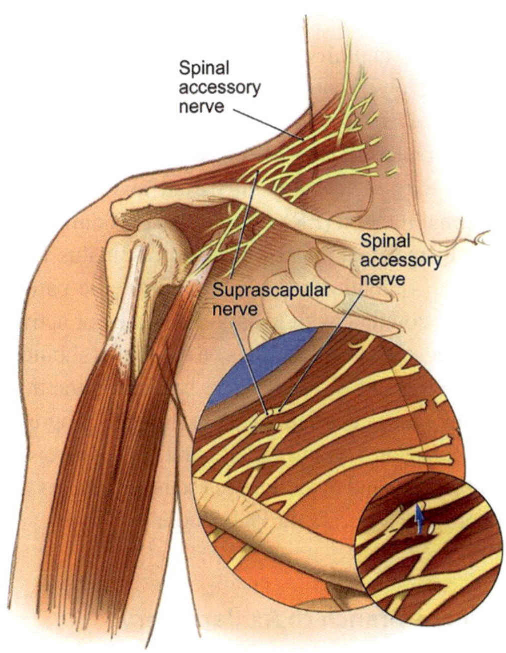

Fig. 39.17 Surgical procedure for spinal accessory to suprascapular nerve transfer

Table 39.1 Spinal accessory nerve to suprascapularnerve

Goal	Restore shoulder external rotation and abduction
Activation technique	Shoulder rolls, shoulder retraction
0–3 weeks after surgery	Shoulder immobilizer/sling for nerve healing
3 weeks after surgery	Maintain passive range of motion to all available joints
	Graded motor imagery
	Perform shoulder rolls or shoulder retraction while visualizing the arm externally rotating or abducting the shoulder
	Strengthen the trapezius
	Actively retract the scapula and passively externally rotate or abduct the shoulder
After EMG confirmation (typically 4–6 months)	Start a gravity-eliminated strengthening program for shoulder external rotation and abduction neuromuscular reeducation
	Begin biofeedback

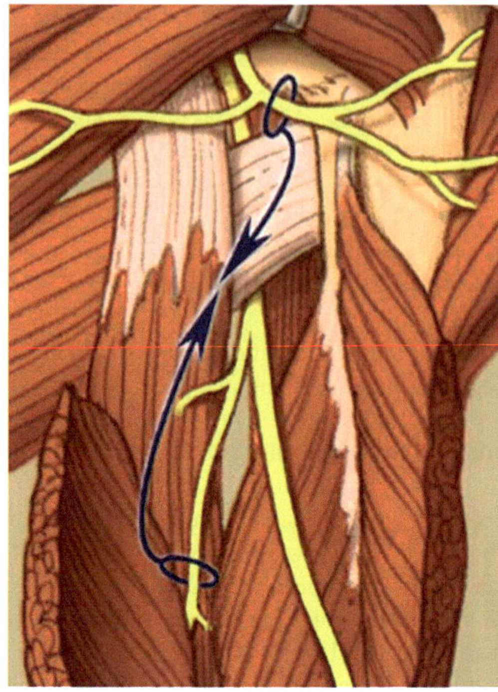

Fig. 39.18 Surgical procedure for triceps branch of the radial nerve to axillary nerve

4–6 months postoperatively. If the patient has an innervated serratus anterior, he/she should work on strengthening this muscle to assist with upward scapular rotation. During active scapular retraction, Kahn and Moore [4] advise the patient to use the uninvolved hand to passively externally rotate the involved arm to assist with developing new motor patterns. They also recommend the patient place the surgical arm in partial abduction and external rotation (ER) for short periods during the day to maintain supraspinatus/infraspinatus ideal length [4]. With further motor return, the patient should continue with gravity-eliminated or active-assisted exercises that focus on combined shoulder abduction and ER with active scapular retraction. As the patient continues to gain strength, progressing to against gravity place and hold exercises, wall slides, and other light resistance exercises are appropriate. See Table 39.1 for our protocol.

Triceps Branch to Axillary Nerve

Triceps branch of the radial nerve to axillary nerve transfer is a common technique to restore deltoid function in an upper trunk injury. This was described by Leechavengvongs in 2003 who transferred the long head of the triceps nerve branch to the anterior division of the axillary nerve [19] (Fig. 39.18). Following surgery, the patient needs to immobilize his/her shoulder and elbow for 3 weeks and work on range of motion of the uninvolved joints. At 3 weeks post-op, passive range of motion to the involved shoulder can begin with an emphasis on shoulder external rotation (ER) and scapular mobilization. Initial neuromuscular rehabilitation starts with activation of the triceps isometrically or with donor/recipient patterning via seated shoulder flexion table slides (Fig. 39.19). Kahn and Moore also instruct the patient to slide his/her affected hand on his/her thigh toward his/her knee from a seated position [4]. In our clinic, we use a light resistance band anchored just above and behind the patient for elbow extension with patterning of shoulder elevation a helpful exercise for reeducation once reinnervation is detected via EMG (typically at 4–6 months) (Fig. 39.20). To reeducate shoulder ER, the patient can be seated with his/her forearm resting on a low friction surface on a

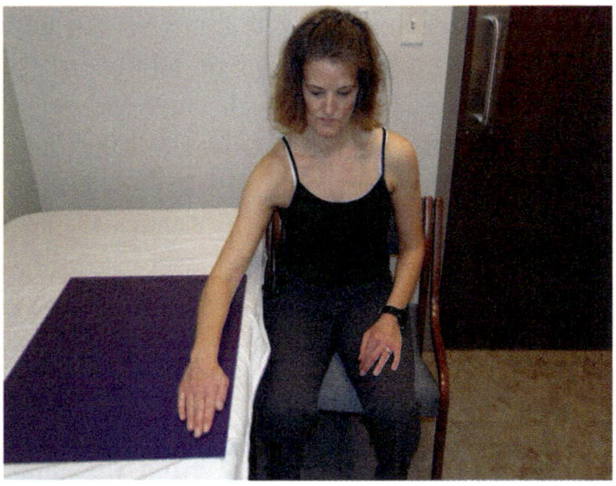

Fig. 39.19 Seated shoulder flexion slides

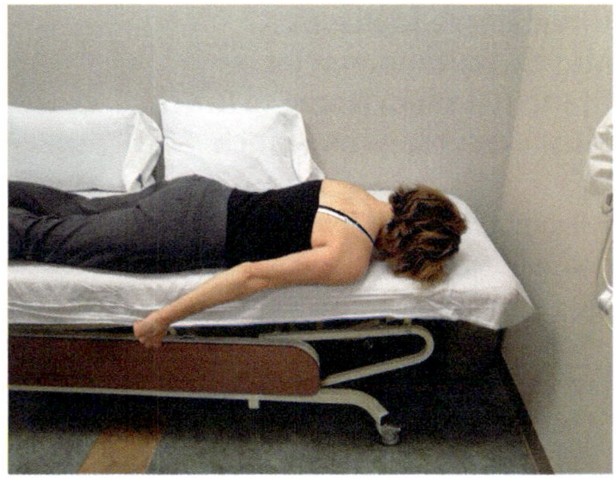

Fig. 39.21 Prone elbow extension with shoulder extension

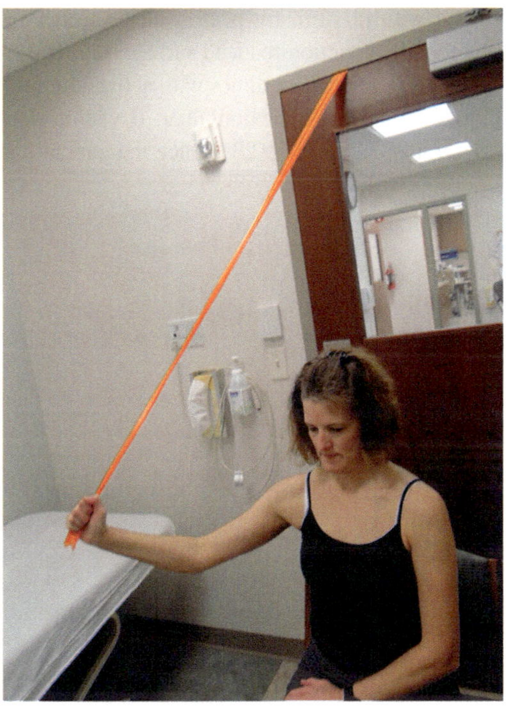

Fig. 39.20 Resistance band triceps activation

Table 39.2 Triceps branch of the radial nerve to axillary nerve

Goal	Restore shoulder forward flexion, abduction, and extension
Activation technique	Activate with elbow extension or wrist extension
0–3 weeks after surgery	Shoulder and elbow immobilization to allow nerves to heal
	Wrist and hand range of motion
3 weeks after surgery	Passive range of motion to shoulder, emphasis on scapular mobilizations, shoulder external rotation
	Graded motor imagery
	Perform elbow extension or wrist extension while visualizing the shoulder moving in forward flexion, abduction, and extension
	Strengthen the triceps and wrist extensors
	Actively extend the elbow or wrist while passively moving the shoulder into forward flexion, abduction, and/or extension
After EMG confirmation (typically 4–6 months)	Start a gravity-eliminated strengthening program for shoulder forward flexion, abduction, and extension neuromuscular reeducation
	Begin biofeedback

table. From here, gentle isometric triceps activation coupled with passive/active assistive ER is begun. Continued reinnervation often begins with the posterior deltoid; therefore, with further motor return, it is helpful to position the patient prone to work on shoulder extension and shoulder abduction. In this position, the patient will co-contract with the triceps to further flood the recipient deltoid (Fig. 39.21). The patient can also be positioned in side-lying on the unaffected side with the surgical arm on a therapy skateboard for gravity-eliminated shoulder flexion reeducation. See Table 39.2 for our protocol.

Ulnar Nerve to Biceps Musculocutaneous Nerve Branch/Median Nerve to Brachialis Musculocutaneous Branch

Restoring elbow flexion is crucial as it helps position the hand for activities of daily living. The most popular nerve transfer to restore elbow flexion in an upper trunk injury with intact C8–T1 function was described by Oberlin in 1994. He transferred ulnar nerve fascicles that primarily innervated the flexor carpi ulnaris (FCU) and to the bicep motor branch of the musculocutaneous nerve [20]. Mackinnon et al. [21] desired to gain further elbow flexion strength and described a double fascicular nerve transfer by adding the transfer of median nerve fascicles to the brachialis motor branch (Fig. 39.22). They reported early reinnervation at 5.5 months after surgery [21]. Similar to the above nerve transfers, the shoulder and elbow are immobilized for 3 weeks with allowed active/passive range of motion to the involved wrist and hand. Kahn and Moore [4] instruct the patient in early activation of the donor muscles through gripping therapy putty and beginning light wrist flexion curls with a 1-pound weight. Once the shoulder immobilizer is discontinued, the patient needs to begin patterning desired elbow flexion with donor activation. This can simply be done with active finger grasp and wrist flexion/ulnar deviation during passive elbow flexion with assistance from the uninvolved arm.

With EMG confirmation of early reinnervation, gravity-eliminated elbow flexion exercises are started with the forearm positioned on a therapy skateboard or friction-reduced surface. It is important that the patient continues with activation techniques using wrist flexion/ulnar deviation and finger grasping (Fig. 39.23). Once the patient has

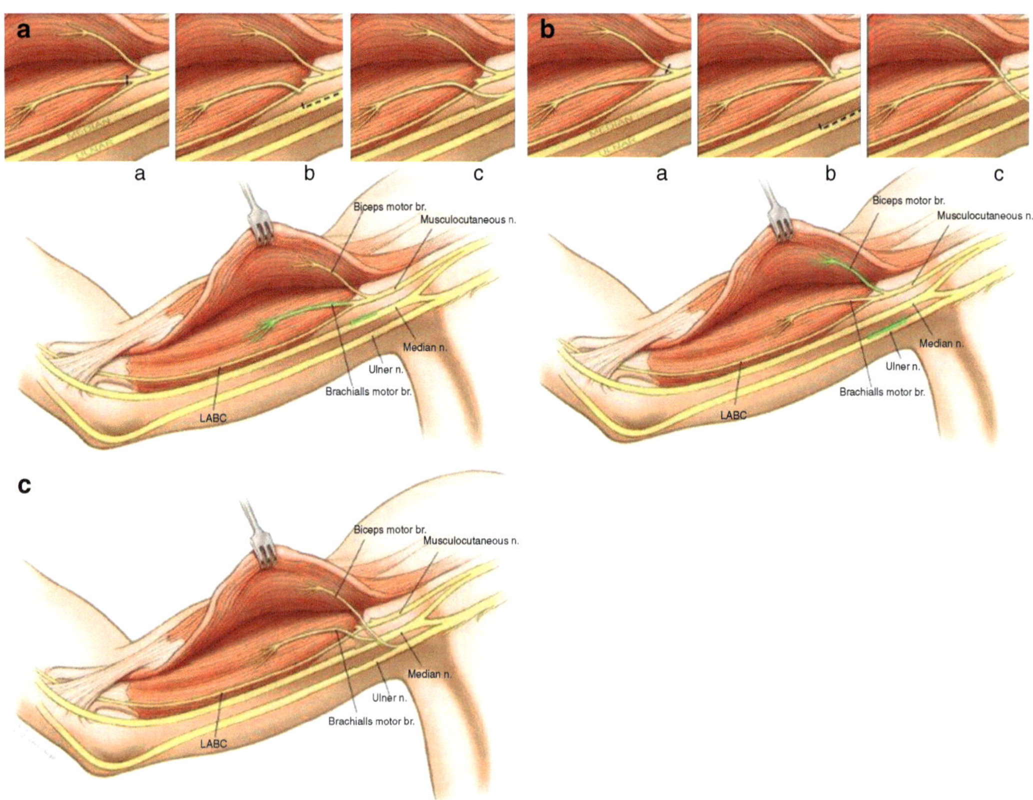

Fig. 39.22 Surgical procedure for double fascicular nerve transfer for elbow flexion. (**a**) Median nerve fascicle to the brachialis motor branch; (**b**) Ulnar nerve fascicle to the biceps motor branch; (**c**) Double fascicular transfer for elbow flexion

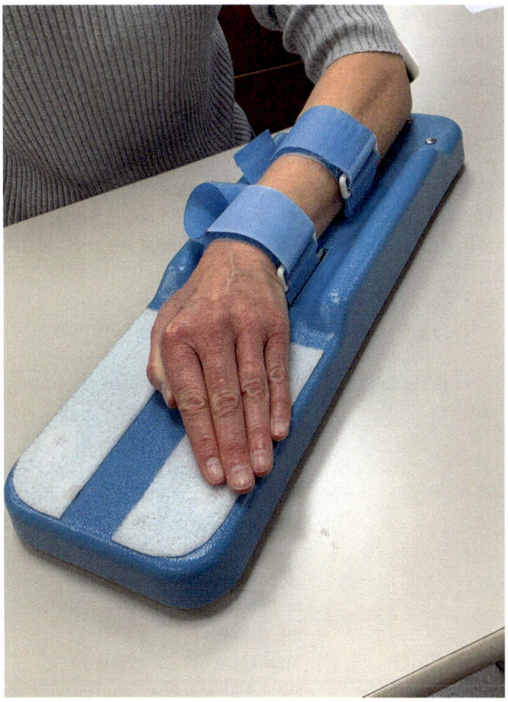

Fig. 39.23 Gravity-eliminated elbow flexion with ulnar deviation of the wrist activation technique while using a skateboard

gained a nearly full arc of elbow flexion in this manner, progressive weight can be added to the skateboard or the patient begins exercising without the aid of the skateboard. The patient can then progress to place and hold elbow flexion exercises against gravity and eventually the use of light handheld weights when they achieve full elbow flexion against gravity. See Table 39.3 for our protocol.

Intercostal Nerve to Musculocutaneous Nerve

If a donor nerve within the brachial plexus is not available for neurotization to restore elbow flexion, intercostal nerves (ICNs) can be transferred to the musculocutaneous nerve (MCN). Typically three to four ICNs are transferred to the MCN or two to three ICNs are directly transferred to the biceps motor branch [22] (Fig. 39.24). The ICN sensory and motor components can be separated during surgery to allow for more pure motor axons being neurotized. If these nerves are transferred, it is important to understand that the patient will have lifelong restrictions regarding shoulder motion. To avoid rupturing the nerve coaptation, the patient needs to avoid shoulder abduction greater than 90°, shoulder flexion greater than 90°, and ER greater than 90°.

Early reeducation begins by instructing the patient in activation techniques for the ICNs to

Table 39.3 Protocol for double fascicular transfer using an ulnar nerve and median nerve fascicle to the musculocutaneous nerve

Ulnar nerve fascicle to biceps musculocutaneous nerve branch	
Goal	**Restore elbow flexion**
Activation technique	Activate with ulnar deviation of the wrist or key pinch
0–3 weeks after surgery	Shoulder immobilizer/sling for nerve healing
3 weeks after surgery	Maintain passive range of motion of all available joints
	Graded motor imagery
	Perform ulnar deviation of the wrist while visualizing elbow flexion
	Strengthen flexor carpi ulnaris
	Actively ulnarly deviate the wrist while passively flexing the elbow
After EMG confirmation (typically 4–6 months)	Start a gravity-eliminated strengthening program for elbow flexion neuromuscular reeducation
	Begin biofeedback
Median nerve fascicle to brachialis musculocutaneous nerve branch	
Goal	**Restore elbow flexion**
Activation technique	Activate with finger flexion
0–3 weeks after surgery	Shoulder immobilizer/sling for nerve healing
3 weeks after surgery	Maintain passive range of motion of all available joints
	Graded motor imagery
	Perform finger flexion while visualizing elbow flexion
	Strengthen grip specifically the flexor digitorum superficialis
	Actively grip while passively flexing the elbow
After EMG confirmation (typically 4–6 months)	Start a gravity-eliminated strengthening program for elbow flexion neuromuscular reeducation
	Begin biofeedback

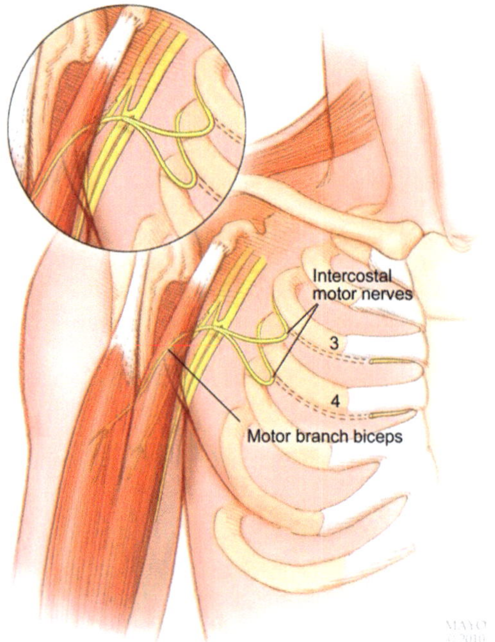

Fig. 39.24 Surgical procedure for intercostal nerve to musculocutaneous nerve transfer

Table 39.4 Intercostal nerve transfer to musculocutaneous nerve

Goal	Restore elbow flexion
Activation technique	Activate with pursed lip breathing, coughing, laughing, breathing in deeply, bearing down, trunk flexion
Permanent restrictions	No shoulder abduction, forward flexion, or external rotation with arm abducted greater than 90°
0–3 weeks after surgery	Shoulder and elbow immobilization to allow nerves to heal
3 weeks after surgery	Maintain passive range of motion of all available joints
	Graded motor imagery
	Perform breathing technique while visualizing elbow flexion
	Spirometer for respiratory exercises
	Actively perform breathing technique while passively flexing the elbow
After EMG confirmation (typically 6–9 months)	Start a gravity-eliminated strengthening program for elbow flexion neuromuscular reeducation
	Begin biofeedback

initiate biceps and brachialis muscle contraction. This would include exhalation, inhalation Valsalva, and trunk flexion. Immediately following surgery, the patient should be educated in the use of a spirometer to complete deep inspiration and exhalation exercises that will help stimulate the new neural pathway. The patient should also promptly start abdominal muscle exercises to help with ICN recruitment. In 2006, Chalidapong et al. [23] reported that patients who had undergone ICN to MCN neurotization had the greatest EMG activity in the elbow flexors during trunk flexion when compared with forced expiration, forced inspiration, and attempted isolated elbow flexion.

Once a palpable twitch is noted in the elbow flexors or with motor unit potentials reported on EMG, the patient's reeducation program needs to progress to GE exercises. These exercises can be done side-lying with the affected extremity on a bolster or a sloped support. If the patient is seated, the affected extremity is placed just below the safe position for shoulder elevation to complete GE exercise. Using low friction surfaces is important to maximize recipient muscle joint motion and minimize fatigue in the beginning. Initiating elbow flexion with donor nerve activation (trunk flexion, pursed-lip breathing, etc.) needs to continue. Once the patient demonstrates a nearly full arc of motion in the GE plane, the therapist can introduce light resistance or increase friction in the GE plane. Advancement of exercises will continue to follow the progressive program and will begin to work on separating the co-contraction of the donor muscle with the target muscle. See Table 39.4 for our protocol.

Free Functioning Muscle Transfers for Elbow Flexion

When the timing from a complete avulsion brachial plexus injury to surgery is greater than 12 months, free functioning muscle transfers (FFMT) are recommended to obtain elbow flexion. In the acute phase, FFMT can be used in

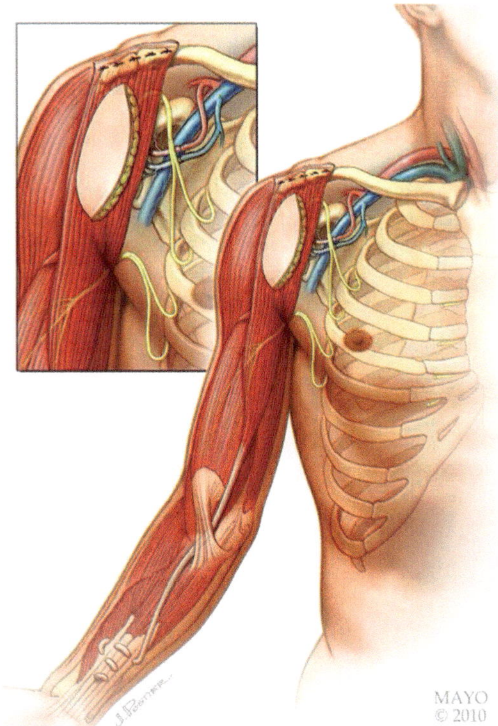

Fig. 39.25 Surgical procedure for free muscle transfer for combined elbow and finger flexion with intercostal nerve transfer

addition to other nerve transfers to restore both elbow flexion and possible graph (Fig. 39.25). The gracilis muscle is often selected because of its proximal neurovascular pedicle that allows more rapid reinnervation and its long tendon length that allows for appropriate tendon excursion [24]. For combined finger flexion and elbow flexion, a Pulvertaft weave is used to secure the gracilis tendon to the flexor pollicis longus tendon and flexor digitorum profundus (FDP) tendons to restore rudimentary grasp. To prevent bowstringing of the distal tendon at the elbow, a pulley mechanism is created by passing the gracilis muscle underneath the biceps tendon and flexor digitorum superficialis (FDS) arch [24, 25]. Nerve innervation can come from the SAN or ICNs. These patients will also have lifetime shoulder motion restrictions if the ICNs are used for reinnervation (avoid shoulder abduction greater than 90°, shoulder flexion greater than 90°, and ER greater than 90°). It is recommended

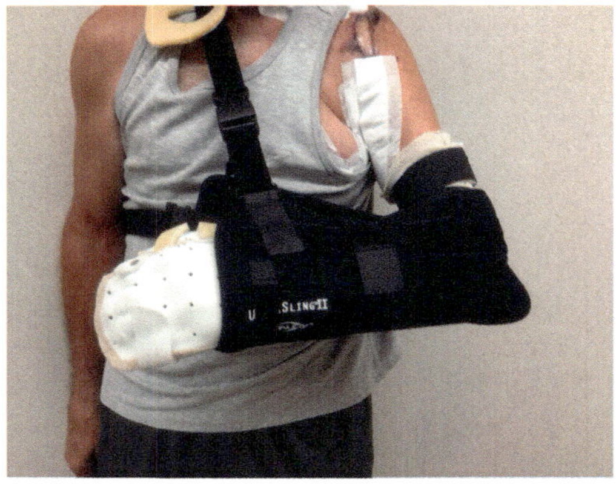

Fig. 39.26 Shoulder immobilizer with posterior elbow orthosis and dorsal blocking orthosis

to avoid any elbow extension less than 30°. This position allows for an ideal angle of pull and more appropriate length-tension relationship of the muscle, making eventual active elbow flexion easier to initiate. A wrist and thumb interphalangeal joint (IP) arthrodesis is performed several months after the FFMT to simplify the wrist/grasp mechanics to allow a single muscle to provide rudimentary grasp.

Postoperatively, the surgical arm is immobilized per surgeon protocol. Often this is with a shoulder immobilizer, posterior 90-degree elbow orthosis, and, if the FFMT was also for combined finger flexion, a dorsal blocking orthosis with the finger metacarpal joints in 70° flexion (Fig. 39.26). Patients should perform passive range of motion to all appropriate joints when it is safe to do so. This includes the shoulder and elbow (within appropriate restrictions), fingers, and thumb carpometacarpal joint (CMC). The fingers need to be moved as a group as during surgery, the finger flexors were sutured together. When the incisions have healed, it is important that the patient begins deep soft tissue mobilization over the anterior cubital fossa three to five times a day. This will minimize adhesions of the tendon and allow for better tendon gliding of the FFMT.

If ICNs are used for reinnervation, early neuromuscular reeducation begins shortly after surgery and is similar to the above ICN to MCN neurotization with various breathing techniques

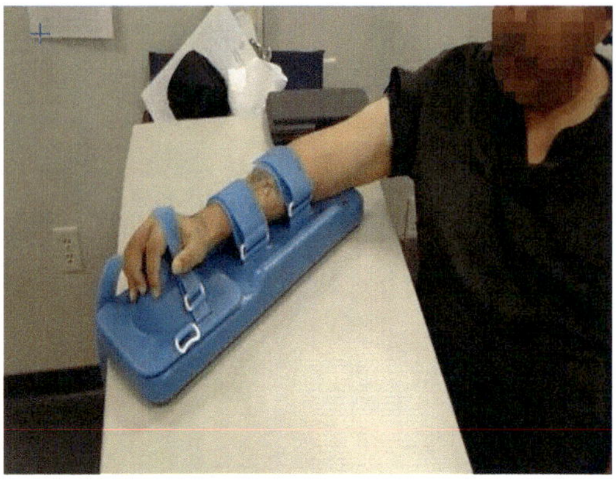

Fig. 39.27 Gravity-eliminated elbow flexion with skateboard

and/or trunk flexion exercises. If the SAN nerve is used, the patient is advised to practice scapular retraction while palpating the biceps/repaired gracilis tendon for tension [25]. Often it takes 6–9 months for early reinnervation to be noted clinically or through an EMG study, and further recovery is a long, slow process. When there is evidence of reinnervation (M1 strength) to the FFMT, it is important that the patient begins a concentrated program of neuromuscular reeducation under the supervision of a physical or occupational therapist. Exercises will follow the progressive GE rehabilitation program on low friction surfaces with continued education in activation techniques for elbow flexion (Fig. 39.27). Initially it may be easiest to generate muscle power in a moderate amount of elbow flexion and gradually work toward less elbow flexion (reminder, patients should have a 30-degree elbow flexion contracture). Resistance can be added into GE exercises when the patient demonstrates a functional arc of elbow flexion, and the program continues to progress as the patient gains muscle strength. See Tables 39.5 and 39.6 for our protocols.

Table 39.5 Free functioning muscle transfer for elbow flexion with intercostal nerve transfer

Goal	Restore elbow flexion
Activation technique	Activate with pursed lip breathing, coughing, laughing, breathing in deeply, bearing down, trunk flexion
Permanent restrictions	No shoulder abduction, forward flexion, or external rotation with arm abducted greater than 90°
	Do not straighten elbow beyond 30° of flexion to create a mild elbow contracture
0–3 weeks after surgery	Shoulder immobilizer
	Passive range of motion to fingers, thumb, wrist, and forearm
3 weeks after surgery	Discontinue shoulder immobilizer and change to a support sling
	Evaluate for glenohumeral support
	90° posterior long arm elbow orthosis
	Begin passive range of motion for shoulder external rotation with the shoulder at 0° of shoulder abduction
	Begin passive range of motion for elbow full flexion to 30° of extension
	If pulley was created at antecubital fossa, place pressure on the antecubital fossa to prevent bow stringing during elbow passive range of motion
	Continue range of motion to the fingers thumb, wrist, and forearm
	Graded motor imagery
	Perform breathing activation technique while visualizing elbow flexion
	Spirometer for respiratory exercises
	Actively perform breathing activation technique while passively flexing the elbow
6 weeks after surgery	Discontinue elbow orthosis and continue with a sling except for exercises
	Initiate scapular mobilizations and continue with above ROM exercises
After EMG confirmation (typically 6–9 months)	Start a gravity-eliminated strengthening program for elbow flexion neuromuscular reeducation
	Begin biofeedback

Surgical Reconstructions that Fall Outside the Norm

At times, a patient may present to therapy following an "uncommon" brachial plexus reconstruction surgery. Other muscles have been used for FFMT such as the rectus femoris and latissimus dorsi for elbow flexion with good outcomes [25].

Table 39.6 Free functioning muscle transfer combined elbow flexion and finger flexion with intercostal nerve transfer

Goal	Restore elbow flexion
Activation technique	Activate with pursed lip breathing, coughing, laughing, breathing in deeply, bearing down trunk flexion
Permanent restrictions	No shoulder abduction, forward flexion, or external rotation with arm abducted greater than 90°
	Do not straighten elbow beyond 30° of flexion to create a mild elbow contracture
0–3 weeks after surgery	Shoulder immobilizer with orthoses worn in the immobilizer
	Forearm-based intrinsic plus orthosis; surgeons prefer this to be *dorsal* based
	90° posterior elbow orthosis
	Passive finger range of motion with the elbow at 90° of flexion
	Move digits as a group, concentrate on intrinsic plus position with MP flexion and IP extension
	Passive elbow range of motion with support over the antecubital fossa to support the tendon transfer limiting elbow extension to 30°. Wrist and digits in flexion
	Wrist and forearm range of motion with elbow at 90° of flexion
	With elbow at approximately 90° of flexion, squeeze the forearm muscle bellies to assist in tendon pull through to the fingers
3 weeks after surgery	Discontinue shoulder immobilizer and change to a support sling
	Evaluate for glenohumeral support
	Continue with elbow orthosis and dorsal blocking orthosis
	Passive range of motion for shoulder external rotation while keeping the shoulder at 0° of shoulder abduction
	Continue with the above 0–3 week exercises
	Graded motor imagery
	Perform breathing activation technique while visualizing elbow flexion and finger flexion
	Spirometer for respiratory exercises
	Actively perform activation breathing technique while passively flexing the elbow and fingers
6 weeks after surgery	Discontinue elbow orthosis and continue with a sling except for exercises
	Continue with forearm based orthosis for night wear
	Initiate scapular mobilizations and continue with above ROM exercises
After EMG confirmation (typically 6–9 months)	Start a gravity-eliminated strengthening program for elbow flexion and finger flexion neuromuscular reeducation
	Begin biofeedback

Rehabilitation would be very similar to a gracilis transfer once it is known what nerve(s) was used for the reinnervation. A branch of the medial pectoral nerve (MPN) can be used with a C5–C6 or C5–C7 brachial plexus injury and still preserve innervation to the pectoralis sternal head. However, drawbacks to using this nerve include its limited length and the nerve diameter difference with the MCN [22]. A branch of the thoracodorsal nerve (TDN) can also be used for neurotization to the MCN due to its sufficient length. Both of these nerves can also be used for triceps reinnervation through the radial nerve [22]. As with other neuromuscular reeducation programs, it begins with understanding the anatomical function of the donor muscle for proper activation of the target muscle. Some surgeries include reinnervation of the triceps (ICNs or SAN) to get added elbow stabilization with biceps restoration. Using the ICNs to reinnervate both biceps and triceps should be avoided [24]. Neuromuscular reeducation for both elbow flexion and extension can get complicated, and the therapist should monitor the patient for co-contraction of both muscles during the desired elbow motion.

Other Rehabilitation Considerations

In addition to previously described neuromuscular reeducation techniques for treatment of nerve repair, various modalities have been encouraged. One of the most commonly suggested modalities is electrical stimulation (functional electrical stimulation or neuromuscular electrical stimulation) following nerve injury. When working with denervated muscle, direct or galvanic stimulation is used to provide an external source of stimulation to the muscles (Fig. 39.28). The hope is that this will prolong the time before the muscle suffers irreversible changes due to denervation [2]. For electrical stimulation to be of most benefit, the parameters need to analogous to a muscle's normal "firing pattern" which has been shown in some animal models using implanted electrodes. Trials have not confirmed the use of surface electrodes for electrical stimulation [18]. However, there is little strong evidence in the literature that supports the use of direct current stimulation in humans [2, 18]. We have abandoned its use in our practice.

Single-channel or dual-channel biofeedback is another modality that is often recommended as part of a neuromuscular rehabilitation program. Biofeedback provides immediate feedback to the patient which helps them understand and learn new motor patterns. Sturma et al. [26] reported surface EMG biofeedback can be used before any noted movements as this device can provide helpful feedback of muscular activity by converting myoelectrical activity into auditory and/or visual cuing. Most often though this modality is not used until the patient begins having positive muscle reinnervation findings clinically or noted on EMG results, but it would be safe to begin much earlier. Surface electrodes are placed on the reinnervated muscle to give real-time information during muscle activation to increase muscle contraction. This tool can also be useful if an antagonistic muscle is overpowering the weaker, reinnervated muscle [18]. Here, the surface electrodes would be placed over the antagonistic muscle, and the patient is educated to decrease muscle activation during the desired motion (e.g., overpowering triceps activity during elbow flexion reeducation following an ulnar nerve fascicle to musculotaneous nerve for elbow flexion). Biofeedback is also a helpful tool if a patient is co-contracting muscles during initiation of movement (Fig. 39.29). Early in the reeducation process, patients may have trouble isolating the weaker reinnervated muscle and accidentally co-contract the stronger antagonistic muscle. Dual-channel biofeedback over both muscle groups provides immediate visual and auditory feedback assists in decreasing antagonistic muscle action while increasing focus to the reinnervated muscle [18]. When the patient can visualize and/or pal-

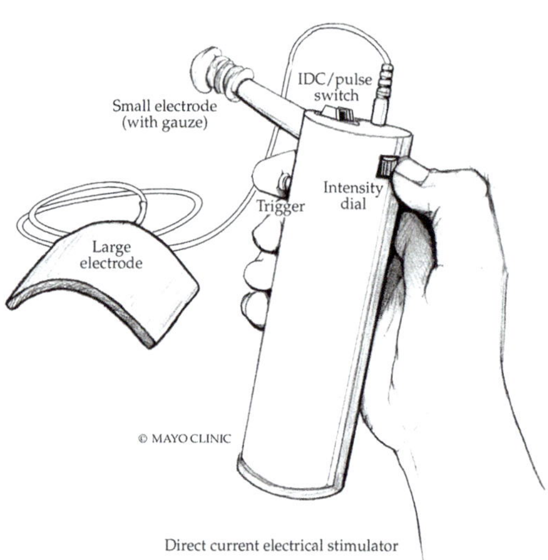

Fig. 39.28 Direct electrical stimulation

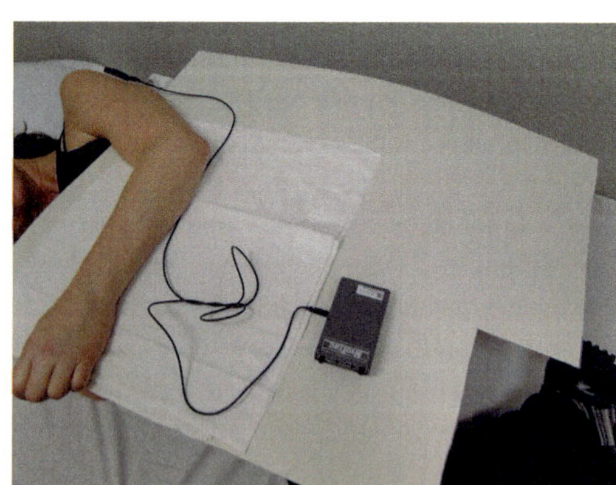

Fig. 39.29 Biofeedback device

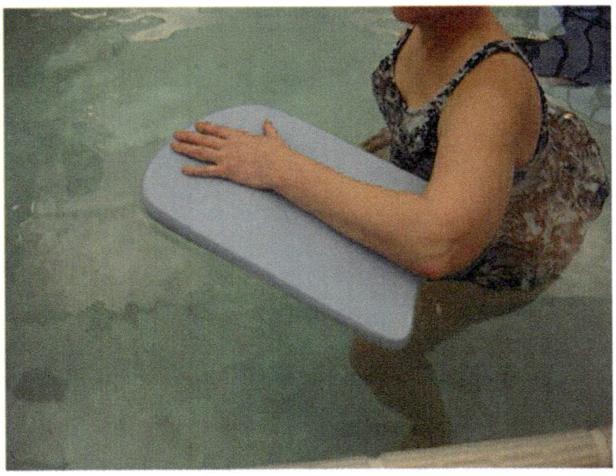

Fig. 39.30 Aquatic therapy for gravity-eliminated elbow extension and flexion

pate their muscle contraction, they can use this option for frequent and useful feedback during exercise. Patients have reported learning how to control the reinnervated muscle and "switch off" the donor muscle to be very challenging [17]. Biofeedback can continue to be used in this later stage of rehabilitation to progressively separate activation of the reinnervated muscle with donor muscle activation [26].

Aqua therapy or pool-based exercises can be helpful in the rehabilitation process. The buoyancy of the water can assist with shoulder flexion, shoulder abduction, and elbow flexion while the patient is using proper donor nerve activation techniques. The patient can also use gravity-eliminated positions for elbow flexion and shoulder external rotation with their affected arm on a swimming kickboard for neuromuscular reeducation (Fig. 39.30). As the patient gains strength in the reinnervated muscle, they can use water for light resistance training.

Neuropathic pain management following surgical reconstruction may be an ongoing concern. Unfortunately, this can limit a patient's therapy tolerance and result in an overall negative outcome [16]. It is important that the patient's pain is managed by a multidisciplinary team approach, including a pain specialist, who can prescribe and monitor a correct medication regime [24]. Non-pharmaceutical treatment choices may include edema control if appropriate, sling use, transcutaneous electrical nerve stimulation, GMI, and relaxation/distraction techniques to name a few (see Chap. 15).

With technological advances, there have been newer therapeutic modalities available to use in rehabilitation. These include the usage of exoskeleton devices. These devices are wearable robotics that can control elbow flexion and extension and a three-point pinch [27]. Exoskeleton-type devices use bioelectric muscle activation signals detected at the surface level. Once the electrodes detect the signal, a motor produces the desired joint motion [27, 28]. These devices can use minimal muscle activation of a twitch to produce the desired motion. Collaboration with a prosthetist/orthotist is recommended. The therapist focuses on function and refining smooth motion, while the prosthetist determines appropriate signal settings, placing the sensors in the optimal positions and refining the fit of the harness and exoskeleton. Once the patient can consistently and smoothly activate the exoskeleton, the therapist will concentrate on bilateral functional movements (Figs. 39.31 and 39.32). Exoskeletons may be a temporary, wearable device until the patient achieves the desired muscle strength or the device may be a lifelong wearable orthosis to assist in activities of daily living.

There are also advances in myoelectric prosthetics and surgical procedures using targeted muscle reinnervation to achieve increased upper extremity function. In a pan-plexal injury pattern, if the patient can achieve grade 4 elbow flexion, there may be a role for an elective forearm amputation and fitting of a myoelectric prosthesis to give the patient hand function. In our experience, we see the patient initially with the prosthetist and focus on bilateral functional movements (Figs. 39.33 and 39.34). Please see Chap. 16 for more information on the use of prosthetics.

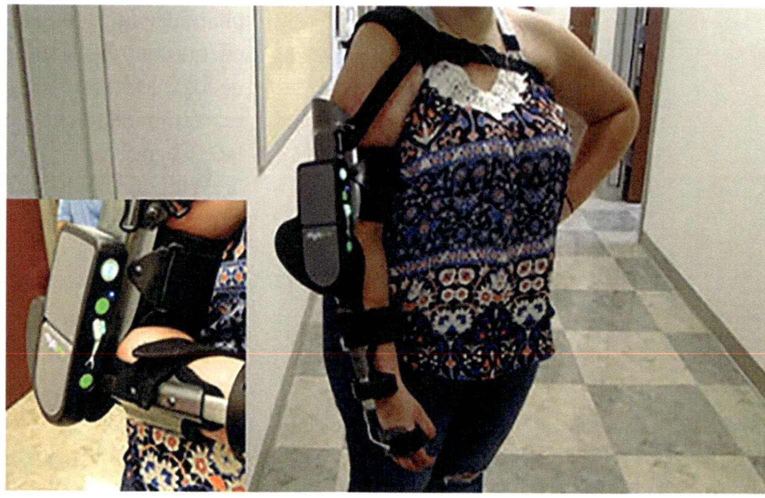

Fig. 39.31 MyoPro in extension and flexion

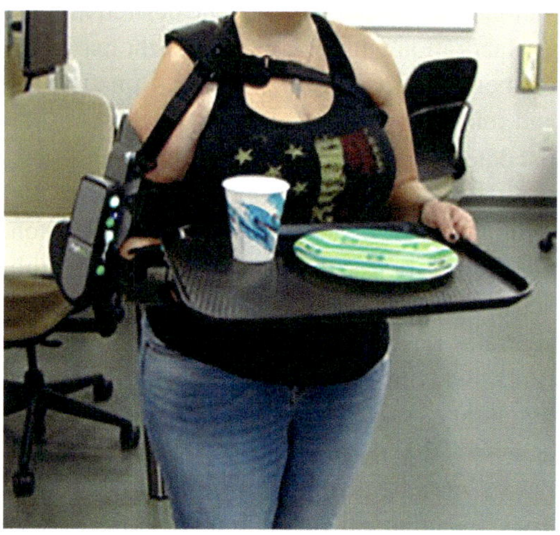

Fig. 39.32 MyoPro use with bilateral hand function: carrying a tray

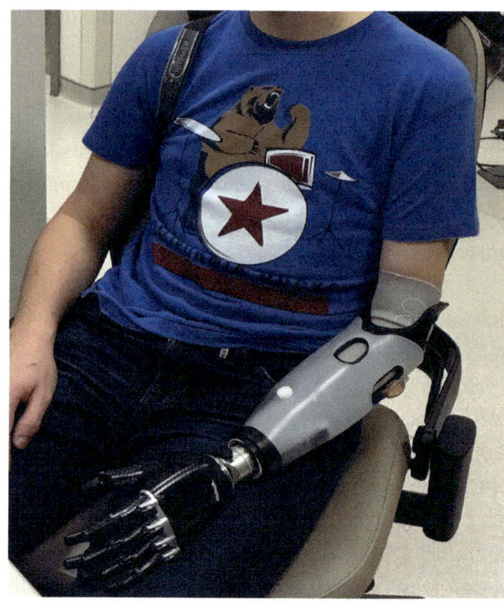

Fig. 39.33 Myoelectric prosthetic after elective amputation

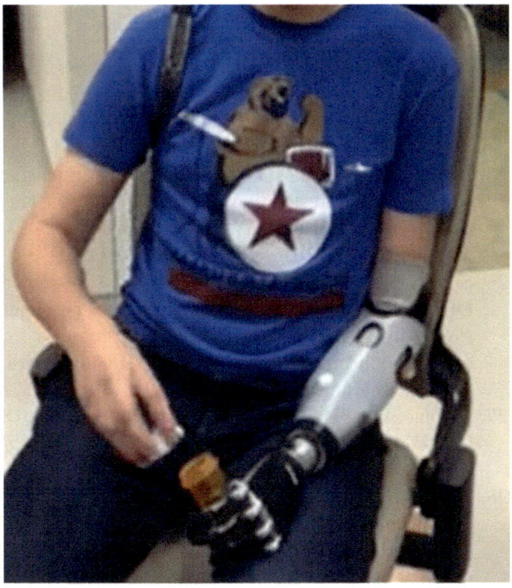

Fig. 39.34 Myoelectric prosthetic use with bilateral hand function: opening a medicine bottle

Conclusion

Traumatic, adult brachial plexus injuries are devastating and life changing. Therapy has a large role in the acute care phase to assist with range of motion, edema control, sling and/or orthotic use, pain management, one-handed ADLs, and addressing psychosocial concerns. Postoperatively, the rehabilitation and recovery will be a long, slow, challenging process. It is imperative to have an integrated team approach between the surgeon and the therapist, to guide the patient toward a successful functional outcome.

References

1. Moran SL, Steinmann SP, Shin AY. Adult brachial plexus injuries: mechanism, patterns of injury and physical diagnosis. In: Bishop AT, Spinner RJ, Shin AY, editors. Brachial plexus injuries in adults. Philadelphia: Elsevier Saunders; 2005. p. 13–24.
2. Novak CB, von der Heyde RL. Evidence and techniques in rehabilitation following nerve injuries. Hand Clin. 2013;29:383–92. https://doi.org/10.1016/j.hcl.2013.04.012.
3. Kinlaw D. Pre-/postoperative therapy for adult plexus injury. In: Bishop AT, Spinner RJ, Shin AY, editors. Brachial plexus injuries in adults. Philadelphia: Elsevier Saunders; 2005. p. 103–8.
4. Kahn LC, Moore AM. Donor activation focused rehabilitation approach: maximizing outcomes after nerve transfers. Hand Clin. 2016;32:263–77. https://doi.org/10.1016/j.hcl.2015.12.014.
5. Am G, Huxley AF, Julian FJ. The variation in isometric tension with sarcomere length in vertebrate muscle fibers. J Physiol. 1966;184:170–92.
6. Anastakis DJ, Malessy MJA, Chen R, Davis KD, Mikulis D. Cortical plasticity following nerve transfer in the upper extremity. Hand Clin. 2008;24:425–44. https://doi.org/10.1016/j.hcl.2008.04.005.
7. Karni A, Meyer G, Jezzard P, Adams MM, Turner R, Ungerleider LG. Functional MRI evidence for adult motor cortex plasticity during motor skill learning. Nature. 1995;14:155–8. https://doi.org/10.1038/377155a0.
8. Priganc VW, Stralka SW. Graded motor imagery. J Hand Ther. 2011;24:164–8. https://doi.org/10.1016/j.jht.2010.11002.
9. Flor H, Denke C, Schaefer M, Grusser S. Effect of sensory discrimination training on cortical reorganization and phantom limb pain. Lancet. 2001;357:163–4.
10. Maihofner C, Hermann O, Handwerker H, Neundorfer B, Birklein F. Patterns of cortical reorganization in complex regional pain syndrome. Neurology. 2003;61:1707–15.
11. Parsons LM, Fox PT. The neural basis of implicit movements used in recognizing hand shape. Cogn Neuropsychol. 1998;15:583–615.
12. Mancuso CA, Lee SK, Dy CJ, Landers ZA, Model Z, Wolfe SW. Compensation by the uninjured arm after brachial plexus injury. Hand. 2016;11:410–5. https://doi.org/10.1177/1558944715627635.
13. Verma CV, Vora T, Thatte M, Yardi S. Patient perception after traumatic brachial plexus injury: a qualitative cast study. J Hand Ther. 2019. https://doi.org/10.1016/j.jht.2019.03.007.
14. Mancuso CA, Lee SK, Dy CJ, Landers ZA, Model Z, Wolfe SW. Expectations and limitation due to brachial plexus injury: a qualitative study. Hand. 2015;10:741–9. https://doi.org/10.1007/s11552-015-9761-z.
15. Udina E, Puigdemasa A, Navarro X. Passive and active exercises improve regeneration and muscle reinnervation after peripheral nerve injury in the rat. Muscle Nerve. 2011;43:500–9. https://doi.org/10.1002/mus.21912.
16. Moore AM, Novak CB. Advances in nerve transfer surgery. J Hand Ther. 2014;27:96–105. https://doi.org/10.1016/j.jht.2013.12.007.
17. Brown H, Johnson K, Gilbert A, Quick TJ. The lived experience of motor recovery of elbow flexion following Oberlin nerve transfer: a qualitative analysis. Hand Ther. 2018;23:130–8. https://doi.org/10.1177/1758998318796010.

18. Novak CB. Rehabilitation following motor nerve transfers. Hand Clin. 2016;24:417–23. https://doi.org/10.1016/j.hcl.2008.06.001.
19. Leechavengvongs S, Witoonchart K, Uerpairojkit C, Thuvasetakul P. Nerve transfer to deltoid muscle using the nerve to the long head of the triceps, part II: a report of 7 cases. J Hand Surg Am. 2003;28:633–8. https://doi.org/10.1016/s0363-5023(03)00199-0.
20. Oberlin C, Beal D, Leechavengvongs S, Salon A, Dauge MC, Sarcy JJ. Nerve transfer to biceps muscle using a part of ulnar nerve for C5–C6 avulsion of the brachial plexus: anatomical study and report of four cases. J Hand Surg. 1994;19:232–7. https://doi.org/10.1016/0363-5023(94)90011-6.
21. Mackinnon SE, Novak CB, Myckatyn TM, Tung TH. Results of reinnervation of the biceps and brachialis muscles with a double fascicular transfer for elbow flexion. J Hand Surg. 2005;30:978–85. https://doi.org/10.1016/j.jhsa.2005.05.014.
22. Bulstra LF, Shin AY. Nerve transfers to restore elbow function. Hand Clin. 2016;32:165–74. https://doi.org/10.1016/j.hcl.2015.12.005.
23. Chalidapong P, Sananpanich K, Klaphajone J. EMG comparison of various exercises to improve elbow flexion following intercostal nerve transfer. J Bone Joint Surg Br. 2006;88:620–2. https://doi.org/10.1302/0301-620X.88B5.17360.
24. Giuffre JL, Kakar S, Bishop AT, Spinner RJ, Shin AY. Current concepts of the treatment of adult brachial plexus injuries. J Hand Surg. 2010;35:678–88. https://doi.org/10.1016/j.jhsa.2010.01021.
25. Estrella EP, Montales TD. Functioning free muscle transfer for the restoration of elbow flexion in brachial plexus injury patients. Injury. 2016;47:2525–33. https://doi.org/10.1016/j.injury.2016.08.011.
26. Sturma A, Hruby LA, Prahm C, Mayer JA, Aszmann OC. Rehabilitation of upper extremity nerve injuries using surface EMG biofeedback: protocols for clinical application. Front Neurosci. 2018. https://doi.org/10.3389/fnins.2018.00906.
27. Myomo. What is a MyoPro orthosis? [Internet]. 2018 [cited 2019 November 7]. Available from: https://myomo.com/what-is-a-myopro-orthosis/.
28. Kubota S, Kadone H, Shimizu Y, Hara Y, Kubo T, Watanabe H, Hada Y, Ochiai N, Sankai Y, Yamazaki M. Robotic rehabilitation training with a newly developed upper limb single-joint hybrid assistive limb (HAL-SJ) for elbow flexor reconstruction after brachial plexus injury: a report of two cases. J Orthop Surg. 2018;26:1–7. https://doi.org/10.1177/2309449901877887.

Part VII

Pediatric Brachial Plexus Injury

Historical Perspectives

40

Willem Pondaag and Howard M. Clarke

A voluminous literature has gathered around this little tragedy in the midwife's art.

– George McFadden 1928

The subject is again brought forward because of the widely divergent opinions which prevail in different groups of the profession, as to the etiology, pathology, and especially the treatment in these cases.

–Taylor 1920

Clinical Description

Although the condition is frequently referred to as Erb-Duchenne paralysis or Erb's palsy, other authors have described the occurrence of an obstetrical brachial plexus palsy earlier than Duchenne (1855) or Erb (1874) [3, 5]. There is a general consensus that the first description of a BPBI was provided by the obstetrician Smellie in 1752 [3, 5–7] (Fig. 40.1). A spontaneously resolving paralysis of both arms was reported that lasted for several days. The cause was assumed to be prolonged compression which had occurred during tedious labor due to a face presentation [8].

In 1851, Danyau presented a case report of a primiparous woman delivering a 3225 g infant after 24 hours of labor [9]. It concerned a face presentation with the right occiput posterior and a difficult delivery. Forceps were used. The newborn appeared dead for about half an hour but recovered slowly. Danyau examined the child at 36 hours and found a partial left facial palsy and a left brachial plexus palsy where the forearm was pronated and the fingers semi-flexed. Apparently, some sensation was preserved, but there was no active movement. The side of the neck showed a mark from the forceps. The child died after 8 days, and an autopsy was performed, which revealed bleeding around the roots of the brachial plexus. The plexus itself was suffused with blood but distally appeared normal. Danyau concluded that the facial nerve palsy and the brachial plexus palsy were both produced by compression from the use of forceps.

Eventually in 1855, Duchenne described four cases as a distinct clinical entity. He described the typical clinical picture of a flaccid palsy in which abduction and external rotation of the arm were paralyzed, together with absent elbow flexion and absent supination of the forearm [10] (Fig. 40.2). He discussed the association of brachial plexus palsy with fractures and dislocations, but he did not wish to speculate on the question of how the paralysis was produced.

Twenty years later, Erb described a similar pattern of paralysis in adults [11]. Using faradic stimulation in healthy subjects, he found a point on the skin of the supraclavicular region, about two fingerbreadths above the clavicle and about one fingerbreadth lateral to the sternocleidomastoid

W. Pondaag (✉)
Department of Neurosurgery, Leiden University Medical Center, Leiden, The Netherlands
e-mail: w.pondaag@lumc.nl

H. M. Clarke
Department of Plastic and Reconstructive Surgery, Hospital for Sick Children, Toronto, ON, Canada

Department of Surgery, University of Toronto, Toronto, ON, Canada

A. Y. Shin, N. Pulos (eds.), *Operative Brachial Plexus Surgery*,
https://doi.org/10.1007/978-3-030-69517-0_40

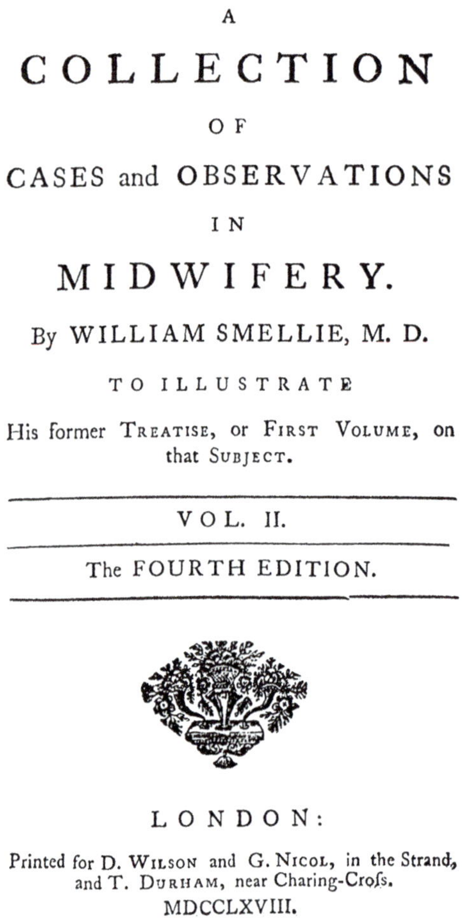

A

COLLECTION

OF

CASES and OBSERVATIONS

IN

MIDWIFERY.

By WILLIAM SMELLIE, M. D.

TO ILLUSTRATE

His former TREATISE, or FIRST VOLUME, on that SUBJECT.

VOL. II.

The FOURTH EDITION.

LONDON:

Printed for D. WILSON and G. NICOL, in the Strand, and T. DURHAM, near Charing-Crofs.

MDCCLXVIII.

Fig. 40.1 Cover of the book that contains the first description by William Smellie

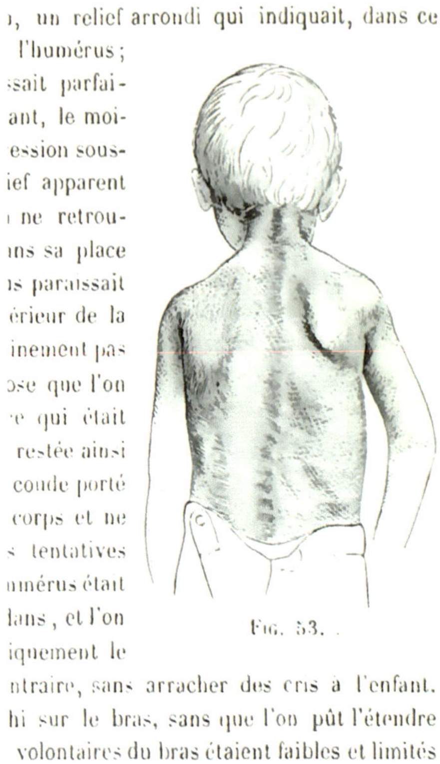

), un relief arrondi qui indiquait, dans ce
l'humérus;
ssait parfai-
ant, le moi-
ession sous-
ief apparent
ne retrou-
ins sa place
is paraissait
érieur de la
inement pas
ose que l'on
e qui était
restée ainsi
coude porté
corps et ne
s tentatives
umérus était
lans, et l'on
iquement le
ntraire, sans arracher des cris à l'enfant.
hi sur le bras, sans que l'on pût l'étendre
volontaires du bras étaient faibles et limités

Fig. 40.2 Drawing by Duchenne of the typical clinical posture of the affected arm [10]

muscle, which evoked a response of all the muscles found to be affected in this specific pattern of paralysis [11]. This point (now called Erb's point) corresponds to the position of the junction of spinal nerves C5 and C6 to form the upper trunk. It was concluded, therefore, that the causative lesion in these patients was probably localized at this point. Erb gave credit to Duchenne for the description of birth paralyses seen in newborns. Besides his adult cases, Erb described the case of an infant born after a difficult delivery with a flaccid upper extremity, and he felt that the version and extraction required in such a difficult delivery (the "Prague manipulation") was the likely cause of the lesion.

Two clinicians reported on Horner syndrome in the clinical picture of BPBI. Seeligmüller described a case of total obstetrical brachial plexus palsy [12]. This child was examined the day after a 12-hour labor at which time the ipsilateral eye was noted "to be smaller." Seeligmüller examined the patient himself at 6 months of age and noted ptosis and miosis and a smaller upper extremity, especially the forearm and hand. The fingers were held in a sweaty fist. Seeligmüller suggested that pupillary changes may have resulted from damage to the cervical sympathetics from trauma or stroke.

Cause of the Lesion

In his original publication, Danyau attributed the palsy to pressure on the nerves by the fingers of the obstetrician or alternatively by forceps during delivery. An alternative explanation was compression of the brachial plexus between the clavicle and the first rib.

To gain insight into the cause of the lesion, biomechanical experiments were performed with stillborn fetuses or infants who died shortly after birth. Fieux was one of the firsts who dissected an undisclosed number of cadavers of otherwise normal newborns and who also undertook experiments in awake rabbits [13]. Forceps applied to the head of the newborn did not reach Erb's point in the neck, and even in a small baby, the forceps could not close tightly enough around the head to apply pressure to the side of the neck. Fieux felt that the constant feature in all cases of obstetrical palsy was traction on the neck. He described the plexus as a cone with its base along the cervical spine and its apex in the axilla. With lateral traction on the head of his dissected specimens, the upper trunk of the brachial plexus came under tension while the lower trunk remained supple. He sectioned the five roots and found that the amount of spatial separation of the stumps with traction was much greater superiorly that inferiorly.

The New York surgeon, Taylor, performed such experiments during 20 dissections of the brachial plexus in 10 infant cadavers within 3–10 days after death and found that "only one thing caused stretching of the nerves, namely, increase in the distance from the neck and head to the shoulder." He concluded that it was evident that such traction was the cause of the lesion. In addition, it was described that the fifth root was ruptured first and then the sixth "and so on down the plexus in regular order if the force used was sufficient." The resulting nerve lesion stretched over a length of several centimeters [3]. Sever also claims to have performed "numerous dissections on infantile cadavers" in which he showed that traction and forcible separation of the head and shoulder puts the upper cords, the fifth and sixth cervical roots of the brachial plexus, "under dangerous tension (...) like violin strings." Furthermore, he described that forcible abduction and elevation of the arm and shoulder stretched the lower cords of the plexus, something which could happen in cases of breech delivery, with the arms extended [5].

In the Dutch medical literature, experiments on 17 stillborn babies were reported by a pediatric surgeon in 1927. The head was fixated, and increasing traction to the arm was performed in different directions with different force. The results support prior notions that an increase in the distance and angle between the cervical spine and shoulder girdle leads to strain on the brachial plexus resulting in the typical lesion pattern of the upper roots of the brachial plexus [14]. Only with increasing traction the lower roots ruptured as well.

Histopathological samples from surgical cases have been described. Torn nerve fibers and hemorrhage in the perineurial sheath of the upper cords of the brachial plexus were observed [3]. This was later confirmed by other authors [15].

Apart from these stretch injuries of the postganglionic nerve and the resulting neuroma formation, avulsion of the nerve roots from the spinal cord was recognized as a specific pathophysiological mechanism. A case was described of bilateral palsy following a difficult breech delivery. The child died on the fifth day due to a cerebral hemorrhage, and at autopsy, the spinal nerves C5 and C6 were found to be avulsed and lying outside the dura [16].

All of the above studies concluded that traction to the nerves, leading to a stretch injury, could explain the observed clinical picture on BPBI. This century-old description of the traction injury can still be considered to be accurate. In the late 1970s, biomechanical studies were again performed where the conclusions were similar to those described in the historical papers [17]. Currently, this pattern of injury is well recognized by nerve surgeons who treat such brachial plexus lesions in infants as well as in adults.

Apart from the stretch to the nerves, further understanding of Horner's syndrome was achieved by Klumpke [18]. She undertook canine experiments to determine the effect of avulsion or section at the intervertebral foramen of C8 and particularly of T1, which produced Horner's sign, while more distal lesions did not. This experimental observation was followed by some very well documented reports of total plexopathies with Horner's sign, which led to an extensive and excellent discussion of the cervical sympathetics and Horner's syndrome.

Emergence of Treatment by Nerve Surgery

In February 1903, Kennedy reported the first description of nerve surgery for a BPBI (the first operation had been performed in 1902 at Glasgow University) [2]. Two of his three cases were surgically treated in early infancy (at 2 and 6 months of age); one case underwent delayed surgery at the age of 14 years. In this older case, the main indication for surgery was torticollis, but the brachial plexus was also repaired during the operation. One year later, Kennedy extended his surgical series to five BPBI cases [19].

The surgical procedure is described in good detail, and the surgical findings were reported as cicatricial changes of the upper trunk. The lesioned upper trunk was resected, and the three distal divisions (suprascapular nerve, anterior division, and posterior division) were sutured with a central suture of "fine chromotized catgut" to the fifth and sixth nerve roots. Because the resection of the upper trunk resulted in a gap, the shoulder of the infant was pushed upward and the head tilted to the operated side in order to be able to suture the stumps together (Fig. 40.3).

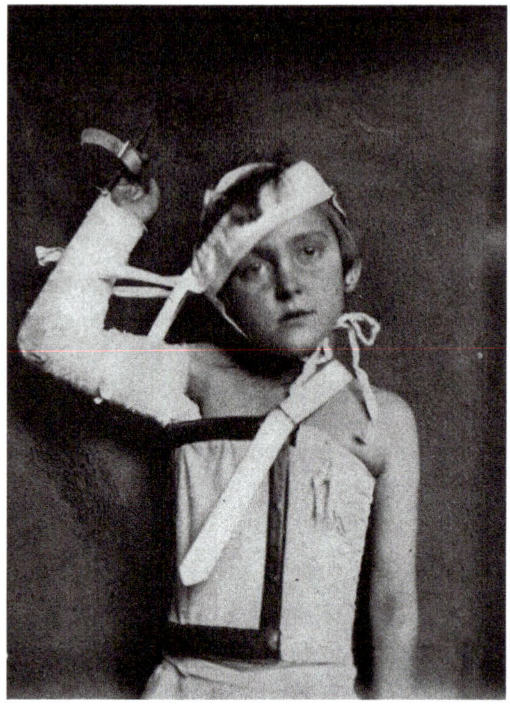

Fig. 40.3 Postoperative splint [16]. Note the abduction of the arm and lateral flexion of the head to the operated side which is necessary for a direct nerve suture

Kennedy claimed that 4–8 months after surgery the infants had fairly good use of their arm. Even the patient operated at the age of 14 showed improvement, although this was not apparent until 2 years after surgery [19] (Fig. 40.4).

In a multidisciplinary collaboration, Clark, a neurologist, Taylor, a surgeon, and Prout, a pathologist, described seven operated children in 1905 [3]. The surgical technique applied was approximately the same as Kennedy's, although the actual nerve repair used "lateral sutures of fine silk involving the nerve sheaths only."

Despite the short operation times required by limited capabilities for prolonged anesthesia, limited illumination, and no surgical magnification, both of these surgeons were able to identify the same findings which are observed today.

In Taylor's patient group, mainly older children (4 1/2 to 11 years) were operated: the three youngest were 8, 16, and 25 months. Of these three younger children, two died within days after the operation, resulting in a mortality rate of almost 30% in his total group. In a 1921 paper, Taylor describes having operated on 76 cases of obstetric palsy in total. In his last 25 patients (surgically treated from 1914 to 1921), only 1 patient "died of hemorrhage on table," and in 1 case, the surgery was stopped because of hemorrhage [16].

One of the difficulties was "to determine (…) whether the lesion will be likely to be spontaneously recovered from or not. In some cases recovery takes place completely, although at birth all the typical signs are exhibited, and it is therefore necessary to wait a reasonable time in all cases before recommending operation" [19]. At that time, electrical muscle testing was already employed to determine prognosis: "If (…) after two months no responses can be got in the muscles with the faradic current, (…) it is safer to proceed with the operation than to put off further time in the hope that recovery will eventually be the result" [2]. This view was shared by Sherren in his 310-page monograph on nerve lesions: "Spontaneous recovery has taken place in about

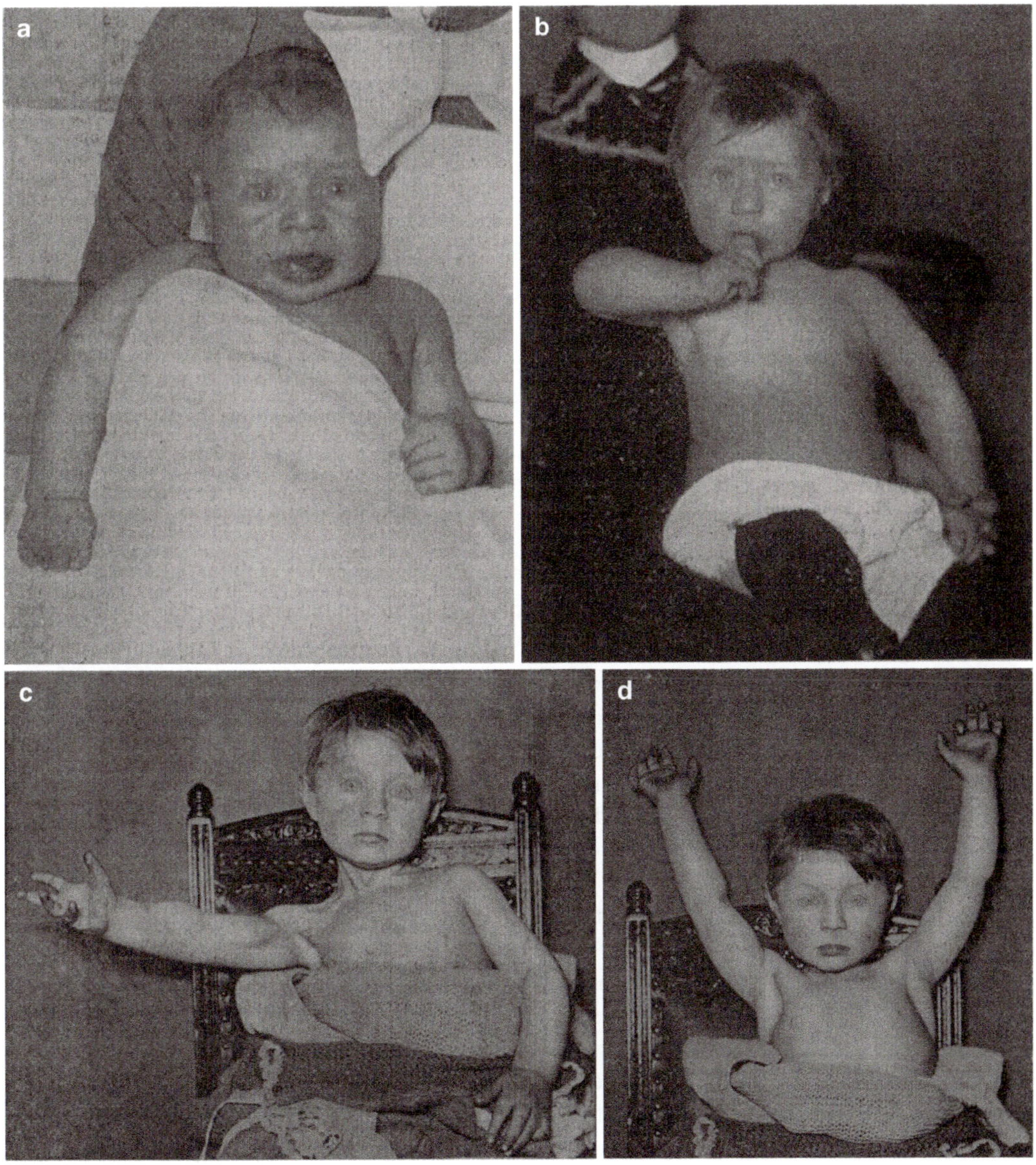

Fig. 40.4 Historic photographs of results from Kennedy [2, 19]. (**a**) Preoperative; (**b**) 9 months postoperative; (**c**, **d**) 2 years postoperative

70 per cent of the cases that have come under my observation. In many the paralysis had completely disappeared by the time the child was brought to have its electrical reactions tested at the age of three months. Complete spontaneous recovery rarely takes place if no improvement is noticed by this date" [20].

Both Kennedy and Clark employed direct suture of the nerve ends after resection of the neuromatous tissue. The nerve ends were positioned next to each other by means of external manipulation (Fig. 40.5).

It is still a matter of debate whether a neurorrhaphy under such tension indeed resulted in good recovery. The current golden standard – using autologous nerve grafts to bridge the defect – was not commonly used in those days, although judging from publications the technique

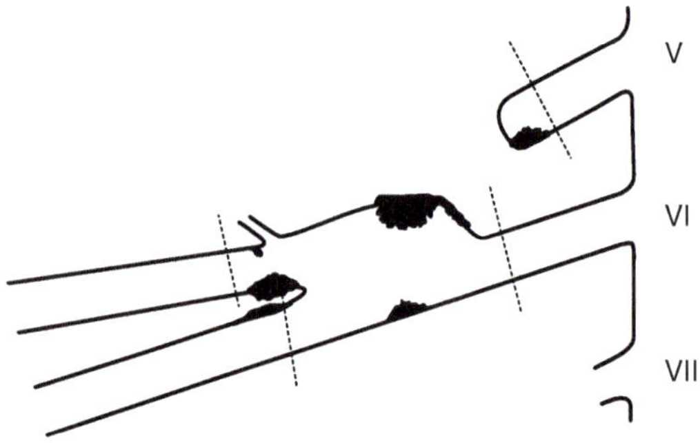

Fig. 40.5 Drawing from a surgical procedure by Taylor [3]

did seem to be known [21, 22]. Apparently nerve transplantation had already been applied in 1876 using a piece of nerve from an amputated limb. Also a dog's sciatic nerve had been sutured in place of a nerve defect. The results of nerve transplantation were poor, and so nerve grafting was not widely applied in clinical practice.

Other reported surgical techniques include nerve transfer (which was then alternatively named nerve crossing), fascicular transfer, and end-to-side repair [21]. All surgical techniques which one might consider to be new and modern were apparently already known one century ago.

The first report, for instance, of end-to-side nerve repair of the brachial plexus in adults appeared in 1903 [23], describing that surgical repair might "be effected by dividing the paralysed fifth cervical root and suturing its distal end into a neighbouring healthy root, the sixth or seventh." To what extent this end-to-side repair yielded any clinical result was not reported. Kennedy was apparently aware of this end-to-side technique but did not use it in BPBI infants: "I should hesitate to implant the ends into one of the neighbouring nerves in this region, on account of the importance of the only nerves into which the implantation could be made with prospects of success; for, in the event of failure, the result might be that additional muscles would participate in the paralysis" [2].

Also, transfer of the accessory nerve to the brachial plexus was already described by Harvey Cushing. "In the upper part of the cord the fifth cervical segment was particularly the seat of injury, the deltoids being absolutely, and the biceps and supinator muscles in large measure paralyzed. The spinal accessory has been sacrificed and transplanted into the upper radicle of the brachial plexus" [24].

The main shortcoming of all surgical papers dating from the early twentieth century is the lack of substantial patient series that were accurately documented postoperatively. In the absence of such information, it is not clear exactly what the results of these surgical treatments were.

Nerve Surgery for BPBI Declines

In 1916, orthopedic surgeon Sever abandoned nerve surgery in a paper in which he presented 471 conservatively treated patients [25]. On the basis of this personal series (which had grown to 617 in 1920 and to 1100 in 1925), he concludes "In regard to the operation on the plexus in the usual upper arm type of case, it might be said that in the experience of this clinic it has not been found necessary. (…) it cannot be too strongly emphasized that no operation on the plexus will be of any great use in restoring functional activity to the arm" [5].

Sever was also pessimistic about nerve surgical treatment of total lesions, usually consisting of the avulsion of multiple lower roots from the spinal cord. He recognized that "the outlook is not so good, although many of the patients regain use of the upper arm in spite of the persistent paralysis of the lower arm and hand." Despite the poor prognosis of spontaneous recovery, nerve surgery did not improve the outlook: "it has been done a number of times without any benefit. The plexus in all cases was found to be so badly torn and so bound down and invaded by scar tissue that any kind of repair was impossible."

Other authors shared this pessimistic view of the results of nerve repair. "There has been no case yet (…) which has shown an anatomic and physiologic cure from the plexus operation. Even marked improvement is usually lacking. (…) Many times the nerve is so badly damaged that it is beyond repair" [26]. Also neurosurgeon Sharpe remarks that "there is not one case of complete recovery of function" in his series of 146 patients [4].

These conclusions are, however, not illustrated by descriptions of the neurological result in patient series which makes it difficult to judge the true results of the nerve surgery, but these were, most probably, poor. It is, therefore, understandable that the voices of the initial enthusiasts simply became weaker and the voices of the opponents of nerve surgery became stronger.

Instead of repair of the nerve lesion, Sever and Jepson advised treating the sequelae of BPBI patients by orthopedic surgery. Sever recommended performing muscle and tendon transfers for improvement of shoulder function, together with release of restricted shoulder mobility [25]. Jepson favored a rotation osteotomy to restore functional use of the limb [26]. The results of these surgical strategies were said to be superior to nerve repair. Modifications of these secondary procedures are still performed today [27].

Another factor which may have led to the decline of nerve surgery was the associated mortality. In those days, ether was used for general anesthesia. In the early series of Taylor, a mortality rate of 2/7 (almost 30%) was reported [3]. Other surgical series do not report such high mortality rates, but there must have been a certain degree of mortality resulting from surgery in such young infants.

Nerve surgery gradually lost popularity. "Taylor, who has had a considerable experience of operations directed to the damaged nerves, now (1938) prefers to wait as long as any improvement is taking place" [28]. Finally, nerve surgery for obstetrical lesions was abandoned for a considerable period.

Fifty years later, peripheral nerve surgery of lesions in adults was renewed by introducing technical improvements including the introduction of the operating microscope [29], better surgical techniques, improved suture material, and in particular the emergence of the use of autologous nerve grafts [30]. These advances, along with the improved safety of anesthesia, made nerve surgery for infants as advocated in 1980 by Alain Gilbert [31] a reality once again.

Summary

At the beginning of the twentieth century, nerve surgery for BPBI was performed for the first time, gaining popularity in the subsequent two decades. The origins of the lesion were investigated and discussed thoroughly. It was recognized that the majority of infants demonstrated spontaneous recovery but that for a small number surgery might be warranted. Additionally, in those patients with a total lesion of the brachial plexus, spontaneous recovery of hand function was known to be poor. The indications for surgery were based on clinical grounds, sometimes together with the results of cutaneous electrical stimulation.

Despite limited illumination, very short operating times, and limitations of anesthesia, these pioneer surgeons were able to deliver an accurate report of the pathology which corresponds to current surgical findings.

Although some papers from that early era systematically summarize cases and the results of surgery, these series lacked valid outcome measures to compare surgical therapy to other treatments or to the outcome of spontaneous recovery. The advocates in favor of surgical treatment, as well as the opponents of surgery, only reported the numbers of patients in order to gain authority as experts. Unfortunately, the detailed results of their treatment were never published. Surgery was abandoned because its usefulness could not be demonstrated, because of the reported mortality, and because alternatives such as secondary surgery became available.

References

1. Thorburn W. A clinical lecture on secondary suture of the brachial plexus. Br Med J. 1900;1(2053):1073–5.
2. Kennedy R. Suture of the brachial plexus in birth paralysis of the upper extremity. Br Med J. 1903;1(2197):298–301.
3. Clark LP, Taylor AS, Prout TP. A study on brachial birth palsy. Am J Med Sci. 1905;130(4):670–707.
4. Sharpe W. End results in neuro-surgery: impressions during decade 1913–123. Ann Surg. 1925;82(5):684–97.
5. Sever JW. Obstetric paralysis. Its cause and treatment. Can Med Assoc J. 1920;10(2):141–61.
6. Harrenstein RJ. De geboorteverlamming van den arm [in Dutch]. Ned Tijdschr Geneeskd. 1922;66:1435–47.
7. Ashhurst APC. Birth injuries of the shoulder. Ann Surg. 1918;67(1):25–50.
8. Smellie W. Smellie's Treatise on the theory and practice of midwifery (edited with annotations by McClintock, A.H.). London: The New Sydenham Society; 1876.
9. Danyau. Séance du 28 mai 1851. Bulletin Société de Chirurgie de Paris B. 1851(2):141–51.
10. Duchenne de Bologne GB. De l'Électrisation Localisée et de son application et a la thérapeutique [in French]. 2nd ed. Paris: J.B. Baillière et fils; 1861.
11. Brody IA, Wilkins RH. Neurological classics: Erb's palsy; "On a characteristic site of injury in the brachial plexus" by W. Erb 1874. Arch Neurol. 1969;21(4):442–4.
12. Seeligmüller A. Zur Pathologie des Sympathicus. Dtsch Arch Klin Med. 1877;20:101–19.
13. Fieux G. De la pathogénie des paralysies brachiales chez le nouveau-né. Paralysies Obstétricales. 1897;47:52–64.
14. Harrenstein RJ. Proefnemingen en practische ervaringen over de geboorteverlamming van de arm [in Dutch]. Ned Tijdschr Geneeskd. 1927;71:828–46.
15. Barlow T, Ballance CA. Rupture of the upper cord of the brachial plexus at birth. Proc R Soc Med. 1908;1(Clin Sect):215–20.
16. Taylor AS. So-called congenital dislocation of the shoulder posterior subluxation. Ann Surg. 1921;74(3):368–75.
17. Metaizeau JP, Gayet C, Plenat F. Brachial plexus birth injuries. An experimental study. [in French]. Chir Pediatr. 1979;20(3):159–63.
18. Klumpke A. Contribution à l'étude des paralysies radiculaires du plexus brachial. Revue de Médicine. 1885;5:739–90.
19. Kennedy R. Further notes on the treatment of birth paralysis of the upper extremity by suture of the fifth and sixth cervical nerves. Br Med J. 1904;2(2286):1065–8.
20. Sherren J. Injuries of nerves and their treatment. London: James Nisbet & Co.; 1908.
21. Sherren J. Some points in the surgery of the peripheral nerves. Edinb Med J. 1906;20:297–332.
22. Huber GC. A study of the operative treatment for loss of nerve substance in peripheral nerves. J Morphol. 1895;11:692–740.
23. Harris W, Low VW. On the importance of accurate muscular analysis in lesions of the brachial plexus and the treatment of Erb's palsy and infantile paralysis of the upper extremity by cross-union of the nerve roots. Br Med J. 1903;2:1035–8.
24. Cushing H. The special field of neurological surgery. Bull John Hopkins Hosp. 1905;16(168):77–87.
25. Sever JW. Obstetric paralysis. An orthopedic problem. J Bone Joint Surg Am. 1916;s2(14):456–75.
26. Jepson PN. Obstetrical paralysis. Ann Surg. 1930;91(5):724–30.
27. Mehlman CT, Koepplinger ME. Hyphenated history: the Sever-L'Episcopo procedure. J Pediatr Orthop. 2007;27(5):533–6.
28. Morison JE. Peripheral brachial paralysis in infants and children. Arch Dis Child. 1938;13(76):310–32.
29. Smith JW. Microsurgery of peripheral nerves. Plast Reconstr Surg. 1964;33:317–29.
30. Millesi H, Ganglberger J, Berger A. Erfahrungen mit der Mikrochirurgie peripherer Nerven. Chir Plast Recontr. 1967;4:47–55.
31. Gilbert A, Khouri N, Carlioz H. Birth palsy of the brachial plexus -surgical exploration and attempted repair in twenty one cases. [in French]. Rev Chir Orthop Reparatrice Appar Mot. 1980;66(1):33–42.

41 Brachial Plexus Birth Injury: Mechanism of Injury

Agnes Z. Dardas and Apurva S. Shah

Introduction

Brachial plexus birth injury presents at a rate of 0.4–4.6 per 1000 births worldwide [1–7]. The prevailing theory regarding mechanism of injury posits the role of mechanical traction to the brachial plexus during birth as a result of the widening of the space between an infant's neck and shoulder. Multiple factors – related to maternal factors and intrauterine environment, fetal anatomy and physiology, and delivery technique – are associated with brachial plexus birth injury and are thought to contribute to increased mechanical traction on the brachial plexus or decreased resistance of the surrounding tissues that allow for increased force transmission on the brachial plexus. However, despite these identified risk factors, up to 55% of births presenting with this condition do not share any identifiable risks [1, 8] and present in the setting of normal birth weights and atraumatic deliveries [9]. The majority of US data, however, stems from the Kids Inpatient Database, which does not include all identifiable factors. International studies and results from other specialties have also typically focused on only a subset of factors. To what degree other as-yet identified factors have not been accounted for remains unknown. Nevertheless the opportunity for comprehensive, high-quality studies remains in order to determine the etiology of this multifactorial disease and implement preventative measures. The remainder of this chapter will focus on the factors that have been published to date and how they are thought to contribute.

Maternal Factors

Gestational diabetes has been among the most common and earliest-published maternal factors associated with brachial plexus birth injury in the literature [10–13]. While the odds ratio of a mother with gestational diabetes delivering an infant with a brachial plexus birth palsy has been reported to range from 1.9 to 4.46, the true odds ratio may be underestimated as the available data stems from a state database [10, 11]. Furthermore, it is not a factor included in the national Kids' Inpatient Database of which several US studies have drawn heavily from [1]. Mechanistically, it contributes to increased fetal birth weight and macrosomia, both of which are explored further below as fetal factors associated with brachial plexus birth palsy [14].

Little is known regarding contributing environmental factors of mothers with children with

A. Z. Dardas
Department of Orthopaedic Surgery, University of Pennsylvania, Philadelphia, PA, USA
e-mail: agnes.dardas@pennmedicine.upenn.edu

A. S. Shah (✉)
Division of Orthopaedic Surgery, Children's Hospital of Philadelphia, Philadelphia, PA, USA
e-mail: shaha6@email.chop.edu

A. Y. Shin, N. Pulos (eds.), *Operative Brachial Plexus Surgery*,
https://doi.org/10.1007/978-3-030-69517-0_41

brachial plexus birth injury. Indeed, only one recent study has examined their demographics and found that in one of the US state registries, mothers that identified as Asian, Black, or Hispanic and, separately, mothers with Medicaid were associated with increased risk of having a child with brachial plexus birth injury [10]. Gestational diabetes may be an underlying confounding factor explaining this as in the same study, mothers who were non-Caucasian or on Medicaid had nearly twice the percentage of gestational diabetes than their Caucasian or non-Medicaid counterparts [10].

Intrauterine Factors

Local intrauterine environmental factors during pregnancy and prior to labor have also been theorized to contribute to brachial plexus birth palsy. Fibroids, presence of a bicornuate uterus, and any other similar chronic compressive scenarios could result in direct pressure to the brachial plexus over a period of time or acute malpositioning such as posterior shoulder impaction against the sacral promontory during a natural birth [15–20].

Multiple births, on the other hand, have presented with conflicting data findings. While several studies present multiple births as a protective mechanism, all three recent prominent ones have used the same US database to present their findings [1, 2, 8]. In a study that used a Colorado state-specific database, however, multiple births were found to be associated with higher odds ratios of brachial plexus birth injury when compared to natural single-infant births [10]. The true answer is likely an interaction of factors that can be hard to delineate from just retrospective reviews of the medical record and large databases.

The metabolic environment of the uterus may also play a previously undetected role in this disease. In comparing infants with brachial plexus birth palsy with and without shoulder dystocia, Gurewitsch et al. found that infants afflicted with the disorder without a record of shoulder dystocia were more likely to be of average weight and experiencing metabolic acidosis ($pH < 7.1$) at birth than those with shoulder dystocia [21]. Similarly, recent research using the Kids' Inpatient Database has introduced birth hypoxia as a possible factor [1]. Hypoxia may result in decreased muscle tone and dampened reflex arcs, which may prevent infants from limiting the amount of shoulder displacement through the birth canal [1]. This may explain why fetal asphyxia has been found to be a risk factor for permanent injury, but not transient brachial plexus birth palsy [22].

Another controversial mechanism of brachial plexus birth injury describes unilateral prolonged ischemia to the brachial plexus stemming from placental insufficiency. This theory was proposed after studying the history of Kaiser Wilhelm whose mother, Princess Royal Victoria, suffered a severe fall during her fourth month of pregnancy. While no birth weight was recorded, it has been reported that Queen Victoria's personal physician, who had overseen the birth of her grandson, later on reported to the Queen that Kaiser Wilhelm was thin at birth and not as large as the Queen's own children, perhaps implicating intrauterine growth restriction [23, 24]. Combining this fact along with the mother's prenatal fall and mathematical modeling of the effects of placental insufficiency on blood shunting in a fetus, it has been hypothesized that Wilhelm's permanent brachial plexus birth injury was due to antenatal ischemia and not his breech positioning during delivery as originally thought [24]. This theory remains controversial, as at least one other study has identified growth restriction to be a protective factor [11].

Fetal Factors

The most commonly studied fetal risk factor for brachial plexus injury relates to macrosomia or large birth weight [2, 3, 6–8, 12, 13, 25]. While there is no specific identified threshold at which the risk of brachial plexus birth injury dramatically increases, the most conservative studies have identified birth weights starting at 4000 g or 90th percentile to be associated with increased risk [3, 7, 12]. Indeed, infants heavier than 4500 g have been reported to be 14–45 times greater risk of being born with brachial plexus birth injury, especially compared to infants less than 3500 g [2, 6]. It is unclear whether birth weight correlates to the severity of the injury as one study reported. In neurosurgically treated conditions, as birth weight increased 1 kg, the odds of a more severe nerve injury identified during surgery increased by 2.7 [25]. However, another study that assessed all brachial plexus injuries, both operative and non-operatively treated, found no correlation between birth weight and level of impairment [6].

Fetal hypotonia has also been identified as a risk factor in a single study [8], possibly due to dampened reflex arcs allowing excessive unilateral traction on the plexus without protective fetal muscle tone to counteract it. Fetal hypotonia and intra-uterine hypoxia, however, have yet to be assessed as possible confounding factors for one another.

In addition, exostosis of the first rib that could cause either compression or stretch on the plexus has only been reported once as a cause of brachial plexus palsy [26]. Last but not least, brachial plexus palsy may have a genetic mechanism in a subset of cases. To date, three familial cases have been reported, with each family having two to eight affected members [27, 28].

Labor-Related Factors

The largest body of literature on this subject examines labor-related factors associated with brachial plexus birth injury with the highest-risk factor identified as shoulder dystocia [1–3, 8, 10, 12, 29]. Infants whose labor is complicated by shoulder dystocia are 76.1–100 times greater risk of being identified with a brachial plexus injury [2, 11]. Shoulder dystocia, however, has not been recorded as a significant labor event in 45–83% of studied cohorts [2, 9, 29], indicating that while a common mechanism, there may be several other factors contributing to this pathology.

Cephalopelvic disproportion may be a broader category that better encompasses size mismatch between the fetus and the birth canal, contributing to shoulder dystocia or other malpositioning associated with brachial plexus birth injury. Current predictive value using MR pelvimetry, however, is limited as the ratio of fetal head volume to soft tissue head volume identifies pregnancies at the greatest risk of shoulder dystocia but cannot accurately determine pregnancies requiring C-section or labor outcomes [30, 31].

Indeed, the etiology of brachial plexus birth palsy at time of delivery likely extends beyond the physical compression of the fetus during labor to include other vectors of force acting upon the fetus to propel it forward in the canal. Historically, iatrogenic force used during labor was commonly thought to contribute to mechanical traction on the brachial plexus resulting in neurapraxia [2, 7, 8, 10, 11]. In certain databases, instrumented forceps and/or vacuum extractor use have been associated with an odds ratio of 2.7–9 times more likely to be associated with infants with brachial plexus birth injury [2, 11, 22]. In another study assessing labors where uninstrumented manual assistance was necessary during the second stage of labor, force applied with downward traction of the head was the only independent risk factor of brachial plexus birth palsy [32]. To prevent this possible cause, several professional societies throughout the world have shared labor delivery guidelines discouraging the use of excessive fetal head traction, fundal pressure, or inverse rotation of the fetal head [33]. In turn, the same societies recommend offering C-section for estimated birth weights >4500 g for diabetic pregnancies and >5000 g for non-diabetic pregnancies, labor induction for pregnancies >39 weeks at risk of fetal macrosomia, and using the McRoberts maneuver with provider proficiency in two or more additional manual maneuvers such as Wood's maneuver or delivery of the posterior arm [33, 34]. Despite these recommendations, labor induction has not been shown to alter the incidence of shoulder dystocia in non-diabetic patients [35], and the incidence of brachial plexus birth injury has persisted despite a large proportional increase in C-sections over time [9].

Intrauterine forces during delivery may contribute to some of this discrepancy, resulting in four to nine times greater force than clinician-applied traction to the fetal head [36]. Forceful contractions may explain the paradoxical association of brachial plexus birth injuries with prolonged extraction times or active phases, or precipitous, breech, or otherwise natural, uncomplicated deliveries [7, 10, 12, 37, 38]. The theory of endogenous forces as a contributing mechanism is further supported by studies demonstrating an association of brachial plexus birth injuries with oxytocin administration or tachysystole occurrence [39].

Lastly, while clavicle fractures were initially posited as a protective factor dissipating labor-related forces due to their higher frequency in transient palsies compared to permanent plexopathies [22, 40], other subsequent studies have demonstrated no difference in outcomes when a clavicle fracture is present [41, 42].

Early Postnatal Brachial Plexus Injury Mechanisms

While this section focuses primarily on brachial plexus birth injury, the predominant pediatric presentation of this pathology, other less-common causes in the perinatal period have been described. Iatrogenic causes include hyperabduction during a prolonged intervention such as a thoracotomy and excessive traction from Pavlik harness straps [43, 44].

In rare cases, the initial physical exam findings of an oncologic condition or infection may be brachial plexus birth injury due to compressive, infiltrative, or metabolic interactions with the brachial plexus. For instance, in one case report, a malignant rhabdoid tumor of the brachial plexus initially presented as a progressive palsy over the first few days of life before a hard palpable supraclavicular mass was recognized [45]. Cervical infantile myofibromatosis has also presented in a similar fashion [46]. In two other cases, a patient with diffuse hemangiomatosis and another with an isolated hemangioma presented with brachial plexus palsy at birth and in the first 5 days of life, respectively [47, 48]. The case of the isolated hemangioma was treated with intravenous corticosteroid therapy with resolution in size and symptoms within 5 days of treatment [48]. The other case, however, experienced persistent symptoms, perhaps indicating an irreversible ischemic injury to those peripheral nerves [47]. Several case reports also write about brachial plexus palsy as a presenting symptom of otherwise asymptomatic humeral or vertebral osteomyelitis [49–52]. Ischemic plexus neuropathy resulting from thrombophlebitis of the vasa nervorum or arterial embolism has been hypothesized as a possible mechanism [52]. Brachial plexopathy has been differentiated from pseudoparalysis from pain due to the absence of deep tendon reflexes and/or significant electromyographic findings [39–52].

References

1. DeFrancesco CJ, Shah DK, Rogers BH, Shah AS. The epidemiology of brachial plexus birth palsy in the United States: declining incidence and evolving risk factors. J Pediatr Orthop. 2019;39(2):e134–40. https://doi.org/10.1097/BPO.0000000000001089.
2. Foad SL, Mehlman CT, Ying J. The epidemiology of neonatal brachial plexus palsy in the United States. J Bone Joint Surg Am. 2008;90(6):1258–64. https://doi.org/10.2106/JBJS.G.00853.
3. Evans-Jones G, Kay SP, Weindling AM, Cranny G, Ward A, Bradshaw A, et al. Congenital brachial palsy: incidence, causes, and outcome in the United Kingdom and Republic of Ireland. Arch Dis Child Fetal Neonatal Ed. 2003;88(3):F185–9. https://doi.org/10.1136/fn.88.3.f185.
4. Dawodu A, Sankaran-Kutty M, Rajan TV. Risk factors and prognosis for brachial plexus injury and clavicular fracture in neonates: a prospective analysis from the United Arab Emirates. Ann Trop Paediatr. 1997;17(3):195–200. https://doi.org/10.1080/02724936.1997.11747886.
5. Hoeksma AF, Wolf H, Oei SL. Obstetrical brachial plexus injuries: incidence, natural course and shoulder contracture. Clin Rehabil. 2000;14(5):523–6. https://doi.org/10.1191/0269215500cr341oa.
6. Bager B. Perinatally acquired brachial plexus palsy--a persisting challenge. Acta Paediatr. 1997;86(11):1214–9. https://doi.org/10.1111/j.1651-2227.1997.tb14849.x.
7. Hudić I, Fatusić Z, Sinanović O, Skokić F. Etiological risk factors for brachial plexus palsy. J Matern Fetal Neonatal Med. 2006;19(10):655–61. https://doi.org/10.1080/14767050600850498.
8. Abzug JM, Mehlman CT, Ying J. Assessment of current epidemiology and risk factors surrounding brachial plexus birth palsy. J Hand Surg

Am. 2019;44(6):515.e1–515.e10. https://doi.org/10.1016/j.jhsa.2018.07.020.
9. Graham EM, Forouzan I, Morgan MA. A retrospective analysis of Erb's palsy cases and their relation to birth weight and trauma at delivery. J Matern Fetal Med. 1997;6(1):1–5. https://doi.org/10.1002/(SICI)1520-6661(199701/02)6:1<1::AID-MFM1>3.0.CO;2-T.
10. Lalka A, Gralla J, Sibbel SE. Brachial plexus birth injury: epidemiology and birth weight impact on risk factors. J Pediatr Orthop. 2019. https://doi.org/10.1097/BPO.0000000000001447.
11. Gilbert WM, Nesbitt TS, Danielsen B. Associated factors in 1611 cases of brachial plexus injury. Obstet Gynecol. 1999;93(4):536–40. https://doi.org/10.1016/s0029-7844(98)00484-0.
12. Mollberg M, Hagberg H, Bager B, Lilja H, Ladfors L. High birthweight and shoulder dystocia: the strongest risk factors for obstetrical brachial plexus palsy in a Swedish population-based study. Acta Obstet Gynecol Scand. 2005;84(7):654–9. https://doi.org/10.1111/j.0001-6349.2005.00632.x.
13. Ecker JL, Greenberg JA, Norwitz ER, Nadel AS, Repke JT. Birth weight as a predictor of brachial plexus injury. Obstet Gynecol. 1997;89(5):643–7. https://doi.org/10.1016/s0029-7844(97)00007-0.
14. Pezzarossa A, Orlandi N, Baggi V, Dazzi D, Ricciarelli E, Coppola F. Effects of maternal weight variations and gestational diabetes mellitus on neonatal birth weight. J Diabetes Complicat. 1996;10(2):78–83. https://doi.org/10.1016/1056-8727(94)00065-4.
15. Jennett RJ, Tarby TJ, Kreinick CJ. Brachial plexus palsy: an old problem revisited. Am J Obstet Gynecol. 1992;166:1673–6. https://doi.org/10.1016/0002-9378(92)91555-o.
16. Gherman RB, Goodwin TM, Ouzounian JG, Miller DA, Paul RH. Brachial plexus palsy associated with cesarean section: an in utero injury? Am J Obstet Gynecol. 1997;177(5):1162–4. https://doi.org/10.1016/s0002-9378(97)70034-6.
17. Gherman RB, Ouzounian JG, Miller DA, Kwok L, Goodwin TM. Spontaneous vaginal delivery: a risk factor for Erb's palsy? Am J Obstet Gynecol. 1998;178(3):423–7. https://doi.org/10.1016/s0002-9378(98)70413-2.
18. Ouzounian JG, Korst LM, Phelan JP. Permanent Erb palsy: a traction-related injury? Obstet Gynecol. 1997;89(1):139–41. https://doi.org/10.1016/s0029-7844(96)00312-2.
19. Dunn DW, Engle WA. Brachial plexus palsy: intrauterine onset. Pediatr Neurol. 1985;1(6):367–9. https://doi.org/10.1016/0887-8994(85)90074-8.
20. Jennett RJ, Tarby TJ. Disuse osteoporosis as evidence of brachial plexus palsy due to intrauterine fetal maladaptation. Am J Obstet Gynecol. 2001;185(1):236–7. https://doi.org/10.1067/mob.2001.110694.
21. Gurewitsch ED, Johnson E, Hamzehzadeh S, Allen RH. Risk factors for brachial plexus injury with and without shoulder dystocia. Am J Obstet Gynecol. 2006;194(2):486–92. https://doi.org/10.1016/j.ajog.2005.07.071.
22. Backe B, Magnussen EB, Johansen OJ, Sellaeg G, Russwurm H. Obstetric brachial plexus palsy: a birth injury not explained by the known risk factors. Acta Obstet Gynecol Scand. 2008;87(10):1027–32. https://doi.org/10.1080/00016340802415648.
23. Rohl JCG. Young Wilhelm: the Kaiser's early life, 1859–1888. Cambridge: Cambridge University Press; 1999.
24. Jain V, Sebire NJ, Talbert DG. Kaiser Wilhelm syndrome: obstetric trauma or placental insult in a historical case mimicking Erb's palsy. Med Hypotheses. 2005;65(1):185–91. https://doi.org/10.1016/j.mehy.2004.12.027.
25. Pondaag W, Allen RH, Malessy MJ. Correlating birthweight with neurological severity of obstetric brachial plexus lesions. BJOG. 2011;118(9):1098–103. https://doi.org/10.1111/j.1471-0528.2011.02942.x.
26. de Turckheim MC, Clavert JM, Paira M. Costal exostoses, complicated in the neonatal period, by brachial plexus paralysis. A distinct entity of exostoses? Ann Pediatr (Paris). 1991;38(1):23–5. French.
27. Mollica F, Li Volti S, Grasso A, De Simone D. Familial congenital brachial palsy. Am J Med Genet. 1991;41(3):322–4. https://doi.org/10.1002/ajmg.1320410312.
28. Zaki MS, el Sabbagh MH, Aglan MS. Familial congenital brachial palsy: a report of two affected Egyptian families. Genet Couns. 2004;15(1):27–36.
29. Chauhan SP, Blackwell SB, Ananth CV. Neonatal brachial plexus palsy: incidence, prevalence, and temporal trends. Semin Perinatol. 2014;38(4):210–8. https://doi.org/10.1053/j.semperi.2014.04.007.
30. Spörri S, Thoeny HC, Raio L, Lachat R, Vock P, Schneider H. MR imaging pelvimetry: a useful adjunct in the treatment of women at risk for dystocia? Am J Roentgenol. 2002;179(1):137–44. https://doi.org/10.2214/ajr.179.1.1790137.
31. Zaretsky MV, Alexander JM, McIntire DD, Hatab MR, Twickler DM, Leveno KJ. Magnetic resonance imaging pelvimetry and the prediction of labor dystocia. Obstet Gynecol. 2005;106(5 Pt 1):919–26. https://doi.org/10.1097/01.AOG.0000182575.81843.e7.
32. Mollberg M, Wennergren M, Bager B, Ladfors L, Hagberg H. Obstetric brachial plexus palsy: a prospective study on risk factors related to manual assistance during the second stage of labor. Acta Obstet Gynecol Scand. 2007;86(2):198–204. https://doi.org/10.1080/00016340601089792.
33. Sentilhes L, Sénat MV, Boulogne AI, Deneux-Tharaux C, Fuchs F, Legendre G, et al. Shoulder dystocia: guidelines for clinical practice from the French College of Gynecologists and Obstetricians (CNGOF). Eur J Obstet Gynecol Reprod Biol. 2016;203:156–61. https://doi.org/10.1016/j.ejogrb.2016.05.047.
34. Schmitz T. Modalités de l'accouchement dans la prévention de la dystocie des épaules en cas de facteurs de risque identifiés [Delivery management for the prevention of shoulder dystocia in case of identified risk factors]. J Gynecol Obstet Biol Reprod (Paris).

2015;44(10):1261–71. https://doi.org/10.1016/j.jgyn.2015.09.051. French.
35. Gherman RB, Chauhan S, Ouzounian JG, Lerner H, Gonik B, Goodwin TM. Shoulder dystocia: the unpreventable obstetric emergency with empiric management guidelines. Am J Obstet Gynecol. 2006;195(3):657–72. https://doi.org/10.1016/j.ajog.2005.09.007.
36. Gonik B, Walker A, Grimm M. Mathematic modeling of forces associated with shoulder dystocia: a comparison of endogenous and exogenous sources. Am J Obstet Gynecol. 2000;182(3):689–91. https://doi.org/10.1067/mob.2000.104214.
37. Allen RH, Gurewitsch ED. Temporary Erb-Duchenne palsy without shoulder dystocia or traction to the fetal head. Obstet Gynecol. 2005;105(5 Pt 2):1210–2. https://doi.org/10.1097/01.AOG.0000141635.94905.21.
38. Lerner HM, Salamon E. Permanent brachial plexus injury following vaginal delivery without physician traction or shoulder dystocia. Am J Obstet Gynecol. 2008;198(3):e7–8. https://doi.org/10.1016/j.ajog.2007.11.018.
39. Louden E, Marcotte M, Mehlman C, Lippert W, Huang B, Paulson A. Risk factors for brachial plexus birth injury. Children (Basel). 2018;5(4):46. https://doi.org/10.3390/children5040046.
40. Wall LB, Mills JK, Leveno K, Jackson G, Wheeler LC, Oishi SN, et al. Incidence and prognosis of neonatal brachial plexus palsy with and without clavicle fractures. Obstet Gynecol. 2014;123(6):1288–93. https://doi.org/10.1097/AOG.0000000000000207.
41. Leshikar HB, Bauer AS, Lightdale-Miric N, Molitor F, Waters PM, TOBI Study Group. Clavicle fracture is not predictive of the need for microsurgery in brachial plexus birth palsy. J Pediatr Orthop. 2018;38(2):128–32. https://doi.org/10.1097/BPO.0000000000000770.
42. Gandhi RA, DeFrancesco CJ, Shah AS. The association of clavicle fracture with brachial plexus birth palsy. J Hand Surg Am. 2019;44(6):467–72. https://doi.org/10.1016/j.jhsa.2018.11.006.
43. Louis D, Sundaram V, Samujh R. An unusual case of Erb's palsy in a neonate: a case report. J Child Neurol. 2010;25(10):1261–4. https://doi.org/10.1177/0883073809356809.
44. Mooney JF 3rd, Kasser JR. Brachial plexus palsy as a complication of Pavlik harness use. J Pediatr Orthop. 1994;14(5):677–9. https://doi.org/10.1097/01241398-199409000-00024.
45. Alfonso I, Papazian O, Prieto G, Alfonso DT, Melnick SJ. Neoplasm as a cause of brachial plexus palsy in neonates. Pediatr Neurol. 2000;22(4):309–11. https://doi.org/10.1016/s0887-8994(99)00144-7.
46. Tierney TS, Tierney BJ, Rosenberg AE, Krishnamoorthy KS, Butler WE. Infantile myofibromatosis: a nontraumatic cause of neonatal brachial plexus palsy. Pediatr Neurol. 2008;39(4):276–8. https://doi.org/10.1016/j.pediatrneurol.2008.06.009.
47. Lucas JW, Holden KR, Purohit DM, Cure JK. Neonatal hemangiomatosis associated with brachial plexus palsy. J Child Neurol. 1995;10(5):411–3. https://doi.org/10.1177/088307389501000516.
48. Naqvi AH, Alfonso DT, Flores P, Grossman JA, Restrepo R, Alfonso I. Resolution of brachial plexus palsy due to hemangioma after intravenous corticosteroid therapy. J Child Neurol. 2008;23(8):956–8. https://doi.org/10.1177/0883073808315346.
49. Dierig A, Ritz N, Tacke U, Heininger U. Group A Streptococcal suppurative arthritis and osteomyelitis of the shoulder with brachial plexus palsy in a newborn. Pediatr Infect Dis J. 2016;35(10):1151–3. https://doi.org/10.1097/INF.0000000000001255.
50. Sadleir LG, Connolly MB. Acquired brachial-plexus neuropathy in the neonate: a rare presentation of late-onset group-B streptococcal osteomyelitis. Dev Med Child Neurol. 1998;40(7):496–9. https://doi.org/10.1111/j.1469-8749.1998.tb15401.x.
51. Gabriel SR, Thometz JG, Jaradeh S. Septic arthritis associated with brachial plexus neuropathy. A case report. J Bone Joint Surg Am. 1996;78(1):103–5. https://doi.org/10.2106/00004623-199601000-00014.
52. Clay SA. Osteomyelitis as a cause of brachial plexus neuropathy. Am J Dis Child. 1982;136(12):1054–6. https://doi.org/10.1001/archpedi.1982.03970480020004.

The Biology of Brachial Plexus Birth Injuries

42

Roger Cornwall

Introduction

Any traumatic event in a child can have deleterious effects on the development of affected organ systems. The occurrence of a brachial plexus birth injury (BPBI) in the perinatal period impacts many aspects of the developing neuromusculoskeletal system, in some ways that are similar to the effects of peripheral nerve injuries in adults and in some ways that are quite different. Optimizing the diagnosis, treatment, and prognosis of brachial plexus birth injuries requires an understanding of the developmental setting and biological effects of BPBI. A detailed review of nerve, muscle, bone, and general developmental biology is beyond the scope of this chapter. Instead, the current chapter will explore the basic principles and relevant advances in our understanding of the biology of BPBI, highlighting where such knowledge has the potential to impact clinical decision-making and to advance care in the future. Much of our knowledge comes from animal models of neonatal nerve injury, but the clinical correlations and relevance of findings from these models will be discussed throughout the chapter.

R. Cornwall (✉)
Orthopaedic Surgery and Developmental Biology, Cincinnati Children's Hospital Medical Center, Cincinnati, OH, USA
e-mail: roger.cornwall@cchmc.org

The Neonatal Nervous System

At full-term birth, the human neuromuscular system is far from fully developed (Fig. 42.1). In contrast to other mammals who can stand and ambulate immediately at birth, human motor control is quite primitive in infancy. Several features of human neurodevelopment are consistent with other neotenous animals (those with an extended juvenile period following birth), including other primates and rodents, in which much of the research on postnatal neuromuscular development has been performed. Many of these features of the incompletely developed state of the human nervous system are pertinent to the evaluation and treatment of a child with BPBI. For instance, in such children, when assessing the degree and recovery of the nerve injury, the primary neurologic output assessed by the provider is limb movement. However, limb movement is affected by many more factors than the structural integrity of the nerves of the brachial plexus. Therefore, aside from the biological effects of the injury on muscles, bones, and joints, the biology of the normal maturing nervous system must be considered when interpreting limb movement in an infant with BPBI. The following sections will therefore cover the developmental dynamics of several key features of the neonatal nervous system.

A. Y. Shin, N. Pulos (eds.), *Operative Brachial Plexus Surgery*,
https://doi.org/10.1007/978-3-030-69517-0_42

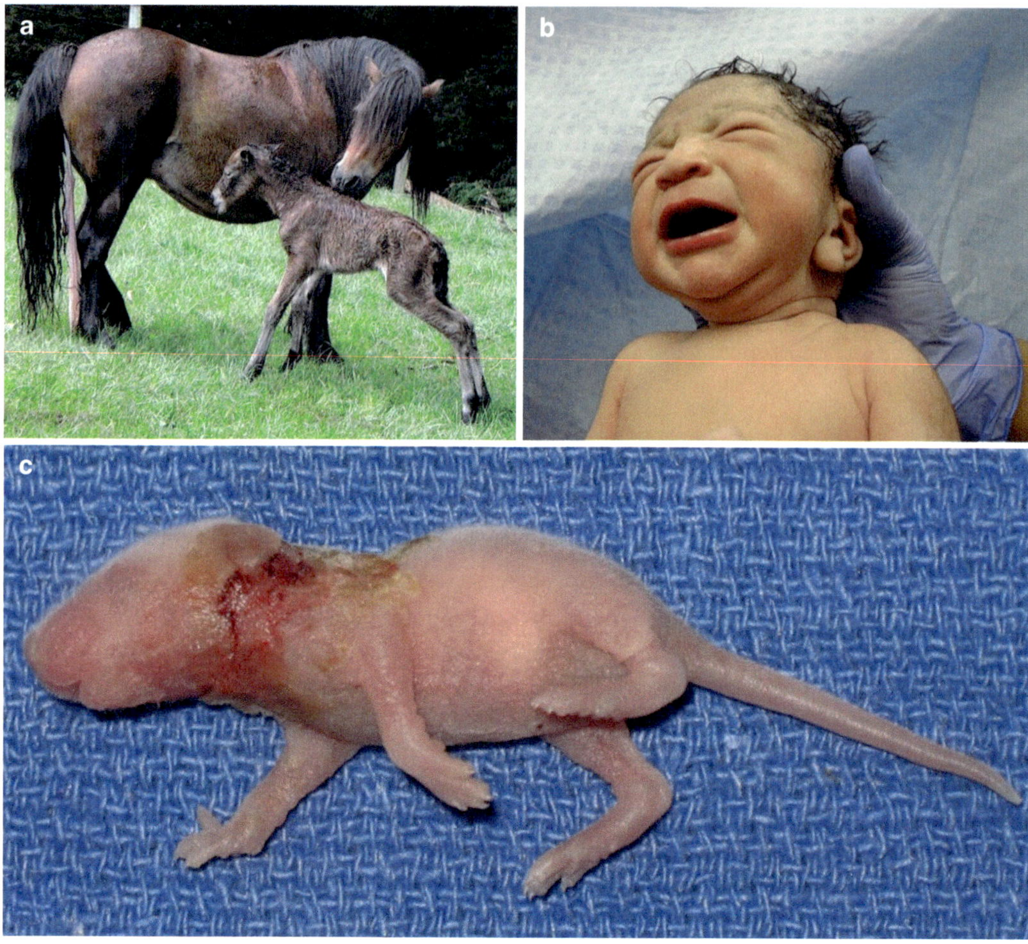

Fig. 42.1 Different species of mammals are born at different stages of neuromuscular development. (**a**) Horses are born with a fully myelinated nervous system and mature neuromuscular control, allowing ambulation immediately at birth. (**b**) Humans are born with incomplete myelination, synaptogenesis, and many other aspects of neuromuscular development and lack even head control at birth. (**c**) Mice and rats are similarly born with immature neuromuscular systems and cannot ambulate or even see at birth. Thus mice are well suited for models of neonatal nerve injury such as BPBI, shown here. (Photo credits: (**a**, **b**) Pixabay. (**c**) Courtesy of Roger Cornwall, MD)

Synaptogenesis

Coordinated movement and integration of sensory input both require cortical and subcortical synaptic connections in the brain. Many or most of these synaptic connections are formed postnatally in many areas of the cerebral cortex, including the sensory and motor cortices [1, 2]. These synapses are formed in response to stimuli and motor learning, both of which are impaired by injury to peripheral mixed motor and sensory nerves. Early experiments in kittens demonstrated that suturing one eyelid closed at birth leads to complete loss of that eye's cortical representation in the visual cortex and that this loss of cortical representation is permanent even when the eye is allowed to open at 3 months [3]. This work, which in part earned David Hubel and Torsten Wiesel a Nobel Prize in Physiology or Medicine, highlights the importance of the interaction between the environment and the developing brain during a critical neonatal window. Similar deprivation experiments have also demonstrated the need for stimulation of many other areas of the brain for proper synaptogenesis during postnatal development [4].

Redundant Innervation

During the same neonatal time period, despite relatively few early synapses, the number of neurons and axons in the central and peripheral nervous system is manyfold greater than in the mature nervous system. These axons get systematically pruned by neuronal apoptosis as the nervous system matures [5]. For instance, in rhesus monkeys, approximately 70% of axons in the corpus callosum are lost in the first few months of life [6]. Similarly, in the peripheral nervous system in rats and humans, skeletal muscle receives innervation from multiple sources at birth, which then become pruned to leave mononeuronal innervation of skeletal muscles in the mature nervous system [7–9] (Fig. 42.2a, b). During the neonatal period then, any given muscle can receive innervation from multiple neuronal sources, so that the activity of one muscle cannot be assumed to represent the function or continuity of the typical nerve pathway innervating that muscle in the adult. This "luxury innervation" has been cited as a primary reason that electromyography cannot be reliably used in BPBI to determine a particular nerve root's status based on the electrical activity of a particular muscle [10]. Furthermore, recruitment of this redundant innervation is assumed to be a cause of agonist/antagonist co-contraction, which is often seen at the elbow in partially resolved BPBI [11]. In the absence of C6 integrity, the elbow flexors can recruit redundant innervation from C7 or lower nerve roots, leading to simultaneous firing of the elbow flexors and triceps muscles [10].

Myelination

Complex coordinated movement requires rapid transmission of neurologic impulses and thus myelination of the axons in the central and peripheral nervous system. Horses have fully myelinated nervous systems at the end of gestation, allowing ambulation immediately at birth [12]. Conversely, in many rodents and in humans, although the process of myelination begins in the third trimester of development, the majority of the process takes place postnatally, well into the third decade of life in humans [13]. Myelination, like synaptogenesis, is activity dependent. Glial cells in the central nervous system and Schwann cells in the peripheral nervous system both respond to electrical impulses [13], although the mechanisms of electrical control of myelination are not fully elucidated. Furthermore, a wide variety of perturbations of the environment, from physical to social, affect the degree of myelination in the brain and spinal cord, much like synaptogenesis is modulated by early postnatal experience [13].

Primitive Reflexes

Normal human infants display several primitive reflexes that diminish with normal development. The provider caring for infants with brachial plexus birth injuries should already be familiar with at least a subset of these reflexes. In the neurological examination of the upper extremity, the grasp reflex can be used to elicit finger flexion, the Moro reflex can be used to elicit shoulder abduction and external rotation, and the asymmetrical tonic neck reflex (ATNR) can be used to elicit elbow flexion on the side away from which the head is turned. However, one must keep in mind the varied implications of abnormal primitive reflexes. In the first 6 months of life, the unmyelinated spinal cord is unable to suppress the reflex arc, leading to easy stimulation of the reflex. Subsequently, as the central nervous system matures, descending inhibition of the reflex arc through interneurons will lead to disappearance of the primitive reflexes [14]. However, persistence of certain primitive reflexes beyond 6 months of age can indicate central nervous system pathology or lack of normal descending inhibition [14]. This mechanism is also responsible for the spasticity of cerebral palsy (CP) only becoming evident after roughly 6 months of age. It is not uncommon for a provider to see asymmetric limb movement or posturing that began at 6 months of age and refer the child for evaluation for a brachial plexus injury. That scenario is much more typical for CP, and not BPBI. Conversely,

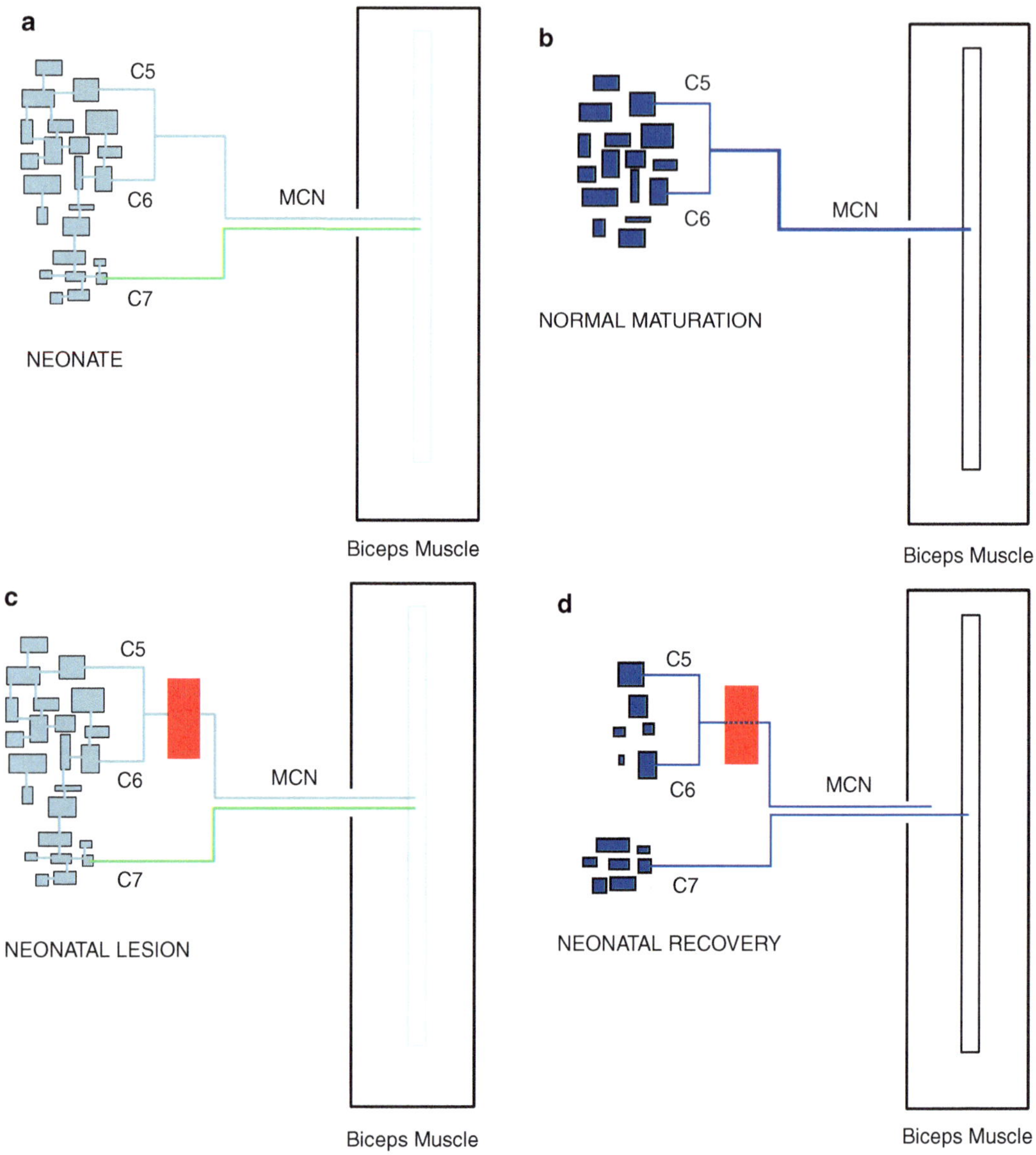

Fig. 42.2 In newborn humans and rodents, skeletal muscles receive polyneuronal innervation (**a**), which gets pruned to mononeuronal inputs postnatally (**b**). (**c**) Neonatal peripheral nerve injury causes persistence of the uninjured redundant innervation, as well as loss of neurons in the spinal cord corresponding to the injured nerve (**d**). (Adapted with permission from Korak et al. [28])

diminished primitive reflexes in the first 6 months of life are also associated with central nervous system dysfunction and can be a very early sign of cerebral palsy [14]. Therefore, in the examination of a newborn with altered limb movement, the failure of a primitive reflex maneuver to elicit the expected movement in a limb is not always indicative of a peripheral nervous system lesion such as a BPBI. A central nervous system lesion can mimic a peripheral nervous system lesion in this way, which is especially important as BPBI and anoxic brain injury can coexist.

Effects of BPBI on the Developing Neuromusculoskeletal System

The primary insult in BPBI is an injury to the nerves of the brachial plexus, most typically at the nerve root level. The injury may be postganglionic, preganglionic, or a combination of both. The degree of nerve injury can range from neuropraxia to axonotmesis to rupture or avulsion. The distribution of the injury can range from upper (C5–C6) to global (C5–T1) plexus involvement. However, regardless of the type of injury, if the duration of paralysis extends beyond the very first few weeks of life, a cascade of secondary events occurs throughout the various organ systems affected. Many of these effects are unique to, or exaggerated in, injuries in the neonatal period as compared to adult or even later childhood injuries. Furthermore, many of these secondary effects are permanent, despite restoration of neurologic connectivity, either by spontaneous recovery or surgical reconstruction, and whether by bridging or bypassing the zone of nerve injury. It has long been thought that most if not all of these secondary effects were the passive mechanical results of altered limb mobility. However, a growing body of evidence now confirms that BPBI causes widespread biological perturbations in the brain, spinal cord, peripheral nerves, muscles, and bones, all of which contribute to the disability caused by BPBI. This paradigm shift from a mechanical to biological realm has opened the door to novel biological strategies to augment our treatment of BPBI. The following sections will review, by organ system, these biological effects and the opportunities they afford for improvements in the care of BPBI.

Peripheral Nerve

The most obvious structure involved in BPBI is the nerve itself. Much of the physiology of nerve injuries has been reviewed in prior chapters. This section, therefore, will focus primarily on the differences in nerve biology following nerve injuries in the neonatal period compared to later nerve injuries. These differences are strikingly distinct when considering the nerve distal to the injury and the nerve proximal to the injury. Distal to a peripheral axotomy, the nerve undergoes the well-known process of Wallerian degeneration, with degradation of the axon and myelin sheath and denervation of the motor endplate in the case of a motor nerve injury [15]. This process begins nearly immediately following axotomy and progresses rapidly thereafter. In an adult mouse model of tibial nerve transection, 89% of motor endplates are denervated, meaning no axons remain present at the neuromuscular junction, within 24 hours following nerve section [16]. Conversely, 24 hours following the same injury in neonatal mice, 86% of motor endplates still remain innervated. This finding suggests that Wallerian degeneration progresses more slowly in the neonatal period. The mechanisms conferring this protective effect of neonatal biology remain to be elucidated, although recent evidence suggests a role for mitochondrial metabolism [17]. It also remains unknown how long a distal axon may survive following neonatal axotomy in humans, but this biological observation in animal models may in part explain the ability to electrically stimulate a nonfunctional muscle upon exposure of the recipient nerve for nerve transfers following BPBI. Knowing that a distal axon downstream from a completely ruptured nerve may survive longer than expected following BPBI could help with the decision to reinnervated a nonfunctional muscle despite the ability to stimulate its nerve intraoperatively.

Substantial biological changes also occur proximal to a peripheral axotomy, with dramatic differences between neonates and adults. In this direction, however, neonates appear uniquely susceptible to the deleterious effects of peripheral nerve injury. Peripheral axotomy in neonatal animal models causes death of approximately half the motor neurons in the spinal cord at the relevant level, while nearly no motor neuron cell death follows adult peripheral axotomy [18, 19]. Nerve root avulsion causes death of 70% of motor neurons in neonates, and although similar losses of motor neurons are seen following adult nerve root avulsion, the neuron loss happens three times faster in neonates than in adults [19]. These findings suggest that neonatal motor neurons are uniquely dependent on connections to their target muscles for survival. This process is thought to involve neurotrophic factors from the target muscles, for which motor neurons compete for survival. This competition is also thought to underlie the normal developmental pruning of neurons from the redundant innervation described previously [20]. Similarly, afferent neurons undergo similar apoptosis in the dorsal root ganglion following peripheral axotomy [21, 22]. These effects are not simply localized to the neuron corresponding to the cut axon, but rather also involve contralateral spinal cord neurons [23] as well as interneurons [24], suggesting complex interactions between neurons and their targets. The biology of these interactions is not completely known but likely involves apoptosis induced by excitotoxicity [23]. Nonetheless, prevention of neuronal cell death following peripheral nerve injury in neonates is a potential opportunity for improving outcomes following nerve reconstruction. Very early studies demonstrated that reinnervation could prevent cell death but that the protective effect of reinnervation was dependent on the length of time between axotomy and reinnervation [25]. Similarly, for at least 25 years since the classic descriptions of this cell death phenomenon, the pharmacologic effects of various neurotrophic factors on motor and sensory neuron survival have been investigated in animal models [18, 24, 26], with promising results in many studies but still no clinically available therapies. Therefore, it remains to be determined if early nerve surgery or adjunctive therapies can become clinically useful in humans with BPBI.

Spinal Cord

Aside from the loss of motor and sensory neuron cell bodies, additional changes occur in the spinal cord following BPBI. As described previously, redundant innervation in the neonatal period can be used to allow persistent innervation of muscles that would become denervated by the same neurologic lesion in adults. For instance, in patients with C5–C6 avulsion injuries in the neonatal period, the biceps can have normal activity and EMG findings unless C7 is also avulsed; conversely, in adults, C5–C6 avulsion injuries lead to complete biceps paralysis [27]. This flexibility of the neonatal nervous system likely involves rerouting of pathways in the spinal cord, as experimental C5–C6 injury in neonatal rats alters the spinal cord architecture with a fourfold increase in C7 neurons innervating the biceps [28] (Fig. 42.2b, c).

Additional alterations in the spinal cord can be seen in the setting of a root avulsion injury. In many respects, a root avulsion injury is analogous to a spinal cord injury. A thorough review of the biology of spinal cord injuries is beyond the scope of this chapter. However, certain aspects must be considered in root avulsion injuries as they impact the feasibility of restoring innervation through root reimplantation. At the site of a root injury, an inflammatory reaction occurs, wherein CNS-specific immune response cells, microglia, and astrocytes are activated and contribute to degeneration of injured neurons [29]. One component of this process, synaptic stripping, involves the selective loss of neurotransmitter receptors on the injured neurons [30]. It is unclear what the function of this synaptic stripping is, although it may serve to protect against excitotoxicity that can lead to motor neuron cell death. Thus, it is unclear if the inflammatory reaction serves a protective or destructive function, or both. Interestingly, both immune suppressors and activators have been shown to have neuroprotective effects [31, 32]. Regardless, the milieu of the injured neuron within the spinal cord undoubtedly plays a complex role in root avulsion injuries.

Brain

As described previously, important processes such as synaptogenesis and myelination are occurring in the brain postnatally and are activity dependent.

It is not surprising then that a brachial plexus birth injury can cause substantial disruption of postnatal brain development. However, before determining the effects of BPBI on brain development, it is important to understand that cortical remodeling occurs after brachial plexus injuries in adults as well. Several studies have investigated cortical remodeling after brachial plexus injuries, mostly using functional magnetic resonance imaging (fMRI). In these studies, fMRI displays regions of activation and connectivity in the cerebral cortex during tasks ranging from resting to active elbow flexion to simply imagining movement. Based on these studies, it is clear that BPI causes reorganization of not only the sensorimotor network (the sensory and motor cortical regions corresponding to the affected upper limb) but also several higher motor areas, such as the frontoparietal network, executive control network, salience network, default mode network, and supplemental motor area [33–35]. Connectivity between some centers is diminished in BPI patients, and some connectivity is increased, suggesting widespread remodeling of the cerebral cortex in response to the injury. The involvement of higher order motor areas suggests changes in motor planning following the peripheral nerve injury. It is not known, however, if these changes are a detrimental result of the injury or if they represent functional adaptation. One study examining patients with unoperated or surgically reconstructed global brachial plexus injuries in adulthood found that those who had functional recovery after surgery had greater connectivity in certain regions compared to unoperated patients, whereas patients without functional recovery after surgery demonstrated no change in connectivity compared to unoperated patients [36]. Again, whether these differences in cortical remodeling are what led to functional improvements following nerve surgery, or if they resulted from successful nerve surgery, has not been determined. However, at least following BPI in adulthood, changes in the brain involve more far-reaching areas than simply the region of the sensorimotor cortex directly involved with function of the affected upper limb.

Similar fMRI studies in patients with BPBI have identified different effects of neonatal injuries on the brain, potentially highlighting different adaptive mechanisms between neonates and adults (Fig. 42.3). Two studies have identified increased activation of the primary sensorimotor cortex corresponding to the affected limb with either imagined limb movement or actual limb movement [37, 38]. This is in contrast to the typically decreased sensorimotor cortex activation following adult BPI. These studies also identified increased activation in higher motor areas, as has been seen in adults, but also increased activation of the contralateral sensorimotor cortex during movement of only the affected limb. Thus, the response to a neonatal injury may involve recruitment of even the contralateral hemisphere sensorimotor cortex, in contrast to decreased interhemispheric connectivity following BPI in adults [39]. Such interhemispheric plasticity is seen following contralateral C7 nerve transfers in adults patients [40] and adult rats [41, 42], although only in rats does the control of the affected limb get fully transferred to the opposite cortex, corresponding to the donor C7 nerve root. Thus the greater ability of children to independently control the treated limb following contralateral C7 transfer may be due to increased capability to remodel across the hemispheres [43]. Finally, the effects of BPBI may extend beyond the regions of the brain responsible for movement and sensation. Typically, in right-handed individuals, the portion of the cortex responsible for language is located in the left hemisphere. However, in 15 patients with right-sided BPBI, fMRI identified a left-to-right shift in language lateralization, with the degree of shift correlating with the degree of impairment in the upper extremity [44]. This finding identifies a connection between upper limb control and language and demonstrates that in the developing brain, isolated peripheral insults can have far-reaching central effects, although the impacts of these effects on our assessment and treatment of BPBI remain to be elucidated.

Nonetheless, it is clear that BPI and its treatments in adults and neonates cause widespread brain remodeling. Therefore, the assessment of limb movement before and after nerve reconstruction is likely affected by the degree and tim-

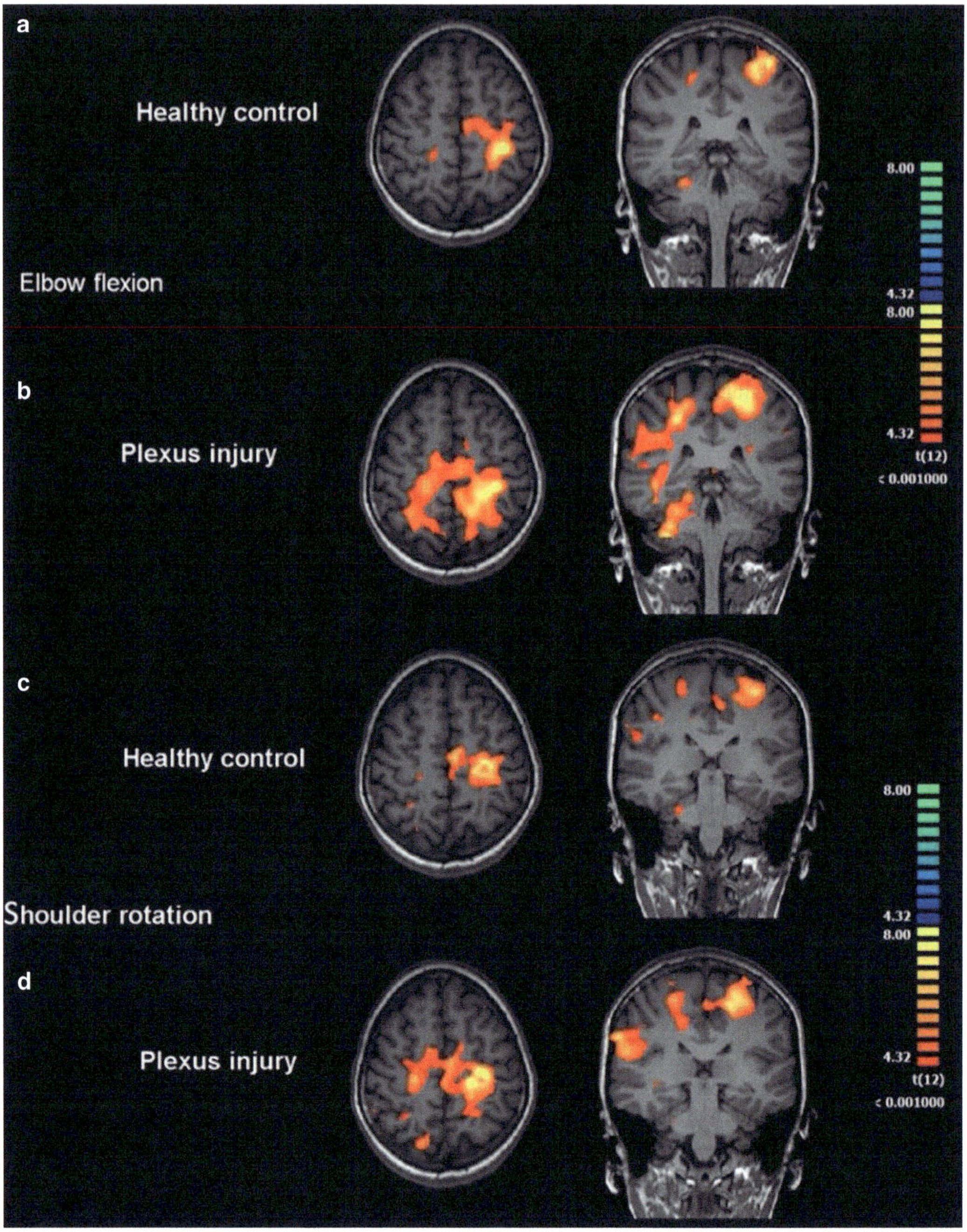

Fig. 42.3 Brain activation demonstrated by fMRI during elbow flexion and shoulder rotation. Compared to healthy controls (**a**, **c**), greater and more widespread brain activation, including activation of the contralateral cortex, is seen following BPBI during elbow flexion (**b**) and shoulder rotation (**d**). (Adapted with permission from Bjorkman et al. [37])

ing of cortical remodeling and its impact on motor learning, as much as it is determined by peripheral connectivity of axons at the site of injury or neurorrhaphy. Furthermore, the treatment of BPI cannot simply rely on technically competent nerve reconstruction but must also involve therapies that promote adapted motor learning.

Muscle

Denervation of skeletal muscle at birth can also have deleterious effects on muscle development, much of which occurs postnatally. Aside from the obvious initial weakness of the muscle from the denervation, additional secondary effects on the development of denervated muscle have important clinical ramifications. The most notable sequela of denervation is the development of contractures, which have recently been demonstrated to be a primarily biological effect of denervation on postnatal muscle growth. The etiology of contractures following BPBI was historically thought to involve purely mechanical processes. A commonly cited mechanism for the development of the shoulder internal rotation contracture has been muscle imbalance between functioning internal rotators and paralyzed external rotators, leading to static internal rotation joint posturing and ultimate joint contracture [45, 46]. However, this muscle imbalance cannot explain the glenohumeral abduction contracture that commonly follows abductor paralysis [47] or the elbow flexion contracture that develops in the setting of elbow flexor paralysis [48–50]. Furthermore, MRI studies have found internal rotation, abduction, and elbow flexion contractures to correspond to atrophy of the subscapularis, abductors, and brachialis, respectively [47, 51, 52], suggesting that contractures may result from tightness of denervated muscles rather than overactivity of functioning muscles.

Recent work in animal models has confirmed that contractures are indeed caused by the biological effect of neonatal denervation on longitudinal muscle growth. Several studies using neonatal lower limb nerve injury in rats previously demonstrated impairment of muscle growth in mass, cross-sectional area, fiber number, and fiber diameter [53–56]. However, the effect of neonatal denervation on longitudinal muscle growth was more recently determined in an animal model of BPBI [57, 58]. In this model, neonatal denervation by C5–C6 nerve root excision led to shoulder internal rotation and elbow flexion contractures with corresponding impaired longitudinal growth in the subscapularis and elbow flexor muscles. Moreover, the elbow flexion contractures could be completely relieved by excising the elbow flexor muscles, leaving the joint capsule intact, suggesting that contractures are due to tight muscles rather than a tight joint capsule. Importantly, these contractures did not occur following excision of the triceps muscle if the elbow flexors remained innervated. Similarly, shoulder internal rotation contractures could not be caused by excision of the external rotators, as long as the subscapularis remained innervated. These data demonstrate that contractures are indeed caused by denervated muscles rather than lack of passive stretch due to muscle imbalance. Furthermore, contractures did not form following denervation in nearly adult animals, confirming the unique susceptibility of neonatal muscle to impaired longitudinal growth, and consistent with clinical observations that BPI in later childhood does not cause contractures [59]. Further experiments in this model [60] investigated the contribution of fibrosis, which had been previously postulated to cause contractures following BPBI [61]. In these experiments, fibrosis occurred after the onset of contractures, and pharmacologic reduction of fibrosis did not prevent contractures, ruling out fibrosis itself as a causative factor in contracture development.

Most recently, the molecular mechanism of impaired longitudinal muscle growth and contractures following BPBI has been identified as increased protein degradation counteracting maintained protein synthesis [62] (Fig. 42.4). Again using an animal model, neonatal denervation was found to increase skeletal muscle protein degradation by the ubiquitin-proteasome system, the main mechanism for protein degradation in adult muscle atrophy. Importantly, pharmacologic inhibition of the proteasome after neonatal BPI was able to completely prevent contractures, despite persistent paralysis. Importantly, in the same experiments, the investigators tracked and manipulated muscle stem cells, known as satellite cells, finding that denervation does not prevent satellite cell function (adding nuclei to the growing multinucleated myofiber) and that preventing satellite cell function does not cause contractures [62]. These data refute previous

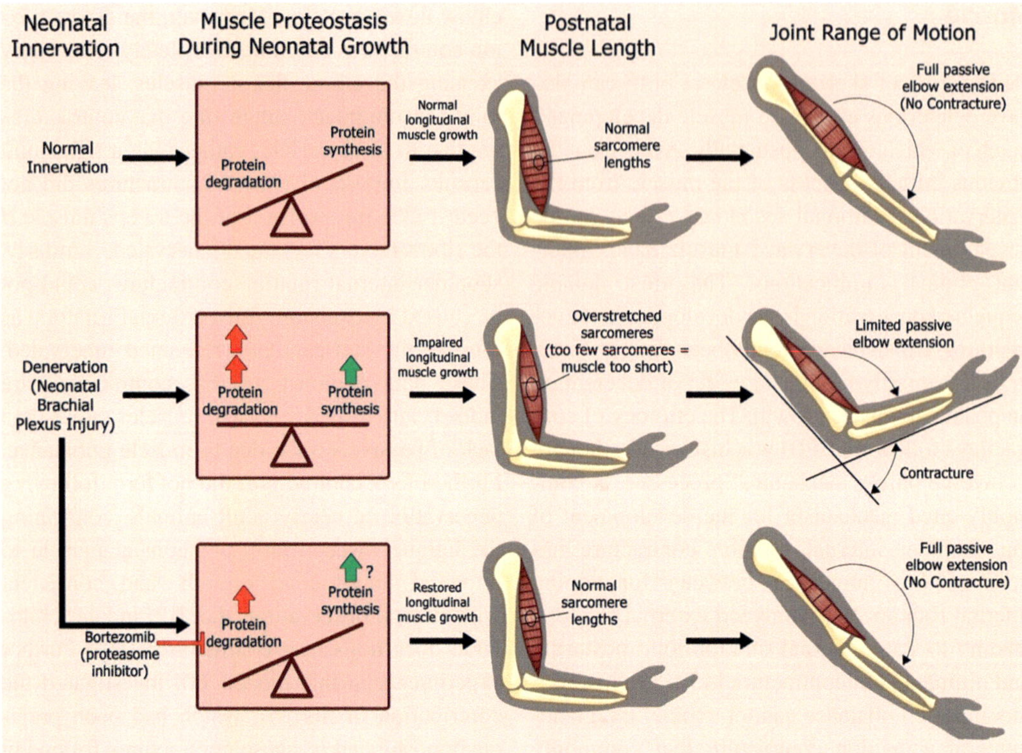

Fig. 42.4 Graphical representation of how BPBI disrupts normal postnatal longitudinal muscle growth by altering the normally anabolic balance between protein synthesis and protein degradation. This impaired growth leads to fewer than normal sarcomeres in series, causing each sarcomere to have to stretch further than normal during muscle stretch (sarcomere elongation) and ultimately limiting the passive motion of the joint (contracture). Inhibition of protein degradation after BPBI restores sarcomere length and range of motion, demonstrating that protein degradation is responsible for contracture formation following BPBI and representing a potential medical strategy to prevent contractures. (Reprinted with permission from Nikolaou et al. [62])

assumptions that postnatal muscle growth requires satellite cell function [63] and that satellite cell dysfunction could be a cause of neuromuscular contractures [64–67]. Therefore, it is unlikely that contractures following BPBI would be amenable to stem cell therapy. Taken together, however, these data shed light on the biological regulation of longitudinal muscle growth and provide a proof of concept that BPBI-induced contractures are amenable to a medical rather than surgical solution by understanding the molecular biological perturbations in neonatally denervated muscles.

In addition to contractures, other perturbations in neonatally denervated muscle can impact assessment and treatment of BPBI. Muscle spindles, specialized muscle fibers that serve as sensory stretch organs, depend on afferent innervation for formation prior to birth and for function and persistence postnatally [68]. In an animal model of BPBI, muscle spindles were found to be degenerated following denervation by postganglionic nerve root excision, but preserved following preganglionic injury, which leaves the afferent neurons in contact with the muscle [69] (Fig. 42.5). Preservation of spindles, which are an important component of coordinated muscle function, may explain the clinical finding that functional recovery of muscle reinnervated by nerve transfer surgery following BPBI nerve root avulsion is superior to that following the same surgery in the setting of BPBI nerve root rupture [70]. Furthermore, contractures did not occur following preganglionic

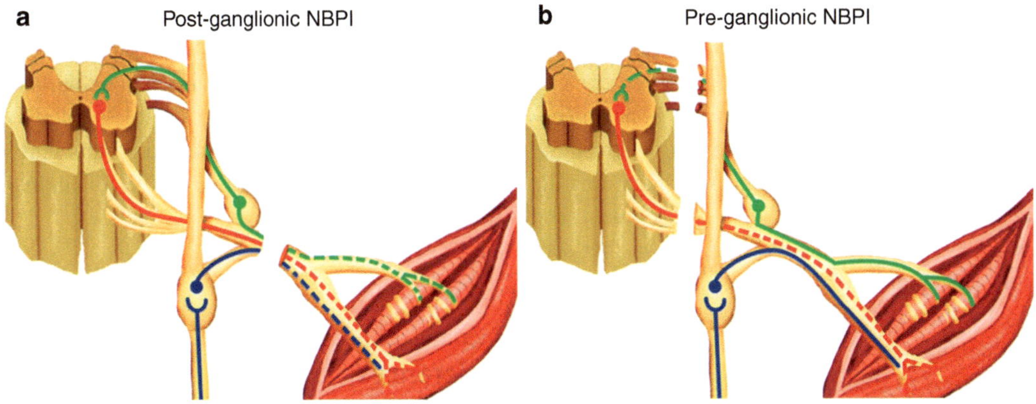

Fig. 42.5 Schematic representation of postganglionic and preganglionic nerve root injuries. In postganglionic injuries (**a**), the cell bodies of the efferent (red), afferent (green), and sympathetic (blue) neurons are disconnected from the muscle, causing complete denervation of the muscle fibers and muscle spindles. In preganglionic injuries (**b**), the cell bodies of the sympathetic and afferent neurons remain connected to the muscle, preserving afferent and sympathetic innervation. This neuroanatomic difference may explain the absence of contractures and better motor recovery after nerve transfer for preganglionic injuries. (Image courtesy of Roger Cornwall, MD)

injury in the animal model [69], consistent with the absence of contractures following C5–C6 nerve root avulsion injuries in BPBI seen clinically [71]. Therefore, afferent innervation may play a role in contracture pathogenesis. However, sympathetic innervation is also preserved following preganglionic injury, and sympathetic neurons have recently been found to innervate the neuromuscular junction between the efferent axon and muscle fiber and play an important role in maintenance and function [72]. Therefore, sympathetic innervation may not only play a role in contracture prevention but may also explain the improved recovery of motor function following nerve transfer surgery for preganglionic versus postganglionic injuries [70]. Nonetheless, the relative roles of afferent and sympathetic innervation in the sequelae of BPBI must be further investigated. Similarly, the expression and behavior of acetylcholine receptors in skeletal muscle have been long known to change during postnatal development and be perturbed by neonatal denervation [73], although the ramifications of this developmental perturbation in BPBI are not known. Finally, the shift in myosin isoform expression (fast to slow) following neonatal denervation is similar to that following adult denervation [74], although again its clinical significance is unknown with respect to BPBI.

Bone

Among the most important sequelae of BPBI is glenohumeral dysplasia. Based on clinical observations before and after shoulder surgery, as well as data from animal and computational models, this dysplasia is widely thought to result from pressure imbalance at the glenoid, where increased posterior pressure from contractures and/or muscle activity imbalance leads to glenoid retroversion, pseudoglenoid formation, and ultimate dislocation [75–82]. However, the biological effects of denervation on bone growth deserve discussion, since the mechanical phenotype of dysplasia may not have a purely mechanical pathophysiology, as exemplified by the muscle contractures discussed above. According to Hilton's law [83], a joint will receive innervation from any nerve that passes it. Therefore, the glenohumeral joint will receive innervation from the suprascapular nerve posteriorly, the axillary nerve inferiorly, and the rest of the brachial plexus anteriorly. Thus the nerves supplying the posterior and inferior glenoid would be denervated in a typical C5–C6 BPBI, whereas intact nerves in the remainder of the brachial plexus would still pass the anterior glenoid. Therefore it is possible that the posterior glenoid insufficiency typical in BPBI-induced dysplasia results in part from denervation-induced impairment of posterior glenoid growth, similar to the denervation-induced impairment of muscle growth.

The direct neuronal regulation of bone homeostasis has been a focus of increasing interest, but much remains unknown, especially regarding the neuronal regulation of bone development and growth [84]. Nonetheless, it is known that sensory and sympathetic neurons innervate developing bones at sites of high osteogenic activity [85]. Although sensory neurons are known to regulate bone mass in adulthood and during development [86, 87], bone development otherwise appears unaltered in the absence of sensory neurons. Similarly, the sympathetic nervous system is known to modulate bone mass and remodeling [88], but its effect on bone growth is unknown. Nonetheless, the longitudinal growth of bone in antlers is slowed by denervation [89], and animal models of BPBI have consistently reported reduced humeral lengths. Furthermore, in human patients with BPBI, bone growth is affected throughout the upper limb, correlating with the distribution and severity of the BPBI [90]. It is unclear whether the bone growth inhibition is modulated directly by innervation or through limb movement, but further research is warranted regarding the role of innervation in bone growth and postnatal development.

Summary

This chapter has reviewed the uniqueness of the neonatal nervous system and how it is perturbed by a peripheral nerve injury. Through clinical observations and experiments in animal models, much has been learned about the biology of various organ systems in the setting of BPBI. However much work remains to be done. Can preservation of the distal axon and motor endplate be extended to allow better reinnervation targets? Can prevention of neuronal cell death improve outcomes of nerve reconstruction? Can cortical plasticity be further harnessed for therapy interventions? Can contractures be prevented in humans by inhibiting muscle protein degradation? Can the protective effect of preganglionic injuries on muscle and possibly bone physiology be harnessed and applied to other types of BPBI? The future of BPBI care will depend not only on improvements in clinical assessment and interventions but also on a deeper understanding of the biology of all of the organ systems that are affected by this injury at a particularly vulnerable stage of human development.

References

1. Bourgeois JP, Rakic P. Changes of synaptic density in the primary visual cortex of the macaque monkey from fetal to adult stage. J Neurosci. 1993;13(7):2801–20.
2. Rakic P, Bourgeois JP, Eckenhoff MF, Zecevic N, Goldman-Rakic PS. Concurrent overproduction of synapses in diverse regions of the primate cerebral cortex. Science. 1986;232(4747):232–5.
3. Wiesel TN, Hubel DH. Comparison of the effects of unilateral and bilateral eye closure on cortical unit responses in kittens. J Neurophysiol. 1965;28(6):1029–40.
4. Rice D, Barone S Jr. Critical periods of vulnerability for the developing nervous system: evidence from humans and animal models. Environ Health Perspect. 2000;108(Suppl 3):511–33.
5. Kim WR, Sun W. Programmed cell death during postnatal development of the rodent nervous system. Develop Growth Differ. 2011;53(2):225–35.
6. LaMantia AS, Rakic P. Axon overproduction and elimination in the corpus callosum of the developing rhesus monkey. J Neurosci. 1990;10(7):2156–75.
7. Gramsbergen A, IJkema-Paassen J, Nikkels PG, Hadders-Algra M. Regression of polyneural innervation in the human psoas muscle. Early Hum Dev. 1997;49(1):49–61.
8. Hesselmans LF, Jennekens FG, Van den Oord CJ, Veldman H, Vincent A. Development of innervation of skeletal muscle fibers in man: relation to acetylcholine receptors. Anat Rec. 1993;236(3):553–62.
9. Brown MC, Jansen JK, Van Essen D. Polyneuronal innervation of skeletal muscle in new-born rats and its elimination during maturation. J Physiol. 1976;261(2):387–422.
10. van Ouwerkerk WJ. Preoperative investigations in obstetric brachial plexus palsy. Semin Plast Surg. 2005;19(1):17–23.
11. Rollnik JD, Hierner R, Schubert M, Shen ZL, Johannes S, Troger M, et al. Botulinum toxin treatment of cocontractions after birth-related brachial plexus lesions. Neurology. 2000;55(1):112–4.
12. Szalay F. Development of the equine brain motor system. Neurobiology (Bp). 2001;9(2):107–35.
13. Fields RD. White matter in learning, cognition and psychiatric disorders. Trends Neurosci. 2008;31(7):361–70.

14. Futagi Y, Suzuki Y. Neural mechanism and clinical significance of the plantar grasp reflex in infants. Pediatr Neurol. 2010;43(2):81–6.
15. Saxena S, Caroni P. Mechanisms of axon degeneration: from development to disease. Prog Neurobiol. 2007;83(3):174–91.
16. Murray LM, Comley LH, Gillingwater TH, Parson SH. The response of neuromuscular junctions to injury is developmentally regulated. FASEB J. 2011;25(4):1306–13.
17. Kline RA, Dissanayake KN, Hurtado ML, Martinez NW, Ahl A, Mole AJ, et al. Altered mitochondrial bioenergetics are responsible for the delay in Wallerian degeneration observed in neonatal mice. Neurobiol Dis. 2019;130:104496.
18. Li L, Oppenheim RW, Lei M, Houenou LJ. Neurotrophic agents prevent motoneuron death following sciatic nerve section in the neonatal mouse. J Neurobiol. 1994;25(7):759–66.
19. Li L, Houenou LJ, Wu W, Lei M, Prevette DM, Oppenheim RW. Characterization of spinal motoneuron degeneration following different types of peripheral nerve injury in neonatal and adult mice. J Comp Neurol. 1998;396(2):158–68.
20. Oppenheim RW. Cell death during development of the nervous system. Annu Rev Neurosci. 1991;14:453–501.
21. Zhou XF, Li WP, Zhou FH, Zhong JH, Mi JX, Wu LL, et al. Differential effects of endogenous brain-derived neurotrophic factor on the survival of axotomized sensory neurons in dorsal root ganglia: a possible role for the p75 neurotrophin receptor. Neuroscience. 2005;132(3):591–603.
22. Schmalbruch H. Loss of sensory neurons after sciatic nerve section in the rat. Anat Rec. 1987;219(3):323–9.
23. Lawson SJ, Lowrie MB. The role of apoptosis and excitotoxicity in the death of spinal motoneurons and interneurons after neonatal nerve injury. Neuroscience. 1998;87(2):337–48.
24. Oliveira AL, Risling M, Negro A, Langone F, Cullheim S. Apoptosis of spinal interneurons induced by sciatic nerve axotomy in the neonatal rat is counteracted by nerve growth factor and ciliary neurotrophic factor. J Comp Neurol. 2002;447(4):381–93.
25. Kashihara Y, Kuno M, Miyata Y. Cell death of axotomized motoneurones in neonatal rats, and its prevention by peripheral reinnervation. J Physiol. 1987;386:135–48.
26. Catapano J, Zhang J, Scholl D, Chiang C, Gordon T, Borschel GH. N-Acetylcysteine prevents retrograde motor neuron death after neonatal peripheral nerve injury. Plast Reconstr Surg. 2017;139(5):1105e–15e.
27. Vredeveld JW, Blaauw G, Slooff BA, Richards R, Rozeman SC. The findings in paediatric obstetric brachial palsy differ from those in older patients: a suggested explanation. Dev Med Child Neurol. 2000;42(3):158–61.
28. Korak KJ, Tam SL, Gordon T, Frey M, Aszmann OC. Changes in spinal cord architecture after brachial plexus injury in the newborn. Brain. 2004;127(Pt 7):1488–95.
29. Penas C, Casas C, Robert I, Fores J, Navarro X. Cytoskeletal and activity-related changes in spinal motoneurons after root avulsion. J Neurotrauma. 2009;26(5):763–79.
30. Emirandetti A, Graciele Zanon R, Sabha M Jr, de Oliveira AL. Astrocyte reactivity influences the number of presynaptic terminals apposed to spinal motoneurons after axotomy. Brain Res. 2006;1095(1):35–42.
31. De Freria CM, Barbizan R, De Oliveira AL. Granulocyte colony stimulating factor neuroprotective effects on spinal motoneurons after ventral root avulsion. Synapse. 2012;66(2):128–41.
32. Scorisa JM, Zanon RG, Freria CM, de Oliveira AL. Glatiramer acetate positively influences spinal motoneuron survival and synaptic plasticity after ventral root avulsion. Neurosci Lett. 2009;451(1):34–9.
33. Lu Y, Liu H, Hua X, Xu WD, Xu JG, Gu YD. Supplementary motor cortical changes explored by resting-state functional connectivity in brachial plexus injury. World Neurosurg. 2016;88:300–5.
34. Feng JT, Liu HQ, Hua XY, Gu YD, Xu JG, Xu WD. Brain functional network abnormality extends beyond the sensorimotor network in brachial plexus injury patients. Brain Imaging Behav. 2016;10(4):1198–205.
35. Qiu TM, Chen L, Mao Y, Wu JS, Tang WJ, Hu SN, et al. Sensorimotor cortical changes assessed with resting-state fMRI following total brachial plexus root avulsion. J Neurol Neurosurg Psychiatry. 2014;85(1):99–105.
36. Bhat DI, Indira Devi B, Bharti K, Panda R. Cortical plasticity after brachial plexus injury and repair: a resting-state functional MRI study. Neurosurg Focus. 2017;42(3):E14.
37. Bjorkman A, Weibull A, Svensson H, Dahlin L. Cerebral reorganization in patients with brachial plexus birth injury and residual shoulder problems. Front Neurol. 2016;7:240.
38. Anguelova GV, Rombouts S, van Dijk JG, Buur PF, Malessy MJA. Increased brain activation during motor imagery suggests central abnormality in Neonatal Brachial Plexus Palsy. Neurosci Res. 2017;123:19–26.
39. Liu B, Li T, Tang WJ, Zhang JH, Sun HP, Xu WD, et al. Changes of inter-hemispheric functional connectivity between motor cortices after brachial plexuses injury: a resting-state fMRI study. Neuroscience. 2013;243:33–9.
40. Yu A, Wang S, Cheng X, Liang W, Bai R, Xue Y, et al. Functional connectivity of motor cortical network in patients with brachial plexus avulsion injury after contralateral cervical nerve transfer: a resting-state fMRI study. Neuroradiology. 2017;59(3):247–53.
41. Jiang S, Li ZY, Hua XY, Xu WD, Xu JG, Gu YD. Reorganization in motor cortex after brachial plexus avulsion injury and repair with the contralateral C7 root transfer in rats. Microsurgery. 2010;30(4):314–20.
42. Stephenson JB, Li R, Yan JG, Hyde J, Matloub H. Transhemispheric cortical plasticity following con-

tralateral C7 nerve transfer: a rat functional magnetic resonance imaging survival study. J Hand Surg Am. 2013;38(3):478–87.
43. Vu AT, Sparkman DM, van Belle CJ, Yakuboff KP, Schwentker AR. Retropharyngeal contralateral C7 nerve transfer to the lower trunk for brachial plexus birth injury: technique and results. J Hand Surg Am. 2018;43(5):417–24.
44. Auer T, Pinter S, Kovacs N, Kalmar Z, Nagy F, Horvath RA, et al. Does obstetric brachial plexus injury influence speech dominance? Ann Neurol. 2009;65(1):57–66.
45. Waters PM. Update on management of pediatric brachial plexus palsy. J Pediatr Orthop. 2005;25(1):116–26.
46. Pearl ML. Shoulder problems in children with brachial plexus birth palsy: evaluation and management. J Am Acad Orthop Surg. 2009;17(4):242–54.
47. Eismann EA, Little KJ, Laor T, Cornwall R. Glenohumeral abduction contracture in children with unresolved neonatal brachial plexus palsy. J Bone Joint Surg Am. 2015;97(2):112–8.
48. Herring JA. In: Herring JA, editor. Tachdjian's pediatric orthopaedics. Philadelphia: WB Saunders; 2002. p. 479–87.
49. Ballinger SG, Hoffer MM. Elbow flexion contracture in Erb's palsy. J Child Neurol. 1994;9(2):209–10.
50. Poyhia TH, Lamminen AE, Peltonen JI, Kirjavainen MO, Willamo PJ, Nietosvaara Y. Brachial plexus birth injury: US screening for glenohumeral joint instability. Radiology. 2010;254(1):253–60.
51. Poyhia TH, Koivikko MP, Peltonen JI, Kirjavainen MO, Lamminen AE, Nietosvaara AY. Muscle changes in brachial plexus birth injury with elbow flexion contracture: an MRI study. Pediatr Radiol. 2007;37(2):173–9.
52. Poyhia TH, Nietosvaara YA, Remes VM, Kirjavainen MO, Peltonen JI, Lamminen AE. MRI of rotator cuff muscle atrophy in relation to glenohumeral joint incongruence in brachial plexus birth injury. Pediatr Radiol. 2005;35(4):402–9.
53. Lowrie MB, Krishnan S, Vrbova G. Recovery of slow and fast muscles following nerve injury during early post-natal development in the rat. J Physiol. 1982;331:51–66.
54. Mousavi K, Miranda W, Parry DJ. Neurotrophic factors enhance the survival of muscle fibers in EDL, but not SOL, after neonatal nerve injury. Am J Physiol Cell Physiol. 2002;283(3):C950–9.
55. Fisher TJ, Vrbova G, Wijetunge A. Partial denervation of the rat soleus muscle at two different developmental stages. Neuroscience. 1989;28(3):755–63.
56. Schmalbruch H. Growth and denervation response of skeletal muscle fibers of newborn rats. Muscle Nerve. 1990;13(5):421–32.
57. Nikolaou S, Peterson E, Kim A, Wylie C, Cornwall R. Impaired growth of denervated muscle contributes to contracture formation following neonatal brachial plexus injury. J Bone Joint Surg Am. 2011;93(5):461–70.
58. Weekley H, Nikolaou S, Hu L, Eismann E, Wylie C, Cornwall R. The effects of denervation, reinnervation, and muscle imbalance on functional muscle length and elbow flexion contracture following neonatal brachial plexus injury. J Orthop Res. 2012;30(8):1335–42.
59. Ho ES. Evaluation of pediatric upper extremity peripheral nerve injuries. J Hand Ther. 2015;28(2):135–42.
60. Nikolaou S, Hu L, Tuttle LJ, Weekley H, Wylie C, Lieber RL, et al. Contribution of denervated muscle to contractures following neonatal brachial plexus injury: not just muscle fibrosis. Muscle Nerve. 2014;49(3):398–404.
61. Hogendoorn S, van Overvest KL, Watt I, Duijsens AH, Nelissen RG. Structural changes in muscle and glenohumeral joint deformity in neonatal brachial plexus palsy. J Bone Joint Surg Am. 2010;92(4):935–42.
62. Nikolaou S, Cramer AA, Hu L, Goh Q, Millay DP, Cornwall R. Proteasome inhibition preserves longitudinal growth of denervated muscle and prevents neonatal neuromuscular contractures. JCI Insight. 2019;4(23):e128454.
63. White RB, Bierinx AS, Gnocchi VF, Zammit PS. Dynamics of muscle fibre growth during postnatal mouse development. BMC Dev Biol. 2010;10:21.
64. Dayanidhi S, Dykstra PB, Lyubasyuk V, McKay BR, Chambers HG, Lieber RL. Reduced satellite cell number in situ in muscular contractures from children with cerebral palsy. J Orthop Res. 2015;33(7):1039–45.
65. Kinney MC, Dayanidhi S, Dykstra PB, McCarthy JJ, Peterson CA, Lieber RL. Reduced skeletal muscle satellite cell number alters muscle morphology after chronic stretch but allows limited serial sarcomere addition. Muscle Nerve. 2017;55(3):384–92.
66. Mathewson MA, Lieber RL. Pathophysiology of muscle contractures in cerebral palsy. Phys Med Rehabil Clin N Am. 2015;26(1):57–67.
67. Smith LR, Chambers HG, Lieber RL. Reduced satellite cell population may lead to contractures in children with cerebral palsy. Dev Med Child Neurol. 2013;55(3):264–70.
68. Zelena J, Soukup T. Ultrastructural changes of developing muscle spindles after denervation. Folia Morphol (Praha). 1975;23(3):275–7.
69. Nikolaou S, Hu L, Cornwall R. Afferent innervation, muscle spindles, and contractures following neonatal brachial plexus injury in a mouse model. J Hand Surg Am. 2015;40(10):2007–16.
70. Little KJ, Zlotolow DA, Soldado F, Cornwall R, Kozin SH. Early functional recovery of elbow flexion and supination following median and/or ulnar nerve fascicle transfer in upper neonatal brachial plexus palsy. J Bone Joint Surg Am. 2014;96(3):215–21.
71. Al-Qattan MM. Obstetric brachial plexus palsy associated with breech delivery. Ann Plast Surg. 2003;51(3):257–64; discussion 65.
72. Khan MM, Lustrino D, Silveira WA, Wild F, Straka T, Issop Y, et al. Sympathetic innervation controls homeostasis of neuromuscular junctions in health and disease. Proc Natl Acad Sci U S A. 2016;113(3):746–50.

73. Brenner HR. Dependence of acetylcholine receptor channel conversion on muscle activity at denervated neonatal rat endplates. Neurosci Lett. 1988;88(2):161–6.
74. Matsuda R, Spector D, Strohman RC. Denervated skeletal muscle displays discoordinate regulation for the synthesis of several myofibrillar proteins. Proc Natl Acad Sci U S A. 1984;81(4):1122–5.
75. Waters PM, Bae DS. The early effects of tendon transfers and open capsulorrhaphy on glenohumeral deformity in brachial plexus birth palsy. Surgical technique. J Bone Joint Surg Am. 2009;91 Suppl 2:213–22.
76. Waters PM, Monica JT, Earp BE, Zurakowski D, Bae DS. Correlation of radiographic muscle cross-sectional area with glenohumeral deformity in children with brachial plexus birth palsy. J Bone Joint Surg Am. 2009;91(10):2367–75.
77. Waters PM, Smith GR, Jaramillo D. Glenohumeral deformity secondary to brachial plexus birth palsy. J Bone Joint Surg Am. 1998;80(5):668–77.
78. Li Z, Ma J, Apel P, Carlson CS, Smith TL, Koman LA. Brachial plexus birth palsy-associated shoulder deformity: a rat model study. J Hand Surg [Am]. 2008;33(3):308–12.
79. Kim HM, Galatz LM, Das R, Patel N, Thomopoulos S. Musculoskeletal deformities secondary to neurotomy of the superior trunk of the brachial plexus in neonatal mice. J Orthop Res. 2010;28(10):1391–8.
80. Kim HM, Galatz LM, Patel N, Das R, Thomopoulos S. Recovery potential after postnatal shoulder paralysis. An animal model of neonatal brachial plexus palsy. J Bone Joint Surg Am. 2009;91(4):879–91.
81. Cheng W, Cornwall R, Crouch DL, Li Z, Saul KR. Contributions of muscle imbalance and impaired growth to postural and osseous shoulder deformity following brachial plexus birth palsy: a computational simulation analysis. J Hand Surg Am. 2015;40(6):1170–6.
82. Crouch DL, Hutchinson ID, Plate JF, Antoniono J, Gong H, Cao G, et al. Biomechanical basis of shoulder osseous deformity and contracture in a rat model of brachial plexus birth palsy. J Bone Joint Surg Am. 2015;97(15):1264–71.
83. Hebert-Blouin MN, Tubbs RS, Carmichael SW, Spinner RJ. Hilton's law revisited. Clin Anat. 2014;27(4):548–55.
84. Brazill JM, Beeve AT, Craft CS, Ivanusic JJ, Scheller EL. Nerves in bone: evolving concepts in pain and anabolism. J Bone Miner Res. 2019;34(8):1393–406.
85. Sisask G, Silfversward CJ, Bjurholm A, Nilsson O. Ontogeny of sensory and autonomic nerves in the developing mouse skeleton. Auton Neurosci. 2013;177(2):237–43.
86. Offley SC, Guo TZ, Wei T, Clark JD, Vogel H, Lindsey DP, et al. Capsaicin-sensitive sensory neurons contribute to the maintenance of trabecular bone integrity. J Bone Miner Res. 2005;20(2):257–67.
87. Fukuda T, Takeda S, Xu R, Ochi H, Sunamura S, Sato T, et al. Sema3A regulates bone-mass accrual through sensory innervations. Nature. 2013;497(7450):490–3.
88. Elefteriou F, Campbell P, Ma Y. Control of bone remodeling by the peripheral sympathetic nervous system. Calcif Tissue Int. 2014;94(1):140–51.
89. Suttie JM, Fennessy PF. Regrowth of amputated velvet antlers with and without innervation. J Exp Zool. 1985;234(3):359–66.
90. Gosk J, Wnukiewicz W, Urban M. The effect of perinatal brachial plexus lesion on upper limb development. BMC Musculoskelet Disord. 2014;15:116.

Epidemiology of Obstetrical Brachial Plexus Injury

43

Lindley Wall and Marie Morris

Introduction

Obstetrical brachial plexus injury (BPBI) remains a source of morbidity and financial burden for the pediatric population, and not all those with a diagnosis of BPBI have identifiable risk factors. Therefore, knowledge of the epidemiology of the condition remains important for identifying potential strategies for prevention.

This chapter will discuss the trends and incidence of BPBI, known risk factors, and methods for prevention.

Incidence

The incidence of BPBI has been estimated at 1.6–5.1 per 1000 live births by population-based studies [1, 2]. Population-based studies examining data from the 1997 to 2012 Kids' Inpatient Database found a decreasing rate of BPBI in the United States. Over this period, the incidence decreased from 1.7 to 0.6 per 1000 live births ($P < 0.001$) [3, 4]. Bager performed a population-based study examining births over a 10-year period, 1980–1989, using the national Swedish Medical Birth Registry and reported an average incidence of BPBI of 1.6 per 1000 [1]. A more recent population-based study in western Sweden examined 38,749 children born between 1999 and 2001 and demonstrated an incidence of BPBI of 2.9 per 1000 live births and an incidence of persistent BPBI at 18 months of age of 0.46 per 1000 live births [5]. The variation in incidence reported across studies can partly be explained by geographic differences in obstetric care and population versus region-based studies.

The majority of BPBI is unilateral with approximately 5% being bilateral.

In unilateral BPBI, the right side is more often affected than the left. In a study of 11, 873 children born in the Netherlands, with 56 suffering BPBI, the ratio of right- to left-sided BPBI was 33:23 [2].

Risk Factors

Risk factors for BPBI include both maternal and fetal factors. Specifically they include shoulder dystocia, fetal macrosomia (>4500 g), a previous child with shoulder dystocia or BPBI, maternal diabetes, assisted vaginal delivery, multiparity, prolonged labor, excessive maternal weight gain, and fetal malposition [6, 7]. There seems to be a higher occurrence in females and black and Hispanic groups than in males or other ethnic

L. Wall (✉) · M. Morris
Department of Orthopaedic Surgery, Washington University School of Medicine, Saint Louis, MO, USA
e-mail: wallli@wustl.edu; marietmorris@wustl.edu

A. Y. Shin, N. Pulos (eds.), *Operative Brachial Plexus Surgery*,
https://doi.org/10.1007/978-3-030-69517-0_43

groups [3]. However, despite these risk factors, more than 80% of BPBI occurs in mothers who do not have known risk factors [6].

Shoulder Dystocia

Shoulder dystocia remains the highest risk factor for BPBI. It is defined as delivery requiring special obstetric maneuvers to deliver the shoulders after gentle downward traction has failed. It is a clinical diagnosis that is made during delivery, and its incidence ranges from 0.2% to 3.0% of all vaginal deliveries. It has been shown to increase the risk of BPBI as high as 166- and 215-fold [8, 9]. The most reliable predictor of shoulder dystocia is a mother's history of prior child with shoulder dystocia [8, 10].

In the setting of shoulder dystocia, the rate of transient BPBI ranges from 1% to 7%, and the rate of persistent BPI (lasting longer than 1 year) ranges from 0.5% to 1.6%. These rates are in comparison to the rate of transient or persistent BPI without shoulder dystocia which is approximately 0.9% [6]. However, despite this increase risk of BPBI with shoulder dystocia, studies have found that only 17–46% of patients with BPBI had a history of shoulder dystocia [4, 8, 11, 12].

Shoulder dystocia also increases the risk of ipsilateral clavicle fractures [13], but the risk of BPBI in the setting of shoulder dystocia and an ipsilateral clavicle fracture is similar to that of shoulder dystocia without a fracture (OR 126.7 versus 112.1, $P = 0.26$) [14]. An ipsilateral clavicle fracture may be protective of the brachial plexus, as neurologic recovery is more likely in the setting of a clavicle fracture than without one (98.1% versus 94.4%, $P = 0.005$) [15]. In difficult deliveries, choices must be made by the treating obstetrician to minimize morbidity and mortality. While we do not necessarily recommend prophylactic clavicle fracture, we believe there is evidence that minimizing shoulder girdle width may be protective for the neurologic function of an infant's upper limb.

Macrosomia

Macrosomia, defined as a birth weight greater than 4500 g, has also been established as a risk factor for BPBI [4]. In the review of data from the Kids' Inpatient Database from 1997 to 2003, a birth weight greater than 4500 g increased the risk of BPBI by 14 times [4]. Examining data from the Swedish Medical Birth Registry, the incidence of BPBI was 45 times higher in neonates with a birth weight greater than 4500 g compared to those with a birth weight less than 3500 g, with an incidence of 18.1 per 1000 births versus 0.4 per 1000 births [1]. A separate population-based study in Sweden found that weight greater than 5000 g increased the risk of BPBI by 34.2 times [8]. In this study, in the setting of shoulder dystocia, the incidence of BPBI in infants with a birth weight between 4500 and 4999 g was 29.5% (OR 2.3) and higher in infants with a birth weight greater than 5000 g with an incidence of 35.3% (OR 3.0). Being heavy for gestational date has also been shown to be a risk factor with [16] an OR of approximately 6.88 [4]. There does not seem to be, however, a correlation between increased birth weight and severity of injury [1]. Consistent with macrosomia being a risk factor of BPBI, prematurity and intrauterine growth restriction appear to be protective against BPBI [17].

Diabetes

Gestational diabetes occurs more commonly in mothers of newborns with BPBI than those without [8, 18]. In a series of patients born in civilian hospitals in California from 1994 to 1995, Gilbert found that gestational diabetes increased the risk of BPBI by 1.9 times. With regard to a diagnosis of gestational diabetes and mode of delivery, the frequency of BPBI was highest in mothers with gestational diabetes and an assisted delivery (vacuum or forceps) and fetal macrosomia (>4500 g) (7.8%) compared to mothers with gestational diabetes and unassisted vaginal delivery which was between 3% and 4% [17].

Assisted Vaginal Delivery

Operative vaginal delivery by forceps or vacuum has also been associated with increased risk of BPBI. Forceps-aided delivery increased the risk of BPBI by nine times and vacuum assisted greater than six times in the series of patients from the Kids' Inpatient Database [4]. As mentioned above, this risk is compounded by a concomitant history of maternal diabetes and fetal macrosomia. Gilbert et al. found that forceps-aided delivery increased the risk of BPBI by 3.4 times and that vacuum-assisted delivery increased the risk by 2.7 times [17].

History of BPBI

Maternal history of an infant with BPBI is also a risk factor for a subsequent infant to be delivered with BPBI. In their series of 59 patients with BPBI, Gordon et al. found 14% of patients were born to a mother who had a prior child with BPBI.

Breech Position

Breech delivery has also been associated with BPBI. After adjusting for other risk factors, Mollberg et al. found breech delivery increased the risk of BPBI by 8.8 times in their series from the Swedish Medical Birth Registry [8]. DeFrancesco et al. found an adjusted odds ratio of 3.65 indicating an increased risk for BPBI in breech delivery by greater than 3 times [3]. Additionally, a diagnosis of "other malpresentation" (ICD-9 code 763.1) has also been associated with an increased risk of BPBI with an estimated OR of 73.6 [17]. There has been suggestion that the event of the brachial plexus injury may sometimes occur from malpresentation prior to labor [17].

Birth Hypoxia

Fetal hypoxia during delivery has been found an independent risk factor for BPBI (OR 3.1, $P < 0.001$) [3]. Along with this risk factor, fetal hypotonia has also been suggested as a possible risk factor with an odds ratio of 1.3 [9]. The decrease in muscle tone and impaired reflexes may prevent the fetus from being able to protect themselves by limiting shoulder displacement during transit through the birth [3]; however, this has not been established as clear mechanism of injury.

Prolonged Labor

Duration of active pushing during vaginal delivery has been associated with a slight increased risk of BPBI [19]. A protracted active phase and secondary arrest of dilatation are also associated with an increased risk of BPBI [8]. Still, several patients with BPBI are delivered without reported difficulties [20].

Multiple Gestation Birth

In review of the Kids' Inpatient Database, multiple gestation birth was associated with a lower risk of BPBI with an adjusted OR 0.45 in the study by DeFrancesco et al. and an adjusted OR of 0.25 in the preceding study by Foad et al. [3, 4]

Prevention

BPBI continues to be a source of morbidity and financial burden for families and the healthcare system. The initial hospital stay for patients with BPBI is longer than for those without it, and hospital stay costs are 40% greater [9]. Only approximately 66% of children with BPBI achieve complete recovery [2, 21], and BPBI continues to be a common reason for litigation for birth complications. Prevention is therefore of paramount importance.

Although identified risk factors do exist for BPBI, the fact that most occur in mothers who do not have risk factors poses a challenge in prevention. Approximately 50–55% of infants with BPBI did not themselves have risk factors or their mothers [3, 4, 18]. In an attempt to predict the occurrence of BPBI, Perlow et al. identified only 19% of cases of BPBI that could be predicted prior to delivery [22].

Induction of Labor

Induction of labor for macrosomia has been suggested as a preventative measure against shoulder dystocia and BPBI. However, the diagnosis of macrosomia poses a challenge, as ultrasound accuracy for estimating fetal weight is approximately 62–66% accurate in measuring weight within 10% of actual birth weight [23].

Cesarean Delivery

Cesarean delivery has been found to be protective of BPBI with an odds ratio of 0.12 [4]. In analysis of the Kids' Inpatient Database, the risk of BPBI was decreased with Cesarean delivery (OR 0.16, $P < 0.001$) [3]. This study also related the decreasing incidence of BPBI from 1997 to 2012 to an increase in the rate of Cesarean section from 20.9% to 34.0% ($P < 0.001$) during this period [3]. Between 2009 and 2017, however, the rate has remained between 31.9% and 32.8% with slight decreases between 2009 and 2016 [24, 25].

The decision to proceed with a Cesarean delivery for BPBI prevention requires shared decision-making between obstetrician and patient, as Cesarean delivery does not always prevent BPBI. BPBI still occurs after Cesarean deliveries, with an incidence of 0.03–0.15% [6]. There is increased risk of shoulder dystocia and BPBI in the setting of maternal diabetes and macrosomia especially in the setting of assisted vaginal delivery. However, Gilbert found that 92% of macrosomic infants born to a mother with diabetes with assisted vaginal delivery did not have BPBI. The routine use of Cesarean section delivery is not recommended, nor is it cost-effective except potentially in the situation of a diabetic mother and fetus with macrosomia [17, 26]. The American College of Obstetricians and Gynecologists (ACOG) practice revised their practice recommendations between 1997 and 2002 to recommend planned Cesarean section for patients with estimated fetal weight greater than 5000 g in women without diabetes and greater than 4500 g in women with diabetes [27, 28]. Unfortunately, the challenge is still to accurately determine fetal weight. However, there may be a benefit to Cesarean section delivery for mothers who have previously given birth to an infant with BPBI [10].

Shoulder Dystocia Training

Some studies have demonstrated a decreased incidence of BPBI after employing dystocia simulation courses for obstetricians [29–31]. After implementing a shoulder dystocia training course for maternity staff, the overall incidence of BPBI after vaginal delivery at one center decreased from 0.40% prior to training down to 0.14% after training ($P < 0.01$). BPBI after shoulder dystocia decreased from 30% to 10.67% ($P < 0.01$) [29].

References

1. Bager B. Perinatally acquired brachial plexus palsy--a persisting challenge. Acta Paediatr. 1997;86(11):1214–9.
2. Hoeksma AF, ter Steeg AM, Nelissen RG, van Ouwerkerk WJ, Lankhorst GJ, de Jong BA. Neurological recovery in obstetric brachial plexus injuries: an historical cohort study. Dev Med Child Neurol. 2004;46(2):76–83.
3. DeFrancesco CJ, Shah DK, Rogers BH, Shah AS. The epidemiology of brachial plexus birth palsy in the United States: declining incidence and evolving risk factors. J Pediatr Orthop. 2019;39(2):e134–e40.
4. Foad SL, Mehlman CT, Ying J. The epidemiology of neonatal brachial plexus palsy in the United States. J Bone Joint Surg Am. 2008;90(6):1258–64.
5. Lagerkvist AL, Johansson U, Johansson A, Bager B, Uvebrant P. Obstetric brachial plexus palsy: a prospective, population-based study of incidence, recovery, and residual impairment at 18 months of age. Dev Med Child Neurol. 2010;52(6):529–34.
6. Executive summary: neonatal brachial plexus palsy. Report of the American College of Obstetricians and Gynecologists' Task Force on Neonatal Brachial Plexus Palsy. Obstet Gynecol. 2014;123(4):902–4.
7. Lindell-Iwan HL, Partanen VS, Makkonen ML. Obstetric brachial plexus palsy. J Pediatr Orthop B. 1996;5(3):210–5.

8. Mollberg M, Hagberg H, Bager B, Lilja H, Ladfors L. High birthweight and shoulder dystocia: the strongest risk factors for obstetrical brachial plexus palsy in a Swedish population-based study. Acta Obstet Gynecol Scand. 2005;84(7):654–9.
9. Abzug JM, Mehlman CT, Ying J. Assessment of current epidemiology and risk factors surrounding brachial plexus birth palsy. Pediatrics. 2018;141(1 Meeting Abstract):661.
10. al-Qattan MM, al-Kharfy TM. Obstetric brachial plexus injury in subsequent deliveries. Ann Plast Surg. 1996;37(5):545–8.
11. Chauhan SP, Rose CH, Gherman RB, Magann EF, Holland MW, Morrison JC. Brachial plexus injury: a 23-year experience from a tertiary center. Am J Obstet Gynecol. 2005;192(6):1795–800; discussion 800–2.
12. Gherman RB, Ouzounian JG, Goodwin TM. Brachial plexus palsy: an in utero injury? Am J Obstet Gynecol. 1999;180(5):1303–7.
13. Lopez E, de Courtivron B, Saliba E. Neonatal complications related to shoulder dystocia. J Gynecol Obstet Biol Reprod (Paris). 2015;44(10):1294–302.
14. Gandhi RA, DeFrancesco CJ, Shah AS. The association of clavicle fracture with brachial plexus birth palsy. J Hand Surg Am. 2019;44(6):467–72.
15. Wall LB, Mills JK, Leveno K, Jackson G, Wheeler LC, Oishi SN, et al. Incidence and prognosis of neonatal brachial plexus palsy with and without clavicle fractures. Obstet Gynecol. 2014;123(6):1288–93.
16. Gordon M, Rich H, Deutschberger J, Green M. The immediate and long-term outcome of obstetric birth trauma. I. Brachial plexus paralysis. Am J Obstet Gynecol. 1973;117(1):51–6.
17. Gilbert WM, Nesbitt TS, Danielsen B. Associated factors in 1611 cases of brachial plexus injury. Obstet Gynecol. 1999;93(4):536–40.
18. Backe B, Magnussen EB, Johansen OJ, Sellaeg G, Russwurm H. Obstetric brachial plexus palsy: a birth injury not explained by the known risk factors. Acta Obstet Gynecol Scand. 2008;87(10):1027–32.
19. Grobman WA, Bailit J, Lai Y, Reddy UM, Wapner RJ, Varner MW, et al. Association of the duration of active pushing with obstetric outcomes. Obstet Gynecol. 2016;127(4):667–73.
20. Jennett RJ, Tarby TJ, Kreinick CJ. Brachial plexus palsy: an old problem revisited. Am J Obstet Gynecol. 1992;166(6 Pt 1):1673–6; discussion 6–7.
21. Foad SL, Mehlman CT, Foad MB, Lippert WC. Prognosis following neonatal brachial plexus palsy: an evidence-based review. J Child Orthop. 2009;3(6):459–63.
22. Perlow JH, Wigton T, Hart J, Strassner HT, Nageotte MP, Wolk BM. Birth trauma. A five-year review of incidence and associated perinatal factors. J Reprod Med. 1996;41(10):754–60.
23. Chauhan SP, Hendrix NW, Magann EF, Morrison JC, Scardo JA, Berghella V. A review of sonographic estimate of fetal weight: vagaries of accuracy. J Matern Fetal Neonatal Med. 2005;18(4):211–20.
24. Martin JA, Hamilton BE, Osterman MJK, Driscoll AK, Drake P. Births: final data for 2016. Natl Vital Stat Rep. 2018;67(1):1–55.
25. Martin JA, Hamilton BE, Osterman MJK, Driscoll AK, Drake P. Births: final data for 2017. Natl Vital Stat Rep. 2018;67(8):1–50.
26. Rouse DJ, Owen J, Goldenberg RL, Cliver SP. The effectiveness and costs of elective cesarean delivery for fetal macrosomia diagnosed by ultrasound. JAMA. 1996;276(18):1480–6.
27. ACOG practice patterns. Shoulder dystocia. Number 7, October 1997. American College of Obstetricians and Gynecologists. Int J Gynaecol Obstet. 1998;60(3):306–13.
28. Sokol RJ, Blackwell SC, Bulletins-Gynecology ACoOaGCoP. ACOG practice bulletin: shoulder dystocia. Number 40, November 2002. (Replaces practice pattern number 7, October 1997). Int J Gynaecol Obstet. 2003;80(1):87–92.
29. Inglis SR, Feier N, Chetiyaar JB, Naylor MH, Sumersille M, Cervellione KL, et al. Effects of shoulder dystocia training on the incidence of brachial plexus injury. Am J Obstet Gynecol. 2011;204(4):322.e1–6.
30. Draycott TJ, Crofts JF, Ash JP, Wilson LV, Yard E, Sibanda T, et al. Improving neonatal outcome through practical shoulder dystocia training. Obstet Gynecol. 2008;112(1):14–20.
31. Crofts JF, Lenguerrand E, Bentham GL, Tawfik S, Claireaux HA, Odd D, et al. Prevention of brachial plexus injury-12 years of shoulder dystocia training: an interrupted time-series study. BJOG. 2016;123(1):111–8.

Associated Concomitant Injuries

44

Ayobami Ward, Brandon Smith, and Lynda Yang

Introduction

The focus of this chapter is to highlight and discuss various concomitant injuries suffered by children with NBPP and their effects on overall recovery and functional outcome. These associated disorders can happen either at the time of the initial nerve injury or in a delayed fashion; they will be presented in relative chronology with some exceptions given the parallel development of many of these conditions.

As clinicians caring for patients with motor deficits, providers tend to focus on motor function in isolation. Single-minded thinking, however, fails to take into account the patient's clinical course as a whole. The WHO-ICF is a useful tool to help us understand that functional classification is much more integrated and also relies heavily on multiple interrelated factors. The injuries and conditions in the following chapter may not directly affect motor function; however, they do have both direct and indirect effects on the other domains of function.

A. Ward · B. Smith · L. Yang (✉)
University of Michigan, Ann Arbor, MI, USA
e-mail: ljsyang@med.umich.edu

Phrenic Nerve Injury

The origin of concomitant injury to the phrenic nerve in NBPP is a result of the same tractional forces on the brachial plexus, which also leads to stretching of the 3rd to 5th cervical nerve root and the associated phrenic nerve [1]. The association of brachial plexus palsy and phrenic nerve injury has been reported as early as the 1950s; it was first described in a patient with "brachial palsy" that demonstrated "dullness at pulmonary base on involved side because of elevation of the diaphragm."

Today, isolated phrenic nerve injury presents in about 1/15,000 to 1/30,000 live births every year [1] but may present more commonly in babies with NBPP. In 1956, the mortality for this injury was reported as 27.6%, whereas now, mortality is almost unheard of. Since the mechanism of injury is similar for the brachial plexus and phrenic nerve, so too are the risk factors.

Diagnosis is based on clinical evaluation at birth. Suspicion of a phrenic nerve injury should increase when a patient with a brachial plexus palsy presents with respiratory distress after birth and often is noticed with difficulty feeding. Fluoroscopy or ultrasound can be used to evaluate, with ultrasound being the preferred modality to avoid radiation exposure. Some centers utilize phrenic nerve stimulation to prognosticate spontaneous recovery [1]. Prolonged latency of the signal would indicate

A. Y. Shin, N. Pulos (eds.), *Operative Brachial Plexus Surgery*,
https://doi.org/10.1007/978-3-030-69517-0_44

that recovery is possible, while absent signal transduction would indicate that the likelihood of spontaneous recovery is low [1–4].

Treatment of phrenic nerve injury is focused on treating the respiratory distress and hemidiaphragmatic failure. Two studies indicate that phrenic nerve injury will spontaneously resolve with conservative management, but for those with recurrent respiratory infections or difficulty feeding, diaphragmatic plication is a viable option [5, 6]. Importantly, Bowerson et al. demonstrated that the severity of respiratory symptoms resulting from phrenic nerve palsy was *not* correlated with the severity of the brachial plexus palsy [5]. One may conclude that functional recovery of neonatal brachial plexus palsy has little value in framing a prognosis in the context of phrenic nerve palsy, and vice versa. If the patient progresses to surgical intervention, the diaphragmatic status is helpful to know from both a surgical and anesthetic standpoint.

Clavicle Fracture

Skeletal birth trauma is a known risk of vaginal delivery. The most common bony injury during delivery is a fracture to the clavicle, which occurs in 0.5–1.6% of neonates [7–9]. There are many risk factors that are associated with clavicle fracture including shoulder dystocia, forceps delivery, vacuum delivery, prolonged labor, gestational diabetes, and increased birth weight. As you have read in earlier chapters, many of these risk factors are the same for NBPP.

Although both are commonly seen in "difficult" deliveries, both NBPP and clavicular fractures have been demonstrated in uncomplicated spontaneous vaginal birth as well as caesarian sections.

After delivery, in the neonatal period, both entities can separately present as decreased limb use and apparent motor asymmetry. A detailed neurologic examination can help to identify the presence and extent of the NBPP, and the presence of a clavicular fracture can be verified with standard radiographs.

Although there is an association between the two injuries, there is no evidence that the severity of fracture is associated with NBPP or vice versa [10–12]. The severity of clavicular fracture can range from asymptomatic and delayed presentation until callus formation in the first weeks of life, to a fully displaced fracture. In either circumstance, the management of clavicle fracture in neonates is generally supportive including pain control and more rarely immobilization with specialized garments.

Other than increased bleeding and scar tissue at the periclavicular area which may impact some surgical planes, the presence of a clavicular fracture should not impact the clinical course or decision-making in nerve reconstruction for NBPP.

Shoulder Dislocation/Subluxation

As with many other joints, friction and pressure are needed in order for the glenohumeral joint to develop into the classic ball and cup formation that we know and depend on for stability [13].

NBPP injuries involve the upper trunk which supplies that main musculature surrounding the glenohumeral joint, regardless of Narakas grade: deltoid, supra-/infraspinatus, teres major and minor, biceps, and coracobrachialis. In patients with NBPP, the muscle imbalances across this joint prevent it from forming the standard 3D architecture that allows the humeral head to articulate securely within a normally configured socket [13].

Joint architecture continues to develop throughout early childhood, and in the shoulder the lack of development often presents issues within the first year of life. The lack of development of the ball and cup architecture lead the joint to subluxate [13]. Many NBPP patients present with subluxations as early as 4–6 months when surgical repairs are occurring. This can be noted when positioning the patient in external rotation needed to access the medial upper arm for the Oberlin procedure. CT scans have been used for grading systems, however, given the increased avoidance of ionizing radiation ultrasound continues to be a mainstay and our preferred method of evaluation. Given that above, exercises to maintain PROM should not be delayed as early joint movement does not seem to increase the incidence of later subluxation [14].

Torticollis

Torticollis is caused by a congenital or secondary shortening of the sternocleidomastoid muscle, resulting in the characteristic tilting/turning of the head to one side. Congenital muscular torticollis is the most common culprit in the neonate affecting 4–16% of all infants. Congenital muscular torticollis differs from the entity we encounter and associate with NBPP, which is classified in the nonmuscular torticollis. Nonmuscular torticollis makes up for 18.4% of all torticollis, and 51% of these patients were found to have a neurological cause including brachial plexus palsy [15, 16].

The nature of the relationship between brachial plexus injury and torticollis is one that has seen only sparse investigation. The true mechanical/physiologic cause has yet to be defined although it is easy to postulate that given their close anatomic proximity, both the nerves and the muscles of the neck can be injured. Kenned in 1903 wrote, "That there may be injury to neighboring structures is to be expected, seeing that force sufficient to rupture the nerves has been exerted…. often very great…as there was at the same time torticollis present due to rupture of the SCM" [16, 17].

NBPP patients present with torticollis in approximately 40% of patients at a single clinic. The distribution of concomitant torticollis and NBPP demonstrates a slight female predominance (58%), as well as a slight left-sided predominance (56%) [16]. In almost all settings, the torticollis will appear on the side ipsilateral to the NBPP (98%). Importantly, there are no studies available that indicate a difference in severity of NBPP between patients with and without torticollis [16].

The diagnosis is most often made by physical exam with the patient assuming the classic posture of a unilateral head tilt/rotation. Further workup is not routinely performed if suspicion is only for torticollis [16]. More than 60% of patients with torticollis and NBPP had spontaneous resolution of the torticollis without other musculoskeletal abnormalities. The presence of torticollis does not pose a major consideration in the treatment of NBPP, nor does it indicate rate or extent of recovery [16]. Similarly, intervention to lengthen or otherwise surgically modify the sternocleidomastoid is not recommended; occupational/physical therapy is the first line of treatment for torticollis associated with NBPP [16].

Plagiocephaly

Neonatal and infantile cranial asymmetry is another intersection between neurosurgery and plastic surgery. Craniosynostosis and plagiocephaly are two causes of cranial asymmetry, with the latter being associated with NBPP.

In one single-center study, positional plagiocephaly was noted in over 60% of children with NBPP representing a likely association between the two entities [18]. As discussed above, torticollis is associated with NBPP and is also associated with positional plagiocephaly. Tang et al. suggest that the increased incidence of plagiocephaly is not fully dependent on the presence of torticollis, but instead due to the motor asymmetry noted in the NBPP patients [18]. In the infant with an asymmetric cranium, close examination and understanding of external forces and bone growth principles helps to diagnose plagiocephaly vs. craniosynostosis.

There is limited data on plagiocephaly and NBPP, but there appears to be a relationship where a worsening severity of NBPP increases the percentage of spontaneous resolution of the plagiocephaly. The authors of this article postulate that patients with more severe NBPP tend to get more physical therapy which could improve their head position, neck musculature, and overall posture [18].

Although plagiocephaly likely does not alter the outcomes of NBPP, it is important to understand its presence and to differentiate this from craniosynostosis. There have been reports of children undergoing unnecessary craniofacial operations since plagiocephaly is not a surgical disease [18].

Contracture

A joint contracture is the pathologic decrease in ROM of a joint as a result of tendon and muscle shortening. In order for the skeletal architecture to remain functional, balance is needed around the joint itself. The balance of agonists, antagonists, and supportive musculature surrounding each joint is of the utmost importance. If there is an imbalance in muscle function, permanent shortening of the tendons and muscles can result in joint contractures. In NBPP the risk factors are twofold with both limited muscle power to maintain active range of motion and dysfunctional joint formation as mentioned above.

The imbalances of muscle strength lead to the classic arm posture for untreated Erb's palsy. Weakness in the external rotors results in an internally rotated shoulder [19], and a lack of repeated ROM causes flexion contractures at the elbow and wrist [20, 21].

Prevention is key when it comes to contracture, since its presence is a formidable foe for the nerve surgeon. Reinnervated musculature often lacks the power of normal musculature, and any hindrance including inflexible joints are difficult to overcome even with successful reinnervation. These issues are one of the major reasons that we suggest early referral to a comprehensive brachial plexus center for all children with brachial plexus palsy [22]. The visits are not only helpful for serial examinations that help decide on surgical intervention but also to initiate therapies to optimize functional outcomes and maintain ROM [14, 23].

In our surgical patients, when early signs of contracture are noted in the pectoralis with internal rotation of the shoulder, we and others utilize botulinum toxin injections of the pectoralis as well as placement in a spica brace post-repair. The surgical repair of contractures will be discussed in other chapters.

Limb Length Differences

In addition to flexion contractures, and joint formation problems, patients with neonatal brachial plexus palsies can have limb length development issues. These issues arise as the growth of bones relies in part on the external forces placed on them by active and intermittently contracting musculature. Many groups have looked at various length and girth measures in both patients who underwent reconstruction and those who did not. The largest series of patient consisted of 179 patents evaluated at McMaster University [24]. They demonstrated that in 95% of patients with NBPP, there is a statistically significant difference in limb length between the affected and unaffected side. These findings were noted at every time points starting at 1 month. In patients with NBPP, the limb girth, due to asymmetric muscle mass, in addition to the limb length also is significantly lower.

Sensation, Proprioception, and Limb Dominance

Sensation in children is difficult to assess and is a current are of research for many programs. There are some beliefs that due to neuroplasticity children seem to be excluded from the pain symptoms after NBPP unlike their adult counterparts [25, 26]. However, autophagy is a not uncommonly seen phenomenon which may argue the counter. Little has been proven in this area given the subjective nature of sensation and pain and the difficulty identifying these symptoms in nonverbal neonates and limitedly verbal infants and toddlers.

It is now well-known that limb preference for the unaffected limb is generally higher in children who suffer from NBPP [27, 28]. Considering that during normal development, the hand/limb dominance presents itself as early as 6–10 months, solidifying between 4 and 10 years of age, it follows that a sufficiently plastic nervous system should be able to adapt to this change, with little issue [27].

Several studies have demonstrated that some children, regardless of severity of injury or repair, continue to demonstrate issues with proprioception and limb placement [28, 29]. Sensation and motor activation/movement are deeply linked neurologically, with proprioception being the critical factor for feedback in motor actions. These deficits have been shown to exist in several areas of the affected limb, including the shoulder, the elbow, and the hand [30–32].

Investigation into the cortical basis of this phenomenon has yielded interesting results. A recent study by Anguelova et al. investigating central activation in motor tasks via fMRI demonstrated that NBPP patients had higher levels of activation in premotor and motor cortices when planning tasks but normal activation when the task was being performed. This suggests that the actual planning of the task requires increased motor planning centrally. This may provide a neurophysiological substrate for the differences seen in limb dominance in patients – higher motor planning "processing" requirements may lead to limb dominance changes in right-handed patients with right NBPP [27, 33].

Cognitive and Psychosocial Effects

Injuries that present with neonatal brachial plexus palsy are not restricted only to physical trauma and anatomic changes. There is also evidence that NBPP may lead to changes in psychosocial adjustment, body image issues, changes in quality of life, as well as cognitive changes that may or may not resolve spontaneously.

When considering the psychosocial effects that NBPP may have on a patient, it is important to make considerations for development. Rehabilitation should include evaluation of early language delay in toddlers, which has been shown to be linked with motor impairment, specifically NBPP [34–36]. Changes in functional limb preference due to NBPP can affect [1] the lateralization of language depending on which limb ends up favored by the child, and thus may delay development of language, and [2] the ability for the child to use environment exploration to build nonverbal communication skills before first speaking [34].

External and internal perception is an important facet of coping with physical impairment. Children and parents generally wish for a form of "external observer normality" when discussing the return of function in a wide range of neonatal pathologies [37]. When we zoom in on neonatal brachial plexus palsy, we see that this holds true. When children with NBPP are asked about their diagnosis and how it had affected their lives, the most likely answers were its impact on recreational activities, activities of daily living (ADLs), as well as techniques involved in maintaining an appearance of normality [38]. Social and emotional health were also frequent topics of discussion.

These results remain consistent into adolescence, where we see that adolescents with previous diagnoses of NBPP were most concerned with their functional limitations [39]. There exists a mountain of evidence which suggests that physical impairment, self-image issues, and self-esteem are closely linked psychologically [40]. It is intuitive to assume that patients who were previously diagnosed with NBPP would have decreased self-esteem, and indeed there is evidence that children with physical disabilities are more likely to suffer from mental health issues while paradoxically tending to be more emotionally happy and self-confident with their condition than their parents [39]. Similarly, despite the difficulties that children with NBPP face, adolescents with NBPP score similarly to their normal counterparts on self-determination assessments, particularly when encouraged by an interdisciplinary program's patient- and family-centered care approach.

Discussion/Conclusion

As you can see from the information in this chapter, although NBPP is technically a focal injury to the nerve roots supplying the brachial plexus, the injuries and conditions associated with NBPP are both unique and numerous. In addition to the direct impact on nerves and muscles of the upper extremity, we see conditions that impact the respiratory system, cranial vault, appendicular skeleton, and even the psychological health of these children. Although as nerve surgeons we tend to focus on the restoration of both the degrees of movement and the power across joints, awareness of many conditions that can also pose as barriers to these children will aid the provider with the overall care of these patients. A focus on the multifactorial nature of function, like that laid out by the WHO-ICF, can help to optimize the overall outcome for children impacted by this condition.

Bibliography

1. Stramrood CAI, Blok CA, Van Der Zee DC, Gerards LJ. Neonatal phrenic nerve injury due to traumatic delivery. J Perinat Med. 2009;37(3):293–6.
2. Imai T, Shizukawa H, Imaizumi H, Matsumoto H. Transient phrenic nerve palsy after cardiac operation in infants. Clin Neurophysiol. 2004;115(6):1469–72.
3. Ross Russell RI, Helms PJ, Elliott MJ. A prospective study of phrenic nerve damage after cardiac surgery in children. Intensive Care Med. 2008;34(4):728–34.
4. Rafferty GF, Greenough A, Dimitriou G, Kavadia V, Laubscher B, Polkey MI, et al. Assessment of neonatal diaphragm function using magnetic stimulation of the phrenic nerves. Am J Respir Crit Care Med. 2000;162(6):2337–40.
5. Bowerson M, Nelson VS, Yang LJS. Diaphragmatic paralysis associated with neonatal brachial plexus palsy. Pediatr Neurol. 2010;42(3):234–6.
6. Al-Qattan MM, Clarke HM, Curtis CG. The prognostic value of concurrent phrenic nerve palsy in newborn children with Erb's palsy. J Hand Surg Eur Vol. 1998;23(2):225.
7. Beall MH, Ross MG. Clavicle fracture in labor: risk factors and associated morbidities. J Perinatol. 2001;21(8):513–5.
8. Hsu TY, Hung FC, Lu YJ, Ou CY, Roan CJ, Kung FT, et al. Neonatal clavicular fracture: clinical analysis of incidence, predisposing factors, diagnosis, and outcome. Am J Perinatol. 2002;19(1):17–21.
9. Lam MH, Wong GY, Lao TT. Reappraisal of neonatal clavicular fracture: relationship between infant size and risk factors. J Reprod Med Obstet Gynecol. 2002;47(11):903–8.
10. Leshikar HB, Bauer AS, Lightdale-Miric N, Molitor F, Waters PM. Clavicle fracture is not predictive of the need for microsurgery in brachial plexus birth palsy. J Pediatr Orthop. 2018;38(2):128–32.
11. Al-Qattan MM, Clarke HM, Curtis CG. The prognostic value of concurrent clavicular fractures in newborns with obstetric brachial plexus palsy. J Hand Surg Am. 1994;19(6):729–30.
12. Wall LB, Mills JK, Leveno K, Jackson G, Wheeler LC, Oishi SN, et al. Incidence and prognosis of neonatal brachial plexus palsy with and without clavicle fractures. Obstet Gynecol. 2014;123(6):1288–93.
13. Pearl ML. Shoulder problems in children with brachial plexus birth palsy: evaluation and management. J Am Acad Orthop Surg. 2009;17(4):242–54.
14. Justice D, Rasmussen L, Di Pietro M, Chang KWC, Murphy SL, Nelson VS, et al. Prevalence of posterior shoulder subluxation in children with neonatal brachial plexus palsy after early full passive range of motion exercises. PM R. 2015;7(12):1235–42.
15. Ballock RT, Song KM. The prevalence of nonmuscular causes of torticollis in children. J Pediatr Orthop. 1996;16(4):500–4.
16. Hervey-Jumper SL, Justice D, Vanaman MM, Nelson VS, Yang LJS. Torticollis associated with neonatal brachial plexus palsy. Pediatr Neurol. 2011;45(5):305–10.
17. Kennedy R. Suture of the brachial plexus in birth paralysis of the upper extremity. Br Med J. 1903;1(2197):298–301.
18. Tang M, Gorbutt KA, Peethambaran A, Yang L, Nelson VS, Chang KWC. High prevalence of cranial asymmetry exists in infants with neonatal brachial plexus palsy. J Pediatr Rehabil Med. 2016;9(4):271–7.
19. Julka A, Vander Have KL. Shoulder sequelae of neonatal brachial plexus injuries: orthopedic assessment and management. J Pediatr Rehabil Med. 2011;4(2):131–40.
20. Wagner ER, Werthel JD, Ansari M, Shaughnessy W, Elhassan BL. Natural history of the elbow bony architecture in patients with obstetric brachial plexus injury and the association with flexion contractures. J Am Acad Orthop Surg. 2018;26(23):e490–5.
21. Sebastin SJ, Chung KC. Pathogenesis and management of deformities of the elbow, wrist, and hand in late neonatal brachial plexus palsy. J Pediatr Rehabil Med. 2011;4(2):119–30.
22. Smith BW, Daunter AK, Yang LJS, Wilson TJ. An update on the management of neonatal brachial plexus palsy-replacing old paradigms a review. JAMA Pediatr. 2018;172(6):585–91.
23. Rasmussen L, Justice D, Chang KWC, Nelson VS, Yang LJS. Home exercise DVD promotes exercise accuracy by caregivers of children and adolescents with brachial plexus palsy. PM R. 2013;5(11):924–30.
24. Bain JR, Dematteo C, Gjertsen D, Packham T, Galea V, Harper JA. Limb length differences after obstetrical brachial plexus injury: a growing concern. Plast Reconstr Surg. 2012;130(4):558e–71e.
25. Anand P, Birch R. Restoration of sensory function and lack of long-term chronic pain syndromes after brachial plexus injury in human neonates. Brain. 2002;125(Pt 1):113–22.
26. Ho ES, Curtis CG, Clarke HM. Pain in children following microsurgical reconstruction for obstetrical brachial plexus palsy. J Hand Surg Am. 2015;40(6):1177–83.

27. Yang LJS, Anand P, Birch R. Limb preference in children with obstetric brachial plexus palsy. Pediatr Neurol. 2005;33(1):46–9.
28. Strömbeck C, Krumlinde-Sundholm L, Remahl S, Sejersen T. Long-term follow-up of children with obstetric brachial plexus palsy I: functional aspects. Dev Med Child Neurol. 2007;49(3):198–203.
29. Palmgren T, Peltonen J, Linder T, Rautakorpi S, Nietosvaara Y. Sensory evaluation of the hands in children with brachial plexus birth injury. Dev Med Child Neurol. 2007;49(8):582–6.
30. Oskay D, Ünal E, Çetinkaya Ş. Do obstetrical brachial plexus injuries affect proprioceptive sense? Neurosciences. 2010;15(4):268–71.
31. Brown SH, Noble BC, Yang LJS, Nelson VS. Deficits in elbow position sense in neonatal brachial plexus palsy. Pediatr Neurol. 2013;49(5):324–8.
32. Brown SH, Wernimont CW, Phillips L, Kern KL, Nelson VS, Yang LJS. Hand sensorimotor function in older children with neonatal brachial plexus palsy. Pediatr Neurol. 2016;56:42–7.
33. Anguelova GV, Rombouts SARB, van Dijk JG, Buur PF, Malessy MJA. Increased brain activation during motor imagery suggests central abnormality in Neonatal Brachial Plexus Palsy. Neurosci Res. 2017;123:19–26.
34. Chang KWC, Yang LJS, Driver L, Nelson VS. High prevalence of early language delay exists among toddlers with neonatal brachial plexus palsy. Pediatr Neurol. 2014;51(3):384–9.
35. Hill EL. Non-specific nature of specific language impairment: a review of the literature with regard to concomitant motor impairments. Int J Lang Commun Disord. 2001;36(2):149–71.
36. Owen SE, McKinlay IA. Motor difficulties in children with developmental disorders of speech and language. Child Care Health Dev. 1997;23(4):315–25.
37. Webbe J, Brunton G, Ali S, Longford N, Modi N, Gale C. Parent, patient and clinician perceptions of outcomes during and following neonatal care: a systematic review of qualitative research. BMJ Paediatr Open. 2018;2(1):e000343.
38. Chang KWC, Austin A, Yeaman J, Phillips L, Kratz A, Yang LJS, et al. Health-related quality of life components in children with neonatal brachial plexus palsy: a qualitative study. PM R. 2017;9(4):383–91.
39. Squitieri L, Larson BP, Chang KWC, Yang LJS, Chung KC. Medical decision-making among adolescents with neonatal brachial plexus palsy and their families: a qualitative study. Plast Reconstr Surg. 2013;131(6):880e–7e.
40. Mentrikoski JM, Duncan CL, Melanson A, Louden E, Allgier A, Michaud L, et al. Factors related to the psychosocial functioning of youth with neonatal brachial plexus injuries. J Pediatr Psychol. 2015;40(3):285–96.

45 Clinical Examination of the Child with Brachial Plexus Birth Injury

Andrea S. Bauer and Peter M. Waters

Introduction

The examination of a child with suspected brachial plexus birth injury (BPBI) can be challenging. Children who have sustained a brachial plexus injury at birth will present to a variety of practitioners, at a variety of ages, with a variety of "chief complaints." Infants often present with "r/o clavicle fracture," while older children may present with scapular winging, limited overhead reach, reaching their hand to mouth with shoulder in abduction and forearm pronated, or an elbow flexion contracture of unknown origin. Further adding to the confusion, patients with many different conditions may present, misdiagnosed, for "evaluation of brachial plexus birth injury." The most common of these rare other conditions is a neonatal stroke. Amidst this confusion, the goals of the clinical evaluation of the infant with a suspect brachial plexus birth injury (BPBI) are straightforward:

1. Establish the correct diagnosis.
2. Evaluate the extent of the nerve injury.
3. Evaluate the extent of glenohumeral dysplasia.

A. S. Bauer (✉) · P. M. Waters
Department of Orthopaedic Surgery, Boston Children's Hospital, Boston, MA, USA
e-mail: andrea.bauer@childrens.harvard.edu; peter.waters@childrens.harvard.edu

This chapter will detail the clinical history and physical examination techniques to effectively evaluate the child with suspected BPBI. Subsequent chapters will describe the use of adjuvant imaging and electrodiagnostics to help with this evaluation.

Taking the History

Specific conditions that must be ruled out include birth fracture, septic shoulder, arthrogryposis, and neonatal stroke or spinal cord injury. It is a medical school adage that "The history is 90% of the history and physical," and this certainly applies to evaluating the infant with suspected BPBI. We begin by asking the parents "What was it like when your child was born?". Although parents may not know the term "shoulder dystocia," those who have experienced this obstetrical emergency will describe doctors and nurses rushing into the room, someone calling a code or starting a large clock on the wall, and maneuvers such as someone pulling their legs over their head (McRoberts maneuver) or someone "jumping" on their stomach (suprapubic pressure). All of these signs of a difficult delivery should heighten suspicion for a brachial plexus birth injury. As the parents are describing the birth history, we continue with questions regarding other traditional risk factors for BPBI including gestational diabetes, fetal macrosomia, and instrumented delivery.

A. Y. Shin, N. Pulos (eds.), *Operative Brachial Plexus Surgery*,
https://doi.org/10.1007/978-3-030-69517-0_45

Up to 50% of BPBI cases, however, are not associated with shoulder dystocia or a difficult delivery, and a recent epidemiological study found that nearly 75% of documented BPBI cases in a large administrative database had no traditional risk factors [1, 2]. So while these questions can help "build the case" for a BPBI diagnosis, negative answers are not exclusionary.

We then ask how the child is doing now and what has changed since birth. The typical timeline of a brachial plexus birth injury is that parents notice immediately that the limb is not moving, followed by a gradual improvement in some movements (or lack thereof). When parents report that a limb was initially moving and is now not moving as well, the differential diagnosis should shift to infection, trauma, and neonatal stroke or cerebral palsy. This is also an opportunity to identify any other medical problems or sequelae of birth trauma, such as birth fractures and respiratory complications. Finally, we ask parents what they are most concerned about for the visit, to help frame the ongoing discussion in ways that matter to the family.

Stages of Child Development

Before approaching the BPBI-specific examination, a review of the stages of child development may be helpful, particularly for those who most commonly see adult patients.

0–3 Months

During this time period, the infant can already turn toward a parent's voice and attend to a human face. But they are still fragile, with open fontanelles and poor head control. If they have sustained a brachial plexus birth injury and/or birth fracture, they may also still be in pain from the birth trauma. The exam should begin with the infant swaddled, either in their parent's arms or on the exam table. Infants of this age will not yet have stranger anxiety, so if a better examination can be performed on the exam table, the infant should be quite comfortable to do so. Young infants will tend to hold both upper extremities with the arms adducted, elbows flexed, forearms pronated, and fists clenched, and they will not yet reach for toys and rattles. Instead, active motion can be elicited by tickling or stroking the area of interest (such as the back of the hand to elicit finger extension). Infant reflexes can also be used to the examiner's advantage (Table 45.1). Infants with BPBI will generally have abnormal Moro and fencing reflexes on the affected side.

3–12 Months

Late infancy is a time of rapid development in both gross and fine motor skills. Although each child's development may progress differently, a 6-month-old should be able to roll over and sit unsupported for at least short periods of time. They should readily put objects in the mouth and transfer objects between hands. By 12 months, infants should pull to stand and start to cruise (walking while holding onto furniture); many are walking by this time as well (average age of walking 13 months).

Toys can be very helpful in the examination of an older infant. It is our practice to allow babies to play with toys in the exam room while discussing the patient's history with the family. This independent play allows for careful inspection of upper extremity function, and the examiner can gradually join in with the play to encourage specific movements. Once infants begin to eat finger foods, around 6 months of age, these finger foods can be very useful in examining the child's ability

Table 45.1 Infant reflexes relevant to the brachial plexus examination

Reflex name	Description	Duration
Moro or startle	Back arches and extremities extend to startling stimulus	4–6 months
Tonic neck or fencing	When the head is turned to one side, the arm on that side will extend, while the opposite arm flexes at the elbow	6 months
Grasp	Infant grasps fingers around an object placed in the palm	3–4 months

to bring the hand to the mouth. Stranger anxiety generally peaks between 6 and 12 months of age. For this reason, more difficult portions of the examination (such as testing passive range of motion) are best accomplished with the child in the parent's lap and at the end of the exam.

1–5 Years

By 18 months, the child should be able to walk independently, say several intelligible words, and feed themselves with a spoon. A 2-year-old can run, speak in two- to three-word sentences, manipulate large buttons and zippers, and scribble with a crayon. A 3-year-old can speak in full sentences, throw and catch a ball, and hold a crayon with a tripod grip. By 5 years old, more complex fine motor skills are acquired, and the child's hand dominance is generally established.

Whenever possible, toddlers and preschoolers should be given choices about the examination. Examples include "Do you want to sit on your mom's lap or on the table?" and "Should we look at this hand first or that one?". Having choices helps the toddler feel in control of the situation while you proceed with the necessary parts of the examination.

5–12 Years

In general, school-aged children are much easier to examine than children less than 5 years. The examination can begin to follow a more adult pattern, and children can follow instructions so that motor strength can be directly examined. However, children at this age often require explanations of the various parts of the examination. To use motor strength testing as an example, most adults will readily comply if you ask them to "bend your elbow and don't let me straighten it." While school-aged children can follow these instructions, the examiner needs to slow down and explain tests more completely. For more complex tests, demonstrating with a parent first can help. For example, you may say something like "Now I need to see how strong you are. Can you bend your elbow? Now hold it bent as strong as you can and don't let me straighten it out."

Modesty develops during the late elementary school and middle school years. Things that adults take for granted, such as men removing their shirts for a shoulder exam, are often much more sensitive concepts for children of this age. This is particularly true for the child with BPBI, who may already be struggling with the cosmetic differences of his or her arm as early as elementary school age. As the chest and shoulders are often an important part of the BPBI exam, the child should be given the opportunity to change into a gown while the examiner waits outside the room. During the exam, only the necessary body part should be exposed from the gown at one time.

13–18 Years

During this time period, children's developmental skills are much like adults, but their social and cognitive skills are still maturing. Modesty remains an issue and should be addressed as above. In addition, there may be certain parts of the examination or interview that are better addressed without the parents in the room. The examination can generally proceed as for adults. However, teenagers are still less accustomed to the doctor's office than are adults, so each part of the examination should be explained, and any tests that may elicit pain should be discussed beforehand. Teenagers, especially females, should either have parent or same-sex professional such as a nurse in room during exam.

Specific Examination for the Child with BPBI

Observation

The child is first observed at rest and at play in the examination room (Fig. 45.1). While the reason for the visit and history are discussed with the parents, the surgeon should keep one eye on the child at play. Through play, you can see

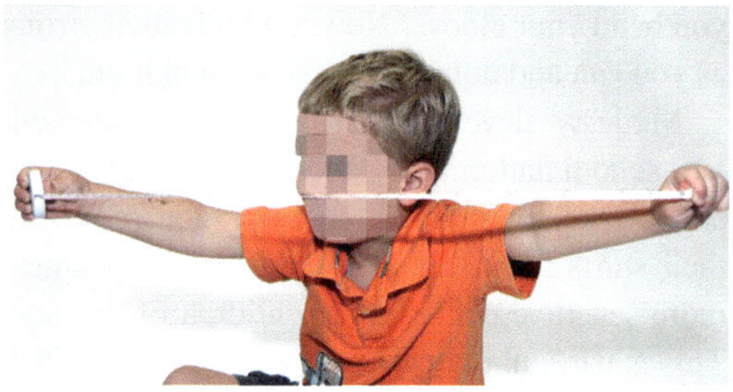

Fig. 45.1 Clinical photo of play-based examination. (Photo courtesy of Shriners Hospitals for Children—Northern California)

whether bilateral upper extremities are symmetric in appearance and whether the child uses both hands equally or tends to favor one over the other.

Inspection

Signs of trauma (ecchymosis, swelling, lacerations, abrasions) and active infection (swelling, erythema) can be detected easily by inspection. In addition, careful inspection should include an assessment of the following:

Overall limb length, hand size, and muscle girth The length and size of the arm is generally smaller than the contralateral side over time (not in infancy), but not necessarily in proportion to the severity of the nerve injury. Bae and colleagues found that the average overall size of the limb is about 95% that of the contralateral side, but that the size did not correlate with active movement scores of the arm [3].

Scapular winging Scapular winging is extremely common in children with BPBI who have had an incomplete upper trunk recovery. This is due in part to variable paralysis of the scapular motors, as well as compensatory use of scapulothoracic motion to make up for limited true glenohumeral motion.

Putti sign The Putti sign describes the obligatory elevation of the medial angle of the scapula that occurs when a child with an abduction contracture attempts to put the arm in full adduction. Often this is associated with posterior glenohumeral instability or dislocation.

Nail deformities/hand wounds Young children with global injuries have altered sensation in the hand. They often respond to this altered sensation with self-mutilating behaviors, including biting and scratching the involved areas. This can result in repeated infections and even autoamputation of fingertips. Parents often do not bring this issue up with surgeons, but close inspection of the fingertips will show signs of this behavior and its extent.

Active Range of Motion

Active range of motion can be observed at play in younger children, as discussed above. The Active Movement Scale and Toronto Test Score, described below, are extensions of this play-based examination that can yield significant information regarding motor function in even young infants with BPBI. By using familiar activities such as a "high five" for finger extension or "fist bump" for finger flexion, active range of motion can be directly tested in children as young as 1–2 years. Children over the age of 3 years can generally participate with testing the more specific movements such as are required for the Mallet score. The AMS, Toronto Test Score, and Mallet score are all performed at this point in the examination.

The Active Movement Scale

The Active Movement Scale (AMS) was developed at The Hospital for Sick Children in Toronto and first published in 2002 [4]. This system is ideal for evaluating infants and young children, as it allows for a rough measurement of muscle strength without requiring the child to follow commands. Rather, through a combination of positioning the child and observing them at play, the examiner records the status of 15 active movements of the upper extremity, each of which is graded on a scale of 0–7 (Fig. 45.2). Each movement is first examined with gravity eliminated, and if full motion (within the child's available

Active Movement Scale

Involved Side (R/L) ____________________

Motion	**Movement Grade**
Shoulder Abduction	____________________
Shoulder Abduction	____________________
Shoulder Flexion	____________________
Shoulder External Rotation	____________________
Shoulder Internal Rotation	____________________
Elbow Flexion	____________________
Elbow Extension	____________________
Forearm Pronation	____________________
Forearm Supination	____________________
Wrist Flexion	____________________
Wrist Extension	____________________
Finger Flexion	____________________
Finger Extension	____________________
Thumb Flexion	____________________
Thumb Extension	____________________

Movement Grade Key

Grade	**Observation**	
0	No muscle tone or contraction	**Gravity eliminated**
1	Muscle contraction, no motion	
2	Joint motion ≤1/2 range	
3	Joint motion >1/2 range	
4	Full joint motion	
5	Joint motion ≤1/2 range	**Against gravity**
6	Joint motion >1/2 range	
7	Full joint range	

Fig. 45.2 Worksheet for active movement scale examination. (Image courtesy of Children's Orthopaedic Surgery Foundation)

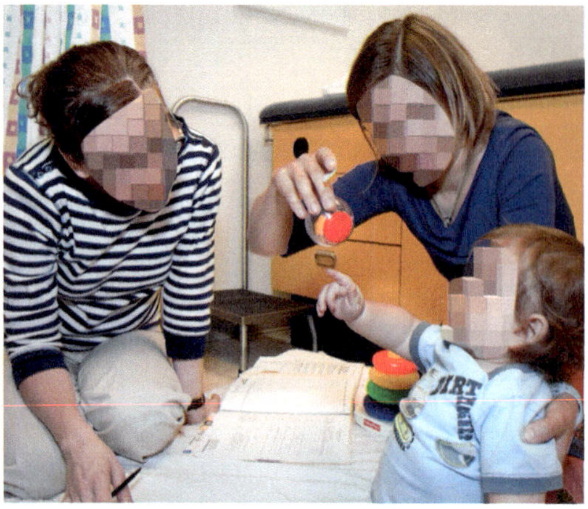

Fig. 45.3 Clinical photo of surgeon and therapist performing active movement scale examination. (Photo courtesy of Shriners Hospitals for Children—Northern California)

range of motion for that joint) is achieved, that movement is then graded against gravity.

During the AMS examination, movement is assessed within the age-appropriate range of motion, using the uninvolved contralateral limb as a control. Wrist extension should be tested while the child is making a fist or holding a small object such as a pencil, so that finger extension cannot be used to substitute for true wrist extension. Finger extension is evaluated as extension of the metacarpophalangeal joints, while finger flexion is evaluated as the distance at rest between the fingertips and the palm.

In our experience, this test is best performed with two examiners, generally a physician and an occupational therapist. This allows one examiner to position the child while the other offers toys (Fig. 45.3). It also allows for flexibility in the examination, as the child may prefer one examiner, or a certain motion might be best observed from one angle in the room versus another.

The Toronto Test Score

Several movements of the AMS have been collected in a simplified manner to create the Toronto Test Score (TTS) [5] (Fig. 45.4). In this score, elbow flexion, elbow extension, wrist extension, finger extension, and thumb extension are each graded on a scale of 0–2, for a total possible combined score of 10. The TTS was designed to predict the need for nerve surgery in BPBI at 3 months of age. In the original study, the authors found that an infant's score on this test at 3 months of age could accurately predict their recovery at 12 months of age. A score at 3 months of less than 3.5 out of 10 predicts poor recovery at 12 months, while a score of greater than 3.5 predicts good recovery. The authors suggest that although all infants should be followed closely as their recovery progresses, those with a score over 3.5 at 3 months are unlikely to need microsurgical intervention. However, because the TTS does not evaluate any movements of the shoulder, it cannot predict those infants who may benefit from nerve surgery to improve a severe, but isolated, upper trunk injury.

The Mallet Score

For older children with BPBI, the Mallet score and the modified Mallet score are commonly used tests of shoulder function. The original Mallet test focuses on functional activities that require shoulder motion and is particularly weighted toward activities involving shoulder external rotation [6]. The Mallet score has been modified over the years by several authors. We favor the modification of Abzug and colleagues, which added an internal rotation measure in an attempt to balance out the movements tested in the Mallet exam [7] (Fig. 45.5). Although younger children can be enticed to perform the movements of the Mallet score using toys and stickers as with the AMS examination, the Mallet score is easiest once a child can actively cooperate, around 2–3 years of age. The specific movements include active global abduction, external rotation (performed at the side), and hand-to-neck, hand-to-mouth, and hand-to-spine movement, with internal rotation added in the modified Mallet score. The score is calculated by grading each activity on a scale of 0–5. It is important to remember that on this scale, a score of 0 indicates that the particular movement was not test-

Toronto Score

Toronto Score	Clinical Grade	Numerical Grade
Elbow Flexion	________	____ . ____
Elbow Extension	________	____ . ____
Wrist Extension	________	____ . ____
Finger Extension	________	____ . ____
Thumb Extension	________	____ . ____

Total Score: ____ ____ . ____

Toronto Score Grading System

Observation (Against Gravity)	Clinical Grade	Numerical Score
No joint movemwnt	0	0.0
Flicker of movement	0 +	0.3
Les than 50% range	1 -	0.6
50% range of movement	1	1.0
More than 50% range	1 +	1.3
Good but not full range	2 -	1.6
Full range of movement	2	2.0

Fig. 45.4 Worksheet for Toronto test score examination. (Image courtesy of Children's Orthopaedic Surgery Foundation)

able, generally because the child was too young or unwilling to cooperate.

The reliability of the AMS, Toronto Test Score, and Mallet examinations was evaluated by Bae et al. [8]. The authors found excellent inter-observer reliability for the individual components of the Mallet score and the AMS score, while inter-observer reliability of the Toronto Test Score was rated as good. The same authors also studied the ability of these exam scores to predict quality of life in children with brachial plexus birth palsy, as measured by the Pediatric Outcomes Data Collection Instrument [9]. They found that all three scores (Mallet, Toronto Test

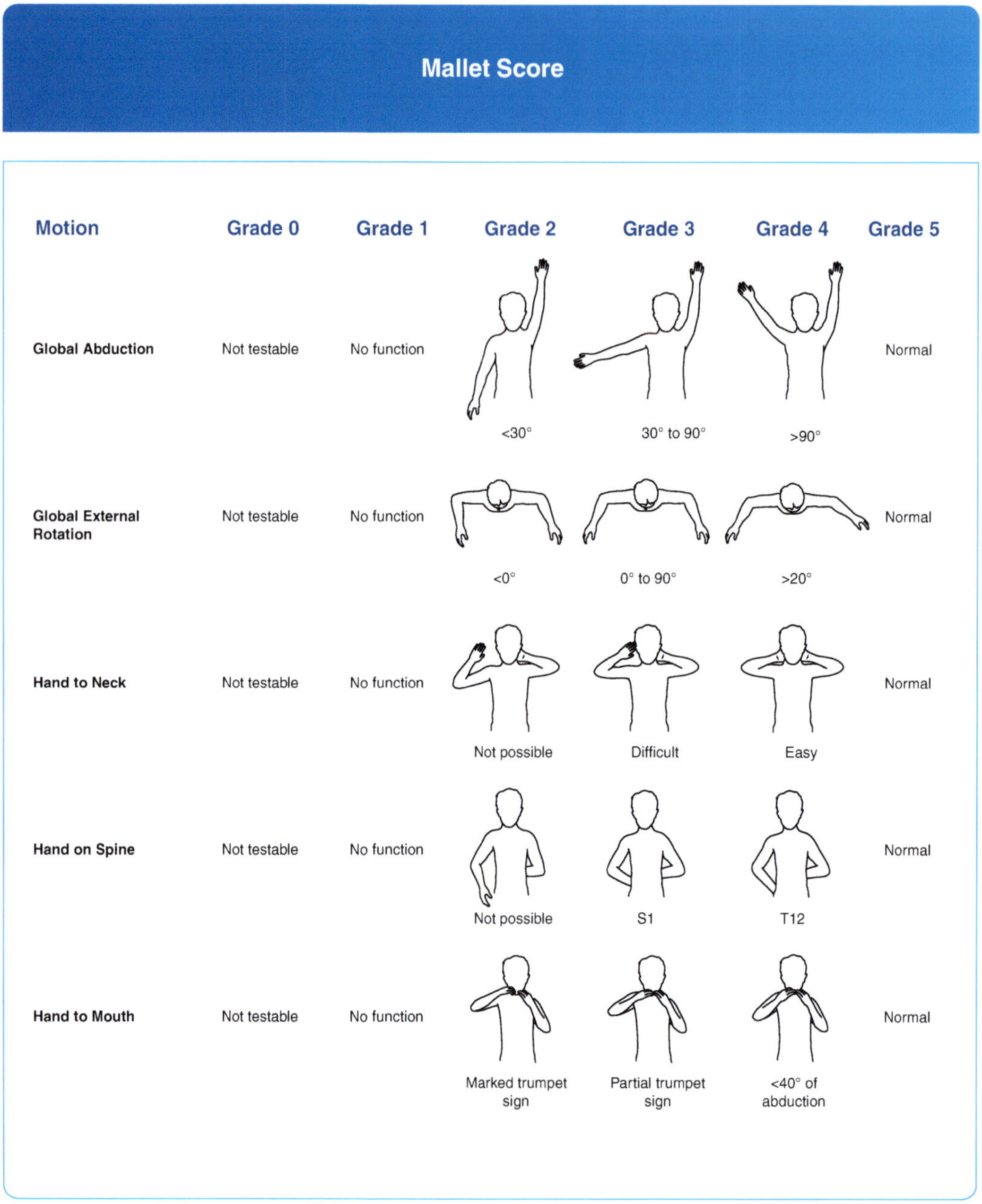

Fig. 45.5 Worksheet for modified Mallet score examination. (Image courtesy of Children's Orthopaedic Surgery Foundation)

Score, and Active Movement Scale) could predict the global function, upper-extremity function, and sports/physical function domains of the Pediatric Outcomes Data Collection Instrument or PODCI. For this reason, it is our practice to continue to collect all three scores throughout childhood.

Passive Range of Motion

Particularly in young children and those with contractures, passive range of motion can be painful and should be saved for the last portion of the examination. We find the following passive range of motion measurements important in children with BPBI. All measurements are repeated on the contralateral side, as normal values can vary widely:

(a) *Scapulohumeral angle.* The arm is extended overhead while stabilizing the position of the scapula. The scapulohumeral angle is the angle between the lateral border of the scapula and the humerus.
(b) *Passive external rotation.* The arm and scapula are stabilized in either full adduction or 90 degrees of abduction and externally rotated as much as possible. The angle between the forearm and the trunk is recorded. In the abducted position, the scapula is stabilized in an attempt to record true glenohumeral rotation.
(c) *Passive adduction.* The arm is brought fully to the side while monitoring the position of the scapula. We record the angle between the lateral scapula and the humerus as an abduction contracture angle in degrees.
(d) *Passive elbow extension.* The elbow is maximally extended. We record the angle between the forearm and humerus as an elbow flexion contracture angle in degrees.
(e) *Passive pronation and supination.* When measuring forearm range of motion, the examiner should stabilize the child's elbow against their side with one hand and rotate the distal forearm with the other hand. This prevents compensatory motion of the shoulder and wrist from affecting the measured rotation.

Synthesis of Clinical Information

As discussed above, the goals of the evaluation of a child with suspected BPBI are to establish the diagnosis and evaluate the extent of both the nerve injury and the glenohumeral dysplasia, if present. It is important to remember that although glenohumeral dysplasia is secondary in etiology to the nerve injury, the issues that arise, and the necessary treatment decisions, are often concurrent in timing. The use of ancillary testing will be discussed in a subsequent chapter, but as there is not yet a single test that can predict the need for surgical intervention, we favor repeated examinations over time to determine which infants will benefit from surgery. Repeated clinical examination ensures that a reasonable approximation of reality is being seen in the clinic room while also allowing the surgeon to monitor the recovery process for plateaus.

In our practice, children with a clearly flail limb are offered surgery after 3 months of age, when it becomes clear that the entire limb is affected with more than a stretch injury. The decision is made at this time because our center is well-equipped for complex surgery in young babies, so we believe we can do so safely. For these reasons, there is no benefit to delaying surgery once the decision is made. For upper trunk injuries, decision-making is more complex. We offer nerve surgery between 5 and 9 months for those infants who have not demonstrated antigravity shoulder abduction and/or elbow flexion. At the same time, we pay careful attention to the passive glenohumeral joint motion on serial physical examination. If the nerve injury appears to be recovering, but passive shoulder motion is limited, we consider shoulder surgery, even at a young age. If there is a plateau in nerve recovery along with limited passive shoulder motion, combined treatment of both the nerve injury and the glenohumeral dysplasia is considered. As will be discussed later, ultrasound and MRI scan exams are helpful in evaluating and quantifying glenohumeral deformity and alignment.

References

1. DeFrancesco CJ, Shah DK, Rogers BH, Shah AS. The epidemiology of brachial plexus birth palsy in the United States: declining incidence and evolving risk factors. J Pediatr Orthop. 2019;39:e134–40.
2. Vakhshori V, Bouz GJ, Alluri RK, Stevanovic M, Ghiassi A, Lightdale N. Risk factors associated with neonatal brachial plexus palsy in the United States. J Pediatr Orthop B. 2020;29(4):392–8.
3. Bae DS, Ferretti M, Waters PM. Upper extremity size differences in brachial plexus birth palsy. Hand (N Y). 2008;3(4):297–303.
4. Curtis C, Stephens D, Clarke HM, Andrews D. The active movement scale: an evaluative tool for infants with obstetrical brachial plexus palsy. J Hand Surg Am. 2002;27(3):470–8.

5. Michelow BJ, Clarke HM, Curtis CG, Zuker RM, Seifu Y, Andrews DF. The natural history of obstetrical brachial plexus palsy. Plast Reconstr Surg. 1994;93(4):675–80; discussion 681.
6. Mallet J. Obstetrical paralysis of the brachial plexus. II. Therapeutics. Treatment of sequelae. Priority for the treatment of the shoulder. Method for the expression of results. Rev Chir Orthop Reparatrice Appar Mot. 1972;58(Suppl 1):166–8.
7. Abzug JM, Chafetz RS, Gaughan JP, Ashworth S, Kozin SH. Shoulder function after medial approach and derotational humeral osteotomy in patients with brachial plexus birth palsy. J Pediatr Orthop. 2010;30(5):469–74.
8. Bae DS, Waters PM, Zurakowski D. Reliability of three classification systems measuring active motion in brachial plexus birth palsy. J Bone Joint Surg Am. 2003;85(9):1733–8.
9. Bae DS, Waters PM, Zurakowski D. Correlation of pediatric outcomes data collection instrument with measures of active movement in children with brachial plexus birth palsy. J Pediatr Orthop. 2008;28(5):584–92.

Operative Brachial Plexus Surgery: Brachial Plexus Birth Injury – Neurodiagnostic Evaluation

46

Willem Pondaag and Martijn R. Tannemaat

Abbreviations

BPBI	Brachial plexus birth injury
CMAP	Compound motor action potentials
EDX	Electrodiagnostic testing
EMG	Electromyography
NAPs	Nerve action potentials
SSEPs	Somatosensory evoked potentials

Introduction

The optimal timing of surgical treatment for BPBI constitutes a major dilemma and is the subject of considerable debate. Data from animal studies suggest that early nerve repair leads to better functional results, but currently, time is needed to clinically distinguish milder lesions, which do not require surgery from more severe lesions, which should be treated as soon as possible. Currently, neurological evaluation at 3 months is generally regarded as the main criterion for the fundamental decision to perform nerve surgery or not. Ideally, the aim of electrodiagnostic testing (EDX) should be to identify injuries that require surgery well before this 3 month time point. Depending on test characteristics, such a test would have two benefits: if the test is specific enough, surgery can be performed on those that require it at the earliest possible time, and a highly sensitive test would reduce uncertainty for parents of children with lesions that are expected to recover spontaneously.

Indeed, in adult patients with a brachial plexus traction injury, EDX is widely used and has been proven a useful tool for diagnosis and prognostication. There is controversy, however, whether the use of EDX is as useful in children with a BPBI. Some argue that EDX has no added value at all [1, 2], whereas others strongly recommend performing EDX on all patients with BPBI [3].

Similarly, the value of intraoperative neurophysiological testing is uncertain. A neurophysiological test that allows the identification of nerve elements or will show spontaneous recovery would greatly enhance surgical decision-making. Intraoperative neurophysiological monitoring is widely used, but its exact effect on the outcome of surgery remains uncertain.

A recent systematic review of the literature identified 16 observational studies with a total sample size of 747 children [4]. A wide variation was found in EDX techniques, outcome algorithms, and decision-making; pooling of data proved impossible. Risk of bias and quality of evidence were rated. Nevertheless, the most

W. Pondaag (✉)
Department of Neurosurgery, Leiden University Medical Center, Leiden, The Netherlands
e-mail: w.pondaag@lumc.nl

M. R. Tannemaat
Department of Neurology and Clinical Neurophysiology, LUMC, Leiden, The Netherlands

A. Y. Shin, N. Pulos (eds.), *Operative Brachial Plexus Surgery*,
https://doi.org/10.1007/978-3-030-69517-0_46

methodologically sound studies were claimed to support the use of EDX, at standardized time frames, as prognostic modality complementing clinical evaluation and neuroimaging.

To understand the difficulties in interpretation of EDX in children with BPBI, it is necessary to consider the specific pathophysiology of BPBI. As in any nerve, the traction injury in BPBI may result in neurapraxia, axonotmesis, neurotmesis, or root avulsion [5]. The main difference between adult traumatic lesions of the brachial plexus and BPBI is that the traction forces are low-velocity and with longer duration, which will probably lead to a different type of traction injury. In effect, during surgical exploration of BPBI, a true rupture as found in adults is encountered seldomly. The key finding of postganglionic injury in BPBI is the *neuroma-in-continuity* in which only impaired, disorganized axonal outgrowth has taken place [6, 7]. It may be more appropriate to classify these neurotmetic lesions between a grade 3 and grade 4 severity according to the Sunderland classification [8]. Some axonal outgrowth is usually encountered through the neuroma. This axonal continuity may result in electrodiagnostic continuity. The related clinical recovery is, however, variable and unpredictable. In this respect a gold standard of the diagnosis to compare neurophysiologic findings is unavailable, and there is a risk of circular reasoning [9]. Additionally, cross-fiber excitation inside the neuroma-in-continuity may further complicate interpretation [10]. Another striking feature in BPBI is axonal misrouting [11]. This may lead to unexpected electromyographic findings in different myotomes. A second difficulty for efficacy of EDX in BPBI is that the resulting nerve injury often consists of a mixture of postganglionic and preganglionic injury, in which the upper nerves (C5 and C6) are more likely to exhibit a postganglionic injury while the lower nerves (C7, C8, and T1) are more likely to be avulsed from the spinal cord, as has been shown in experimental settings and in imaging studies [12, 13]. The mixed character of the injury may complicate the interpretation of EDX findings. Due to these pathophysiologic mechanisms, the utility of electrodiagnostic continuity for prognostication is uncertain in children with BPBI.

The value and difficulties of different EDX modalities will be discussed for needle electromyography (EMG), nerve conduction studies, and intraoperative neurophysiology.

Electromyography

One specific feature of needle EMG is that spontaneous muscle activity (denervation) is not as often found in BPBI as in adults. In view of the short length and smaller diameter of the axon, it is logical to expect signs of denervation earlier than in adults, and after restoration of some axonal continuity, denervation will disappear more quickly than in adults [14]. In fact, we found denervation activity starting after as few as 5 days, which contrasts with many textbooks indicating that denervation activity starts from 10 to 14 days after axonal discontinuity in adults. At the age of 1 month, two-thirds of children showed denervation in the deltoid muscle, which lasted through the age of 3 months in only 14% of children [15]. Other authors found that all denervation activity had disappeared after week 19 [16].

A traditional timing to decide whether surgical repair of BPBI is necessary was defined by Alain Gilbert as absent biceps muscle recovery at the age of 3 months [17]. EMG performed at that age usually shows a discrepancy: in the majority of patients, motor unit potentials are seen in clinically paralyzed muscles [18]. This can be explained in five ways: an overly pessimistic clinical examination; overestimation of EMG recruitment due to small muscle fibers; persistent fetal innervation; developmental apraxia; and misdirection, in which axons reach inappropriate muscles [14]. If the presence of motor unit potentials is interpreted as the start of recovery, and a nonsurgical treatment strategy is chosen, the eventual clinical recovery is often disappointing.

We prospectively studied a consecutive group of 48 infants with BPBI at the age of 1 week, 1 month, and 3 months and gathered clinical data and EMG at these 3 time points [19]. As endpoints in this study, we defined a dichotomous outcome as either a severe lesion, i.e., the surgical findings of neurotmesis of root avulsion, or favorable neurological recovery after 2 years without nerve reconstruction. We could make a useful prediction of outcome already at the age of 1 month based on clinical recovery of elbow flexion and extension, aided with needle EMG of the biceps. This signifies that complete axonal discontinuity to the biceps muscle at the age of 1 month is a good predictor of eventual outcome. EMG of the biceps lost its predictive value at 3 months of age. In clinical practice this simple test enables early prognostication, which is of great value in early counseling the parents already at 1 month of age to express an optimistic or pessimistic expectation of outcome (Fig. 46.1). In our institution, neurological evaluation at 3–4 months remains the main indicator at which the fundamental decision to perform nerve surgery or not is taken.

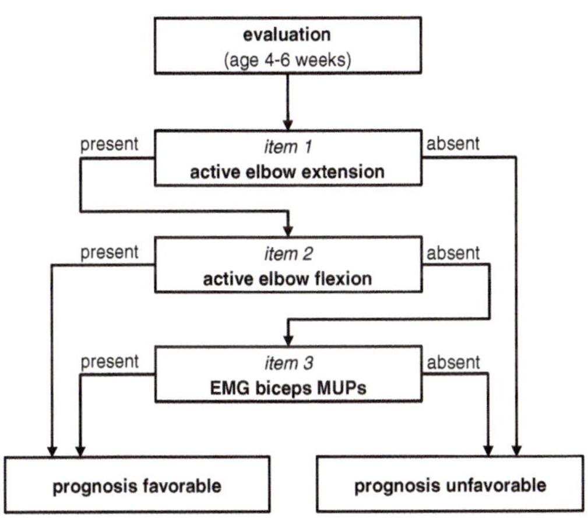

Fig. 46.1 Our proposed algorithm to evaluate the prognosis of a BPBI at the age of 4–6 weeks. An absent elbow extension against gravity reflects a lesion with involvement of the lower roots, so on clinical grounds it concerns a severe lesion with unfavorable prognosis. When both active elbow extension flexion and elbow extension demonstrate movement against gravity, the prognosis is favorable. When elbow flexion is not strong enough for movement gravity (with the child in supine position and the arm brought in 90 degrees abduction), an EMG is performed. The absence or presence of MUPs determines prognosis

Nerve Conduction Studies

One of the earlier papers that promoted the use of nerve action potentials (NAPs) dates from 1996 [20]. NAPs were recorded using surface (skin) electrodes from the median and the ulnar nerves in both forearms, with percutaneous stimulation at the wrist and recording at the elbow. A favorable nerve lesion was defined as a normal NAP amplitude (i.e., >50% of the uninjured side). This diagnostic algorithm was employed in a cohort of 73 children [3]. Based on a combination of NAP results and EMG findings, the authors predicted outcome correctly for C6 and C7 in 92% and 96% of the cases, respectively. The inability to record nerve action potentials for C5 led to a predictive value in a smaller proportion of cases (78%).

The use of sensory NAPs has been advocated as a diagnostic method for detecting root avulsions. The presence of a normal sensory NAP or an amplitude greater than 50% of normal compared to the uninvolved site together with EMG abnormalities in the corresponding muscles is accepted as a main criterion for avulsion. One patient series that promotes the use of NAPs examined 13 infants and claims that electromyography can be of great value to identify patients with a poor prognosis [21]. In this study, however, all children with an upper-type lesion recovered well, and all children with a total lesion had a poor outcome, suggesting that in this patient series, clinical outcome was determined by the extent of the lesion and the added value of NAP measurements to clinical evaluation was limited. Another study in 54 patients claimed an overall accuracy of the detection of preganglionic lesions of 74% for EDX (a combination of sensory NAPs and EMG) for all nerve roots [22]. The presence of a preganglionic injury implies an indication for surgery, as spontaneous recovery does not occur in these avulsion injuries. The actual diagnosis was made during surgery. The overall sensitivity of detecting preganglionic lesions by EDX was low (31%), but the specificity was high (90%). The authors compared EDX to imaging, where they found an overall sensitivity of detecting preganglionic lesions of 66%, and an overall specificity was 70%. The low sensitivity to identify preganglionic lesions limits NAP use as a sole diagnostic entity, although the combination of NAP and needle EMG is of use to detect root avulsions.

Intraoperative Neurophysiology

Direct stimulation of nerves during surgery and evaluation of elicited muscle contractions and strength is widely performed, but no clinical studies have evaluated the effectiveness of this qualitative evaluation. Intraoperative NAP recording was introduced by Kline in 1969 [23]. It was employed in BPBI, specifically to decide whether a neuroma in continuity should be resected or that simple neurolysis was sufficient [24]. When an amplitude decrease of 50% or more across the neuroma was present, neuroma excision and grafting was performed. This threshold has never been validated, which was the reason for us to perform a study in 95 infants [25]. We measured NAPs and elicited compound motor action potentials (CMAP) during surgery and classified the severity of the nerve lesion irrespective of the EDX findings. Although axonotmesis, neurotmesis, and avulsion could be distinguished on group level, we were unable to identify valid cutoff points for the individual patient to facilitate the decision of whether to resect a neuroma-in-continuity and graft or leave the nerve-in-continuity and perform neurolysis.

Intraoperative EDX was also advocated by Chin et al. They used CMAP recordings after direct intraoperative stimulation, but instead of comparing the amplitude resulting from stimulation proximal and distal to the neuroma, they looked at the morphology of the CMAP to help in the decision-making process [26]. Roughly two-thirds of their surgically treated patients (22 of 32) underwent neurolysis only, which resulted in good recovery of abduction and elbow flexion but poor recovery of external rotation. In our opinion, external rotation is the hallmark function of recovery in BPBI patients, and therefore their algorithm was unable to predict poor shoulder recovery, which makes it less useful.

Another modality that has been used intraoperatively is the somatosensory evoked potential (SSEP) to detect root avulsions. The combination of an intact sensory nerve action potential with an absent cortical SSEP is indicative of a dorsal root avulsion lesion. However, data on the clinical utility of this technique is very limited [26].

SSEPs cannot be used to evaluate integrity of motor pathways. In adults, motor evoked potentials have been used to identify root avulsion injuries [27], but to our knowledge, this technique has not been used in BPBI patients.

Conclusion

Although EDX is often performed for the evaluation of lesion severity, the added value to a proper serial neurological evaluation is uncertain. Needle EMG at 3 months, the timing when a decision has to be taken to perform nerve reconstruction or not, is often too optimistic. Nerve conduction studies to detect root avulsions have a high specificity but low sensitivity. Moreover, as root avulsions primarily occur in the lower roots, the added value to neurological evaluation is questionable. Intraoperative neurophysiology was, in our hands, insufficient to aid in intraoperative decision-making. The main indication for EDX in our view is needle EMG at 4–6 weeks of age which expresses an optimistic or pessimistic prognosis for outcome, which is helpful for counseling parents at an early stage and enables timely referral to a specialized center.

References

1. Gilbert A, Razaboni R, Amar KS. Indications and results of brachial plexus surgery in obstetrical palsy. Orthop Clin North Am. 1988;19(1):91–105.
2. Clarke HM, Curtis CG. An approach to obstetrical brachial plexus injuries. Hand Clin. 1995;11(4):563–80.

3. Bisinella GL, Birch R, Smith SJ. Neurophysiological prediction of outcome in obstetric lesions of the brachial plexus. J Hand Surg Br. 2003;28(2):148–52.
4. van der Looven R, Le Roy L, Tanghe E, van den Broeck C, de Muynck M, Vingerhoets G, Pitt M, Vanderstraeten G. Early electrodiagnosis in the management of neonatal brachial plexus palsy: A systematic review. Muscle Nerve. 2020;61(5):557–66. https://doi.org/10.1002/mus.26762. Epub 2019 Dec 9.
5. Seddon HJ. A classification of nerve injuries. Br Med J. 1942;2(4260):237–9.
6. Chen L, Gao SC, Gu YD, Hu SN, Xu L, Huang YG. Histopathologic study of the neuroma-in-continuity in obstetric brachial plexus palsy. Plast Reconstr Surg. 2008;121(6):2046–54.
7. van Vliet AC, Tannemaat MR, van Duinen SG, Verhaagen J, Malessy MJ, De Winter F. Human neuroma-in-continuity contains focal deficits in myelination. J Neuropathol Exp Neurol. 2015;74(9):901–11.
8. Sunderland S. Nerve injuries and their repair: a critical appraisal. Edinburgh, London, Melbourne, New York: Churchill Livingstone; 1991. p. 1991.
9. Malessy MJ, Pondaag W, van Dijk JG. Electromyography, nerve action potential, and compound motor action potentials in obstetric brachial plexus lesions: validation in the absence of a "gold standard". Neurosurgery. 2009;65(4 Suppl):A153–9.
10. Seltzer Z, Devor M. Ephaptic transmission in chronically damaged peripheral nerves. Neurology. 1979;29(7):1061–4.
11. Anguelova GV, Malessy MJ, van Zwet EW, van Dijk JG. Extensive motor axonal misrouting after conservative treatment of obstetric brachial plexus lesions. Dev Med Child Neurol. 2014;56(10):984–9.
12. Metaizeau JP, Gayet C, Plenat F. Brachial plexus birth injuries. An experimental study. [in French]. Chir Pediatr. 1979;20(3):159–63.
13. Steens SC, Pondaag W, Malessy MJ, Verbist BM. Obstetric brachial plexus lesions: CT myelography. Radiology. 2011;259(2):508–15.
14. van Dijk JG, Pondaag W, Malessy MJ. Obstetric lesions of the brachial plexus. Muscle Nerve. 2001;24(11):1451–61.
15. Van Dijk JG, Pondaag W, Buitenhuis SM, Van Zwet EW, Malessy MJ. Needle electromyography at 1 month predicts paralysis of elbow flexion at 3 months in obstetric brachial plexus lesions. Dev Med Child Neurol. 2012;54(8):753–8.
16. Paradiso G, Granana N, Maza E. Prenatal brachial plexus paralysis. Neurology. 1997;49(1):261–2.
17. Gilbert A, Tassin JL. Surgical repair of the brachial plexus in obstetric paralysis. [in French]. Chirurgie. 1984;110(1):70–5.
18. van Dijk JG, Malessy MJ, Stegeman DF. Why is the electromyogram in obstetric brachial plexus lesions overly optimistic? Muscle Nerve. 1998;21(2): 260–1.
19. Malessy MJ, Pondaag W, Yang LJ, Hofstede-Buitenhuis SM, le Cessie S, van Dijk JG. Severe obstetric brachial plexus palsies can be identified at one month of age. PLoS One. 2011;6(10):e26193.
20. Smith SJ. The role of neurophysiological investigation in traumatic brachial plexus lesions in adults and children. J Hand Surg Br. 1996;21(2):145–7.
21. Yilmaz K, Caliskan M, Oge E, Aydinli N, Tunaci M, Ozmen M. Clinical assessment, MRI, and EMG in congenital brachial plexus palsy. Pediatr Neurol. 1999;21(4):705–10.
22. Smith BW, Chang KWC, Yang LJS, Spires MC. Comparative accuracies of electrodiagnostic and imaging studies in neonatal brachial plexus palsy. J Neurosurg Pediatr. 2018;23(1):119–24.
23. Kline DG, Hackett ER, May PR. Evaluation of nerve injuries by evoked potentials and electromyography. J Neurosurg. 1969;31(2):128–36.
24. Laurent JP, Lee R, Shenaq S, Parke JT, Solis IS, Kowalik L. Neurosurgical correction of upper brachial plexus birth injuries. J Neurosurg. 1993;79(2):197–203.
25. Pondaag W, van der Veken LP, van Someren PJ, van Dijk JG, Malessy MJ. Intraoperative nerve action and compound motor action potential recordings in patients with obstetric brachial plexus lesions. J Neurosurg. 2008;109(5):946–54.
26. Chin KF, Misra VP, Sicuri GM, Fox M, Sinisi M. Intra-operative neurophysiological prediction of upper trunk recovery in obstetric brachial plexus palsy with neuroma in continuity. Bone Joint J. 2013;95(B(5)):699–705.
27. Oberle J, Antoniadis G, Rath SA, Richter HP. Intraoperative electrophysiological diagnosis of spinal root avulsion during surgical repair of brachial plexus stretch injuries. Acta Neurochir. 1997;139(3): 238–9.

Brachial Plexus Birth Injuries: Evaluation—Radiologic Evaluation

47

Felix E. Diehn, Julie B. Guerin, V. Michelle Silvera, and Laurence J. Eckel

Introduction

Imaging is critical in the evaluation of preganglionic brachial plexus birth injury (BPBI). As in adults, the timely identification of nerve root avulsions is a vital component of prognostication and surgical decision-making. The primary modalities used to assess injuries proximal to the dorsal root ganglia in children are computed tomography myelography (CTM) and magnetic resonance imaging (MRI), including myelography-type MRI sequences. Please refer to the chapter on adult BPI radiologic evaluation for details on these modalities, the normal imaging anatomy, and the findings of preganglionic BPI in non-penetrating trauma. This brief chapter is complementary, addressing unique considerations for the pediatric patient, with a focus on the choice of CTM vs. MRI in BPBI. Similar to the chapter on adult imaging, additional radiological evaluation for postganglionic injuries, with not only MRI and radiographs but also ultrasound in the neonate, is beyond the scope of this chapter and well-covered by other references [1–4]. Note that the findings of preganglionic injury in children, including but not limited to the primary findings of nerve root avulsions and pseudomeningoceles (Figs. 47.1 and 47.2), are the same as in the adult.

F. E. Diehn (✉) · J. B. Guerin · V. M. Silvera
L. J. Eckel
Department of Radiology, Division of Neuroradiology, Mayo Clinic, Rochester, MN, USA
e-mail: diehn.felix@mayo.edu

CTM vs. MRI in Pediatric Patients

In adults, as covered in the prior chapter, CTM is the imaging gold standard and probably the first choice for advanced imaging of preganglionic BPI at most institutions. But MRI also performs very capably in this clinical scenario. Due to their differing advantages and disadvantages, CTM and MRI are considered by many to be complementary. Especially in pediatric patients, the minimal risks of CTM are more carefully considered. Specifically, minimizing radiation dose is a higher priority; in fact, the principle is to keep radiation dose to the patient as low as reasonably achievable (ALARA) [5, 6]. A guiding principle in pediatric care is also to avoid invasive procedures when possible, even if they are only minimally invasive. Thus, all other factors being equal, MRI would be preferred over CTM. However, given the complementary nature of the modalities, several nuanced aspects are worth highlighting.

In the evaluation of pediatric preganglionic BPI, particularly in the setting of BPBI, currently CTM is still technically considered by many to be the gold standard advanced imaging test (Fig. 47.1) [7–11]. However, there is a significantly growing trend toward MRI (Fig. 47.2)

A. Y. Shin, N. Pulos (eds.), *Operative Brachial Plexus Surgery*,
https://doi.org/10.1007/978-3-030-69517-0_47

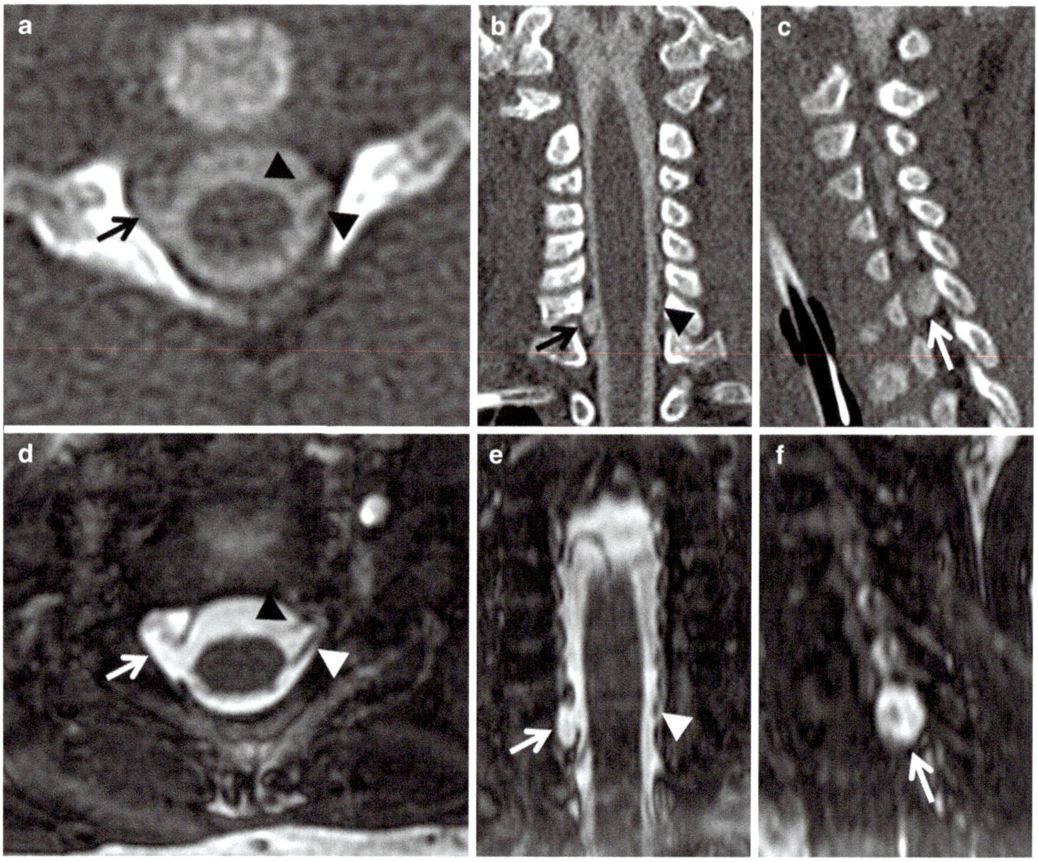

Fig. 47.1 Complete ventral and dorsal nerve root avulsions and pseudomeningocele in a 5 month-old male. CTM (**a**–**c**) and heavily T2-weighted three-dimensional gradient echo MR images, FIESTA sequence (GE) (**d**–**f**). On both examinations, images were acquired in the axial plane (**a**, **d**) and reformatted in oblique coronal (**b**, **e**) and sagittal (**c**, **f**) planes. A right C7–T1 pseudomeningocele (arrows in **a**–**f**) mildly deforms the right lateral aspect of the thecal sac. Neither the right C8 ventral nor dorsal nerve roots are evident. In contrast, the normal left C8 ventral and dorsal roots are well visualized (arrowheads in **a**, **d**). The normal C8 dorsal root on the left is shown in the coronal plane (arrowheads in **b**, **e**). Both modalities depict the abnormalities similarly well

[7, 9, 11–13]. The earlier data on MRI was variable, with relatively low diagnostic performance in identifying preganglionic injuries in babies in some studies [14]. Other authors published more encouraging data of the utility of MRI [15], including when heavily T2-weighted (T2/T1) three-dimensional gradient echo sequences with very high contrast to noise ratio and fewer flow artifacts were added [16]. Several more recent publications demonstrate relatively high sensitivity, specificity, and accuracy for MRI in this setting [12, 17]. Indeed, some centers now use MRI as their first-line imaging examination and predict that it will widely replace CTM [7, 11]. For some physicians or in some cases, the images produced by MRI may be more confidently interpreted than those produced by CTM, including for the diagnosis of nerve root avulsions (Fig. 47.2).

It is notable that large studies and robust head-to-head comparisons of the modalities are lacking in the birth trauma-related brachial plexus injury setting. For example, a 2014 study by Somashekar demonstrated MRI sensitivity and specificity for preganglionic root avulsion of 75% and 82%, respectively, numbers which are comparable to the performance of CTM reported in the literature. However,

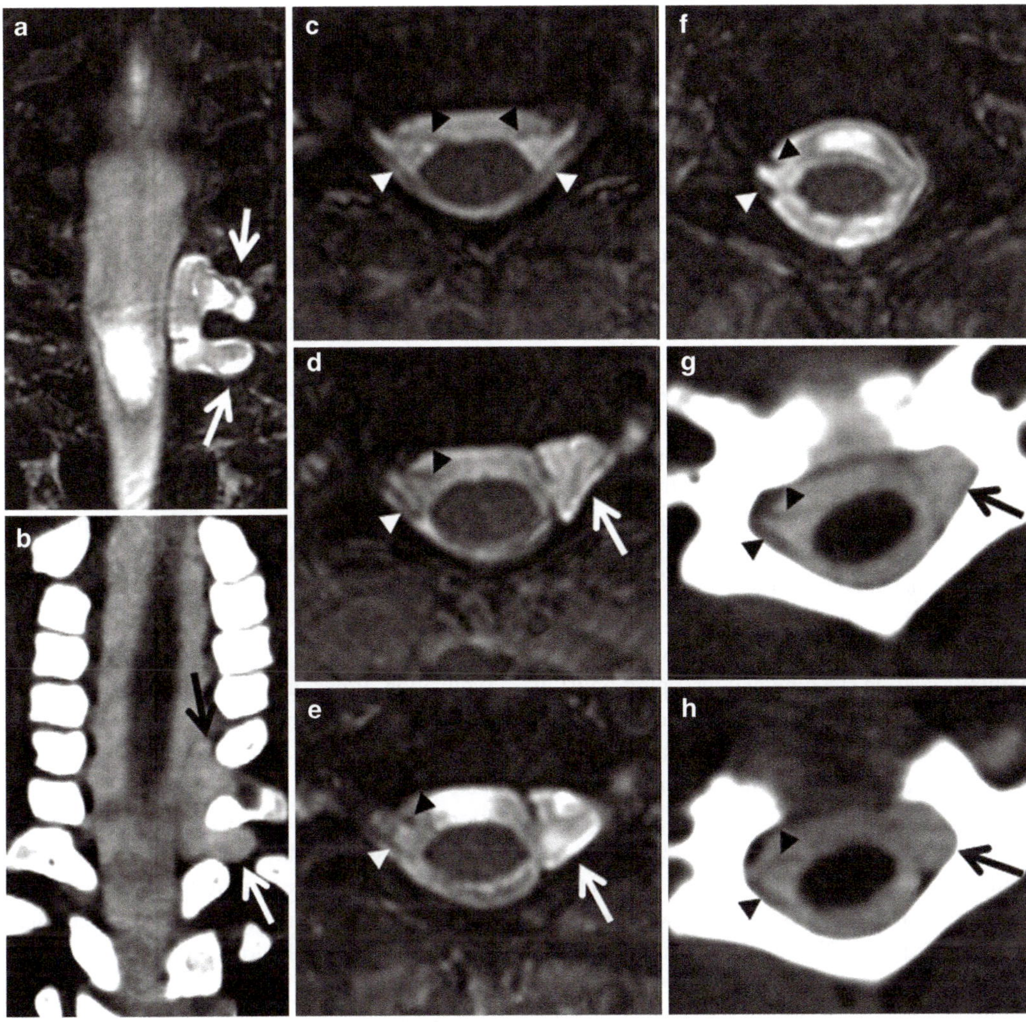

Fig. 47.2 Complete ventral and dorsal nerve root avulsions and pseudomeningoceles in a 7 month-old male. Heavily T2-weighted three-dimensional gradient echo MR images, FIESTA sequence (GE) (**a**, **c**–**f**) and CTM (**b**, **g**, **h**) in the coronal (**a**, **b**) and axial (**c**–**h**) planes. Axial images are at the normal C5–C6 level (**c**) and at the abnormal C6–C7 (**d**, **g**), C7–T1 (**e**, **h**), and T1–T2 (**f**) levels. Communicating left C6–C7 and C7–T1 pseudomeningoceles are readily seen on both modalities (arrows in **a**, **b**, **d**, **e**, **g**, **h**), with mild deformation of the left lateral aspect of the thecal sac. The presence/absence of nerve roots is slightly better appreciated on MR than CTM. Normal nerve roots (arrowheads in **c**–**h**) are present ventrally and dorsally at C5–C6 bilaterally (**c**) but only on the right at C6–C7 (**d**, **g**), C7–T1 (**e**, **h**), and T1–T2 (**f**). The neuroradiologist in this case felt more confident diagnosing complete ventral and dorsal C7, C8, and T1 nerve root avulsions on the left at C6–C7, C7–T1, and T1–T2 on MRI than on CTM. The CTM was performed after the MRI, did not significantly affect interpretation, and could have been obviated by the diagnostic quality MR images

the study did not have CTM as a comparison and included only 13 patients who underwent MRI, with just six undergoing comparison to the ultimate reference standard of surgery [17]. Radiologists may also be less confident in interpreting MRI examinations than CTM [11], and MRI is more likely to be degraded by artifact or be otherwise nondiagnostic [16]. Indeed, just as for adults, surgeon and/or radiologist preference as well as patient-specific factors may also factor heavily into the choice of modality [18].

Rational Approach to Modality Choice in Pediatric Patients

Head-to-head studies comparing MRI to CTM may never be done, for bioethical reasons, since CTM is invasive and exposes the child to ionizing radiation. In addition, a 2014 study by Tse showed that using both modalities did not increase diagnostic accuracy [11]. In the past both CTM and MRI in a baby generally required general anesthesia, or at a minimum sedation [8]. However, in current clinical practice, MRI in newborns and young infants can often be accomplished without sedation, with feeding and swaddling of the baby sufficing. After 3 months of age, this technique is less reliably successful and sedation may be necessary. If practically feasible, one potential approach that factors in the preference for MRI in children and the relative risks of anesthesia and CTM to the baby, is to start with an MRI without sedation (feeding and wrapping only). If the study is equivocal or nondiagnostic (e.g., if it suffers from significant artifact at the relevant side/levels) and if resource utilization allows, this attempt of avoiding sedation could be repeated. If the MRI is still not of diagnostic quality, one could proceed with repeat MRI under sedation/anesthesia and then proceed only with immediately subsequent CTM under anesthesia if the MRI remains equivocal or nondiagnostic. Such an approach could reduce the number of CTMs performed in these pediatric patients and would limit the need for multiple sessions of sedation/anesthesia. This tactic has been used at our center on occasion, but it has not been formally validated. It would align with the suggestion by some advocates of MRI that CTM should no longer be routinely performed in addition to MRI in this clinical scenario [7, 11].

Pediatric Imaging Technical Considerations

Several technical considerations enable optimal imaging evaluation of pediatric preganglionic BPI. Unlike in adults, for CTM, the volume of iodinated contrast administered into the thecal sac is calculated based on a weight-based protocol. Multidetector CT scanners (e.g., 64-slice or 128-slice) are ideal, enabling optimal submillimeter slice thickness of approximately 0.625 mm [1]. In addition to the acquired axial images, reformatted sagittal and coronal images are critical to visualize the small caliber nerve roots. For myelographic MR technique, it is essential to employ heavily T2-weighted three-dimensional gradient echo sequences with very high contrast to noise ratio and fewer flow artifacts. Trade names for such sequences include fast imaging employing steady-state acquisition (FIESTA) on General Electric (GE) magnets, constructive interference in steady state (CISS) on Siemens machines, and balanced FFE on Philips magnets. Generally, 3 Tesla field strength is preferable over 1.5 Tesla due to the former's higher signal-to-noise ratio [1]. A slice thickness of approximately 0.5–0.9 mm is preferred [1, 11]. Acquisition times are variable (approximately 2–8 minutes) [11] and increased by thinner slice thickness. Imaging can be performed in any plane (axial, sagittal, and coronal). Which acquisition plane is optimal may be vendor, sequence, and patient dependent, and more than one plane of acquisition may be required in a given patient. Once acquired, the images are typically reformatted in both of the orthogonal planes.

Summary

Advanced imaging with either CTM or MRI plays a critical role in the evaluation of pediatric preganglionic BPBI. The imaging findings of pediatric preganglionic BPBI do not differ from those in adults, with the primary goal of imaging being to detect nerve root avulsions and pseudomeningoceles. CTM is historically considered the imaging gold standard and remains the first choice for advanced imaging at some centers. However, in pediatric patients, it is important to minimize exposure to ionizing radiation and avoid anesthesia and even minimally invasive procedures when possible. Thus, there is a growing trend toward MRI, which also offers excellent diagnostic performance for the evaluation of brachial plexus birth palsy. A rational approach would be to start imaging in this clinical scenario with MRI and only move on to CTM if the MRI findings are less than definitive.

References

1. Menashe SJ, Tse R, Nixon JN, Ishak GE, Thapa MM, McBroom JA, et al. Brachial plexus birth palsy: multimodality imaging of spine and shoulder abnormalities in children. AJR Am J Roentgenol. 2015;204(2):W199–206.
2. Gunes A, Bulut E, Uzumcugil A, Oguz KK. Brachial plexus ultrasound and MRI in children with brachial plexus birth injury. AJNR Am J Neuroradiol. 2018;39(9):1745–50.
3. Somashekar DK, Di Pietro MA, Joseph JR, Yang LJ, Parmar HA. Utility of ultrasound in noninvasive preoperative workup of neonatal brachial plexus palsy. Pediatr Radiol. 2016;46(5):695–703.
4. Stilwill SE, Mills MK, Hansford BG, Allen H, Mahan M, Moore KR, et al. Practical approach and review of brachial plexus pathology with operative correlation: what the radiologist needs to know. Semin Roentgenol. 2019;54(2):92–112.
5. Cohen MD. ALARA, image gently and CT-induced cancer. Pediatr Radiol. 2015;45(4):465–70.
6. Applegate KE, Cost NG. Image gently: a campaign to reduce children's and adolescents' risk for cancer during adulthood. J Adolesc Health. 2013;52(5 Suppl):S93–7.
7. Somashekar DK, Wilson TJ, DiPietro MA, Joseph JR, Ibrahim M, Yang LJ, et al. The current role of diagnostic imaging in the preoperative workup for refractory neonatal brachial plexus palsy. Childs Nerv Syst. 2016;32(8):1393–7.
8. Steens SC, Pondaag W, Malessy MJ, Verbist BM. Obstetric brachial plexus lesions: CT myelography. Radiology. 2011;259(2):508–15.
9. Vanderhave KL, Bovid K, Alpert H, Chang KW, Quint DJ, Leonard JAJ, et al. Utility of electrodiagnostic testing and computed tomography myelography in the preoperative evaluation of neonatal brachial plexus palsy. J Neurosurg Pediatr. 2012;9(3):283–9.
10. Chow BC, Blaser S, Clarke HM. Predictive value of computed tomographic myelography in obstetrical brachial plexus palsy. Plast Reconstr Surg. 2000;106(5):971–7; discussion 8–9.
11. Tse R, Nixon JN, Iyer RS, Kuhlman-Wood KA, Ishak GE. The diagnostic value of CT myelography, MR myelography, and both in neonatal brachial plexus palsy. AJNR Am J Neuroradiol. 2014;35(7):1425–32.
12. Grahn P, Pöyhiä T, Sommarhem A, Nietosvaara Y. Clinical significance of cervical MRI in brachial plexus birth injury. Acta Orthop. 2019;90(2):111–8.
13. Smith BW, Chang KWC, Yang LJS, Spires MC. Comparative accuracies of electrodiagnostic and imaging studies in neonatal brachial plexus palsy. J Neurosurg Pediatr. 2018;23(1):119–24.
14. Medina LS, Yaylali I, Zurakowski D, Ruiz J, Altman NR, Grossman JA. Diagnostic performance of MRI and MR myelography in infants with a brachial plexus birth injury. Pediatr Radiol. 2006;36(12):1295–9.
15. Abbott R, Abbott M, Alzate J, Lefton D. Magnetic resonance imaging of obstetrical brachial plexus injuries. Childs Nerv Syst. 2004;20(10):720–5.
16. van Ouwerkerk WJ, Strijers RL, Barkhof F, Umans U, Vandertop WP. Detection of root avulsion in the dominant C7 obstetric brachial plexus lesion: experience with three-dimensional constructive interference in steady-state magnetic resonance imaging and electrophysiology. Neurosurgery. 2005;57(5):930–40; discussion -40.
17. Somashekar D, Yang LJ, Ibrahim M, Parmar HA, High-resolution MRI. evaluation of neonatal brachial plexus palsy: a promising alternative to traditional CT myelography. AJNR Am J Neuroradiol. 2014;35(6):1209–13.
18. Duff SV, Dematteo C. Clinical assessment of the infant and child following perinatal brachial plexus injury. J Hand Ther. 2015;28(2):126–33; quiz 34.

Priorities of Treatment and Rationale (Babies Are Not Small Adults)

48

Scott H. Kozin, Dan A. Zlotolow, and Francisco Soldado

Diagnosis and Classification

Injury severity is measured using the Narakas classification that divides brachial plexus birth injuries (BPBI) into four groups (Table 48.1) [1]. Group 1 is the classic Erb-Duchenne palsy (C5 and C6). Group 2 is the extended Erb-Duchenne palsy (C5, C6, and C7). Groups 3 and 4 are total plexus palsies separated by the absence (Group 3) or presence of a Horner syndrome (Group 4). The presence of a Horner syndrome (drooped eyelid, constricted pupil, and sweating deficiency along the affected side of the face) suggests an avulsion injury at C8 and T1 (Fig. 48.1). This finding portends an unfavorable independent prognostic value for recovery [2, 3]. The Narakas 1, 2, and 3/4 groupings have been shown to have prognostic power, with dramatically lower rates of full recovery for Narakas 3 and 4 patients compared to both 1 and 2 [2, 4, 5].

Active motion is graded according to the Active Movement Scale (AMS) developed at The Hospital for Sick Children in Toronto, Canada (Table 48.2) [6]. A key rule during the scoring of the AMS is that a motion cannot be graded as 5 or higher unless the movement is full against gravity first (grade 4). For example, elbow flexion must be full with gravity minimized before achieving a grade of 5, 6, or 7. We have applied a similar concept to our grading during manual muscle testing in older children. In other words, a patient must achieve full motion against gravity (grade 3) in our adapted MRC grading before being granted a grade 4 or 5. The AMS is an invaluable tool to assess infants before and after surgery and has been validated for reliability between adequately trained observers [7].

Physical examination is necessary and sufficient for determining the Narakas classification and the AMS, relying on the practical anatomy of the brachial plexus to determine the injury pattern and root involvement. Examination begins as early as the first day of life, with serial examinations every 4–6 weeks to monitor recovery [8]. Neonates clearly cannot obey commands nor respond reliably to environmental stimuli. The principal component of the physical examination is observations of the patient's active movements. In addition, a neonate will move toward gentle stimuli. Stroking the dorsal forearm will

We obtain photo consent on all of our patients as part of their Conditions of Care. Scott

Supplementary Information The online version of this chapter (https://doi.org/10.1007/978-3-030-69517-0_48) contains supplementary material, which is available to authorized users.

S. H. Kozin (✉) · D. A. Zlotolow
Shriners Hospitals for Children, Philadelphia, PA, USA
e-mail: skozin@shrinenet.org

F. Soldado
Barcelona Childrens HM nens, HM Hospitals, Barcelona, Spain
e-mail: drsoldado@cirugiamanoinfantil.com

A. Y. Shin, N. Pulos (eds.), *Operative Brachial Plexus Surgery*,
https://doi.org/10.1007/978-3-030-69517-0_48

Table 48.1 Practical anatomy for brachial plexus injury pattern

Narakas classification[a]	Nerves involved	Muscles or functions	Sensation
Grade 1	Upper trunk (C5 and C6)	Shoulder (rotator cuff and deltoid) Forearm supination (biceps and supinator) Elbow flexion (biceps and brachialis) Wrist extension (extensor carpi radialis longus)	Median nerve sensibility thumb and index finger
Grade 2	Middle trunk (C7)	Elbow extension (triceps) Latissimus dorsi Forearm pronation (pronator teres) Wrist extension (extensor carpi radialis longus) Digital extension (MCP joints) Wrist flexion (flexor carpi radialis)	Median nerve sensibility long finger
Grade 3	Lower trunk (C8 and T1)	Forearm pronation (pronator quadratus) Extrinsic finger and thumb flexors (flexor digitorum profundus and flexor pollicis longus) Wrist flexion (flexor carpi ulnaris) Digital extension (IP joints) Intrinsic muscles	Ulnar nerve sensibility (ring and small fingers)
Grade 4	Sympathetic nerves	Pupillary dilation Facial sweating Eye opening	Not applicable

Adapted from Kozin [40]
MCP metacarpophalangeal, *IP* interphalangeal
[a]Narakas grades are additive: grade 2 includes grade 1; grade 3 includes grades 1 and 2; grade 4 includes grades 1, 2, and 3

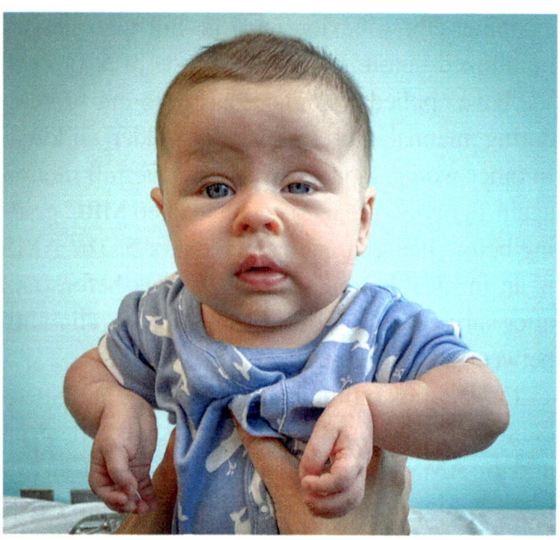

Fig. 48.1 Three-month-old with left sided Horner syndrome with ptosis (drooped eyelid) and miosis (constricted pupil). (Courtesy of Shriners Hospital for Children, Philadelphia). (Courtesy of Dan A. Zlotolow, MD, with permission)

Table 48.2 Active Movement Scale (AMS)

Shoulder abduction	________		
Shoulder adduction	________	*Gravity eliminated*	*Score*
Shoulder flexion	________	No contraction	0
Shoulder external rotation	________	Contraction, no motion	1
Shoulder internal rotation	________	<50% motion	2
Elbow flexion	________	>50% motion	3
Elbow extension	________	Full motion	4
Forearm supination	________	*Against gravity*[a]	
Forearm pronation	________	<50% motion	5
Wrist flexion	________	>50% motion	6
Wrist extension	________	Full motion	7
Finger flexion	________		
Finger extension	________		
Thumb flexion	________		
Thumb extension	________		
Total	________		

Adapted from Clarke and Curtis [6]
[a]A score of 4 must be achieved before a higher score can be assigned. Movement grades are within available range of motion

often produce shoulder external rotation, while volar forearm contact will elicit internal rotation; radial forearm contact will provoke elbow flexion and ulnar forearm elbow extension; stroking the back of the hand may elicit finger and wrist extension. Reflexive grasp (palmar grasp reflex) lasts until about 5–6 months of age and is a reliable test for lower trunk function via finger and thumb flexion [9]. As the neonate becomes an infant, toys and props can be used to elicit the AMS scores (Video 48.1).

Sensibility cannot be assessed in an infant. Clinical clues are finger moistness and withdrawal from a gentle pinch. Pruning of the fingers in the bathtub is another indication of intact nerve supply.

Timing of Recovery

The timing of recovery is dependent upon the degree and extent of injury. The mildest plexus injuries, pure neurapraxia injuries, are common and recover spontaneously and completely by 6–8 weeks of life via remyelination alone. Because the axons remain intact, Wallerian degeneration does not occur. When some but not all axons within a nerve root are axotomized (motor and sensory neurons disconnected from their target organs by nerve injury), the timing and degree of recovery are highly variable and depend principally upon the percentage of axotomy [10]. Mixed injuries with a neurapraxia and axonotmetric components can recover spontaneously, but recovery may be slower and incomplete. Proximally demyelinated axons undergo remyelination, and at the same time, these intact axons have begun terminal and nodal sprouting to expand their control over muscle fibers that were previously controlled by axons that have undergone Wallerian degeneration from upstream axotomy (Fig. 48.2). If the ratio of axotomy to neurapraxia is low, with restoration of innervation dependent primarily on remyelination and not on terminal/nodal sprouting, recovery will be complete and nearly as rapid as for a pure neurapraxia. As more and more axons are axotomized, and the ratio of axotomy to neurapraxia increases, recovery becomes more and more reliant on terminal/nodal sprouting. While sprouting has been shown to begin within 24 hours of muscle denervation, the process is not complete until at least 3 months from injury [11].

Animal studies have shown that sprouting can make up for the loss of a staggering 80% of axons to any particular muscle. This recovery is because each muscle fiber innervated by any single axon is surrounded by between five and eight muscle fibers innervated by other axons [12]. Schwann cell mediated axonal sprouting can therefore reach these fibers and reinnervate them. Loss of fewer than 80% of motor axons (80% axotomy/20% neurapraxia) will therefore

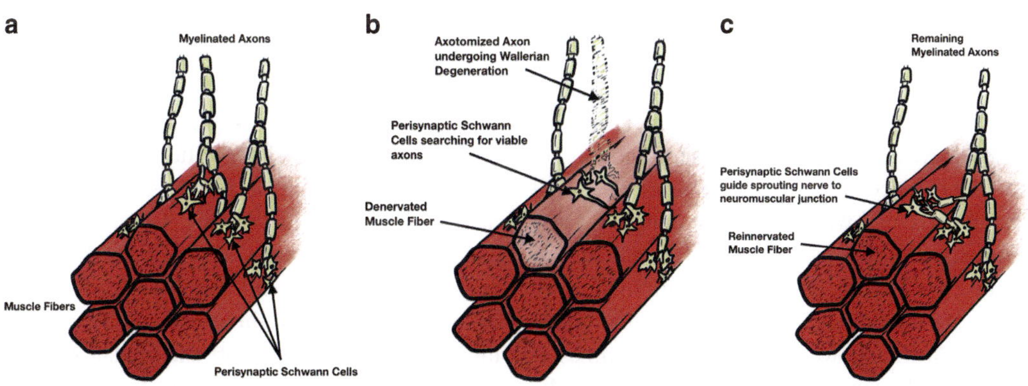

Fig. 48.2 Myelinated efferent axons typically innervate several hundred muscle fibers throughout a muscle, with perisynaptic Schwann cells (PSCs) maintaining and facilitating the neuromuscular junction (**a**). Following nerve injury, any axotomized axons undergo Wallerian degeneration, leading to extension of cytoplasmic processes by the PSCs (**b**). Terminal and nodal sprouting from nearby intact axons are led by the PSCs that bridge between the innervated and denervated muscle fibers to reinnervate the denervated muscle end plate (**c**) (Modified from Gordon and Borschel [12]). (Courtesy of Dan A. Zlotolow, MD, with permission)

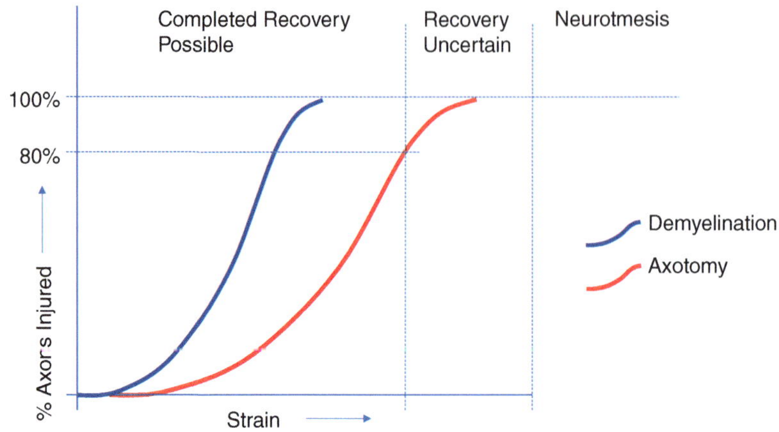

Fig. 48.3 Nerves subjected to small levels of strain (longitudinal deformation) will initially just stretch and return to their original length. With increasing strain, the myelin sheaths will begin to be disrupted (demyelination), followed by injury to the axons themselves (axotomy). Even when up to 80% of axons are axotomized, normal or near normal function can be expected via remyelination and terminal/nodal axonal sprouting. More than 80% axotomy requires regrowth of the axons from the site of injury to their target organs, followed by terminal/nodal sprouting of those regenerative axons and then cortical (brain) reorganization. If all of the axons are demyelinated and themselves disrupted, the endoneurial tubes may remain in continuity, allowing but not guaranteeing functional recovery. Once the nerve is completely ruptured (neurotmesis), there is no continuity of the endoneurial tubes, and recovery is unlikely. (Courtesy of Dan A. Zlotolow, MD, with permission)

recover within 3–4 months of injury from sprouting and remyelination, without the need for axonal regeneration from the proximal axonotmetric injured nerve stumps (Fig. 48.3) [13]. Evidence of sprouting can be seen on electromyography (EMG) as higher amplitude but fewer motor units, often referred to on EMG reports as "signs of reinnervation." A motor unit is comprised of one axon and up to several hundred muscle fibers distributed widely throughout the cross section of the muscle. In a normally innervated muscle, only four to six muscle fibers of a particular motor unit are typically within the pickup range of an EMG needle. Each of these normal motor units, when activated, will have an amplitude of just under 2 mV with a 5–10 ms duration. Once terminal sprouting has completed, amplitudes of up to 20 mV with 20–30 ms durations may be seen. The larger amplitudes suggest that some axons can expand to control five to ten times as many muscle fibers within the range of the EMG needle compared as they did prior to the injury [14, 15]. Other studies have cited between a four- and sixfold expansion of single axon control over additional motor fibers in a variety of human and animal models [16–20]. Beyond that limit, muscle strength decreases proportionally and the weakness begins to become noticeable clinically. Fewer but larger motor units may not result in weakness below the four- to sixfold threshold, but fine muscle control is progressively compromised. In a neonate, a loss of less than 80% of motor axons to the most affected muscle after a BPBI will therefore recover clinically by 3 months via sprouting and remyelination alone. Beyond this threshold, recovery will take longer and rely increasingly on axonal regeneration crossing the upstream injury site.

At the injury site, Wallerian degeneration begins within 24–36 hours after axotomy, with degeneration of the axon progressing in a proximal to distal direction. Within 3 weeks, macrophages and the Schwann cells degrade the axons and myelin. Schwann cells take on a different role once the axon and myelin have degenerated, proliferating to provide support and guidance to the regenerating axons as they cross the injury site and enter the empty endoneurial sheathes [21].

Meanwhile, the axons have begun to sprout from the proximal nerve stump in a staggered and disorganized fashion over 3–4 weeks, with very few axons making the initial leap. Many axons are misdirected backward, back into the proximal nerve stump. Once the Schwann cells align in parallel at the injury site and into the endoneurial tubes, about 10 days after injury, the axonal outgrowth becomes more purposeful, and the axons are led into the endoneurial tubes [22]. Initially, there is no discrimination from the motor axons between motor and sensory endoneurial tubes. Preferential motor reinnervation increases gradually over the first month after injury [23]. Nodal sprouting can also redirect misdirected motor axons into motor endoneurial tubes at or further downstream from the injury site [24].

As regenerating axons reach their target muscle fibers, they are led by Schwann cells to find available motor end plates and begin establishing a new neuromuscular junction. Nodal and terminal sprouting then increases the number of muscle fibers under that axon's control. Because axonal regeneration is staggered over a month, and because distal axonal growth occurs at a variable rate between 1 and 3 mm per day, the first axons to cross the injury site and enter the distal endoneurial tubes will arrive at the target muscle at least 1 month before the last axons arrive. For injuries where more than 80% of axons have been axotomized, clinically evident recovery can therefore range from months to years depending on the distance from the axotomy site to the muscle target and the percentage of axotomy. Cortical plasticity is then required to relearn which axons control which muscles and is dependent on the amount of misalignment of outgrowing axons [4].

In a complete axonotmetric injury where 100% of the axons have been axotomized, but there is still some structural continuity between the proximal and distal ends of the nerve, clinically evident recovery requires at least 20% of the motor axons travelling down the endoneurial tubes to reach their target muscles. The proximal muscles will recover first followed by the more distal muscles. The more axons that reach the muscle and the less reliance on sprouting, the faster and more robust the recovery.

Timing of recovery is therefore dependent on the percentage of neurapraxia vs. axotomy, the distance between the injury site and the muscle target, the speed of axonal regeneration, the percentage of axotomized axons that reach the target, and the cortical plasticity required to purposefully engage the newly rewired motor units.

Neurotmesis via rupture, where the peripheral nerve is ruptured distal to the dorsal root ganglion (postganglionic injury), is unlikely to recover spontaneously. Avulsion injuries, where the nerve root is avulsed from the cervical spine proximal to the dorsal root ganglion (postganglionic injury), will not recover spontaneously. Due to strong fibrous bands that connect the nerve sheaths of C5 and C6 to the periosteum of the transverse processes at the neuroforamen of the spinal column, avulsions at these nerve roots are rare [25]. Clarke and colleagues reported on 63 patients that underwent surgical exploration for BPBI [26]. There were no root avulsions encountered at surgical exploration of C5, and only eight root avulsions at C6 (21%). Because the fibrous anchors at C7 are less robust and nearly absent at the lower trunk roots of C8 and T1, the rate of avulsions for the middle and lower trunks was much higher (both at 34%) [26]. Our experience has been similar, with frequent avulsions of C7 and C8/T1 seen during surgical exploration for global injuries. Other factors in whether or not any particular root is avulsed include the direction, magnitude, and speed of the traction force applied. The more direct, forceful, and rapid the nerve root is pulled, the more likely to sustain an avulsion [25].

Because recovery of axotomy progresses in a proximal to distal direction, proximal muscles will typically recover first. By contrast, remyelination and sprouting are not influenced by the distance from injury to muscle, so recovery is based on the extent of demyelination or percentage of axotomy. Since the upper roots tend to sustain the most stress and therefore a larger component of axotomy, and the upper roots innervate the most proximal muscles, more proximal muscles will recover last if primarily dependent on axonal sprouting. Therefore, it is typical for a global injury without avulsion or rupture of the middle and lower trunk to recover hand function first, followed by finger extension, wrist extension, and elbow extension. Upper trunk function (elbow flexion and shoulder abduction/external rotation), if it is to recover, will recover last. Again, if the upper trunk axotomy was below 80%, recovery will be evident by 3 months. Greater degrees of axonotmetric injury will recover more slowly in a proximal to distal direction, with greater reliance on regrowth of axons from the injury site. In a 3-month-old child, who has recovered lower trunk function, followed by upper trunk recovery, with no middle trunk recovery, C7 is likely an avulsion injury. If only the upper trunk of a global injury recovers by 3 months, it is likely that both the lower and middle trunks have sustained an avulsion. Using this thought process, the surgeon can discern the likely type of injury sustained by each root based on the timing and direction (proximal to distal direction or distal to proximal) of recovery.

Diagnostic Tests

Imaging and electrodiagnostic studies have limited ability to discriminate between axonotmetric and neurotmetric injuries. The determination of the degree of axotomy is even more difficult, especially in mixed neurapraxic/axonotmetric injuries [27]. Electromyography (EMG) has been shown to be overly optimistic in predicting recovery, identifying "inactive motor unit potentials (MUPs)," which appear normal but do not correlate with recovery [28]. The reason for inactive MUPs is not clearly understood but may be related to co-contraction or incomplete cortical reorganization of re-routed axons [4]. An alternate explanation based on our experience is that motor axons remain viable and do not undergo Wallerian degeneration in some C7 avulsion injuries. These axons will eventually be pruned over the first 12–18 months of life but stimulate intraoperatively despite having no continuity with the spinal cord (Video 48.2).

Magnetic resonance imaging (MRI) or computed tomography myelography (CTM) can demonstrate pseudomeningoceles consistent with nerve root avulsion injuries. The presence of a pseudomeningocele, a meningeal pouch filled with cerebrospinal fluid that extends through the intervertebral foramen into the paraspinal area, suggests a nerve root avulsion (Fig. 48.4). This pouch represents an extraction of the dural and arachnoidal sleeve through the intervertebral foramen that often occurs during a root avulsion injury. CTM and MRI have greater than 90% true positive rates for determining avulsion injuries correlated at surgery when pseudomeningoceles are seen [29, 30]. Smaller pseudomeningoceles may represent a false positive with preservation of nerve root integrity [29].

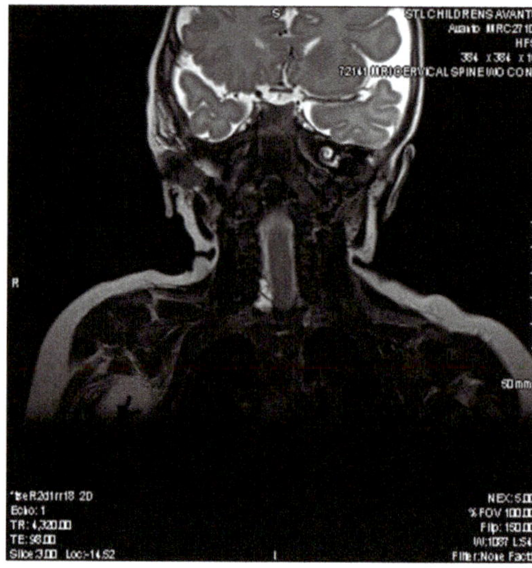

Fig. 48.4 Coronal MRI reveals right-sided pseudomeningoceles that have formed outside the intervertebral foramen indicative of root avulsion injury. (Courtesy of Shriners Hospital for Children, Philadelphia). (Courtesy of Dan A. Zlotolow, MD, with permission)

Vanderhave and colleagues have questioned the efficacy of advanced imaging studies to differentiate between avulsions and ruptures [31]. In their study, CTM was able to detect avulsions with a sensitivity of 50% in the upper trunk roots, 80% in the middle trunk, and 75% in the lower trunk. The addition of electrodiagnostic studies actually decreased the sensitivity compared to CTM alone, reducing the sensitivity to detect avulsions to 20% in the upper trunk roots and approximately 30% in the middle and lower trunks. Current imaging studies are also unable to assess whether the neuroma has axons in continuity or if there has been complete axonal disruption. The clinical examination using the AMS scoring system has been shown to be superior to MRI and EMG in the neonatal period at predicting the child's prognosis by 12 months of age [32].

Timing of Surgical Reconstruction

The quandary in brachial plexus birth injuries is determining when to explore the plexus. Surgery must have a positive effect compared to the natural history of recovery. Global injuries with a Horner syndrome (Narakas 4) usually require early surgery within the first 3 to 4 months of life [33]. The injury pattern is likely a combination of ruptures and avulsions that requires surgical reconstruction with an amalgamation of nerve grafting and nerve transfers.

The Narakas 1 (C5 and C6) and 2 (C5, C6, and C7) injury patterns are more controversial regarding timing and techniques of nerve reconstruction. There is no universal consensus regarding indications and timing of surgical intervention. Failure to demonstrate noteworthy signs of recovery by 5–8 months has been cited as an indication for surgery [6, 34]. Injuries with no recovery or minimal recovery require surgery. In addition, injuries that demonstrate some early recovery but the process subsequently stagnates require surgical intervention.

Priorities of Surgical Reconstruction

The priorities of brachial plexus reconstruction are different in children compared to adults. In adults, repairing injuries to the lower trunk (avulsions or ruptures) is futile; the distance from the injury and the slow nerve regeneration preclude useful hand recovery. In children, the distance is less and the regeneration is quicker. Hence, useful hand function is obtainable in a majority of cases and is the primary goal [35]. After hand function, the priorities, in order, are as follows: (1) elbow flexion for hand-to-mouth function, (2) shoulder stability and motion, and (3) elbow extension to allow for overhead function and increased workable reach space. The surgical plan should consider this hierarchy during the decision-making process.

In global palsies, the surgical focus is on reanimation of the hand. In extended and upper palsies, the priorities are elbow and shoulder motion. The surgical procedures are divided into two types: nerve grafting and nerve transfers. Nerve grafting utilizes a viable ruptured root to restore downstream function. Nerve transfers utilize a functioning expendable nerve or portion of a nerve to restore downstream function [63, 35]. Nerve transfer options are more available and work better for more proximal muscles about the shoulder and elbow compared to more distal muscles of the wrist and hand. Distal nerve transfers are hampered by the limited number of potential donors and the complexity of hand function.

Global Brachial Plexus Birth Palsies

Global palsies (aka total or pan-plexus injuries) are the most challenging surgical reconstructions. The surgical exposure is more difficult, the degree of damage imposing, and the reconstructions more complex. Despite advances in imaging techniques, surgical exploration remains the gold standard to assess the degree of damage and the number of nerve root ruptures and avulsions.

For any global injury, the surgery is scheduled for the entire day, as the exact reconstruction is a "game time" decision-making process. The surgery begins via a thorough exposure of the brachial plexus. The exposure is performed in a stepwise fashion to avoid missing critical steps. Table 48.3 lists the key elements of the exposure (Video 48.3). The principal goal of the surgical exposure is to tally the number of nerve root ruptures and the number of nerve root avulsions. As described previously, the upper nerve root (C5) or upper nerve roots (C5 and C6) and lower nerve roots (C7, C8, and T1) tend to avulse. However, the surgeon must be prepared to find different patterns dependent upon the force and vector applied. Once the injury pattern has been established, the surgical strategy is developed considering the number of viable axons available for reconstruction and the priorities of reconstruction. The number one priority is the hand and the

Table 48.3 Brachial plexus exposure

Step	Rationale and comments
Draw transverse skin incision about clavicle	Langer's line and heals with imperceptible scar. Avoid longitudinal limb over sternocleidomastoid
Infiltrate skin incision with dilute epinephrine (0.5 mg/100 ml normal saline solution)	Weight-based administration, confer with anesthesia. Lessens bleeding and facilitated dissection
Incise skin with scalpel blades and use bovie electrocautery down to fat pad	
Reflect fat pad from medial to lateral	Retain fat pad for vascularity after reconstruction
Identify phrenic nerve on anterior scalene	Must identify and protect phrenic nerve, C5 contribution can be within upper trunk neuroma
Identify and ligate transverse cervical vessels across the upper trunk	Ligaclips® (Ethicon, Johnson and Johnson, Belgium)
Identify nerve roots from cephalad to caudad (C5 through T1)	
C7 nerve root has overlying dorsal scapular artery that requires ligation	C7 is inferior and posterior to C5/C6 nerve roots
C8 and T1 nerve roots have overlying subclavian artery that must be protected	
Determine the number of nerve root rupture(s) and nerve root avulsion(s)	
Plan surgical reconstruction and execute	

best root is designated as inflow to the lower trunk [36]. The recent advent of the pre-spinal route for the contralateral C7 (CC7) nerve transfer has changed the paradigm [37]. The CC7 offers an extensive number of axons for reconstruction. We currently reserve CC7 transfers for avulsions of three to five nerve roots leaving only up to two viable roots for reconstruction. If two roots are available, reconstruction can be performed by graft reconstruction only (Fig. 48.5) or by adding CC7 for additional axonal inflow. The availability of only one nerve root leaves a paucity of viable axons for reconstruction. In these scenarios, the limited numbers of axons warrants the risk/benefit ratio associated with CC7 nerve transfer. Three viable roots can satiate the reconstructive goals following a global plexus injury, especially with the addition of local nerve transfers (intercostal nerves and spinal accessory nerve).

Nerve grafting and CC7 transfer to the lower trunk require nerve graft material in most cases. In babies, the CC7 nerve transfer will not reach the lower trunk but rather only the anterior triangle of the neck adjacent to the carotid sheath of the injured side. Therefore, a short nerve graft segment is necessary. Similarly, mobilization of the lower trunk lessens the distance to the C5 or C6 nerve root; however, a small gap may remain requiring nerve grafting. We strongly favor autograft over allograft for reconstruction, as there is a preponderance of animal data that supports the use of autograft and there is a dearth of human studies to support the use of allograft [38, 39]. Potential donors include bilateral sural nerves, medial antebrachial cutaneous nerve, and radial sensory nerve.

For elbow function, we prioritize flexion over extension. We will graft from viable C6 nerve root or perform a nerve transfer (three intercostal nerves to the musculocutaneous nerve). During intercostal nerve harvest, we will also assess the status of the long thoracic nerve. A viable long thoracic nerve can add an additional nerve transfer for elbow extension.

For global injuries with one viable root, we will perform a spinal accessory to suprascapular nerve transfer for shoulder function, three intercostal nerves to the musculocutaneous nerve for elbow flexion, and grafting from the one root and the CC7 to the middle and lower trunks. This reconstruction allows for recovery of hand function, elbow flexion, elbow extension, and shoulder stability. There are insufficient axons to reinnervate the deltoid, teres minor, upper subscapularis, and upper pectoralis.

Two available roots, combined with the CC7, allow a more complete reconstruction. After we

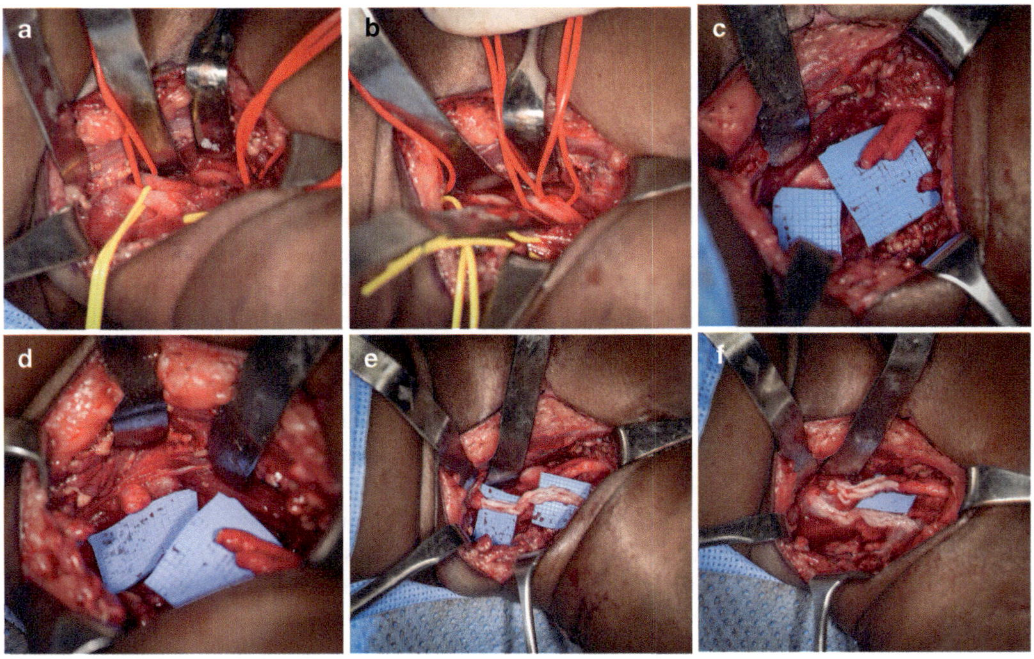

Fig. 48.5 Five-month-old female child with right global brachial plexus injury. (Courtesy of Shriners Hospital for Children, Philadelphia). (**a**) Right brachial plexus exploration with C5 and C6 nerve root ruptures (yellow loop around C5 and red loop around C6). (**b**) Intraforaminal avulsion of C8 and T1. (**c**) Preparation of lower trunk (C8 and T1) and upper trunk. (**d**) Preparation of C5 and C6 nerve roots. (**e**) Nerve grafts from C5 to upper trunk. (**f**) Nerve grafts from C6 to lower trunk. (Courtesy of Dan A. Zlotolow, MD, with permission)

have selected the donor for lower trunk reanimation, usually the C6 nerve root, we can obtain a primary coaptation without graft or with only a short graft. We then move on to the next priorities. For shoulder function, we will graft from C5 nerve root to the posterior division of the upper trunk (suprascapular nerve and axillary nerve) and/or perform a nerve transfer for rotator cuff function (spinal accessory to suprascapular nerve transfer). For elbow flexion, we will transfer three intercostal nerves to the musculocutaneous nerve. The CC7 is then grafted to the ipsilateral middle trunk. This reconstruction allows the possibility of reinnervation of all major muscles of the arm. A three-root plexus is reconstructed in the same manner as a two-root plexus, with the extra available ipsilateral root taking the place of the CC7.

Extended Upper Brachial Plexus Birth Palsies

Brachial plexus palsies with sparing of the lower trunk (C8 and T1 nerve roots) offer additional nerve transfer options. If the lower trunk was working at birth, we can infer that the lower trunk has inherent axonal redundancy and is therefore available as a source of axons for nerve transfer. A global injury at birth that quickly recovers lower trunk function is likely related to remyelination. In contrast, a global injury at birth that slowly recovers lower trunk function is likely related to an axonotmetric injury and distal sprouting. In this scenario, the lower trunk may not have redundant axons and is not an available donor for nerve transfer. The distinction is critical, as we will only use a normal ulnar nerve (C8, T1) as a donor for nerve transfer. A history of a never-injured or rapidly recovered lower trunk verified by electrical stimulation at surgery provides evidence that the ulnar nerve has its full or near-full count of axons. Using the Checkpoint® (Checkpoint Surgical, Cleveland, Ohio) stimulator on a viable ulnar nerve at 0.5 milliamps and mid-pulse width will generate a "manicule sign" (Video 48.4). The manicule sign is generated by stimulation of the C8 and T1 axons in the ulnar nerve and not the C8 and T1 axons in the median nerve (anterior interosseous and recurrent branch). This stimulation yields flexion of the long, ring, and small fingers interphalangeal joints from the flexor digitorum profundus (FDP); flexion of the index, long, ring, and small fingers metacarpophalangeal joints from the intrinsic muscles; extension of the index and thumb interphalangeal joints from the unopposed interossei and adductor pollicis; and thumb adduction from the adductor pollicis.

When considering the median nerve as a potential donor, the surgeon must understand that median nerve motor function is primarily derived from the lower trunk (C8/T1). There is some middle trunk (C7) contribution (mainly the flexor digitorum superficialis, the flexor carpi radialis, and the pronator teres muscles). We only use the median nerve as a donor if the C7, C8, and T1 nerve roots are uninjured. Hence, we avoid using the median nerve as a donor in extended upper brachial plexus injuries for fear of losing useful function.

The surgical exposure for extended upper brachial plexus injuries is less difficult, the degree of damage less daunting, and the reconstructions more straightforward compared to global palsies. Surgical exploration remains the gold standard to assess the degree of damage and the number of nerve root ruptures and avulsions. The surgery is scheduled for 4–6 hours, as the lower trunk does not require reconstruction and CC7 transfer is unnecessary. The surgical priorities are similar to global injuries without the need to address the lower trunk.

In cases with three nerve root ruptures, the goal is anatomic reconstruction using autograft to bridge the gaps between the roots and divisions (Fig. 48.6). Nerve grafts are placed from the C5 nerve root to the suprascapular nerve and/or axillary nerve (posterior division of the upper trunk); C6 nerve root to the anterior division of the upper trunk (musculocutaneous nerve); and C7 nerve root to the middle trunk. Subtle deviations in the surgical reconstruction may be necessary depending upon the quality of each nerve root as a donor. The clavicle may hamper exposure of the divisions (distal targets). Inferior retraction improves distal exposure; however, inadequate visualization for grafting requires clavicular osteotomy. We prefer subperiosteal isolation of the clavicle and performing a greenstick fracture of the clavicle. A bone bitter cuts the inferior half or two thirds of the clavicle, and downward traction completes the fracture yielding distal exposure. Following the procedure, the clavicle is not repaired and quickly heals within its preserved periosteal sleeve (Video 48.5).

In cases with one or two avulsions, surgical creativity is necessary. The donor nerve root is usually the C5 nerve root ± C6 nerve root. The upper trunk is more amenable to nerve transfer reconstruction using the spinal accessory nerve, intercostal nerves, and the ulnar nerve as potential donor sources. In contrast, the middle trunk is less amenable to nerve transfer other than restoration of elbow extension. Therefore, the middle trunk is prioritized for graft reconstruction. The upper trunk is reconstructed with nerve grafts and/or nerve transfers depending upon the number of roots available. In dire straits, the upper trunk can be entirely reconstructed with nerve transfers (spinal accessory to suprascapular nerve transfer, intercostal nerves to musculocutaneous nerve transfer, and ulnar nerve fascicle to axillary nerve).

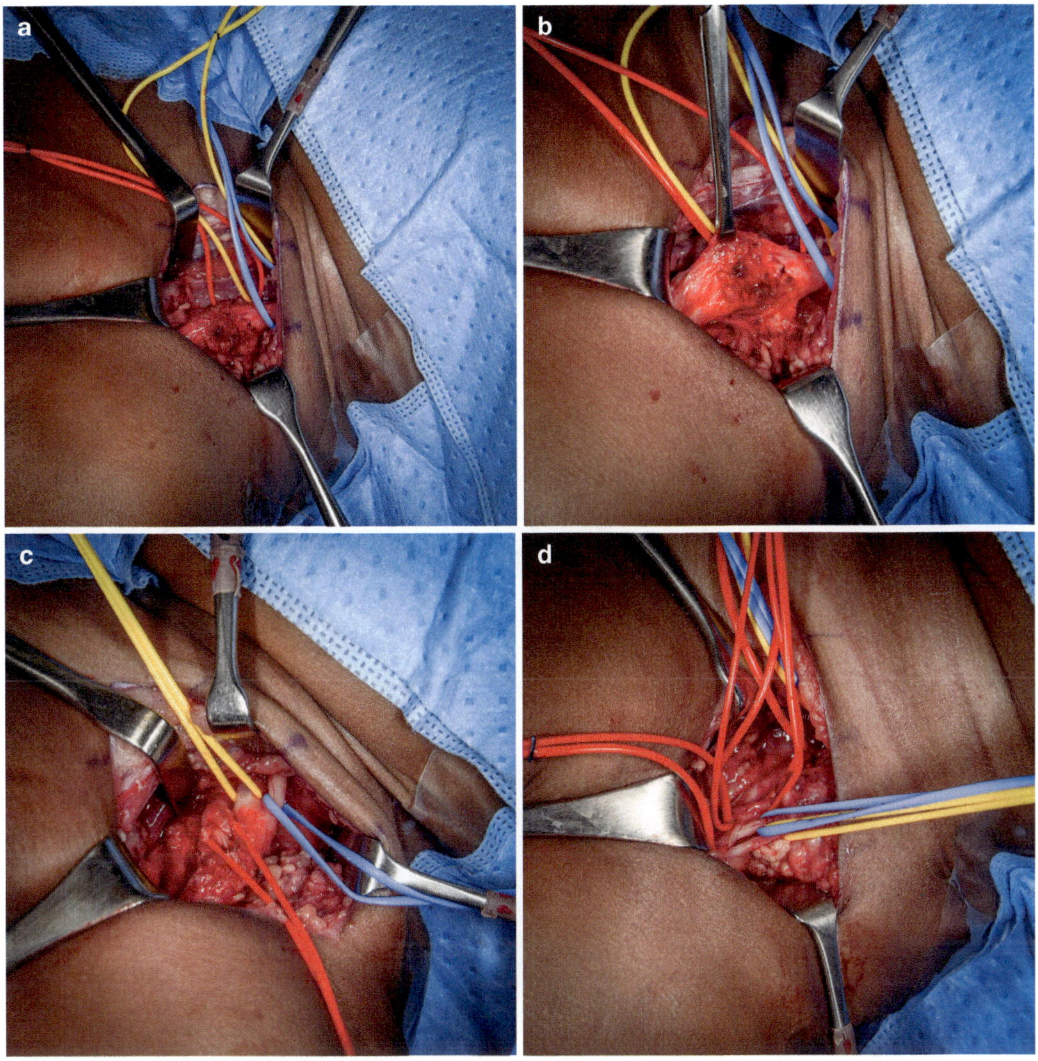

Fig. 48.6 Six-month-old male child with left extended Erb's brachial plexus injury. (Courtesy of Shriners Hospital for Children, Philadelphia). (**a**) Surgical exposure of left brachial plexus. (**b**) Large neuroma. (**c**) Three viable nerve roots (C5, C6, and C7). (**d**) Distal targets to receive autografts from C5, C6, and C7. (Courtesy of Dan A. Zlotolow, MD, with permission)

Upper Brachial Plexus Birth Palsies

Upper brachial plexus injuries are the most straightforward reconstructions as there are a plethora of surgical options available. In addition, the injury is less severe and the entire operation less intimidating and less demanding. The C5 and C6 roots are isolated and the reconstruction options assessed. Nerve grafting alone is appropriate for C5 and C6 nerve root ruptures (Fig. 48.7). Alternatively, except for cases where wrist extension is C6 dependent, an upper plexus injury (C5 and C6 nerve roots) can be entirely reconstructed via a series of nerve transfers. For shoulder reconstruction, spinal accessory nerve to suprascapular nerve transfer combined with a radial nerve triceps branch to the anterior division of the axillary nerve transfer restores the majority of rotator

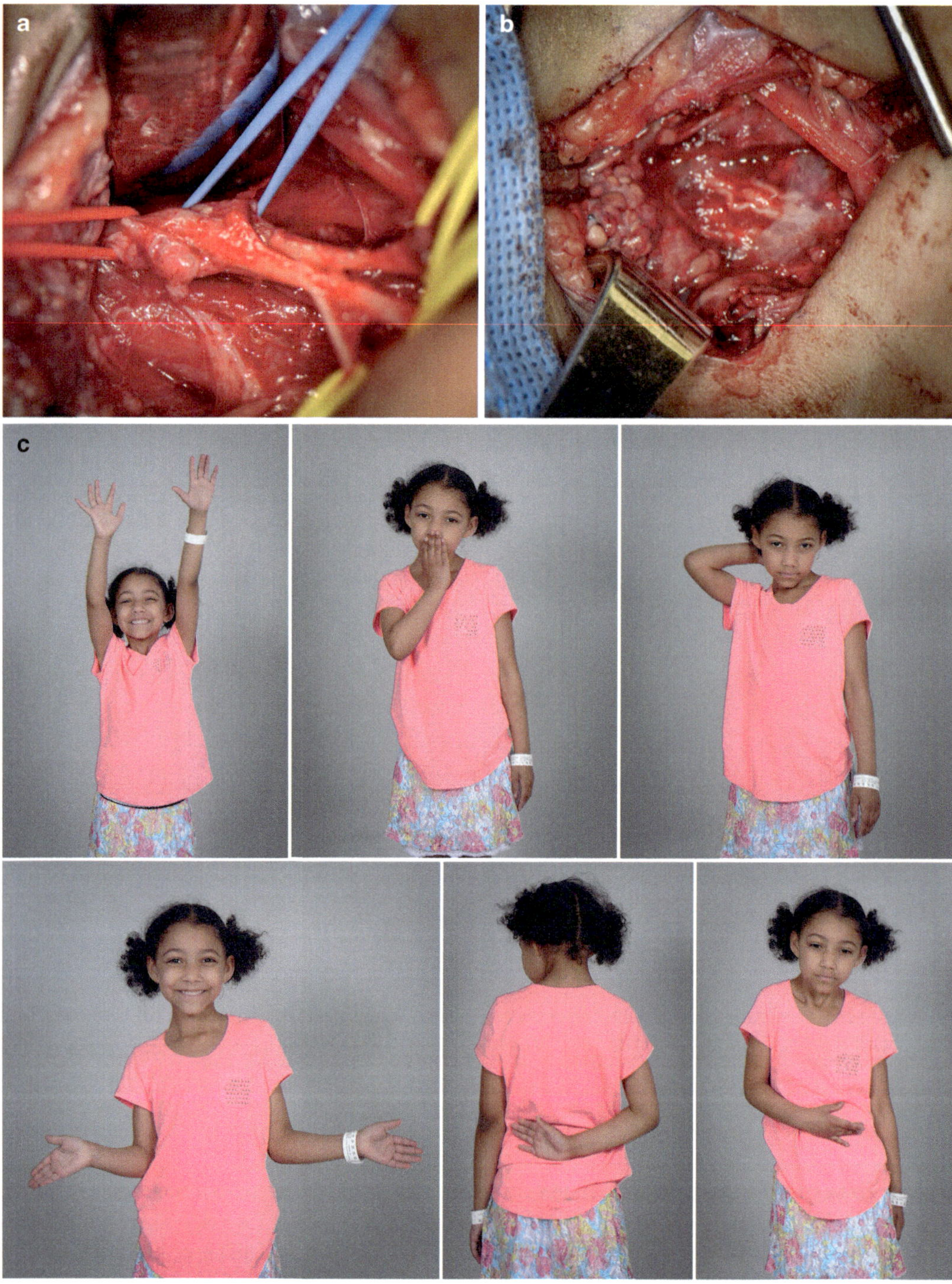

Fig. 48.7 Six-month-old male child with right Erb's (C5 and C6 nerve roots) brachial plexus injury. (Courtesy of Shriners Hospital for Children, Philadelphia). (**a**) Right brachial plexus exploration with upper trunk neuroma and isolation of divisions. (**b**) Nerve grafting from C5 and C6 to upper trunk secured with fibrin glue. (**c**) Outcome at 7 years of age. (*a*) Abduction. (*b*) Hand to mouth. (*c*) Hand to neck. (*d*) External rotation. (*e*) Hand to spine. (*f*) Hand to belly. (Courtesy of Dan A. Zlotolow, MD, with permission)

cuff and deltoid function. For elbow flexion and forearm supination, a double nerve transfer can be performed. A fascicle of the ulnar nerve can be transferred to the biceps motor nerve, and a fascicle of the median nerve can be transferred to the brachialis motor nerve. This series of quadruple nerve transfers can achieve a remarkable result in children (Fig. 48.8).

Surgical Options to Obtain Priorities

Nerve Grafting

Nerve grafting requires neuroma excision back to proximal and distal viable fascicles followed by cable grafting [40]. We use a circumferen-

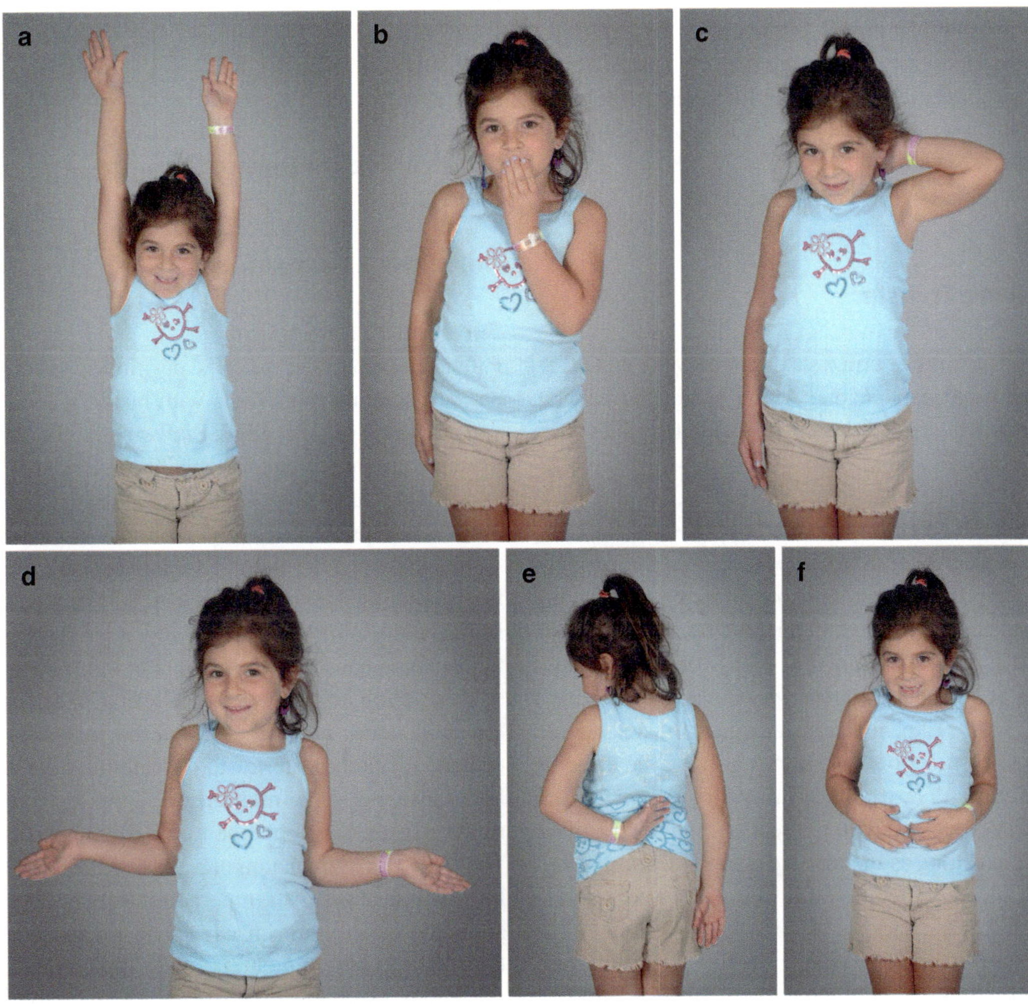

Fig. 48.8 Five-year-old girl with left Erb's (C5 and C6 nerve roots) brachial plexus injury s/p quadruple nerve transfers (spinal accessory nerve to suprascapular nerve, radial nerve triceps branch to the anterior division of the axillary nerve transfer, fascicle of the ulnar nerve to the biceps motor nerve, and fascicle of the median nerve to the brachialis motor nerve). (Courtesy of Shriners Hospital for Children, Philadelphia). (**a**) Abduction. (**b**) Hand to mouth. (**c**) Hand neck. (**d**) External rotation. (**e**) Hand to spine. (**f**) Hand to belly. (Courtesy of Dan A. Zlotolow, MD, with permission)

tial nerve cutting device (Accurate Surgical & Scientific Instrument (ASSI) Corporation, Westbury, New York) to generate an even cut and lessen the trauma to the nerve compared to scissors [41]. Nerve grafting that interposes multiple strands of donor nerve to bridge the defect is referred to as cable grafting. The goal is to place enough cables to satisfy the caliber of the proximal (root) and distal (trunk, division, or branch) recipients. The cable can be secured with microsuture or fibrin glue. The grafts are placed slightly loose without any tension across the coaptation sites. This looseness will lessen the chances of the awake child tearing the repair apart.

Nerve Transfer

Nerve transfer utilizes a donor nerve that is available and expendable, which is transferred to a recipient nerve in need of axons to achieve the desired function.

Selection of the Donor Nerve

The donor nerve has to be available and expendable [40, 63, 35]. Available implies a functioning and normal nerve that can sustain loss of a portion of its axons. Fortunately, many nerves have built in redundancy in their proximal aspect within the arm. Expendable means that if there is some loss of function from donor harvest, the effect is minimal. For example, harvesting the intercostal nerves has negligible effect on pulmonary function as long as the phrenic nerve is working [42]. Similarly, selection of a radial nerve to a single head of the triceps has miniscule effect on elbow extension as long as the other two heads are preserved [43].

An additional consideration during nerve transfer is synergism. Logically, using a donor nerve that provides synergistic function with the intended action would facilitate relearning after reinnervation. For example, when selecting an ulnar nerve fascicle for elbow flexion, selecting the fascicle that innervates the flexor carpi ulnaris would ease relearning.

Selection of the Recipient Nerve

The recipient nerve should be chosen to achieve the desired function. The motor nerve recipient should be close to the end plate to minimize reinnervation time. When selecting recipient motor nerves, there is a trend to provide dual reinnervation to achieve a desired function. For example, nerve transfers for elbow flexion attempt to reinnervate both the biceps and brachialis muscles. Similarly, nerve transfers for shoulder motion try to reinnervate both deltoid and rotator cuff function.

Surgical Techniques to Obtain Priorities

Nerve Graft Harvesting

Sural Nerve Harvesting

Patient position: The baby is positioned supine on the operating room table with his or her feet at the distal edge (Fig. 48.9). Sitting at the foot of the table provides a comfortable harvesting position for the surgeon to harvest the sural nerves under tourniquet control (Fig. 48.8).

Incision: A longitudinal incision along the full course of the sural nerve course can result in a hypertrophic scar in infancy. A long zigzag incision can solve this problem, but parents still complain about the unsightly scar. We prefer sural nerve harvesting via three incisions: oblique incision posterior to the lateral malleolus, transverse in the midportion of the leg, and transverse at the popliteal fossa (Fig. 48.10). The transverse incisions are along Langer's lines and heal with an imperceptible scar. This approach is no more invasive than endoscopic harvesting, which requires additional equipment and usually is performed in the prone position.

Sural Nerve Anatomy

The sural nerve is formed by a connection between the medial sural nerve (MSN, tibial nerve branch) and lateral sural nerve (LSN, common peroneal nerve branch) in approximately two thirds of cases (Huelke type A) [44]. The

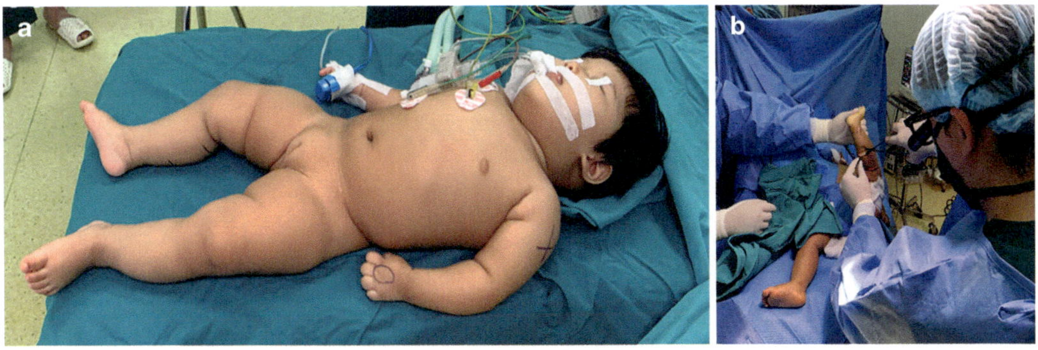

Fig. 48.9 The baby is placed at the end of the table. Sural nerve harvesting is more comfortable if the surgeon faces the baby's lower limbs. The assistant is located lateral to the operating table to hold the infant's lower limbs in a raised position. (Courtesy of Shriners Hospital for Children, Philadelphia). (Courtesy of F. Soldado, MD PhD, with permission)

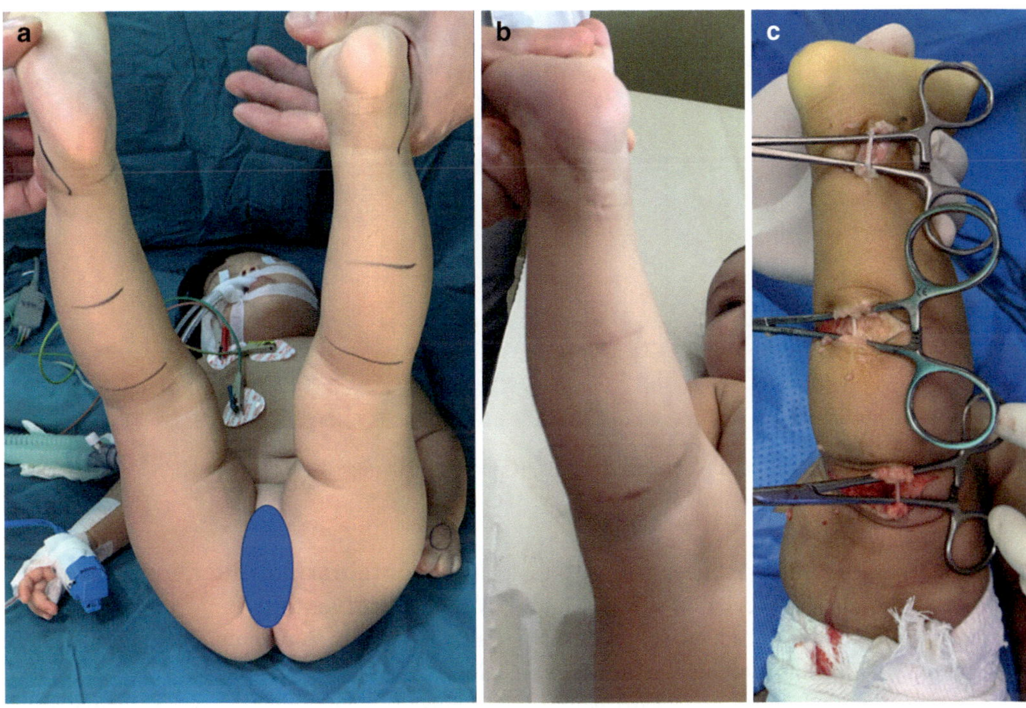

Fig. 48.10 The use of three incisions (**a**) to harvest the sural nerve (**b**) leads to a more aesthetically acceptable result (**c**). (Courtesy of Shriners Hospital for Children, Philadelphia). (Courtesy of F. Soldado, MD PhD, with permission)

connection commonly (80%) occurs in the lower half of the leg. In 30% of cases, the LSN does not contribute to formation of the sural nerve (Huelke type B) (Fig. 48.11). Uncommonly, the sural nerve is formed only by the LSN (Huelke type C). The sural nerve is accompanied by the lesser saphenous vein, which must be protected during harvesting.

Technique: Dissection begins in the distal incision posterior to the malleolus. The sural nerve and lesser saphenous vein are identified in the subcutaneous tissue. The nerve is traced in a proximal direction to the midportion of the leg. Angled retractors of varying sizes assist in the elevation of the skin from the underlying nerve. The investing fascia must be released. Via the

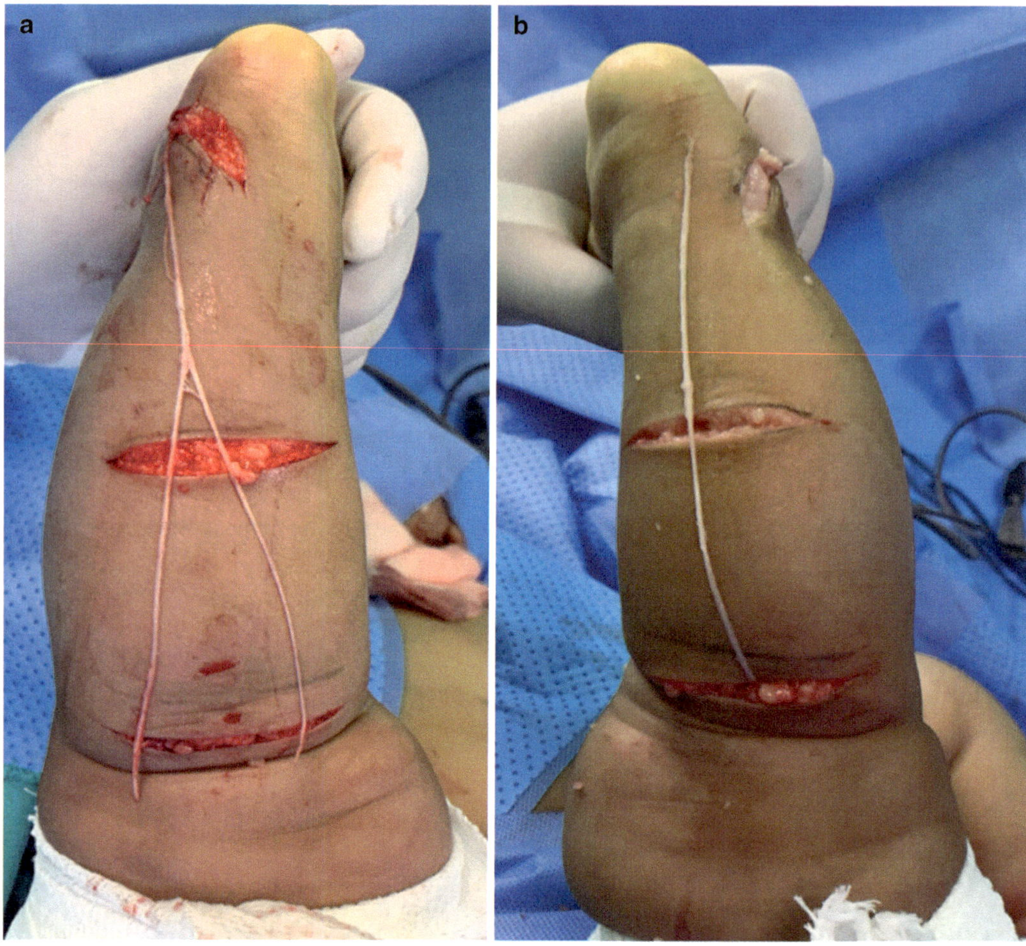

Fig. 48.11 Huelke type A (**a**) and type B sural nerves. (Courtesy of Shriners Hospital for Children, Philadelphia). (Courtesy of F. Soldado, MD PhD, with permission)

middle incision, the MSN is identified deep to the fascia within the gastrocnemius sulcus. More lateral dissection allows for identifying the LSN contribution. Within the popliteal incision, the MSN is also identified deep in the gastrocnemius sulcus and is followed in a proximal direction to its origin from the tibial nerve. When an LSN is present, the nerve is followed to its origin from the common peroneal nerve. The sural nerves must be completely free between the incisions before harvest. Once the sural nerve is cut, all tension is lost, and dissection of any remaining connections within the leg becomes tedious and frustrating.

Medial Antebrachial Cutaneous Nerve (MABCN) Harvesting

Patient position: Supine on the operating room table.

Incision: Longitudinal along the medial arm.

Technique: The MABCN is identified deep to the brachial fascia. The nerve is the most superficial nerve in the brachium and travels with the basilic vein. Harvesting in the arm is straightforward. The nerve is traced in a proximal direction as far as possible toward its origin from the medial cord. Distal dissection is continued in a distal direction including into its two to three terminal branches to optimize graft length.

Radial Sensory Nerve

Patient position: Supine on the operating room table.

Incision: Three transverse forearm incisions with the proximal incision more medial compared to the distal incision (Fig. 48.12).

Technique: The radial sensory nerve is isolated in the distal incision within the subcutaneous tissue. The distal branches of the nerve are followed in a more distal direction to maximize length. Within the middle and proximal incisions, the nerve is localized deep to the fascia, under the deep surface of the brachioradialis muscle. The nerve is dissected as proximal as possible, coagulating branches from radial recurrent vessels and avoiding the posterior interosseous nerve. The nerve is cut distal and retrieved proximal.

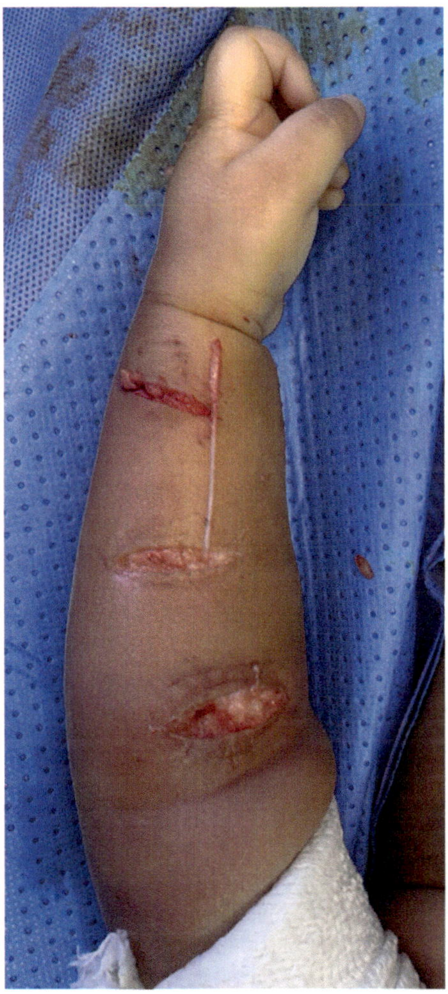

Fig. 48.12 Incisions for harvest of the radial sensory nerve. (Courtesy of Shriners Hospital for Children, Philadelphia). (Courtesy of F. Soldado, MD PhD, with permission)

Nerve Transfer [40, 63, 35]

Spinal Accessory Nerve (SAN) to Suprascapular Nerve (SSN) Transfer

Anterior Approach

Patient position: Use a standard supraclavicular approach for brachial plexus birth palsy exploration. The patient is supine with a rolled towel placed between the scapulae. The baby's head is turned toward the opposite side.

Incision: A transverse incision is made 1 cm above the clavicle similar to brachial plexus exploration (Fig. 48.13a). Another option is a more sagittal incision at the midlevel of the supraclavicular fossa for an isolated SAN to SSN transfer (Fig. 48.13b).

Anatomy: The spinal accessory nerve travels in the window between the levator scapulae and trapezius muscles. The spinal accessory nerve often resides deep to the fascia overlying the anterior surface of the trapezius [45]. A nerve stimulator can help identify the nerve in times of struggle. True landmarks are the cervical transverse vessels entering the muscle. The SAN is isolated adjacent to these vessels and traced in a distal direction. Proximal dissection is also important to move the pivot point closer to the suprascapular nerve. The most superior motor branches to the trapezius muscle must be preserved. The SAN is cut as distal as possible.

The suprascapular nerve exits the upper trunk as a trifurcation along with the anterior and posterior divisions of the upper trunk [46]. The suprascapular nerve travels deep to the suprascapular notch. The lateral head of the omohyoid muscle is a useful landmark for localizing the SSN. Once identified, the SAN is traced in

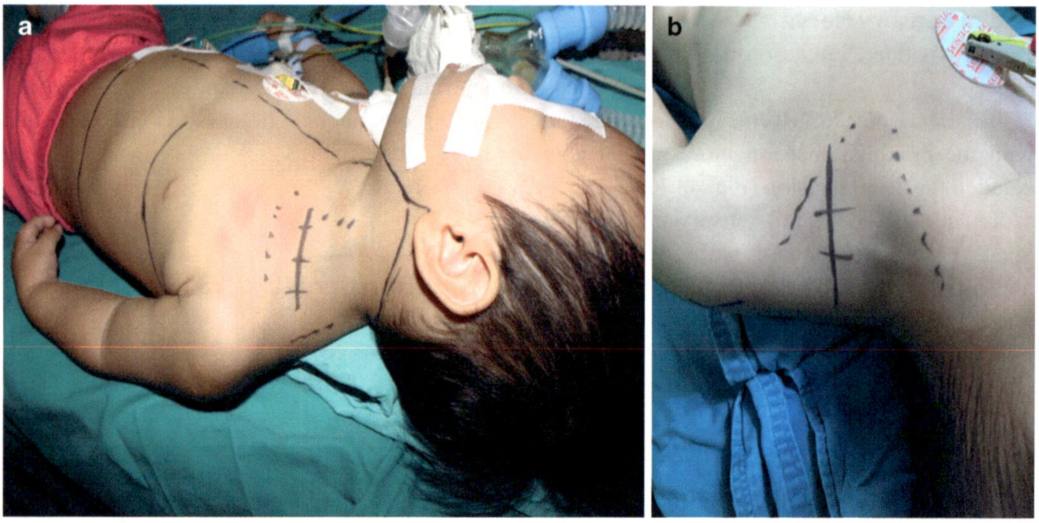

Fig. 48.13 Position and incision options for spinal accessory nerve (SAN) to suprascapular nerve (SSN) transfer. (Courtesy of Shriners Hospital for Children, Philadelphia). (Courtesy of F. Soldado, MD PhD, with permission)

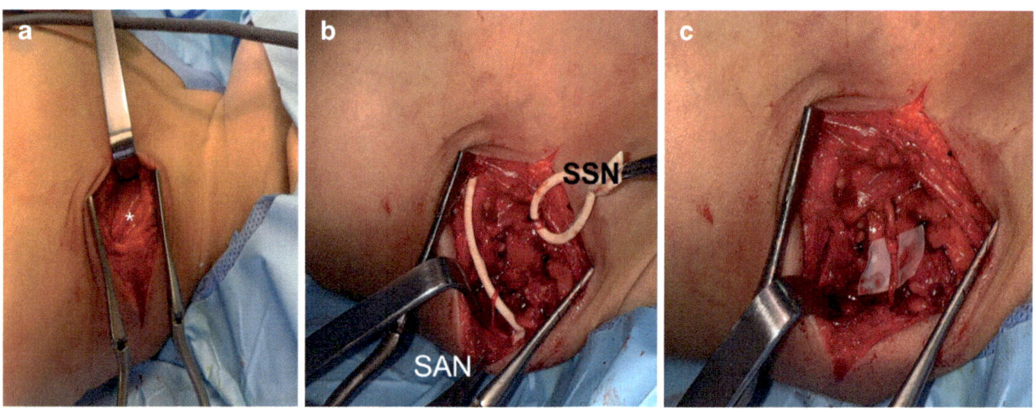

Fig. 48.14 The omohyoid (*) (**a**) is the landmark to find the SSN (**b**); the nerves are coapted without tension (**c**). (Courtesy of Shriners Hospital for Children, Philadelphia). (Courtesy of F. Soldado, MD PhD, with permission)

a proximal direction and cut at its origin in the upper trunk (Fig. 48.14). The SAN and SSN are coapted and secured with fibrin glue.

Additional note: Although there is no supportive evidence published in the literature, some surgeons cut the suprascapular ligament via the anterior approach. The suprascapular nerve is traced in a distal direction with the aid of angled retractors. The trapezius muscle is elevated or detached from the lateral clavicle to facilitate distal dissection. The scapular notch is identified and the ligament is released [47].

Posterior Approach [48]

Patient position: Lateral decubitus or prone on the operating room table.

Incision: A transverse incision just above the spine of the scapula (Fig. 48.15).

Technique: The upper trapezius muscle is elevated from the scapular spine with electrocautery (Video 48.6) (Fig. 48.15). The underlying supraspinatus muscle is identified and is often pale secondary to denervation. The trapezius is elevated in a cephalad direction and supraspinatus retracted in a caudad position. The omohyoid

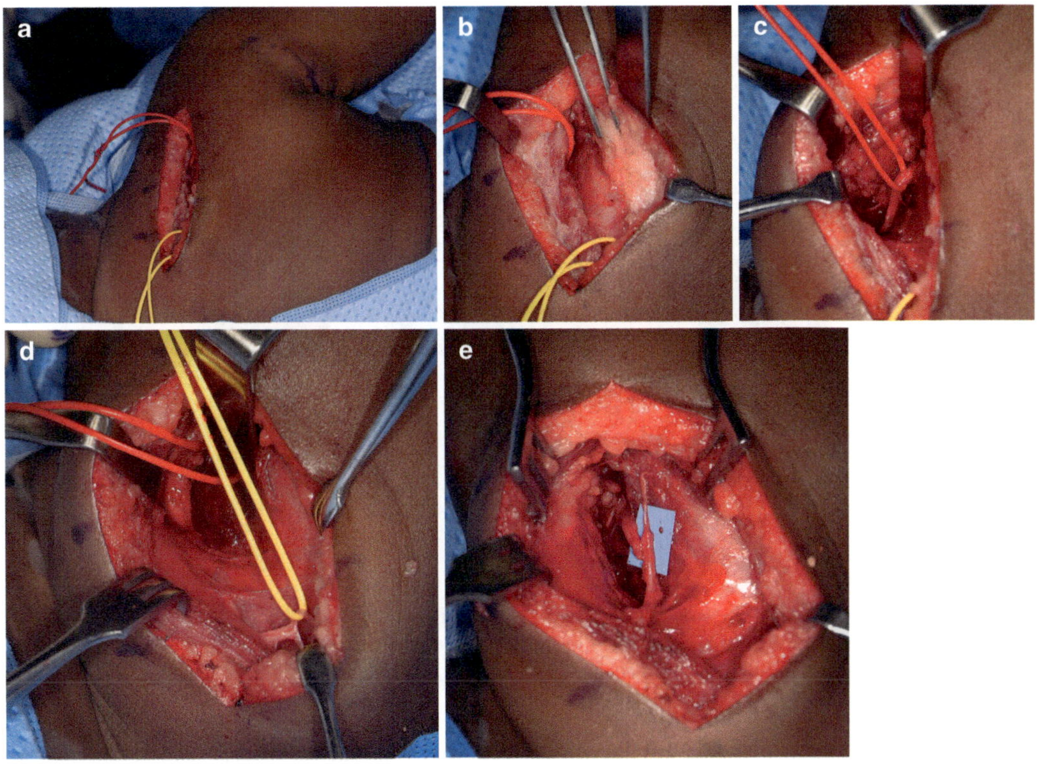

Fig. 48.15 Spinal accessory to suprascapular nerve transfer via posterior surgical approach. (Courtesy of Shriners Hospital for Children, Philadelphia). (**a**) Infant positioned in the lateral decubitus position. (**b**) Trapezius muscle elevated from scapular spine (forceps). (**c**) Suprascapular nerve identified and traced through the scapular notch with release of the superior transverse scapular ligament. (**d**) Spinal accessory nerve isolated deep to the trapezius muscle. (**e**) Spinal accessory transferred to suprascapular nerve with excessive length to allow for nerve trimming and tension-free coaptation. (Courtesy of Dan A. Zlotolow, MD, with permission)

muscle is identified inserting on the top of the scapula just medial to the suprascapular notch. The notch and ligament are isolated. The suprascapular nerve is deep to the ligament and the suprascapular vessels pass over the spinous ligament. The ligament is sectioned while protecting the underlying nerve. The suprascapular nerve is traced in a proximal direction to its trifurcation from the upper trunk. The spinal accessory nerve is localized deep to the trapezius muscle, running in a vertical direction just lateral to the medial border of the scapula. The spinal accessory nerve is traced in a distal direction, deep to the inferior trapezius, and divides into two main terminal branches, which are cut as distal as possible for tensionless coaptation with the suprascapular nerve.

Spinal Accessory Nerve to the Infraspinatus Motor Nerve [48, 49]

Patient position: Lateral decubitus or prone position on the operating room table.

Incision: Transverse along the scapular spinous process (Fig. 48.16).

Technique: The spinal accessory is localized identical to the posterior approach described above. The infraspinatus motor branch is isolated at spinoglenoid notch. The infraspinatus muscle is partially detached from the scapular spine and retracted in an inferior direction. The infraspinatus motor nerve is identified at the spinoglenoid notch (Fig. 48.16). The suprascapular vessel courses with the nerve and must be protected to avoid bleeding. The infraspinatus motor branch is

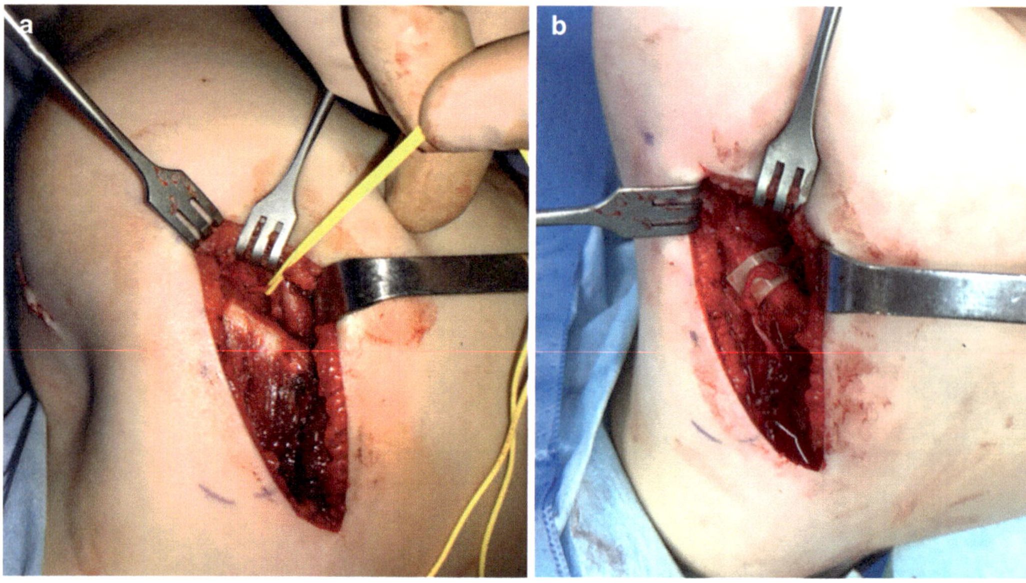

Fig. 48.16 The infraspinatus nerve is identified arriving from the spinoglenoid notch (**a**) to be transferred to the spinal accessory nerve (**b**). (Courtesy of Shriners Hospital for Children, Philadelphia). (Courtesy of F. Soldado, MD PhD, with permission)

sectioned as proximal as possible and the nerves are coapted using fibrin glue.

Ulnar to Biceps Motor Nerve [50, 51, 52]

Patient position: Supine on the operating room table with the arm on a hand table.

Incision: Longitudinal incision along the middle half of the brachium.

Technique: The skin is incised and the dissection is carried out deep to the fascia (Fig. 48.17) (Video 48.7). The medial antebrachial cutaneous nerve and basilic vein are isolated and mobilized. The musculocutaneous nerve (MCN) is identified between the coracobrachialis and biceps muscles. The nerve is traced in a distal direction eyeing for motor branches entering the biceps muscle. In two thirds of patients, the MCN provides one branch to the biceps muscle in the proximal half of the arm and one branch to the brachialis muscle in the distal part [54].

After biceps motor nerve dissection, the MCN is followed in a distal direction until its division into the lateral antebrachial cutaneous nerve and brachialis motor branch. The brachialis branch is more medial. The lateral antebrachial cutaneous nerve continues in a distal direction to enter the forearm (lateral antebrachial cutaneous nerve). The motor branches (biceps and brachialis) are dissected under magnification in a proximal direction by intraneural dissection to gain length and mobility (usually 1–2 cm).

The median nerve is isolated medial to the brachial vessels, while the ulnar nerve is located posterior to the medial intermuscular septum. Under magnification, a longitudinal epineurotomy is performed to identify a donor motor fascicle. The chosen fascicle must be redundant and expendable. A nerve stimulator on low amplitude is necessary to demonstrate redundant extrinsic and intrinsic musculature. Although obtaining fascicles that preferentially activate extrinsic muscles (FCR for median nerve and FCU for ulnar nerve) has been recommended, there is no evidence to support its benefit [55]. Before fascicle sectioning, the surgeon must understand that the median nerve glides in a distal direction with elbow extension, while the ulnar nerve glides in a distal direction with elbow flexion. The donor fascicles of the ulnar nerve and median nerves are traditionally transferred to the biceps and brachialis motor nerves, respectively. However, the donor-recipient combination can be performed in the opposite direction depending upon the surgeon preference and patient's anatomy.

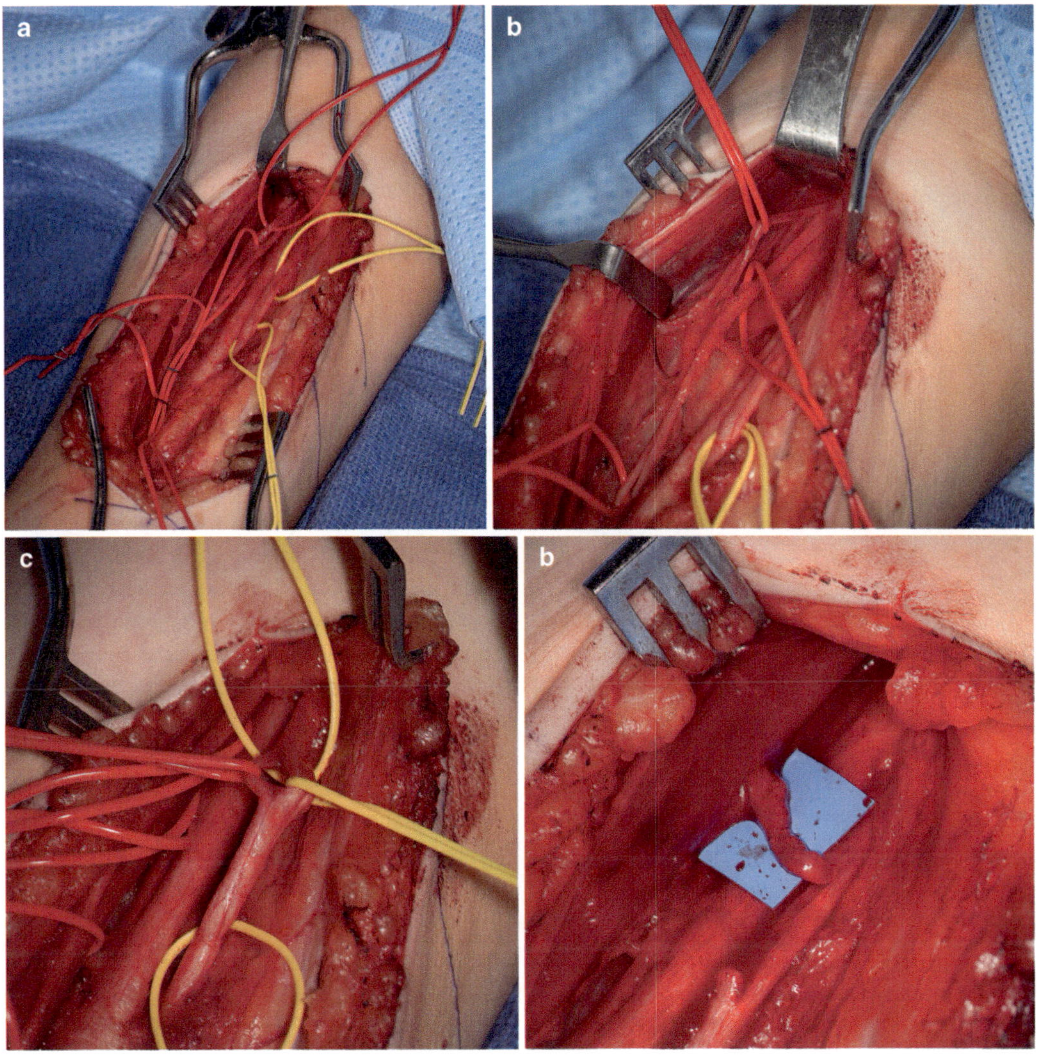

Fig. 48.17 Ulnar motor fascicle transfer to the bicep's motor nerve. (Courtesy of Shriners Hospital for Children, Philadelphia). (**a**) Medial arm exposure. Yellow loops around ulnar nerve and red loops around musculocutaneous nerve. (**b**) Bicep's motor nerve isolated from musculocutaneous nerve. (**c**) Isolation of a fascicle from the ulnar nerve. (**d**) Transfer of the fascicle from the ulnar nerve to the bicep's motor nerve. (Courtesy of Dan A. Zlotolow, MD, with permission)

Triceps to Axillary and Triceps to Teres Minor Transfer [53]

Patient position: Supine.

Incision: We prefer the axillary approach [56]. The axillary crease skin is incised in a triangle configuration with an extension along the medial arm (Fig. 48.18a).

Dissection: The latissimus dorsi tendon is the main anatomical landmark to identify motor branches from the posterior cord [56] (Fig. 48.18b). The radial nerve is identified running above the latissimus dorsi tendon. The motor nerve branches to the long head of the triceps (LHTc), lateral head of the triceps, and the medial head (UMTc) are identified (Fig. 48.19). The axillary nerve is located proximal to the proximal border of the latissimus dorsi tendon along with the posterior circumflex humeral vessels (medial with relationship to the arm) entering the quadrangular space. The axillary nerve divides into an anterior division (lateral with relationship to the arm) and a posterior division (medial with relationship to the arm). The posterior division provides a medial motor nerve branch to the teres minor (medial with relationship to the arm).

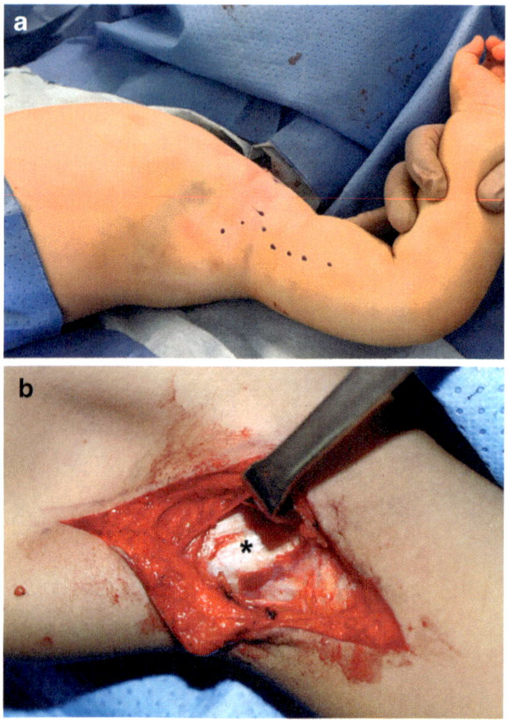

Fig. 48.18 Axillary approach using an inverted V-shaped incision (**a**). The latissimus dorsi tendon (**b**) is the landmark used to identify the radial and axillary nerves. (Courtesy of Shriners Hospital for Children, Philadelphia). (Courtesy of F. Soldado, MD PhD, with permission)

Both triceps branches and axillary divisions are dissected under magnification by intraneural dissection to obtain as much length to achieve tensionless coaptation. During triceps to axillary transfers, the long head of the triceps (LHTc) and the medial head (UMTc) are transferred to the anterior division of the AxN and teres minor motor branch [56]. The donor-recipient combination is dependent upon the surgeon's preference.

Intercostal to Musculocutaneous Nerve Transfers [42, 57]

Patient position: Supine on the operating room table with the baby's shoulder in abduction.

Incisions: A thoracic incision is planned along the ribs from the posterior axillary line to the costochondral junction. In babies, the future inframammary crease can be produced by pushing the breast tissue in a downward direction (Fig. 48.20). This incision ultimately will be well-concealed. The brachial incision is placed along the proximal medial arm (Fig. 48.21a). A subcutaneous tunnel is created between the two incisions to bring the intercostal nerve (ICN) to the MCN, or the two incisions can be connected with an intervening axillary incision (Fig. 48.21c).

The anterior surfaces of the ribs are exposed by elevation of the pectoralis major and minor mus-

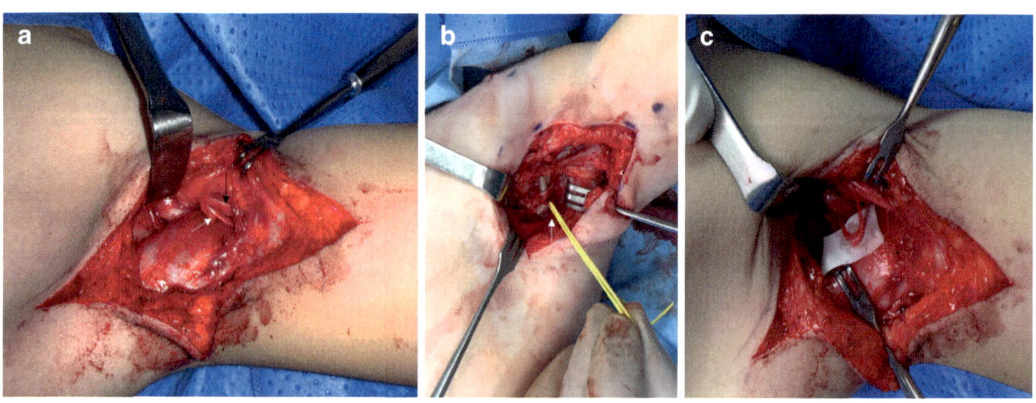

Fig. 48.19 (**a**) The motor branch to the long head of the triceps (white arrow) is identified following the medial side of the radial nerve (black arrow). The axillary nerve is marked with *. (**b**) The motor branch to the teres minor (white arrow) originates from the posterior division of the axillary nerve. (**c**) Both nerves are coapted. (Courtesy of Shriners Hospital for Children, Philadelphia). (Courtesy of F. Soldado, MD PhD, with permission)

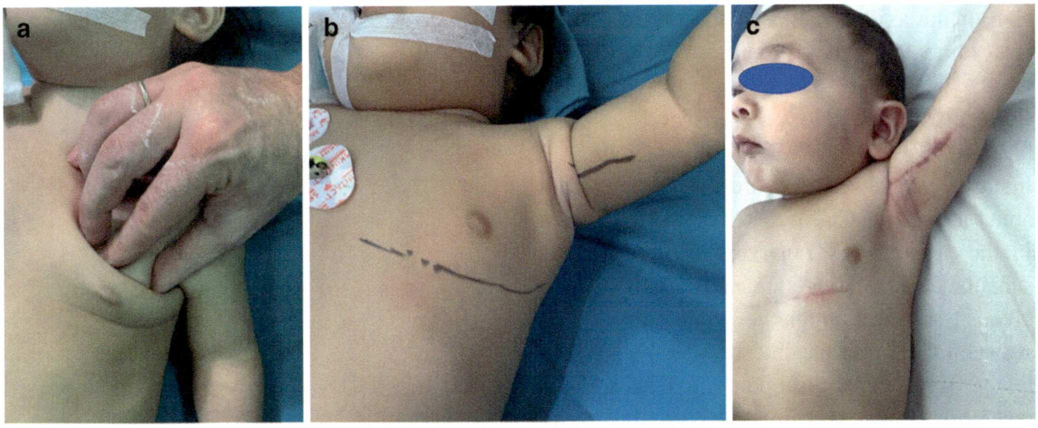

Fig. 48.20 A thoracic incision in the future inframammary crease will improve the aesthetic appearance (**a**). This incision is extended from the costochondral junction to the posterior axially line. Brachial incision (**b**). Healed incision 4 weeks after surgery (**c**). (Courtesy of Shriners Hospital for Children, Philadelphia). (Courtesy of F. Soldado, MD PhD, with permission)

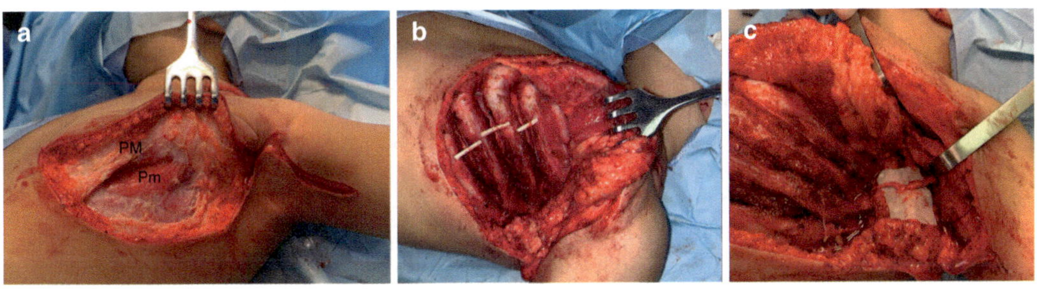

Fig. 48.21 The origins of the pectoralis major (PM) and minor (Pm) are detached. In this case, the thoracic incision is connected to the brachial incision (**a**), with intercostal nerves 3–5 dissected (**b**). The ICN are coapted to the musculocutaneous nerve (**c**). (Courtesy of Shriners Hospital for Children, Philadelphia). (Courtesy of F. Soldado, MD PhD, with permission)

cles (Fig. 48.21b). Between the ribs, the intercostal nerves are isolated. The identification begins at the most cephalad rib and proceeds in a caudad direction. The superficial intercostal muscle is released from the inferior aspect of the rib. Using gentle spreading dissection with a small hemostat and upward traction on the rib, the intercostal nerve and artery are isolated (Video 48.8). We do not use subperiosteal dissection as this technique increases surgical time, bleeding, and morbidity. Once the nerve is located, the nerve is dissected from the costochondral junction to the posterior axillary line to avoid any need for an intervening nerve graft. The third, fourth, and fifth intercostal nerves (or fourth, fifth, and sixth) are harvested in a similar fashion.

Through the medial arm incision, the MCN is isolated between the coracobrachialis and biceps muscles. The nerve is dissected in a proximal direction through the coracobrachialis muscle, ensuring the coracobrachialis has been completely released. The musculocutaneous nerve is traced as proximal as possible toward the lateral cord.

The intercostal nerves are passed to the MCN and coapted with epineural sutures or fibrin glue. Coaptation should be completed with the shoulder in maximum abduction to prevent disruption of the coaptation during passive shoulder exercises.

Intercostal to Axillary Nerve Transfers

Patient position: Supine on the operating room table with the baby's shoulder in abduction.

Incisions: The axillary and thoracic incisions are performed as described above. Three intercostal nerves are transferred to the anterior division of the axillary nerve and the branch to the teres minor.

Contralateral C7 Nerve Transfer [37, 58, 59]

In cases with fewer than three nerve roots available for grafting, CC7 transfer can be considered. In the past, the CC7 nerve root was tunneled subcutaneously across the neck to the injured plexus [58, 59]. Long nerve grafts were required between CC7 and the intended recipients (e.g., lower trunk) with disappointing results. More recently, a passage behind the esophagus has been utilized to shorten the distance and lessen the graft length [37]. This approach requires surgical expertise as the vertebral artery and carotid sheath are in harm's way. We utilize the assistance of our cervical spine surgeons who are comfortable with the exposure for anterior cervical spine procedures. The procedure requires proficiency and meticulous technique to avoid consequential mishaps.

All global injuries with no recovery of lower and middle trunk function by 3 months are potential candidates for a CC7 transfer. We begin this procedure with the patient prone. Both sural nerves are harvested and placed on ice in a saline-soaked nonadhesive dressing inside a specimen cup. The spinal accessory to suprascapular nerve transfer is performed from the posterior approach while prone. The patient is then repositioned supine with an A-frame under the shoulders (Fig. 48.22). The intravenous catheter and monitoring equipment are moved to the legs. The arms, neck, and chest are prepped and draped in one field.

If intraoperative dissection of the plexus yields two or fewer viable nerve roots for grafting, the decision is made to use the CC7 as a donor. In the past, we utilized two separate supraclavicular incisions. Currently, we simply extend the supraclavicular incision along Langer's lines to the contralateral neck to the level of the trapezius (Fig. 48.23). This allows an extensile approach to both the injured and uninjured brachial plexus and the entire neck. The dissection is carried down to the plexus, which should be normal (Fig. 48.24). A nerve stimulator (Checkpoint®, Checkpoint Surgical, Cleveland, Ohio) is used to confirm the redundancy of the middle trunk: stimulation of the posterior division of the lower trunk should produce elbow and finger extension, and stimulation of the posterior division of the upper trunk should produce wrist extension. The entire C7 root and middle trunk are isolated to the level where the divisions merge with the divisions of the other two trunks. It is critically important to make sure that both the anterior division of the upper trunk and the posterior divisions of the upper and lower trunks are visualized and isolated from the divisions of the middle trunk prior to cutting the middle trunk. The lateral pectoral nerve has a takeoff at the point where the anterior divisions of the upper and middle trunks meet. Proximally, the C7 contribution to the long thoracic nerve may need to be divided to provide greater mobility of the root, depending on its branch point.

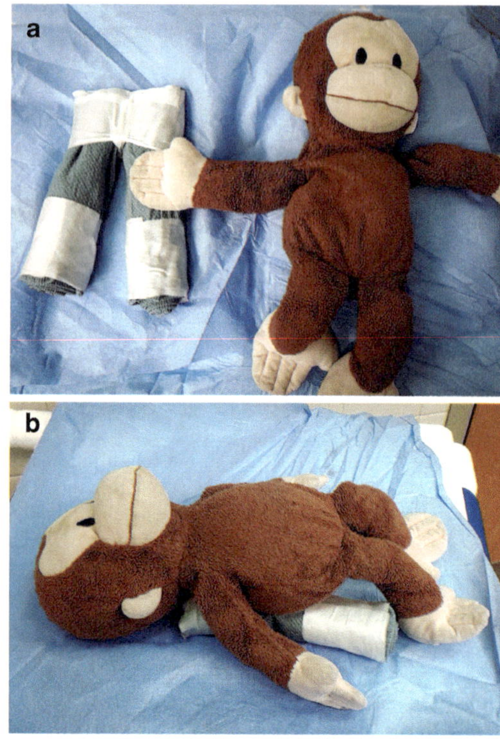

Fig. 48.22 A-frame comprised of two rolled towel taped together (**a**) stabilizes infant on operating room table (**b**) and allows access to both sides. (Courtesy of Shriners Hospital for Children, Philadelphia). (Courtesy of Dan A. Zlotolow, MD, with permission)

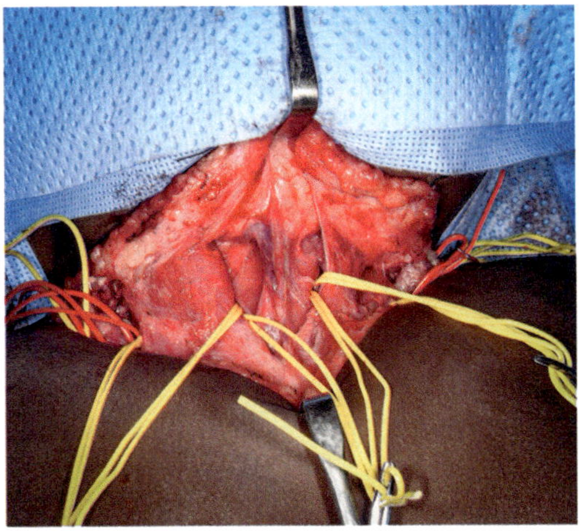

Fig. 48.23 Contralateral C7 transfer can be performed using a supraclavicular incision along Langer's lines from the injured side to the contralateral neck to the level of the trapezius. (Courtesy of Shriners Hospital for Children, Philadelphia). (Courtesy of Dan A. Zlotolow, MD, with permission)

We prefer to keep the anterior scalene intact to protect the phrenic nerve. A right angle is passed from the neuroforamen directly anterior through the interval between the longus coli and the anterior scalene muscles, and a looped vessel loop is passed from anterior to posterior around the C7 root. This loop helps to pass the CC7 medial to the scalene muscle to shorten the distance without dividing the anterior scalene. Further dissection is carried out anterior to the scalene muscle. The interval is between the phrenic nerve and the carotid sheath. We try not to violate the carotid sheath, as none of its contents are relevant to the operation and these only increase the risks of surgery when exposed. With blunt dissection in a lateral to medial direction, the vertebral artery is identified and the space directly superior developed. We have had to pass the CC7 inferior to the vertebral artery in some cases to create a more direct (shorter) path, but this should be done with extreme caution. Injury to the vertebral artery is difficult to manage and typically requires an emergent transfer to interventional radiology for embolization.

Another window is created in the anterior triangle of the injured side of the neck. The skin of the neck is sutured to the chin for temporary retraction (Fig. 48.23). Dissection is carried down to the prevertebral space through the interval between the carotid sheath and the esophagus, which can look remarkably similar. There are multiple vessels in this interval, which we try to preserve whenever possible.

A dissection on the injured side of the neck between the phrenic nerve and the carotid sheath is then performed bluntly to connect the ipsilateral plexus window with the ipsilateral anterior triangle window and the contralateral plexus window. Again, the vertebral artery is at risk. Another looped vessel loop is passed from the ipsilateral to the contralateral side.

The CC7 is then re-explored and division points reconfirmed. Lidocaine is injected into the epineural space with a 1 cc 27-gauge insulin needle at the root of the C7 to limit trauma to the motoneuron cell bodies. We use a circumferential nerve cutting device (Accurate Surgical & Scientific Instrument (ASSI) Corporation, Westbury, New York) to generate an even cut and lessen the trauma to the nerve compared to scissors [41].

The CC7 is then passed between the anterior scalene and longus coli muscles and across the neck into the anterior triangle window using the preplaced vessel loops. The target trunk on the injured side is mobilized as medial as possible, and autograft nerve is interposed between the CC7 and the target trunk. Fixation at the coaptation sites is achieved with fibrin glue or a combination of glue and suture.

Rehabilitation

Nerve Grafting

Nerve rehabilitation following nerve grafting is divided into an immobilization phase followed by a mobilization phase awaiting nerve regeneration (Protocol 1). The immobilization position varies with the tightness of any joint. Supple joints allow immobilization in a swathe wrapping the arm against the body. A tight joint, such as a shoulder internal rotation contracture, requires immobilization in a shoulder spica cast stretching

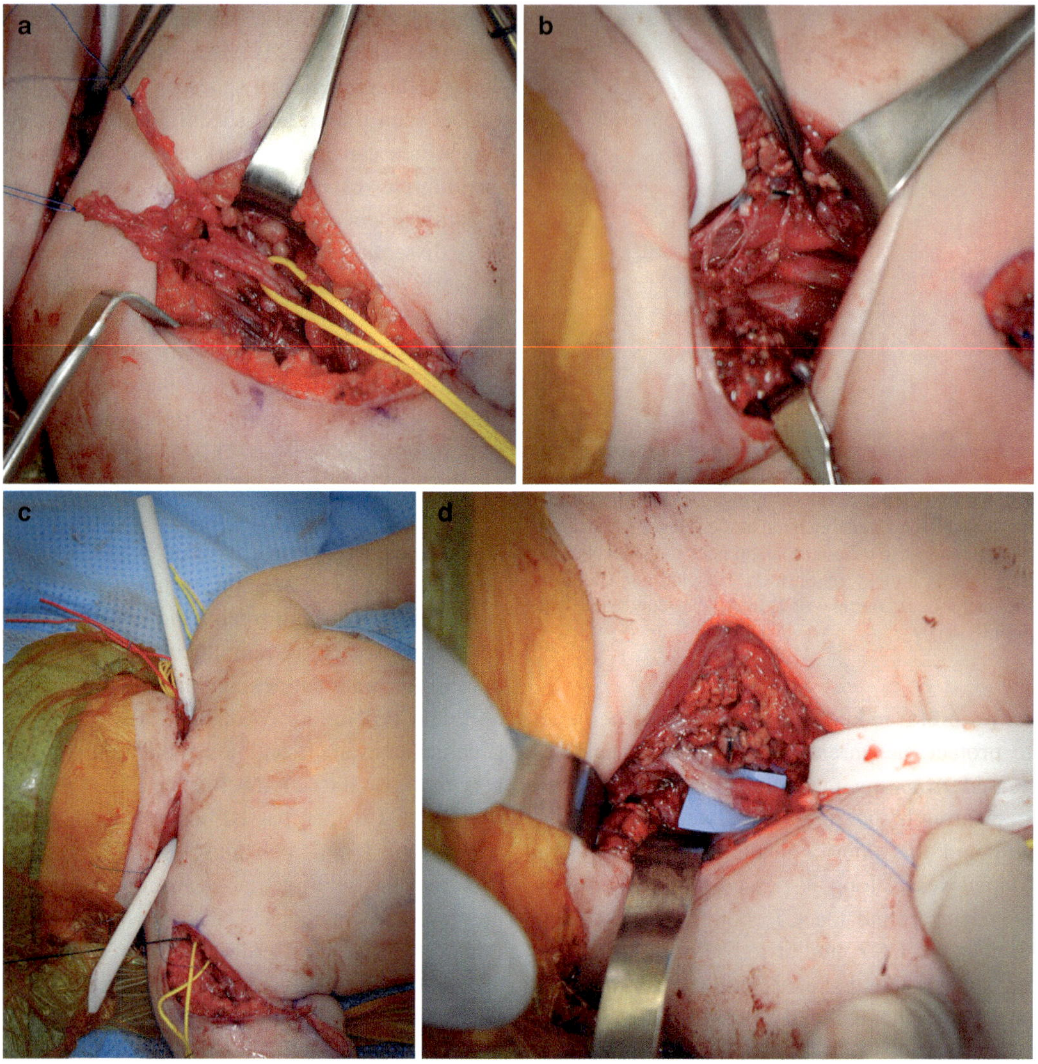

Fig. 48.24 Three-month-old child with right global brachial plexus palsy, Horner's syndrome, and pseudomeningoceles at C8 and T1. (Courtesy of Shriners Hospital for Children, Philadelphia). (**a**) Exploration revealed frank ruptures of C5 and C6 without continuity. (**b**) Examination of the lower trunk (C8 and T1) beneath the subclavian artery revealed intraforaminal avulsions. (**c**) Passage developed behind the esophagus from the normal left brachial plexus to the injured right brachial plexus. (**d**) Contralateral left C7 nerve trunk grafted to right C8 and T1 nerve roots using 2.5 cm sural nerve grafts. (Courtesy of Dan A. Zlotolow, MD, with permission)

the glenohumeral joint. Immobilization is continued for 3–4 weeks.

The mobilization phase is initiated in therapy and continued at home via a home exercise program (HEP). The joints are stretched to maintain suppleness awaiting nerve regeneration. Incisional care is also instructed. The therapist must educate the parents on nerve regeneration as months will pass before active motion is seen. In addition, sensory recovery can result in hyperesthesia in infants that manifests as scratching or biting (Fig. 48.25). The biting can be severe and result in infection and even nibbling away of the affected fingertips. Regrettably, there is no

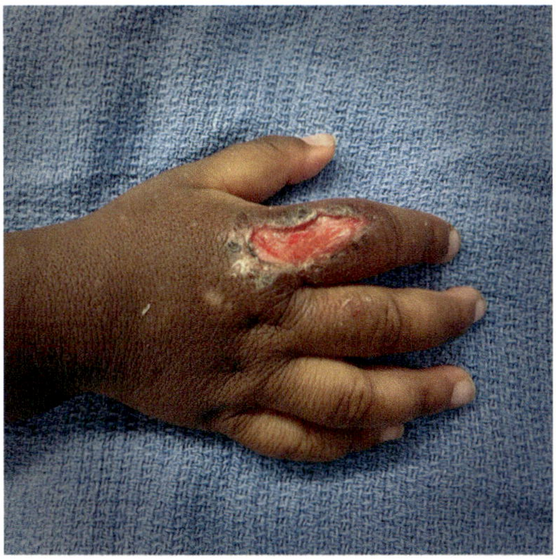

Fig. 48.25 Tactile hyperesthesia in babies with brachial plexus palsies manifests as biting that can be severe. (Courtesy of Shriners Hospital for Children, Philadelphia). (Courtesy of Dan A. Zlotolow, MD, with permission)

intellectual reasoning with infants and the parents feel horrible about the biting. We have tried numerous medical and home remedies to no avail as the infants continue to gnaw at their digits. Fortunately, as the sensory recovery progresses and the tactile hyperesthesia lessens, the biting diminishes. The result is often physical scarring to the child and emotional scarring to the parents.

Nerve Transfer

Nerve rehabilitation following nerve transfer is straightforward. Following a brief period of immobilization to allow for wound healing, the arm is mobilized. Certain nerve transfers allow unrestricted motion, while other nerve transfers have postoperative limitations (e.g., intercostal nerve transfer – Protocol 2). Nerve regeneration occurs at a rate of 1 mm/day. The patients are instructed to link their donor and recipient nerve function (e.g., flexor carpi ulnaris wrist flexion and elbow flexion following ulnar to bicep's motor nerve transfer) to promote cortical learning. This combined movement pattern is performed numerous times per day awaiting nerve regeneration. When the donor nerve regenerates to the recipient muscle, the patient will "learn" to fire his or her recipient movement independent of donor function.

Outcomes

Nerve Grafts

Reported outcomes following nerve grafting are difficult to decipher. There are variable injury patterns, varying surgical approaches, and different methods of assessing outcome. The shared theme is that the outcome varies directly with the number of nerve roots ruptured and avulsed. In addition, avulsion of the lower roots portends the worst functional outcome.

Gilbert reported on 436 patients who underwent surgical reconstruction [60, 61]. Follow-up was a minimum of 4 years and included those patients who had undergone secondary reconstructive procedure. Assessment of outcome and function utilized the Mallet scale. For children with C5–C6 injuries, 80% of patients achieved good or excellent shoulder function. In C5–C7 injuries, 61% attained good or excellent shoulder function. For C5–T1 injuries, only 25% recovered useful hand function.

Clarke and colleagues at The Hospital for Sick Children reported important data regarding the role of neurolysis [62]. The cohort consisted of 108 patients with long-term follow-up (minimum of 4 years). Sixteen underwent neurolysis of conducting neuromas-in-continuity compared to 92 (48 with C5–C6 injuries and 44 with total plexus palsies) that were treated with neuroma resection and nerve grafting. The authors concluded that early functional improvements following neurolysis were not sustained over time. In contrast, neuroma resection and nerve grafting produced significant functional improvement for both C5–C6 injuries and total plexus palsies. Hence, neurolysis should be abandoned in favor of neuroma resection and nerve grafting.

Nerve Transfers

The published reports for nerve transfer in brachial plexus birth palsy have focused on the shoulder and elbow [63]. Many series include variable injury patterns, concomitant nerve grafting, and secondary procedures that confound the results. The spinal accessory to suprascapular nerve transfer has discrepancies in the published outcome, especially concerning external rotation [64, 65]. Malessy and colleagues rigorously assessed the results following nerve grafting of C5 to the suprascapular nerve (n = 65) or nerve transfer of the accessory nerve to the suprascapular nerve (n = 21) in a retrospective analysis 3 years after surgery [65]. Outcome was expressed in degrees of true glenohumeral external rotation, which can be only performed by infraspinatus muscle. Only 17 (20%) of the 86 patients reached more than 20 degrees of external rotation, whereas 35 (41%) were unable to perform true external rotation. There was no statistically significant difference between nerve grafting from the C5 nerve root and nerve transfer using the spinal accessory nerve. Functional scores were better with 88% of children able to reach their mouth and 75% could touch their head. The authors concluded that restoration of true glenohumeral external rotation after nerve graft or nerve transfer to the suprascapular nerve in brachial plexus birth palsies was suboptimal. However, compensatory techniques allow a considerable range of functional motion.

Nerve transfers for elbow flexion for elbow in children brachial plexus birth palsy have more positive outcomes. Nerve donors have included the medial pectoral nerve, ulnar nerve, and median nerve. Blaauw and Slooff published a large series of 25 children that underwent transfer of the pectoral nerves to the musculocutaneous nerve [66]. Results were reported as excellent in 17 children and fair in five patients with two failures. A small series by Noaman and a larger series by Little and colleagues have reported excellent results with the ulnar and/or median nerve [50, 67]. Noaman reported a series of seven children that underwent ulnar nerve transfer to the biceps at an average of 16 months of age. Five children recovered M3 or greater elbow flexion, while two children recovered less than M3 strength [67]. Little and colleagues reviewed 31 patients that underwent nerve transfer for elbow flexion using the ulnar and/or median nerve fascicle transfer to the biceps and/or brachialis branches of the musculocutaneous nerve [50]. The primary outcome measure was elbow flexion and supination as measured on the Active Movement Scale (AMS). Of the 31 patients, 27 (87%) obtained functional elbow flexion (AMS $\geq$ 6) and 24 (77%) had full flexion recovery (AMS = 7). Of the 24 patients for whom supination recovery was recorded, only 5 (21%) obtained functional recovery (AMS $\geq$ 6). Single fascicle transfer resulted in functional flexion (AMS $\geq$ 6) in 85% (22/26) and functional supination (AMS $\geq$ 6) in only 15% (3/20). Combined ulnar and median nerve fascicle transfers were performed in five patients. This combination resulted in full elbow flexion (AMS = 7) and supination (AMS $\geq$ 5) in all patients.

References

1. Narakas AO. Obstetric brachial plexus injuries. Chapter 9. In: Lamb DW, editor. The paralyzed hand. Edinburgh: Churchill Livingstone; 1987. p. 117–22.
2. Al-Qattan MM, El-Sayed AAF, Al-Zahrani AY, Al-Mutairi SA, Al-Harbi MS, Al-Mutairi AM, Al-Kahtani FS. Narakas classification of obstetric brachial plexus palsy revisited. J Hand Surg. 2009;34E:788–91.
3. Foad SL, Mehlman CT, Foad MB, Lippert WC. Prognosis following neonatal brachial plexus palsy: an evidence-based review. J Child Orthop. 2009;3:459–63.
4. Malessy MJA. Obstetric brachial plexus injuries. Neurosurg Clin NA. 2009;20(1):1–14.
5. Sibinski M, Synder M. Obstetric brachial plexus palsy-risk factors and predictors. Orthop Traumatol Rehabil. 2007;9:569–76.
6. Clarke HM, Curtis CG. An approach to obstetrical brachial plexus injuries. Hand Clin. 1995;11:563–81.
7. Bae DS, Waters PM, Zurakowski D. Reliability of three classification systems measuring active motion in brachial plexus birth palsy. J Bone Joint Surg Am. 2003;85:1733–8.
8. Curtis C, Stephens D, Clarke HM, Andrews D. The active movement scale: an evaluative tool for infants with obstetrical brachial plexus palsy. J Hand Surg Am. 2002;27:470–8.

9. Schott JM, Rossor MN. The grasp and other primitive reflexes. J Neurol Neurosurg Psychiatry. 2003;74:558–60.
10. Fu SY, Gordon T. The cellular and molecular basis of peripheral nerve regeneration. Mol Neurobiol. 1997;14:67–116.
11. Pamphlett R. Early terminal and nodal sprouting of motor axons after botulinum toxin. J Neurol Sci. 1989;92:181–92.
12. Gordon T, Borschel GH. The use of the rat as a model for studying peripheral nerve regeneration and sprouting after complete and partial nerve injuries. Exp Neurol. 2017;287(Pt 3):331–47.
13. Rogozhin AA, Pang KK, Bukharaeva E, Young C, Slater CR. Recovery of mouse neuromuscular junctions from single and repeated injections of botulinum neurotoxin A. J Physiol Lond. 2008;586: 3163–82.
14. Mills KR. The basics of electromyography. J Neurol Neurosurg Psychiatry. 2005;76(suppl 2):32–5.
15. Lispi L, Leonardi L, Petrucci A. Longitudinal neurophysiological assessment of intramuscular type-A botulin toxin in healthy humans. Neurol Sci. 2018;39(2):329–32.
16. Gordon T, Tyreman N. Sprouting capacity of lumbar motoneurons in normal and hemisected spinal cords of the rat. J Physiol. 2010;588:2745–68.
17. Tam SL, Archibald V, Tyreman N, et al. Increased neuromuscular activity reduces sprouting in partially denervated muscles. J Neurosci. 2001;21:654–67.
18. Rafuse VF, Gordon T, Orozco R. Proportional enlargement of motor units after partial denervation of cat triceps surae muscles. J Neurophysiol. 1992;68:1261–75.
19. Yang JF, Stein RB, Jhamandas J, et al. Motor unit numbers and contractile properties after spinal cord injury. Ann Neurol. 1990;28:496–502.
20. Gordon T, Yang JF, Ayer K, et al. Recovery potential of muscle after partial denervation: a comparison between rats and humans. Brain Res Bull. 1993;30:477–82.
21. Gordon T. Nerve regeneration: understanding biology and its influence on return of function after nerve transfers. Hand Clin. 2016;32:103–17.
22. Witzel C, Rohde C, Brushart TM. Pathway sampling by regenerating peripheral axons. J Comp Neurol. 2005;485:183–90.
23. Brushart TM. Motor axons preferentially reinnervate motor pathways. J Neurosci. 1993;13:2730–8.
24. Tomatsuri M, Okajima S, Ide C. Sprout formation at nodes of Ranvier of crush-injured peripheral nerves. Restor Neurol Neurosci. 1993;5(4):275–82.
25. Terzis JK, Novikov ML. Radiological and electrophysiological detection of nerve roots avulsion in patients with birth-related brachial plexus paralysis. Semin Plast Surg. 2005;19:24–41.
26. Chow BCL, Blaser S, Clarke HM. Predictive value of computed tomographic myelography in obstetrical brachial plexus palsy. Plast Reconstr Surg. 2000;106:971–9.
27. Shenaq SM, Berzin E, Lee R, et al. Brachial plexus birth injuries and current management. Clin Plast Surg. 1998;25(4):527–36.
28. van Dijk JG, Pondaag W, Malessy MJ. Obstetric lesions of the brachial plexus. Muscle Nerve. 2001;24:1451–61.
29. Steens SCA, Pondaag W, Malessy MJA, Verbist BM. Obstetric brachial plexus lesions CT myelography. Radiology. 2011;259:508–15.
30. Kawai H, Tsuyuguchi Y, Masada K, Heise CO, Siqueira MG, Martins RS. Identification of the lesion in brachial plexus injuries with root avulsion: a comprehensive assessment by means of preoperative findings, myelography, surgical exploration and intraoperative diagnosis. Neuro-Orthop. 1989;7: 15–23.
31. Vanderhave KL, Bovid K, Alpert H, Chang KW, Quint DJ, Leonard JAJ, Yang LJ. Utility of electrodiagnostic testing and computed tomography myelography in the preoperative evaluation of neonatal brachial plexus palsy. J Neurosurg Pediatr. 2012;9:283–9.
32. Yilmaz K, Calişkan M, Oge E, Aydinli N, Tunaci M, Ozmen M. Clinical assessment, MRI, and EMG in congenital brachial plexus palsy. Pediatr Neurol. 1999;705–710(1999):21.
33. Al-Qattan MM, Clarke HM, Curtis CG. The prognostic value of concurrent Horner's syndrome in total obstetric brachial plexus injury. J Hand Surg Br. 2000;25:166–7.
34. Waters PM. Comparison of the natural history, the outcome of microsurgical repair, and the outcome of operative reconstruction in brachial plexus birth palsy. J Bone Joint Surg Am. 1999;85:649–59.
35. Kozin SH. Nerve transfers in brachial plexus birth palsies: indications, techniques, and outcome. Hand Clin. 2008;24:363–76.
36. Pondaag W, Malessy MJA. Recovery of hand function following nerve grafting and transfer in obstetric brachial plexus lesions. J Neurosurg. 2006;105: 33–40.
37. Wang SF, Li PC, Xue YH, Yiu HW, Li YC, Wang HH. Contralateral C7 nerve transfer with direct coaptation to restore lower trunk function after traumatic brachial plexus avulsion. J Bone Joint Surg Am. 2013;95:821–7.
38. Moore AM, MacEwan M, Santosa KB, et al. Acellular nerve allografts in peripheral nerve regeneration: a comparative study. Muscle Nerve. 2011;44:221–34.
39. Pang D, Mackinnon SE, Wood MD. Advances in the repair of segmental nerve injuries and trends in reconstruction. Muscle Nerve. 2019; https://doi.org/10.1002/mus.26797. (Epub ahead of print).
40. Kozin SH. Nerve repair manual. Beachwood: Checkpoint Surgical; 2016.
41. Smetana B, Wolfmeyer K, Lovett S, Romot B, Orrico M, Greenberg JA. Improving nerve end preparation for neurorrhaphy through use of a circumferentially constraining surgical device. Presented at the 2018 Annual Meeting of the American Association for Hand Surgery, 10–13 Jan 2018, Phoenix, Arizona.

42. Malessy MJ, Thomeer RT. Evaluation of intercostal to musculocutaneous nerve transfer in reconstructive brachial plexus surgery. J Neurosurg. 1998;88:266–71.
43. Leechavengvongs S, Witoonchart K, Uerpairojkit C, Thuvasethakul P, Malungpaishrope K. Combined nerve transfers for C5 and C6 brachial plexus avulsion injury. J Hand Surg Am. 2006;31:183–9.
44. Ramakrishnan PK, Henry BM, Vikse J, et al. Anatomical variations of the formation and course of the sural nerve: a systematic review and meta-analysis. Ann Anat – Anat Anzeiger. 2015;202:36–4.
45. Bertelli JA, Ghizoni MF. Improved technique for harvesting the accessory nerve for transfer in brachial plexus injuries. Oper Neurosurg. 2006;58:366–70.
46. Leung S, Zlotolow DA, Kozin SH, Abzug JM. Surgical anatomy of the supraclavicular brachial plexus. J Bone Jt Surg Am. 2015;97(13):1067–73.
47. Zlotolow DA, Low SL, Lin IC, Williamson C, Tinsley B, Kozin SH. Suprascapular ligament release from an anterior approach: an anatomic feasibility study. J Hand Surg Am. 2019;44:900.e1–4.
48. Colbert SH, Mackinnon S. Posterior approach for double nerve transfer for restoration of shoulder function in upper brachial plexus palsy. Hand. 2006;1:71–7.
49. Bhandari PS, Deb P. Posterior approach for both spinal accessory nerve to suprascapular nerve and triceps branch to axillary nerve for upper plexus injuries. J Hand Surg Am. 2013;38:168–72.
50. Little KJ, Zlotolow DA, Soldado F, Cornwall R, Kozin SH. Early functional recovery of elbow flexion and supination following median and/or ulnar nerve fascicle transfer in upper neonatal brachial plexus palsy. J Bone Joint Surg Am. 2014;96:215–21.
51. Oberlin C, Béal D, Leechavengvongs S, Salon A, Dauge MC, Sarcy JJ. Nerve transfer to biceps muscle using a part of ulnar nerve for C5-C6 avulsion of the brachial plexus: anatomical study and report of four cases. J Hand Surg Am. 1994;19:232–7.
52. Mackinnon SE, Novak CB, Myckatyn TM, Tung TH. Results of reinnervation of the biceps and brachialis muscles with a double fascicular transfer for elbow flexion. J Hand Surg Am. 2005;30A:978–85.
53. Leechavengvongs S, Witoonchart K, Uerpairojkit C, Thuvasethakul P. Nerve transfer to deltoid muscle using the nerve to the long head of the triceps, part II: a report of 7 cases. J Hand Surg Am. 2003;28:633–8.
54. Soldado F, Ghizoni MF, Bertelli J. Thoracodorsal nerve transfer for elbow flexion reconstruction in infraclavicular brachial plexus injuries. J Hand Surg Am. 2014;39:1766–70.
55. Smith BW, Chulski NJ, Little AA, Chang KWC, Yang LJS. Effect of fascicle composition on ulnar to musculocutaneous nerve transfer (Oberlin transfer) in neonatal brachial plexus palsy. J Neurosurg Pediatr. 2018;22(2):181–8.
56. Bertelli JA, Kechele PR, Santos MA, Duarte H, Ghizoni MF. Axillary nerve repair by triceps motor branch transfer through an axillary access: anatomical basis and clinical results. J Neurosurg. 2007;107(2):370–7.
57. El-Gammal TA, Abdel-Latif MM, Kotb MM, et al. Intercostal nerve transfer in infants with obstetric brachial plexus palsy. Microsurgery. 2008;28(7):499–504.
58. Chen L, Gu Y-D, Hu S-N, Xu J-G, Xu L, Fu Y. Contralateral C7 transfer for the treatment of brachial plexus root avulsions in children—a report of 12 Cases. J Hand Surg Am. 2007;32(1):96–103.
59. Gu YD, Zhang GM, Chen DS, Yan JG, Cheng XM, Chen L. Seventh cervical nerve root transfer from the contralateral healthy side for treatment of brachial plexus root avulsion. J Hand Surg Br. 1992;17:518–21.
60. Gilbert A. Long-term evaluation of brachial plexus surgery in obstetrical palsy. Hand Clin. 1995;11:583–94.
61. Gilbert A, Pivata G, Kheiralla T. Long-term results of primary repair of brachial plexus lesions in children. Microsurgery. 2006;26:334–42.
62. Lin J, Schwentker-Colizza A, Curtis CG, Clarke HM. Final results of grafting versus neurolysis in obstetrical brachial plexus palsy. Plast Reconstr Surg. 2009;123:939–48.
63. Clarke H, Tse R, Malessy M, Kozin S. The role of nerve transfers in the treatment of neonatal brachial plexus palsy, International Federation of Societies for Surgery of the Hand (IFSSH) Scientific Committee on neonatal brachial plexus palsy. IFSSH ezine. 2015;5:17–25.
64. Kawabata H, Kawai H, Masatomi T, Yasui N. Accessory nerve neurotization in infants with brachial plexus birth palsy. Microsurgery. 1994;15:768–72.
65. Pondaag W, de Boer R, van Wijlen-Hempel MS, Hofstede-Buitenhuis SM, Malessy MJ. External rotation as a result of suprascapular nerve neurotization in obstetric brachial plexus lesions. Neurosurgery. 2005;57:530–7.
66. Blaauw G, Slooff AC. Transfer of pectoral nerves to the musculocutaneous nerve in obstetric upper brachial plexus palsy. Neurosurgery. 2003;53:338–41.
67. Noaman HH, Shiha AE, Bahm J. Oberlin's ulnar nerve transfer to the biceps motor nerve in obstetric brachial plexus palsy: indications, and good and bad results. Microsurgery. 2004;24:182–7.

49 Specificity and Controversies in the Management of Obstetric Brachial Plexus Lesions

Jörg Bahm

Introduction

After 20 years of regular clinical and scientific experience with all surgical aspects of brachial plexus birth injury (BPBI), I was allowed by the editors of this book to give in this chapter a personal and synoptic view on specific achievements and still existing controversies about this fascinating field of functional reconstructive surgery.

I combine my acquired surgical expertise with a literature review, influenced and weighted by my active participation in a lot of congresses and symposia dedicated to peripheral nerve surgery and especially obstetric palsy.

As many and even very recent articles describe the general features of BPBI [12], and as the overall strategy is also detailed by other authors in the present book (see chapters written by Gilbert, Kozin, Muset, et al.), we concentrate on specific details, relevant for the surgical treatment, expanding thereby the description of our center's strategy and experience [1].

J. Bahm (✉)
Section for Plexus Surgery, Clinic for Plastic, Hand and Burn Surgery, RWTH University Hospital Aachen, Aachen, Germany
e-mail: jorg.bahm@belgacom.net

A. Y. Shin, N. Pulos (eds.), *Operative Brachial Plexus Surgery*,
https://doi.org/10.1007/978-3-030-69517-0_49

Causation, Risk Factors, and Types

Obstetric causation mainly concerns relevant traction on a heavy child (macrosomia, feto-maternal disproportion, peripartum emergency) or a breech delivery (shearing of rootlets).

Non-obstetric circumstances for upper limb weakness and thus diagnostic alternatives are:

- Atypical upper limb arthrogryposis (without relevant joint ankylosis).
- Transient upper limb weakness, well-known by neuropediatricians (this condition doesn't need more than physiotherapy as it resolves within months).

Types: In our unit, we easily distinguish the frequent *upper* type (involving the roots C5 and C6 – extended upper when C7 is also affected), the more rare but impressive *total* palsy (flail limb, no hand function, all roots involved), and the exceedingly rare *C7-centered* lesion (Fig. 49.1) with the typical posture of a medially rotated and elbow flexed arm.

Natural History

The natural evolution is conditioned by the *extent and severity of the initial nerve lesion* and the ongoing activity of biological nerve regeneration and its speed, allowing a progressive

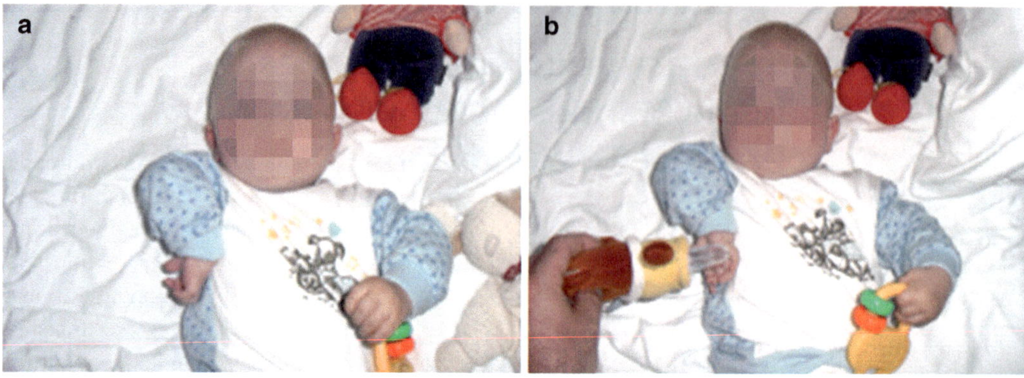

Fig. 49.1 C7 centered lesion

proximal-to-distal functional recovery both for sensation and motion. Motor recovery is limited by the capacity of muscle denervation atrophy to reverse and motor end plate survival. Little is known about the exact behavior of the latter under variable denervation conditions [6] and the functional prognosis, but some information helps our clinical decision-making:

1. After 18 months, severe muscle denervation might not be overcome by reinnervation. A commonly accepted sign of functional muscle death is the extinction of spontaneous fibrillation activity in the electromyogram (EMG).
2. Sensory end organs seem to survive longer periods of denervation and may be targeted even later on.

The timing of any early nerve reconstruction surgery is thus conditioned by our knowledge of the biology of regenerating cones and the target organs.

Clinically, our observation focuses on the *muscle imbalance between agonists and antagonists* and the biomechanical consequence of *impaired growth and development* – both affecting functional limb integration.

Most importantly, we frequently observe medial rotation imbalance of the shoulder joint, evolving into glenohumeral dysplasia, as well as, but more rarely, complex radial head imbalance in elbow flexion-supination resulting in a radial head anterior subluxation or even dislocation and eventually associated elbow flexion contracture. Fortunately, wrist or finger joint deformities are very rare but existent (e.g., ulnar head dysplasia associated with an ulnar deviated wrist; [3, 4]).

Thus, any clinical observation of a child affected by BPBI must be interdisciplinary and not driven only by nerve concerns (as it is initially a nerve trauma) but also include all orthopedic aspects (deformity, growth) and the goal of functional reintegration, even when anatomy might not be normalized.

Therapy

Neurophysiology-based physiotherapy is routinely prescribed at least for 12–18 months for every child with an initial severe lesion, undergoing nerve regeneration and progressive functional recovery. "Neurophysiology-based" means with detailed understanding of the regeneration process, target recovery, and the relearning of the complex but physiologic motion pattern during the first years of life. Special attention is given to all muscle imbalances, the development of soft tissue contractures, and orthopedic deformities at the shoulder, elbow, and wrist level.

Task-oriented *occupational therapy* is started later on in preschool age and focuses on daily activities for social independence and leisure.

Splinting is recommended in specific situations, either supportive-corrective or as a preventive tool:

- Corrective splint: for wrist drop, elbow extension lag.
- Preventive splint: like the lateral rotation-supination dynamic (night) splint.

Diagnostic Ancillary Procedures

We do not rely on electrodiagnostic tools in little children, as in our country only very few neurologists are qualified and the examination is potentially painful and mainly because a good correlation between the findings and their prognostic value (estimation of the amount of root damage) may only be validated in teams with long-term skills [5].

Concerning lesion imagery, we ask for a magnetic resonance imaging (MRI) if root avulsion is suspected (like in breech presentation or when the muscle waste is very fast and spectacular). Perhaps in the near future, high-resolution ultrasound (being noninvasive, needing no sedation) may define the type and ultrastructure of neuromas or rupture sites in the supraclavicular area. This exam demands miniaturized probes and standardized examination conditions.

Timing and Surgical Strategy

Timing

Any total lesion without hand recovery in the first 2 months and any proven root avulsion will need an early surgical exploration and repair, generally before 3 months. There might be a decision conflict with anesthesiology about safety and risks [13, 14]. Newborns under 5 kg, babies with a "poly-trauma" history of birth, and especially those with weakened respiratory function (diaphragm palsy by phrenic nerve damage, bronchiolitis, airway problems) must be evaluated and discussed carefully.

In our unit, all subtotal (meaning with preserved hand function) cases with insufficient functional recovery are operated between 6 and 9 months (or even older) to expose and repair the common root or trunk ruptures and neuroma. In an unpublished cohort comparison of upper BPBI children operated before or after 12 months, there was no significant difference in the postoperative outcome for shoulder and biceps function [8] – that does not mean that we would wait all that time, but that we consider for primary surgery also children presenting the first time older than 9 months, if the shoulder or elbow flexion function is definitely too weak.

Surgical Strategy

The primary aim of any BPBI reconstructive surgery of the brachial plexus itself is to re-establish a near to normal anatomy, i.e., a root to trunk continuity. This requires a minimum of three good-quality roots available and the direct coaptation of the proximal and distal stumps, best by suture – which is possible for some short neuroma under 15 mm and after extensive distal dissection [3, 4] – or by routine fascicular grafting.

If upper root quality is bad, either considering their number or histologic tissue quality, meaning an insufficient motor fiber source, additional nerve transfers must be considered.

With two or less available roots, a priority list of functional targets must be followed (Table 49.1) and includes absolute priority of the hand, the focus on a basic limb function including active elbow flexion and shoulder stability with sufficient active abduction (60°), forward flexion (30°), and active lateral rotation. In these cases, additional donors for extraplexic neurotization must be considered like the spinal acces-

Table 49.1 Major targets for primary reconstruction surgery

Hand first: Sensation and finger (thumb) flexion
Elbow flexion
Shoulder stability and motion (including a stable scapula)
Elbow and wrist extension
Forearm prosupination

sory nerve (for suprascapular nerve or biceps motor branch) or intercostal nerves (for biceps or triceps targeting).

We don't use contralateral C7 transfers in children, unlike other teams with good results [9] and never use the phrenic nerve in children.

In some specific conditions (more than two root avulsions), we actually stress a transdisciplinary paradigm, thinking out of the "nerve-only" box, and target additional distal nerves like the thoracodorsal and long thoracic nerve in the primary setting with intercostal nerves, in anticipation of potential late surgery: a reinnervated latissimus dorsi muscle is always a good secondary donor, and a stabilized scapula by means of basic serratus and trapezius muscle function allows further motion reconstruction by means of muscle transfers.

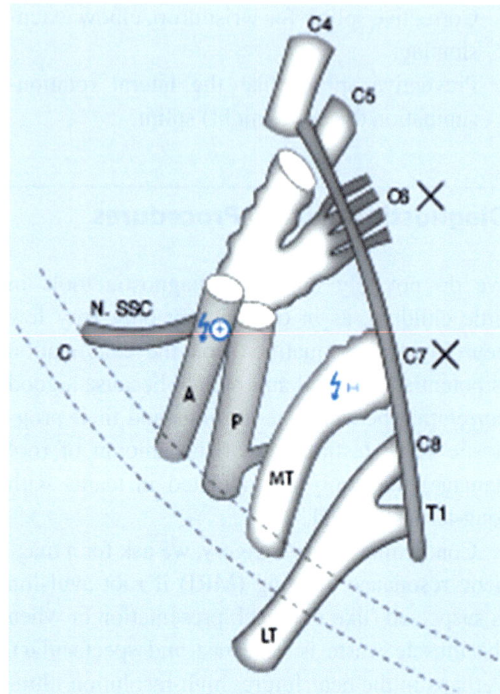

Fig. 49.2 Intraoperative drawing

Technique

Child supine, head turned to the contralateral side, neck-arm and one leg sterilized and draped. Suprascapular transverse approach, adipolymphatic fat pad retraction, exposure of the interscalene triangle, supra- and retroclavicular dissection, identification of the lesion, resection of scar and neuroma, proximal and distal stump assessment by instant neuropathologic examination of the stump slices, intraplexic reconstruction.

Documentation in a drawing (Fig. 49.2); 3 weeks of immobilization (Fig. 49.3).

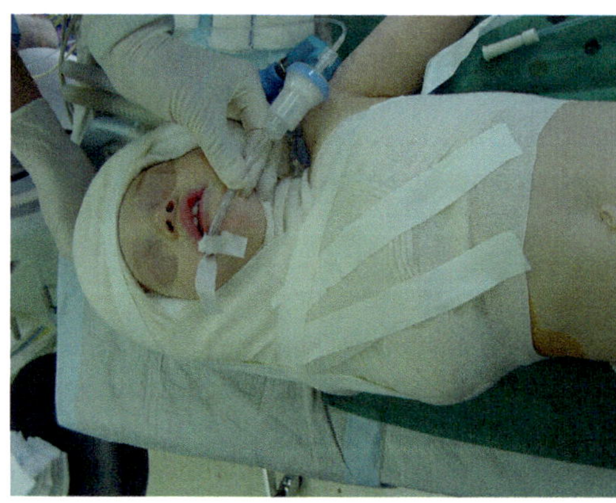
Fig. 49.3 Immobilization

Nerve Transfer Techniques (Table 49.2)

When performing a nerve transfer, one has to consider the frequent difference in tissue quality of the healthy donors and the demyelinated recipients: difficult (interfascicular) suture, implying high quality of the microsurgical technique in nerve coaptation.

Our most frequent transfer aims to re-establish the shoulder rotational balance, by transferring the distal branch of the spinal accessory nerve onto the suprascapular nerve, generally nonselective, but in specific cases on the motor branch to the infraspinatus muscle or teres minor muscle. This contributes to our regimen of early treatment of shoulder medial rotation contracture (MRC; Table 49.3).

In C5 and C6 root avulsions, we restore biceps and deltoid/spinati activity by commonly used nerve transfers onto the motor branches of the

Table 49.2 Nerve transfer techniques

For elbow flexion, targeting the motor branches of biceps and brachialis muscle: Donors are motor fascicles from ulnar and median nerve, intercostals, 11th nerve
For arm abduction, targeting the axillary motor branches: Donors are motor branches to the triceps muscle
For shoulder external rotation, targeting infraspinatus muscle: By the 11th nerve
For latissimus dorsi and serratus m. activity: By intercostals

Table 49.3 Medial rotation contracture (MRC) of the shoulder: treatment options for a rotational rebalance

Closed relocation of a dorsally subluxated humeral head and immobilization for 4 weeks
Passive ROM exercises (arm adducted – Perform lateral rotation – Stretching anterior capsule and soft tissues, especially subscapularis muscle)
LR-supination splint at night
Botulinum toxin injection in subscapularis muscle
Anterior shoulder release: Coracoid shortening, section of coracohumeral and coracoacromial ligaments, lengthening of subscapularis tendon, section of anterior glenohumerale capsule
Nerve transfer of the distal spinal accessory nerve to the suprascapular nerve (± selective)

musculocutaneous, axillary, and suprascapular nerve (Table 49.2).

Analysis of the Lesion (Drawings)

A basic drawing realized just at the end of the surgical procedure gives a long-lasting compilation of important information about the lesion: root avulsion(s) or traction-induced trunk rupture(s), the neuroma in (dis)continuity. More traction may result in avulsion with ganglion exposure in the extraforaminal interscalene operative field.

Figure 49.2 gives an example; the drawing is further annexed to the patient's chart.

Secondary Surgery

Secondary procedures are either aimed to improve motor function (and then they should not be indicated before the nerve regeneration – with or without nerve reconstructive surgery – is completed, i.e., about 2 years) or to interfere with the global limb architecture (joint relocation, bone correction).

Ideally, these operations should be completed before school age, although some muscle transfers and their specific reeducation clearly need a good compliance.

Concerning muscle (tendon) transfers, we summarize our strategy in a table with a topographic classification (Table 49.4). Always consider that the donor might have been affected by the initial nerve lesion and thus is a reinnervated, less powerful muscle, which will lose an additional MRC grade with transposition.

Any joint relocation should be addressed very early, first by therapy (exercises and splint; Fig. 49.4) and then by open surgery, to prevent dysplasia and associated joint incongruity.

Osteotomies are regularly late and last steps, as they change a global arm or forearm position and should be performed after taking the patient's own wishes into consideration. For example, the decision to correct a late medial rotation position anomaly often is only taken

Table 49.4 Secondary surgery

Topographic classification of muscle transfers, according to the aim
Shoulder:
LR in an *abd*ucted arm: LD and TM
LR in an *add*ucted arm: Horizontalized TM, PecM rerouting or lower trapezius
Elbow:
Flexion or extension: LD
Forearm:
Correction of supination deformity:
Biceps tendon rerouting (Zancolli)
BR rerouting (Özcan)
Wrist:
Extension: FCU or PT
Radial deviation: Özkan sling procedure
Hand:
Thumb opposition: PL, abductor V
Clawing: Zancolli lasso

LR lateral rotation of the shoulder, *LD* latissimus dorsi muscle, *TM* teres major muscle, *PecM* pectoralis major muscle, *BR* brachioradialis muscle, *FCU* flexor carpi ulnaris muscle, *PT* pronator teres muscle, *PL* palmaris longus tendon after puberty or in the young adult, when the shift of decision has occurred from the parents to the patient himself. There is no argument in the literature showing that the results of this procedure are influenced by the age at the time of surgery.

Recently, we focused on more rare deformities with multifactorial, often unknown pathophysiology, like radial head subluxation (Table 49.5 summarizes our surgical strategy) and ulnar wrist deviation (Table 49.6; [3, 4]).

Here follows a list of still unsolved and debated issues:

- Finger flexion weakness: transfer of latissimus dorsi down to finger flexion tendons or free gracilis muscle transfer [2] – unpredictable functional results.
- Loss of intrinsic finger extension (at the PIP and DIP level).
- Radial head dynamics.
- Late GH deformity.
- Glenoid reconstruction by means of neck angulation correction (opening wedge osteotomy), dorsal capsule tightening.

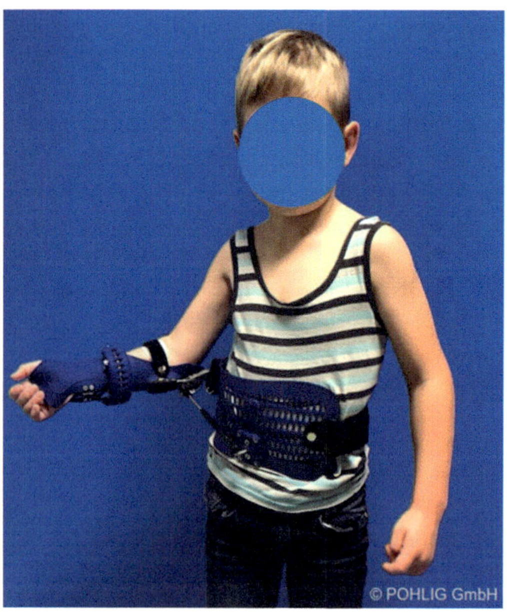

Fig. 49.4 ER-sup splint

Table 49.5 Radial head (volar) subluxation

Aim: Prevent dislocation and elbow ankylosis
Rationale: Open joint relocation with radius shortening osteotomy, allowing the radial head to drop again into the capitellar fossa, reconstruction of the annular ligament, change of the supinating lever arm by biceps tendon rerouting or transposition onto the proximal ulna
Caveats: Proximity of posterior interosseous nerve, radial head vascularization, recurrent subluxation

Table 49.6 Ulnar wrist deviation

Aim: Understand and rebalance the wrist axis before growth disturbance arrives
Classification on radiologic standard views [3, 4]
Tendon rerouting: Özkan "switch" procedure [11]
Bone correction, e.g., Sauvé-Kapandji leveling

Results and Outcome Measures

We use active and passive ROM measurements as they are simple and reliable.

They are mostly target-focused (joint motion in one plane).

There exist a lot of functional, global assessment questionnaires and scales, which are beyond our competence and scope in this chapter. The perception of the functional improvement by the parents is an important factor and might be visualized by amateur photographs sent back to the surgical team (Fig. 49.5).

Prevention and Medicolegal Issues

The intraoperative precise description of the lesion itself is the best diagnostic assessment we may provide so far, to parents, doctors, therapists, and lawyers. Our additional role, beside our surgical work, is to enhance awareness concerning the reality of BPBI among obstetricians and midwives but also pediatricians and neurologists.

Further Developments

Some mandatory improvements may arise from new technologies:

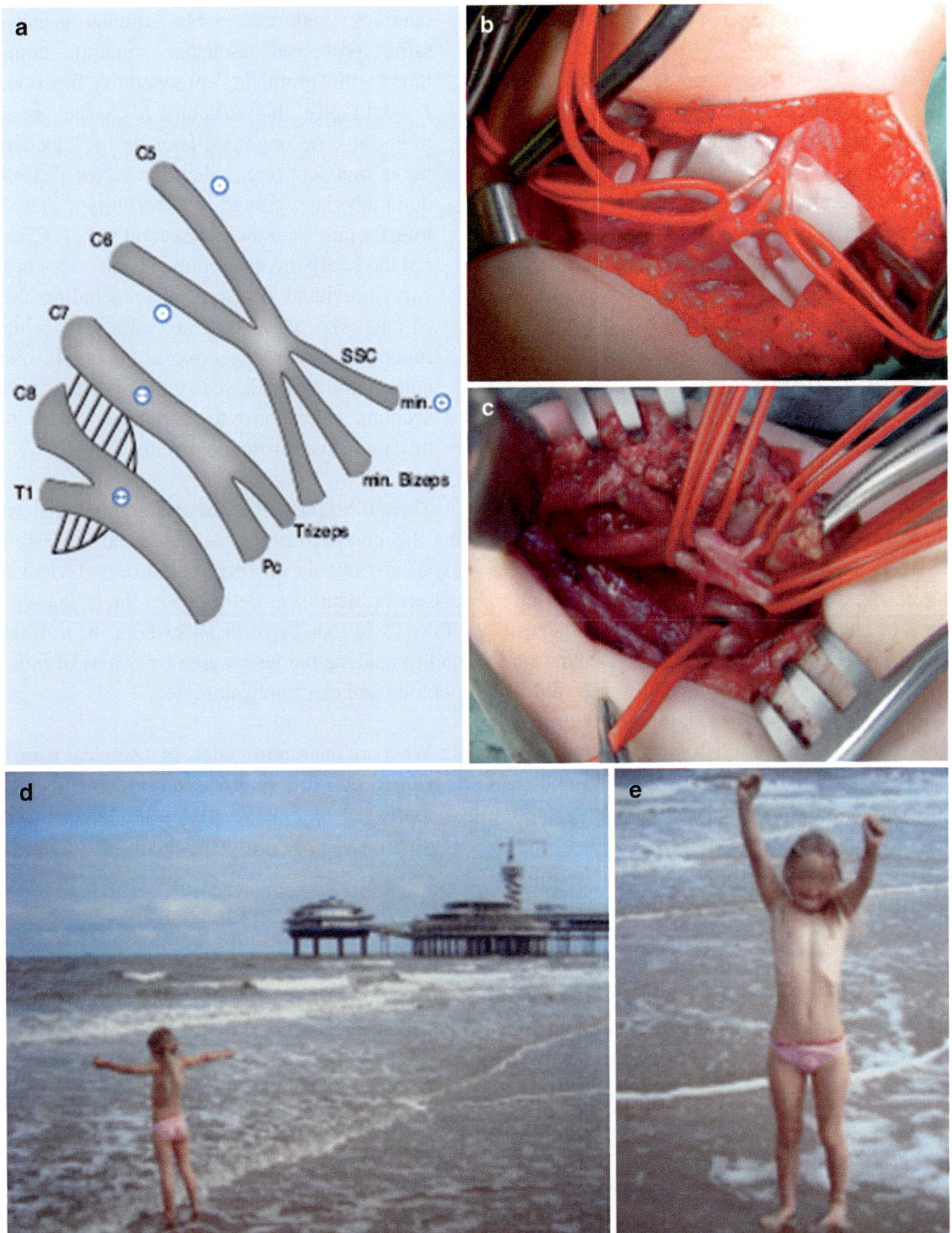

Fig. 49.5 Global result: photos sent from parents

- A better preoperative imaging: high-resolution ultrasound?
- Intraoperative functional testing by electrostimulation (nerve conduction studies better than a simple motor response to electric stimulation?)
- Biologic enhancement of nerve regeneration capacity, influencing the speed of nerve regeneration, or motor target (end plate) preservation.

Ongoing Controversy

1. Is neurolysis still an option in severe lesions, despite Clarke's paper [10]?

Most of the BPBI observed at birth recover so well that their morphologic nerve lesion is never exposed surgically or precisely viewed on any imaging technique. But we hypothesize that besides rare simple elongation injury causing transient neurapraxia, most of these "hidden" lesions are neuromas in continuity. As they give good function, we don't bring them to surgery. Those with bad function are exposed and then the paradigm of the resection of a nonconducting neuroma in continuity applies.

The dilemma is within the evaluation of that neuroma and the criteria set for conductivity.

Distal to the lesion, one frequently gets good muscle contraction upon 1–2 mA stimulation, but often the proximal stimulation is needing higher intensity to elicit muscle activity, and then the decision about neuroma resection is purely subjective:

- Some resect all neuromas whenever the patient is indicated for surgery and then a graft repair is done.
- Grossman [7] proposes the jump-graft procedure, where only the badly conducting areas are excised and grafted. This needs careful epineurotomy and interfascicular dissection within a neuromatous environment, made of mingled minifascicles.
- "Never say never": If the intraoperative exposure and nerve cleaning show a neuroma in continuity with "acceptable" stimulation and a rather preserved fascicular structure, combined with "promising" preoperative function, I would give this structure a chance, as it might also be upgraded later on by selective nerve transfers (e.g., when the elbow flexion definitely lays behind, a Oberlin-type nerve transfer may be done as a second step, if C7 is not too badly involved in the lesion). This is a very individual decision, also including the parents who argue they are afraid of losing functions that have recovered so far. In our consent policy, we have to take this aspect into account, and we have to accept restrictive permissions given from the parents.

There is no 100% rule about neuroma excision, but this emphasizes the absolute need for lesion exposure, as only this supra- and retroclavicular dissection with clear definition of the lesion will allow to further perform an external neurolysis and to analyze the lesion area by means of morphology and electrophysiology.

2. What are the requirements of a surgical team? Countries with referral centers (BPBI programs), center building? Including neuropediatrician, PT/OT, psychologists?

When meeting colleagues from other countries, we notice how differently caregivers are organized. BPBI surgery seems to stay concentrated in few colleagues' hands; and the claim for "specialized centers" is maintained. The medical view should be *interdisciplinary*, and a constant exchange with physiotherapists and occupational therapists is mandatory, also because treatment plans last for the whole growing period.

3. Importance of counselling and nonmedical measures (mother's trauma therapy, school integration, sports, adult life, and especially work adaptation).

Over the years, we learned a lot from parents and other, nonmedical professionals.

For some mothers and parents, the birth event is a long-lasting physical and psychological trauma affecting the whole family setting but mostly the mother, with a lot of feelings of guilt. Trauma therapy might be an issue, when everyday life gets too influenced by coping mechanisms that affect the relationship with the child, school environment, etc.

School integration among peers and sport activities are not always self-explanatory, as only few people are really aware what BPBI sequelae mean with respect to function, posture, psychological impact, and self-image changes.

Patients and parents choosing education and a work profile may need good explanations about limited range of motion and strength and further degenerative changes due to unfavorable biomechanics – especially at the shoulder level.

4. Neglect, pain, and sensation deficit.

Neglect might be seen early in the severe and complete cases. It may be explained by a preference given by the cortical decision-making toward the unaffected arm and may be addressed by physiotherapy, e.g., specifically in a setting of constrained-induced movement therapy (CIMT). We need to clearly define these settings, the time and logistic frame; we also need to explain the logics of neglect (which is not the same than "laziness").

Pain is more often referred when the child is prone to infectious disease and febrile; and very little is known about the impact and extent of sensation deficit in small children, although good measurement tools do exist for pressure and thermoception. Probably, physiotherapy in the future should look even more on somatosensory reeducation.

5. Limb development and length discrepancy.

Clinical experience shows that especially complete lesions and severe lower root involvement lead to limb shortening. Historic pictures like German emperor Wilhelm II with a hidden hand are becoming rare, because total palsies are nowadays operated and nerve lesions reconstructed. However, a severe lack of nerve fiber sources will not only end up with muscle weakness but also with various aspects of impaired development (muscle imbalance, joint incongruency) and, more visible, with long bone shortening [15].

In exceptional cases, diaphyseal distraction surgery may be indicated to correct limited bone shortening, although no functional benefit is gained after those corrections – making a very strict education and informed consent procedure absolutely mandatory.

Conclusion

Severe BPBI lesions nowadays benefit from early microsurgical nerve repair and a huge variety of secondary procedures. Decision-making and operative skills remain individual, but the function may be improved and, hence, the negative impact on growth, self-image, and functional use. The generation of pioneers taught us a valuable reconstructive strategy we are still busy to spread and refine.

Surgery alone is not an option; and interdisciplinary approach is mandatory, including all therapeutic options, splints, counselling, and incentives for sport and professional activity.

A confirmed diagnosis of BPBI will never be erased from patient's history, but we are privileged to own an extensive toolbox to allow acceptable living conditions for this patient group.

References

1. Bahm J, Becker M, Disselhorst–Klug C, Williams S, Meinecke L, Müller H, Sellhaus B, Schröder JM, Rau G. Surgical strategy in obstetric brachial plexus palsy: the Aachen experience. Semin Plast Surg. 2004;18(4):285–99.
2. Bahm J, Ocampo-Pavez C. Free functional gracilis muscle transfer in children with severe sequelae from obstetric brachial plexus palsy. J Brach Plex Periph Nerve Inj. 2008;3(1):23.
3. Bahm J, Esser T, Sellhaus B, El-kazzi W, Schuind F. Tension in peripheral nerve suture. In: Vanaclocha V, Saiz-Sapena N, editors. Treatment of brachial plexus injuries. London: IntechOpen; 2019.
4. Bahm J, Bouslama S, Hagert EM, Andersson JK. Ulnar wrist deviation in children with obstetric brachial plexus palsy: a descriptive study of clinical

and radiological findings of impaired ulnar growth and associated incongruence of the distal radio-ulnar joint. Hand. 2019; https://doi.org/10.1177/2F1558944719831243.
5. Bisinella GL, Birch R, Smith SJM. Neurophysiological prediction of outcome in obstetric lesions of the brachial plexus. J Hand Surg Eur Vol. 2003;28(2):148–52.
6. Gordon T, Wood P, Sulaiman OAR. Long-term denervated rat Schwann cells retain their capacity to proliferate and to myelinate axons in vitro. Front Cell Neurosci. 2019; https://doi.org/10.3389/fncel.2018.00511.
7. Grossman JA, DiTaranto P, Yaylali I, Alfonso I, Ramos LE, Price AE. Shoulder function following late neurolysis and bypass grafting for upper brachial plexus birth injuries. J Hand Surg. 2004;29B(4):356–8.
8. Hütt B. Microsurgical nerve reconstruction after obstetrical brachial plexus lesions: post-operative evaluation of children aged 9 months or older. Thesis, Aachen. 2011.
9. Leblebicioglu G, Ayhan C, Firat T, Uzumcugil A, Yorubulut M, Doral MN. Recovery of upper extremity function following endoscopically assisted contralateral C7 transfer for obstetrical brachial plexus injury. J Hand Surg Eur Vol. 2016;41(8):863–74.
10. Lin JC, Schwentker-Colizza A, Curtis CG, Clarke HM. Final results of grafting versus neurolysis in obstetrical brachial plexus palsy. Plast Reconstr Surg. 2009;123(3):939–48.
11. Özkan T, Aydin HU, Berköz Ö, Özkan S, Kozanoglu E. "Switch" technique to restore pronation and radial deviation in 17 patients with brachial plexus birth palsy. J Hand Surg Eur Vol. 2019;44(9):905–12.
12. Russman B. Neonatal brachial plexus palsy. www.uptodate.com; 2019.
13. Saricaoglu F, Sahin A, Yukselen MA, Leblebicioglu G, Aypar U. Anesthesia and perioperative care of newborns with obstetrical brachial plexus injuries. Neurosciences (Riyadh). 2005;10(1):44–6.
14. Sauerzapfe B: Anaesthesia in newborn and small children with obstetric brachial plexus palsy (in German) In: Bahm J: Movement disorders of upper extremity in children (in German) Springer Berlin 2017.
15. Terzis JK, Kokkalis ZT. Bone discrepancy as a powerful indicator for early surgery in obstetric brachial plexus palsy. Hand. 2010;5(4):386–96.

Surgical Approaches for Brachial Plexus Birth Injuries

50

José L. Borrero

Introduction

By definition, a surgical approach has two components. One is the description of the path or access to the operative site. The other is the description of the surgical plan: the strategy and method of reconstruction.

Both components are affected by perioperative factors such as risks, vital signs, or fluid replacement. These factors are important and pertinent to surgery in babies under 1 year of age. To be complete, the chapter begins with a brief review of some of those factors.

Perioperative Factors Pertinent to Surgery on an Infant

Anesthesia Risk

Surgical risks include operative risks and anesthesia risks. Anesthesia risks are most important in defining timing of surgery. Anesthesia risks relate to patient's age and weight. Age is calculated as time since conception (post-conceptual age, PCA) or gestation (gestation age, GA). A term baby is between 37 and 42 weeks PCA or GA.

Anesthesia risks are based on a number of adverse events. Neonates (patients age 1–30 days) have the highest number of intraoperative adverse events. Anesthesia-related adverse events are less frequent in ages 1–12 months than ages 1–5 years [1, 2].

Anesthesia risks are most commonly related to the respiratory system. Apnea (absence of breathing for 20 seconds or longer) is the most common and most important anesthesia risk factor [2, 3].

Central apnea relates to respiratory system immaturity. This is usually no longer a factor after 50–60 weeks PCA, or about 2 ½ months since birth for a term baby.

Obstructive apnea relates to upper respiratory tract infections (URI), which is more frequent after 1 year in age. In a term baby, with no URI, anesthesia risks are not higher at 3 months than at 6, 9, or 11 months of age [2–4].

Vital Signs

Generally, patients undergoing primary brachial plexus exploration and reconstruction are under 1 year in age, weighting 5–12 Kg (11–26 lbs.). For this group, the average respiratory rate is 20–40 breaths per minute, with a tidal volume of 7 ml/Kg (about 40–80 ml. for a 12 lbs. baby).

J. L. Borrero (✉)
University of Central Florida, College of Medicine, Orlando, FL, USA

Arnold Palmer Hospital for Children, Orlando Health, Orlando, FL, USA

A. Y. Shin, N. Pulos (eds.), *Operative Brachial Plexus Surgery*,
https://doi.org/10.1007/978-3-030-69517-0_50

The average heart rate and blood pressure are 110–180 beats/min and 90/60 mmHg, respectively. Blood volume averages 80 ml/Kg.

Hypothermia is an important factor since infants have decreased ability to regenerate heat and have a faster heat loss rate due to the higher ratio of surface area to weight. Hypothermia is associated with hypoxia, acidosis, hypercapnia, and hypoglycemia. Normal core temperatures are 36.4–37.7 °C (97.5–100.0 °F). Core temperature below 35 °C is considered hypothermia [2, 5].

Fluids

Infants, having a faster metabolic rate and a larger body surface per weight, become dehydrated faster than adults. Fluid loss due to fasting over 3–4 h. Must be considered and replaced. Insensible water loss is not important in small neck incisions. It is important with prolonged operative time and exposure of long leg incisions for sural nerve harvesting and large chest incisions for intercostal nerve retrieval. Maintenance fluid requirements for infants up to 10 Kg in body weight are estimated at 4 ml/Kg. For this group, normal urine output is 0.5–1.5 ml/kg /h. Inhalation anesthesia, hypoperfusion, and hypothermia are causes of decreased urine output [2, 5].

Unrecognized hypoglycemia due to pre-op fasting and long operating time must be anticipated. Maintenance fluid of 5% dextrose in 0.45% normal saline can prevent hypoglycemia.

Classification

Access and path to the operative field varies depending on the injury. To make it simple, consider only two types of brachial plexus injuries in the newborn: (1) injuries affecting the *upper plexus (partial)* and (2) injuries affecting the *lower plexus (total)*.

Injuries Affecting the Upper Plexus (Partial)

Upper plexus injuries involve roots C5, C6, and/or C7. Roots can be avulsed, torn or partially torn, and stretched. A neuroma-in-continuity involving the upper and middle trunks may be present. The degree or injury extent is quite variable.

Deficits manifested are also variable yet almost always include poor or absent shoulder motion with weak external rotation, excessive internal rotation, and poor or absent elbow flexion and forearm supination. Elbow extension and finger grasp are usually normal (normal wrist, thumb, and finger flexion). Wrist, finger, and thumb extension may be normal or absent. Making it simple, upper plexus injuries can be considered as displaying a *"good hand, bad shoulder, and poor elbow flexion"* (Fig. 50.1).

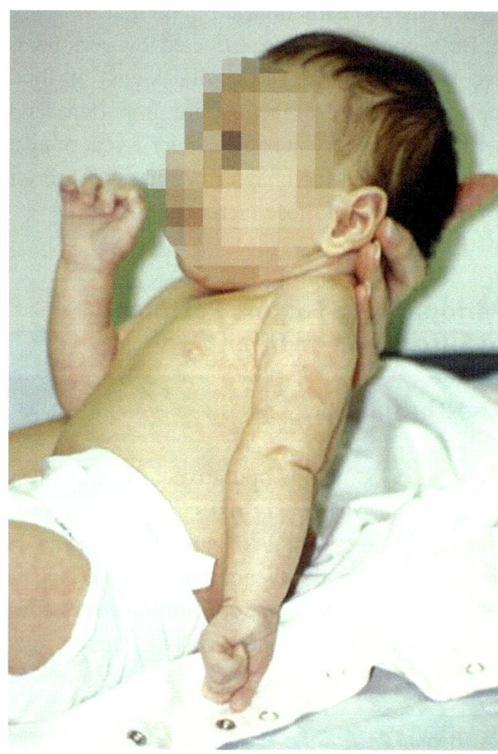

Fig. 50.1 Upper (partial) plexus: Characteristic presentation for patients with upper plexus injuries: "*good hand, bad shoulder and poor elbow flexion*"

Injuries Affecting the Lower Plexus (Total)

Injuries affecting the lower plexus are most commonly associated with a total plexus palsy as isolated lower plexus injuries are rare. Lesions affecting the lower or total plexus injuries are severe injuries, and the C8 and T1 roots are predominantly affected.

In total injuries, deficits range from a complete flail extremity to one with some shoulder activity and minimal elbow, wrist, or finger motion. Since lower roots are affected, fingers and thumb are usually flail, supple, or cupped with zero flexion or extension. Horner's syndrome is usually present on that same side. The presentation is variable, depending on severity of injury. It also changes rapidly with time. To make it simple, lower total injuries can be described as *"bad hand, some shoulder, maybe Horner's"* (Fig. 50.2).

For these injuries the strategy and method of reconstruction is both variable and complex. Recovery is usually incomplete. Permanent residual deficits usually remain.

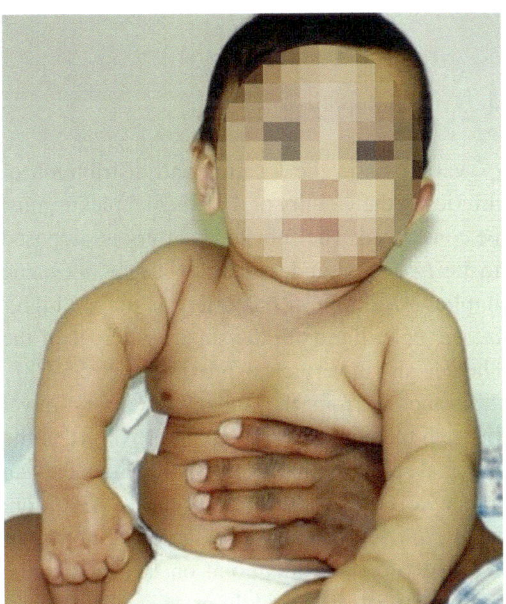

Fig. 50.2 Lower (total) plexus: Characteristic presentation for patients with total plexus injury: "*bad hand, some shoulder, maybe Horner's*"

Surgical Approach

Anatomy

1. Posterior Triangle

Upper plexus injuries are contained within the posterior triangle bordered by the trapezius *(Tz)*, sternocleidomastoid *(SCM)*, and clavicle. The surface anatomy has been described in Chapt. 2 and 20.

2. Cervical Plexus

The cervical plexus, formed from cervical roots 1–4, is anatomically closely related to posterior triangle and the brachial plexus. A brief simplified review follows.

The cervical plexus has two components: a superficial (sensory) and a deep (motor). The *sensory component* emerges deep but becomes anterior and superficial as it drapes over the posterior border of the SCM, almost at its midpoint, between clavicle and mastoid. The sensory component of the cervical plexus *is an important landmark* for it represents the upper limit of exposure during surgical exploration of the brachial plexus.

As it drapes over the SCM, the cervical plexus branches into *posterior auricular*, *lesser occipital*, *transverse cervical* (also called cutaneous cervical), and *supraclavicular*. These are purely sensory branches. The supraclavicular branch ramifies over the posterior triangle toward the clavicle. These cervical plexus supraclavicular branches need to be displaced or divided during brachial plexus exposure. They can, if necessary, serve as nerve grafts. *Motor* branches from roots C1, C2, C3, and C4, of the cervical plexus, emerge *below, deep to the SCM*. Posterior fibers join the *spinal accessory nerve*. Anterior fibers form the *ansa cervicalis* (supplying the "strap" muscles in the neck) and the *phrenic nerve*. These branches are mostly motor (Fig. 50.3).

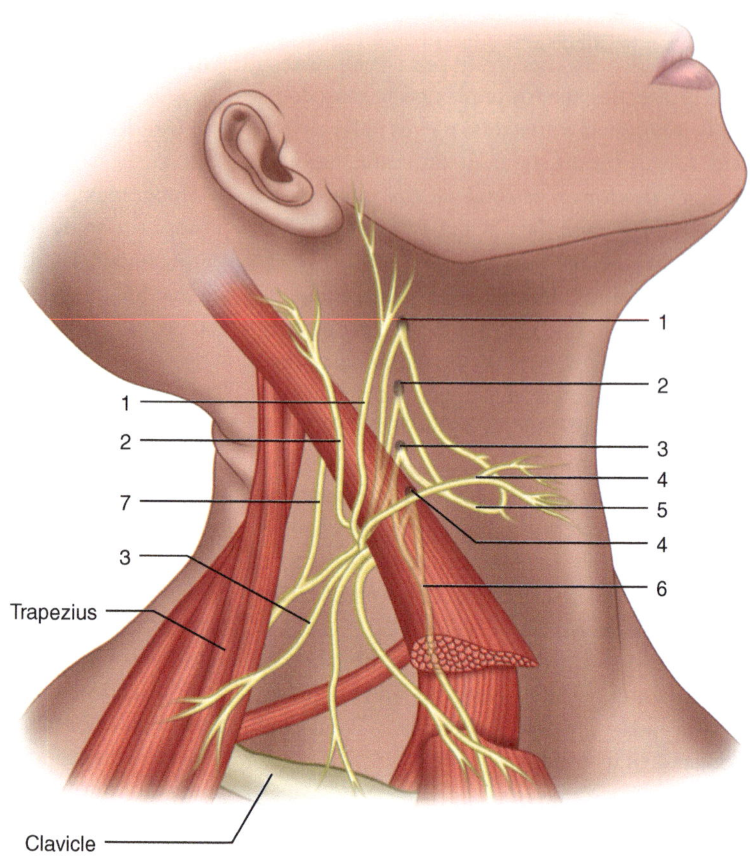

Fig. 50.3 The cervical plexus and posterior triangle: Roots C1, C2, C3, and C4 form the cervical plexus and split into two components: a superficial sensory (in yellow) and a deep motor (in blue). Superficial sensory nerves enter the posterior triangle and drape over the sternocleidomastoid muscle: (1) greater auricular, (2) lesser occipital, (3) supraclavicular, and (4) transverse cervical. Deep motor nerves form the (5) ansa cervicalis, (6) phrenic, and (7) spinal accessory nerves

3. Lymphatics

Numerous lymph nodes are found under the deep cervical fascia within the supraclavicular fat pad in the posterior triangle. They are abundant along the posterior border of the sternocleidomastoid muscle and surround the cervical plexus as it surfaces to drape over this muscle.

On both right and left sides, thin friable lymphatics join the junction of jugular and subclavian veins. Lymphatic ducts, on the right side, drain the right side of the face, right hemithorax, and right upper extremity. On the left side, the larger thoracic duct drains both lower extremities, abdomen, and remaining left side of the body (Fig. 50.4).

4. Arterial Supply

Variations in the location and distribution of arteries in the vicinity of the brachial plexus must be considered. The subclavian artery is supposed to lie *below* or under the clavicle, as its name implies. Oftentimes, this artery is noted "high," *above,* or in line with the superior border of the clavicle and in very close proximity of root C8.

Branches from the subclavian artery travel through the posterior triangle in proximity to the brachial plexus. Anatomically, the subclavian artery is divided into three portions. The more distal, *third portion* ends at the lateral border of the first rib. From this point on, it becomes the axillary artery. The middle or *second portion* of the subclavian artery lies under the anterior sca-

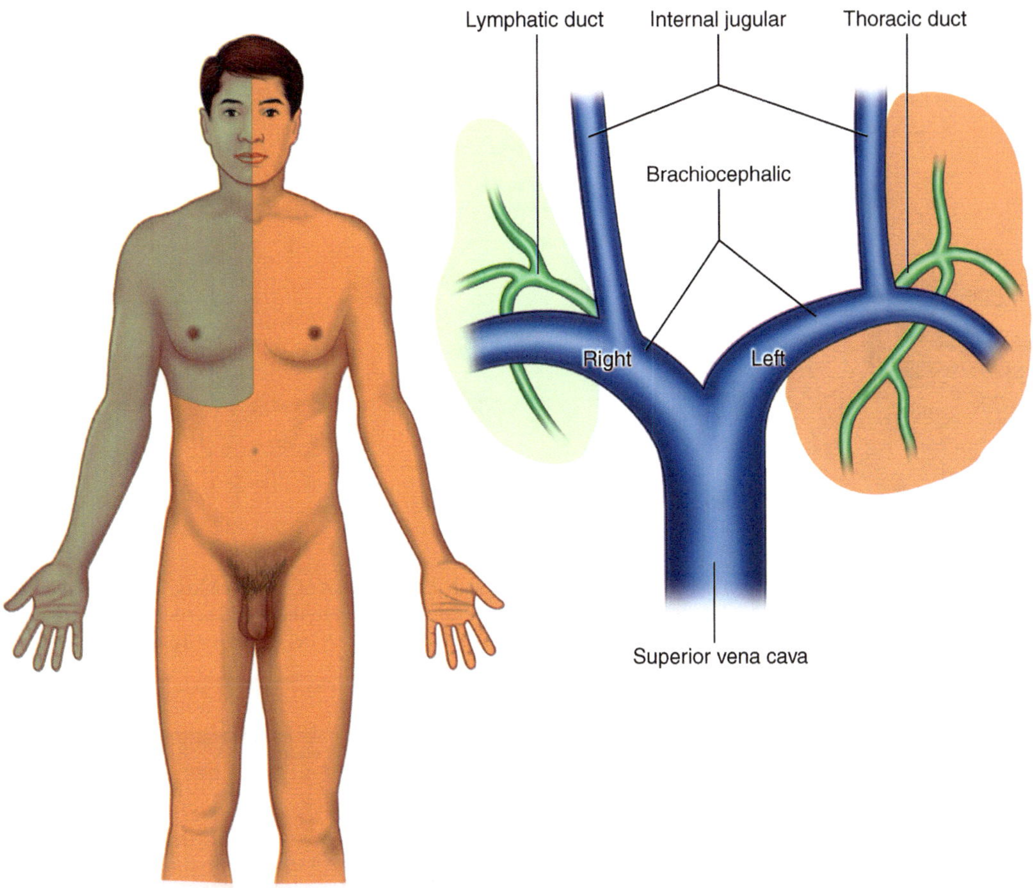

Fig. 50.4 Lymphatic drainage: Lymphatic drainage from right side of face, right upper extremity and right hemi thorax drain to the right side of the supraclavicular region. The rest of the body drains via the thoracic duct to the left side

lene muscle and is defined by the lateral and medial borders of this muscle.

The *thyrocervical trunk* originating from the first portion, but very close to the medial border of the anterior scalene, is of importance to the brachial plexus surgeon. Its lateral branches, *transverse cervical* and *suprascapular* (also known as transverse scapular), pass through the posterior triangle and must be identified during brachial plexus dissection.

Variations in arterial distribution must be considered. The *dorsal scapular* artery is a branch of the transverse cervical, which originates at the thyrocervical trunk. Frequently, however, it can originate *directly from the subclavian* artery. The dorsal scapular artery travels *under* the middle trunk or *between* middle and upper trunks [6] (Fig. 50.5).

Two examples illustrate the need to understand the arterial supply through the plexus. (1) Serious bleeding can occur if the dorsal scapular artery is injured during exposure of the upper and middle trunks. Both trunks can be part of a large neuroma enveloped in scar tissue. Dissection to separate scarred trunks can result in injury to the dorsal scapular artery traveling between them. (2) Oftentimes the transverse scapular artery, when crossing over the upper trunk, becomes a tight vascular leash. This leash can cause nerve compression when the angle between head and shoulder is increased.

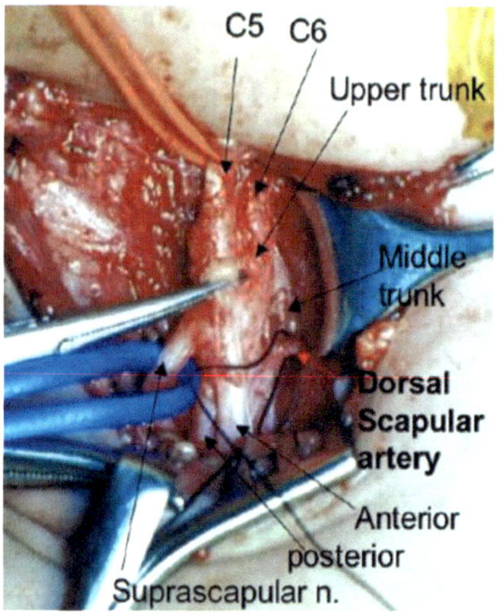

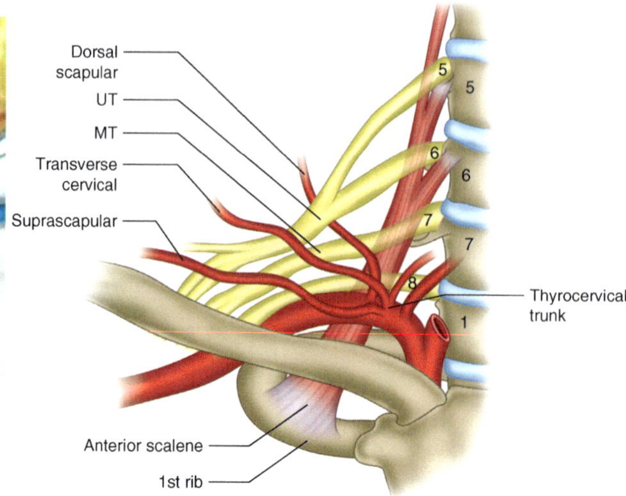

Fig. 50.5 Arteries in the vicinity of the brachial plexus: When both trunks are part of a large neuroma enveloped in scar tissue, dissection to separate scared trunks is dangerous and can result in injury to the dorsal scapular artery traveling between them. The dorsal scapular artery may originate from the subclavian artery (as shown) or from the thyrocervical trunk (UT upper trunk, MT middle trunk)

Surgical Approach (Path and Access) for Upper (Partial) Plexus Lesions

1. Incision, Exposure, Technique

Exposure for upper plexus exploration and reconstruction is usually obtained through a transverse supraclavicular incision above, and parallel to the clavicle. It extends from the posterior border of the SCM to the medial border of the Tz (about 5 cm long in a 4-month-old baby) (Fig. 50.6).

The incision is deepened through the platysma. The *subplatysmal* plane is identified and bluntly developed. This maneuver exposes the *deep cervical fascia* which is also part of the posterior triangle. The *posterior triangle* should be exposed in all four directions: *superiorly* to identify the emergence of the cervical plexus, *laterally* (or posterior) to the medial border of the Tz, *medially* (or anterior) to the posterior border of the SCM, and *inferiorly* to expose the clavicle. External jugular veins in this area, over the cervical fascia, can be ligated (Fig. 50.7).

When addressing the inferior border of the posterior triangle, divide the insertion of the SCM over the clavicle using the cautery leaving the superior border of the clavicle bare. In babies, this insertion may include a good portion of the clavicle. Anterior and medial retraction of the SCM (toward the sternum) allows exposure of the anterior scalene muscle above and under the clavicle. The *phrenic nerve* lies over this muscle. Direct nerve stimulation will confirm its identity.

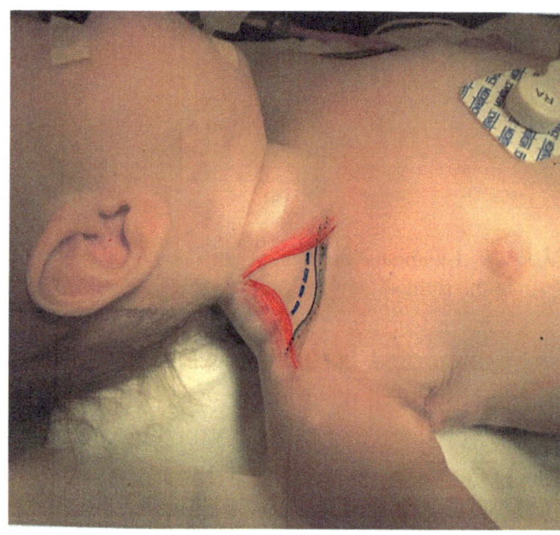

Fig. 50.6 Incision, upper plexus: Transverse supraclavicular incision for upper (partial) plexus exploration and reconstruction. It extends from the posterior border of the sternocleidomastoid to the median border of the trapezius across the posterior triangle

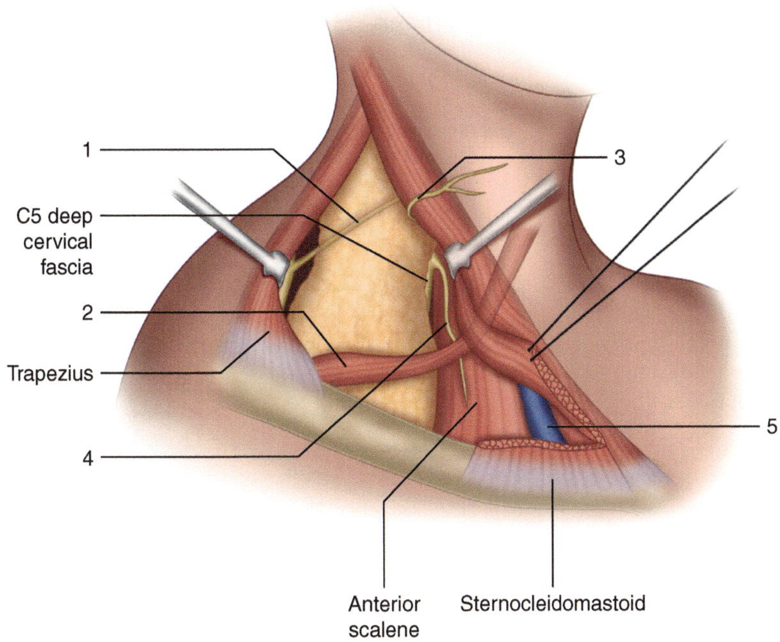

Fig. 50.7 Subplatysmal exposure of the posterior triangle: 1. Spinal accessory nerve, 2. omohyoid muscle, 3. cervical plexus, 4. phrenic nerve, 5. internal jugular vein

One must remember that this point, over the anterior scalene and deep to where the clavicle and sternum meet, the *internal jugular* vein joins the *subclavian* vein.

The *omohyoid muscle* is another important landmark. It travels from the superior border of the scapula to the hyoid bone and crosses the posterior triangle obliquely, superficial to the deep cervical fascia. It divides the posterior triangle into two triangles: one superior and one inferior. The superior one (the *occipital triangle*) is larger and contains fat and lymphatics and the *spinal accessory nerve*. The smaller, inferior triangle over the clavicle (the omoclavicular or *supraclavicular triangle*) contains portions of the *upper trunk* and *lower plexus*. The omohyoid can be divided, not forgetting that its location serves as a reference point. Most surgeons do not repair this muscle.

Now the anterior border of the posterior triangle must be addressed. Remember that the *anterior border of the posterior triangle* is the *posterior border of the SCM*. Make a shallow incision along the posterior border of the SCM and mobilize this muscle edge. The dissection is extended superiorly as far as the *cervical plexus* as it drapes over the SCM. Inferiorly, it is extended as far as the clavicle.

The incision along the posterior border of the SCM is deepened to include the border with the *anterior scalene*. This maneuver permits elevation and mobilization of the *fat pad* in the posterior triangle. It allows for the creation of a *flap, hinging posteriorly,* toward the trapezius. This flap is part of the *supraclavicular fat pad* with its lymphatics. When lifting the flap, the *transverse cervical artery* is exposed. It can be ligated and divided. Mobilization of the flap exposes the *upper trunk*, *upper roots,* and the *phrenic nerve*. During wound closure this flap may serve to cover nerve grafts, if used to bridge the gap after neuroma resection (Fig. 50.8).

The phrenic nerve is traced proximally to the point where it communicates with *brachial plexus root C5*. Since this communication is quite constant, it serves to positively identify root C5. It is important, however, to *expose root C5 proximal to its communication with the phrenic nerve.* If necessary, the dissection may continue proximally toward C5 vertebra and its root foramen, the origin of *C5 plexus root*.

Exposure of the superior border of the clavicle requires dissection of the *subclavius muscle*, although at times this muscle is not very promi-

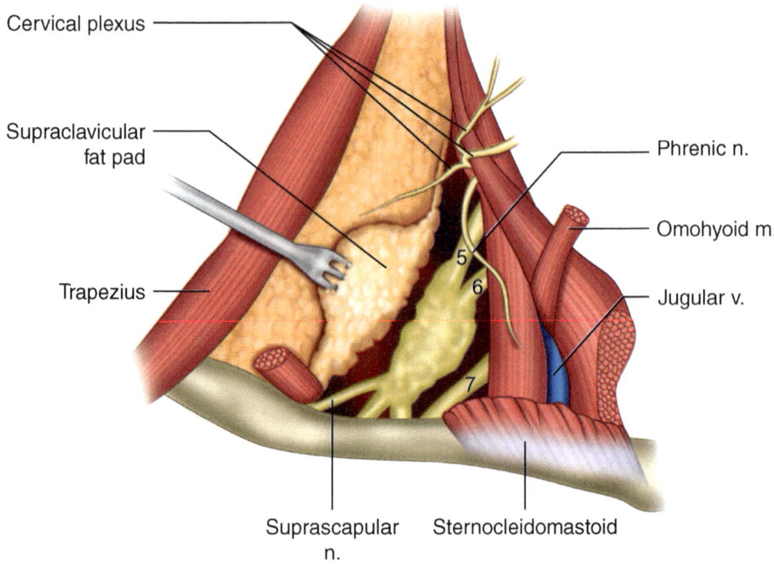

Fig. 50.8 Mobilization of the supraclavicular fat pad: An incision along the posterior border of the sternocleidomastoid muscle allows mobilization of the supraclavicular fat pad as a flap, hinging posteriorly

nent. The *suprascapular artery* may be within this muscle and must be kept in mind. When dissecting the superior border of the clavicle *medially*, toward the sternoclavicular joint, a *high-riding subclavian artery* or branches of the *thyrocervical trunk* may come into view.

Dissection *laterally*, along the superior border of the clavicle, allows visualization of the *distal upper trunk* and its branches (the *suprascapular nerve* and the *anterior and posterior divisions* of the *upper trunk*). The suprascapular nerve should be dissected as far distally as possible and tagged.

At times, clear visualization of the distal upper trunk divisions may not be possible for they lie *under the clavicle*. Extended exposure can easily be obtained by dividing the clavicle which allows its inferior retraction.

A simple longitudinal incision dividing the periosteum over the clavicle allows exposure of a small central area of bare bone. Transection of the clavicle at its midpoint should follow. *Downward retraction* of the divided clavicle and periosteum allows inferior angulation and provides *additional exposure* of the distal upper trunk and its divisions. If maintained within its periosteum, the divided clavicle does not need fixation. Suture approximation of periosteal edges, maintaining clavicular bone ends in alignment, is sufficient [8, 9] (Fig. 50.9).

Surgical Approach for Lower (Total) Lesions

1. Incision, Exposure, Technique

Total (lower) lesions may require exposure and exploration of the entire plexus. Proximally, the surgeon must be able to directly observe and inspect all plexus roots and, if necessary, all five vertebral foramina. Distally, components of the plexus within the infraclavicular or retroclavicular areas may need exposure.

For total injuries, the "Z-shaped or L-shaped" incision along the posterior border of the SCM and superior border of the clavicle is best suited. *Note* that this incision can also be used as an approach for just an upper plexus problem (Fig. 50.10).

To expose the retro- and infraclavicular areas, the neck and supraclavicular incision can be extended obliquely across the clavicle.

For a more "complete" exposure of the entire plexus, the same incision is continued parallel to and below the clavicle toward the *coracoid* process ending at the deltopectoral groove. This incision allows exposure of *cords*, branches from cords, and terminal nerves. This incision also *facilitates division of the clavicle*.

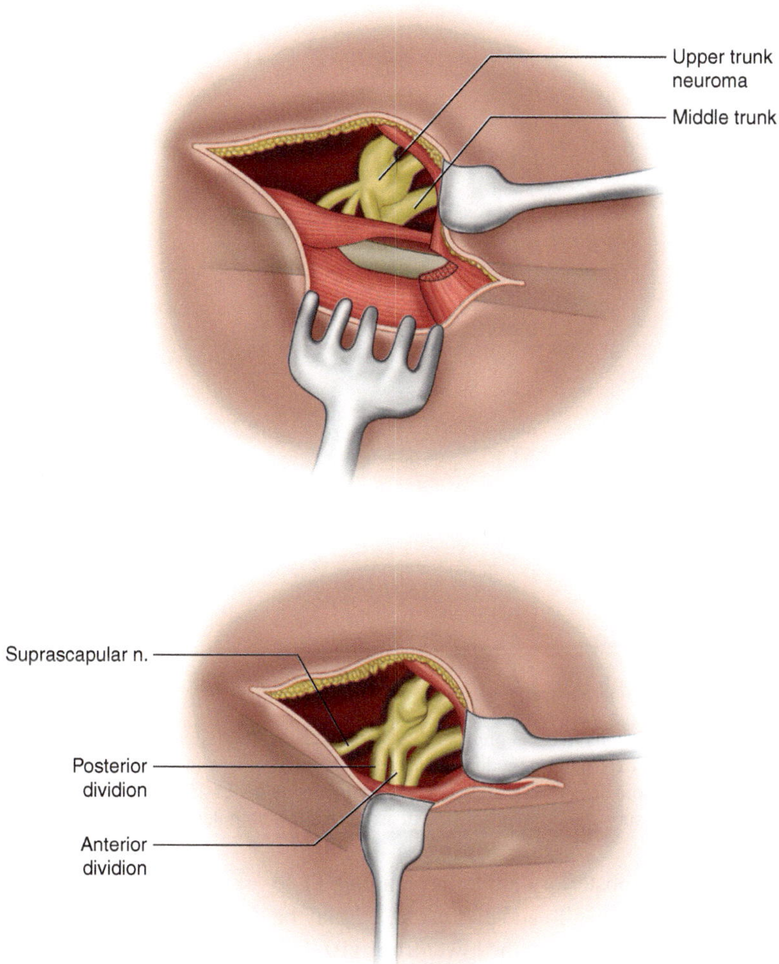

Fig. 50.9 Simple clavicular osteotomy for extended exposure: Division of clavicle after a longitudinal periosteal incision followed by inferior retraction allows extended exposure of the distal upper and middle trunks

Approach for total injuries begins with a supraclavicular exposure of the upper plexus. As described earlier, this can be done through a simple transverse incision or through the "L-shaped or Z-shaped" incision. Lower plexus roots, (C8, T1) are found close to, or under, the superior border of the clavicle under the anterior scalene muscle. The anterior scalene continues under the clavicle to its insertion in the first rib.

In total plexus injuries, spinal nerves could be avulsed or involved in a *neuroma-in-continuity*. When upper roots are avulsed and scarred, upper and middle trunks may retract toward the clavicle. When there is no continuity with the spinal cord, the expected location for upper and middle trunks is found devoid of normal nerve fibers. Rather, interscalene muscle fibers mixed with scar tissue are encountered.

Special attention must be paid when dissecting the superior border of the clavicle, and proceeding medially, toward the sternoclavicular joint, to expose the lower plexus. Important structures are found in this area. The *phrenic nerve* and *jugular vein* are *in front* of the scalene muscle. Plexus roots *and T1, the lower trunk,* and *subclavian artery lie behind* the anterior scalene and drape over the first rib.

Anatomical variations must be kept in mind. A lower trunk *may not* exist. Instead, T1 may join C8 quite distal, under the clavicle, or C8 may

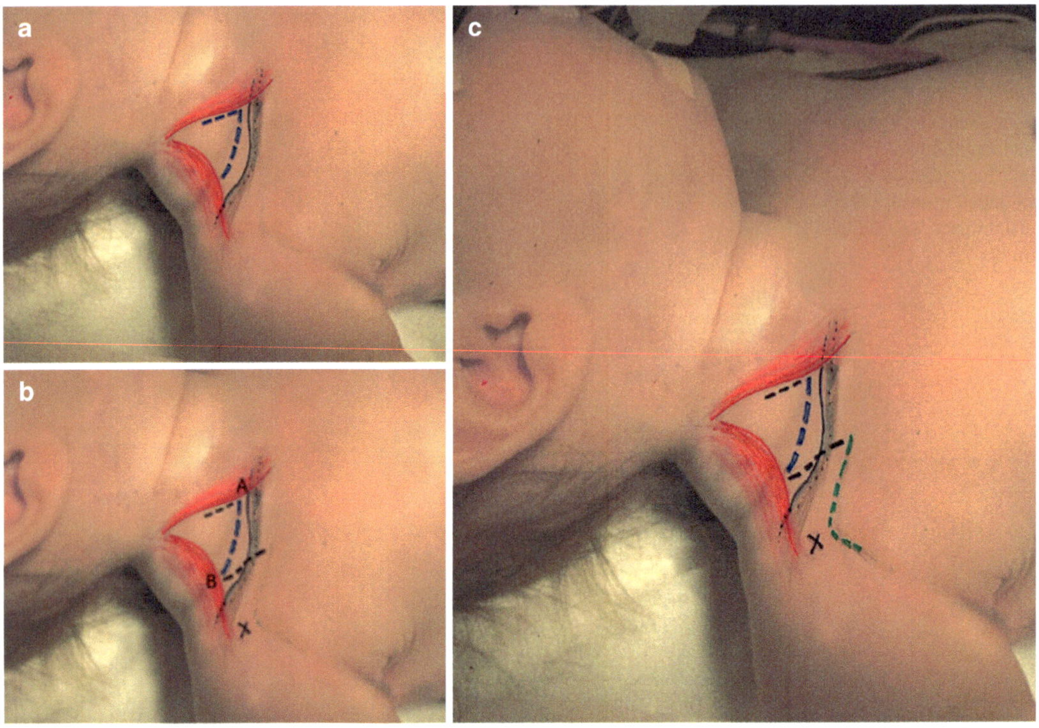

Fig. 50.10 Incisions for total plexus: (**a**) Classic incision. (**b**) Extension of classic incision. The Incision is continued over clavicle to expose retro- and infraclavicular areas. It is important to make incision angles labeled A, B, 45 degrees or greater to avoid devascularization of these triangular skin areas. The "X" marks the location of the coracoid process. (**c**) Complete exposure. Infraclavicular extension to allow complete exposure of the plexus

branch to the posterior cord before joining T1 to form a lower trunk. To add confusion, T2 may be involved, contributing to the lower trunk [10, 11].

To make matters worse, C8 may be avulsed and lie in this area. It may be engulfed in scar tissue, involving the *anterior scalene* and the *subclavian artery*. Extreme care must be used during this dissection in trying to define the anatomy. *Magnification* and *good light* are essential. To improve exposure and expand the field, clavicular osteotomy should be considered. One *should not hesitate* in doing so.

(a) Clavicular Osteotomy

The *lower plexus, divisions forming cords,* and the *lower trunk* may be found in the retroclavicular area. Access and safe exposure are readily obtained by *dividing the clavicle.*

Clavicular osteotomy begins by first exposing the *superior border* of the clavicle. Portions of the subclavius muscle under this border may need resection. As mentioned earlier, exercise caution, for the *suprascapular artery*, if large and injured, may cause unnecessary bleeding. In addition, injury to a *"high-riding" subclavian artery*, if present, can be a serious life-threatening complication.

Next, expose the *inferior border* of the clavicle by stripping the clavicular portion of the pectoralis major muscle. As needed, the inferior border can be exposed from coracoid to claviculosternal junction.

Complete transection of the clavicle is best done by first creating periosteal flaps. Once the bone is exposed, clavicle osteotomy site is marked. Small, 1 mm drill holes are made approximately 1 cm from the osteotomy mark. The clavicle is then cut. Retraction of divided ends allows full exposure and access to the lower plexus as well as important structures in the retroclavicular area (Fig. 50.11).

Once exploration and reconstruction are completed, anatomical approximation of the divided clavicle ends should be done. Absorbable monofilament sutures can be used for this. The clavicle is aligned, and once tied, the suture maintains alignment and fracture-site approximation. After that, periosteal flaps are approximated to cover the fracture line.

2. Approach to Infra- and Retroclavicular Areas (with or Without Osteotomy) [12]

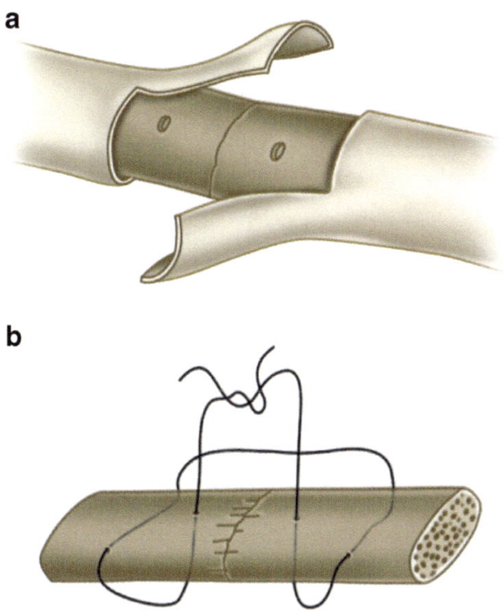

Fig. 50.11 Clavicular osteotomy: (**a**) Clavicular osteotomy. It is suggested to create periosteal flaps, mark the osteotomy site, and drill holes before dividing the clavicle. (**b**) Approximation of divided clavicular ends. Anatomical rigid fixation can be obtained with a single, monofilament, absorbable suture placed through small drill holes as illustrated

Close to the clavicle, muscle fibers of the clavicular portion of the pectoralis major are split, and the *interpectoral space* is entered. The *coracoid process*, an important landmark, is palpated. The *pectoralis minor* is identified and traced to its insertion at the coracoid process (Fig. 50.12).

Both lateral and medial borders of the pectoralis minor muscle are dissected free. Bluntly, the posterior surface of this muscle, enveloped by its fascia, is separated from underlying fat. The muscle is mobilized and then is cut at its insertion in the coracoid process. *Downward retraction,* of the pectoralis minor (together with portions of the overlying pectoralis major), exposes the axilla and its contents. That is why the pectoralis minor is considered as *"the gateway to the axilla."* Important components of the brachial plexus are found under the pectoralis minor. These include *cords,* formation of cords, *branches* from cords, and *terminal nerves*, all surrounding the *axillary artery*. The pectoralis minor also defines the second portion of the axillary artery with its two branches (thoracoacromial and lateral thoracic) (Fig. 50.13).

If needed, improved access to structures in this area is obtained by lateral retraction of the deltoid muscle edge. It may be necessary to divide and ligate the cephalic vein. To gain even better exposure, at times, a tight or foreshortened pectoralis major requires partial division of musculotendinous fibers near its insertion into the humerus.

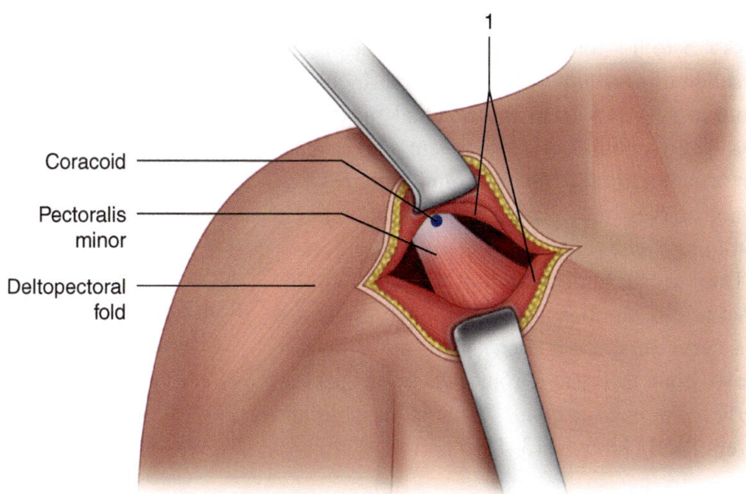

Fig. 50.12 Approach to infra- and retroclavicular areas: [1] Close to the clavicle, muscle fibers of the clavicular portion of the pectoralis major are split and retracted exposing the pectoralis minor, dividing the pectoralis minor muscle at the coracoid allows access to the axilla and its contents. The pectoralis minor muscle is considered as "the gateway to the axilla"

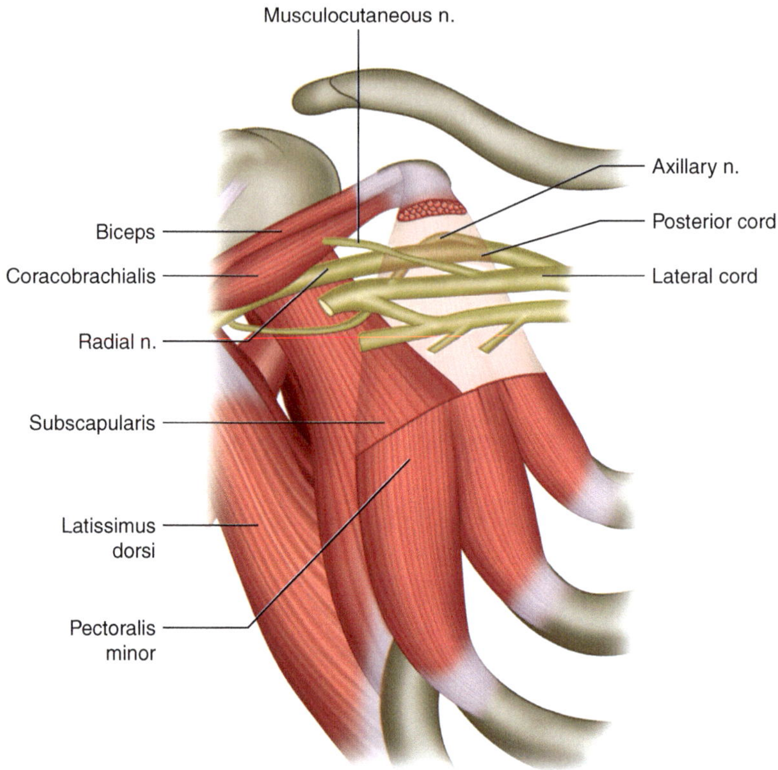

Fig. 50.13 The infraclavicular plexus under the pectoralis minor: Important components of the brachial plexus are found under the pectoralis minor. These include cords, formation of cords, branches from cords, and terminal nerves; all surrounding the axillary artery. Notice that on many occasions, the axillary nerve and posterior cord are superior and slightly deeper than the lateral cord and musculocutaneous nerve

Nerve Transfers

In a nerve transfer (neurotization), a non-injured nerve (*donor nerve*) serving a muscle with normal function (*native muscle*) is directed to an injured nerve (*recipient nerve*) serving a non-functioning muscle (*target muscle*). Transfers where donor and recipient nerves are served from roots C5 to T1 forming the brachial plexus are considered *intraplexual*. Transfers including donor nerves not from the brachial plexus are considered *extraplexual*. Recipient nerves contain *nonfunctioning fibers* from *injured roots*. Donor nerves must contain *functioning fibers* from *unaffected roots*.

Due to variability in root distribution, the exact origin, number, and type of fibers contained in a nerve (*the nerve content*) are never known. Nerve content varies from person to person. *Nerve content in a donor nerve* is variable and never exactly known [13–15].

For a nerve transfer to be successful, the origin, number, and type of fibers (nerve content), within the donor nerve, must be *adequate*. With adequate nerve fiber content, a donor nerve becomes capable of eliciting *useful contraction* in the target muscle. But exactly how many fibers are needed for a nerve to be "adequate" is not known. *"Adequacy"* of a donor nerve is but an intelligent guess based on inexact information [16]. During surgery, electrical stimulation can be of help in determining adequacy of a donor nerve.

Intraoperative electrical stimulation of a donor nerve should result in a "normal" or "acceptable" muscle contraction: considered an *acceptable response*. In contrast, stimulation of a recipient nerve produces absent or weak muscle contraction: *a non-acceptable response*.

Though subjective and inexact, response to nerve stimulation is of help in determining adequacy of donor nerves, non-adequacy of recipient nerves, and success of a nerve transfer.

Nerve Transfers to Restore Shoulder Function

Shoulder motion, stability, and control are a complex function. It is mediated by several muscles, all acting in synchrony, and supplied by different nerves served from all roots of the brachial plexus. In order to restore normal function, muscles have to regain appropriate contractile strength, coordinated contractions have to occur, and joint incongruences must be reduced and contractures or laxity of supporting ligaments corrected. All of this must take place in the absence of pain or compensatory habits. Restoration of *normal* shoulder function *is not simple!*

For the more common upper (partial) plexus injury, adequate (not perfect) shoulder *stability, abduction,* and *external rotation* can be obtained with nerve transfers. Function needs to be restored in two nerves: the *axillary nerve* and the *suprascapular nerve.* "Adequate" activity must be restored to the three muscles they serve: (1) the *deltoid,* (2) the *infraspinatus*, and (3) the *supraspinatus*.

1. Nerve Transfer to the *Suprascapular* Nerve *(SSN)*

The most common extraplexual transfer is transferring the spinal accessory nerve *(SAN)* to the suprascapular nerve *(SSN).*

(a) Approach for the *Spinal Accessory Nerve (SAN)*

When performing exploratory plexus surgery, one should anticipate the possibility of needing to perform a nerve transfer utilizing the *SAN.* Identification and isolation of this nerve is easier if done early, when the posterior triangle is defined and before formal plexus exposure.

The *SAN* enters the posterior triangle deep to the SCM, a bit superior, but very close to where the cervical plexus drapes over the SCM. The *SAN* travels obliquely in a posterior direction toward the trapezius.

To expose the *SAN*, first identify muscle fibers forming the anterior border of the trapezius. Lift this muscle border and its fascia and retract it posteriorly, exposing the underlying deep cervical fascia. The *SAN* is within this fascia. Direct nerve stimulation serves to confirm *SAN* identification.

Tagging for future identification should be done at this time. This author prefers to use a loop of black silk secured with a vessel clip instead of a vessel loop with a hemostat. (In one occasion the pull from the heavier vessel loop and clamp produced significant damage to this small nerve.)

For nerve transfer, *SAN* to *SSN*, the *SAN* needs be dissected distally as it sends branches into the trapezius muscle, forming small fragile arcades. *SAN* transection is done distal to these arcades and their accompanying fragile vessels. This is important, for it ensures that innervation to the *proximal trapezius is preserved.* It also provides sufficient donor nerve length so it reaches the recipient suprascapular nerve. Caution: to ensure adequate length, it may be safer to wait until the *SSN* is exposed before cutting the *SAN.*

(b) Approach for the *Suprascapular Nerve: Anterior Supraclavicular*

The suprascapular nerve is most commonly approached through a supraclavicular incision exposing the posterior triangle and the upper trunk as described earlier in the section for upper plexus exposure. Lateral and posterior dissection of the superior border of the clavicle allows clear visualization of the distal upper trunk. The suprascapular nerve is identified as it comes off the distal end of the upper trunk. It continues laterally diving under the clavicle to the superior border of the scapula, toward the scapular notch. It is dissected as far distal (lateral, posterior) as possible. It is then transected proximally, close to the upper trunk. After ensuring that the nerve is a suitable receptor, it should be routed to meet the spinal accessory nerve which was previously isolated under the anterior border of the trapezius. For this, the suprascapular nerve is passed

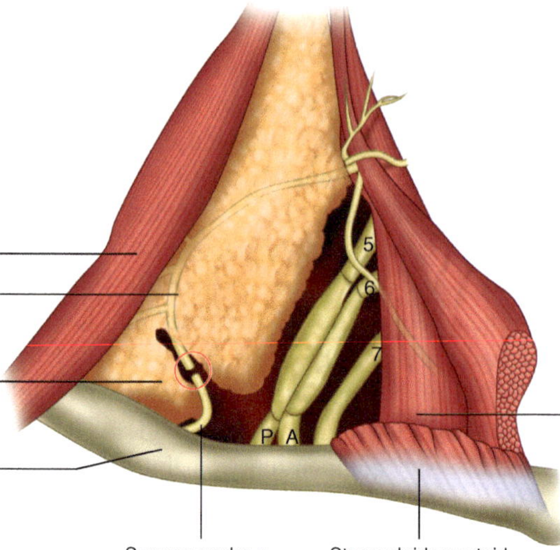

Fig. 50.14 Nerve, transfer, spinal accessory to suprascapular: anterior, supraclavicular approach
The suprascapular nerve is cut away from an upper trunk neuroma. It is routed to meet the spinal accessory nerve through a tunnel in the supraclavicular fat pad or after a wedge is cut through the fat pad as shown. The neuroma has been resected and the gap between roots C5 and C6 bridged with nerve grafts

through a tunnel in the fat pad. As an alternative, a wedge is cut in the supraclavicular fat pad allowing unobstructed passage of the suprascapular nerve [17, 18] (Fig. 50.14).

(c) Approach for the *Suprascapular Nerve*: *Posterior, Suprascapular*

A posterior shoulder incision allows access to the *SSN* and in addition permits exposure of the *SAN*. With this approach, nerve transfer, *SAN* to *SSN*, can be performed without the need to expose the brachial plexus in the posterior triangle.

Prior to incision making, appropriate skin marks should be made identifying the *superior angle* of the scapula and the *acromion*. Another mark should be made above and slightly medial to the superior angle of the scapula. This is the approximate location of the *SAN*. One last mark is made for the *scapular notch*. The notch is found about midpoint between the superior angle of the scapula and the acromion, along the superior border of the scapula. This also marks the approximate location of the *SSN* (Fig. 50.15).

A linear incision is made above and parallel the spine of the scapula from below the superior angle of the scapula to the mark made for the scapular notch. Trapezius muscle fibers are identified below the subcutaneous plane and followed to the spine of the scapula. The trapezius is elevated after detaching it from the scapular spine. The intermuscular space between trapezius and supraspinatus is exposed. In this thin layer, in the direction of the superior border of the scapula and close to the anterior border of the trapezius, lies the *SAN*.

This same plane is followed anteriorly and laterally over the supraspinatus muscle toward the anterior border of the scapula. The supraspinatus muscle is retracted inferiorly to expose the anterior border of the scapula. The suprascapular notch is identified by palpation or by observing the whitish suprascapular ligament over it. The suprascapular artery, superficial to this ligament, is ligated and divided. The ligament is then divided with care not to injure the nerve that enters and travels through the notch. Proximal to the notch, the *SSN* is exposed and isolated. The nerve is mobilized and traced proximally. Nerve transfer *SAN* to *SSN* can be accomplished by direct end to end coaptation at this level [19–21] (Fig. 50.16).

2. Nerve Transfers to the *Axillary Nerve*

Donor nerves commonly used for this intraplexual transfer include *branches from the radial nerve to the triceps* muscle or *branches from the*

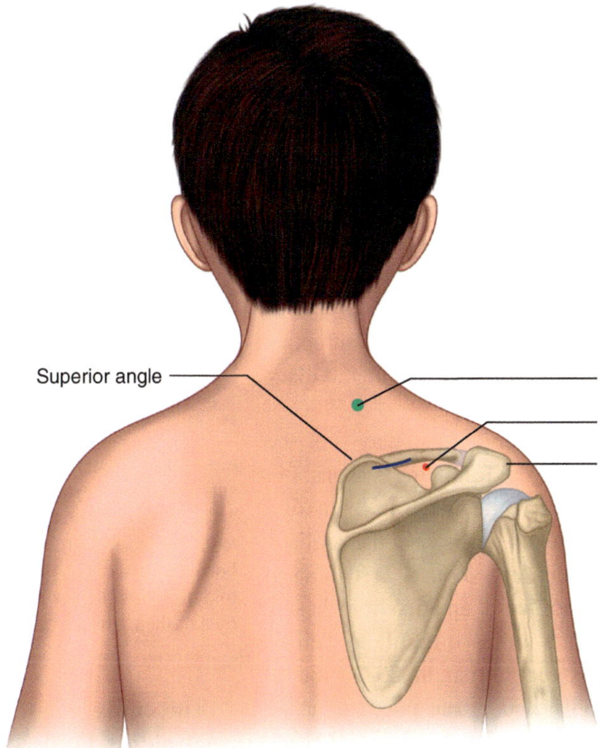

Fig. 50.15 Nerve transfer, spinal accessory to suprascapular: posterior suprascapular approach

The Incision is illustrated by the *blue* dashed line. The *green* dot is the approximate location of the spinal accessory nerve (superior and slightly medial to the superior angle of the scapula).

The *red* dot is the approximate location of the scapular notch and the suprascapular nerve: (midpoint between acromion and superior angle of the scapula along superior border of scapula)

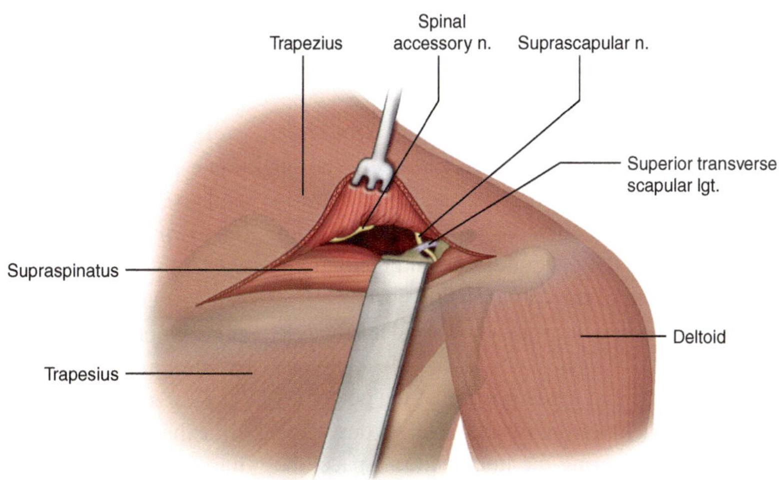

Fig. 50.16 Posterior exposure of spinal accessory and suprascapular nerves

The trapezius muscle is detached from the scapular spine and elevated to find the spinal accessory nerve under its fascia

The supraspinatus muscle is retracted inferiorly to expose the anterior border of the scapula and the suprascapular notch

posterior cord. The axillary nerve can be exposed via different routes: (1) *anteriorly, in the axilla* (before the axillary nerve enters the quadrilateral space) or (2) *posteriorly* (after the axillary nerve exits the quadrilateral space).

The anterior exposure can be through three different approaches: (a) an *infraclavicular approach*, (b) an *axillary approach,* and a (c) *deltopectoral approach.* The deltopectoral approach is a variant of the infraclavicular approach.

(a) Approach for the *Axillary Nerve*: *Anterior, Infraclavicular*

An anterior infraclavicular approach is necessary when branches of the posterior cord (upper or lower subscapular, thoracodorsal) are to be used as donor nerves. It is the best route to expose the axillary nerve origin. It permits direct exposure of other posterior cord branches as they emerge from the posterior cord. This approach is well-known and common for vascular surgeons for it allows proximal control of the axillary artery.

Unfortunately, this approach may not be familiar or popular for the following reasons:

(1) The axillary nerve lies deep in the axilla, adjacent to other plexus cords and the axillary artery, making dissection tedious. (2) The anatomy of the posterior cord and its branches is quite variable and at times difficult to define. Bonnel and others report that in 50 newborns examined, only 33% had a true posterior cord. Hollinshead reports that in 36 of 163 cases (21%), there was no posterior cord as such. Instead, the axillary nerve originated from the posterior division of the upper trunk (roots C5 and C6) and remained with the subscapular nerves as an independent unit. The anatomist Walsh considered the usual configuration of the brachial plexus was not having a posterior cord [11].

Incision, Approach, Technique (Anterior, Infraclavicular) The *coracoid process* is an important landmark. The infraclavicular incision centers below the coracoid process and extends laterally to the deltopectoral line and medially to the midportion of the clavicle (Fig. 50.17).

The infraclavicular incision is deepened to expose the *pectoralis major* fascia. Muscle fibers are split or the clavicular portion of the pectoralis major is detached from the clavicle. As described earlier, after entering the interpectoral space, the pectoralis minor is identified. Both medial and lateral borders of the pectoralis minor as well as its insertion into the *coracoid process* should be mobilized with blunt dissection. Its insertion to the coracoid process is then divided. The muscle is retracted inferiorly exposing the axilla and its contents (Fig. 50.18).

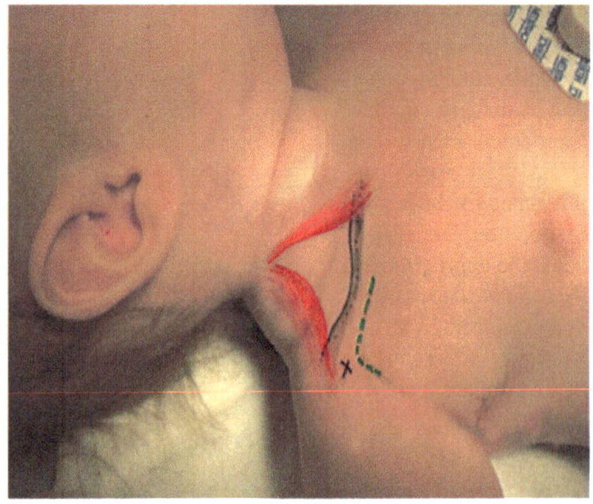

Fig. 50.17 Anterior, infraclavicular incision for exposure of the axillary nerve

The coracoid process (marked with an X) is an important land mark. Borders of the posterior triangle (anterior border of trapezius, posterior border of sternocleidomastoid and clavicle) are highlighted. The incision is marked by a dashed, green line

The cords and terminal nerves of the brachial plexus lie deep in this area. Commonly the lateral cord is found superficial to the posterior cord. Both the *musculocutaneous nerve* and the *axillary nerve* originate from their respective *lateral* and *posterior cords* at about the same level in reference to the coracoid though on average the *axillary nerve is in line* with the coracoid and the *musculocutaneous is a bit more proximal*. In many instances, contrary to some anatomical drawings, the posterior cord and *axillary nerve* are found more *lateral* and *superior* (though deeper or posterior) than the *musculocutaneous* nerve. Also, one must remember that a common variation is for the musculocutaneous nerve to arise from the *median nerve* instead of the lateral cord [22].

The *axillary nerve* travels deep and lateral over the *subscapularis* muscle and goes through the quadrilateral space. The *musculocutaneous nerve* travels lateral and anterior and pierces the *coracobrachialis* muscle.

Due to the variability of the posterior cord and its branches, when transferring branches of the posterior cord to the axillary nerve, it is necessary to verify that the donor and recipient nerves are not served by fibers coming from the same,

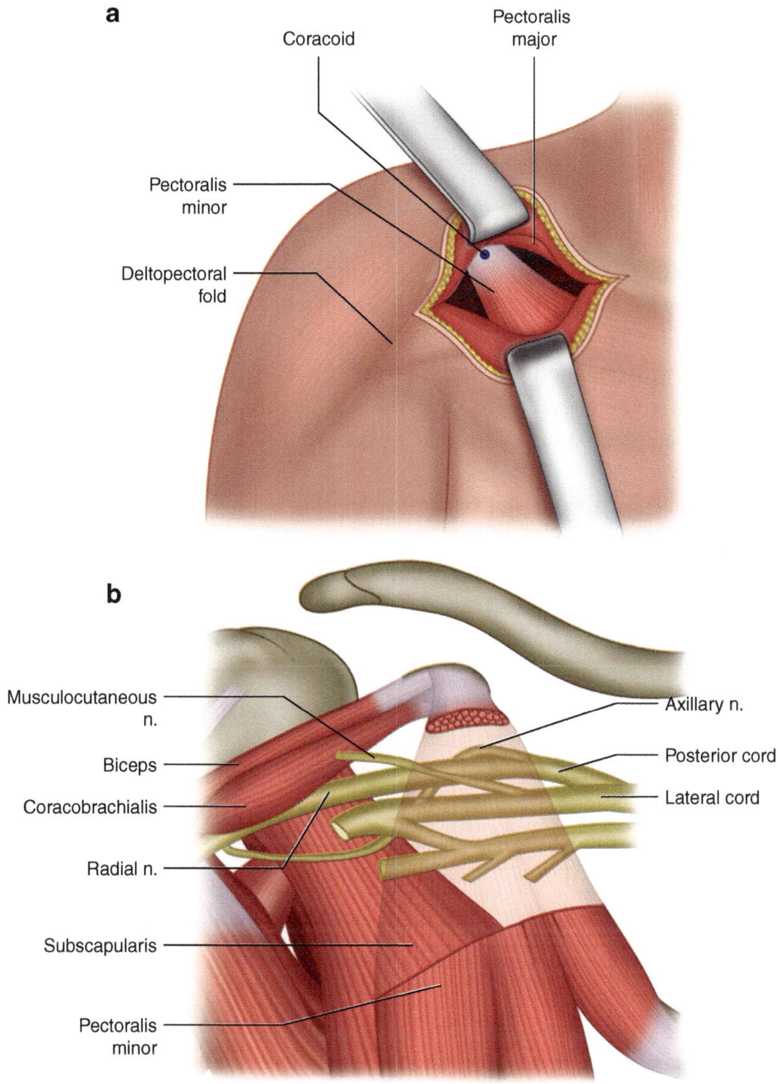

Fig. 50.18 Approach for the axillary nerve: anterior, infraclavicular exposure. (**a**) Close to the clavicle, muscle fibers of the clavicular portion of the pectoralis mayor are split and retracted exposing the pectoralis minor. (**b**) The pectoralis minor is divided at the coracoid process and retracted inferiorly exposing the axilla and its contents. Notice that, as shown, on many occasions, the *axillary nerve* and posterior cord are superior (closer to the coracoid or clavicle) and *slightly deeper* than the lateral cord and musculocutaneous nerve

injured plexus root. (*Nerve fiber content* for donor and recipient nerves must be *different*.) [23].

Response to nerve stimulation is of help in defining suitability of a donor nerve. Active, obvious muscle contraction should be noted in response to stimulation of a donor nerve. In contrast, no muscle response should be noted when the recipient nerve is stimulated. Although highly subjective and inaccurate, this method is widely accepted. It is fast and simple and, most times, sufficient.

If there is a good muscle response when thoracodorsal or subscapular nerves are stimulated and no response when the axillary nerve is stimulated, transferring thoracodorsal or subscapularis branches to the axillary nerve is expected to be successful.

In eight different cases, this author has used this approach to transfer branches of the posterior cord to the axillary nerve in children under 2 years of age. Clinical and electromyographic return of strong, useful deltoid function was obtained in all eight. When the subscapularis muscle was used, added benefit due to lessening the exaggerated, unopposed tendency for internal rotation was noted. When the thoracodorsal nerve was used, no ill effect from a denervated latissimus was noted during a 4-year follow-up period [8, 24].

(b) Approach to the *Axillary Nerve*: *Anterior, Deltopectoral*

This exposure is similar to the infraclavicular exposure described earlier. But being a bit more lateral (or distal), it does not lend itself for clear, easy exposure of the proximal posterior cord and its emerging branches. It is not the best for accessing proximal portions of the axillary artery in case of emergency. It does allow for a clear view of the distal axillary nerve and the quadrilateral space.

The incision for the deltopectoral approach follows the pectoral fold at the deltopectoral groove. The incision exposes the cephalic vein, which can be reflected or transected. The deltoid muscle edge is reflected laterally and the coracoid exposed medially. Splitting or displacing fibers of the pectoralis major allows exposure of the pectoralis minor. Blunt dissection of the pectoralis minor borders and coracoid process insertion allows its elevation off the coracoid. Medial and inferior retraction of the pectoralis minor exposes the axilla and its contents [25, 26].

(c) Approach to the *Axillary Nerve*: *Anterior, Axillary*

This approach allows excellent exposure of the axillary nerve in the axilla, just before it enters the quadrilateral space. It also permits clear view of the proximal portion of the radial nerve. It is therefore excellent when performing a radial nerve to axillary nerve transfer anterior to the quadrilateral space. Since the axillary nerve splits into branches as it enters the quadrilateral space, this approach permits selective transfer to anterior and posterior branches of the axillary nerve. It also allows exclusion of recipient sensory fibers. This exposure does not permit clear dissection of the posterior cord or its branches. It is not suited for exposure of the axillary nerve as it emerges from the posterior cord [27].

Incision, Exposure, Technique (Anterior Axillary)

An incision is made along the posterior axillary fold over the lateral border of the latissimus dorsi (Fig. 50.19).

With the arm abducted to 90°, the incision is deepened and extended to follow the axillary fold for a short distance. The lateral border of the latissimus is first identified and then traced proximally to its tendon of insertion at the humerus. This white, broad, and glistening tendon is an important landmark. Together with the teres major muscle, it defines the lateral border of the quadrilateral space.

Retracting the teres major laterally (toward the elbow in the abducted arm) opens the quadrilateral space and allows palpation of the axillary nerve as it dives into the space in a posterior direction. The teres minor and subscapularis muscle lie medially forming the medial border of the quadrilateral space.

The axillary nerve is found in the superior border of the quadrilateral space [28].

Using a right-angle clamp and blunt dissection, the nerve can be isolated and tagged. The axillary nerve usually begins to separate into

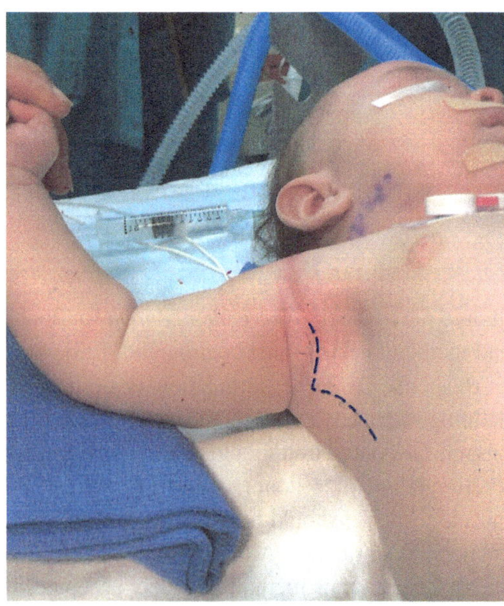

Fig. 50.19 Incision for anterior, axillary approach for the axillary nerve: The incision, along the posterior axillary fold, over the lateral border of the latissimus dorsi, is extended proximally, for a short distance along the axillary fold

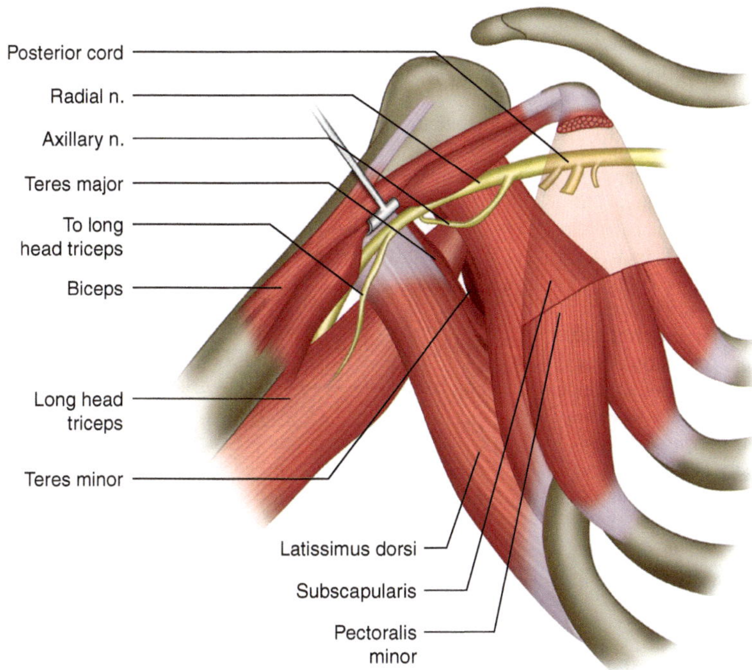

Fig. 50.20 Anterior, axillary exposure for the axillary nerve

This exposure permits a clear view of the axillary nerve, the quadrilateral space, the radial nerve, and the long had of the triceps branch. It *does not* provide good exposure for the origin of the axillary nerve from the posterior cord or for the complete posterior cord and its branches

branches as it enters the space. The posterior circumflex humeral artery also penetrates this space along with the nerve.

Superior and anterior to the quadrilateral space, just below the coracobrachialis, runs the radial nerve. Once the nerve is identified, it is traced distally to expose its branches. Usually, close to the teres major, the first branch is to the long head of triceps *(LHT)* (Fig. 50.20).

At times, a single common branch supplying both the lateral and long heads of triceps is found. If this is the case, careful dissection of the common branch and nerve stimulation allows proper identification of the *LHT*. One of the two nerves can serve as donor.

Attention is then paid to the tagged axillary nerve. Dissection to define its branches is now done proximal to the quadrilateral space. This allows selection of desired recipient fibers.

(d) Approach to the *Axillary Nerve*: *Posterior*

A posterior approach to the axillary nerve allows exposure of the nerve as it exits the quadrilateral space. When a long, posterior incision is used, this approach also permits access to the radial nerve within the triangular space. This long incision allows *nerve transfer: radial nerve branches to axillary nerve branches*. This nerve transfer, to restore axillary nerve function, provides the shortest distance to the deltoid (the target recipient muscle), which correlates with shorter reinnervation time. It also permits exclusion of recipient sensory fibers which reduces donor motor fiber dispersion [29].

The long incision is centered at the *triangular space between lateral* and *long* heads of the triceps muscle. It follows the lateral border of the deltoid ending distally at the *deltoid insertion* at mid arm. Proximally, it ends just *posterior to the acromion*. A *shorter incision* over the quadrilateral space can be used if the intention is just to identify the axillary nerve posteriorly, and a nerve transfer using the long head of the triceps *is not planned* (Fig. 50.21).

Reflecting the lateral border of the deltoid anteriorly allows exposure of teres minor and major muscles. The cleavage between these two is developed toward the humerus. The teres *minor* is *above* and more *superficial*. It passes *over* the long head of the triceps and *covers* the insertion of the lateral head of the triceps, where it terminates on the *lat-*

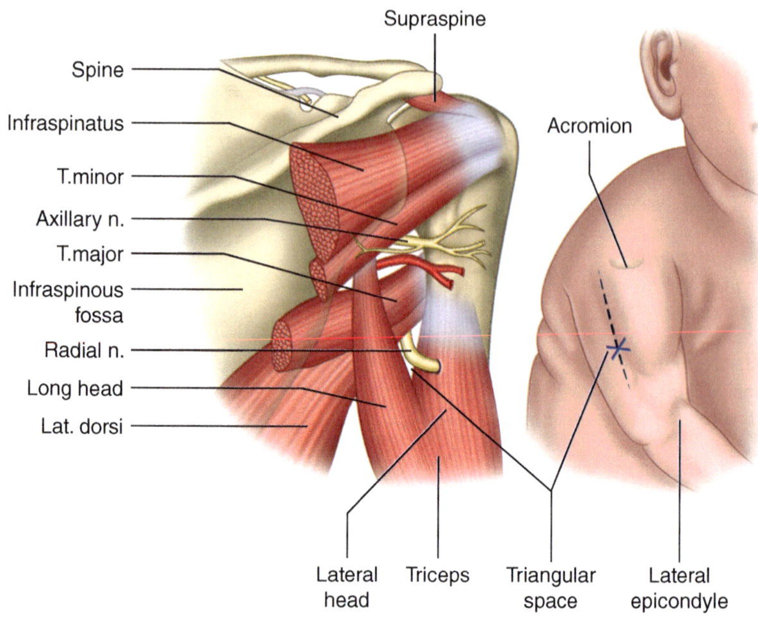

Fig. 50.21 Incision and anatomy: posterior exposure of the axillary nerve

The X marks the space between *lateral* and *long* heads of the triceps muscle (the *triangular* space). The incision follows the lateral border of the deltoid ending distally at the deltoid insertion at mid arm. Proximally, it ends at the posterior acromion

The axillary nerve exits the *quadrilateral* space. The radial nerve is found deep in the *triangular* space

eral border of the *humerus*, *above* the *surgical neck*. The teres *major* is larger and bulkier and lies *below* and *deeper*. It passes *under* the long head of the triceps before it terminates in the *medial border* of the humerus, *below* its *surgical neck.*

The *axillary nerve,* usually found in the *superior-medial* portion of the quadrilateral *space,* close to the teres minor and humerus, is bluntly separated and identified. Once looped, the nerve is skeletonized, allowing clear separation and identification of its branches (anterior, posterior, and sensory).

If a nerve transfer using branches of the radial nerve is planned, the interval between *lateral* and *long* heads of the triceps is developed proceeding distally along the arm. The triangular space is exposed and the radial nerve is identified within. The nerve is isolated and traced proximally up to the teres minor. Radial nerve branches to the lateral and long heads of the triceps are found at this level. The branch to the long head of the triceps is usually the most proximal [30–32].

Nerve Transfers to Restore Elbow Flexion

1. Nerve Transfer to the *Musculocutaneous Nerve*
   (a) Approach to Portions of Ulnar or Median Nerve in Upper Arm *(Oberlin Transfer)*

Transferring portions of ulnar and/or median nerves to musculocutaneous nerve (MCN) branches to the biceps and brachialis muscles is known to yield predictable successful restoration of elbow flexion [31, 33].

The approach calls for an incision in the medial aspect of the arm. It extends linearly toward the elbow, in the upper half of the arm width, from the pectoral fold or axillary fold to mid arm (Fig. 50.22).

The biceps muscle is found superior to the incision, above the brachialis muscle. The interval between the two muscles is developed and the musculocutaneous nerve (MCN) comes into view. Continue by isolating the MCN. The biceps branch (at times two branches) is identified and separated from the MCN. One must remember that variations are common and the MCN may arise from the median nerve [34].

With frequency, a vascular pedicle providing blood supply to the biceps crosses over the nerve. The nerve branch to the biceps from the MCN arises proximal to this pedicle.

At that same level, but inferior to the median nerve and brachial artery, the ulnar nerve is found contained within the neurovascular bundle. Stimulation confirms its identity and allows isolation and dissection. A portion of the nerve corresponding to the *flexor carpi ulnaris*, matching in size with the branch to the biceps, is selected.

This ulnar nerve portion is cut distally and mobilized to meet the branch of the biceps, which was cut proximally. This procedure is considered a *"selective single nerve transfer."* It is aimed to *restore biceps muscle function* (elbow flexion and forearm supination) (Fig. 50.23).

If a *selective double transfer is intended*, a portion of the median nerve is transferred to the brachialis branch of the MCN *in addition to* the ulnar nerve portion transferred, just mentioned.

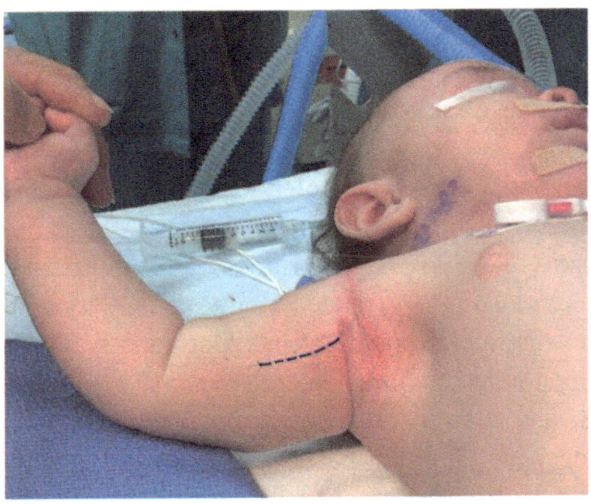

Fig. 50.22 Incision, nerve transfer: portions of ulnar or median nerves to branches of musculocutaneous nerve

The incision extends from the pectoral fold to mid arm on its upper half. It is important not to cross the axillary fold

For this, the MCN is exposed *distal* to the vascular pedicle previously mentioned. The branch to the brachialis is separated from the cutaneous terminal branch of the MCN and cut proximally. At this level, but inferiorly, the median nerve, within the neurovascular bundle, is found. The nerve is isolated and a portion corresponding to wrist flexors is selected as donor, for transfer. This portion is cut distally, at appropriate length to meet the branch for the brachialis [35].

Some surgeons prefer to alter the sequence and instead transfer portions of the median nerve to the biceps branch and portions of the ulnar nerve to the brachialis branch.

(b) Approach to *Intercostal Nerves*

For severe brachial plexus injuries, the use of intercostal nerves (ICN) to innervate the musculocutaneous nerve (MCN) has been of value. Incision and approach usually combine access to both, ICN and MCN [36, 37].

For exposure of the ICN, the incision extends along the posterior axillary line, curving anteriorly along the mammary fold to the mammary line.

The incision is deepened over the latissimus dorsi to expose the chest wall. The long thoracic nerve should be protected. The inframammary incision is also deepened proceeding anteriorly

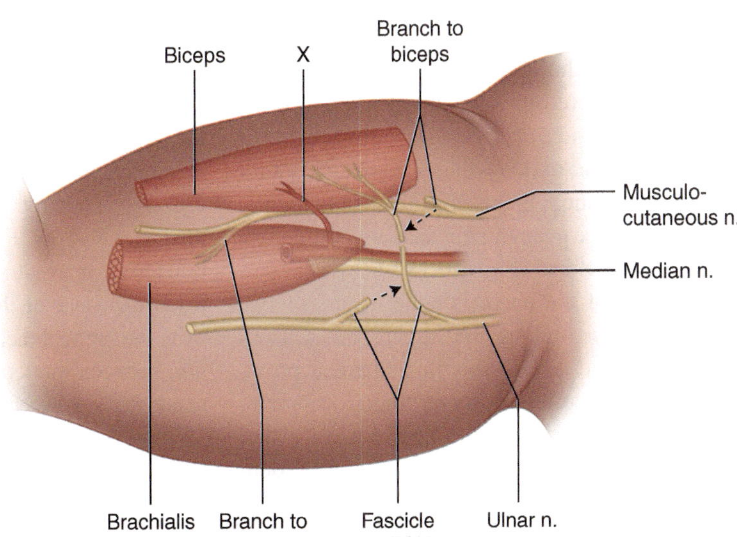

Fig. 50.23 Approach for nerve transfer: portions of median and/or ulnar nerve to branches of musculocutaneous nerve

The musculocutaneous nerve is found between biceps and brachialis muscles. The branch to the biceps is proximal to a vascular pedicle (*X*) providing blood supply to the biceps. The ulnar nerve is inferior to the median nerve within neurovascular bundle

A portion of the ulnar nerve is mobilized to meet the cut branch to the biceps. A selective single nerve transfer is shown

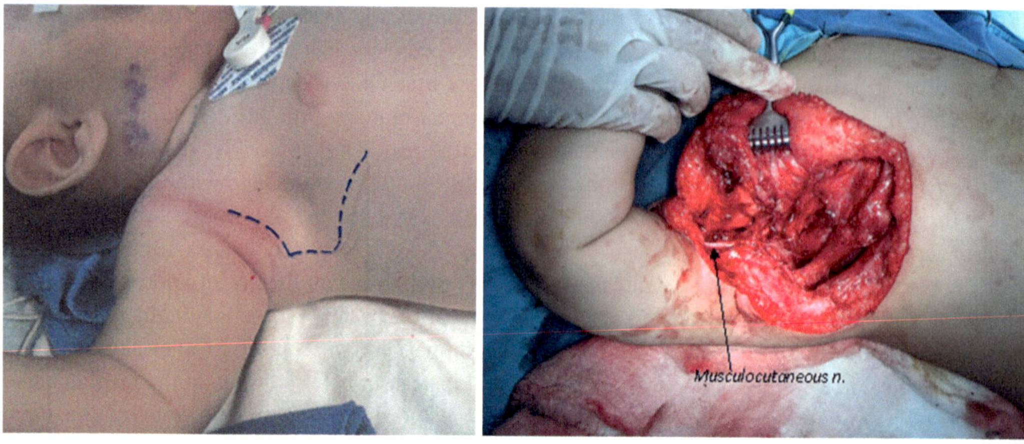

Fig. 50.24 Incision and flap mobilization for intercostal nerve harvesting
A large flap containing the pectoralis major and mammary gland is mobilized. This exposes the chest wall and ribs. This incision also allows access to the proximal portion of the musculocutaneous nerve

along the chest wall. Portions of serratus and pectoralis major muscle fibers attachments to ribs may need to be divided. Mobilization of a large flap containing the pectoralis major and mammary gland exposing the chest wall follows. Ribs 3, 4, and 5 are identified (Fig. 50.24).

For each rib, an incision is made over the rib and a subperiosteal plane is developed to its inferior border. Muscle fibers from both *internal* and *externa*l *intercostal muscles* are bluntly spread apart from the inferior border of the rib. Gently grasping, retracting, and elevating the rib helps to bring the intercostal nerve into view. Thin, *innermost intercostal* muscle fibers and the almost transparent *pleura* lay underneath separating the nerve from the thoracic cavity.

The thin intercostal nerve divides into a superficial sensory and a deep motor component at the level of the mid-axillary line. The deeper motor branch continues between intercostal muscle fibers, while the even thinner sensory component becomes superficial (Fig. 50.25).

Isolation of the nerve is done in one of two ways: (1) by finding the superficial sensory component and tracing this thin filament proximally to the common nerve fiber, containing motor and sensory components, or (2) by first finding the common nerve fiber [38]. Once identified and isolated, the nerve is mobilized proximally and distally from the posterior axillary line to the costochondral junction, where it is cut. The nerve now can be swung toward the axilla.

Some surgeons prefer to expose the MCN before isolation of intercostal nerves. For exposure of the MCN, the arm is abducted 90°, and the incision is extended along the axillary fold to the lateral border of the pectoralis major. It then may continue laterally, for a short distance, along the upper arm. The incision is deepened and the pectoralis major is retracted medially. This allows exposure of the coracobrachialis muscle and the MCN as it pierces the muscle.

The MCN is traced proximally, as close to its emergence from the lateral cord, as possible. Transection of the nerve at this level allows for direct coaptation (without the need of nerve grafts) with ICN 3, 4, and 5, without tension.

As an alternative, a skin bridge is maintained at the axillary fold, and a separate incision is made along the mid arm, as previously illustrated in Fig. 50.22, when transferring portions of ulnar or median nerves to musculocutaneous nerve branches (Oberlin transfer). This allows for a more distal exposure of the MCN (after it pierces and exits the coracobrachialis muscle). Direct coaptation between intercostal nerves and musculocutaneous nerve is possible at this level (Fig. 50.26).

Nerve Transfer for Elbow Extension

Restoration of elbow extension is of importance. Useful function can be obtained by transferring

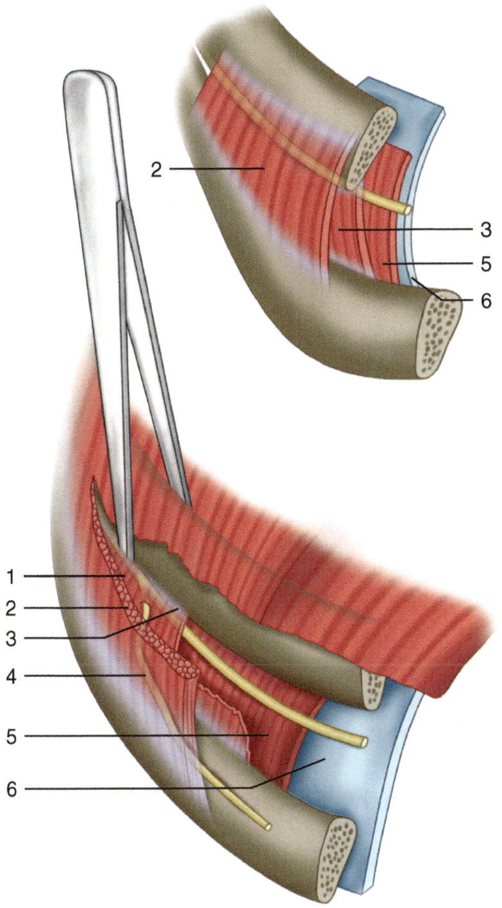

Fig. 50.25 Exposure of intercostal nerve and anatomy of intercostal space: Graphic illustration of intercostal space showing relationship between (2) external, (3) internal, and (5) innermost intercostal muscles and (6) pleura. The intercostal nerve lies inferior to the rib between interior and innermost intercostal muscles
An incision directly over the rib and mobilization of the periosteum allows exposure of bare rib. Internal and external muscle fibers are bluntly spread. Grasping, retracting, and elevating the rib help to bring the intercostal nerve into view. Thin innermost intercostal muscle fibers and the almost transparent pleura lie underneath the nerve, separating the nerve from the thoracic cavity
1. Division of intercostal into sensory and motor, at mid axillary line; 2. external intercostal m; 3. internal intercostal m; 4. sensory (superficial) portion of intercostal n; 5. innermost intercostal m; 6. pleura

portions of the ulnar nerve to *branches of the radial nerve* supplying the triceps muscle.

Of the three heads forming the triceps muscle, the long head arises from the inferior glenoid in the scapula and, thus, crosses the shoulder joint. Contraction of the long head produces elbow extension and shoulder extension and adduction. The long head is considered a weak elbow extensor. The medial head arising most distal from the humerus is thought to be the strongest elbow extensor [39].

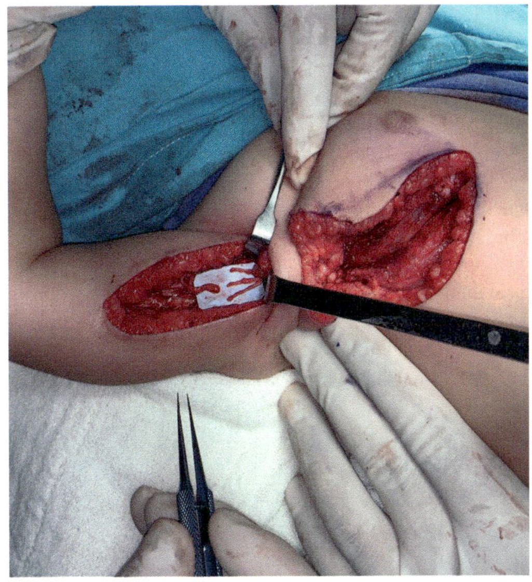

Fig. 50.26 Nerve transfer, intercostals 3, 4, 5 to distal musculocutaneous nerve at upper arm level with a skin bridge at the axillary fold
Intercostal nerves can reach the musculocutaneous at the proximal portion of the upper arm. Notice that the skin bridge preserves the axillary fold

(a) Approach to Branches of Radial Nerve to Triceps

Approach for this transfer in the upper arm is similar to the approach used for elbow flexion transfer (Oberlin), described earlier. A longitudinal incision in the medial upper arm, distal to the pectoral fold, is used. The incision is deepened to expose the neurovascular bundle just distal to the attachment of latissimus dorsi and teres major muscles into the humerus. At this point, radial and ulnar nerves lie close to each other within the neurovascular bundle. The radial and ulnar nerves are isolated. Branches from the radial nerve are identified.

The branch to the long head of the triceps is usually the most proximal branch. Branches to the medial and lateral heads are more distal. The medial head is most commonly served by *two branches* from the radial nerve: one more proximal or *superior* and one more distal or *inferior*.

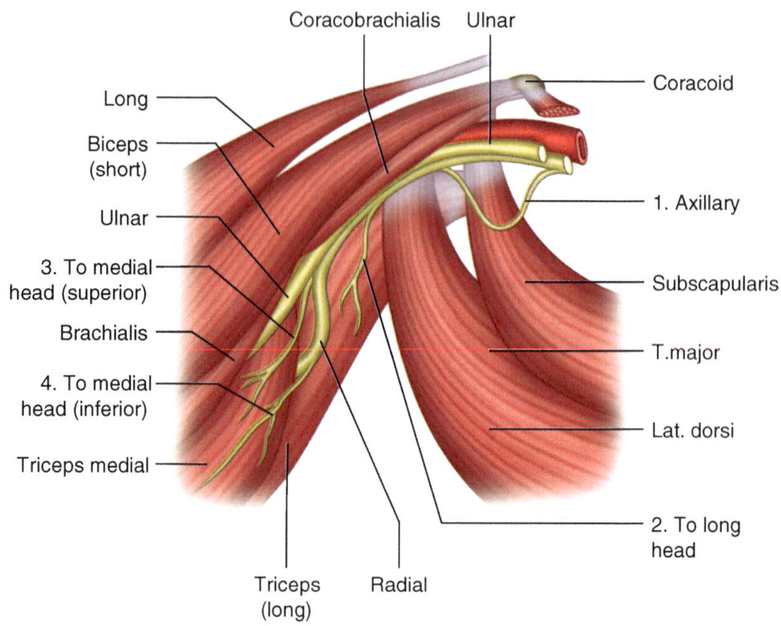

Fig. 50.27 Radial nerve branches in the proximal arm

The branch to the long head of the triceps is usually the most proximal branch. The medial head is most commonly served by two branches: one more proximal or superior and one more distal or inferior which continues to supply the anconeus muscle

The *superior branch* accompanies the ulnar nerve and may be joined by enveloping connective tissue. It has been referred as the *ulnar collateral nerve* (Fig. 50.27).

The *inferior branch* remains close to the radial nerve yet apart from the ulnar nerve before it branches out to innervate the medial head of the triceps and the anconeus muscle [40].

Either one of these two branches, superior or inferior, can become the *recipient nerve* for elbow extension. Bear in mind that the inferior branch innervates two muscles that extend the elbow: the medial head of the triceps and the anconeus. It follows that the inferior branch should be the *preferred recipient nerve* to restore elbow extension [41].

Similar to the Oberlin transfer, a *portion of the ulnar nerve not serving* hand intrinsic muscles is selected and cut distally to serve as *donor nerve*. *Inferior* or *superior* motor branch to medial head of triceps is selected as *receptor nerve* and cut proximally. End to end coaptation between a portion of the ulnar nerve *(donor)* and a branch to the medial head of the triceps *(recipient)* follows.

Bibliography

Perioperative Factors

1. Cohen MM, Cameron CB, Duncan PG. Pediatric anesthesia: morbidity, and mortality in the perioperative period. Anesth Analg. 1990;70:160–7.
2. Cladis F, Anixter M. Anesthesia for pediatric plastic surgery. In: Bentz ML, Bauer BS, Zuker RM, editors. Pediatric plastic surgery: principles and practice. 2nd ed. New York: Thieme; 2016. p. 31–72.
3. Tait AR, Malviya S, Voepel-Lewis T. Risk factors for perioperative respiratory adverse events in children with upper respiratory tract infections. Anesthesiology. 2001;95:299–306.
4. Welborn LG, Rice EJ, Hanallah RS. Postoperative apnea in former preterm infants: prospective comparison of spinal and general anesthesia. Anesthesiology. 1990;72:838–84.
5. Lerman JL, Cote CJ, Steward DJ. Manual of pediatric anesthesia. 6th ed. Philadelphia: Elsevier; 2010. p. 10–42.

Anatomy Arteries

6. Huelke D. A study of the transverse cervical and dorsal scapular arteries. Anat Rec. 1990;132:233–5.

Surgical Approach Technique

7. Cooper DE, Jenkins RS, Bready L, Rockwood CA Jr. The prevention of injuries of the brachial plexus secondary to malposition of the patient during surgery. Clin Orthop Relat Res. 1998;288(228):33–41.
8. Borrero JL. Obstetrical brachial plexus palsy. Orlando: Progressive Communications, (Xerographics); 2007. p. 53.
9. Borrero JL. Surgical technique. In: Gilbert A, editor. Brachial plexus injuries. London: Martin Dunitz; 2001. p. 191.

Variations, Lower Trunk

10. Tubbs RS, Shoja MM, Loukas M, editors. Bergman's comprehensive encyclopedia of human anatomic variations. New Jersey: Wiley Blackwell; 2016. p. 1074.
11. Hollinshead WH. Anatomy for surgeons. In: The back and limbs, vol. 3. 2nd ed. Hagerstown: Harper & Row; 1969. p. 236–48.

Infraclavicular Exposure

12. Baltzer HL, Spinner RJ, Bishop AT, Shin AY. Axillary nerve reconstruction: anterior-posterior exposure with sural nerve cable graft pull-through technique. Tech Hand Up Extrem Surg. 2015;19(4):168–75.

Nerve Transfer Root Contribution Variations; Thoughts

13. Zhong L-y, Wang A-p, Li-Hong. Microanatomy of the brachial plexus root and its clinical significance. Surg Radiol Anat. 2017;39:601–10.
14. Slingluff CL, Terzis JK, Edgerton MT. The quantitative microanatomy of the brachial plexus in man: reconstructive relevance. In: Terzis JK, editor. Microreconstruction of nerve injuries. Philadelphia: W. B. Saunders; 1987. p. 285–325.
15. Tubbs RS, Shoja MM, Loukas M, editors. Bergman's comprehensive encyclopedia of human anatomic variations. New Jersey: Wiley Blackwell; 2016. p. 1073–6.
16. Narakas AO. Thoughts on neurotization or nerve transfers in irreparable nerve lesions. Clin Plastic Surg. 1984;11(4):153–9.

Anterior Approach to SAN to SSN

17. Bertelli JA, Ghizoni MF. Transfer of the accessory nerve to the suprascapular nerve in brachial plexus reconstruction. J Hand Surg Am. 2007;32(7):989–98.
18. Bertelli JA, Ghizoni MF. Reconstruction of C5 and C6 brachial plexus avulsion injury by multiple nerve transfers: spinal accessory to suprascapular, ulnar fascicles to biceps branch and triceps long or lateral head branch to axillary nerve. J Hand Surg. 2004;29A:131–9.

Posterior Approach to SAN to SSN

19. Colbert SH, Mackinnon SE. Posterior approach for double nerve transfer for restoration of shoulder function in upper brachial plexus palsy. Hand. 2006;1(2):71–7.
20. Bahm J, Naoman H, Becker M. The dorsal approach to the suprascapular nerve in neuromuscular reanimation for obstetric brachial plexus lesions. Plast Reconstr Surg. 2005;115:240–4.
21. Bhandari MS, Prabal D. Posterior approach for both spinal accessory nerve to suprascapular nerve and triceps branch to axillary nerve for upper plexus injuries. J Hand Surg. 2013;38A:168–72.

Axillary Nerve: Anterior Infraclavicular Approach

22. Pandey SK, Shukla VK. Anatomical variations of the cords of brachial plexus and the median nerve. Clin Anat. 2007;20(2):150–6.
23. Bhat KMR, Girijavallabham V. Variations in the branching pattern of the posterior cord of the brachial plexus. Neuroanatomy. 2008;7:10–1.
24. Dai SY, Lin DX, Han Z, Zhong SZ. Transference of thoracodorsal nerve to musculocutaneous or axillary nerve in old traumatic injury. J Hand Surg [Am]. 1990;15:36–7.

Anterior Deltopectoral Approach

25. Wheelock M, Clark TA, Giuffre JL. Nerve transfer for treatment of isolated axillary nerve injuries. Plast Surg. 2015;23(2):77–80.
26. Baltzer HL, Spinner RJ, Bishop AT, Shim AY. Axillary nerve reconstruction: anterior-posterior exposure with sural nerve cable graft pull-through technique. Tech Hand Surg. 2015;19:168–75.

Approach to the Axillary Nerve: Anterior, Axillary

27. Bertelli JA, Kechele PR, Santos MA, Duarte H, Ghizoni MF. Axillary nerve repair by triceps motor branch transfer trhough an axillary access: anatomical basis and clinical results. J Neurosurg. 2007;107:370–7.
28. Tubbs RS, Tyler-Kabara EC, Aikens AC. Surgical anatomy of the axillary nerve within the quadrangular space. J Neurosurg. 2005;102:912–4.

Posterior Approach to Axillary Nerve

29. Leechavengvongs S, Witoonchart K, Uerpairojkit C, Thuvasethakul P. Nerve transfer to deltoid muscle using the nerve to the long head of the triceps, part II: a report of 7 cases. J Hand Surg. 2003;28A:633–8.
30. Zuckerman SL, Eli M, Shah MN, Bradley N, Stutz CM, Park TS, et al. Radial to axillary nerve transfers; a combined case series in children. J Neurosurg Pediatr. 2014;14(5):518–26. 22
31. Maldonado AA, Bishop AT, Spinner RJ, Shin AY. Five operations that give best results after brachial plexus injury. Plast Reconstr Surg. 2017;140(3):545–56.
32. Jacome DT, Alencar FHU, Lemos MVV. Axillary nerve neurotization by triceps motor branch: comparison between axillary and posterior arm approaches. Rev Bras Ortop. 2017;12:53(1):15–21.

Nerve Transfer for Elbow Flexion

33. Oberlin C, Beal D, Leechavengvongs S, Salon A, Dauge MC, Sarcy JJ. Nerve transfer to biceps muscle using part of the ulnar nerve for C5-C6 avulsion of the brachial plexus: anatomical study and report of four cases. J Hand Surg. 1994;19A(2):232–7.
34. Guerri-Guttenberg RA, Ingolotti M. Classifying musculocutaneous nerve variations. Clin Anat. 2009;22:671–83.
35. Tung TH, Novak PT, Mackinnon SE. Nerve transfer to the biceps and brachialis to improve elbow flexion strength after brachial plexus injuries. J Neurosurg. 2003;98:313–8.

Intercostal Nerve Transfer for Elbow Flexion

36. Kabawata H, Shibata T, Matsui Y. Use of intercostal nerves for neurotization of the musculocutaneous nerve in infants with birth-related brachial plexus palsy. J Neurosurg. 2001;94(3):386–91.
37. El Gammal TA, Abdel-Latif MM, Kotb MM. Intercostal nerve transfer in infants with obstetric brachial plexus palsy. Microsurgery. 2008;28(7):499–504.
38. Freilinger G, Holle J, Sulzgruber SC. Distribution of motor and sensory fibers in the intercostal nerves: significance in reconstructive surgery. Plast Reconstr Surg. 1978;62:240–4.

Nerve Transfer for Elbow Extension

39. Hollinshead WH. Anatomy for surgeons. In: The back and limbs, vol. 3. 2nd ed. Hagerstown: Harper & Row; 1969. p. 367.
40. Cho SH, Chung IH, Lee UY. Relationship between the ulnar nerve and the branches of the radial nerve to the medial head of the triceps brachii muscle. Clin Anat. 2019;32:137–42.
41. Flores LP. Transfer of a motor fascicle from the ulnar nerve to the radial nerve destined to the long head of the triceps for restoration of elbow extension in brachial plexus surgery: technical case report. Neurosurgery. 2012;70(2):16–20.

Management of Brachial Plexus Birth Injuries: Erbs and Extended Erbs Palsy

51

Chris Stutz

Introduction

Currently, there is no clear consensus on the surgical treatment of the nerve injury in infants with Erb's palsy (C5–C6) and extended Erb's palsy (C5–C7) who fail to attain adequate spontaneous recovery. In fact, with the rise in utility of extraplexal nerve transfers, the definition of "adequate spontaneous recovery" is beginning to blur. Some authors advocate for microsurgical intervention with no recovery of antigravity elbow flexion by 3 months of age [1]. Others have advocated for microsurgical intervention if no antigravity elbow flexion is present by 6 months of age [2], while still others use 9 months of age without antigravity elbow flexion as a surrogate for adequate spontaneous recovery [3]. And if the variability of surgical timing is not confounding enough, the variability in surgical procedures is enough to confuse even the savviest of those who treat these patients. Neurolysis, neuroma excision and nerve grafting, nerve transfer, and some combination of all have been reported in the literature as acceptable means of treatment in this patient population. Moreover, the use of intraoperative electrodiagnostic testing and performing concomitant procedures for shoulder reconstruction continue to be debated topics.

Nonoperative Management

Nonsurgical care is the initial treatment for all infants with brachial plexus birth palsy. The nonsurgical care is often initiated prior to evaluation in a surgeon's office by the newborn nursery or pediatrician. The care is centered on stretching and range of motion exercises focusing on the shoulder to preserve motion and prevent contracture and joint deformity. Infants with Erb's and extended Erb's palsy most often present with an adducted, internally rotated limb at the glenohumeral joint, extension of the elbow, pronation of the forearm, and flexion of the wrist. Hence, passive range of motion and stretching regimens should consist of external rotation of the glenohumeral joint with the scapula stabilized, abduction or overhead stretching, elbow flexion, forearm supination, and wrist extension. As spontaneous recovery of muscle function progresses, the regimen is modified to fit the persistent deficits. The stretching and range of motion exercises can be associated with diaper changes in an effort to remind caretakers and improve compliance. In addition to passive range of motion and stretching regimens, some have advocated the use of the static splinting techniques to improve patient recovery and musculoskeletal alignment [4].

C. Stutz (✉)
Department of Orthopedics, Pediatric Orthopedic, Hand, and Microvascular Surgery, Texas Scottish Rite Hospital for Children, UT Southwestern School of Medicine, Dallas, TX, USA
e-mail: Chris.Stutz@tsrh.org

A. Y. Shin, N. Pulos (eds.), *Operative Brachial Plexus Surgery*,
https://doi.org/10.1007/978-3-030-69517-0_51

Surgical Management

The indications for microsurgical brachial plexus reconstruction continue to be an area of debate among surgeons caring for infants with a brachial plexus birth palsy. From surgical timing to surgical procedure, the care of these infants continues to evolve with improved understanding of the natural history of spontaneous recovery to the advancement of surgical techniques. With that, almost all will agree that surgical intervention is indicated when surgical outcomes are expected to be better than natural history.

Indications

Spontaneous recovery in infants with Erb's or extended Erb's palsy is quite good, ranging from 60% to 80%. Early recovery of antigravity biceps function (before 3 months of age) often results in full neurologic recovery with no functional deficits [5]. The recovery of antigravity biceps function between 3 and 6 months of age also shows good upper extremity function in long-term follow-up but may necessitate the need for secondary reconstructive procedures to augment shoulder function [2, 6]. Furthermore, evaluating the need for microsurgical intervention based solely on the antigravity function of the biceps may lead to an incorrect prediction of poor outcome [7]. Including additional assessments of elbow, wrist, finger, and thumb extension may increase the evaluator's ability to predict long-term recovery of upper limb function and determine the need for microsurgical reconstruction. A Toronto Test Score less than 3.5 at 3 months of age and failure to improve from 3 months to 6 months of age are both indications for microsurgical reconstruction [3, 8]. Additionally, failure of the "cookie test" at 9 months of age can also be used as an indication for microsurgical reconstruction [3]. Even more recently, the technique of single muscle or single muscle group innervation with extra-plexal nerve transfers has further shifted the ambiguity of "indications" for primary nerve surgery. This technique can allow the surgeon the ability to treat persistent deficits in function with targeted microsurgical interventions at later time points in infancy when spontaneous recovery might have plateaued.

Imaging

Preoperative imaging of the brachial plexus in infants remains an imperfect science. Plain radiographs provide little to no diagnostic or treatment assisting information; hence these are not routinely obtained. The use of MRI or CT myelogram can be useful for identifying the presence of root avulsions by demonstrating the presence of pseudomeningoceles or diverticula (Fig. 51.1). However, their utility for assessing the location or severity of postganglionic injuries remains limited. The use of these imaging modalities also requires a general anesthetic to obtain quality images in most institutions. There are MRI protocols described that obviate the need for sedation, but their utility and usefulness have yet to be fully determined [9].

When treating infants with Erb's and extended Erb's palsy, MRI is a useful modality for identification of the presence of pseudomeningoceles indicating a nerve root avulsion while concomitantly allowing for the visualization of musculoskeletal sequelae from the brachial plexus injury, such as glenohumeral dysplasia, which is common in these patients. Ultrasound has also been used successfully utilized for the evaluation of glenohumeral articular anatomy [10] (Fig. 51.2).

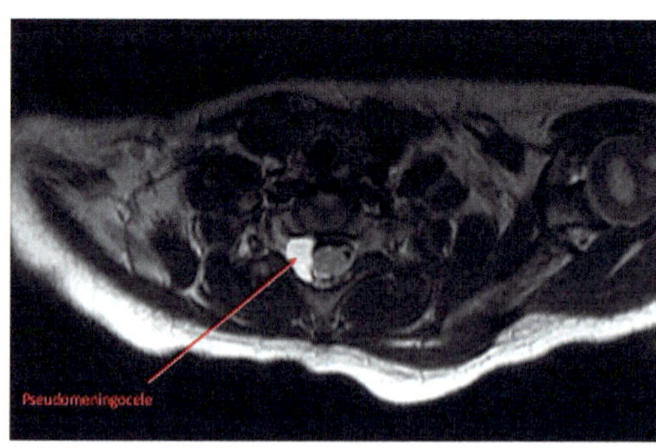

Fig. 51.1 Magnetic resonance image of an infant with a cervical root avulsion and an associated pseudomeningocele

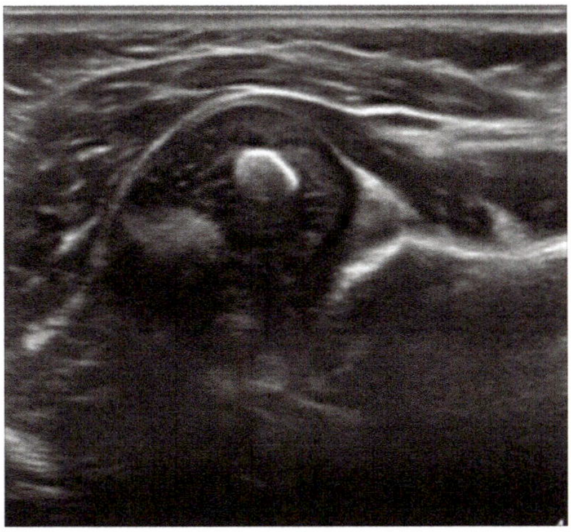

Fig. 51.2 Ultrasound image of an infant with posterior glenohumeral dysplasia and humeral head positioned posteriorly within the glenoid fossa

When performing brachial plexus microsurgery in combination with procedures for the treatment of the musculoskeletal sequelae, one or both of these imaging modalities can be useful for preoperative planning.

Electrodiagnostics

The use of preoperative electrodiagnostics in brachial plexus birth palsy is less useful than its use in the treatment of adult injuries. The underestimation of injury severity and overestimation of potential recovery along with the plasticity of the infant neurologic system make the results extremely difficult to interpret.

The use of intraoperative electrodiagnostics is highly variable between institutions and surgeons. Interpretation inconsistencies make studying the effectiveness of their use difficult across institutional practices. Surgeons with well-established electrodiagnostic programs often employ the use of intraoperative electromyography to determine conductivity through neuromas-in-continuity by using compound muscle activation potentials (CMAPs). Others prefer the use of handheld nerve stimulators to determine conductivity. In addition to distal testing, electrodiagnostics can be used to determine the presence or absence of nerve root avulsions by utilizing somatosensory evoked potentials (SSEPs). Currently, succinct recommendations or standards concerning electrodiagnostic use intraoperatively for decision-making during microsurgical management of brachial plexus birth palsy do not exist. Rather, their use is guided by institutional availability and surgeon preference.

Surgical Procedures

Neurolysis

The use of neurolysis alone for treatment of brachial plexus birth palsy and its associated neuromas-in-continuity has declined in most brachial plexus treatment protocols in favor of neuroma excision and nerve grafting and/or nerve transfers. Lin et al. published a manuscript in 2009 stating "neurolysis as a complete surgical treatment for obstetrical brachial plexus palsy should be abandoned in favor of neuroma resection and nerve grafting." [11] This view has subsequently been supported by others [12]. That being said, some still argue the benefit of neurolysis alone in a certain subset of infants who meet clinical indications for microsurgical exploration. Those who support the use of neurolysis maintain that some "conducting" neuromas-in-continuity supply sufficient axonal function to alleviate the need to complete excision and grafting. The operative decision to neurolyse versus excise a neuroma-in-continuity is based on the use of intraoperative electromyography. Andrisevic et al. support the use of neurolysis alone when >50% conduction is seen across the neuroma during intraoperative testing citing an improvement in shoulder and elbow function postoperatively [13].

Neuroma Excision and Nerve Grafting

Neuroma excision and nerve grafting remain the gold standard in treatment for infants with Erb's and extended Erb's palsy who do not recover satisfactory function spontaneously. The concept of neuroma excision rests on the principle of proximal and distal resection to healthy fascicles. In most infants, the proximal resection is at the root level, while the distal resection usually falls at the divisional level. In a less common scenario, the nerve roots have been avulsed from the spinal cord leaving no healthy fascicles proximally. In these instances, alternative anatomic reconstructions have been described, as well as the use of extra-plexal nerve transfers.

Surgical approach to the brachial plexus is commonly done through a V-shaped incision along the posterior border of the sternocleidomastoid muscle extending along the superior clavicle to the trapezius insertion or alternatively through a supraclavicular transverse incision from the posterior border of the sternocleidomastoid to the anterior border of the trapezius. Regardless of incision, the omohyoid muscle is transected and retracted medially to identify the anterior scalene. The phrenic nerve is intimately associated with the anterior surface of the anterior scalene and is a consistent surgical landmark. The phrenic nerve can then be traced proximally to identify the C5 nerve root. Once identified, the transversely oriented C5 nerve root can be traced distally to identify the neuroma most often located at Erb's point – the junction of the C5 and C6 nerve roots. From this point, proximal dissection is used to identify the more vertically oriented and deeper C6 nerve root. In an isolated Erb's palsy, this may be the extent of root exposure necessary. In the extended Erb's palsy, C7 root identification is necessary. Retraction of the C5–C6 neuroma in a superolateral direction will facilitate the exposure of C7. Care is taken during C7 exposure to protect the transverse scapular artery as it often crosses the nerve root at the trunk transition. With the proximal plexus dissection complete, the focus turns to distal aspect of the neuroma. The distal aspect of the neuroma most often lies at the division or cord level. Given the amount of scar present, planning the reconstruction at the cord level can simplify the surgical reconstruction of the upper plexus.

After isolation of the neuroma is completed, the surgeon must then determine the quantity and quality of proximal fascicles available for reconstruction. Sectioning of the nerve roots proximal to the neuroma should reveal healthy fascicles with absence of scarring and the presence of slight fascicular extrusion from the epineurial sheath secondary to elevated intraneural pressure. If healthy fascicles are not evident, sequential proximal sectioning should be completed until healthy fascicles are exposed. The failure to expose healthy fascicles prior to encountering the vertebral foramen represents the presence of a neural avulsion and prevents the associated nerve root from being useful in surgical reconstruction. As an alternative or in addition to sequential sectioning, some surgeons utilize the presence of SSEPs to determine the viability of a nerve root.

After the inventory of available proximal fascicles is complete, the surgical reconstruction plan can be delineated. Priorities in reconstruction for infants with Erb's and extended Erb's palsy are (1) elbow flexion, (2) shoulder abduction and external rotation, and (3) wrist extension. Distal targets often include the lateral cord for restoration of elbow flexion and suprascapular nerve for restoration of abduction and external rotation. This can be accomplished in a variety of ways based on availability of proximal fascicles (Fig. 51.3). When an extended Erb's palsy is present, C7 grafting to the posterior cord or posterior division of the middle trunk is performed to try and achieve wrist extension (Fig. 51.4). Again, variability in the reconstruction pattern is depen-

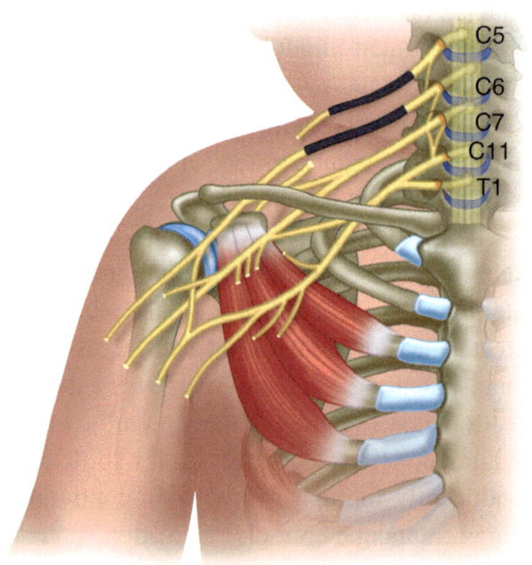

Fig. 51.3 Brachial plexus reconstruction using C5 nerve root to provide fascicles to the suprascapular nerve and the C6 nerve root to provide fascicles to the anterior division of the lateral cord

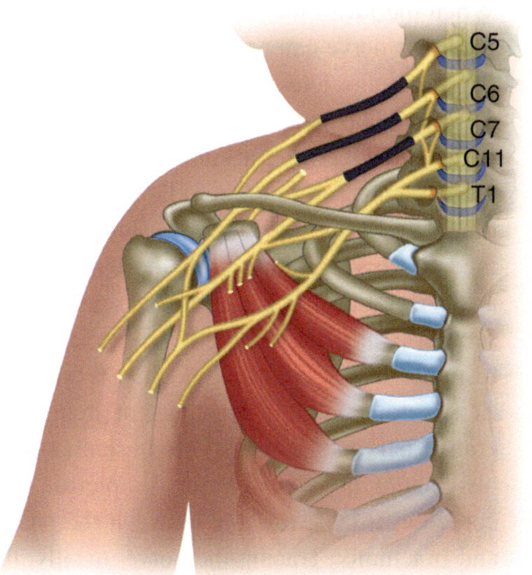

Fig. 51.4 Brachial plexus reconstruction using C5 nerve root to provide fascicles to the suprascapular nerve, the C6 nerve root to provide fascicles to the anterior division of the lateral cord, and the C7 nerve root to provide fascicles to the posterior cord

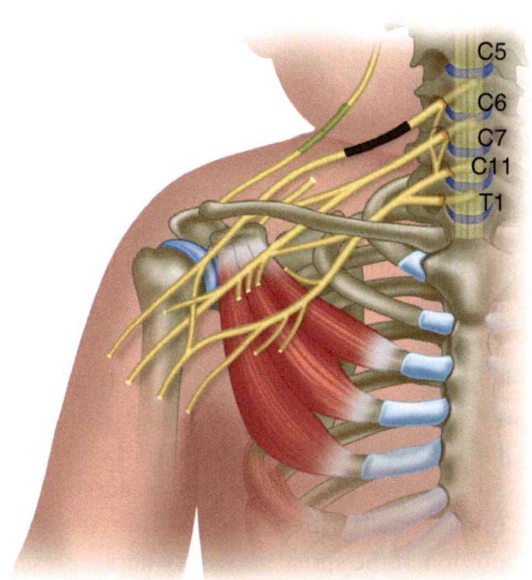

Fig. 51.5 Hybrid brachial plexus reconstruction with C5 nerve root avulsed; therefore C6 nerve root is used to provide fascicles to the lateral cord, and the spinal accessory nerve is used to provide fascicles to the suprascapular nerve

dent on the availability of healthy proximal fascicles. In fact, neuroma excision and nerve grafting are often combined with nerve transfer techniques to maximize fascicles available for functional restoration (Fig. 51.5).

Autologous sural nerve graft remains the gold standard for surgical reconstruction of nerve defects in brachial plexus surgery. Although there are reports outlining the use of nerve allograft and nerve conduit for primary reconstruction in brachial plexus birth palsy, these techniques need considerable more study prior to becoming first-line treatments [14]. Neurorrhaphy is most commonly completed with 8–0 or 9–0 nylon suture. This is then reenforced with fibrin glue. Some authors have advocated for the use of fibrin glue alone in an effort to decrease intraneural scarring as well as decrease total surgical times. The differences in these techniques have yet to be explicitly studied in this patient population.

Nerve Transfer

The technique of nerve transfer surgery continues to offer an alternative as well as an adjunct to the traditional technique of neuroma excision and nerve grafting. Since its inception, the technique of nerve transfer has been rapidly expanding in regard to the number of nerves potentially useful as available transfers. In brachial plexus birth palsy, nerve transfer techniques have been found effective for late presentation, isolated deficits, failed primary reconstruction, and multiple nerve root avulsions in addition to their expanding use for primary reconstruction [15].

Several nerve transfers are commonly used in the treatment of infants with Erb's and extended Erb's palsy. Despite neuroma excision and nerve grafting still being the gold standard for primary reconstruction, nerve transfer has become increasingly popular in the reconstruction of these upper trunk lesions. The proposed benefits include avoidance of surgery in a scarred surgical field, targeted reinnervation of certain muscle/muscle groups in the setting of mosaic recovery where neuroma excision may not be indicated, late presentation, and in those situations where proximal fascicles may not be available for reconstruction secondary to root avulsion. In addition to their exclusive use for primary reconstruction, nerve transfer is also used alongside neuroma excision and nerve grafting in hybrid reconstructions aimed at maximizing functional limb recovery.

1. Spinal Accessory Nerve to Suprascapular Nerve Transfer
   The suprascapular nerve innervates the supraspinatus and the infraspinatus muscles of the rotator cuff. Effective abduction and external rotation of the glenohumeral joint is largely dependent on their function. The suprascapular nerve arises from the superior trunk and is often involved in the neuroma associated with an Erb's and extended Erb's palsy. With available proximal fascicles, the suprascapular nerve can be reinnervated with grafting from the cervical nerve roots (C5 or C6). Alternatively, the suprascapular nerve can be reinnervated with fascicles from the distal portion of the spinal accessory nerve, preserving cervical root fascicles for reconstruction of other plexus structures. This nerve transfer has been reported by multiple authors to be effective for restoration of abduction and external rotation in the setting of brachial plexus birth palsy [16, 17]. Anterior and posterior approaches have been described for completion of this nerve transfer. In infants, especially those undergoing concomitant brachial plexus exploration and possible neuroma excision and nerve grafting, the anterior approach through a supraclavicular incision is often most useful.
2. Ulnar Nerve Fascicle to Biceps Branch of the Musculocutaneous Nerve

When the lower plexus is spared from injury, the ulnar nerve can provide a valuable source of healthy fascicles for transfer to gain biceps function. This nerve transfer is often referred to as the Oberlin transfer [18]. Through a medial approach to the middle brachium, the ulnar nerve is identified posterior to the median nerve running with the basilic vein. After isolating the nerve, intrafascicular dissection is utilized to isolate the fascicle most responsible for flexor carpi ulnaris function. This is done with the assistance of an intraoperative nerve stimulator. The musculocutaneous nerve is found after it pierces the coracobrachialis, running between the biceps and brachialis. Tracing the nerve distally, the branch to the biceps is found in the middle/distal third of the brachium. Using the "donor-distal, recipient-proximal" technique, the fascicle of the ulnar nerve and the branch of the musculocutaneous nerve to the biceps are cut. Coaptation in the medial arm is then easily achieved in tension-free fashion (Fig. 51.6).

Multiple modifications of the original technique have been introduced in the recent past. The double fascicular transfer uses a fascicle from the median nerve to innervate the brachialis in addition to an ulnar nerve fascicle for transfer to the biceps branch of the musculocutaneous nerve [19]. Others have used median nerve fascicles alone to achieve elbow

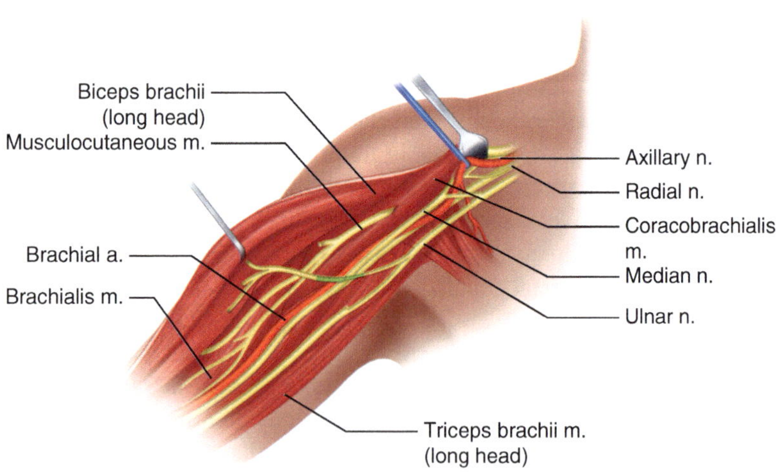

Fig. 51.6 Transfer of a fascicle of the ulnar nerve to the biceps branch of the musculocutaneous nerve

flexion via innervation of the biceps branch of the musculocutaneous nerve [20]. The specific technique chosen is tailored to each patient based on available healthy fascicles.

3. Radial Nerve Fascicle to Axillary Nerve
   Described by Leechavengvongs and colleagues, the transfer of long head of triceps branches from the radial to nerve to the motor branches of the axillary nerve has proven a useful technique for achieving deltoid function in those infants with persistent C5–C6 dysfunction [21]. As with other nerve transfers, a mandatory prerequisite for transfer is a functioning radial nerve; hence those infants with an extended Erb's palsy may not be the best candidates for this procedure. This operation is typically described through a posterior approach to the brachium. Recently, an anterior approach has been described [22]. In infants, this approach is often easily incorporated with additional procedures, including additional nerve transfers and/or open procedures for treatment of glenohumeral dysplasia.

Concomitant Surgery

Shoulder Realignment for Treatment of Glenohumeral Dysplasia

The care of children with persistent Erb's and extended Erb's palsy is rarely limited to decisions involving microsurgical nerve reconstruction. In fact, the majority of children experience spontaneous recovery sufficient to preclude the need for nerve intervention, while many without complete motor recovery will have some degree of glenohumeral dysplasia. When taking care of infants who meet the indications for microsurgical nerve reconstruction and have clinical and/or imaging findings of glenohumeral dysplasia, the decision-making regarding surgical timing becomes more complicated. In an effort to limit anesthetic exposure to infants, surgical planning to accomplish multiple procedures under a single anesthesia is preferable. The earliest reports of glenohumeral dysplasia occur in infants as young as 2–3 months of age [23]. Delaying intervention for the glenohumeral dysplasia is warranted pending the determination of sufficient neurologic recovery to preclude microsurgical nerve reconstruction. In those infants who meet the clinical indications for both microsurgical nerve reconstruction and treatment of glenohumeral dysplasia, concomitant procedures can be safely performed under a single anesthetic. For those infants whose glenohumeral deformity is reducible by closed means under anesthesia, chemodenervation of the internal rotators of the shoulder and placement in an external rotation cast may prove sufficient for treatment of the dysplasia. For those who have an irreducible deformity, an open procedure with transfer of the latissimus dorsi tendon (and/or teres major) to the infraspinatus footprint is indicated.

Postoperative Care

Following microsurgical nerve reconstruction involving surgical dissection in the posterior triangle of the neck, infants are generally admitted for overnight observation. Although the risk of developing a hematoma that may compromise the infant's airway is small, overnight observation is warranted following neck exploration and an often-extended anesthetic time in an infant less than 12 months of age. Those who do not require concomitant intervention for glenohumeral dysplasia have incisions dressed with simple gauze dressings. When postoperative discomfort has subsided and the wounds have healed (usually ~ 1 week postoperatively), the infants resume external rotation, overhead and supination stretching exercises under the direction of the caretaker at home. Those who do require intervention for glenohumeral dysplasia are immobilized in an external rotation cast for 6 weeks.

The timing of neurologic recovery is dependent on the type of microsurgical reconstruction performed, the level of the lesion, the age of the infant, and possibly other factors. In general, close monitoring for neurologic recovery begins around 6 months after surgery and can be seen as late as 18 months.

References

1. Gilbert A, Whitaker I. Obstetrical brachial plexus lesions. J Hand Surg Br. 1991;16(5):489–91.
2. Waters PM. Comparison of the natural history, the outcome of microsurgical repair, and the outcome of operative reconstruction in brachial plexus birth palsy. J Bone Joint Surg Am. 1999;81(5):649–59.
3. Clarke HM, Curtis CG. An approach to obstetrical brachial plexus injuries. Hand Clin. 1995;11(4):563–80; discussion 580-561.
4. Verchere C, Durlacher K, Bellows D, Pike J, Bucevska M. An early shoulder repositioning program in birth-related brachial plexus injury: a pilot study of the Sup-ER protocol. Hand (N Y). 2014;9(2):187–95.
5. Narakas AO. Injuries of the brachial plexus and neighboring peripheral nerves in vertebral fractures and other trauma of the cervical spine. Orthopade. 1987;16(1):81–6.
6. Al-Qattan MM. The outcome of Erb's palsy when the decision to operate is made at 4 months of age. Plast Reconstr Surg. 2000;106(7):1461–5.
7. Michelow BJ, Clarke HM, Curtis CG, Zuker RM, Seifu Y, Andrews DF. The natural history of obstetrical brachial plexus palsy. Plast Reconstr Surg. 1994;93(4):675–80; discussion 681.
8. Fisher DM, Borschel GH, Curtis CG, Clarke HM. Evaluation of elbow flexion as a predictor of outcome in obstetrical brachial plexus palsy. Plast Reconstr Surg. 2007;120(6):1585–90.
9. Shen PY, Nidecker AE, Neufeld EA, Lee PS, James MA, Bauer AS. Non-sedated rapid volumetric proton density MRI predicts neonatal brachial plexus birth palsy functional outcome. J Neuroimaging. 2017;27(2):248–54.
10. Vathana T, Rust S, Mills J, et al. Intraobserver and interobserver reliability of two ultrasound measures of humeral head position in infants with neonatal brachial plexus palsy. J Bone Joint Surg Am. 2007;89(8):1710–5.
11. Lin JC, Schwentker-Colizza A, Curtis CG, Clarke HM. Final results of grafting versus neurolysis in obstetrical brachial plexus palsy. Plast Reconstr Surg. 2009;123(3):939–48.
12. Hale HB, Bae DS, Waters PM. Current concepts in the management of brachial plexus birth palsy. J Hand Surg Am. 2010;35(2):322–31.
13. Andrisevic E, Taniguchi M, Partington MD, Agel J, Van Heest AE. Neurolysis alone as the treatment for neuroma-in-continuity with more than 50% conduction in infants with upper trunk brachial plexus birth palsy. J Neurosurg Pediatr. 2014;13(2):229–37.
14. Ashley WW Jr, Weatherly T, Park TS. Collagen nerve guides for surgical repair of brachial plexus birth injury. J Neurosurg. 2006;105(6 Suppl):452–6.
15. Tse R, Kozin SH, Malessy MJ, Clarke HM. International Federation of Societies for Surgery of the Hand Committee report: the role of nerve transfers in the treatment of neonatal brachial plexus palsy. J Hand Surg Am. 2015;40(6):1246–59.
16. Segal D, Cornwall R, Little KJ. Outcomes of spinal accessory-to-suprascapular nerve transfers for brachial plexus birth injury. J Hand Surg Am. 2019;44(7):578–87.
17. Kostas-Agnantis I, Korompilias A, Vekris M, et al. Shoulder abduction and external rotation restoration with nerve transfer. Injury. 2013;44(3):299–304.
18. Oberlin C, Beal D, Leechavengvongs S, Salon A, Dauge MC, Sarcy JJ. Nerve transfer to biceps muscle using a part of ulnar nerve for C5-C6 avulsion of the brachial plexus: anatomical study and report of four cases. J Hand Surg Am. 1994;19(2):232–7.
19. Goubier JN, Teboul F. Technique of the double nerve transfer to recover elbow flexion in C5, C6, or C5 to C7 brachial plexus palsy. Tech Hand Up Extrem Surg. 2007;11(1):15–7.
20. Al-Qattan MM, Al-Kharfy TM. Median nerve to biceps nerve transfer to restore elbow flexion in obstetric brachial plexus palsy. Biomed Res Int. 2014;2014:854084.
21. Leechavengvongs S, Witoonchart K, Uerpairojkit C, Thuvasethakul P. Nerve transfer to deltoid muscle using the nerve to the long head of the triceps, part II: a report of 7 cases. J Hand Surg Am. 2003;28(4):633–8.
22. Bauer AS, Rabinovich RV, Waters PM. The anterior approach for transfer of radial nerve triceps fascicles to the axillary nerve. J Hand Surg Am. 2019;44(4):345 e341–6.
23. Moukoko D, Ezaki M, Wilkes D, Carter P. Posterior shoulder dislocation in infants with neonatal brachial plexus palsy. J Bone Joint Surg Am. 2004;86(4):787–93.

Management of Brachial Plexus Birth Injuries: Pan Plexus

52

Alejandro Muset Lara, Anil Bhatia, Jorge Clifton Correa, Tarek Abdalla El Gammal, Ana Moratona, and Daniel Oliveras

Total brachial plexus palsies represent severe traction injuries to all the five roots of the brachial plexus. In the context of brachial plexus birth injuries (BPBI), they imply babies being born with complete disconnection of the brain and spinal cord from the affected upper limb. Given the small size of the baby's neck and the slow speed of injury during delivery, the broken ends of the roots are said to lie close to the proximal stumps. The short lengths of these nerve defects and the high potential for neural regeneration in the ruptured roots lead to spontaneous appearance of function in the paralysed upper limbs with time. However, this is usually limited to the proximal muscles and is, almost never, coordinated enough to permit use of the arm in any activity. There is a consensus that such a severe deficit is an automatic indication for surgical exploration and reconstruction. The quality of function achieved will depend considerably on the strategy employed in nerve reconstruction. Over the years, we have realized that nerve repairs in BPBI yield much better results than those seen in similar post-traumatic cases. In addition, such patients need prolonged care and supervision as well as periodic secondary operations to improve the shoulder and elbow functions that contribute towards better use of the hand. We would like to propose this aggressive strategy to achieve independent function in total palsies rather than merely a helping hand.

Initial Management

Total BPBI have been reported to be more frequent in the presence of predisposing factors such as high birth weight [1–7], prolonged labour necessitating application of external force in the form of forceps or vacuum to assist delivery, induction of labour with medication while progress is impeded by shoulder dystocia, etc.

The arm lies insensate and flaccid by the side of the trunk. The presence of a Horner's sign provides testimony to the severity of the injury [8, 9]. Fractures of the humerus (particularly epiphyseal separation at the upper end) and other causes of pseudo-paralysis should be ruled out by suitable investigations.

A. M. Lara (✉)
Department of Brachial Plexus and Birth Palsy Surgery, Muset Institute and Brachial Plexus International School, Barcelona, Spain
e-mail: dr.muset@musetinstitute.com

A. Bhatia
Deenanath Mangeskan Hospital, Pune, India

J. C. Correa
Instituto Mielinade Guadalajara, Guadalajara, Mexico

T. A. E. Gammal
Microsurgery Unit Assiut University, Assiut, Egypt

A. Moratona · D. Oliveras
Muset Institute, Barcelona, Spain

A. Y. Shin, N. Pulos (eds.), *Operative Brachial Plexus Surgery*,
https://doi.org/10.1007/978-3-030-69517-0_52

The parents are informed about the injury and the care necessary to avoid excess manipulation of the affected arm as that will not be resisted by the baby.

Most surgeons agree that infants with T1 involvement who fail to show rapid recovery, and/or presence of Horner's syndrome, should undergo early surgical intervention at 3 months of age or younger. The presence of Horner's syndrome, alone, is not pathognomonic of root avulsions of the C8–T1 roots (unlike in post-traumatic palsies), and cases with preserved or recovered hand functions have been reported in presence of Horner's syndrome. However, its association with a total paralysis at 3 months and even complete absence of hand functions despite recovery of shoulder antepulsion and elbow flexion are considered absolute indications for early microsurgical reconstruction. The child's condition, need for surgery, outcomes anticipated, the prolonged physical therapy and possibility of secondary operations at periodic intervals are all part of the counselling required in such cases.

Preoperative Evaluation

The diagnosis of a serious injury is usually evident clinically and the decision to operate is automatic. Of course, one has to rule out other causes of weakness such as arthrogryposis. Concomitant defects and anomalies must be noted. Clinical assessment is the basis for considering microsurgical repair. The extent of the lesion is evaluated from the features at presentation, while the type of nerve injury is determined by the clinical improvement, if any, within the first few months after birth [10].

Pondaag [11] has published on the utility of an EMG of the biceps that can point towards a severe injury as early as a month. However, the search for a gold standard continues. It has not been possible to determine conclusively the difference between avulsions and extra-foraminal ruptures of individual roots. Various units have reported systematic evaluation of the intraspinal course of the roots using CT myelography under general anaesthesia [12–19] or 1.5 Tesla MRI [20]. As mentioned above, the short distance between the ruptured ends of the roots and the trunks results in appearance of function in the proximal muscles, e.g. pectoralis major and triceps within 3–4 months. Dissection of the roots to their ruptured ends would inevitably involve loss of these primitive functions. The parents have to be informed that the arm will be in the condition seen at birth immediately after the operation. Also, management of a larger child is more difficult after the operation, and, hence, we prefer to operate upon such babies as early as possible. Three months is considered a suitable age from the perspective of anaesthetic risks.

A concomitant phrenic nerve injury may jeopardize the recovery from general anaesthesia and precludes harvesting intercostal nerves, and, hence, evaluation of the movements of the domes of the diaphragm by sonography and an x-ray of the chest is essential [21–23].

Surgical Treatment

The decision to do nerve surgery in BPBI is based on the premise that spontaneous recovery is unlikely to restore useful function. In cases of total lesions, all the five roots are affected, and that automatically implies a severe stretching injury. Inevitably, such lesions include avulsions at several levels with complete interruption of continuity at intraspinal levels. Experience has shown that such injuries, if left alone, will not resolve spontaneously and, ultimately, the child will be left with a deformed, non-functional upper limb [24–31]. Hence, it is imperative to explore the brachial plexus and attempt to restore function of the paralysed arm. Such a procedure would involve excision of the scarred remnants of the nerve ends in the neck so that viable proximal and distal stumps can be reconnected. Evidently, the function anticipated would depend on the strategy employed during the nerve operation.

Surgical repairs of these injuries were attempted as early as the beginning of the twentieth century [32]. Initial efforts aimed at direct repairs across the injured segments with immobilization of the head, neck and trunk in awkward positions of lateral flexion. The morbidity of these operations and the poor outcomes led to progressive disinterest in primary treatment, and the focus shifted to correction of deformities and addressing residual motor deficits. The utility of nerve grafting in bridging nerve defects brought back interest in reconstruction of brachial plexus injuries and BPBI. Gilbert [33–37] is, often, cited as having pioneered the strategy of early nerve repairs in children with extensive palsies and in those with delayed spontaneous return of functions. He also showed that nerve repairs in the neck do provide useful hand function in BPBI unlike the disappointing experience in post-traumatic situations in adults.

The principles of peripheral nerve surgery for closed injuries are all applicable in these operations. Formal exploration of the injured brachial plexus is essential. All the roots must be examined. It is important to distinguish between ruptured roots (described occasionally as neurotmetic roots) that have the potential for regrowth and can serve as nerve donors and root avulsions that have no capacity for spontaneous regeneration. In general, the upper roots (C5 and C6) are more likely to be ruptured, while the lower roots are more susceptible to intra-foraminal lesions and avulsions. Unlike high-velocity injuries associated with post-traumatic brachial plexus lesions, the slow speed of injury during delivery implies that the ruptured root stumps most often contain higher percentages of healthy nerve ends that can be harnessed for repair. The paucity of nerve axons in available extra-plexal donors such as intercostals and the spinal accessory nerve make the search for these ruptured roots essential. Experience helps to determine the condition of the available root stumps before using them for grafting. Roots of dubious quality should be directed to least important functions. Surgeons who commit to care of infants with NBPP need to avoid an over-reliance on brachial plexus exploration and nerve grafting and should have the capability and inclination for nerve transfer reconstruction [38, 39].

Surgical Technique

The child is laid supine with a pad between the scapulae to produce neck extension with the head turned to the opposite side. The field is prepared to include the contralateral side of the neck; ipsilateral hemi-chest for intercostal nerves and both legs are prepared for harvest of the sural nerves. We do not prefer to infiltrate saline adrenaline in the surgical field prior to incision although that has been the practice in some units [38]. Bleeding in the subdermal and subcutaneous planes can be readily controlled.

The supraclavicular brachial plexus is exposed via an incision along the sternocleidomastoid and along the clavicle. The external jugular vein is retracted and suitable tributaries are clipped and divided. The omohyoid muscle and the transverse cervical vessels are divided. The phrenic nerve is identified on the anterior surface of the scalenus anterior muscle and protected. The carotid sheath (particularly the internal jugular vein) often overlies the scalenus anterior and has to be retracted gently in the medial direction. The C5 root can be usually identified at the lateral border of the scalenus anterior as it is crossed by the phrenic nerve. The root can be traced medial to the phrenic nerve and into the intervertebral foramen. The scalenus anterior muscle fibres can be divided to facilitate this dissection. The branch to the serratus anterior can usually be seen leaving the posterior aspect of the root at this level. It traverses the scalenus medius muscle joining other branches from the C6 and C7 roots to form the long thoracic nerve. Dissection then proceeds inferiorly in the plane deep to the scalenus anterior. The C6 and C7 roots are explored at the respective intervertebral foramina, the latter being slightly inferior and posterior to the upper root.

The trunks are usually found encased in dense scar tissue in the interscalene area. The key to the distal dissection is identification of the suprascapular nerve close to the notch. The insertion of the omohyoid at the superior border of the scapula helps in this [38]. The nerve normally lies along the lateral border of the plexus as it arises from the upper trunk and courses inferiorly and laterally towards the suprascapular notch. This site of origin gets distorted as the upper trunk is stretched, torn and scarred. The suprascapular nerve must be handled carefully as it is traced proximally to the upper trunk and the posterior and anterior divisions are separated. The middle trunk is then identified behind the clavicle and traced superiorly to the scarred area. The dorsal scapular artery is found either between the upper and middle trunks or between the middle and lower trunks and should be divided to facilitate exposure. The C8 and T1 roots lie deep in the operative field but, with retraction of the clavicle, can be readily visualized without dividing the clavicle. The T1 root lies immediately superficial to the parietal pleura. If the pleura is violated, as demonstrated by air bubbles in a saline-flooded field, it may be possible to seal the leak with fibrin glue (Tisseel; Baxter International, Deerfield, IL), or it may become necessary to insert a chest tube. An osteotomy of the clavicle after raising periosteal flaps was often used to facilitate exposure of the trunks and divisions. However, we observed failure of union in some of our patients. This did not affect the outcome. We now choose to approach this area by extending the wound to the deltopectoral groove and dissecting the medial cord proximally. Dissection continues distal to the neuroma to define where the nerve appears undamaged. The lower trunk can be visualized only after retracting the middle trunk laterally. It lies inferiorly and medially behind the subclavian artery. The artery and its branches are carefully identified and retracted and the lower trunk traced to the C8 and T1 roots. Usually the avulsed ends are found outside the foramina. However, occasionally, the trunk may appear smooth and the roots seem intact. In the absence of clinical function and with no response on stimulation at 3–4 months of age, good spontaneous recovery in the hand cannot be reasonably expected in such cases. So, we prefer to disregard this apparent continuity and plan for reconstruction of hand function by grafting from distinctly ruptured upper roots to the lower trunk.

The quality of the ruptured roots is then examined. They are sectioned close to the neuroma and, then, serially, towards the foramina. In general, as mentioned above, the upper roots tend to be ruptured, while the lower roots are more susceptible for avulsions. If the root appears intact within the foramen, the branch to the serratus anterior gives a good response on stimulation (provided it remains in continuity with the long thoracic nerve), and the cut section shows healthy fascicles with minimal scar tissue, the root may be utilized for reconstruction. We have not used intraoperative electrophysiological evaluation or somatosensory evoked potentials to determine the proximal continuity of these roots.

The strategy for restoration of maximal function in the paralysed upper limb depends upon the number of roots available. Unlike partial palsies where hand function is preserved and there are alternative procedures for reconstruction of shoulder and elbow functions, the final utility of the totally paralysed arm would depend upon the decisions made during the primary nerve operation. Surgeons across the globe agree that hand functions should receive priority [36, 40–49]. The objective of surgical treatment of OBPP is to establish the ability to use the affected hand to assist in bimanual activity. Strong finger flexion, in combination with good elbow flexion, is mandatory for a supportive role in the bimanual execution of activities of daily living. Without reanimation of the hand, the maximal function that can be obtained for the affected limb is that of a hook.

The mainstay of brachial plexus reconstruction in OBPP is neuroma excision and interpositional nerve grafting. Extra-plexal nerve transfers are performed if there are insufficient cervical roots to act as donors for nerve grafting or for specific functions for which the transfers have proved to be very efficient [38, 40, 44, 50]. Specific reconstructive algorithms vary between surgeons and institutions, but there is overall consensus that the primary target for reinnervation in a total plexus injury is the lower trunk and that the reconstruction should be anatomic when possible.

The technique of redirecting growing axons from ruptured upper roots towards the hand via the avulsed lower roots has existed for a long time. Gilbert [33–37] recommended this strategy while demonstrating good return of distal functions in BPBI unlike the disappointing outcomes seen in post-traumatic palsies in adults. Pondaag and Malessy [44] referred to the different sites of distal repairs. Utilization of the avulsed ends of the C8 and T1 (after trimming to excise the damaged intra-foraminal elements including the dorsal root ganglia) would have the advantage of short nerve grafts (and also greater numbers of cables to act as conduits for the growing axons). However, this had to be balanced with the loss of axons along unwanted proximal pathways. Using longer nerve grafts to the medial cord would mean greater concentration of axons towards the hand but fewer cables. They also felt that it was unreasonable to expect useful restoration of ulnar intrinsic functions and preferred to direct the axons towards the median nerve for reinnervation of the forearm flexors and sensation over the thumb, index and middle fingers. In fact, they even reported use of the ulnar nerve as a graft in three cases. On the other hand, they have also referred to the practice of direct approximation of the lower trunk to the C6 root as that would avoid axon loss at two repair sites and, also, help to deploy the available nerve grafts for the other root reconstructions.

We have followed a systematic protocol for reinnervation of the lower trunk. So, if there are one or two ruptured roots, they are bridged to the lower trunk using multiple short cables of nerve grafts. We must remember that the lower trunk, through the posterior division, contributes to innervation of the latissimus dorsi, long head of the triceps and the extrinsic extensors of the fingers. Hence, diversion of maximum numbers of axons to the lower trunk in the neck helps in restoring not just flexion of the wrist and fingers and of the intrinsics but also extension of the elbow and fingers. This is extremely significant for the eventual utilization of the recovered arm in daily activities. In BPBI, innervation of the C8 and T1 roots in the neck can lead to independent flexion and extension of the fingers. The importance of the PDLT (posterior division of the lower trunk) was evident from Wang's study of innervation of the posterior division of the lower trunk using the phrenic nerve in post-traumatic total palsies [51]. If three or more ruptured roots are found, the best quality root stump (usually C5) is used for the hand, while the lower ruptured roots are directed towards the upper and middle trunks. If there is a doubt about the quality of one or more of the stumps, we can ensure elbow flexion using intercostals for the musculocutaneous nerve and utilize the best available root for the hand. The less useful roots can then be grafted to the posterior division of the upper trunk and the middle trunk.

In the rare cases with extra-foraminal injuries of all five roots, we have to be circumspect about the quality of each of the stumps. Of course, if all or four of them are of good quality, we can attempt anatomical reconstruction. If, eventually, the biceps does not recover well or within a reasonable period after the operation, we can always salvage by transferring intercostals to the musculocutaneous nerve.

In this context, the importance of innervation of the deltoid must be mentioned. When we have only one or two ruptured roots, the hand gets priority. So, only the rotator cuff can be served with a nerve transfer from the spinal accessory to the suprascapular. With time, the supraspinatus proves to be insufficient to maintain abduction as the child grows older. So, we have to divert axons for the posterior division of the upper trunk. The contralateral C7 root could prove to be valuable for this purpose with the grafts being laid via the prespinal route.

Extra-Plexal Nerve Transfers

The spinal accessory nerve is usually intact and can be identified as it enters the trapezius. Care is taken to preserve the branches to the upper part of the trapezius. The nerve is divided distally and transferred to the suprascapular nerve. This is done systematically in all cases of total birth palsies [52]. Innervation of the rotator cuff is essential and is the only control of the shoulder possible when only one ruptured root is found. The posterior approach for this transfer does not carry a significant additional advantage since both the spinal accessory and the suprascapular nerves can be readily accessed through the same approach used for exploration of the brachial plexus.

Use of the intercostal nerves for restoration of elbow flexion in BPBI has been reported on several occasions [53–55].

Although direct transfer to the terminal motor branches of the musculocutaneous nerve has been reported in post-traumatic brachial plexus injuries, the general protocol in BPBI has been to separate the musculocutaneous nerve as proximally as possible from the lateral cord and to approximate three or four intercostal nerves directly to the entire stump (without effort to separate the motor and sensory components) with the help of fibrin glue, the shoulder in 90° of abduction. Approximation to the trunk of the MCN results in innervation of the biceps and brachialis that augments the strength of elbow flexion. We prefer to transfer four intercostal nerves for restoration of elbow flexion (third–sixth). The technique of harvest differs from that employed in adults as circumferential separation of the periosteum at multiple levels carries the risk of deformities of the chest wall as the child grows. That technique became popular as it reduced the bleeding associated with dissection between the layers of intercostal muscles. We have not encountered this problem in infants. The intercostal muscles are carefully separated from the lower margin of the rib anteriorly, and the intercostal nerve is identified at the level of the costochondral junction. It is then separated from the pleura and dissection proceeds proximally. The tiny branches to the intercostal muscles can be readily divided. The motor component is traced to the common trunk, and further separation from the sensory branch to the anterior chest wall is possible till sufficient length is obtained for direct approximation to the musculocutaneous nerve in abduction. Preservation of the sensory branch of the fourth intercostal nerve is particularly important in girls as that would provide sensibility to the nipple area. This method has proved to restore elbow flexion in >90% of cases. Approximation to the trunk of the MCN results in innervation of the biceps and brachialis that augments the strength of elbow flexion. It also allows us to reserve the available root stumps for the hand. This is particularly relevant when we consider the situation where more than two ruptured root stumps are found. In such cases, we have to direct the axons from the two best roots to the lower trunk. However, it is not prudent to rely on the remaining ruptured root stump(s) for the most important function of elbow flexion. Years of experience with intercostal nerve transfers have shown consistent restoration of elbow flexion with negligible or no side effects. Hence, we recommend the use of this extra-plexal transfer when doubts exist about some of the available root stumps (in cases of three roots ruptured).

The strategy that is currently adopted in each situation is summarized in Table 52.1.

Table 52.1 Strategies for nerve reconstruction practiced currently based on the findings during exploration of the brachial plexus in the neck

Intraoperative findings	Strategy
C5 rupture, C6–T1 avulsions (one root available)	XI–SS; ICN 3456–MCN, C5–nerve grafts–lower trunk + CC7–nerve grafts–posterior division of upper trunk and middle trunk
C5–C6 ruptures, C7–C8–T1 avulsions (two roots available)	XI–SS; ICN 3456–MCN; best root lower trunk. The other root to posterior division of upper (and middle) trunk
C5–C7 ruptures, C8–T1 avulsions (three roots available)	XI–SS; best two roots–nerve grafts–lower trunk; remaining root–nerve grafts to the upper trunk; if the third root is doubtful, intercostals to the MCN and use the root for the posterior division of the upper trunk and the middle trunk
4 and 5 roots available	XI–SS; nerve grafting or direct approximation of two best roots to the lower trunk and grafting from the remaining roots to the upper and middle trunks

XI, Spinal accessory nerve; *SS*, suprascapular nerve; *ICN 3456*, third to sixth intercostal nerves; *MCN*, musculocutaneous nerve

Post-Operative Care

As is evident, the arm will be flail at the end of the operation. Hence it needs to be supported against the trunk with the elbow flexed in front. This can be achieved with the help of a stockinet sling as reported by the unit from Toronto [40]. They do not feel it necessary to immobilize the head as most of the movements occur at the atlanto-occipital and atlanto-axial junctions. They keep this support for 2 weeks. The unit in Leiden prefers to add a prefabricated splint to prevent movements of the head for 2 weeks, while the arm immobilization continues for 2 weeks more. Passive mobilization of the arm starts at 6 weeks. Leblebicioglu [20] has published on his experience with the use of the opposite C7 transfers in the treatment of total birth palsies. The position of splintage of the upper extremity at the injured side was determined intraoperatively by checking the position of the least tension at the neural coaptation sites, especially the CC7. The stabilization of the injured upper extremity was typically with the shoulder in 90° of abduction and external rotation and the elbow in 90° flexion. After 6 weeks of immobilization, rehabilitation was initiated.

We prefer to place the forearm across the abdomen, the arm adjacent to the trunk and elbow flexed. The head and trunk are wrapped with padding cotton, and a plaster cask is applied to maintain the position of the head relative to the shoulder. Care is taken to avoid pressure points over the insensate upper limb. Access for feeding and periodic cleaning and wound inspection is arranged. The parents are instructed in handling the child during the month in this support and to avoid excess mobilization for the month after the plaster is removed.

Reinnervation of the supraspinatus and the biceps from the nerve transfers happens rapidly, and some primitive movements can be observed by 3 months.

It is essential to maintain the passive mobility of the shoulder, elbow, wrist and hand. Particular attention is paid to external and internal rotation with the elbow against the trunk and pronation and supination with the elbow supported.

The parents are instructed to encourage the active movements as they appear in order to make the child aware of the arm. As the child grows older and reaches out for objects, games have to be designed to encourage use of the affected arm as well in spite of the absence of distal functions. Active flexion of the wrist and fingers takes at least 7–8 months to appear (in general at the age of 12–14 months). The ability to hold objects has to be demonstrated to the child with the wrist supported. Care to encourage bimanual functions has to be continued daily for several years.

Strengthening of the triceps is essential but very difficult to execute. This can be achieved by constantly encouraging the child to reach out while the shoulder and arm are supported. We have found it effective in helping to stretch the biceps as the child grows and, thus, reducing the severity of the ultimate flexion deformity of the elbow.

Secondary Reconstruction

In general, there is a need to augment shoulder abduction and external rotation. This is achieved by coraco-humeral release by shortening of the tip of the coracoid process as well as subscapularis release from the anterior surface of the body of the scapula. Muscle transfers using the latissimus dorsi +/– teres major [56] may be added if their function in them has been restored. This is generally necessary before the age of 3 years. It improves the utility of the regained functions and the ability of the child to use the arm in bimanual activities. This also serves to encourage the progress in hand functions that continues, in our experience, until the age of 7–8 years.

A third stage for surgery is often necessary at the age of 5 years to correct the persistent supination. This happens due to the unrestrained action of the shortened biceps and poor recovery in the pronators of the forearm. Although muscle transfers using the brachioradialis [57] or re-routing the biceps [58, 59] have been described, they are feasible only when passive pronation is retained or can be achieved by surgical release. In addition, splitting and re-routing the biceps serves to weaken the elbow flexion further. We prefer to perform a corrective osteotomy of the forearm bones. Initially, an osteotomy of the proximal third of the ulna is done with plate fixation after correction. If the deformity recurs or correction is inadequate, an osteotomy of the radius is added at a later stage. The forearm is thus brought to a more functionally useful position that encourages use of the hand. We have to remember that simple actions such as closure and opening of the fist are activities that the child is incapable of performing for the first 5 years of his or her life. Hence, the child's brain has to be trained afresh to learn these actions. The position of the forearm and of the wrist (with a thermoplastic splint) has to be maintained throughout the first 5 years of live. The two main factors that contribute to achieving the best outcomes are co-operative and diligent parents and a compliant patient.

The eventual hand function is achieved at the age of 6–8 years. We have found the Raimondi scale [60] very useful for this assessment. Wrist dorsiflexion and palmar flexion, flexion and extension of the fingers, intrinsic functions and abduction and opposition of the thumb are observed. Feasibility of further action in terms of a palliative transfer for extension of the wrist and fingers is determined and discussed with the parents. Traditionally, the presence of wrist palmar flexion and finger flexion is considered favourable for further reconstruction. However, we have observed that the regular transfers of wrist flexors for finger extension do not work as well in BPBI as in regular peripheral nerve injury indications. This is partly because the donor muscles are not strong enough. Also, the source of innervation of the wrist and finger flexors is the same, i.e. the intraplexal nerve transfer of the upper roots to the lower trunk in the neck. The child cannot dissociate these two actions to achieve the desired objective of finger extension. Free functioning muscle transfers have been used in post-traumatic cases for restoration of finger extension. The lack of suitable nerve donors hinders the use of this option. The brachialis muscle can be detached from the ulna and transferred to the wrist or finger extensors with a tendon graft. The use of intercostals to innervate the biceps also supplies the brachialis. Of course, the automatic flexion of the elbow must be countered by independent function of the triceps, which is fortunately achieved by innervation of the lower trunk in the neck.

Derotation Osteotomy of the Humerus

After 8–10 years, there is a plateau in the hand function. The ability to reach the abdomen, chest and face is established. However, the ability to reach out above the level of the shoulder is limited by the lack of external rotation of the shoulder. This is, particularly, important when the latissimus dorsi is not innervated and cannot be utilized as a muscle transfer. An osteotomy of the humerus with plate osteosynthesis has proved to be invaluable. Traditionally, a transverse osteotomy is performed between the insertions of the deltoid and pectoralis major via an anterolateral approach, and the distal fragment is rotated externally. This has to be done judiciously to avoid losing the ability to reach the midline [61–68].

Results

We reviewed the cases operated upon in our service up to 2015. Between 1995 and 2015, we operated upon 509 cases of BPBI for primary nerve reconstruction. Of these, 147 patients had injuries to all 5 roots. In each case, the operation was performed as early as possible, usually at 3 months of age. Follow-up longer than 4 years was available for each of the 147 patients.

Raimondi Scale (Modified and Updated by Dr. Alex Muset).

0: Complete paralysis or slight finger flexion of no use, useless thumb, no pinch, some or no sensation.
1: Limited active flexion of fingers, no extension of wrist or fingers, lateral pinch of thumb present or absent.
2: Active extension of wrist with passive flexion of fingers (by means of tenodesis), passive lateral pinch of thumb (by means of pronation).
3: Active complete flexion of wrist and fingers, mobile thumb with partial abduction-opposition, intrinsic balance, no active supination.

3A: Fingers stay flexed with no active interphalangeal extension-uncertain prognosis for improvement with secondary surgery.
3B: Fingers can be held away from the palm due to some recovery of interphalangeal extension – good potential for secondary surgery.
4: Active complete flexion of wrist and fingers, active wrist extension, weak or absent finger extension, good thumb opposition with active ulnar intrinsics, partial pronation/supination.
5: All function described in grade 4 plus finger extension and almost complete pronation/supination.

Raimondi described a scale to achieve uniformity in reporting the function observed following early microsurgical reconstruction in total birth palsies. According to this system, types 0, 1 and 2 referred to no or minimal functions that are not useful, while types 4 and 5 are close to normal hands. Type 3 function implied restoration of wrist and finger flexion with minimal or no intrinsic activity and the poor thumb abduction and opposition. This type was considered as the benchmark of success for microsurgical reconstruction as it could be improved using secondary muscle transfers so that the child could grasp and release objects.

We could consider our outcomes in two significant phases. The early cases involved utilization of the available root stumps for all the desired functions of the shoulder, elbow and the hand. The hand function could be classified as type 4 in 12.2% cases, which was possible only when four or five roots could be grafted.

In 79.6% cases, the function was limited to flexion of the wrist and fingers of varying strengths, no intrinsic recovery and weak abduction and opposition of the thumb, i.e. type 3 hand. However, attempts to improve the function with secondary procedures were not uniformly successful. Further analysis of this group showed that there was wide variation even among these patients. The strength of flexion of the fingers and wrist differed. The key difference appeared to be in the ability to extend the fingers at interphalangeal joints away from the palm. In the absence of suitable donor muscles, fusion of the wrist in the neutral position or in 10° of palmar flexion has been found useful, particularly in patients who have regained some extension of the interphalangeal joints.

Correlation with findings during exploration revealed that the numbers of available root stumps (that were utilized for nerve grafting to the target nerves described above) were 3 in 46 cases and 4 in 36 cases and all 5 roots appeared ruptured in 29 patients. Thus in 111 out of the 147 cases, we had been able to achieve significant innervation of the lower trunk. Yet, the ultimate result of the nerve procedure was a type 3 hand in 117 cases.

This has led us to suspect that our impression of the quality of the root stump was not uniformly accurate. Inadvertent grafting from roots of poorer quality to the lower trunk could account for the frequency of unsatisfactory results.

In addition, the reliance on intraplexal nerve donors (ruptured roots) for most functions at the shoulder and elbow led to insufficient innervation distal to the elbow. We also noted that secondary operations for extension of the fingers were more successful when some degree of interphalangeal extension was already present. The possibilities for secondary tendon transfers for restoration of extension of the fingers are limited in total palsies. This is because the wrist flexors are innervated from the same source as the finger flexors (reconstruction of the lower trunk in the neck). Also, these are re-innervated muscles and, hence, do not behave in the same way as the donor muscles for tendon transfers in peripheral nerve injuries. So, the only possibilities in the absence of interphalangeal extension would be use of the brachialis with a tendon graft or a free functioning muscle transfer.

Thus, type 3 hands should be further subclassified as type 3A where the fingers stay flexed against the palm and type 3B when the child can hold the fingers away from the palm to a certain extent. This study is being prepared for publication.

The objective of primary nerve reconstruction in the complete BPBI should not be limited to restoring flexion of the wrist and fingers but should aim to regain at least some interphalangeal extension as well. In other words, the available nerve donors should be utilized to maximize hand functions.

This can be best achieved by careful intraoperative evaluation of the root stumps and utilizing the best root to innervate the lower trunk while addressing the shoulder and elbow functions by using other available roots or extra-plexal donors.

The progress in the distal functions also correlated well with the quality of the results at the shoulder and elbow. So, we had to tailor our primary strategy according to the outline described above. When we depended entirely on spinal accessory to suprascapular for the rotator cuff and intercostals to the musculocutaneous nerve for the biceps (as in the cases with only one ruptured root), we found that the patients consistently regained 45°–60° abduction [52, 69, 70] and almost full elbow flexion. Innervation of the lower trunk with a good root also provided triceps function so that the patient could reach out in space.

With growth, however, the range of abduction appeared to diminish as the supraspinatus could not cope with the increasing weight of the arm.

Augmentation of shoulder abduction would necessitate innervation of the deltoid and, if possible, the posterior axillary fold muscles. Grafting from the available root stumps would decrease the number of axons destined to the lower trunk and would result in a weak, functionless hand. In this case, we prefer innervation of the posterior division of the upper trunk or the middle trunk using the contralateral C7.

Series	No. of cases	Nerve strategy	Outcome measurement	Results
Haerle and Gilbert [36]	73	Upper roots to lower trunk grafting	Raimondi scale	Useful hand in 73%
Pondaag and Malessy [44]	13	Upper roots to lower trunk grafting or direct repairs	Raimondi scale	Type 3 hand in 9/13 cases
Birch et al. [71]	47	Grafting to the lower trunk	Raimondi scale	Type 4 or 5 in 57% and type 3 in 36% cases
El-Gammal [72]	35	Grafting to the lower trunk from the upper roots	Raimondi scale	Type 3 in 18 cases (53%)
Chen [73]	7	CC7–VUNG–median nerve in 6 cases, radial nerve in 1 case	Motor function restored	Strong flexion of wrist and fingers in 3 of 6 cases; strong wrist extension and triceps in one case
Leblebicioglu [20]	18	Nerve grafting from CC7 to lower trunk in 7 cases and upper + lower trunks in 11 cases	Raimondi scale	Type 3 hand in 5/7 in the lower trunk series and 4/11 cases in the upper + lower trunk series
Vu et al. [74]	5	CC7–nerve grafts–lower trunk	Active motion scale	Strong flexion of thumb and fingers in 2 cases; 3/7 fingers and thumb flexion in 2 cases with strong wrist flexion in one case; intrinsic function in one case

Haerle and Gilbert [36] reported on a series of 73 patients followed for an average period of 6.4 years. Nerve reconstruction was performed mainly by intraplexal grafting. 77% of cases had good and average shoulder outcomes, while 81% of cases regained useful elbow flexion following primary nerve repairs and secondary muscle transfers. The hand function was reported upon after completion of secondary procedures whenever they were possible. 73% of cases regained useful hand function. However, the degree of recovery of hand function was not correlated with the type of primary reconstruction. They described continued improvement of the hand functions even up to the age of 8–10 years.

Pondaag and Malessy [44] reported on a smaller series of 16 patients operated upon at a mean age of 4.4 months. In their report, they focused on the results of nerve reconstruction only. The number of available roots was one in three cases, three in six cases and four in three cases. The shoulder function was achieved mainly by transfer of the spinal accessory to the suprascapular nerve, while elbow flexion was achieved by using intraplexal grafting in 12 of the 16 cases and 3 intercostal nerve transfers in 4 cases. The hand function was entirely achieved by grafting from proximal root stumps to the medial cord or lower trunk in 13 of the 16 patients, and direct approximation of the C8 and T1 roots to the C6 root stump. Follow-up ranged from 24 to 105 months (mean 50 months). The Raimondi scale was used to evaluate the hand outcomes with type 3 or better function being rated as a success. This was noted in 9 of the 13 cases (69%).

Birch et al. [71] reported the outcome of surgical treatment of BPBI in 93 infants.

In patients with C8–T1 lesion, repair was performed in 47 patients with no demonstrable intraoperative function, and the results were good (Raimondi grade 4 or 5) in 57% of repairs and fair (Raimondi grade 3) in 36% of repairs.

Shenaq et al. [41] briefly presented their results of 282 infants with BPBI with a mean follow-up of 5 years. Good to excellent hand function was reported in 62% of patients.

El-Gammal et al. [72] reported on a series of 35 cases total birth palsies that underwent exploration and nerve reconstruction. However, the age at surgery ranged from 3 to 60 months. The follow-up ranged from 2.5 to 7.3 years (mean 4.2 years). They reported Raimondi type 3 hand in seven cases (20%), type 4 in seven cases (20%) and type 5 in four cases (13%). They did mention a preference for nerve transfers for the rotator cuff and biceps functions. Also, they referred to the frequent need for additional procedures to augment shoulder external rotation.

The use of the contralateral C7 transfer in BPBI has been reported by a few authors over the past 10 years. Chen [73] described the Shanghai experience in a series of 12 cases of the paediatric age group of which 7 were patients with total birth palsies. However, they preferred to transfer the contralateral C7 via a vascularized ulnar nerve graft to the median nerve, and, so, the ulnar territory was not innervated. They confirmed the worldwide experience of the futility of nerve reconstruction beyond 12 months from the injury. Good flexion of the wrist and fingers was restored, but these movements were associated with significant synchronous movements of the donor arms. Similarly, triceps, wrist and finger extension were restored when the ulnar nerve graft was connected to the radial nerve. Although the follow-up was long enough (38–55 months for the BPBI cases), the utility of the recovered hand function was not referred to.

Leblebicioglu [20] has reported on 20 cases in which the contralateral C7 was transferred to the lower trunk or upper and lower trunks. The contralateral C7 transfer was done using sural nerve grafts via the prespinal route. In nine patients the distal repair was done to the lower roots, and in nine other patients, it was done to both the upper and lower roots. However, the T1 root was left in continuity in several cases. Raimondi type 3 hand was achieved in 5 of 7 patients in whom the transfer was done to the lower root and in 4 of 11 patients in whom transfer was done to both the upper and lower roots. The presence of significant synchronous movements in the opposite upper limb was not mentioned.

Vu et al. [74] reported on their experience in a series of five patients in whom the contralateral C7 was transferred to the lower trunk with sural nerve grafts by the prespinal route. The average follow-up was 3.3 years. The outcomes were described using the Toronto Active Motion Scale [75]. They reported recovery of ulnar intrinsic functions in one patient and strong flexion of the fingers and thumb in another patient. The overall utility of the hand was not described.

However, we do not consider it useful for augmenting hand function as synchronous movements in the donor limbs can never be eliminated and incorporation of the recipient hand movements in daily activities is very difficult. On the other hand, the results for proximal control are far more predictable and useful. Hence, we currently prefer to bridge the opposite C7 root to the posterior division of the upper trunk or to the middle trunk.

The regained latissimus dorsi and teres major muscles could be transferred to provide external rotation of the shoulder by strengthening the rotator cuff.

The utility of the function regained following microsurgical reconstruction is an important consideration as it requires sustained efforts over several years. Uniformity in presenting outcomes is necessary for comparison of various nerve strategies. The Toronto unit has described a method of measurement based on the use of the affected hand (independently or assisted by the normal hand or in helping the normal hand) in three activities that can be taught to a child of 6–7 years. This scale has been validated for consistency between observers [75].

Indications for Free Functioning Muscle Transfers

Free functioning gracilis transfers have been in use in the treatment of post-traumatic palsies. However, we find very limited use for this operation in BPBI. This is primarily because we tend to use most available nerve donors in the primary operation. Hence, we find application for free muscle transfers for salvage when the biceps regained is too weak or for the treatment of a type 3A hand for restoration of extension of the fingers.

Future Prospects Observations of our results over the past 20 years have prompted periodic alterations in our strategies. The gratifying results of nerve repairs in BPBI allow us to predict the functions that can be achieved. Hence, we can hope to improve the shoulder and elbow functions further by the modifications that we are using now. Innervation of the deltoid using the opposite C7 for the posterior division of the upper trunk is one such procedure whose outcomes are awaited. Similarly, one can attempt a double innervation of the rotator cuff by transferring the spinal accessory to the suprascapular nerve and adding a nerve graft cable from the C5 or C7 root to the suprascapular nerve distal to the supraspinatus. These steps do not interfere with the fundamental principle maximizing innervation of the lower trunk. The shoulder function is augmented with the hope of encouraging the use of the hand so that the threshold of type 3B function is achieved in a consistent manner.

Conclusions Early exploration and microsurgical reconstruction are essential in the treatment of complete BPBI. All available nerve donors must be evaluated and harnessed in a judicious manner. The priority is restoration of hand functions. Hence, the best available ruptured root must be utilized for reinnervation of the lower trunk. Extra-plexal nerve transfers are an integral part of the operation. Use of the opposite C7 needs further evaluation. Sustained and diligent therapy with active participation of the parents and of the patient are necessary over several years. Close supervision and periodic review for supplementary surgical procedures are often necessary.

Nerve repairs give consistent results in BPBI. Hence, a correct reconstruction is likely to provide function at the shoulder and elbow in most cases. Properly planned secondary operations serve to augment the ability to place the arm in space and contribute to improvement in distal functions. This sustained and aggressive approach is essential for restoration of independent prehension in these devastating injuries.

Illustrative Cases

Case 1 C5–C7 ruptures, C8–T1 avulsions: primary reconstruction at 3 months of age – spinal accessory to suprascapular and intercostals 3, 4, 5 and 6 to musculocutaneous nerve; nerve grafting from C5–C6 to C8–T1, nerve grafting from C7 to posterior division of upper and middle trunks. At 3 years of age, release of internal rotation contracture of the shoulder with transfer of the latissimus dorsi and teres major to the rotator cuff to augment abduction and external rotation; at 5 years of age, osteotomy of the ulna to correct the supination deformity of the forearm. Videos showing functions at the shoulder, elbow and hand at 12 years

Case 2 C5 rupture, C6–T1 avulsions: primary reconstruction – spinal accessory to suprascapular and intercostals 3, 4, 5 and 6 to the musculocutaneous nerve; nerve grafting from the C5 root to C8–T1 including the posterior division of the lower trunk; nerve grafting from the opposite C7 to the posterior division of the upper trunk. Videos showing functions at the elbow and hand

References

1. Jolly MC, Sebire NJ, Harris JP, Regan L, Robinson S. Risk factors for macrosomia and its clinical consequences: a study of 350,311 pregnancies. Eur J Obstet Gynecol Reprod Biol. 2003;111(1):9–14.
2. Araujo Júnior E, Peixoto AB, Zamarian ACP, Elito Júnior J, Tonni G. Macrosomia. Best Pract Res Clin Obstet Gynaecol. 2017;38:83–96.
3. Mayer C, Joseph KS. Fetal growth: a review of terms, concepts and issues relevant to obstetrics. Ultrasound Obstet Gynecol. 2013;41(2):136–45.
4. Mollberg M, Hagberg H, Bager B, Lilja H, Ladfors L. High birthweight and shoulder dystocia: the strongest risk factors for obstetrical brachial plexus palsy in a Swedish population-based study. Acta Obstet Gynecol Scand. 2005;84(7):654–9.
5. Pondaag W, Allen RH, Malessy MJA. Correlating birthweight with neurological severity of obstetric brachial plexus lesions. BJOG. 2011;118(9):1098–103.
6. Beta J, Khan N, Fiolna M, Khalil A, Ramadan G, Akolekar R. Maternal and neonatal complications of fetal macrosomia: cohort study. Ultrasound Obstet Gynecol. 2019;54(3):319–25.
7. Wilson TJ, Chang KWC, Chauhan SP, Yang LJS. Peripartum and neonatal factors associated with the persistence of neonatal brachial plexus palsy at 1 year: a review of 382 cases. J Neurosurg Pediatr. 2016;17(5):618–24.
8. Amonoo-Kuofi HS. Horner's syndrome revisited: with an update of the central pathway. Clin Anat. 1999;12(5):345–61.
9. Al-Qattan MM, Clarke HM, Curtis CG. The prognostic value of concurrent Horner's syndrome in total obstetric brachial plexus injury. J Hand Surg (Br Eur Vol). 2000;25B(2):166–7.
10. Bisinella GL, Birch R, Smith SJM. Neurophysiological prediction of outcome in obstetric lesions of the brachial plexus. J Hand Surg Am. 2003;28(B(2)):148–52.
11. Malessy MJA, Pondaag W, Yang LJS, Hofstede-Buitenhuis SM, le Cessie S, van Dijk JG. Severe obstetric brachial plexus palsies can be identified at one month of age. PLoS One. 2011;6(10):1–6.
12. Somashekar DK, Di Pietro MA, Joseph JR, Yang LJS, Parmar HA. Utility of ultrasound in noninvasive preoperative workup of neonatal brachial plexus palsy. Pediatr Radiol. 2016;46(5):695–703.
13. Somashekar DK, Wilson TJ, DiPietro MA, Joseph JR, Ibrahim M, Yang LJS, et al. The current role of diagnostic imaging in the preoperative workup for refractory neonatal brachial plexus palsy. Childs Nerv Syst. 2016;32(8):1393–7.
14. Somashekar D, Yang LJS, Ibrahim M, Parmar HA. High-resolution MRI evaluation of neonatal brachial plexus palsy: a promising alternative to traditional CT myelography. Am J Neuroradiol. 2014;35(6):1209–13.
15. Malessy MJA, Pondaag W, Van Dijk JG. Electromyography, nerve action potential, and compound motor action potentials in obstetric brachial plexus lesions: validation in the absence of a "gold standard". Neurosurgery. 2009;65(Suppl. 4):1–14.
16. König RW, Antoniadis G, Börm W, Richter HP, Kretschmer T. Role of intraoperative neurophysiology in primary surgery for obstetrical brachial plexus palsy (OBPP). Childs Nerv Syst. 2006;22(7):710–4.
17. Vanderhave KL, Bovid K, Alpert H, Chang KWC, Quint DJ, Leonard JA, et al. Utility of electrodiagnostic testing and computed tomography myelography in the preoperative evaluation of neonatal brachial plexus palsy: clinical article. J Neurosurg Pediatr. 2012;9(3):283–9.
18. Kline DG, Hackett ER, May PR. Evaluation of nerve injuries by evoked potentials and electromyography. J Neurosurg. 1969;31(2):128–36.
19. Tse R, Nixon JN, Iyer RS, Kuhlman-Wood KA, Ishak GE. The diagnostic value of CT myelography, MR myelography, and both in neonatal brachial plexus palsy. Am J Neuroradiol. 2014;35(7):1425–32.
20. Leblebicioglu G, Ayhan C, Firat T, Uzumcugil A, Yorubulut M, Doral MN. Recovery of upper extremity function following endoscopically assisted contralateral C7 transfer for obstetrical brachial plexus injury. J Hand Surg Eur Vol. 2016;41(8):863–74.
21. Yoshida K, Kawabata H. The prognostic value of concurrent phrenic nerve palsy in newborn babies with neonatal brachial plexus palsy. J Hand Surg Am. 2015;40(6):1166–9.
22. Friedenberg SM, Hermann RC. The breathing hand: obstetric brachial plexopathy reinnervation from thoracic roots? J Neurol Neurosurg Psychiatry. 2004;75(1):158–60.
23. Rizeq YK, Many BT, Vacek JC, Reiter AJ, Raval M V, Abdullah F, et al. Diaphragmatic paralysis after phrenic nerve injury in newborns- ClinicalKey. J Pediatr Surg. 2019;55(2):240–44.
24. Boome RS, Kaye JC. Obstetric traction injuries of the brachial plexus. Natural history, indications for surgical repair and results. J Bone Joint Surg Ser B. 1988;70(4):571–6.

25. Hardy AE. Birth injuries of the brachial plexus. Incidence and prognosis. J Bone Joint Surg Ser B. 1981;63(1):98–101.
26. Chauhan SP, Blackwell SB, Ananth CV. Neonatal brachial plexus palsy: incidence, prevalence, and temporal trends. Semin Perinatol. 2014;38(4):210–8.
27. Waters PM. Comparison of the natural history, the outcome of microsurgical repair, and the outcome of operative reconstruction in brachial plexus birth palsy. J Bone Joint Surg. 1999;81-A(5):649–59.
28. Foad SL, Mehlman CT, Foad MB, Lippert WC. Prognosis following neonatal brachial plexus palsy: an evidence-based review. J Child Orthop. 2009;3(6):459–63.
29. Gilbert A, Pivato G. Obstetrical palsy: the French contribution. Semin Plast Surg. 2005;19(01):5–16.
30. Pondaag W, Malessy MJA, Van Dijk JG, Thomeer RTWM. Natural history of obstetric brachial plexus palsy: a systematic review. Dev Med Child Neurol. 2004;46(2):138–44.
31. Buterbaugh KL, Shah AS. The natural history and management of brachial plexus birth palsy. Curr Rev Musculoskelet Med. 2016;9(4):418–26.
32. Clark L, Taylor A, Prout TA. Study on brachial birth palsy. Am J Med Sci. 1905;4(10):670–707.
33. Gilbert A, Tassin JL. Obstetrical palsy: a clinical, pathologic, and surgical review. In: Microreconstruction of nerve injuries. Philadelphia: Saunders; 1987. p. 529.
34. Gilbert A. Long-term evaluation of brachial plexus surgery in obstetrical palsy. Hand Clin. 1995;11: 583–95.
35. Gilbert A, Tassin JL. Surgery repair of the brachial plexus after obstetric paralysis. Chirurgie. 1984;110:70–5. (Fr)
36. Haerle M, Gilbert A. Management of complete obstetric brachial plexus lesions. J Pediatr Orthop. 2004;24:194–200.
37. Gilbert A, Brockman R, Carlioz H. Surgical treatment of brachial plexus birth palsy. Clin Orthop Relat Res. 1991;264:39–47.
38. Davidge KM, Clarke HM, Borschel GH. Nerve transfers in birth related brachial plexus injuries: where do we stand? Hand Clin. 2016;32:175–90.
39. Tse R, Kozin SH, Malessy MJ, Clarke HM. International federation of societies for surgery of the hand committee report: the role of nerve transfers in the treatment of neonatal brachial plexus palsy. J Hand Surg Am. 2015;40(6):1246–59.
40. Borschel GH, Clarke HM. Obstetrical brachial plexus palsy. Plast Reconstr Surg. 2009;124(1 Suppl):144–55.
41. Shenaq SM, Kim JYS, Armenta AH, Nath RK, Cheng E, Jedrysiak A. The surgical treatment of obstetric brachial plexus palsy. Plast Reconstr Surg. 2004;113(4):54–67.
42. Chuang DCC, Mardini S, Ma HS. Surgical strategy for infant obstetrical brachial plexus palsy: experiences at Chang gung memorial hospital. Plast Reconstr Surg. 2005;116(1):132–42.
43. Wilson TJ, Chang KWC, Yang LJS. Prediction algorithm for surgical intervention in neonatal brachial plexus palsy. Clin Neurosurg. 2018;82(3):335–41.
44. Pondaag W, Malessy MJA. Recovery of hand function following nerve grafting and transfer in obstetric brachial plexus lesions. J Neurosurg. 2006;105(PEDIAT(SUPPL. 1)):33–40.
45. Squitieri L, Steggerda J, Yang LJS, Kim HM, Chung KC. A national study to evaluate trends in the utilization of nerve reconstruction for treatment of neonatal brachial plexus palsy. Plast Reconstr Surg. 2011;127(1):277–83.
46. Hale HB, Bae DS, Waters PM. Current concepts in the Management of Brachial Plexus Birth Palsy. J Hand Surg Am. 2010;35(2):322–31.
47. Waters PM. Update on management of pediatric brachial plexus palsy. J Pediatr Orthop B. 2005;14(4):233–44.
48. Swan MC, Clarke HM. Microsurgery for obstetrical brachial plexus palsy. Pediatr Up Extrem. 2015:607–30.
49. Nelson MR, Armenta AH. Birth brachial plexus palsy update. Curr Phys Med Rehabil Rep. 2014;2(2):79–85.
50. Malessy MJA, Pondaag W. Nerve surgery for neonatal brachial plexus palsy. J Pediatr Rehabil Med. 2011;4(2):141–8.
51. Wang SF, Li PC, Xue YH, Zou JY, Li WJ, Li Y. Direct coaptation of the phrenic nerve with the posterior division of the lower trunk to restore finger and elbow extension function in patients with Total brachial plexus injuries. Neurosurgery. 2016;78(2):208–15.
52. Kawabata H, Kawai H, Masatomi T, Yasui N. Accessory nerve neurotization in infants with brachial plexus birth palsy. Microsurgery. 1994;15:768–72.
53. Tarek AE-G, Mohamed MA-L. Intercostal nerve transfer in infants with obstetric brachial plexus palsy. Microsurgery. 2009;10:504–6.
54. Kawabata H, Shibata T, Matsui Y, et al. Use of intercostal nerves for neurotization of the musculocutaneous nerve in infants with birth-related brachial plexus palsy. J Neurosurg. 2001;94:386–91.
55. Luo PB, Chen L, Zhou CH, Hu SN, Gu YD. Results of intercostal nerve transfer to the musculocutaneous nerve in brachial plexus birth palsy. J Pediatr Orthop. 2011;31(8):884–8.
56. Hoffer MM, Wickenden R, Roper B. Brachial plexus birth palsies. Results of tendon transfers to the rotator cuff. J Bone J Surg Ser A. 1978;60(5):691–5.
57. Ozkan T, Aydin A, Ozer K, Ozturk K, Durmaz H, Ozkan S. A surgical technique for pediatric forearm pronation: brachioradialis rerouting with interosseous membrane release. J Hand Surg Am. 2004;29(1):22–7.
58. Zancolli EA, Zancolli ER. Palliative surgical procedures in Sequelae of obstetric palsy. Hand Clin. 1988;4(4):643–69.
59. Zancolli EA, Zancolli ER. Reconstructive surgery in brachial plexus Sequelae. In: The growing hand; 1999. p. 805–23.

60. Raimondi P. Evaluation of results in obstetric brachial plexus palsy. The hand. Presented at the International Meeting on Obstetric Brachial Plexus Palsy, Heerlen, The Netherlands, 1993.
61. Waters PM, Bae DS. The effect of derotational humeral osteotomy on global shoulder function in brachial plexus birth palsy. J Bone Joint Surg. 2006;88-A:1034–42.
62. Abzug JM, Chafetz RS, Gaughan JP, Ashworth S, Kozin SH. Shoulder function after medial approach and derotational humeral osteotomy in patients with brachial plexus birth palsy. J Pediatr Orthop. 2010;30(5):469–74.
63. Al-Qattan MM. Total obstetric brachial plexus palsy in children with internal rotation contracture of the shoulder, flexion contracture of the elbow, and poor hand function improving the cosmetic appearance of the limb with rotation osteotomy of the humerus. Ann Plast Surg. 2010;65(1):38–42.
64. Al-Qattan MM, Al-Husainan H, Al-Otaibi A, El-Sharkawy MS. Long-term results of low rotation humeral osteotomy in children with Erb's obstetric brachial plexus palsy. J Hand Surg Eur Vol. 2009;34(4):486–92.
65. Al-Qattan MM. Rotational osteotomy of the humerus for Erb's palsy in children with humeral head deformity. J Hand Surg Am. 2002;27:479–83.
66. Waters PM, Bae DS. The effect of derotational humeral osteotomy on global shoulder function in brachial plexus birth palsy. J Bone Joint Surg Am. 2006;88:1035–42.
67. Kirkos JM, Papadopoulos IA. Late treatment of brachial plexus palsy secondary to birth injuries: rotational osteotomy of the proximal part of the Humerus. J Bone Joint Surg Am. 1998;80A:1477–83.
68. Kozin SH. The evaluation and treatment of children with brachial plexus birth palsy. J Hand Surg Am. 2011;36(8):1360–9.
69. Pondaag W, De Boer R. Van Wijlen-Hempel MS, Hofstede-Buitenhuis SM, Malessy MJA. External rotation as a result of suprascapular nerve neurotization in obstetric brachial plexus lesions. Neurosurgery. 2005;57(3):530–6.
70. Tse R, Marcus JR, Curtis CG, Dupuis A, Clarke HM. Suprascapular nerve reconstruction in obstetrical brachial plexus palsy: spinal accessory nerve transfer versus C5 root grafting. Plast Reconstr Surg. 2011;127(6):2391–6.
71. Birch R, Ahad N, Kono H, Smith S. Repair of obstetric brachial plexus palsy. Results in 100 children. J Bone Joint Surg Br. 2005;87(8):1089–95.
72. El-Gammal TA, El-Sayed A, Kotb MM, Ragheb YF, Saleh WR, Elnakeeb RM, Semaya AES. Total obstetric brachial plexus palsy: results and strategy of microsurgical reconstruction. Microsurgery. 2010;30:169–78.
73. Liang Chen L, Yu-Dong Gu Y-D, Shao-Nan Hu S-N, Jian-Guang Xu J-G, Lei Xu L, Contralateral FY. C7 transfer for the treatment of brachial plexus root avulsions in children—a report of 12 cases. J Hand Surg. 2007;32A:96–103.
74. Vu AT, Sparkman DM, van Belle CJ, Yakuboff KP, Schwentker AR. Retropharyngeal Contralateral C7 nerve transfer to the lower trunk for brachial plexus birth injury: technique and results. J Hand Surg Am. 2018;43(5):417–24.
75. Curtis C, Stephens D, Clarke HM, Andrews D. The active movement scale: an evaluative tool for infants with obstetrical brachial plexus palsy. J Hand Surg Am. 2002;27(3):470–8.

Expected Outcomes of Surgical Treatment in Obstetrical Brachial Plexus Injuries

53

M. Claire Manske and Michelle A. James

Introduction

Increased experience in surgical intervention for brachial plexus birth injuries (BPBI) has improved understanding of outcomes and allowed surgeons to abandon techniques with inferior results in favor of more successful alternatives. Historically, operative management of BPBI consisted of brachial plexus exploration, neuroma resection, and direct nerve approximation [1–3]; however, given the poor results of primary repair and the advent of microsurgical techniques, alternative surgical strategies have been developed, including neuroma excision and nerve grafting, neurolysis, and nerve transfers. Neuroma excision and nerve grafting are considered the mainstay of surgical treatment and are often performed concomitantly with neurolysis. Neurolysis is a frequent adjunct to other techniques, but its use as a stand-alone treatment is controversial. More recently, nerve transfers using intraplexal donor nerves from the lower plexus when available have increased in popularity with good results. Extraplexal donor nerves are considered when intraplexal donors are not available, as in global brachial plexus injuries. The current literature indicates the outcomes of brachial plexus nerve grafting, neurolysis, and nerve transfers are superior to nonoperative treatment in infants with absent or delayed spontaneous nerve recovery or in infants with global injuries [4, 5]. Regardless of surgical technique, however, surgery usually does not "normalize" upper extremity strength and function, and secondary reconstructive surgeries and ongoing physical therapy are commonly needed. Currently, the surgeon's biggest challenges are determining the optimal surgical strategy and timing for an individual infant's unique injury to optimize function, limit musculoskeletal sequelae, and minimize the need for further interventions.

Studies of outcomes of brachial plexus surgery in infants are limited by (1) heterogeneity of injury patterns, surgical indications, timing of surgery, and operative techniques within the same study, (2) selection bias introduced by surgeon preference in surgical indications and technique, (3) lack of long-term follow-up, (4) inconsistent outcome measures between studies, (5) limited understanding of the role of rehabilitation and adjunctive treatments, and (6) a focus on clinician-derived measures of motor function and less attention devoted to patient-reported outcomes. Moreover, there are few studies comparing the outcomes of the most common surgical techniques. Long-term, multicenter prospective studies addressing these methodological deficiencies are needed to provide further insight and improve care of infants with BPBI.

M. C. Manske (✉) · M. A. James
Department of Orthopedic Surgery, Shriners Hospital for Children—Northern California, University of California, Davis, Sacramento, CA, USA
e-mail: mcmanske@shrinenet.org; mmanske@ucdavis.edu; mjames@shrinenet.org

A. Y. Shin, N. Pulos (eds.), *Operative Brachial Plexus Surgery*,
https://doi.org/10.1007/978-3-030-69517-0_53

This chapter summarizes the available evidence regarding outcomes of the most commonly performed surgical techniques: nerve grafting, neurolysis, and nerve transfers.

Outcomes of Nerve Grafting

Since Narakas [6, 7] and Gilbert [8] began reporting outcomes of neuroma resection with nerve grafting in the early 1980s, this technique has become the mainstay of surgical treatment. Sural nerve autograft is the most commonly reported graft source, and although alternatives to autograft have been proposed (including nerve allograft, synthetic conduit tubes, vein graft, and human amniotic membrane), few have been evaluated in human or infant subjects [9].

Understanding of surgical outcomes of neuroma resection and nerve grafting comes principally from heterogeneous, retrospective cohort studies that include a variety of surgical indications and techniques, including brachial plexus exploration, neurolysis, neurorrhaphy, nerve grafting, nerve transfer, and various combinations thereof [10–13]. These studies report reliable recovery of deltoid and biceps function [4, 10, 14–16] with less predictable recovery of shoulder external rotation (SER) [10, 11, 14, 17–19]. In infants with global palsies, for whom the reconstructive priority is recovery of hand function followed by elbow and shoulder function, results are more variable. Infants undergoing these procedures commonly recover some hand motor function, but there is no clear consensus that they recover meaningful hand use [20–25].

Upper and Middle Trunk BPBI

Two recent studies evaluated the outcomes of neuroma resection and nerve grafting in a cohort treated with a uniform surgical technique and consistent surgical indications. Lin et al. [17] evaluated 92 infants at a minimum of 4 years of follow-up. Infants with upper and middle trunk injuries experienced significant improvement in 7 of the 15 motions measured by the Active Movement Scale (AMS) (Fig. 53.1), including shoulder abduction, flexion, and external rotation, elbow flexion, and forearm supination. At final follow-up, >60% of infants demonstrated functionally useful motor function (defined as AMS score ≥ 6) for shoulder abduction and flexion, elbow flexion and extension, forearm pronation and supination, and wrist flexion and extension. Infants with global injury significantly improved in 13 of the 15 AMS motions (all except shoulder internal rotation and pronation), and the majority (>50%) demonstrated functionally useful shoulder adduction and internal rotation, elbow flexion and extension, wrist flexion, finger flexion, and thumb flexion. They concluded that neuroma resection and nerve grafting resulted in significant improvements in AMS scores and in the proportion of patients demonstrating functional motor use. Manske et al. [14] reported the outcomes of this procedure in 43 infants at a mean age of 7 months with a minimum of 18 months' follow-up. Using the Active Movement Scale, 91% of infants recovered antigravity elbow flexion, and 67% recovered antigravity shoulder abduction. Fewer infants recovered SER (19%) and wrist extension (37%). The mean duration until antigravity strength was observed was >12 months for all evaluated motions. Secondary reconstructive procedures were common, including tendon transfers for SER (49% of children), biceps rerouting (21%), and tendon transfer for wrist extension (21%).

Despite the postoperative improvements in upper limb function following neuroma resection

The Active Movement Scale	
Observation	*Muscle Grade*
Gravity eliminated	
No contraction	0
Contraction, no motion	1
Motion ≤ 1/2 range	2
Motion > 1/2 range	3
Full motion	4
Against gravity	
Motion ≤ 1/2 range	5
Motion > 1/2 range	6
Full motion	7

Fig. 53.1 Active movement scale. (With permission from Curtis et al. [26])

and nerve grafting compared to preoperative function, impairments commonly persist, and secondary reconstructive surgeries are often necessary. Up to 70% of children may undergo multiple secondary procedures, including tendon transfers for SER, biceps rerouting, tendon transfer for wrist extension, and forearm or humerus osteotomies [14]. One-third of patients may require assistance with activities of daily living, with the extent of persistent impairment correlating with the extent and severity of injury [21]. Impairments due to a BPBI, however, may not limit participation and health-related quality of life. Children with BPBI participate in sports at the same rate as unaffected children without increase in rate of injury [27] and report peer relationships similar to an age-matched population [28].

Global BPBI

Several studies have specifically evaluated recovery of hand function in infants with global BPBI [14, 21–23, 25, 29], most commonly using the modified Raimondi scale, which rates hand motor function from 0 (no function) to 6 (normal function) (Fig. 53.2). Most indicate that hand motor recovery is commonly observed, but may not result in meaningful hand use (Raimondi score ≥ 3). Pondaag and Malessy [23] reported that 69% of infants who underwent brachial plexus reconstruction at approximately 4.4 months old had Raimondi scores of 3 or greater. Similarly, Terzis et al. reported Raimondi scores of 4 or better in 16 BPBI infants with poor hand function preoperatively who underwent neuroma resection and nerve grafting in the first 3 months of life [24]. In contrast, Kirjavainen et al. reported a mean Raimondi score of 2.2 (range: 0–5) in 25 infants with global BPBI who underwent a wide variety of procedures, compared to mean scores of 4.6 in infants with upper trunk palsies and 4.3 in infants with upper and middle trunk palsies [21]. Kirjavainen also reported abnormal sensation using Semmes-Weinstein monofilament testing in 76% of infants with global injuries who underwent nerve grafting, half of whom lacked protective sensation or worse. Additionally, 40% of these children demonstrated abnormal stereognosis using the Moberg-Dellon pickup test, with 16% unable to identify any of the six items tested [21]. Lower plexus avulsion injuries were associated with a lower Raimondi score.

Hand 0	Total palsy
Hand 1	No sensibility; possible tropic disturbance Some finger flexion (useless); useless thumb; no lateral pinch
Hand 2	Protective sensibility Some active useful finger flexion; no extension of wrist or fingers Weak lateral pinch with thumb; supinated forearm
Hand 3	Protective sensibility (some discrimination) Active extension of wrist with passive flexion of fingers (tenodesis) Lateral pinch with thumb; pronated forearm
Hand 4	Protective sensibility (some discrimination) Active useful flexion of wrist and fingers; intrinsic balance Mobile active thumb with some oppoition-adduction Pronated foream (no active supination)
Hand 5	Discriminative sensibility Active complete wrist and finger flexion Active extension of wrist but weak or absent finger extension Good intrinsic (median and ulmar)
Hand 6	Active pronosupination (even partial) As in hand 5 but with active extension of fingers and quite normal pronosupination

Fig. 53.2 Modified Raimondi scale. (With permission from Terzis and Kokkalis [24])

Outcomes of Neurolysis

Neurolysis is often performed in conjunction with nerve grafting, and evaluation of outcomes is often included in retrospective reviews of a variety of procedures as described above. Neurolysis as a stand-alone treatment for BPBI is controversial. Andrisevic et al. [30] reviewed 17 infants treated with isolated neurolysis of the upper trunk neuroma-in-continuity for whom intraoperative nerve conduction studies demonstrated >50% conduction across the neuroma. The authors reported significant postoperative improvement in shoulder abduction, flexion, external rotation, and internal rotation; elbow flexion; forearm supination; and wrist extension. Among children with 2 years of follow-up, the majority recovered "useful function," defined as AMS score ≥ 6, for elbow flexion (14/16), shoulder abduction (11/16) and shoulder flexion (11/15), but not external rotation (5/15). The authors concluded that infants with >50% conduction across the neuroma-in-continuity benefit from neurolysis, as an alternative to neuroma excision and nerve grafting [31]. However, the lack of a control group makes it difficult to prove that this recovery was due to the neurolysis and would not have occurred without surgery. Similarly, Chin et al. [32] described the outcomes of brachial plexus exploration and isolated neurolysis in 32 infants with favorable intraoperative EMG findings (absence of spontaneous insertional activity and normal compound motor action potential (CMAP) morphology) and also reported good recovery of shoulder abduction and elbow flexion but limited recovery of SER.

Other studies have reported less encouraging results from isolated neurolysis [17, 32–34]. Lin et al. [17] compared the outcomes of 92 infants who underwent neuroma resection and reconstruction with sural nerve grafting to 16 infants who underwent neurolysis alone. Among those who had neurolysis alone, significant postoperative increases in AMS scores were seen only for forearm supination in infants with upper and middle trunk palsies. In infants with global injury, significant improvement was observed in elbow flexion, supination, finger extension, and thumb extension. In comparison, infants with all types of BPBI who underwent grafting experienced significant improvement in nearly all motions measured by the AMS. Additionally, a greater proportion of infants who underwent nerve grafting showed functional recovery (AMS score ≥ 6) compared to those undergoing neurolysis alone. The authors concluded that, while nerve resection and grafting results in functional AMS scores, the inferior outcomes seen with neurolysis alone support abandoning neurolysis as a stand-alone treatment. König et al. [33] performed intraoperative nerve conduction studies in ten infants undergoing brachial plexus exploration for BPBI and performed an isolated neurolysis for the five infants who demonstrated conduction across the neuroma and neuroma resection and nerve grafting for the remainder. The outcomes of neurolysis alone were "disappointing" compared to those of resection and grafting.

Lastly, several studies [32, 34, 35] evaluated the ability of intraoperative electrodiagnostic studies to predict lesion severity, but none identified clinically useful criteria to differentiate avulsion, neurotmesis, and axonotmesis from normal nerves to guide intraoperative decision-making.

Outcomes of Nerve Transfer

Extrapolating from experience in adult brachial plexus injuries, use of nerve transfers (neurotization) for the management of BPBI has become increasingly popular. These are particularly useful in the setting of isolated deficits, late presentation, failed nerve grafting, and multiple root avulsions [36, 37]. Intraplexal donors are used most commonly in isolated upper and middle trunk injuries, while extraplexal donors are useful in global plexus injuries and isolated upper trunk injuries.

Upper and Middle Trunk BPBI

Multiple nerve transfers are often performed concomitantly. One common combination of transfer for upper trunk injuries is the "triple nerve transfer": (1) spinal accessory to suprascapular nerve for SER, (2) long or medial branch of triceps to axillary nerve for shoulder abduction, and (3) median or ulnar nerve fascicle to the biceps or brachialis branch of the musculocutaneous nerve for elbow flexion [38, 39].

Ladak et al. [40] presented the outcomes of triple nerve transfer in ten infants with isolated upper trunk injuries between 10 and 18 months of age. Mean AMS score for shoulder abduction, flexion, and external rotation, elbow flexion, and forearm supination all improved significantly between preoperative evaluation and exams performed at 1 and 2 years postoperatively. Mean scores at final follow-up demonstrated antigravity strength for shoulder abduction (AMS = 5.0), shoulder flexion (AMS = 5.4), elbow flexion (AMS = 6.2), and forearm supination (AMS = 5.9). While improved from preoperative exam, SER recovery was more limited (AMS = 4.3). McRae and Borschel [41] looked at the results of shoulder function following nerve transfers for pediatric brachial plexus injuries, including two infants with BPBI. Both of the infants with BPBI recovered functional shoulder abduction (AMS = 6), with less robust recovery of SER (AMS = 2, AMS = 3). To evaluate elbow flexion recovery, Little and colleagues [42] conducted a multicenter, retrospective review of 31 infants with BPBI who underwent either a single (median or ulnar) or double fascicle transfer to the biceps and/or brachialis branch of the musculocutaneous nerve. They found that 87% of infants recovered functional elbow flexion strength (defined as AMS score ≥6) and 21% had functional supination at a minimum 2 years' follow-up. It remains unclear if a double fascicular transfer results in superior elbow flexion and forearm supination recovery compared to single fascicle transfer. Alternative intraplexal nerve transfers to the musculocutaneous nerve, including the medial pectoral nerve [43, 44], have also been described with encouraging results.

O'Grady and colleagues [45] compared the outcomes of triple nerve transfer to nerve grafting for isolated upper trunk injuries in infants with similar preoperative AMS scores and age at time of surgery. Both groups demonstrated similar improvement in postoperative shoulder flexion, shoulder abduction, and elbow flexion, but the nerve transfer group had significantly better SER (AMS = 4.3 vs AMS = 2.9) and forearm supination (AMS = 5.6 vs AMS = 4.4) at 2-year follow-up. Nerve transfer was also associated with decreased operative time, shorter length of hospital stay, and lower costs.

Several studies compared the outcomes of spinal accessory nerve (SAN) to suprascapular nerve (SSN) transfer to nerve grafting for SER recovery and demonstrated similar findings in favor of the SAN to SSN transfer [18, 46–48]. Pondaag et al. [18] retrospectively evaluated SER recovery in 86 infants who underwent grafting of C5 to the SSN (n = 65) or transfer of the SAN to the SSN (n = 21). They identified no differences in postoperative SER AMS scores between the two techniques and reported that only 20% of the entire cohort recovered >20° of true SER. Similarly, Seruya et al. [47] evaluated the long-term outcomes of 74 infants with BPBI who underwent grafting (n = 28) or transfer of the SAN to the SSN (n = 46). Although there was no difference in postoperative AMS SER scores between the two techniques, there was a significantly higher rate of secondary reconstructive shoulder procedures in the grafting group compared with the transfer group. Interpretation of these studies is limited by baseline differences in AMS scores, injury severity, number of avulsion injuries, and age at the time of surgery. In a multicenter cohort of infants with similar injury severity, AMS scores, and age at surgery, Manske and colleagues [48] compared infants who underwent nerve grafting to the SSN (n = 59) or SAN to SSN transfer (n = 86) with a minimum follow-up of 18 months. The authors found that although there was no difference in mean postoperative AMS scores for SER (AMS = 3 in both groups), a greater proportion of infants who underwent nerve transfer achieved functional strength (AMS score ≥6) and the nerve transfer cohort had fewer secondary shoulder reconstruction procedures (hazards ratio 0.58 (95% CI 0.35–0.95)). Several approaches have been described for both the SAN to SSN transfer [49, 50] and triceps to axillary nerve [49, 51] transfer, but no comparative studies have demonstrated the optimal surgical strategy.

Lastly, Tora et al. [52] conducted a meta-analysis of nerve grafting versus nerve transfers to evaluate elbow flexion recovery and found comparable recovery of functional recovery in the nerve transfer and nerve graft groups (93% vs 96%, odds ratio = 1.15, 95% CI 0.19–7.08).

Global BPBI

In global BPBI, nerve transfers are used in conjunction with nerve grafting to provide an additional source of axonal inflow, especially in the setting of multiple nerve root avulsions. As in upper trunk injuries, the SAN is commonly transferred to the SSN for recovery of SER. Intercostal nerves are common donors to the musculocutaneous nerve for elbow flexion recovery [43, 53–55], and contralateral C7 nerve root transfer has been described for treatment of injuries with four or more root avulsions. Although these techniques are well-described in traumatic adult brachial plexus injuries, there is less information available regarding indications and outcomes for infants with birth injuries.

Luo et al. [54] evaluated the outcomes of transferring 3 or 4 intercostal nerves to the anterior division of the upper trunk or musculocutaneous nerve in 24 infants (16 global BPBI, 8 C5–C7 BPBI) and reported reliable recovery of elbow flexion using the Medical Research Council (MRC) scale; 92% of infants recovered ≥M3 elbow flexion and 71% recovered M4 strength. The authors found no difference in motor recovery between three and four intercostal nerve transfers, and transfer directly to the musculocutaneous nerve resulted in shorter reinnervation time (7.8 vs 9.3 months) compared to transfer to the upper trunk.

An alternative donor in brachial plexus injury with multiple avulsions is the contralateral C7 nerve root. Lin et al. [56] evaluated 9 infants with global BPBI with ≥ 4 root avulsions treated with contralateral C7 nerve transferred to the musculocutaneous and median nerve via a vascularized ulnar nerve graft. Seven of the nine infants recovered M3 or M4 elbow flexion strength, and five of nine recovered M3 or M4 wrist and finger flexion. The authors did not discuss donor side deficits or hand function on the affected side.

Contralateral C7 transfers were originally described with long cable grafts or vascularized ulnar nerve grafts, but more recent studies have used a retropharyngeal approach which decreases the amount of nerve graft needed.

Vu et al. [57] reported the outcomes of contralateral C7 transfer to the lower trunk using a retropharyngeal approach in five infants. At minimum 2-year follow-up, all children recovered sensation in the ulnar nerve distribution, but motor recovery did not often result in functional strength; one child recovered full wrist flexion strength (AMS = 7), while all other motions in all five patients were ≤3.

Conclusions

Nerve surgery for infants with BPBI has progressed since the initial description of primary nerve repairs. Newer techniques, including nerve grafting and nerve transfers, improve upper extremity function compared to nonoperative treatment in appropriately indicated patients, especially with regard to biceps and deltoid function. Despite these successes, persistent impairments and the need for additional operative and nonoperative treatment are common throughout childhood. Moreover, restoration of hand function in global injuries, recovery of SER, and mitigation of the musculoskeletal sequelae of BPBI remain challenging. Importantly, the effect of these interventions on patients' quality of life is not known. Methodologically rigorous studies are needed to advance understanding of surgical outcomes and improve care of infants with BPBI.

References

1. Clark LP, Taylor AS, Prout TP. A study on brachial plexus birth palsy. Am J Med Sci. 1905;130(4):670.
2. Thorburn W. A clinical lecture on secondary suture of the brachial plexus. Br Med J. 1900;1(2053):1073–5. https://doi.org/10.1136/bmj.1.2053.1073.
3. Kennedy R. Suture of the brachial plexus in birth paralysis of the upper extremity. Br Med J. 1903;1(2197):298–301. https://doi.org/10.1136/bmj.1.2197.298.
4. Waters PM. Comparison of the natural history, the outcome of microsurgical repair, and the outcome of operative reconstruction in brachial plexus birth palsy. J Bone Joint Surg Am. 1999;81(5):649–59. https://doi.org/10.2106/00004623-199905000-00006.
5. Smith NC, Rowan P, Benson LJ, Ezaki M, Carter PR. Neonatal brachial plexus palsy. Outcome of absent biceps function at three months of age. J Bone Joint Surg Am. 2004;86(10):2163–70.
6. Narakas A. Brachial plexus surgery. Orthop Clin North Am. 1981;12(2):303–23.
7. Narakas AO. Obstetrical brachial plexus injuries. In: Lamb DW, editor. Hand and upper limb: the paralyzed hand, vol. 2. Edinburgh: Churchill Livingstone; 1987. p. 116–35.

8. Gilbert A, Tassin JL. Surgical repair of the brachial plexus in obstetric paralysis. Chirurgie. 1984;110(1):70–5.
9. Ashley WW, Weatherly T, Park TS. Collagen nerve guides for surgical repair of brachial plexus birth injury. J Neurosurg. 2006;105(6 Suppl):452–6. https://doi.org/10.3171/ped.2006.105.6.452.
10. Gilbert A, Pivato G, Kheiralla T. Long-term results of primary repair of brachial plexus lesions in children. Microsurgery. 2006;26(4):334–42. https://doi.org/10.1002/micr.20248.
11. Boome RS, Kaye JC. Obstetric traction injuries of the brachial plexus. Natural history, indications for surgical repair and results. J Bone Joint Surg Br. 1988;70(4):571–6.
12. Kirjavainen M, Remes V, Peltonen J, et al. Long-term results of surgery for brachial plexus birth palsy. J Bone Joint Surg Am. 2007;89(1):18–26. https://doi.org/10.2106/JBJS.E.00430.
13. Strömbeck C, Krumlinde-Sundholm L, Forssberg H. Functional outcome at 5 years in children with obstetrical brachial plexus palsy with and without microsurgical reconstruction. Dev Med Child Neurol. 2000;42(3):148–57. https://doi.org/10.1017/s001216220000027x.
14. Manske MC, Bauer AS, Hentz VR, James MA. Long-term outcomes of brachial plexus reconstruction with Sural nerve autograft for brachial plexus birth injury. Plast Reconstr Surg. 2019;143(5):1017e–26e. https://doi.org/10.1097/PRS.0000000000005557.
15. Laurent JP, Lee R, Shenaq S, Parke JT, Solis IS, Kowalik L. Neurosurgical correction of upper brachial plexus birth injuries. J Neurosurg. 1993;79(2):197–203. https://doi.org/10.3171/jns.1993.79.2.0197.
16. Hentz VR, Meyer RD. Brachial plexus microsurgery in children. Microsurgery. 1991;12(3):175–85. https://doi.org/10.1002/micr.1920120307.
17. Lin JC, Schwentker-Colizza A, Curtis CG, Clarke HM. Final results of grafting versus neurolysis in obstetrical brachial plexus palsy. Plast Reconstr Surg. 2009;123(3):939–48. https://doi.org/10.1097/PRS.0b013e318199f4eb.
18. Pondaag W, de Boer R, van Wijlen-Hempel MS, Hofstede-Buitenhuis SM, Malessy MJA. External rotation as a result of suprascapular nerve neurotization in obstetric brachial plexus lesions. Neurosurgery. 2005;57(3):530–7; discussion 530–537. https://doi.org/10.1227/01.neu.0000170557.13788.d2.
19. Malessy MJA, Pondaag W. Neonatal brachial plexus palsy with neurotmesis of C5 and avulsion of C6: supraclavicular reconstruction strategies and outcome. J Bone Joint Surg Am. 2014;96(20):e174. https://doi.org/10.2106/JBJS.M.00547.
20. Gilbert A, Whitaker I. Obstetrical brachial plexus lesions. J Hand Surg Edinb Scotl. 1991;16(5):489–91. https://doi.org/10.1016/0266-7681(91)90100-3.
21. Kirjavainen M, Remes V, Peltonen J, Rautakorpi S, Helenius I, Nietosvaara Y. The function of the hand after operations for obstetric injuries to the brachial plexus. J Bone Joint Surg Br. 2008;90(3):349–55. https://doi.org/10.1302/0301-620X.90B3.19830.
22. Haerle M, Gilbert A. Management of complete obstetric brachial plexus lesions. J Pediatr Orthop. 2004;24(2):194–200. https://doi.org/10.1097/00004694-200403000-00012.
23. Pondaag W, Malessy MJA. Recovery of hand function following nerve grafting and transfer in obstetric brachial plexus lesions. J Neurosurg. 2006;105(1 Suppl):33–40. https://doi.org/10.3171/ped.2006.105.1.33.
24. Terzis JK, Kokkalis ZT. Outcomes of hand reconstruction in obstetric brachial plexus palsy. Plast Reconstr Surg. 2008;122(2):516–26. https://doi.org/10.1097/PRS.0b013e31817d6139.
25. Maillet M, Romana C. Complete obstetric brachial plexus palsy: surgical improvement to recover a functional hand. J Child Orthop. 2009;3(2):101–8. https://doi.org/10.1007/s11832-009-0161-1.
26. Curtis C, Stephens D, Clarke HM, Andrews D. The active movement scale: an evaluative tool for infants with obstetrical brachial plexus palsy. J Hand Surg Am. 2002;27(3):470–8.
27. Bae DS, Zurakowski D, Avallone N, Yu R, Waters PM. Sports participation in selected children with brachial plexus birth palsy. J Pediatr Orthop. 2009;29(5):496–503. https://doi.org/10.1097/BPO.0b013e3181aa9583.
28. Manske MC, Abarca NE, Letzelter JP, James MA. Patient-reported outcomes measurement information system (PROMIS) scores for children with brachial plexus birth injury. J Pediatr Orthop. 2021;41(3):171–6. https://doi.org/10.1097/BPO.0000000000001754. PMID: 33448721.
29. El-Gammal TA, El-Sayed A, Kotb MM, et al. Total obstetric brachial plexus palsy: results and strategy of microsurgical reconstruction. Microsurgery. 2010;30(3):169–78. https://doi.org/10.1002/micr.20726.
30. Andrisevic E, Taniguchi M, Partington MD, Agel J, Van Heest AE. Neurolysis alone as the treatment for neuroma-in-continuity with more than 50% conduction in infants with upper trunk brachial plexus birth palsy. J Neurosurg Pediatr. 2014;13(2):229–37. https://doi.org/10.3171/2013.10.PEDS1345.
31. Van Heest AE, Andrisevic E, Agel J. Neurolysis and upper trunk brachial plexus birth palsy. Response. J Neurosurg Pediatr. 2014;14(3):324–7. https://doi.org/10.3171/2014.3.PEDS14163.
32. Chin KF, Misra VP, Sicuri GM, Fox M, Sinisi M. Intra-operative neurophysiological prediction of upper trunk recovery in obstetric brachial plexus palsy with neuroma in continuity. Bone Joint J. 2013;95-B(5):699–705. https://doi.org/10.1302/0301-620X.95B5.30948.
33. König RW, Antoniadis G, Börm W, Richter H-P, Kretschmer T. Role of intraoperative neurophysiology in primary surgery for obstetrical brachial plexus palsy (OBPP). Childs Nerv Syst. 2006;22(7):710–4. https://doi.org/10.1007/s00381-005-0033-z.
34. Pondaag W, van der Veken LPAJ, van Someren PJ, van Dijk JG, Malessy MJA. Intraoperative nerve action and compound motor action potential record-

ings in patients with obstetric brachial plexus lesions. J Neurosurg. 2008;109(5):946–54. https://doi.org/10.3171/JNS/2008/109/11/0946.

35. Malessy MJA, Pondaag W, van Dijk JG. Electromyography, nerve action potential, and compound motor action potentials in obstetric brachial plexus lesions: validation in the absence of a "gold standard". Neurosurgery. 2009;65(4 Suppl):A153–9. https://doi.org/10.1227/01.NEU.0000338429.66249.7D.
36. Shah AS. Are nerve transfers supplanting nerve grafting as the primary treatment strategy for brachial plexus birth palsy? Poster 404 presented at the: American Society for Surgery of the Hand Annual Meeting; September 13, 2018; Boston. https://www.asshannualmeeting.org/servlet/servlet.FileDownload?file=00P0a00000jN7YMEA0.
37. Tse R, Kozin SH, Malessy MJ, Clarke HM. International Federation of Societies for surgery of the hand committee report: the role of nerve transfers in the treatment of neonatal brachial plexus palsy. J Hand Surg. 2015;40(6):1246–59. https://doi.org/10.1016/j.jhsa.2015.01.027.
38. Oberlin C, Béal D, Leechavengvongs S, Salon A, Dauge MC, Sarcy JJ. Nerve transfer to biceps muscle using a part of ulnar nerve for C5-C6 avulsion of the brachial plexus: anatomical study and report of four cases. J Hand Surg. 1994;19(2):232–7. https://doi.org/10.1016/0363-5023(94)90011-6.
39. Mackinnon SE, Novak CB, Myckatyn TM, Tung TH. Results of reinnervation of the biceps and brachialis muscles with a double fascicular transfer for elbow flexion. J Hand Surg. 2005;30(5):978–85. https://doi.org/10.1016/j.jhsa.2005.05.014.
40. Ladak A, Morhart M, O'Grady K, et al. Distal nerve transfers are effective in treating patients with upper trunk obstetrical brachial plexus injuries: an early experience. Plast Reconstr Surg. 2013;132(6):985e–92e. https://doi.org/10.1097/PRS.0b013e3182a97e13.
41. McRae MC, Borschel GH. Transfer of triceps motor branches of the radial nerve to the axillary nerve with or without other nerve transfers provides antigravity shoulder abduction in pediatric brachial plexus injury. Hand N Y. 2012;7(2):186–90. https://doi.org/10.1007/s11552-012-9398-0.
42. Little KJ, Zlotolow DA, Soldado F, Cornwall R, Kozin SH. Early functional recovery of elbow flexion and supination following median and/or ulnar nerve fascicle transfer in upper neonatal brachial plexus palsy. J Bone Joint Surg Am. 2014;96(3):215–21. https://doi.org/10.2106/JBJS.L.01405.
43. Pondaag W, Malessy MJA. Intercostal and pectoral nerve transfers to re-innervate the biceps muscle in obstetric brachial plexus lesions. J Hand Surg Eur Vol. 2014;39(6):647–52. https://doi.org/10.1177/1753193413501588.
44. Blaauw G, Slooff ACJ. Transfer of pectoral nerves to the musculocutaneous nerve in obstetric upper brachial plexus palsy. Neurosurgery. 2003;53(2):338–41; discussion 341–342. https://doi.org/10.1227/01.neu.0000073420.66113.66.
45. O'Grady KM, Power HA, Olson JL, et al. Comparing the efficacy of triple nerve transfers with nerve graft reconstruction in upper trunk obstetric brachial plexus injury. Plast Reconstr Surg. 2017;140(4):747–56. https://doi.org/10.1097/PRS.0000000000003668.
46. Tse R, Marcus JR, Curtis CG, Dupuis A, Clarke HM. Suprascapular nerve reconstruction in obstetrical brachial plexus palsy: spinal accessory nerve transfer versus C5 root grafting. Plast Reconstr Surg. 2011;127(6):2391–6. https://doi.org/10.1097/PRS.0b013e3182131c7c.
47. Seruya M, Shen SH, Fuzzard S, Coombs CJ, McCombe DB, Johnstone BR. Spinal accessory nerve transfer outperforms cervical root grafting for suprascapular nerve reconstruction in neonatal brachial plexus palsy. Plast Reconstr Surg. 2015;135(5):1431–8. https://doi.org/10.1097/PRS.0000000000001096.
48. Manske MC, Kalish LA, Cornwall R, Peljovich AE, Bauer AS, TOBI Study Group. Reconstruction of the Suprascapular nerve in brachial plexus birth injury: a comparison of nerve grafting and nerve transfers. J Bone Joint Surg Am. 2019. https://doi.org/10.2106/JBJS.19.00627.
49. Kozin SH. Nerve transfers in brachial plexus birth palsies: indications, techniques, and outcomes. Hand Clin. 2008;24(4):363–76. https://doi.org/10.1016/j.hcl.2008.04.002.
50. Rui J, Zhao X, Zhu Y, Gu Y, Lao J. Posterior approach for accessory-suprascapular nerve transfer: an electrophysiological outcomes study. J Hand Surg Eur Vol. 2013;38(3):242–7. https://doi.org/10.1177/1753193412447495.
51. Bauer AS, Rabinovich RV, Waters PM. The anterior approach for transfer of radial nerve triceps fascicles to the axillary nerve. J Hand Surg. 2019;44(4):345.e1–6. https://doi.org/10.1016/j.jhsa.2018.10.019.
52. Tora MS, Hardcastle N, Texakalidis P, Wetzel J, Chern JJ. Elbow flexion in neonatal brachial plexus palsy: a meta-analysis of graft versus transfer. Childs Nerv Syst. 2019;35(6):929–35. https://doi.org/10.1007/s00381-019-04133-z.
53. Kawabata H, Shibata T, Matsui Y, Yasui N. Use of intercostal nerves for neurotization of the musculocutaneous nerve in infants with birth-related brachial plexus palsy. J Neurosurg. 2001;94(3):386–91. https://doi.org/10.3171/jns.2001.94.3.0386.
54. Luo P-B, Chen L, Zhou C-H, Hu S-N, Gu Y-D. Results of intercostal nerve transfer to the musculocutaneous nerve in brachial plexus birth palsy. J Pediatr Orthop. 2011;31(8):884–8. https://doi.org/10.1097/BPO.0b013e318230a783.
55. El-Gammal TA, Abdel-Latif MM, Kotb MM, et al. Intercostal nerve transfer in infants with obstetric brachial plexus palsy. Microsurgery. 2008;28(7):499–504. https://doi.org/10.1002/micr.20545.

56. Lin H, Hou C, Chen D. Modified C7 neurotization for the treatment of obstetrical brachial plexus palsy. Muscle Nerve. 2010;42(5):764–8. https://doi.org/10.1002/mus.21752.
57. Vu AT, Sparkman DM, van Belle CJ, Yakuboff KP, Schwentker AR. Retropharyngeal contralateral C7 nerve transfer to the lower trunk for brachial plexus birth injury: technique and results. J Hand Surg. 2018;43(5):417–24. https://doi.org/10.1016/j.jhsa.2017.12.001.

Brachial Plexus Birth Injury: Late Complications and Treatment (Shoulder, Forearm, and Hand)

54

Tim Hems

Introduction

Long-term outcomes after brachial plexus birth injury (BPBI) are variable. In many cases, where the paralysis is transient with recovery of biceps and other muscle groups before the age of 2 months, normal upper limb function is likely to be regained. However, if biceps recovery does not occur until 3 months or later, then there will be some functional limitation in the longer term [1–4]. In general, the later the recovery of biceps and the greater the extent of the initial paralysis, the greater the residual deficit in the upper limb. It is very rare for elbow flexion not to recover spontaneously [1, 5, 6]. Longer-term deficits most often include limitation of shoulder movement, fixed flexion of the elbow, and reduction in forearm rotation [1, 7–9]. Hand function usually recovers well except in the most severe total palsies. As well as the amount of neurological recovery, the limitations and deformities in the upper limb are influenced by the effects of the nerve injury on the growing musculoskeletal structures.

This chapter is concerned with the assessment and treatment of the upper limb after the initial neurological recovery, which mostly occurs by the age of 2 years.

T. Hems (✉)
Scottish National Brachial Plexus Injury Service, Queen Elizabeth University Hospital and Royal Hospital for Children, Glasgow, UK
e-mail: t.e.j.hems@doctors.org.uk

Clinical Assessment

Clinical assessment of a child with BPBI starts by obtaining a history from the parents and medical records including details of the birth, the extent of the initial paralysis of the upper extremity, and how quickly improvement of movements, in particular recovery of active elbow flexion, occurred. This should enable a classification of the initial injury to be made using the Narakas groups [6]. Details of any previous operative and nonoperative treatment should be noted. The parents should be asked what functional limitations the child has and how these have changed with time. Hand dominance should be noted once the child reaches an age when this becomes established. In most cases of BPBI, the contralateral limb becomes dominant. It is important to check the child's overall development and whether there are any other medical problems.

Examination is carried out first by observing play. When possible, the child is asked to perform active movements, and then passive movements are assessed. The assessment sheet, which is currently used in our service, is shown in Fig. 54.1. This includes a detailed assessment of shoulder, elbow, and forearm rotation movements. Our form allows for successive measurements to be recorded over time and compared. The components of the Mallet score for active shoulder movement including abduction, external rotation, hand to head, hand to back, and hand mouth (1–5) are noted together with the total score (5–25) [4, 10].

A. Y. Shin, N. Pulos (eds.), *Operative Brachial Plexus Surgery*,
https://doi.org/10.1007/978-3-030-69517-0_54

Children's Brachial Plexus Injury Service

Email: brachial.plexus@ggc.scot.nhsuk Web: www. brachiaplexus.scot.nhs.uk

NAME:

CHI:

Patient Label

Date:										
Active Elevation										
Passive Elevation										
Active Inf. GH Angle										
Passive Inf. GH Angle										
Passive Post. GH Angle										
Opposite Post. GH Angle										
Active ER (in adduction)										
Passive ER (in adduction)										
Active ER (in abduction)										
Passive ER (in abduction)										
Active Medial Rotation										
Passive Medial Rotation										
Active Forearm Pronation										
Passive Forearm Pronation										
Active Forearm Supination										
Passive Forearm Supination										
Mallet Score* (see below)										
Fixed Elbow Flexion										
Range of Active Elbow Flexion										
Shoulder Stability										
Total Arc of Rotation										
BP Outcome Measure Score										
BrAT Score										

***Mallet Score:**	Abduction	/ 5	External Rotation	/ 5	Hand to Head	/ 5	Hand to Back	/ 5	Hand to Mouth	/ 5

Fig. 54.1 Form for assessment of upper limb movement in children with BPBI used by the Scottish National Brachial Plexus Injury Service

The shoulder is examined for evidence of posterior subluxation or dislocation. With the child facing him/her, the clinician's thumbs are placed over the superior aspect of the acromion of both shoulders. The posterior aspect of the shoulder is palpated with the fingers. There is a hollow below the posterior aspect of the acromion in the normal shoulder, whereas in posterior dislocation or subluxation, the humeral head fills the hollow and may project behind the acromion.

Additional subjective observations may be made regarding deformities and the use of the limb can be made. Formal task-based assessment of function using the Brachial Plexus Outcome Measure is possible after the age of 5 years [11].

Shoulder Deformity

In nearly all cases of continuing deficit after BPBI, there is delayed and incomplete recovery of active shoulder external rotation, a movement powered by infraspinatus and teres minor, innervated by the suprascapular and axillary nerves (C5–C6). This presumably represents a failure of neurological recovery in these nerves. In addition, other limitations may occur to varying degrees, including [12]:

- Range of active elevation (abduction/flexion) of the shoulder. This is likely to be related to the amount of neurological recovery in the supraspinatus and deltoid muscles.
- Degree of internal rotation contracture of the shoulder (loss of passive as well as active external rotation). It is classically believed that internal rotation contracture develops as a result of relative weakness of the shoulder external rotators compared with internal rotators which occurs in many cases of BPBI. However, the cause is probably more complex, and it is unclear why some cases develop more severe contractures (Fig. 54.2).
- The ranges of active and passive shoulder movements, other than external rotation, are often reduced, including internal rotation (Fig. 54.3). There is commonly some degree of abduction contracture of the glenohumeral joint [13].
- Bony deformity of the proximal humerus, glenoid, and scapula (see below).
- "Trumpeting". This is the tendency to abduct the shoulder while flexing the elbow, for example, when bringing the hand to the mouth. It may result from weakness of the shoulder external rotators or from co-contraction of shoulder abductors and elbow flexors after nerve regeneration.

Bony Deformity

In the shoulder affected by BPBI, the size of the humeral head is almost universally reduced. This may contribute to the reduction in range of rotation as impingement of the small humeral head on the glenoid could reduce the possible freedom of movement of the joint. There are variable amounts of retroversion of the humeral neck and glenoid, which increase during growth [14–16]. Posterior subluxation or dislocation of the shoulder may develop and is thought to be secondary to internal rotation contracture [16, 17]. The degree of glenohumeral deformity has been classified on the basis of computed tomography (CT) and magnetic resonance imaging (MRI) by Waters et al. [16] (Table 54.1) and Birch [18, 19]. Birch described posterior subluxation (simple), posterior dislocation (simple), and complex subluxation/dislocation on the basis of clinical and radiographic findings.

For the purposes of this chapter, posterior dislocation is defined as complete displacement of the humeral head from the true glenoid into a "false" glenoid, which cannot be reduced without soft tissue releases. Subluxation refers to a situation where the glenoid is flattened and retroverted. There may be two glenoid facets, with the humeral head subluxing into the posterior one on internal rotation but reducible to the true anterior facet with external rotation.

Nath and Paizi emphasised that the deformity after BPBI involves the whole shoulder girdle [20]. Based on CT imaging, hypoplasia of the scapula and clavicle, elongation of the acro-

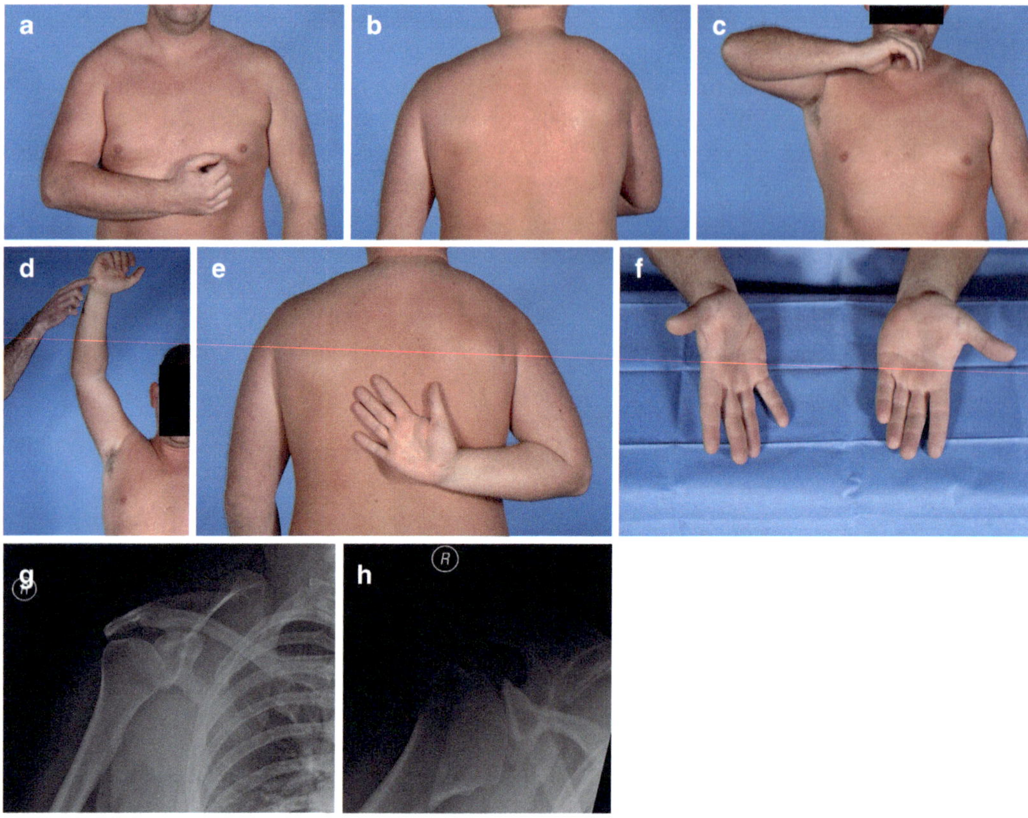

Fig. 54.2 (**a**–**f**) Clinical photographs of an adult patient with a history of right BPBI affecting the upper roots. He has had no surgical intervention. There has been good recovery of elbow flexion, but he has a minor flexion contracture of the elbow. While there is almost full shoulder abduction, he has a marked internal rotation contracture of the shoulder and trumpeting. There is prominence of the superior angle of the scapula indicating an abduction contracture of the shoulder (Putti sign). Internal rotation of the shoulder is adequate. There is limitation of forearm supination. (**h**–**i**) Anteroposterior and axillary lateral radiographs of the shoulder show no evidence of posterior subluxation

mion, and downward rotation of the scapula were described as well as subluxation of the humeral head. Downward rotation of the scapula results from abduction contracture of the glenohumeral joint and has been shown to be associated with atrophy of abductor muscles on MRI [13].

Pathogenesis of Contractures and Bony Deformity

Traditionally it has been believed that soft tissue contractures develop at the shoulder after BPBI as a result of muscle imbalance. Hence relative weakness of the external rotators of the shoulder, innervated by C5 and C6, compared with subscapularis and other internal rotators, innervated by C6, C7, and C8, in many cases of BPBI might allow an internal rotation contracture of the shoulder to develop. In a recent review of clinical and experimental evidence, Olofsson et al. concluded that muscle imbalance is not the only factor generating contractures [21]. Changes resulting from denervation which lead to impaired muscle growth appear to have an influence [22]. This mechanism is more consistent with the finding of a global reduction in shoulder movement seen in many cases of BPBI. Further experimental work has suggested that degeneration of muscle spindles has a role in development of contractures. When comparing the effects of pre- and postganglionic injury to nerve roots, there was less severe muscle contracture after preganglionic injury where afferent innervation is partially preserved and muscle spindles do not degenerate [23]. The exact mechanism of development of bony defor-

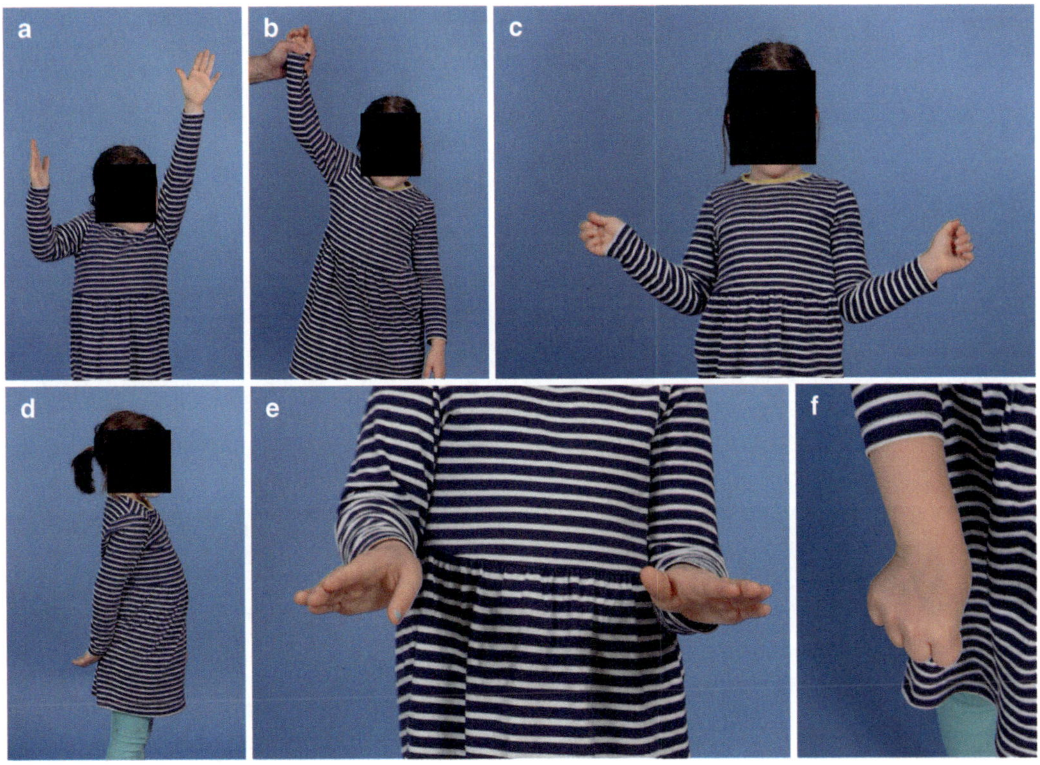

Fig. 54.3 Clinical photographs of a child aged 6 years with a history of right BPBI, Narakas group 2 with biceps recovery at age 6 months. No surgery has been carried out. Active and passive shoulder abduction (**a**, **b**). There is good external rotation of the shoulder but limited internal rotation (**c**, **d**). Forearm pronation is reduced and there is ulnar deviation of the wrist (**e**, **f**)

Table 54.1 Classification of glenohumeral deformity in BPBI based on CT or MRI findings (Waters et al. [16])

Type	
I	Normal glenoid (less than a 5-degree difference in retroversion compared with that on the normal, contralateral side)
II	Minimum deformity (more than a 5-degree difference in retroversion compared with that on the normal side, with no posterior subluxation of the humeral head)
III	Moderate deformity (posterior subluxation of the humeral head, defined as less than 35% of the head anterior to the bisecting line)
IV	Severe deformity (a false glenoid)
V	Severe flattening of the humeral head and glenoid, with progressive or complete posterior dislocation of the head
VI	Dislocation of the glenohumeral joint in infancy
VII	Growth arrest of the proximal aspect of the humerus

mity at the shoulder is also unknown. Although soft tissue contractures and bony deformities are linked, there is not a close correlation between the severity of the two pathologies. Significant contracture can occur with little glenohumeral deformity.

Investigations

Plain radiographs of the shoulder, both in antero-posterior and axillary lateral views, help to define the degree of bony deformity. Both shoulders are imaged for comparison. The anteroposterior views will typically show hypoplasia of the proximal humerus and downward rotation of the scapula, with more of the superior and medial borders of the scapula visible above the clavicle. On the axillary lateral of a normal shoulder, the centre of the humeral head (epiphysis) lies below the acromio-clavicular joint. Displacement pos-

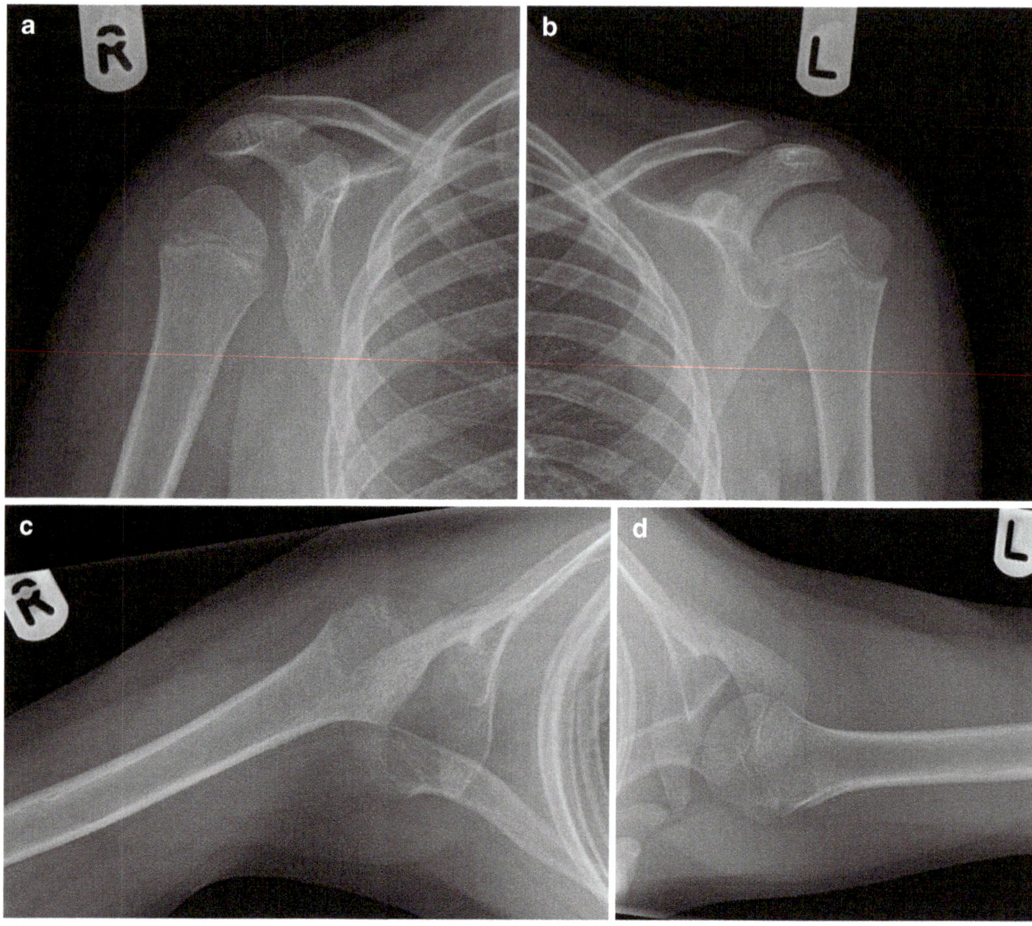

Fig. 54.4 Anteroposterior (**a**, **b**) and axillary lateral radiographs (**c**, **d**) of both shoulders in a child with BPBI at age 12 years. There is posterior dislocation of the right shoulder which has not been treated

teriorly indicates subluxation or dislocation, and there may be a windswept appearance of the humeral head (Fig. 54.4).

If operative intervention is being considered, then CT or MR scans may be obtained. Measurements of the degree of retroversion of the glenoid and subluxation of the humeral head can be made on axial images. For glenoid version a line is drawn parallel to the blade of the scapula and a second line along the line of the joint. To calculate the glenoid version, the angle in the posteromedial quadrant is measured and 90° subtracted. Normal glenoid version is approximately –5° [16]. The percentage of the humeral head anterior to the middle of the glenoid fossa is calculated by drawing a line along the greatest diameter of the humeral head. The distance from the scapular line to the anterior margin of the humeral head is divided by the diameter of the head and expressed as a percentage. This measurement is approximately 50% in a normal shoulder. The lower the percentage, the greater the degree of posterior subluxation (Fig. 54.5).

Nonoperative Treatment

Physiotherapy is usually recommended for all children with BPBI and is aimed at maintaining the range of movement in the shoulder and other joints. Although there is no definite evidence, I have the impression in our service that

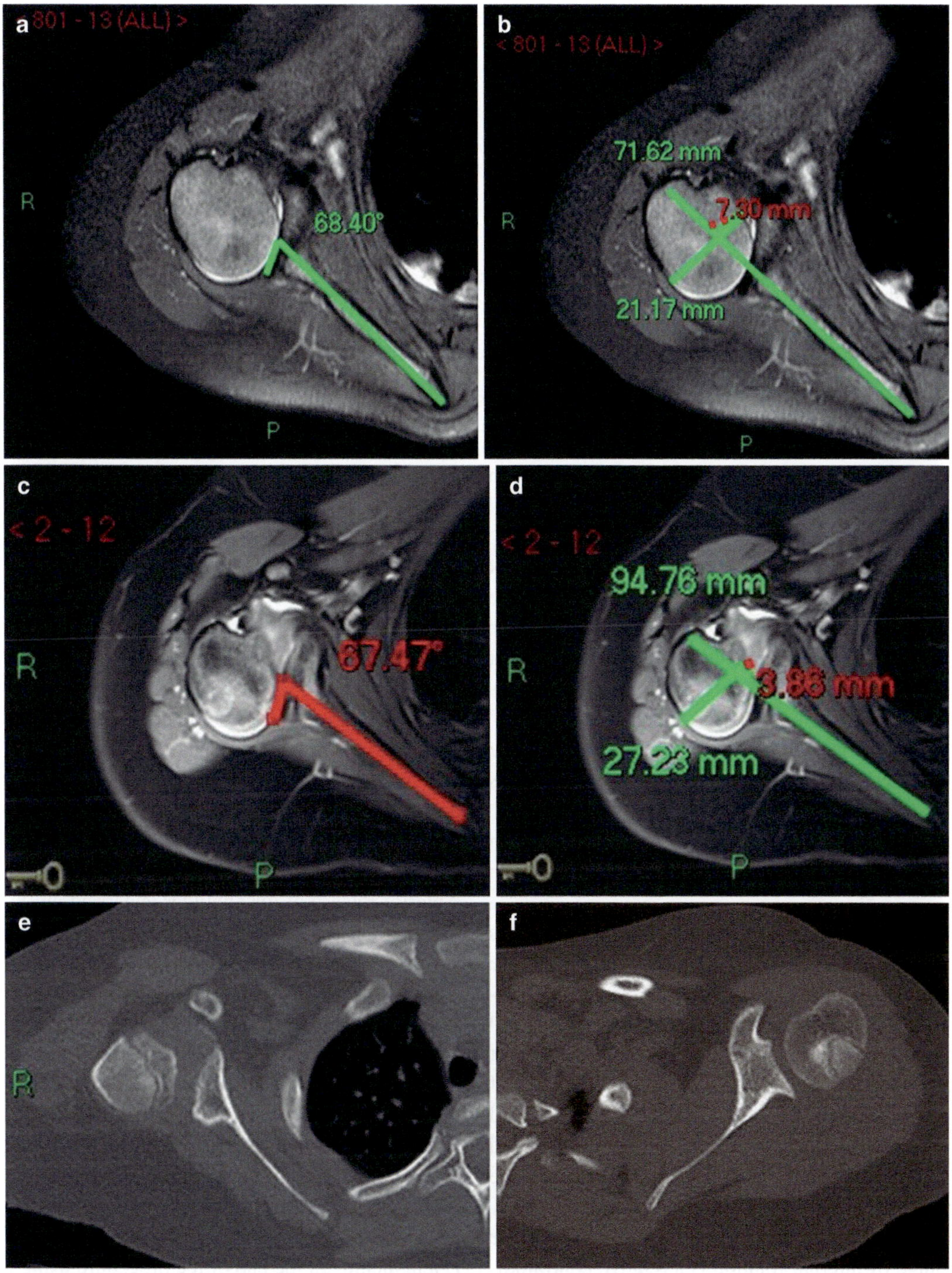

Fig. 54.5 Axial MR images of the right shoulder: at age 16 months, (**a**) glenoid version = 68–90 = −22°, (**b**) percentage of humeral head anterior to the middle of the glenoid fossa = 7/21 × 100 = 33%; the same child at age 6, (**c**) glenoid version = −23°, (**d**) percentage of humeral head anterior to the middle of the glenoid fossa = 4/27 × 100 = 15%, indicating that there has been increase in the degree of posterior subluxation; CT scan at age 8 comparing (**e**) affected shoulder with (**f**) the normal side

when physiotherapy is started within the first few weeks of life, the chance of a fixed internal rotation contracture of the shoulder and hence the need for surgery is lowered. After initial assessment children are followed up to monitor whether the range of movement is improving or deteriorating. While manipulation under anaesthetic and botulinum toxin injection into the internal rotator muscles of the shoulder is an option before the age of 1 year, it is unlikely that this procedure will be effective in older children.

Indications for Surgery

Indications for soft tissue rebalancing surgery on the shoulder up to the age of 5 or 6 years include:

- Internal rotation contracture with evidence of posterior subluxation or dislocation of the shoulder.
- Internal rotation contracture which is not improving or is deteriorating despite physiotherapy. Active external rotation less than 0° (with the shoulder adducted) and passive external rotation less than 20° are thresholds at which to consider operation.
- Marked weakness of active external rotation in the presence of a good passive range.

It should be appreciated that surgery to increase the range of external rotation of the shoulder is likely to reduce the range of internal rotation, which may have major functional implications if the child cannot reach their waist or buttock [12, 24, 25]. Therefore, the range of active internal rotation should be assessed and taken into account in the decision to operate and the type of surgery performed. In cases where the degree of internal rotation contracture and bony deformity is less severe, then limitation of the range of internal rotation is a relative contraindication for operation. Hultgren et al. [26, 27] recommended that subscapularis lengthening should not be performed if the child has less than 70° of internal rotation. When posterior dislocation of the shoulder is identified at a young age, I would recommend operation for reduction, regardless of the range of internal rotation, as there is a good chance that a congruent joint can be obtained and hence more normal development of the shoulder. However, a simultaneous internal rotation osteotomy of the humeral head is performed (see surgical techniques) [12].

If dislocation is not identified until the age of 6 because of late referral, then reduction is unlikely to be successful because of the extent of secondary bony deformity. Palliative external rotation osteotomy of the humerus may be considered.

Author's Preferred Surgical Techniques

For children undergoing soft tissue rebalancing for the shoulder, an "à la carte" approach can be applied to manage variable indications. If there is an internal rotation contracture of the shoulder, the child is positioned supine with a sandbag under the chest on the affected side.

A deltopectoral incision is made. As well as developing the interval between the deltoid and pectoralis major to expose the coracoid and conjoint tendon, the pectoralis major tendon is divided near its insertion (if latissimus dorsi transfer or humeral osteotomy is to be performed). Working on the lateral side of the conjoint tendon, the proximal humerus and subscapularis are exposed. Anterior release of the shoulder is carried out by dividing the coraco-acromial ligament, the shoulder capsule in the rotator interval, and the upper half of the subscapularis tendon as far medially as can be safely exposed. In most cases, where the shoulder is stable, this release is adequate to gain full external rotation. If a contracture remains or there is posterior dislocation of the shoulder, the lower half of the subscapularis tendon is divided more laterally near its insertion so making a Z-shaped tenotomy. The anterior shoulder capsule is opened. The subscapularis tendon is repaired by Z-lengthening at the end of the procedure using a non-absorbable suture.

If dislocated, the shoulder is reduced from the false glenoid to the true glenoid by externally rotating the humerus. The shoulder is then examined to establish the stable range. Often the humeral head is stable on the true glenoid in external rotation but re-dislocates with internal rotation past neutral. In order that the stable arc of shoulder rotation is in the functional range, approximately 60° internal rotation to 30° external rotation, an internal rotation osteotomy of the proximal humerus may be necessary. The periosteum of the proximal humeral shaft is incised longitudinally taking care to remain below the proximal humeral epiphysis. The osteotomy site is selected and a four-hole 2 mm or 2.7 mm mini-plate positioned. K-wires are inserted proximal and distal to the osteotomy site. The distal wire is angled laterally by the predicted amount of rotation, usually 40°–60°. An oscillating saw is used to make the osteotomy, and then the K-wires are lined up by internally rotating the distal segment. The amount of internal rotation is checked. It should be possible to internally rotate the shoulder so that the forearm will rest on the abdomen without posterior subluxation or dislocation of the humeral head. The plate is then reapplied and secured with screws.

In order to strengthen external rotation, the latissimus dorsi is transferred onto infraspinatus. When an anterior approach has been made, the latissimus dorsi tendon is detached from the humerus through this exposure. A vertical incision is made on the posterior aspect of the shoulder running into the skin crease in the axillary fold. The posterior edge of deltoid is identified and mobilised to expose infraspinatus. The latissimus dorsi tendon is passed into the posterior incision and the muscle mobilised. The tendon is then attached near the insertion of infraspinatus with non-absorbable sutures.

If the child has no fixed internal rotation of the shoulder, then latissimus dorsi transfer may be performed to strengthen active external rotation. In these cases the entire procedure can be accomplished through a posterior incision.

The pectoralis major tendon is repaired before skin closure. In order to maintain the release of the internal rotation contracture and reduction of the shoulder joint and protect the tendon transfer, a lightweight shoulder spica is applied with the shoulder just short of maximal external rotation, usually about 40°, and 45° abduction. The cast is removed after 6 weeks and physiotherapy started to mobilise the shoulder.

Alternative Techniques

Arthroscopic Release

An alternative to the open subscapularis release is arthroscopic release [25, 28]. With the child in a lateral position, posterior and anterior portals are established. The anterior capsular ligaments are released from their attachment to the glenoid and then the subscapularis tendon. Pearl found that tenotomy of the subscapularis and overlying capsule was adequate to restore full passive external rotation in younger children [28]. For severe contractures and older children, release of the rotator interval was necessary. Kozin followed up 44 children with MRI and clinical measurements a year after arthroscopic capsular release and subscapularis tenotomy with or without tendon transfers [25]. There were significant improvements in external rotation, Mallet scores, glenoid retroversion, and the degree of posterior subluxation.

Subscapularis Slide

An alternative to release or lengthening of the subscapularis tendon is release of the origin of the muscle from the blade of the scapula [18, 29, 30]. The muscle is exposed through an axillary incision and then detached from the inner face of the scapula without opening the shoulder capsule. The shoulder is stretched into full external rotation. The technique appears to be effective where there is mild limitation of external rotation and no bony deformity. However, it is difficult to see how this approach can address the capsular tightness, which appears to make a significant contribution to the contracture and bony deformity. Gilbert et al. reported a greater gain in external rotation and more reliable maintenance of the correction in children under the age of 2 years [30]. Some cases failed because of unrecognised articular deformities. Birch reported that the procedure failed in the longer term in about a third of cases with recurrence of the internal rotation contracture and development of bony deformities [18].

Glenoid Osteotomy

Traditionally soft tissue rebalancing procedures are not attempted for older children with posterior dislocation or severe subluxation of the shoulder. A palliative external rotation osteotomy of the humerus may be considered. An alternative approach is an osteotomy of the glenoid to correct the retroversion [31, 32]. The procedure is usually combined with lengthening of the subscapularis, if there is limited passive external rotation, and transfer of latissimus dorsi to infraspinatus.

Dodwell et al. recommend operation with the patient in a lateral position [31]. An extensive posterior exposure of the shoulder is made including elevation of the posterior edge of the deltoid, to expose infraspinatus and teres minor. The interval between infraspinatus and teres minor is developed to expose the posterior aspect of the shoulder joint. Subperiosteal exposure of the neck of the scapula is performed preserving the suprascapular nerve. The joint capsule is opened vertically to visualise the alignment of the glenoid articular surface. An osteotomy is made in the neck of the scapula parallel to and 1 cm from the articular surface and deepened to just short of the anterior cortex. The osteotomy is then opened hinging the whole glenoid on the intact anterior cortex by an amount required to correct the glenoid retroversion to neutral. This can be determined by measuring preoperative CT or MR scans. A bone block of appropriate size to fit the opening of the posterior cortex is obtained from the medial aspect of the scapular spine and wedged into the osteotomy. The capsule is closed. Di Mascio et al. reported a slightly different technique, described as a glenoplasty, where the osteotomy is made through the posterior cortex and the posterior glenoid margin is elevated bending articular surface to mould it to the humeral head [32].

There was an improvement in glenoid version of 26° in the series of 32 children with a median age of 6.8 years (range, 2.1–16.2) reported by Dodwell et al. [31]. The procedure is likely to be most applicable to a situation where the glenoid is flattened and retroverted allowing subluxation of the shoulder but without the false and true glenoid facets seen in true dislocation. These cases often respond poorly to soft tissue balancing alone. Reorientation of the glenoid can potentially stabilise the joint.

Salvage Procedures

If posterior dislocation of the shoulder is identified over the age of 6, then reduction is not usually attempted as the extent of bony deformity makes a successful outcome unlikely. Even in the absence of dislocation, internal rotation contracture in older children is less likely to respond well to soft tissue rebalancing procedures. External rotation osteotomy of the humerus to move the arc of rotation of the shoulder into a more functional range may be recommended (the patient illustrated in Fig. 54.2 could benefit from external rotation osteotomy). There will be some loss of internal rotation, and therefore the range of internal rotation should be carefully assessed to check that a reduction will not have major functional consequences.

The osteotomy is performed in the midshaft of the humerus. A posteromedial approach to the humerus allows the incision to be made of the medial aspect of the arm where the scar is less visible. A longitudinal incision is made on the medial aspect of the upper arm. The ulnar nerve is identified, carefully dissected from the medial border of the triceps muscle, and retracted anteriorly. The shaft of the humerus is then exposed taking care to identify the radial nerve in the proximal part of the exposure. A plate is selected depending on the size of the patient and temporarily positioned. After marking the osteotomy site, K-wires are inserted above to guide the amount of rotation. A transverse osteotomy is performed with an oscillating saw. The distal segment is externally rotated, usually by 30°–40° before reapplying and securing the plate with screws.

Outcomes

Waters and Bae reported a series of mild-to-moderate glenohumeral dysplasia treated with transfer of latissimus dorsi and teres major and extra-articular soft tissue releases in children with mean age of 42 months [33]. At a minimum of 2 years of follow-up, there were a global improvement in shoulder function and a slight improvement in the degree of glenoid retroversion and posterior subluxation. None of the patients had progression of the glenohumeral deformity. Therefore, soft tissue rebalancing appears to prevent progression of the deformity.

For more severe glenohumeral deformity, Kambhampati et al. reported outcomes for surgery on 101 cases of posterior subluxation and 83 of dislocation [34]. Operation included excision of the coracoid, Z-lengthening of the subscapularis tendon, and medial rotation osteotomy of the humerus in selected cases. The mean range of active external rotation increased by 58°. There was failure of reduction of the joint in 20 cases. Avascular necrosis of the humeral head, confirmed radiologically, occurred in six children who presented with an irritable and stiff shoulder. Pain resolved within 6 months in all these cases.

In a series of 25 children who had an operation using the soft tissue rebalancing technique described above in the author's unit, 9 shoulders were dislocated and 7 subluxed before operation [12]. Reduction was maintained at a mean follow-up of 3.8 years in all cases except one, who had a full passive range of movement but continued to sublux on internal rotation. Mean active external rotation for the whole group increased from −21° to 32°, passive external rotation from 26° to 67°, and total Mallet score from 12.8 to 17.5. Mean active abduction was 111° and did not significantly improve after operation. Using a similar surgical approach, Hultgren et al. reported a series of 270 children with 1-year follow-up. Mean active external rotation increased by 85° [26]. Of the 105 patients with subluxed or dislocated shoulders, 6 could not be reduced and 3 required further surgery.

Although reduction of the shoulder at an early age allows more normal development of the shoulder joint (Fig. 54.6), shoulder function in the longer term is generally poorer than in cases where subluxation or dislocation did not occur (Personal observation) [26, 27]. There is no definitive evidence that eventual shoulder function is better than palliative external rotation osteotomy alone. However, an adult patient who develops shoulder pain associated with chronic dislocation represents an insoluble problem.

The author recommends simultaneous transfer of latissimus dorsi +/− teres major in most cases in order to strengthen external rotation [12]. This appears to help stabilise the joint in cases where reduction is necessary. Pearl et al. found more reliable maintenance of external rotation after arthroscopic release of internal rotation contracture if latissimus dorsi transfer was used [28]. However, Hultgren et al. found no greater improvement in external rotation if latissimus dorsi transfer was used over subscapularis lengthening alone [26].

Sibinski et al. emphasised the risk of deterioration in internal rotation as a result of surgery to increase external rotation, which may have significant functional consequences (Fig. 54.7, [12]). Out of 25 cases, active internal rotation was worse in 9. Five, who had not had simultaneous internal rotation osteotomy, had significant functional impairment, and this was sufficiently severe in three to justify later humeral osteotomy. The risk of this problem appeared to be highest in cases who had a good passive range of external rotation, and muscle transfer alone was performed to increase active external rotation. Hultgren et al. did not recommend simultaneous internal rotation osteotomy, but at longer-term follow-up, 23 of 63 patients who had reduction of the shoulder had required delayed osteotomy [26, 27]. Abdel-Ghani et al. reported a higher incidence of external rotation contracture of the shoulder (defined as inability to touch the abdomen with the wrist extended) if teres major and latissimus dorsi are transferred rather than latissimus dorsi alone and recommended that only latissimus dorsi should be transferred [24].

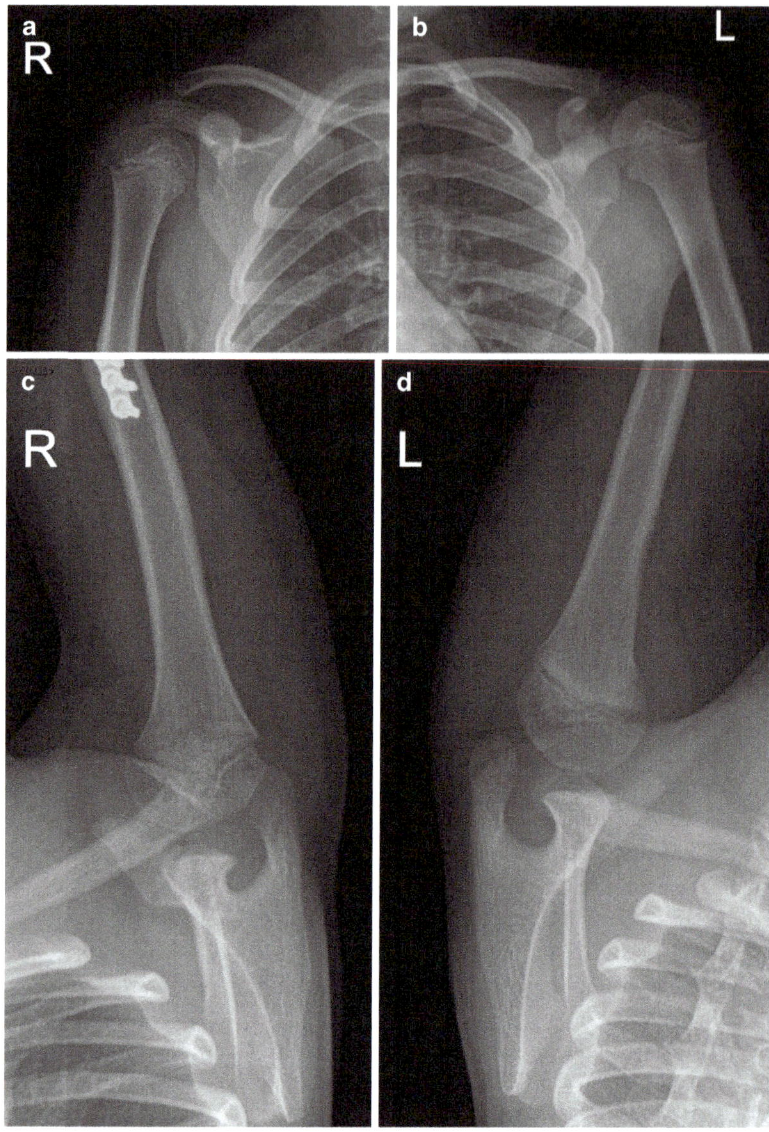

Fig. 54.6 Anteroposterior (**a**, **b**) and axillary lateral radiographs (**c**, **d**) of both shoulders in a child with right BPBI at age 7. Open reduction for posterior dislocation of the right shoulder had been carried out at age 1 year. The procedure included subscapularis lengthening, transfer of latissimus dorsi and teres major, and internal rotation osteotomy of the proximal humerus. There has been good remodelling of the glenoid, and the humeral head is centred beneath the lateral clavicle similar to the normal side. There is still a degree of downward rotation of the scapula as a result of abduction contracture of the shoulder

Eismann et al. studied glenohumeral abduction contracture before and after soft tissue rebalancing surgery. The contracture was unchanged, but greater glenoid retroversion was associated with worse abduction contracture after operation [13].

Longer-term outcomes suggest that there may be some deterioration of the gains in shoulder movement after soft tissue rebalancing procedures. Kirkos et al. reported outcomes of ten cases of anterior release and transfer of teres major and latissimus dorsi with a mean follow-up of 30 years [35]. The mean gain of 36.5° in active external rotation after operation was maintained for 10 years but then deteriorated in eight patients to a mean of 10.5°. There was radiographic evidence of degenerative change in the glenohumeral joint at long-term follow-up in some cases. Hultgren et al. reported outcomes of subscapularis lengthening with or without reduction of the shoulder with minimum follow-up of 7 years [27]. A useful gain in external rotation had been maintained although the mean improvement from presurgery of 66.5° was less than that at 1-year follow-up. The range of active abduction did not change at longer follow-up.

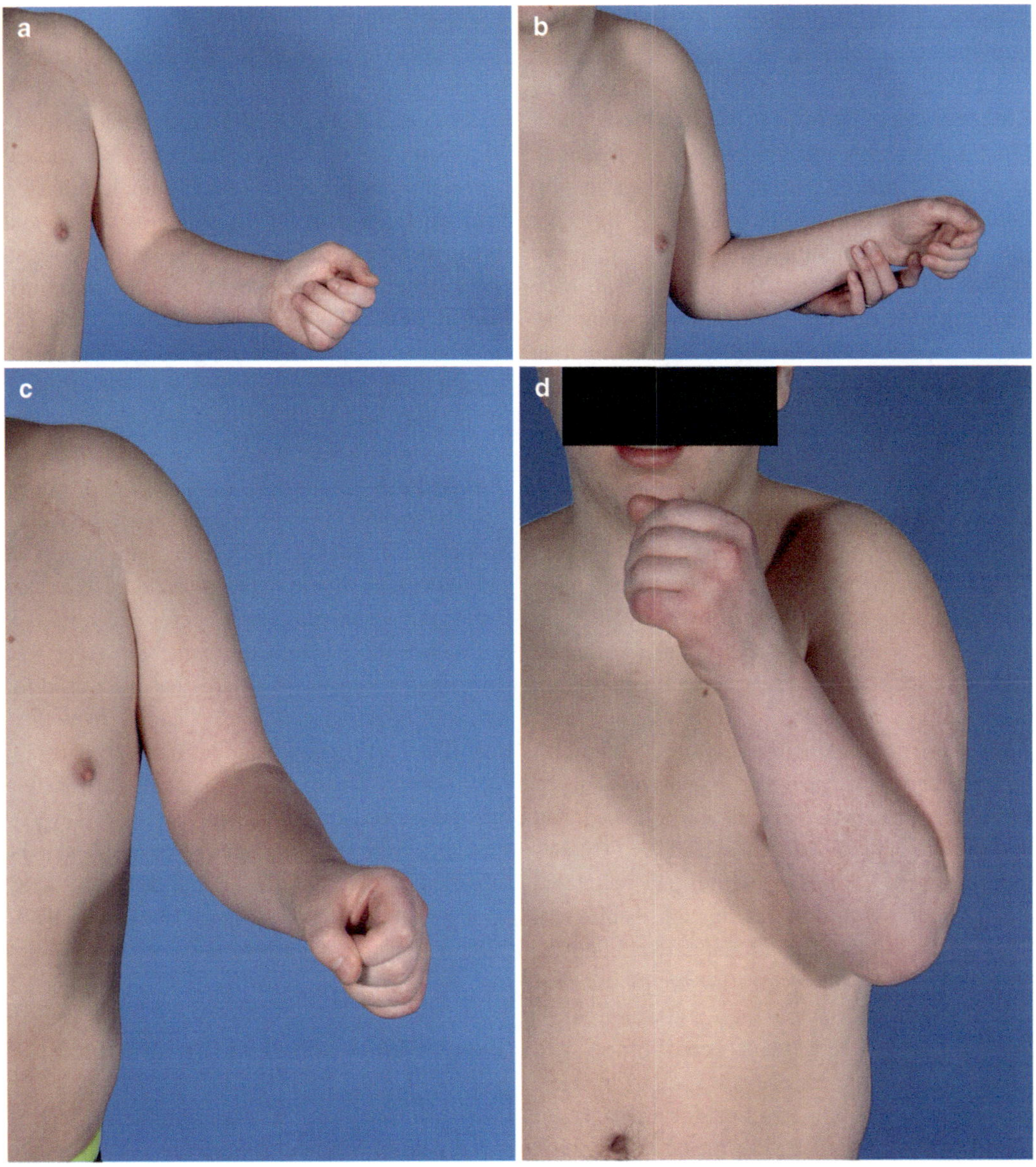

Fig. 54.7 Clinical photographs of an adult with a history of left BPBI. Open reduction of the shoulder had been carried out at age 15 months. There are 30° active shoulder external rotation (**a**) and almost full passive external rotation (**b**). However, he is unable to internally rotate past neutral (**c**) and consequently cannot get his hand to his mouth (**d**)

For isolated external rotation osteotomy of the humerus, a number of authors have reported improved function. In a series of 22 osteotomies through the humeral neck with mean follow-up of 14 years, there was a mean increase in active shoulder abduction of 27° and the arc of rotation of 25°. Ability to bring the hand to the mouth was improved [36]. Waters and Bae also performed the osteotomy through the humeral neck in children with severe glenohumeral deformity with a mean improvement in external rotation of 64° and in aggregate Mallet score from 13 to 18 [37]. The greatest gains were in hand-to-mouth, hand-to-neck, and external rotation movement. Al-Qattan et al. reported that the gain in external rotation after low rotation osteotomy was maintained in the long term, but there was deterioration in shoulder abduction [38].

Restoration of Shoulder Abduction

Most series reporting outcomes of surgery to increase external rotation of the shoulder, including Sibinski et al. and Hultgren et al., have not shown a significant improvement in the range of active abduction [12, 26]. Vekris et al. have recommended transfer of the trapezius onto the lateral aspect of the humerus, suggesting that more than 90° abduction can be achieved if some supraspinatus function is present [39].

Elbow Deformity

Failure of recovery of the adequate elbow flexion is unusual after spontaneous recovery of BPBI [1, 5, 6]. In the author's unit, Hems et al. [5] studied children born before the service routinely offered nerve reconstruction for BPBI. Excluding cases who had made a full recovery within 1–2 months, 152 children with persisting deficit were identified from the service database. Five had had undergone nerve exploration and repair. All children managed without operation had recovered elbow flexion with only one having insufficient flexion to reach their mouth. None were considered to require late reconstruction to improve elbow flexion. In 130 cases the age at which elbow flexion started to recover had been recorded, with a mean of 4 months for Narakas group 1 injuries, 6 months for group 2, 8 months for group 3, and 12 months for group 4. The mean active range of elbow flexion measured in 44 cases was 138° and was similar between groups. Mean isometric elbow flexion strength at long-term follow-up, in 39 patients, was 63% of the normal side and again was similar in different groups. This cohort study shows that almost all cases of BPBI treated nonoperatively regain functional elbow flexion, although recovery occurs later in more severe lesions. The author's service has continued to see new cases of older children and adults with a history of BPBI, who have not had access to nerve repair surgery. A similar pattern has been observed with only one child presenting with absence of active elbow flexion. Therefore reconstruction to improve active elbow flexion is rarely required.

For cases where elbow flexion remains weak, reconstructive options include free vascularised transfer of the gracilis muscle, Steindler transfer, and bipolar transfer of latissimus dorsi [40] and pectoralis minor transfer. Gilbert et al. reported the long-term results of a modified Steindler procedure carried out for poor active elbow flexion in 27 cases [41]. There were good results in 67% with a mean active elbow flexion of 97°. Results were more reliable if active wrist extension was present or had been restored by tendon transfer. For pectoralis minor transfer, Costil et al. found an improvement in the mean range of elbow flexion from 81° to 111° [42]. They concluded that the procedure was reliable in children who had weak, but not absent flexion, before operation.

Within the author's unit, microvascular free functioning transfer of gracilis has been used for cases of BPBI who have insufficient elbow flexion after nerve reconstruction, using the method described by Kay et al. [43]. The muscle transfers are innervated by intercostal nerves (III–V) or fascicles from the ulnar nerve. For free functioning transfer of gracilis, Kay et al. achieved MRC grade 4 elbow flexion in 12 of 13 cases of BPBI although the range of flexion was unclear [43].

Flexion Contracture of the Elbow

Many children with a history of BPBI develop fixed flexion of the elbow. There is no contracture at birth, but it develops during childhood. In most cases there is only a minor contracture of 10°–20°, but some children develop a more severe limitation of elbow extension of more than 30°. Although function is not usually directly impaired, the elbow contracture affects the cosmetic appearance of the upper limb with apparent shortening. Anterior or posterior dislocation of the radial head occasionally occurs in association with flexion contracture of the elbow (see forearm section below).

Sheffler et al. investigated the occurrence and progression with age of elbow flexion contracture in a large cohort of 319 patients with BPBI [44]. A contracture of ≥10° occurred in 152 (48%) with a median age of onset of 5.1 years. The contracture was ≥30° in 54 cases. The prevalence of contracture increased with age but was not significantly associated with the extent of the brachial plexus injury. Experience from the author's unit suggests that children with more extensive brachial plexus lesions and those with poorer recovery of shoulder movement are at greater risk of severe contracture ≥30° (Unpublished data).

The cause of the elbow flexion contracture remains uncertain. Experimental work in a mouse model suggests that impaired growth of the denervated biceps and brachialis muscle is a contributing factor [22]. If afferent innervation and hence muscle spindles are preserved after a preganglionic injury, the severity of contracture appears to be reduced [23]. Ballinger and Hoffer have discussed the possibility of flexion-extension muscle imbalance at the elbow, but this seems unlikely to be a cause of contracture as triceps is rarely paralysed initially and regains good power in all except the most severe cases of BPBI [45]. Pöyhiä demonstrated in an MRI-based study that elbow flexion contracture is associated with atrophy of the brachialis, brachioradialis, and supinator muscles [46].

Nonoperative treatments including splinting or serial casting are sometimes recommended for flexion contracture of the elbow after BPBI. Sheffler et al. treated children with a contracture of more than 30° with serial casting and reported a 31% improvement, but the contracture continued to progress after treatment was stopped [44]. For less severe contractures, night time splinting was used. While not improving the contracture, the rate of progression was significantly reduced.

Surgical release for severe elbow contracture may be considered although it is important that the strength and range of active flexion of the elbow is not compromised. Garcia-Lopez et al. reported a small series of ten patients with contractures of more than 35° treated by fractional lengthening of the anterior brachialis and biceps tendons. A mean gain in extension of 28° was maintained after a mean follow-up of 3 years [47].

Observations by Price et al. indicate that, in addition to the soft tissue contracture, there are secondary changes in the bones of the elbow [48]. Bony overgrowth causes elongation, widening, and flattening of the olecranon. The enlarged olecranon then doesn't fit into the shallow olecranon fossa creating a block to full extension. As a result, they have developed a modified Outerbridge-Kashiwagi procedure in which the tip of the olecranon is shortened and narrowed. If the olecranon fossa is too shallow, it is deepened by making a hole through the distal humerus. If the anterior structures are tight, then intramuscular lengthening of biceps, release of the fascia over brachialis, and anterior capsulotomy of the elbow is performed. In a series of ten patients of mean age of 14 years with severe contractures (mean 51°) of the elbow, mean fixed flexion 3 years after operation was 21°. Mean DASH scores improved from 39 to 22. All except one patient had an increase in the flexion arc of the elbow.

Vekris et al. have recommended arthrodiastasis of the elbow using an external fixator in adult patients with flexion contracture of the elbow after BPBI [39, 49]. The soft tissues are gradually distracted without opening the elbow. In a series of ten patients with mean fixed elbow flexion of 55°, full extension was gained after distraction. At final follow-up (minimum 1 year), the mean contracture was maintained at 8°.

Restriction of Forearm Rotation

Although there is a full range of passive movement after birth, most children with any remaining deficit in the upper limb after BPBI develop some degree of limitation of forearm rotation during childhood, even when recovery of muscle function appears good. In most cases this is a minor loss of pronation and supination which has little functional consequence. A few children develop a more severe restriction which becomes progressively more fixed. This is more commonly a supination contracture which causes significant functional compromise. Sibinski et al. studied 56 patients at a mean age of 8 years who had incomplete recovery after BPBI [8]. Active forearm rotation was more limited than passive movement, with active pronation less than normal in 48 children, active supination reduced in 36, passive pronation in 22, and passive supination in 9. Greater limitations of active pronation and active and passive supination were significantly associated with worse Mallet scores for shoulder function and Narakas group 4 lesions. Although supination is initially paralysed in most cases of BPBI, pronation is more often reduced in the longer term. In an MRI study, Pöyhiä found that reduced forearm rotation was associated with more atrophy of pronator teres [46].

Supination Deformity

In a large cohort of cases, Yam et al. reported that supination deformity of the forearm occurred in 6.9%, but was not seen in children with Narakas group 1 lesions [50]. There was an increasing incidence in more severe lesions, 5.7% for Narakas group 2, 9.6% for group 3, and 23.4% for group 4. The deformity was first recorded at a median age of 5 years. The exact cause of supination deformity remains unclear, but it appears to be associated with poor recovery in C7 innervated muscles including pronators of the forearm and the radial wrist flexors and extensors. As a consequence, there is often an associated ulnar deviation deformity of the wrist [50]. There may be secondary shortening of the interosseous membrane [51]. There is occasionally dislocation of the radial head or distal radio-ulnar joint [50, 51].

Clinical assessment of the forearm includes careful measurement of the range of active and passive pronation and supination. This is done with the elbow flexed at 90° and the arm held against the trunk in order to exclude the influence of shoulder movement. A fixed supination contracture compromises function of the hand as many activities are performed with the forearm in neutral or pronated position. Cosmesis of the limb is also affected as the hand normally rests in neutral or slightly pronated position. Therefore, surgical intervention may be considered in order to improve the range of pronation if there is absence of active pronation beyond a neutral position and if the deformity is progressing. Surgery to strengthen pronation before the supination deformity becomes fixed may be advantageous, but it is difficult to predict the extent to which the deformity will progress without intervention [40]. Before making a decision, an occupational therapy assessment is carried out to define what functions are impaired and how these might be improved by surgery. It is also important to assess overall wrist and hand function, particularly to check that active wrist extension is adequate if the hand is brought into a pronated position.

The most commonly reported surgical option for improving active pronation of the forearm is lateral rerouting of the distal biceps [52]. If there is sufficient passive pronation, then this procedure can be performed in isolation. If there is fixed supination, then rotation osteotomy of the radius is necessary. Release of the interosseous membrane has also been described.

Author's Preferred Technique

The child is placed supine on the operating table with the affected arm on a hand table. A tourniquet is applied to the upper arm. An S-shaped incision about 10 cm in length is made on the anterior aspect of the elbow centred on the elbow crease, with the proximal limb medially. The distal biceps tendon is exposed down to its insertion together with the radial neck, carefully preserving the lateral cutaneous nerve of the forearm and the radial nerve. The biceps tendon is split longitudinally over a length of 5–6 cm. One half is then detached from its insertion and the other half divided as high as possible. A passage is made around the neck of the radius. A suture is placed in the half which remains attached to the radial tuberosity, and the free end is passed behind the radial neck and retrieved on the lateral side (Fig. 54.8).

If an osteotomy of the radius is required, then a longitudinal incision is made over the anterolateral aspect of the forearm centred on the junction of the middle and distal thirds. A standard approach is made to the radius between bra-

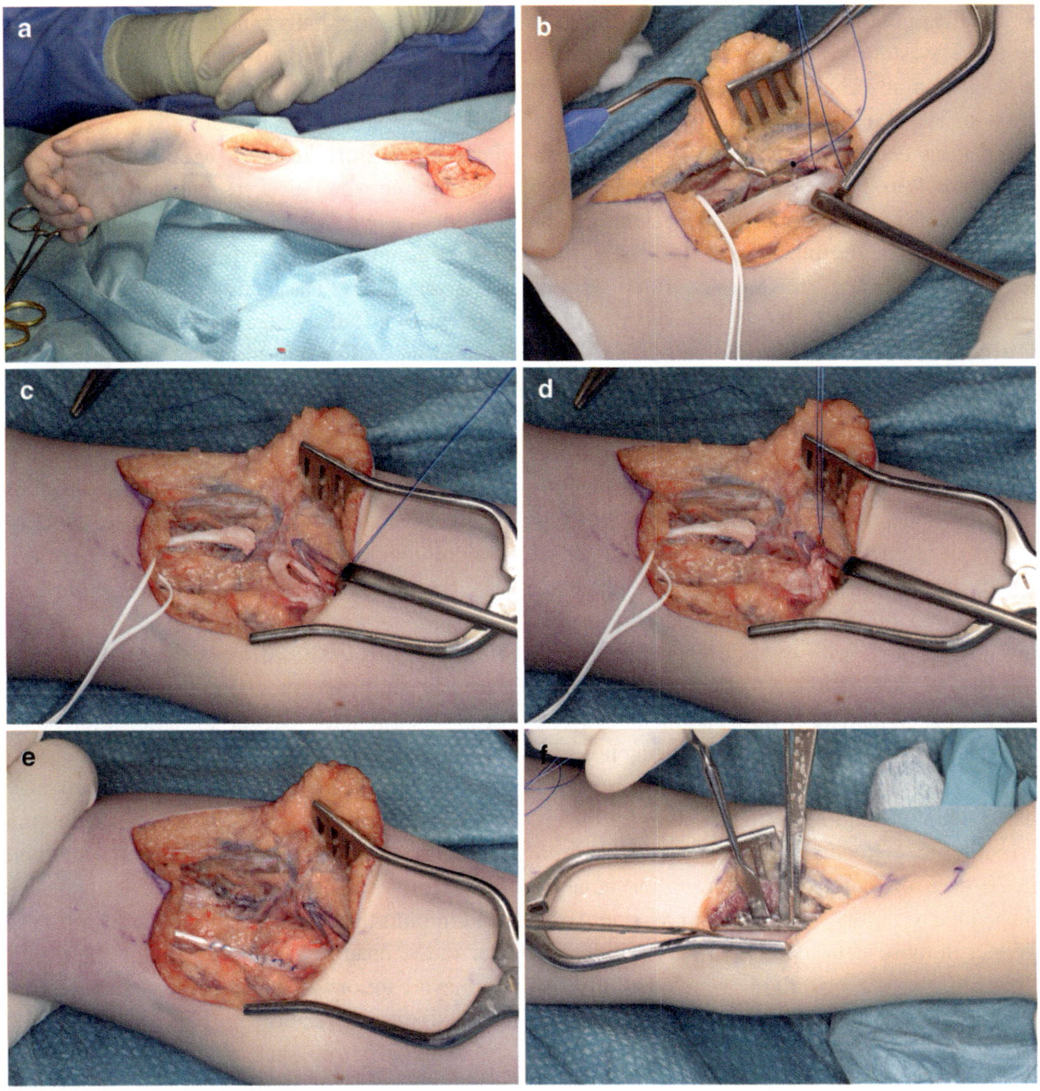

Fig. 54.8 Operative photographs of correction of supination deformity of the forearm. (**a**) Incisions. (**b**) The insertion of the biceps tendon is exposed at the elbow, and a suture is passed around the radial neck (in this case using a curved suction tube) (the hand is indicated on the right of the photograph). (**c**) The tendon is split longitudinally and divided leaving one half attached distally. (**d**) The distal tendon is passed around the radial neck, using the suture, to lie on the lateral side. (**e**) Continuity of the biceps is restored using a tendon weave and side by side suture. (**f**) Pronation osteotomy of the radius. Provisional positioning of the plate. K-wires are used as an indicator of the rotation

chioradialis and the radial artery. The superficial radial nerve is identified. An osteotomy site is planned at the junction of the middle and distal thirds of the radius. The periosteum is incised longitudinally and elevated. A four- or five-hole plate is temporarily positioned and a screw inserted proximal to the osteotomy site. A quarter tubular plate with 2.7 mm screws is usually an appropriate size for children aged 5–8 years. K-wires are inserted perpendicular to the bone above and below. The plate is removed and the osteotomy made with a small oscillating saw. The distal segment of the radius is then rotated using the K-wires as markers to achieve about 30–40° of pronation at the wrist. The plate is reapplied and secured with screws proximally and distally.

Finally, continuity of the biceps tendon is restored by suturing the two halves side to side with a non-absorbable suture under moderate tension. The skin is closed. An above elbow plaster of Paris or lightweight splint is applied with the elbow flexed at 90° and the forearm held in pronation and is retained for 4–6 weeks. Gradual mobilisation of the elbow and forearm is then allowed.

Outcomes

In a series of 42 cases, Yam et al. found that pronation osteotomy of the radius alone placed the hand in a more functional position and increased the arc of forearm rotation [50]. However, the supination deformity recurred in 40%. For radial osteotomy or osteoclasis, Bahm and Gilbert reported mean intraoperative rotation of 78° bringing the forearm into 29° pronation, with 17° pronation at mean 4 years' follow-up [51]. There was recurrence of the supination deformity in 7 out of 23 cases. In a systematic review and meta-analysis, Metsaars et al. found a 75° gain in resting position and 65° in passive pronation for osteotomy compared with 79° gain in resting position for biceps rerouting [53]. Recurrence of deformity occurred in 20–40% of the osteotomy group but none of the tendon rerouting group. The improvement was greater in those with more severe deformities. In the author's unit operation, which has usually included biceps rerouting and radial osteotomy, has been successful in achieving a stable resting position of the forearm in about 30° pronation, but there is little active pronation or supination movement from this position.

Alternative Surgical Approaches

Özkan et al. have described an alternative procedure for children with loss of active pronation, but full passive range, combined with ulnar deviation of the wrist [54]. The brachioradialis is transferred to abductor pollicis longus to strengthen radial deviation of the wrist and the extensor carpi ulnaris (ECU) onto the distal tendon of brachioradialis to create a pronation force. Active pronation improved from -29° to 33° at mean follow-up of 21 months.

Pronation Deformity

For children who lack active supination past neutral, but have a full passive range, Amrani et al. have recommended operation to reroute the pronator teres [55]. The tendon of pronator teres is divided in a Z-fashion, and distal end is passed behind the radius and through a window in the interosseous membrane, before suturing it to the proximal end. This manoeuvre converts the pronator into a supinator muscle. Amrani et al. reported an improvement of the median range of active supination from 5° to 75° in a series of 14 children who underwent operation at a mean age of 7.6 years [55]. There was no loss of pronation.

Radial Head Dislocation

Anterior or posterior dislocation of the radial head occasionally occurs in association with restriction of forearm rotation and flexion contracture of the elbow. The dislocation itself may not cause additional symptoms. Open reduction or excision of the radial head has been suggested [40]. Hoffer recommended transfer of the biceps tendon onto the proximal ulna for cases of anterior radial head dislocation [56]. However, others have cautioned against surgical intervention because of poor results [19, 57]. Excision of the radial head before skeletal maturity should be avoided because of the effect on growth [19].

Wrist and Hand

Issues which can arise in the wrist after more severe cases of BPBI include failure of recovery of active extension and ulnar deviation deformity. Although wrist extension is paralysed initially in cases of BPBI involving the C7 and C8 roots, in the author's experience, failure to recover adequate active extension is unusual. Careful assessment often reveals relative weakness of the radial wrist extensors. Extension may be relying on the action of the finger extensors, but function is satisfactory. Ulnar deviation of the wrist can result from this muscle imbalance and may be associated with supination deformity of the forearm (see above). If there is no active wrist extension, then digital extension may also be absent. Chuang et al. identified weak digital (metacarpophalangeal joint) and wrist extension among the most common deficits in their series of late presenting cases of forearm and hand deformities [58].

Wrist and Digital Extension

If wrist extension is not adequate, then function of the hand is substantially impaired, and patients will usually benefit from surgery. Options are likely to be limited because few muscles in the forearm have sufficient strength for transfer. If flexor carpi ulnaris (FCU) is strong, then it may be transferred to extensor carpi radialis longus or brevis (ECRL or ECRB) to strengthen wrist extension [59]. This procedure may also have the advantage of correcting ulnar deviation of the wrist.

If wrist and digital extension are absent, then wrist arthrodesis is a more predictable option. Consideration should be given to the consequences of wrist fusion on digital extension, since hand opening may rely on wrist flexion. However, fusion of the wrist may make wrist motors available for transfer for digital extension, e.g. transfer of FCU to extensor digitorum communis (EDC) and palmaris longus to extensor pollicis longus (EPL). Where possible, fusion should be delayed until or close to skeletal maturity to minimise any effect on growth [40].

A standard technique is used for wrist fusion. The articular cartilage and subchondral bone are thoroughly removed from the surfaces of the radiocarpal and midcarpal joints. The fusion is then stabilised with a plate from the third metacarpal to the radius. The author usually positions the wrist in a neutral position rather than extended as this favours hand opening if digital extensors are weak. If tendon transfers are planned for digital extension, then these can be performed at the same time, avoiding direct contact of the tendon junctions with the fusion plate.

Ulnar Deviation of the Wrist

If passively correctable, then this deformity may be controlled with a brace. For surgical correction Zancolli recommended tendon transfer for children who are still growing [40]. The ECU tendon is released from its insertion and passed through the interosseous membrane around the anterior aspect of the radius, deep to the radial neurovascular bundle, and sutured to the ECRL tendon. Özkan et al. have described a similar technique using brachioradialis and ECU (see above, supination deformity of the forearm) (Fig. 54.9, [54]).

Hand Function

Fortunately, digital flexion and some intrinsic function are present in all but the most extensive BPBI cases. When impaired, reconstructive options are often limited as there are few available motors with sufficient strength for tendon transfers and there are few published reports of outcomes. Possibilities for improving thumb adduction deformity include transfer of ECU to abductor pollicis longus [39]. For finger interphalangeal extension, distal advancement of the digital extensor mechanism or a "Lasso" procedure may be considered. Weak finger flexion may be reinforced with transfer of a wrist extensor, if available; otherwise free muscle transfer may be the only option.

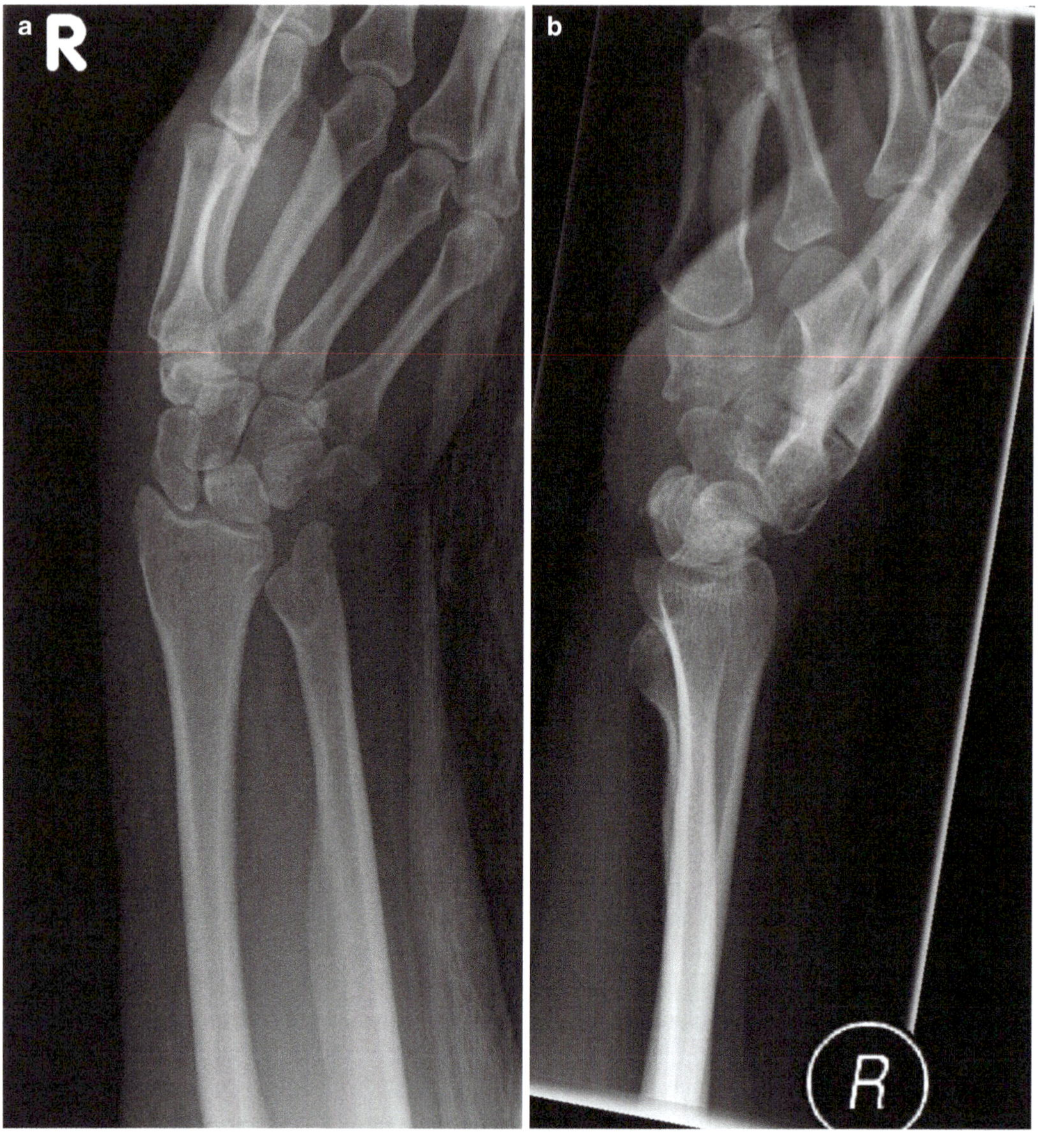

Fig. 54.9 Anteroposterior (**a**) and lateral (**b**) radiographs of the wrist in an adult with a history of BPBI. There are ulnar deviation of the wrist and relative shortening of the ulna

Acknowledgements I would like to acknowledge the help of David Sherlock, former Paediatric Orthopaedic Surgeon, for encouraging long-term follow-up and study of the natural history of BPBI; Andrew Hart, Plastic Surgeon, and Claire Murnaghan, Paediatric Orthopaedic Surgeon, for their involvement in cases on which my experience is based; John McCrum, Service Administrator for careful maintenance of the service database recording outcomes; the Departments of Medical Illustration in Royal Hospital for Children and New Victoria Hospital, Glasgow; and Janice Hems for proofreading the drafts.

References

1. Gilbert A, Tassin JL. Obstetrical palsy: a clinical, pathologic, and surgical review. In: Terzis JK, editor. Microreconstruction of nerve injuries. Philadelphia: WB Saunders; 1987. p. 529–53.
2. Pondaag W, Malessy MJA, Gert van Dijk J, Thomeer RTWM. Natural history of obstetric brachial plexus palsy: a systematic review. Dev Med Child Neurol. 2004;46:138–44.

3. Smith NC, Rowan P, Benson LJ, Ezaki M, Carter PR. Neonatal brachial plexus palsy. Outcome of absent biceps function at three months of age. J Bone Joint Surg Am. 2004;86:2163–70.
4. Waters P. Comparison of the natural history, the outcome of microsurgical repair, and the outcome of operative reconstruction in brachial plexus birth palsy. J Bone Joint Surg. 1999;81-A:649–59.
5. Hems TEJ, Savaridas T, Sherlock DA. The natural history of recovery of elbow flexion after obstetric brachial plexus injury managed without nerve repair. J Hand Surg Eur Vol. 2017;42(7):706–9.
6. Narakas AO. Obstetrical brachial plexus injuries. In: Lamb DW, editor. The paralysed hand. Edinburgh: Churchill Livingstone; 1987. p. 116–35.
7. Hulleberg G, Elvrum AKG, Brandal M, Vik T. Outcome in adolescence of brachial plexus birth palsy. Acta Orthop. 2014;85:633–40.
8. Sibinski M, Sherlock D, TEJ H, Sharma H. Forearm rotational profile in obstetric brachial plexus injury. J Shoulder Elb Surg. 2007;16:784–7.
9. Sever JW. Obstetric paralysis: report of eleven hundred cases. JAMA. 1925;85:1862–5.
10. Mallet J. Paralysie obstétricale du plexus brachial. Traitement des sequelles. Rev Chir Orthop. 1972;58(Supplement 1):166–8.
11. Ho ES, Curtis CG, Clarke HM. The brachial plexus outcome measure: development, internal consistency, and construct validity. J Hand Ther. 2012;25(4):406–17.
12. Sibinski M, Hems TEJ, Sherlock DA. Management strategies for shoulder reconstruction in obstetric brachial plexus injury with special reference to loss of internal rotation after surgery. J Hand Surg Eur Vol. 2012;37:772–9.
13. Eismann EA, Little K, Laor T, Cornwall R. Glenohumeral abduction contracture in children with unresolved neonatal brachial plexus palsy. J Bone Joint Surg Am. 2015;97(2):112–8.
14. Terzis JK, Vekris MD, Okajima S, Soucacos PN. Shoulder deformities in obstetric brachial plexus paralysis: a computed tomography study. J Pediatr Orthop. 2003;23:254–60.
15. Van Der Sluijs JA, Van Ouwerkerk WJ, de Gast A, Wuisman P, Nollet F, Manoliu RA. Retroversion of the humeral head in children with an obstetric brachial plexus lesion. J Bone Joint Surg Br. 2002;84:583–7.
16. Waters PM, Smith GR, Jaramillo D. Glenohumeral deformity secondary to brachial plexus birth palsy. J Bone Joint Surg Am. 1998;80:668–77.
17. Gudinchet F, Maeder P, Oberson JC, Schnyder P. Magnetic resonance imaging of the shoulder in children with brachial plexus birth palsy. Pediatr Radiol. 1995;25(Suppl 1):125–8.
18. Birch R, Bonney G. Birth lesions of the brachial plexus. In: Birch R, Bonney G, Wynn Parry C, editors. Surgical disorders of the peripheral nerves. 1st ed. Edinburgh: Churchill Livingstone; 1998. p. 209–33.
19. Birch R. Birth lesions of the brachial plexus. In: Surgical disorders of the peripheral nerves. 2nd ed. London: Springer-Verlag; 2011. p. 429–81.
20. Nath RK, Paizi M. Scapular deformity in obstetric brachial plexus injury: a new finding. Surg Radiol Anat. 2007;29(2):133–40.
21. Olofsson PN, Chu A, McGrath AM. The pathogenesis of glenohumeral deformity and contracture formation in obstetric brachial plexus palsy-a review. J Brachial Plex Peripher Nerve Inj. 2019;14(1):e24–34.
22. Nikolaou S, Peterson E, Kim A, Wylie C, Cornwall R. Impaired growth of denervated muscle contributes to contracture formation following neonatal brachial plexus injury. J Bone Joint Surg Am. 2011;93(5):461–70.
23. Nikolaou S, Hu L, Cornwall R. Afferent innervation, muscle spindles, and contractures following neonatal brachial plexus injury in a mouse model. J Hand Surg Am. 2015;40(10):2007–16.
24. Abdel-Ghani H, Hamdy KA, Basha N, Tarraf YN. Tendon transfer for treatment of internal rotation contracture of the shoulder in brachial plexus birth palsy. J Hand Surg Eur Vol. 2012;37(8):781–6.
25. Kozin S. The evaluation and treatment of children with brachial plexus birth palsy. J Hand Surg Am. 2011;36(8):1360–9.
26. Hultgren T, Jönsson K, Pettersson H, Hammarberg H. Surgical correction of a rotational deformity of the shoulder in patients with obstetric brachial plexus palsy: short-term results in 270 patients. Bone Joint J. 2013;95-B:1432–8.
27. Hultgren T, Jönsson K, Roos F, Järnbert-Pettersson H, Hammarberg H. Surgical correction of shoulder rotation deformity in brachial plexus birth palsy: long-term results in 118 patients. Bone Joint J. 2014;96-B:1411–8.
28. Pearl ML, Edgerton BW, Kazimiroff PA, Burchette RJ, Wong K. Arthroscopic release and latissimus dorsi transfer for shoulder internal rotation contractures and glenohumeral deformity secondary to brachial plexus birth palsy. J Bone Joint Surg Am. 2006;88:564–74.
29. Carlioz H, Brahimi L. La place de la disinsertion interne du sous-scapulaire dans le traitement de la paralysie obstetricale du member superieur chez l'enfant. Chirurgie Pediatrique. 1986;12:159–67.
30. Gilbert A, Brockman R, Carlioz H. Surgical treatment of brachial plexus birth palsy. Clin Orthop Relat Res. 1991;264:39–47.
31. Dodwell E, O'Callaghan J, Anthony A, Jellicoe P, Shah M, Curtis C, Clarke H, Hopyan S. Combined glenoid anteversion osteotomy and tendon transfers for brachial plexus birth palsy. J Bone Joint Surg Am. 2012;94(2):2145–52.
32. Di Mascio L, Chin K-F, Fox M, Sinisi M. Glenoplasty for complex shoulder subluxation and dislocation in children with obstetric brachial plexus palsy. J Bone Joint Surg Br. 2011;93-B(1):102–7.

33. Waters PM, Bae DS. Effect of tendon transfers and extraarticular soft-tissue balancing on glenohumeral development in brachial plexus birth palsy. J Bone Joint Surg Am. 2005;87:320–5.
34. Kambhampati SB, Birch R, Cobiella C, Chen L. Posterior subluxation and dislocation of the shoulder in obstetric brachial plexus palsy. J Bone Joint Surg Br. 2006;88:213–9.
35. Kirkos JM, Kyrkos MJ, Kapetanos GA, Haritidis JH. Brachial plexus palsy secondary to birth injuries. J Bone Joint Surg Br. 2005;87(2):231–5.
36. Kirkos JM, Papadopoulos IA. Late treatment of brachial plexus palsy secondary to birth injuries: rotational osteotomy of the proximal part of the humerus. J Bone Joint Surg Am. 1998;80(10):1477–83.
37. Waters PM, Bae DS. The effect of derotational humeral osteotomy on global shoulder function in brachial plexus birth palsy. J Bone Joint Surg Am. 2006;88(5):1035–42.
38. Al-Qattan MM, Al-Husainan H, Al-Otaibi A, El-Sharkawy MS. Long-term results of low rotation humeral osteotomy in children with Erb's obstetric brachial plexus palsy. J Hand Surg Eur Vol. 2009;34(4):486–92.
39. Vekris MD, Papadopoulos DV, Gelalis ID, Kontogeorgakos V, Tsantes AG, Gkiatas I, Kostas-Agnantis I, Kosmas D. Secondary procedures for restoration of upper limb function in late cases of neonatal brachial plexus palsy. Eur J Orthop Surg Traumatol. 2019;29:329–36.
40. Zancolli EA, Zancolli ER. Palliative surgical procedures in sequelae of obstetric palsy. Hand Clin. 1988;4(4):643–69.
41. Gilbert A, Valbuena S, Posso C. Obstetrical brachial plexus injuries: late functional results of the Steindler procedure. J Hand Surg Eur Vol. 2014;39:868–75.
42. Costil V, Romana C, Fitoussi F. Pectoralis minor transfer for elbow flexion restoration in late obstetric brachial plexus palsy. Int Orthop. 2018;42(5):1137–41.
43. Kay S, Pinder R, Wiper J, Hart A, Jones F, Yates A. Microvascular free functioning gracilis transfer with nerve transfer to establish elbow flexion. J Plast Reconstr Aesthet Surg. 2010;63(7):1142–9.
44. Sheffler LC, Lattanza L, Hagar Y, Bagley A, James MA. The prevalence, rate of progression, and treatment of elbow flexion contracture in children with brachial plexus birth palsy. J Bone Joint Surg Am. 2012;94(5):403–9.
45. Ballinger SG, Hoffer MM. Elbow flexion contracture in Erb's palsy. J Child Neurol. 1994;9(2):209–10.
46. Pöyhiä TH, Koivikko MP, Peltonen JI, Kirjavainen MO, Lamminen AE, Nietosvaara AY. Muscle changes in brachial plexus birth injury with elbow flexion contracture: an MRI study. Pediatr Radiol. 2007;37(2):173–9.
47. Garcia-Lopez A, Sebastian P, Martinez-Lopez F. Anterior release of elbow flexion contractures in children with obstetrical brachial plexus lesions. J Hand Surg Am. 2012;37(8):1660–4.
48. Price AE, Chim H, Valencia H, Grossman JAI. Result of modified Outerbridge-Kashiwagi procedure for elbow flexion contractures in brachial plexus birth injury. J Hand Surg Eur Vol. 2019;44(3):242–7.
49. Vekris MD, Pafilas D, Lykissas MG, Soucacos PN, Beris AE. Correction of elbow flexion contracture in late obstetric brachial plexus palsy through arthrodiatasis of the elbow (Ioannina method). Tech Hand Up Extrem Surg. 2010;14(1):14–20.
50. Yam A, Fullilove S, Sinisi M, Fox M. The supination deformity and associated deformities of the upper limb in severe birth lesions of the brachial plexus. J Bone Joint Surg Br. 2009;91(4):511–6.
51. Bahm J, Gilbert A. Surgical correction of supination deformity in children with obstetric brachial plexus palsy. J Hand Surg Br. 2002;27(1):20–3.
52. Zancolli EA. Paralytic supination contracture of the forearm. J Bone Joint Surg Am. 1967;49(7):1275–84.
53. Metsaars WP, Nagels J, Pijls BG, Langenhoff JM, Nelissen RG. Treatment of supination deformity for obstetric brachial plexus injury: a systematic review and meta-analysis. J Hand Surg Am. 2014;39(10):1948–1958.e2.
54. Özkan T, Aydin HU, Berköz Ö, Özkan S, Kozanoğlu E. 'Switch' technique to restore pronation and radial deviation in 17 patients with brachial plexus birth palsy. J Hand Surg Eur Vol. 2019;44(9):905–12.
55. Amrani A, Dendane MA, El Alami ZF. Pronator teres transfer to correct pronation deformity of the forearm after an obstetrical brachial plexus injury. J Bone Joint Surg Br. 2009;91(5):616–8.
56. Hoffer HM. Assessment and natural history of brachial plexus injury in children. In: Gelberman RH, editor. Operative nerve repair and reconstruction. Philadelphia: J.B. Lippincott Company; 1991. p. 1361–8.
57. Huo CW. Radial head dislocation as a rare complication of obstetric brachial plexus palsy: literature review and five case series. Hand Surg. 2012;17(1):33–6.
58. Chuang DC, Ma HS, Borud LJ, Chen HC. Surgical strategy for improving forearm and hand function in late obstetric brachial plexus palsy. Plast Reconstr Surg. 2002;109(6):1934–46.
59. Waters PM. Pediatric brachial plexus palsy. In: Green DP, Hotchkiss RN, Pederson WC, Wolfe SW, editors. Green's operative hand surgery. Philadelphia: Elsevier; 2005. p. 1297–318.

Index

A. Y. Shin, N. Pulos (eds.), *Operative Brachial Plexus Surgery*,
https://doi.org/10.1007/978-3-030-69517-0

GPSR Compliance

The European Union's (EU) General Product Safety Regulation (GPSR) is a set of rules that requires consumer products to be safe and our obligations to ensure this.

If you have any concerns about our products, you can contact us on ProductSafety@springernature.com

In case Publisher is established outside the EU, the EU authorized representative is:

Springer Nature Customer Service Center GmbH
Europaplatz 3
69115 Heidelberg, Germany

Batch number: 10732805

Printed by Printforce, the Netherlands